D1609520

The Spine in Sports

The Spine in Sports

Robert G. Watkins, M.D.

Spine Surgeon,
Kerlan-Jobe Orthopaedic Clinic;
Codirector, Minimally Invasive Surgery Institute,
Arthroscopic Spine Surgery,
Centinela Hospital Medical Center;
Clinical Associate Professor of Orthopaedics,
University of Southern California School of Medicine,
Los Angeles, California;
Spine Consultant to the Los Angeles Dodgers, California Angels, Los Angeles Lakers, Los Angeles
Kings, Mighty Ducks of Anaheim, and the Professional Golf Association

Associate Editors

Lytton Williams, M.D.

Orthopaedic Surgeon,
Kerlan-Jobe Orthopaedic Clinic,
Centinela Hospital Medical Center;
Assistant Professor of Orthopaedics,
University of Southern California School of Medicine,
Los Angeles, California

Paul Lin, M.D.

Sun Orthopaedic and Sports Medicine,
Lewisberg, Pennsylvania

Burton Elrod, M.D.

Southern Sports Medicine,
Nashville, Tennessee

Neil Kahanovitz, M.D.

Director, Spine Surgery,
The Anderson Clinic,
Washington Hospital Center,
Arlington, Virginia

with 1102 illustrations

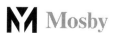 Mosby

St. Louis Baltimore Boston Carlsbad Chicago Naples New York Philadelphia Portland
London Madrid Mexico City Singapore Sydney Tokyo Toronto Wiesbaden

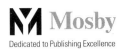

Mosby
Dedicated to Publishing Excellence

A Times Mirror
Company

Publisher: Anne S. Patterson
Editor: Robert Hurley
Developmental Editor: Lauranne Billus
Project Manager: Deborah L. Vogel
Production Editor: Judith Bange
Manufacturing Manager: Theresa Fuchs
Design Manager: Pati Pye
Book and Cover Design: Preface, Inc.

Copyright © 1996 by Mosby–Year Book, Inc.

All rights reserved. No part of this publication may be reproduced,
stored in a retrieval system, or transmitted, in any form or by any
means, electronic, mechanical, photocopying, recording, or otherwise,
without prior written permission from the publisher.

Permission to photocopy or reproduce solely for internal or personal
use is permitted for libraries or other users registered with the Copyright
Clearance Center, provided that the base fee of $4.00 per chapter plus $.10
per page is paid directly to the Copyright Clearance Center, 27 Congress
Street, Salem, MA 01970. This consent does not extend to other kinds
of copying, such as copying for general distribution, for advertising or
promotional purposes, for creating new collected works, or for resale.

Printed in the United States of America
Composition by Graphic World, Inc.
Printing/binding by Maple-Vail Book Mfg. Group

Mosby–Year Book, Inc.
11830 Westline Industrial Drive
St. Louis, Missouri 63146

Library of Congress Cataloging in Publication Data
The spine in sports / [edited by] Robert G. Watkins ; associate
   editors, Lytton Williams . . . [et al.].
        p.   cm.
     Includes bibliographical references and index.
     ISBN 0-8016-7502-2 (hard cover : alk. paper)
     1. Spine—Wounds and injuries. 2. Sports injuries.   I. Watkins.
   Robert G.
     [DNLM: 1. Spinal Injuries—diagnosis. 2. Spinal Injuries—
   therapy. 3. Athletic Injuries—diagnosis. 4. Athletic Injuries—
   therapy.   WE 725 S7597 1995]
   RD533.S69   1995
   617.3′75044′088796—dc20
   DNLM/DLC
   for Library of Congress   95-41097
                                                                    CIP

95 96 97 98 99 / 9 8 7 6 5 4 3 2 1

Contributors

Michael A. Abdenour, A.T.C.
Head Athletic Trainer,
Detroit Pistons,
Detroit, Michigan

Dvera Berson, M.S.
Author and Lecturer,
Boca Raton, Florida

James P. Bradley, M.D.
Clinical Assistant Professor,
University of Pittsburgh Medical Center;
Director, Sports Medicine Center,
St. Margaret Memorial Hospital,
Pittsburgh, Pennsylvania

Salvador A. Brau, M.D.
Clinical Instructor in Surgery,
University of California—Los Angeles;
Centinela Hospital Medical Center,
Los Angeles, California

Courtney W. Brown, M.D.
Assistant Clinical Professor of Orthopaedic Surgery,
University of Colorado,
Denver, Colorado;
Orthopaedic Surgeon,
Lakewood Orthopaedic Clinic,
Lakewood, Colorado

William Buhler, A.T.C
Head Athletic Trainer,
Los Angeles Dodgers,
Los Angeles, California

Edmund R. Burke, Ph.D.
Associate Professor,
Biology Department,
University of Colorado at Colorado Springs,
Colorado Springs, Colorado

David R. Campbell, M.D.
Spine Surgeon,
Palm Beach Orthopaedic Institute,
Palm Beach Gardens, California

Andrew J. Cole, M.D.
Clinical Assistant Professor,
Physical Medicine and Rehabilitation, and Physical Therapy,
University of Texas Southwestern Medical Center;
Director, Spine Rehabilitation Services,
Baylor University Medical Center,
Dallas, Texas

Tammy Rubenstein de Koekkoek, D.C., D.A.B.C.O.
Associate Professor,
Los Angeles College of Chiropractic,
Los Angeles, California;
Chiropractic Orthopaedist,
Soest, The Netherlands

Steven C. Dennis, M.D.
Orthopaedic Spine Surgeon,
Hoag Memorial Hospital,
Newport Beach, California

William H. Dillin, M.D.
Senior Associate Surgeon,
Kerlan-Jobe Orthopaedic Clinic,
Centinela Hospital Medical Center,
Los Angeles, California

Jocylane M. Dinsay, R.N.
Research Nurse,
Kerlan-Jobe Orthopaedic Clinic,
Los Angeles, California

Lawrence D. Dorr, M.D.
Professor, Orthopaedic Surgery,
University of Southern California School of Medicine;
Director, The Center for Arthritis and Joint Implant
  Surgery,
Los Angeles, California

Andrew B. Dossett, M.D.
Assistant Clinical Professor,
University of Texas Southwestern;
Spine Consultant,
Texas Rangers Baseball Club;
Dallas Spine Group,
Dallas, Texas

Gary L. Douglas, M.D.
Cook Children's Medical Center,
Fort Worth, Texas

Michele Toomay Douglas, D.S.N., M.A.
University of Hawaii,
Honolulu, Hawaii

Richard A. Eagleston, M.A., P.T., A.T.C.
Owner/Clinical Supervisor,
S.T.A.R. Physical Therapy,
Redwood City, California

Christopher R. Edwards, M.D.
Clinical Assistant Professor of Surgery,
Morehouse School of Medicine;
Resurgens Orthopaedic P.C.,
Atlanta, Georgia

Bruce C. Elliott, Ph.D., M.Ed.
Professor and Head,
Department of Human Movement,
University of Western Australia,
Perth, Western Australia, Australia

Jeremy C.T. Fairbank, M.D., F.R.C.S.
Clinical Senior Lecturer in Orthopaedics,
Oxford University;
Consultant Orthopaedic Surgeon,
Nuffield Orthopaedic Centre,
John Radcliffe Hospital,
Oxford, United Kingdom

†Harry F. Farfan, M.D.
St. Mary's Hospital;
Jewish General Hospital,
Quebec, Montreal, Canada

Joseph P. Farrell, P.T., M.S.
Senior Clinical Faculty,
Kaiser Hayward Physical Therapy Residency Program in
   Advanced Manual Therapy,
Kaiser Permanente Medical Center,
Hayward, California;
Director, Redwood Orthopaedic Physical Therapy, Inc.,
Castro Valley, California

Brett Fischer, A.T.C.
Registered Physical Therapist;
Certified Strength and Conditioning Specialist;
Consultant to European Golf Tour;
Formerly Physical Therapist/Athletic Trainer for U.S.
   PGA Tour,
Phoenix, Arizona

Joseph D. Fortin, D.O.
Medical Director,
Rehabilitation Hospital of Fort Wayne,
Fort Wayne, Indiana;
Formerly Assistant Professor,
University of Colorado Health Sciences Center,
Denver, Colorado;
Formerly Clinical Assistant Professor,
Louisiana State University Medical Center,
New Orleans, Louisiana

Daryl Hugh Foster, M.Ed.
Department of Human Movement,
University of Western Australia,
Perth, Western Australia, Australia

Martin Francis Gargan, M.A., F.R.C.S.
Consultant Senior Lecturer,
University of Bristol;
Consultant Orthopaedic Surgeon,
Bristol Royal Infirmary,
Bristol, United Kingdom

Scott Haldeman, M.D., Ph.D.
Associate Clinical Professor of Neurology,
University of California—Irvine,
Irvine, California

Hamilton Hall, M.D., F.R.C.S.
Professor of Surgery,
University of Toronto;
Director of Spine Surgery;
Deputy Chief of Surgery,
Orthopaedic and Arthritic Hospital;
Orthopaedic Consultant,
National Ballet of Canada;
Toronto Raptors, NBA,
Toronto, Ontario, Canada

Mark F. Hambly, M.D.
Spine Surgeon,
Northern California Spine and Rehabilitation Associates,
Sacramento, California

†Deceased.

Philip Hobson Hardcastle, M.B.B.S., F.R.C.S.
Department of Human Movement,
University of Western Australia;
Sir George Beobrook Spinal Unit,
Perth, Western Australia, Australia

Harry N. Herkowitz, M.D.
Chair, Department of Orthopaedic Surgery,
William Beaumont Hospital,
Royal Oak, Michigan

Stanley A. Herring, M.D.
Pugent Sound Sports and Spine Physicians;
Clinical Associate Professor, Rehabilitation Medicine;
Clinical Associate Professor, Orthopaedics;
University of Washington,
Seattle, Washington

Timothy M. Hosea, M.D.
Clinical Assistant Professor of Surgery,
Division of Orthopaedic Surgery,
UMDNJ–Robert Wood Johnson Medical School,
New Brunswick, New Jersey

Douglas W. Jackson, M.D.
Medical Director, Southern California Center for Sports
    Medicine;
Medical Director, Orthopaedic Research Institute,
Long Beach, California

David Jaffray, F.R.C.S.
Consultant Spine Surgeon;
Senior Lecturer,
Keele University;
Orthopaedic Hospital,
Oswestry, Shropshire, United Kingdom

Michael E. Janssen, D.O.
Associate Clinical Professor,
University of Colorado,
Denver, Colorado;
Center for Spinal Disorders,
Thorton, Colorado

R. Scott Kingston, M.D.
Director of Magnetic Resonance Section,
Centinela Hospital Medical Center;
Clinical Instructor,
University of Southern California School of Medicine,
Los Angeles, California

Irv Klein, M.D.
Senior Staff Anesthesiologist,
Centinela Hospital Medical Center,
Los Angeles, California

Peter R. Kurzweil, M.D.
Orthopaedic Surgeon,
Southern California Center for Sports Medicine,
Long Beach, California

Philip Kwong, M.D.
Kerlan-Jobe Orthopaedic Clinic,
Los Angeles, California

Nathan H. Lebwohl, M.D.
Associate Professor of Orthopaedics and Rehabilitation,
University of Miami School of Medicine;
Jackson Memorial Hospital,
Miami, Florida

Claire F. McCarthy, P.T., M.S.
Associate Professor,
MGH Institute of Health Professionals;
Instructor in Orthopaedic Surgery,
Harvard Medical School;
Research Associate Professor,
Boston University Research Center;
Director, Department of Physical Therapy and Occupational
    Therapy,
Children's Hospital,
Boston, Massachusetts

Edward J. McPherson, M.D.
Assistant Professor of Orthopaedic Surgery,
University of Southern California School of Medicine;
Assistant Director,
University of Southern California Center for Arthritis and
    Joint Implant Surgery,
Los Angeles, California

Michael F. Mellman, M.D.
Team Physician,
Los Angeles Dodgers, Los Angeles Kings, and Los Angeles
    Lakers;
Centinela Hospital Medical Center,
Los Angeles, California

Lyle J. Micheli, M.D.
Associate Clinical Professor of Orthopaedic Surgery,
Harvard Medical School;
Director, Division of Sports Medicine,
Children's Hospital,
Boston, Massachusetts

Marilou Moschetti, B.Sc., P.T.A.
Physical Therapy Assistant,
AquaTechnics Consulting Group/NovaCare,
Watsonville, California

James M. Odor, M.D.
Associate Clinical Faculty,
Department of Orthopaedics,
University of Oklahoma Health Sciences Center;
Orthopaedic Spine Surgeon,
Spine Surgery, Inc.,
Baptist Medical Center,
Northwest Surgical Hospital,
Mercy Health Center,
Oklahoma City, Oklahoma

Mary O'Toole, Ph.D.
Associate Professor and Director,
Human Performance Laboratory,
University of Tennessee–Campbell Clinic,
Department of Orthopaedic Surgery,
Memphis, Tennessee

Benjamin J. Paolucci, D.O.
Clinical Associate Surgeon,
Michigan State University College of Osteopathic
    Medicine,
Detroit, Michigan

Richard D. Peek, M.D.
Clinical Assistant Professor,
University of Arkansas;
Arkansas Spine Center,
St. Vincent Infirmary,
Little Rock, Arkansas

Jo-Anne Piccinin, B.Sc., P.T.
Staff Physiotherapist,
Orthopaedic and Arthritic Hospital,
Toronto, Ontario, Canada

Joel M. Press, M.D.
Associate Clinical Professor,
Physical Medicine and Rehabilitation,
Northwestern University Medical School;
Medical Director,
Center for Spine, Sports, and Occupational Rehabilitation,
Rehabilitation Institute of Chicago,
Chicago, Illinois

Glenn R. Rechtine, M.D., F.A.C.S.
Florida Orthopaedic Institute,
Tampa, Florida

W. Carlton Reckling, M.D.
Spinal Unit,
Queen's Medical Centre,
Nottingham, United Kingdom

Michael W. Reed, M.D.
Orthopaedic Surgeon,
Gulf Coast Hospital,
Panama City, Florida

Jeffrey A. Saal, M.D., F.A.C.P.
Associate Clinical Professor,
Stanford University Medical Center;
SOAR, Physiatry Group,
Menlo Park, California

Joel S. Saal, M.D.
Clinical Instructor,
Department of Functional Restoration,
Stanford University,
San Francisco, California

Michael B. Schlink, M.A., P.T.
Clinical Director/Owner,
Schlink and Associates Physical Therapy,
Los Angeles, California

Terry A. Schroeder, D.C.
North Ranch Chiropractic,
Westlake Village, California

Curtis W. Spencer III, M.D.
Director of Spine Surgery,
Southern California Sports Medicine Center,
Long Beach Memorial Hospital,
Long Beach, California

Raymond W. Steffanus, B.A.
Health/Fitness Instructor,
Pasadena Athletic Club,
Pasadena, California

Steven A. Stratton, Ph.D., P.T., A.T.C.
Associate Professor,
University of Texas Health Science Center;
President,
Alamo Physical Therapy Resources, Inc.,
San Antonio, Texas

James E. Tibone, M.D.
Clinical Professor of Orthopaedics,
University of Southern California School of Medicine;
Associate,
Kerlan-Jobe Orthopaedic Clinic,
Centinela Hospital Medical Center,
Los Angeles, California

Linda C. Tiefel, P.T.
Lakewood Center for Physical Therapy,
Lakewood, Colorado

Thomas C. Tolli, M.D.
Spine Surgeon,
Kerlan-Jobe Orthopaedic Clinic,
Los Angeles, California

Terry R. Trammell, M.D.
Clinical Instructor,
Department of Orthopaedics,
Indiana University Residency Program;
Director of Medical Services, CART/Indy Car;
Methodist Graduate Medical Center,
Indianapolis, Indiana

Masamitsu Tsuchiya, M.D.
Associate Professor of Orthopaedic Surgery,
Tokyo Medical and Dental University;
Chair, Department of Orthopaedic Surgery,
Doai Memorial Hospital,
Tokyo Japan

Gurvinder S. Uppal, M.D.
Clinical Assistant Professor,
Loma Linda University,
Loma Linda, California;
Orthopaedic Medical Group of Riverside,
Riverside, California

Pieter F. van Akkerveeken, M.D., Ph.D.
Orthopaedic Surgeon,
Rug Advies Centrum,
Zeist, The Netherlands

Robert Ward, P.Ed.
Sports Research Director,
Emprise International,
Dallas, Texas

Robert G. Watkins, M.D.
Spine Surgeon,
Kerlan-Jobe Orthopaedic Clinic;
Codirector, Minimally Invasive Surgery Institute,
Arthroscopic Spine Surgery,
Centinela Hospital Medical Center;
Clinical Associate Professor of Orthopaedics,
University of Southern California School of Medicine,
Los Angeles, California;
Spine Consultant to the Los Angeles Dodgers, California
    Angels, Los Angeles Lakers, Los Angeles Kings, Mighty
    Ducks of Anaheim, and the Professional Golf Association

Christopher R. Weatherley, M.D., F.R.C.S.
Consultant Spinal Surgeon,
Princess Elizabeth Orthopaedic Hospital,
Exeter, United Kingdom

John K. Webb, F.R.C.S.
Spinal Unit,
Queen's Medical Centre,
Nottingham, United Kingdom

Arthur H. White, M.D.
Medical Director,
SpineCare Medical Group,
San Francisco Spine Institute,
Daly City, California

Lytton Williams, M.D.
Orthopaedic Surgeon,
Kerlan-Jobe Orthopaedic Clinic,
Centinela Hospital Medical Center;
Assistant Professor of Orthopaedics,
University of Southern California School of Medicine,
Los Angeles, California

Leon L. Wiltse, M.D.
Clinical Professor of Orthopaedic Surgery,
University of California — Irvine,
Irvine, California;
Long Beach Memorial Hospital,
Long Beach, California

Jeffrey L. Young, M.D.
Assistant Professor, Physical Medicine and Rehabilitation,
Northwestern University Medical School;
Codirector, Sports Rehabilitation Program,
Rehabilitation Institute of Chicago,
Chicago, Illinois

Norman P. Zemel, M.D.
Associate Clinical Professor,
Department of Orthopaedic Surgery,
University of Southern California School of Medicine;
Associate,
Kerlan-Jobe Orthopaedic Clinic,
Los Angeles, California

To my wife, Kaytie, and my children, Andy, Robert, Susan, Claire, and Emily

Preface

The Spine in Sports is a detailed, concise approach to the management of spinal problems in athletes. It attempts to be comprehensive in that it includes a great variety of athletic and sports activities, yet it still presents a very straightforward approach to using the appropriate diagnostic and therapeutic techniques for dealing with specific spinal injuries in athletes. This work is a compilation of my 15 years of specialization in spinal problems in athletes, as well as a product of the work of a great number of specialists in this area. While there is a strong scientific foundation for the work presented, the backbone of this material is the hands-on, practical experience of the many trainers and physical therapists dealing with these athletes. These are skilled professionals who continually teach physicians what can and should be done in the management of the complex rehabilitation problems of professional athletes. There are many physicians who specialize in the medicine and surgery of athletic injuries. The difficulty lies in finding physicians who specialize in spinal medicine and surgery and still have the exposure and expertise in sports medicine that is necessary to provide athletes with comprehensive knowledge and comprehensive treatment for their spinal injuries.

The Spine in Sports points the way for spinal specialists to become involved in the science and practical applications of sports medicine as it pertains to athletes with spinal problems. Spinal specialists need to understand the sport just as they need to understand any patient's occupation. Time spent understanding patients is time well spent.

Robert G. Watkins

Acknowledgment

Special thanks to Kathy Williams, who prepared the entire manuscript, organized illustrations, handled all correspondence, and without whom there would be no *The Spine in Sports*.

Robert G. Watkins

Contents

The Spine in Sports

Section One

◆

Anatomy and Biomechanics

Chapter One

◆

Anatomy of the Spine

Martin Francis Gargan
Jeremy C.T. Fairbank

Accurate anatomic knowledge is crucial to understanding the diagnosis, investigation, and treatment of all types of sports injuries. It is relevant, not only to the orthopaedic specialist, but also to members of other disciplines involved in the care of athletes. This chapter outlines the general principles of the spine's anatomy, detailing the specifics of the cervical, thoracic (dorsal), and lumbar sections. Particular emphasis is given to the ligaments and muscles, which are often overlooked. A short review of specialized areas, including the sacroiliac joints, is also given.

Structurally, the vertebral column, or backbone, forms the central axis of the primate skeleton. Fig. 1-1 shows the lateral, anterior, and posterior views of the human vertebral column. It is divided into five regions: cervical, thoracic, lumbar, sacral, and coccygeal. There are 24 individual bony segments—7 cervical, 12 thoracic, and 5 lumbar—and the sacral and coccygeal segments are fused. Congenital anomalies and minor variations in segmentation are common.

The functions of the vertebral column are as follows:
1. Protection for the spinal cord within

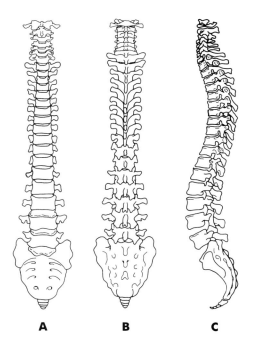

Fig. 1-1. Anterior (**A**), posterior (**B**), and lateral (**C**) views of the spinal column.

2. Support for the head and neck structures
3. Point of attachment for the thoracic cage (and thus the upper limbs via the pectoral girdle)
4. Support of the abdominal contents and pelvic girdle
5. Transmission of weight to the lower limbs

In general, the individual vertebrae are increasingly large moving down the column, which confers increased strength (although it should be noted that the fifth lumbar vertebra is often smaller than the fourth[6]). The configuration of multiple bony segments also confers great flexibility. In the developing fetus the column assumes a flexed position, producing a forward concavity that is maintained in adult life in the thoracic and sacral regions. In adults the two regions not supporting a bony cage (the cervical and lumbar regions) assume a secondary curve that is lordotic (i.e., a forward convexity).

Each vertebra consists of an anterior (ventral) body and a posterior neural arch that enclose the vertebral canal. Three processes develop from this neural arch: the spinous process posteriorly and paired transverse processes laterally. The part of the neural arch between the transverse and spinous processes is called the lamina, and that between the transverse process and the body is called the pedicle. Developmentally, part of the body (dorsolaterally) is in fact part of the neural arch, and the costal element, which all vertebrae possess (and which forms the ribs in the thoracic region) articulates with the neural arch, not with the vertebral body.

Blood is supplied to the back from large regional vessels. In the cervical region, branches from the occipital, vertebral, deep, and ascending cervical arteries supply the spine. The posterior intercostal arteries and subcostal and lumbar arteries from the aorta supply the lower spinal regions.

Venous drainage is via two freely communicating systems: the internal and external vertebral venous plexuses, which extend from the coccyx to the skull. The venous relations of the spinal nerves are of great importance to the spinal surgeon, since their conservation avoids troublesome hemorrhage perioperatively.[5] The lymphatic drainage follows that of the veins.

The blood supply for the spinal cord itself arises from the vertebral arteries. The anterior spinal artery runs within the anterior median fissure, and the posterior spinal arteries descend as two arteries on each side of the cord—one anterior and one posterior to the posterior nerve roots.

SPINAL CORD

The spinal cord lies within the bony vertebral canal and is continuous proximally with the medulla oblongata of the brainstem. It extends from the foramen magnum to the lower part of the first lumbar vertebra, although this varies. The cord is enclosed in three protective membranes: the pia, arachnoid, and dura maters. The pia and arachnoid maters are separated by the subarachnoid space, which contains cerebrospinal fluid. The arachnoid mater terminates at the level of the second sacral segment. The subdural space is merely a potential space, since, unlike the dual layer of dura mater lining the cranial bones, the spinal dura is a single layer. The space between the dura mater and the wall of the vertebral canal is filled with fat, loose connective tissue and a plexus of veins; this is the epidural space.

The spinal cord is approximately cylindric, although the transverse diameter is always greater than the anteroposterior diameter. The cord is incompletely divided into two symmetric halves by an anteroposterior longitudinal fissure connected by a transverse commissure. A less distinct posterolateral fissure is found along the line of the posterior nerve roots.

The cord has two pronounced swellings: the cervical enlargement gives rise to the brachial plexus, and the lumbar enlargement gives rise to the lumbosacral plexus. The spinal cord terminates as the conus medullaris at the level of the second lumbar vertebra in the adult and at the level of the third lumbar vertebra in the neonate. From this a fibrous cord—the filum terminale—extends to the dorsum of the first coccygeal segment. The nerves below the conus medullaris are said to resemble a horse's tail and are known as the cauda equina.

SPINAL NERVES

At each level the cord gives off paired dorsal and ventral roots of spinal nerves (Fig. 1-2). The roots cross the subarachnoid space and pierce the dura before uniting close to their respective intervertebral foramina to emerge as a mixed spinal nerve. The dura of the dural sac is prolonged around the emerging roots as a dural sleeve, which blends with the epineurium of the spinal nerve. The dorsal root of each spinal nerve, with its cell body in the dorsal root ganglion, transmits sensory fibers from the spinal nerve to the spinal cord; the ventral root transmits mainly motor fibers to the spinal nerve but may also contain some sensory fibers. Since the vertebral column is longer than the cord, the path of each of these nerves becomes increasingly more vertical in the caudal segments.

As each spinal nerve leaves the intervertebral foramen, it divides into anterior (ventral) and posterior (dorsal) primary rami. The posterior primary rami

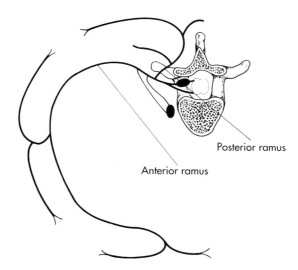

Fig. 1-2. Schematic view of the principal nerves of a spinal segment.

supply the erector spinae muscles (i.e., all the muscles deep to the splenius in the neck and to the thoracolumbar fascia more distally). They also supply the facet joints and the overlying skin to varying degrees. The anterior primary rami provide a segmental nerve supply to the skin of the neck and to the front and sides of the thoracic and abdominal walls and the associated musculature (intercostal and abdominal recti muscles) as far posteriorly as the prevertebral recti (longus capitis, psoas).

The anterior primary rami of C5 to C8 and T1 form the brachial plexus to supply the upper limb, and the rami of L1 to L5 and S1-2 form the lumbosacral plexus to supply the lower limb. The sympathetic chains lie on the anterolateral aspect of the vertebral column adjacent to the aorta and supply autonomic innervation to the anterior primary rami by means of gray rami communicantes. All spinal nerves receive gray rami, whereas only those from T1 to L2 supply white rami communicantes to the sympathetic chain. This is because the cell bodies of the sympathetic fibers lie in the lateral horns of the spinal cord gray matter between these levels. The recurrent nerve of Luschka supplies the posterior longitudinal ligament and the posterior part of the annulus fibrosis of the intervertebral discs. It is connected directly to the dorsal root ganglion and the sympathetic chain.

BONY VERTEBRAL COLUMN
Cervical Vertebrae

The typical cervical vertebrae are the third, fourth, fifth, and sixth vertebrae (Fig. 1-3). They possess a foramen transversarium, and the spinous process is bifid. The body is reniform and broader from side to side than from front to back and is generally smaller than the triangular spinal canal. Posterolaterally in the region of

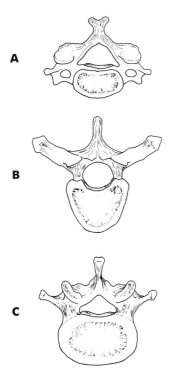

Fig. 1-3. Axial view (from the head) of typical cervical (**A**), thoracic (**B**), and, lumbar (**C**) vertebrae. Note the increasing cross-sectional area of the vertebral bodies from the cervical to the lumbar spine. In contrast, the vertebral canal is relatively constant in the cross-sectional area.

the body, which is a derivative of the neural arch, there is a ridge that articulates, as a synovial joint, with a reciprocal beveled area of the vertebrae above—this is the neurocentral joint. The pedicle is attached below this ridge, and a bar of bone extends laterally from this and ends as the anterior tubercle. The true transverse element extends from the pedicle more posteriorly and ends as the posterior tubercle. These tubercles are joined by the costotransverse lamellae to form the foramen for the vertebral artery. At the junction of the lamina and pedicle are the articular surfaces, which are oval; the superior processes face upward and backward, and the lower processes face forward and downward.

The first, second, and seventh cervical vertebrae are atypical. The atlas, or first cervical vertebra, has no body and no spinous process. It consists of two lateral masses that carry the weight-bearing articular processes, connected by anterior and posterior arches. The superior articular processes are concave to receive the convex occipital condyles in a synovial joint; these joints allow flexion and extension, as well as lateral flexion of the skull on the neck. The inferior articular surfaces are circular and flat and articulate with the superior articular surfaces of the axis.

The axis, or second cervical vertebra, is characterized by the dens, or odontoid process, which is in fact the body of the atlas, which has become incorporated into the body of the axis. The dens articulates with the posterior aspect of the anterior arch of the atlas by a small synovial joint. The lateral masses of the axis have superior articular processes to form synovial joints with the atlas. This atlantoaxial joint complex allows lateral rotation of the neck. Weight bearing is taken through the lateral masses, but the inferior surface of the axis is that of a typical cervical vertebra, and weight is transmitted via the vertebral bodies throughout the rest of the column. This specialization of the atlas and axis confers an enormous range of motion to the head and neck. The vertebra prominens, usually the seventh cervical vertebra, is atypical inasmuch as it has a very prominent spinous process that is not bifid and the foramen transversarium does not transmit the vertebral artery.

Thoracic Vertebrae

There are 12 thoracic vertebrae, all of which follow a set pattern except the first, eleventh, and twelfth (see Fig. 1-3). There is a gradual increase in size moving down the column, although the height of the discs in the thoracic region is generally less than in the cervical and lumbar regions because of the relative lack of movement in this region.

The body of a typical thoracic vertebra is heart shaped, and the spinal canal is circular. The most conspicuous feature is the presence of costal facets. Demifacets are found on the posterolateral aspects of the body to articulate with the heads of the ribs. The larger, superior facet is semicircular and faces laterally; the smaller, inferior facet faces downward. The facet for articulation with the tubercle of the rib lies at the tip of the transverse process anteriorly. The upper six costal facets are concave; the lower four are flat. T11 and T12 have no costal facet on the transverse processes. Each rib therefore forms three synovial joints with the vertebra with which it articulates.

The intervertebral apophyseal joints lie at the junction of the pedicle and lamina. They are oval and set very steeply. The facets of the superior articular processes face backward and laterally, and the facets of the inferior articular processes face forward and medially.

The spinous processes slope steeply downward from the junction of the laminae.

The first thoracic vertebra is atypical inasmuch as the body is broader, resembling a cervical vertebra. There is a large facet on the posterolateral aspect of the body to articulate with the single articular facet of the head of the first rib, although there is a normal thoracic inferior demifacet for the superior articular surface of the head of the second rib.

The eleventh thoracic vertebra has no costal facet on the transverse process, and a single facet for the head of the eleventh rib on its pedicle.

The twelfth thoracic vertebra also has one facet, for the head of the twelfth rib, which again lies on the pedicle. The inferior surface resembles a lumbar vertebra with a short, stout transverse process (with no costal facet), which is projected backward to form a mamillary process and downward to form an accessory tubercle. The facet of the superior articular process faces backward (thoracic), whereas the facet of the inferior articular process faces laterally (lumbar).

Lumbar Vertebrae

A typical lumbar vertebra has large transverse processes that are costal elements (see Fig. 1-3). The true transverse elements are contracted to form the mamillary processes, which project posteriorly from the superior articular process and the accessory tubercle lying below. They are the surface landmarks of the pedicles and the point of entry of pedicle screws. The articular processes lie on the lamina. The facets of the superior articular processes face medially to allow articulation with the laterally facing facets of the inferior articular surface of the vertebra above. Commonly there are variations in the orientation of the lumbar apophyseal joints, and asymmetry between the left and right is not infrequent.

The vertebral body is reniform, and the spinal canal is triangular. The vertebral body is shaped for weight-bearing purposes, to accommodate longitudinal loads. The design of the body, with a shell of cortical bone and a cancellous cavity of vertically and horizontally arranged trabeculae, confers the added advantage of suitability for dynamic load bearing. This configuration does not, however, confer any stability in the horizontal plane.

The posterior elements are important in considerations of horizontal stability. The orientation of the articular facets allows adjacent vertebrae to lock into one another to prevent sliding and twisting. The numerous processes of the posterior elements serve to allow muscular and ligamentous attachment, and the longer processes (e.g., transverse) act as levers to enhance the actions of the attached muscles.

One portion of the lamina, the pars interarticularis, which lies at the junction of the vertical lamina and horizontal pedicle, has to withstand higher stresses, and microscopic examination of the bone in that region reveals an increased proportion of cortical bone. This region is particularly vulnerable to stress fracture.

The pedicles transmit the forces of the posterior elements to the body, and their cross-sectional design as thick-walled cylinders confers a maximal mechanical advantage for this role.

Sacrum

The five sacral segments are fused to form the sacrum, the inverted triangular bone that is wedged between the two halves of the pelvis and that forms the posterosuperior wall of the pelvic cavity. Developmentally, the fused vertebral bodies form the median portion, and the transverse and costal elements form the lateral masses. The two parts are separated by four pairs of intervertebral foramina on both the pelvic and the dorsal surfaces.

The base is directed upward and forward, with its anterior edge projecting as the sacral promontory. There is an oval articular facet on the base for the lumbosacral disc, and behind the triangular sacral canal the concave superior articular processes form synovial joints with the inferior articular processes of L5.

The dorsal surface is irregular. The laminae are fused to enclose the cauda equina, and the spinous processes form the median sacral crest. The transverse elements form the lateral sacral crest. The erector spinae arise from the area between the two, with the posterior layer of thoracolumbar fascia attaching to both crests.

The lateral mass bears a roughened area for articulation with the ilium. The area between the auricular surface and the lateral crest has a number of deep fossae for attachment of the weight-bearing sacroiliac ligaments.

The posterior wall of the sacral canal is deficient inferiorly to form the sacral hiatus, which is the entry site for caudal epidural injection.

JOINTS

The individual vertebrae are connected by joints between the bodies and between the neural arches.

Joints Between the Vertebral Bodies

The interbody joints need to be able to transfer weight, as well as allow movement, and herein specialized structures—the intervertebral discs—are found. These discs are found throughout the vertebral column except between the first and second cervical vertebrae. The discs are designed to accommodate movement, weight bearing, and shock by being strong but deformable.

Each disc contains a central nucleus pulposus and a peripheral ring of annulus fibrosus sandwiched between a pair of vertebral end-plates. They form a secondary cartilaginous joint or symphysis at each vertebral level.

The nucleus pulposus is a semifluid mass of mucoid material, 70% to 90% water with proteoglycan constituting 65% of the dry weight and collagen constituting 15% to 20% of the dry weight.

The annulus fibrosus consists of a dozen concentric lamellae, with alternating orientation of collagen fibers in successive lamellae to withstand multidirectional strain. The annulus is 60% to 70% water, with 50% to 60% collagen and 20% proteoglycan dry weight. The proportion of proteoglycan (and hence water) falls with increasing age.[7]

There is no strict demarcation between the annulus

and the nucleus; rather, the two merge in a junctional zone.

The vertebral end-plates are 1-mm-thick sheets of cartilage, both fibrocartilage and hyaline cartilage, with an increased ratio of fibrocartilage with increasing age.

The discs are the largest avascular structures in the body and for their nutrition depend on diffusion from a specialized network of end-plate blood vessels.

Joints Between the Posterior Elements

The joints of the posterior elements are the facet joints or, more correctly, the zygapophyseal joints, between the inferior articular processes of one vertebra and the superior articular processes of that immediately below. These are synovial joints, with the surfaces covered by articular cartilage, a synovial membrane bridging the margins of the articular cartilage, and a joint capsule enclosing them. The innervation of these joints is via branches of the posterior primary rami.

There are three types of intraarticular structures in the zygapophyseal joints.[2] They are best known in the lumbar region, and it is postulated that they may be responsible for some of the conditions of the lumbar spine. The largest is the fibroadipose meniscoid, a leaflike fold of synovium that enclosed fat, collagen, and blood vessels and projects from the superior and inferior capsules. The other structures are the adipose tissue pad and the connective tissue rim.

LIGAMENTS (Fig. 1-4)

The ligaments of the spine can be classified into those connecting the bodies, those connecting the posterior elements, and the others, including "false" ligaments.

Ligaments Connecting the Vertebral Bodies

Anterior longitudinal ligament. The anterior longitudinal ligament extends from the cervical region to the front of the sacrum and is well developed in the lumbar region. The ligament consists of several sets of collagen fibers attached to the anterior margins of the vertebral bodies and connecting adjacent bodies, and of longer sets of fibers spanning up to five vertebral bodies. The ligament functions to resist vertical separation of the anterior margins of the bodies. They may also function to prevent bowing of the lumbar spine on extension but are less important in this action than the annulus fibrosis.

Posterior longitudinal ligament. The posterior longitudinal ligament extends the length of the column and forms a narrow band over the backs of the vertebral bodies. The ligament fans out over the discs and penetrates the annuli to gain attachment to the posterior margin of the body. The individual fibers are primarily attached over three vertebrae and thus span two interspaces, but longer fibers spanning up to five vertebrae can be identified. The fibers act to resist separation of the posterior ends of the bodies.

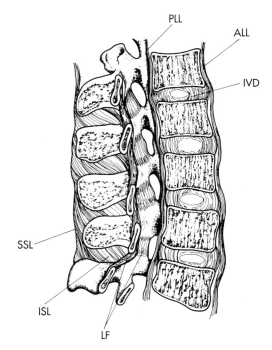

Fig. 1-4. Schematic lateral view of the principal ligaments of the spine. *SSL,* Supraspinous ligament; *ISL,* interspinous ligament; *LF,* ligamentum flavum; *PLL,* posterior longitudinal ligament; *IVD,* intervertebral disc; *ALL,* anterior longitudinal ligament.

Posterior Element Ligaments

Ligamentum flavum. The ligamentum flavum is a paired structure at each level, joining the laminae of consecutive vertebrae. It acts to resist separation of the laminae. Interestingly, the ligament contains up to 80% elastic fibers, which makes it unique among the ligaments of the spine, although the functional significance of this is not clear.

Interspinous ligaments. The interspinous ligaments connect adjacent spinous processes. Three separate parts of this ligament can be identified: ventral, middle, and dorsal. The fibers lie obliquely.

Supraspinous ligament. The supraspinous ligament lies in the midline and is attached to the posterior edges of the spinous processes. Some of the fibers of this ligament are derived from the dorsal fibers of the interspinous ligament. The lower limit of the supraspinous ligament is the spinous process of the fifth lumbar vertebra. These two ligaments act to prevent separation of the spinous processes.

SPECIALIZED AREAS

Specialized areas include the region of the atlas and axis, the region between the thoracic vertebrae and the ribs, the lumbosacral junction and the iliolumbar ligament complex, and the sacroiliac joints.

Atlantoaxial Joints

The atlantoaxial joints are three synovial joints between the dens and the anterior arch of the atlas and the lateral masses of the two bones. They are supported by strong ligaments. The apical ligament connects the apex of the dens to the anterior margin of the foramen magnum, and although this is a rather weak structure, two very strong ligaments lie on each side—the alar, or check, ligaments, which run obliquely from the dens to the margins of the foramen magnum. The alar ligaments act to limit rotation of the head at the atlantoaxial joint.

The cruciate ligament consists of a strong transverse band that attaches on each side to the inner aspect of the lateral mass of the axis, and of a weaker vertical component from the posterior aspect of the body of the axis that attaches to the anterior margin of the foramen magnum. This ligament holds the dens against the anterior arch of the atlas.

The membrana tectoria is the upward continuation of the posterior longitudinal ligament; it attaches to the inner margin of the foramen magnum and covers the posterior surface of the dens and the apical, alar, and cruciate ligaments. It is anterior, but firmly adherent, to the dura mater.

Costovertebral Joints

Each rib articulates with a typical thoracic vertebra in two places: the head of the rib with the costal facet on the body and the tubercle of the rib with the costal facet on the transverse process. These joints are supported by rugged ligaments that are stronger than the ribs themselves. The head of the rib has two articular facets: the lower facet articulates with the costal facet of its own vertebra, and the upper facet articulates with the costal facet of the vertebra above. They form synovial joints. The ridge between the two rib-head facets attaches to the disc by means of a fibrous connection. The ligament supporting these joints has three components from the head of the rib: one passes upward to the body of the vertebra above; one passes downward to the body of the corresponding vertebra; and the middle element runs horizontally in continuity with the disc, deep to the anterior longitudinal ligament to merge with fibers from the opposite side. This is the triradiate ligament.

The tubercle of the rib has a medial facet that forms a synovial joint with a facet on the transverse process of the corresponding vertebra. This joint is supported by the superior and inferior costotransverse ligaments.

The superior costotransverse ligament attaches the crest of the neck of the rib to the lower aspect of the transverse process of the vertebrae above. Two layers can be identified: an anterior layer and a posterior layer that is inclined more medially. The first rib has no superior costotransverse ligament, and the twelfth rib has a lumbocostal ligament inferiorly. An accessory ligament can be identified more medially and is separated from the major part of the ligament by the posterior primary ramus of the spinal nerve and its vessels.

The inferior costotransverse ligament joins the neck of the rib to the transverse process of its own vertebrae. The medial portion joins the neck of the rib to the anterior surface of the transverse process, and the lateral part attaches the tubercle of the rib to the tip of the transverse process.

These are strong ligaments that limit movement of the costotransverse joint to slight gliding as dictated by the shapes of the articular facets.

Lumbosacral Junction and Lumbar Lordosis

As the base of the sacrum is inclined forward and downward, the lumbar spine assumes a lordotic curve to maintain the overall alignment of the vertebral column. Numerous factors interact to achieve this effect.[4] The lumbosacral disc is wedge shaped; its anterior height is 7 mm more than its posterior height. The fifth lumbar vertebra is also wedge shaped; its anterior height exceeds its posterior height by 3 mm. The other lumbar vertebrae are each inclined backward with respect to the vertebra below. In the upright position the L1 vertebra lies directly above the sacrum.

The area is supported by strong ligamentous structures. The iliolumbar ligaments consist of five parts[11] and connect the tip of the transverse process of L5 to the anteromedial surface of the ilium and the inner lip of the iliac crest. This ligament is extremely strong and thus helps to prevent forward displacement of the L5 vertebra on the sacrum (spondylolisthesis). This ligament is fully ligamentous only in adult life; in children and adolescents it is a true muscle.[4]

Sacroiliac Joints

The sacroiliac joints are considered plane joints, although the articular surfaces are irregular; interestingly, the sacral surface is covered with hyaline cartilage, and the iliac surface is covered with fibrocartilage.[10] The joints are very strong to allow weight transmission to the lower limbs. This strength is due almost entirely to its ligamentous supports. These ligaments are ventral, interosseous, and dorsal.

Accessory Ligaments

A number of other structures are called "ligaments" in the lumbar spine. The intertransverse "ligaments" connect adjacent transverse processes but more closely resemble a membrane. The transforaminal "ligaments" bridge the outer aspects of the intervertebral foramina, but their structure is more like that of strips of fascia, and they are not a constant feature. The mamillary accessory "ligaments" connect the ipsilateral mamillary and accessory tubercles of each lumbar vertebra. They resemble tendons in structure and connect two points on the same bone; thus they are not true ligaments.

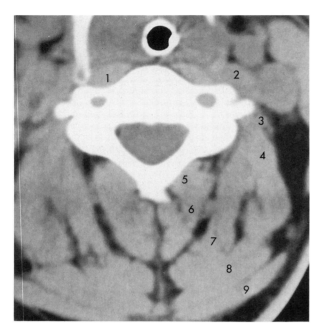

Fig. 1-5. CT scan of a typical cervical segment. *1,* Longus colli; *2,* scalenus anterior; *3,* scalenus medius; *4,* longissimus capitis; *5,* multifidus; *6,* semispinalis capitis; *7,* semispinalis capitis; *8,* splenius; *9,* trapezius.

MUSCLES OF THE VERTEBRAL COLUMN

The muscles acting on the vertebral column can be divided into four groups:

1. *Anterior group*—These muscles lie anterior to the plane of the transverse processes and are supplied segmentally by the anterior primary rami.
2. *Middle group*—These muscles are attached in the plane of the transverse processes.
3. *Posterior group*—These are the true back muscles, known in standard anatomy texts, collectively, as the erector spinae. They lie behind the plane of the transverse processes and receive their nerve supply from the posterior primary rami. They can be subdivided into three groups.
4. *Accessory muscles*—These muscles exert an effect on the vertebral column without being directly attached to it. Muscles in this group have varied origins as reflected in their innervation—cranial and upper limb innervation, as well as body wall innervation. This group includes the sternomastoid, intercostal, latissimus dorsi, and oblique abdominal muscles.

Figs. 1-5 to 1-7 show cross-sectional CT scans at each level of the vertebral column to depict the muscular levels: cervical (Fig. 1-5), thoracic (Fig. 1-6), and lumbar (Fig. 1-7).

Anterior Group

Cervical region. In the cervical region several weak, prevertebral flexor muscles extend from the base of the skull to the superior mediastinum. They are separated

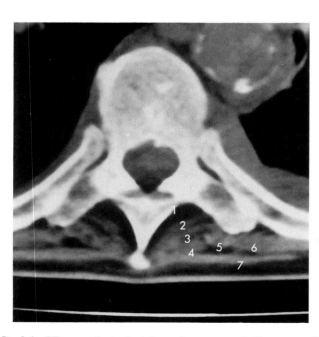

Fig. 1-6. CT scan of a typical thoracic segment. *1,* Rotatores; *2,* multifidus; *3,* semispinalis; *4,* spinalis; *5,* longissimus; *6,* iliocostalis; *7,* latissimus dorsi.

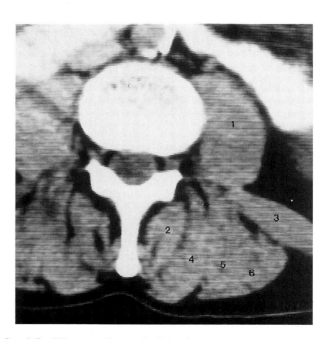

Fig. 1-7. CT scan of a typical lumbar segment. *1,* Psoas; *2,* multifidus; *3,* quadratus lumborum; *4,* spinalis; *5,* longissimus; *6,* iliocostalis.

from the cervical viscera by the strong prevertebral fascia.

The rectus capitis anterior muscle passes from the lateral mass of the atlas to the foramen magnum. The rectus capitis lateralis lies next to this and passes to the jugular process of the occiput. The anterior primary ramus of C1 supplies both muscles.

The longus capitis arises from the anterior tubercles of the typical cervical vertebrae (C3 to C6) and inserts into the basiocciput. It acts to flex the skull and upper cervical spine and is supplied by the anterior primary rami of C1 to C4.

The longus cervicis (colli) muscle has three parts. The upper part connects the anterior tubercle of the atlas to the anterior tubercles of the third, fourth, and fifth cervical vertebrae. The central part connects the bodies of the second, third, and fourth cervical vertebrae to the bodies of the upper three thoracic vertebral bodies. The lower part connects the anterior tubercles of the fifth and sixth cervical vertebrae to the upper three thoracic vertebral bodies. They act to flex the cervical spine and are supplied segmentally by the anterior primary rami.

The scalenus anterior muscle arises from four tendons in line with those of the longus capitis but passes inferiorly to the scalene tubercle of the first rib. It acts to flex the cervical spine forward and laterally. It is supplied by the anterior primary rami of C5 and C6.

Thoracic region. There is no anterior group of muscles in the thoracic spine.

Lumbar region. The anterior group includes the psoas major and minor. The psoas major arises from the anterior aspect of the transverse process, the intervertebral disc, the margin of the vertebral body, and the fibrous arch connecting the upper and lower margins at each level. The fibers form a tendon that traverses the pelvic brim to be inserted into the lesser trochanter of the femur. Its action is to flex the hip, but if the lower limbs are fixed, it acts as a primary flexor of the lumbar spine. The psoas muscles are supplied by the anterior primary rami of the lumbar plexus, which are contained within its mass. The muscle is invested in the strong psoas fascia, which is attached to the discs, the vertebral bodies, and the fibrous arches and extends to the pelvic brim along the iliopectineal line.

The psoas minor muscle is found in 70% of people and arises from the T12-L1 disc; it blends in with the psoas fascia distally.

Middle Group

Cervical region. The scalenus medius muscle arises from the posterior tubercles and costotransverse lamellae of all the cervical vertebrae and is inserted into an area between the neck and subclavian groove of the first rib. It is supplied by the anterior primary rami of C3 to C8.

The scalenus posterior muscle arises from the poste-

rior tubercles of the lower cervical vertebrae and is inserted into the second rib. It is supplied by the anterior primary rami of C4 to C8. The scalene muscles flex the neck forward and laterally or, if the neck is fixed, elevate the ribs as accessory muscles of respiration.

The intertransversarii—small muscles connecting the transverse processes—are best developed in the cervical region. They are divided into anterior and posterior slips by the anterior rami of the spinal nerves. The posterior slips are further divided into medial and lateral components. The anterior and lateral components of the posterior intertransversarii connect the true costal elements and are supplied by the anterior primary rami. The medial components of the posterior intertransversarii connect the true transverse elements and are "true" back muscles, supplied by the posterior primary rami. These muscles have a high density of muscle spindles, and it is postulated that they act as proprioceptive transducers to monitor the movement of the cervical spine and provide feedback to influence the action of the surrounding, more powerful muscles.[1]

Thoracic region. There is no middle group of muscles in the thoracic spine.

Lumbar region. The middle group of muscles includes the quadratus lumborum, which arises from the anterolateral aspects of the transverse processes, the twelfth rib superiorly, and the iliolumbar ligament and ilium inferiorly. The quadratus lumborum acts to flex the lumbar spine laterally and also to fix the twelfth rib on inspiration. It is supplied by the anterior primary rami of T12 and the upper three or four lumbar nerves. Lateral flexion of the lumbar spine is assisted by the intertransversarii laterales, which connect the transverse and accessory processes of one vertebra with the transverse process of the vertebra directly below. These muscles are supplied segmentally by the anterior primary rami.

Posterior Group

The posterior back muscles are the "true" back muscles, which lie behind the plane of the transverse processes and are supplied segmentally by the posterior primary rami. They can be divided into three groups: superficial, middle, and deep.

Deep cervical region. The deep cervical muscles are specialized to effect movements of the head on the neck.

The superior oblique muscle attaches from the lateral aspect of the superior nuchal line of the occiput to the lateral mass of the atlas. It acts to extend the skull and flex it laterally.

The inferior oblique muscle attaches the lateral mass of the atlas to the spine of the axis. It acts to rotate the atlas laterally.

The rectus capitis posterior major and minor muscles both insert into the occiput below the inferior nuchal line; the minor rectus inserts into the posterior arch of the atlas and extends the head; the major rectus originates from the spine of the axis and extends the head and rotates it laterally.

The oblique and recti muscles are supplied by the posterior primary rami of C1.

The cervical intertransversarii posterior mediales are "true" back muscles on the basis of their innervation. The high density of muscle spindles is discussed earlier.

The interspinales are short, paired fasciculi between adjacent vertebral spines, flanking the interspinous ligaments.

There are six pairs of muscles in the cervical region between the axis and the first thoracic vertebra. The rotatores cervicis are irregular and variable. The function of the interspinales and rotator muscles in the cervical region is unknown.

Deep thoracic region. The thoracic region is the only region where true rotation occurs, and here the rotatores spinae are best developed. There are 11 pairs of rotators connecting the upper posterior part of the transverse process to the lateral surface of the root of the spinous process of the vertebra above. The direction of the fibers is thus transverse, conferring maximum leverage.

The levator costae muscles are fan shaped and spread from the tip of each transverse process to insert into the upper border of the rib below, lateral to the tubercle. They act to elevate the ribs.

The thoracic intertransversarii are found between the last three thoracic and the first lumbar vertebrae.

Deep lumbar region. In the lumbar region the deepest layer of "true" back muscles consists of the intertransversarii mediales, which connect the accessory process of one vertebra with the mamillary process of the one below, and the interspinales, which flank the interspinous ligaments.

Middle (Transversospinalis) Muscles

The multifidus is the largest of the back muscles. It consists of a repeating series of fascicles from the lamina of one vertebra to the spinous process two or three levels higher. The multifidus commences at the level of the first dorsosacral foramen and terminates at the C2 level. It is a primary sagittal rotator of the vertebral column.

The semispinalis muscle, which lies on the multifidus from the lower thoracic region to the skull, consists of three parts. The semispinalis capitis is the most powerful part and originates from the transverse processes of the lower four cervical and upper six thoracic vertebrae and inserts into the occiput between the superior and inferior nuchal lines. The semispinalis cervicis connects the transverse processes of the upper six thoracic vertebrae to the spines of the second to fifth cervical vertebrae. The semispinalis thoracis connects the transverse processes of T6 to T10 to the spinous processes of the lower two cervical and upper four thoracic spines. The semispinalis muscles extend the regions of the vertebral column for which they are named.

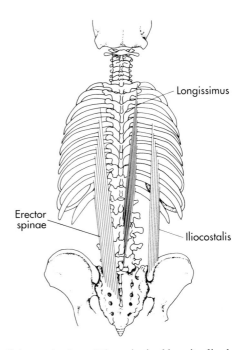

Fig. 1-8. Schematic view of the principal longitudinal muscles of the spine.

Superficial (Sacrospinalis) Muscles (Fig. 1-8)

The sacrospinalis muscles are the long polysegmental muscles, which are the most powerful of the back muscles. There are three muscles—iliocostalis, longissimus, and spinalis—from lateral to medial.

The iliocostalis has three parts, which act to extend the vertebral column and flex it laterally. The iliocostalis cervicis arises from the angles of the third to sixth ribs and ascends to the posterior tubercles of the fourth to sixth cervical transverse processes. The iliocostalis thoracis arises from the upper borders of the angles of the lower ribs and ascends to the upper borders of the angles of the upper ribs and the back of the transverse process of C7. The iliocostalis lumborum is now recognized as having two components[8]: thoracic and lumbar. The thoracic part arises from the angles of the lower eight ribs and attaches distally to the dorsal surface of the sacrum, the erector spinae aponeurosis, and the posterosuperior iliac spine. This part of the muscle spans the lumbar spine without gaining attachment to it and so can act to increase the lumbar lordosis. The lumbar part arises from the posterior aspects of the first to fourth lumbar transverse processes and from the middle layer of the thoracolumbar fascia, and inserts into the lateral aspect of the posterosuperior iliac spine. This part of the muscle can also produce axial rotation of the lumbar spine.

The longissimus muscle also has three parts, which act to extend the vertebral column and flex it laterally. The longissimus capitis arises from the transverse processes of the upper five thoracic vertebrae and the articular processes of the lower four cervical vertebrae and inserts into the posterior margin of the mastoid process. It can also act to extend the head and rotate it laterally. The longissimus cervicis arises from the upper five thoracic transverse processes and attaches to the posterior tubercles of the transverse processes of the second to sixth cervical vertebrae. The longissimus thoracis is recognized as having two parts.[8] A thoracic part arises as fascicles from the ribs and transverse processes from T1 to T12; the fascicles are inserted progressively more caudally to the spinous processes. The fibers from higher levels run more medially. The caudal tendons, along with those of the thoracic part of the iliocostalis lumborum, form what is commonly termed the erector spinae aponeurosis. A lumbar part arises from the accessory tubercle and transverse process of each lumbar vertebra; the fibers converge to form the lumbar intermuscular aponeurosis, which attaches to the medial aspect of the posterosuperior iliac spine. This part of the muscle can also act to translate the lumbar vertebrae posteriorly. The lumbar fibers of the longissimus thoracis and iliocostalis lumborum do not attach to the erector spinae aponeurosis. The attachments and orientation of the individual fascicles of these muscles have recently been studied in great detail and have been found to be relatively constant.[9]

The spinalis muscle is arbitrarily divided into three parts. The spinalis capitis is variably blended with the semispinalis capitis. The spinalis cervicis is often absent. The spinalis thoracis lies superficial to the semispinalis thoracis and medial to the longissimus thoracis and is blended with both muscles.

FASCIA

In the neck the underlying muscles are bound down by the splenius muscle. This muscle arises from the spinous processes and supraspinous ligaments of the upper six thoracic vertebrae and inserts into the superior nuchal line of the occiput and the mastoid process.

The thoracolumbar fascia covers the "true" back muscles more distally. In the cervical region it is continuous with the superficial lamina of the deep posterior cervical fascia. In the thoracic region it is a thin layer between the back muscles and the superficial muscles connecting the upper limbs to the vertebral column.

In the lumbar region the fascia is trilaminar.[3,4] The anterior layer, consisting of vertical fibers, is derived from the fascia of the quadratus lumborum and is attached medially to the anterior surface of the lumbar transverse processes. It separates the anterior and middle groups of back muscles. The middle layer of thoracolumbar fascia separates the middle and posterior groups of back muscles, although its identity is debatable.

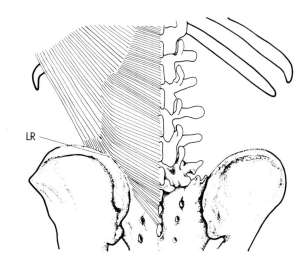

Fig. 1-9. Superficial fibers of the posterior leaf of the thoracolumbar fascia (aponeurosis of latissimus dorsi). *LR,* Lateral raphe.

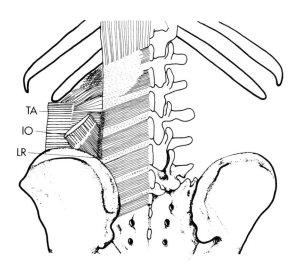

Fig. 1-10. Middle fibers of the posterior leaf of the thoracolumbar fascia. *LR,* Lateral raphe; *IO,* internal oblique; *TA,* transversus abdominis.

The three layers of the thoracolumbar fascia unite to form a dense raphe at the lateral border of the iliocostalis muscle (the most lateral of the erector spinae muscles); this is termed the lateral raphe.

The posterior layer of the thoracolumbar fascia is itself bilaminar (Fig. 1-9) and has a cross-hatched appearance because the fibers in the superficial lamina are oriented caudomedially and those in the deep lamina are oriented caudolaterally.

The superficial lamina of the posterior layer of the thoracolumbar fascia is derived from the aponeurosis of the latissimus dorsi muscle. The arrangement of the fibers and their contribution to the fascia are relatively constant. The fibers from the most lateral portion of the latissimus dorsi insert directly into the iliac crest and do not contribute to the fascia. The fibers adjacent to this reach the iliac crest near the lateral raphe and then skirt around to reach the sacral spinous processes. The next fibers become aponeurotic at the level of the lateral raphe and then deflect medially to reach the spinous processes of the lower lumbar vertebrae. The most rostral fibers do not become aponeurotic until they are much closer to the midline and form the superficial lamina of the posterior layer at the upper lumbar and thoracic levels.[4]

The deep lamina of the posterior layer of the thoracolumbar fascia consists of discrete bands of collagen fibers arising from the lumbar and upper sacral spinous processes (Fig. 1-10); it is not found in the thoracic region. The most caudal bands attach to the posterosuperior iliac spine, whereas the more rostral bands fuse at the lateral raphe with the other layers of the fascia and with the aponeurosis of the transversus abdominis (and also with at least part of the internal oblique muscle). It is thought that the posterior layer of the thoracolumbar fascia, especially, is important in stabilizing the flexed lumbar in the act of lifting.[12]

REFERENCES

1. Abrahams CV: Sensory and motor specialization in some muscles of the neck, *Trends Neurosci* 4:24, 1981.
2. Bogduk N, Engel R: The menisci of the lumbar zygapophyseal joints: a review of their anatomy and clinical significance, *Spine* 9:454, 1984.
3. Bogduk N, Macintosh JE: The applied anatomy of the thoracolumbar fascia, *Spine* 9:164, 1984.
4. Bogduk N, Twomey LT: *Clinical anatomy of the lumbar spine*, 1987, Churchill Livingstone.
5. Crock HV: *Practice of spinal surgery*, New York, 1983, Springer-Verlag.
6. Davis PR: Human lower lumbar vertebrae: some mechanical and osteological considerations, *J Anat* 95:337, 1961.
7. Gower WE, Pedrini V: Age-related variation in protein polysaccharides from human nucleus pulposus, annulus fibrosus and costal cartilage, *J Bone Joint Surg* 51A:1154, 1969.
8. Macintosh JE, Bogduk N: The morphology of the lumbar erector spinae, *Spine* 12:658, 1987.
9. Macintosh JE, Bogduk N: The attachments of the lumbar erector spinae, *Spine* 16:783, 1991.
10. Schunke GB: The anatomy and development of the sacroiliac joint in man, *Anat Rec* 72:313, 1938.
11. Shellshear JL, Macintosh NWG: The transverse process of the fifth lumbar vertebra. In Shellshear JL, Macintosh NWG: *Surveys of anatomical fields,* Sydney, 1980, Grahame.
12. Tesh KM et al: The abdominal muscles and vertebral stability, *Spine* 12:501, 1987.

Chapter Two

◆

Biomechanics of the Spine in Sports

Harry F. Farfan

We may divide sports into two main categories: those in which the lower extremities play a primary (though not necessarily the only) role in attaining the objective (e.g., walking, running, and jumping) and those in which the upper extremities play a primary role (e.g., tennis, pitching or batting in baseball, and golf).

We make our efforts against a fixed base, whether this is the ground or a parallel bar that is itself fixed to the ground. We exert an effort, a shear, a compression, or a twist against the ground, which reacts against our body in exactly the opposite direction according to Newton's third law of motion: to every action there is an equal and opposite reaction. The reaction against our body may be transferred to other parts of the body in accordance with the objective to be accomplished. If the objective is to throw a ball, then the speed and direction of the ball ultimately depend on the action developed by ground contact and the efficiency with which this is transferred by the hand to the ball.

In foot sports, the ground furnishes the action, which is transmitted by the lower extremities to the pelvis. The back transmits the action to the shoulders and upper extremities. From there it is transmitted back along the spine to the pelvis and lower extremities, resulting in greater speed.

In sports where some of the energy is put into the acceleration of an object, such as a javelin, the efficiency of the transmission of efforts by the spine is crucial to achieving the objective, which usually involves speed, distance, and direction.

Therefore in all sports the spine plays a central role in accomplishing the objective of the sport. In certain sports, it is this objective that furnishes the limitations that may result in back injury. For instance, as discussed later, downhill skiing causes fewer back problems than cross-country skiing. In many sports, such as swimming, rowing, and weight lifting, the upper and lower extremities seem equally involved. The spine is obviously involved with the transmission of action and the coordination of activities between the upper and lower extremities. However, from a practical point of view, the artificial division of sports is useful because sports requiring exertion of the upper extremities generally cause most of the back injuries.

The key to understanding injuries to the low back is a knowledge of normal spinal functions. In recent years it has become increasingly evident that the fundamental law controlling normal spinal motion is that our bodies are tuned to our gravitational field, so that the integrated muscular effort results in minimal stress at the intervertebral joints. Depending on the objective, the muscles work to minimize the stress at the joints.

The spine is made up of bones, joints, and ligaments, which are all passive structures and therefore cannot directly affect the movement of the spine. The spinal joints all have muscles, which guide and control the movement. The variable effort of the muscles can change the angle of the joint and activate ligament tensions to support loads.

Although muscles can support loads, there is a finite limit to what they can do. For instance, a weight lifter can support, by muscular effort alone, about 130 pounds. However, by bringing his ligaments into play, he can support loads of three times his weight. Thus, the passive structures of the spine permit action with less muscular effort.

MOTIONS OF THE SPINE
Flexion/Extension in the Sagittal Plane

Flexion and extension are the only movements that are free and can occur without other movements. An individual may bend forward 90 to 100 degrees. The spine can flex forward about 50 degrees, and the rest of the motion is accomplished by rotation of the pelvis about the hips. The angle of flexion of the lumbar spine at the end of range is called λ_0 degrees.[1]

Lateral Bending to Either Side in the Coronal Plane

Free motion in the coronal plane is blocked by the facet joints. Thus as the spine bends laterally, it must also rotate along the axis of the spine. As the spine bends to the left, it rotates to the right. When the spine is flexed, the range of lateral rotation becomes restricted. In extension, the spine permits about 30 degrees of lateral bend.

Axial Rotation

Axial rotation is also a motion greatly affected by the facet joints and by the degree of spinal flexion. The range of axial rotation of the lumbar spine in extension is about 15 to 20 degrees. In full flexion this motion is reduced to zero.

Thus at full flexion at λ_0 degrees, a person cannot bend sideways or rotate the vertebral joints. In this

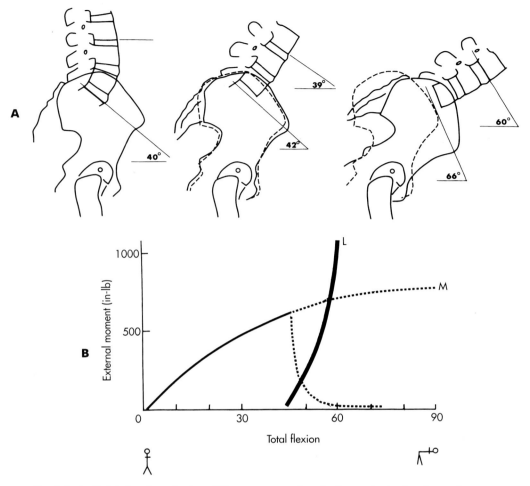

Fig. 2-1. A, Pelvic-lumbar rhythm. When a person bends forward, the lumbar spine rotates forward through an angle of about 50 degrees; the remainder of the motion is from rotation of the pelvis about the hips. When the person returns to the upright position, the pelvis rotates backward first, carrying the bent spine. At about 50 degrees, the spine starts to extend. **B,** The turning moments change with the degree of flexion, increasing as one flexes forward and decreasing as one returns to the upright position. The ligaments tighten at about 50 degrees when the spine is fully flexed. After this, the spine does not flex further. The moment is completely supported by the ligament, and the muscles do not have to work. (**A** from Farfan HF: *Orthop Clin North Am* 6:135, 1975.)

position the back is "locked" and in absolutely the best position to accept axial loading. In this position the spine can function at its maximum capacity.

The reader must understand that full flexion does not mean a forward flexion angle of 90 degrees (Fig. 2-1). As stated above, full flexion occurs naturally in flexing to touch the toes, but it occurs in this movement at about 50 degrees of flexion. However, if the pelvis is rotated backward and then held there, the spine will move through its range of motion of 50 degrees, and full flexion of the spine will be achieved while the person is still standing almost upright.

Full flexion may be achieved by the body weight alone, without active contraction of the abdominal muscles. It may be brought about by active abdominal contraction, as in the performance of a curl-up, or it may be accomplished by tilting the pelvis upward (or forward) by the extensors of the hips.

Full flexion of the spine without muscle activity does not provide active muscle control or produce the stabilizing activity of the lumbodorsal fascia and abdominal muscles. Flexion of the spine accomplished with the hip extensors prevents the full use of the hip extensors. It interferes with the use of the hips for walking. However, when one is not walking, extension at the hips is necessary to remove the lordosis and gain the λ_0-degree position. Thus the best alternative is active muscle control, which occurs naturally: any exertion of the back equivalent to a lift of 50 pounds demands abdominal contraction.

MUSCULAR SYSTEM

Muscle activity means expenditure of energy because of the high metabolic rate of active muscle. Muscle is one of the very few tissues that can store energy for instant release without oxygen. (Compare this with brain tissue, which depletes its stored energy and cannot tolerate anoxia for more than 2 minutes.) The muscles of the trunk, both extensors and flexors, are arranged and balanced so that the extensor moment is the same as the flexor moment. The size of this moment increases gradually in proportion to the area of the disc, which increases from L5 to L1. This arrangement makes it easier to equalize the stress at each intervertebral joint.

Muscle tissue may have a direct effect on a joint. By exerting a force on one of the vertebrae adjoining a joint, it may produce a movement at the joint or, if it cannot produce a movement, it will change the stress at the joint. Muscle tissue may also produce an indirect effect on a joint by affecting the tension in a ligament attached to one of the vertebrae. Muscles at a distance from the joint may also affect the lumbar intervertebral joint. A nod of the head is sufficient to affect the stress at the lumbar spine.

LIGAMENT SYSTEMS

The two types of ligament systems in the lumbar spine are the posterior midline and lateral posterior systems.

Posterior Midline Ligament System

The tensions developed in the midline ligaments result totally from the angle of flexion (Fig. 2-2). These ligaments are attached to the spinous processes and to the neural arch. As the spine is flexed forward, these structures become more and more separated, until the ligament starts to become stretched. This occurs at the same degree (or slightly before) as full spinal flexion: at λ_0 degrees. The weight of the upper body produces a slight extension of the ligament. The degree of stretch depends on the extra load. Thus the degree of stretch of the midline posterior ligament system controls the amount of tension in this ligament and therefore the amount of load it can support.[5]

As a person bends forward, the increasing moment of body weight is supported by muscle, until the ligament stretch is sufficient for the moment. From this point on, the ligament supports the moment while the muscles relax. Moving from the full-flexed to the upright position, the pelvis is rotated backward first, raising the spine and stretching the ligaments to the tension required to support the moment. At λ_0 degrees, if the muscle is able to support the moment, then the back can be straightened and lumbar lordosis restored. If the weight is increased by a person's picking up an object, the pelvis

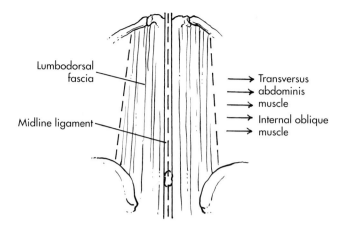

Fig. 2-2. The distance between the dorsal spines increases by 50% or more with flexion. Therefore both the midline ligament and the lumbodorsal fascia are stretched by this change in geometry. In addition, the lumbodorsal fascia provides attachment for the internal oblique and transversus abdominis muscles, which permits these muscles to affect the tension of the lumbodorsal fascia. (From Farfan HF, Gracovetsky S, Lamy C: *Spine* 6:249, 1981.)

is rotated back further, to the angle at which the muscles can take over the increased moment. λ_0 degrees comes at a reduced angle of forward flexion.

Lateral Posterior Ligament System (Lumbodorsal Fascia)

The lumbodorsal fascia, a broad sheet of ligament in the same anatomic plane and continuous with the posterior midline ligament, is attached securely to bone at the upper and lower ends. The middle of this sheet can be activated by muscle attached to its lateral free margin, or it can be stretched by the muscles underlying the fascia. Therefore the tensions in this fascial sheet are affected by the angle of flexion of the spine, as well as by muscle contraction.

The muscles attached to the lateral margin of this sheet are the internal oblique and the transversus abdominis, two of the abdominal muscles.

The ligament systems—one under the sole control of changing geometry and one controlled partly by geometry and partly by muscle—must combine in careful coordination with the angle of flexion. In normal use, each ligament system and the muscular system must contribute about one third of the effort. It is evident that this is so because when one is lifting an object of 50 pounds or even less, the abdominal muscles can be felt to be working. Although it is possible to lift this weight without contraction of these muscles, the fact that a person is not using the abdominal muscles is often a first sign of lost coordination.

The ultimate aim, for maximum effort, is the λ_0-degree angle of the spine. In this position the spine becomes a solid link between the pelvis and shoulders,

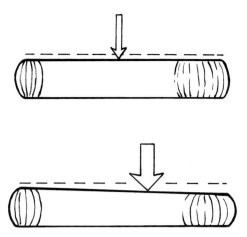

Fig. 2-3. The disc supports compression load. With a compression load, both the back and the front of the disc are compressed. As the load is increased, the disc must flex, and the load is shifted anteriorly.

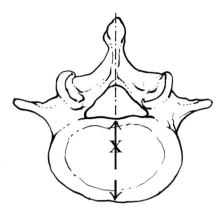

Fig. 2-4. The movement of the instantaneous center of motion is forward with increased compression, toward the facet joints with axial rotation.

and this is the best position for transmitting maximum effort from the ground to the upper extremities. The significance for upper extremity sports is obvious.

INTERVERTEBRAL JOINT

To reduce lumbar lordosis to λ_0 degrees, the compressive load must be increased. This can be achieved either by increasing the muscular effort or by increasing the load on the spine. The disc supports all of the compression load, and the facet joint creates all of the shear (Fig. 2-3).

Under normal circumstances the disc annulus and the nucleus both contribute to the support of the load, but the annulus can support the load without the nucleus. The nucleus appears to be a stress-distributing device. As the load is increased, the pressure in the disc slowly rises. This requires the disc to be unloaded because high pressures in the disc nucleus may cause a problem in the joint. The unloading mechanism is a change in the angle at the joint.

The center of rotation in neutral position is at the geometric center of the disc[4] (Fig. 2-4). In most discs this is at the center of the nucleus. In wedged discs this center is located more posteriorly. When the joint is subjected to a compression load, there is flexion at the joint and the center of motion moves forward with the increasing degree of flexion. The effective lengths of the lever arm of the erector spinae and the ligament system are thereby increased. The effective distance to the facet joints is also increased and more compressed, thereby increasing the effectiveness of the facets in resisting or transmitting torque.

With axial rotation in the neutral position, the instantaneous center of motion moves toward one facet joint, causing a shearing motion at the disc, which is damaging because the disc is constructed to withstand

compression, not shear. It is poorly designed to resist shear.

With the joint in neutral position, the fibers of the annulus are not under undue stress. However, as the joint becomes flexed, the fibers of the annulus become stretched by a lateral bulging of the disc. This also adds to the torque strength of the unit.

Again, we can see that the strength and thus the safety of the intervertebral joint depend on the degree of flexion of the lumbar spine. Some misguided amateurs will stand upright, holding a barbell on their shoulders, and do repeated rotations of the trunk or repeated side bends. The potential for injury with these movements is great. Because of the increased torque due to the added compression, it is better to do these rotations with a light weight on the shoulders.

INJURIES TO THE LOW BACK
Torsional Injury

The most common injury is due to an overload in axial torsion. A single episode of overwhelming force may be required to cause this overload, but more frequently it results from several minor episodes.[2]

The three-joint complex that makes up an intervertebral joint is injured in all its members. The disc annulus is stretched and torn off its attachment to the vertebral end-plate. One facet joint is compressed and suffers damage to its articular surface on one side, whereas the ligaments of the other facet joint are subjected to traction injury.

The symptoms derive from the facet joints, from the disc, and from the deformity of the neural contents. The facet joints cause pain in the buttocks and down the lateral side of the thigh and knee, to the ankle. These pains come in recurrent attacks, and symptoms progress to include irritation of the nerve root with numbness on the outer side of the foot and weakness of dorsiflexion of the great toe.

Because a right-handed person habitually twists to the left when throwing or when swinging a racquet, the torsional injury occurs to the disc and facet joints, blocking movement to the left. The symptomatic leg is usually, but not invariably, on the left for right-handed persons. For left-handed persons, the reverse is true.

The victim may suffer for a long while with back pain and sciatica but may show no evidence of impaired nerve function and thus is denied surgery.

Compression Injury

A compression injury results from an unexpected overload in compression, such as occurs with an unexpected fall on the backside or with unexpectedly receiving a load in the arms. The result is a fracture of the end-plate, or a burst disc. The goalie in ice hockey is prone to falling in this way, but disc problems do not often occur.

With fracture of the end-plate not detectable by simple radiographs, the facet joint and annulus remain relatively little affected. The complaints of persons with these injuries are usually transient. Only years later do they develop symptoms, when the facet joints become arthritic after loss of disc thickness. Still later, they may develop a true nerve root irritation from stenosis of the intervertebral canal.

In the relatively rare instance of a burst disc, much of the disc content may be forced out into the canal and cause immediate lower extremity signs and symptoms.

Compression injuries are seen commonly in the seated sports, such as horseback riding and motorcycle or bicycle riding, and in luge and bobsled enthusiasts. The energy of the repeated axial load on the buttocks is only partially dissipated by the buttocks and pelvis; the lowest joint of the spine receives the overload and may fail.

INJURIES ASSOCIATED WITH SPECIFIC SPORTS
Walking and Running

A person walks by rotating the hips and shoulders in opposite directions. During this motion lumbar lordosis and the degree of flexion increase and decrease. As walking speed is increased, the amplitude of these oscillations decreases, until at running speed the oscillations are very small and the lordosis is reduced to near λ_0 degrees.[4]

The initial power comes from the extensors of the hip and spine. By raising the trunk, a person increases the potential energy at each oscillation. The potential energy is converted to kinetic energy at heel strike. The counter-oscillating masses of shoulders and hips form a device like a pendulum, which can store and release energy with each oscillation. For increasing speed, to transmit the rotatory forces of these oscillations, the

torque strength of the spine must increase. This is automatically provided by the increased flexion (or decreased lordosis) produced by muscular action.

In a sprint we recognize the λ_0-degree position of the runner. At a slow walking pace the lordosis is easily recognized. At intermediate speeds the spinal lordosis is reduced just enough for the torque transmission required to accomplish the objective. Thus if the lordosis is not corrected for the speed and remains excessive, then the torsional strength of the joint can easily be exceeded. The situation is clearly demonstrated when a person suddenly steps into a pothole while walking. The energy released by the larger drop of the foot to the ground may suddenly exceed the resistance to rotation of the spine in extension, resulting in back strain.

Skiing

In cross-country skiing, the foot is fixed to the ski at the toe. This reduces the effectiveness of heel strike, lowering the torque delivered to the spine. Normally, this would cause the skier to progress with a lordosis. However, the skier also uses ski poles, which force the shoulders to rotate through a larger arc than usual. The potential for injury remains high.

Downhill skiers, on the other hand, have their feet fixed to the skis with a certain degree of flexion at the ankle. This in turn causes the abdominal muscles to tighten and reduces the lordosis, protecting the back. Barring accidental spills, very few downhill skiers have back problems caused by skiing.

Baseball Pitching

Fig. 2-5 shows a pitcher throwing a baseball. Fig. 2-5, A, shows the pitcher just before, and Fig. 2-5, B, shows him just after, the release of the ball. In Fig. 2-5, A, the pelvis is almost in line with the pitch. The back is extended, and the right arm and elbow are cocked at about 100 degrees of flexion, with the arm behind the shoulder. The weight of the body is being transferred to the left foot, which is about to touch the ground. The trunk position is upright without flexion to one side or the other. In Fig. 2-5, B, the pelvis has turned through 90 degrees to the frontal plane. The back is in full flexion and is still upright with the shoulder in the same plane. The arm is still in flexion at the elbow but is in front of the shoulder. The left foot is firmly planted on the ground.

The power behind the pitch is due to the movement of the spine from extension to full flexion, but the torsion, although adding to the power, is important for a different reason. The rotatory acceleration, which is transmitted from the ground to the pelvis, must be transmitted to the shoulders and arms. If this acceleration is not properly transmitted, the shoulders will not be synchronized.

To transmit a maximal rotation up through the spine,

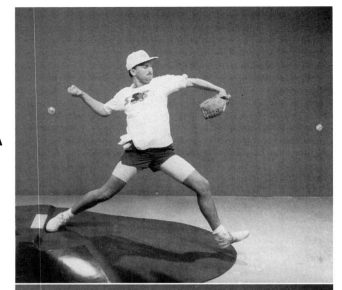

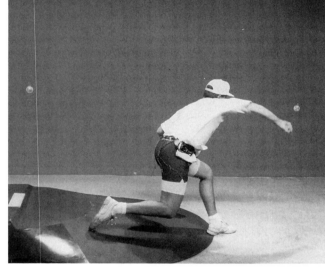

Fig. 2-5. Pitcher. **A,** Just before ball release. Note the degree of back extension and the alignment between the pelvis and the shoulder girdle. **B,** Just after ball release. Note, in particular, the flexion of the spine and the frontal alignment of the pelvis and shoulder girdle.

the joints at L5 of the lumbar spine must be stabilized. Without active musculature, the normal spine can transmit about 750 pounds of torque. However, if the spine is compressed axially, its torque strength is greatly increased. Compression of the joints at L5 forces the facet joints to be more closely engaged, thereby increasing the torque strength of the spine. Therefore, to increase the torque strength of the spine, the muscles must pull the back from extension to flexion. If this does not occur, the torque strength of the joints at L5 in extension can easily be exceeded by the rotating shoulders. Injury to the low back may result.

If the spine is imperfectly flexed to withstand the rotation of the pelvis, then there will be a lag between the shoulders and the pelvis, and ball release will come either earlier or later than intended, making the throw erratic. This fault can be recognized as the pitcher becomes tired. His lordosis increases as the abdominal muscle becomes unable to keep pace. He pitches to the right side of the plate with an early ball release, and as he tries to correct this, he pitches his ball too far to the left.

A torsional injury in the spine is usually ascribable to twisting forcibly when the spine is not sufficiently flexed to withstand the torque. In right-handed players, the twist usually occurs as the body twists to the left side. Symptoms commonly arise first from damage to the facet joints and usually, but not invariably, occur in the left hip and thigh. These injuries are very hard to treat adequately. Because of the recurrent problem, the player continues to twist to the damaged side, and the injury tends to progress. It is interesting to note that the batter is often in the same position and is often injured under the same circumstances.

A pitcher who habitually does not release the ball at the right moment (either early or late) may learn to correct his aim but will develop another problem (e.g., a joint injury or ligamentous strain) with the upper back.

Upper dorsal injury. To lift the arms, the shoulder blades must be stabilized. This is done by the levator scapulae, the rhomboids, and the lower part of trapezius, which are posteriorly attached around the periphery of the shoulder blade. Anteriorly, the serratus anterior muscle holds the rim of the scapula against the back and sides of the chest.

As the arms are extended forward at shoulder height, the levator scapulae attached to the upper angle and the rhomboids along the medial border of the scapulae contract. The lower portion of the trapezius also contracts to prevent the scapulae from rotating[3] (Fig. 2-6).

These muscles set up a contractive force between C1 and T9 or T10. This force tends to increase the lordosis of the cervical spine and the kyphosis of the dorsal spine. The upper dorsal spine is relatively rigid, so it can give only at its joints. The smallest joint—usually the fifth dorsal (D5-6)—suffers the largest compression force and is often the first to fail.

The pain radiates from D5 to both shoulders and up into the neck, and it is usually more pronounced on one side. With pitching a baseball, the asymmetric motion produces an element of torsion, which aggravates the tendency toward shoulder pain.

In addition to the transient stiff neck, with pain radiating to the shoulder, the individual can suffer an intercostal neuralgia or may develop numbness in the upper extremities, usually in the ulnar distribution.

The mechanism by which numbness is produced in the upper extremity is interesting. As the shoulder moves forward, normally it drops. In persons with supraclavic-

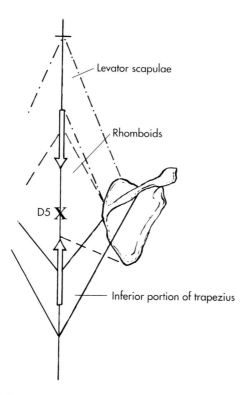

Fig. 2-6. Source of pitcher's shoulder. Compression and torsional overload of D5-6.

ular (or cervical) ribs, this drop in height is sufficient to produce an irritation of the lower two cords of the brachial plexus, often resulting in numbness or tingling in the fingers.

When the movements of the arm become uncoordinated with the movements of the hips, the baseball pitcher tries to correct the throw by either early or late ball release. The resulting overswing of the shoulders produces symptoms in the upper back, shoulder, and upper extremity—the "pitcher's shoulder." The basic cause is poor coordination of the abdominal muscles. The degree of lumbar flexion must be adjusted to the acceleration demands on the spine to transmit this increased torsion.

Thus the increasing lordosis, combined with erratic pitches, is a sign that a pitcher is out of control. A prolonged warm-up in the bull pen may actually work against the player.[6,7]

Golf

The golfer stands astride and hits a ball with a club with a long handle. The long handle allows the golfer to stand with a forward flexion angle of about 40 degrees. The direction of the ball is decided by the alignment of the pelvis and shoulders with the line of flight. The ball must be hit at the bottom of the swing, when the club is traveling at maximum velocity. The length of the drive depends on the velocity of the club head at the time of contact with the ball. The acceleration of the club head also is maximum at the time of ball contact. To achieve this acceleration, the shoulder must swing through an arc of 80 to 90 degrees for best distance. For lesser distances the rotation of the shoulder need not be as great.

To achieve the desired result, several different factors must be taken into account, depending on the distance desired. The first factor is the degree of rotation of the shoulder. Standing upright, the shoulder can be rotated through about 30 degrees while the pelvis is held steady. Thus for a person to achieve 90 degrees of rotation at the shoulders, the pelvis must also be rotated. The five joints of the lumbar spine can supply only about 10 to 15 degrees of motion, the thoracic spine can provide another 5 to 6 degrees, and the shoulders must provide the rest.

This amount of rotation depends critically on the degree of lumbar flexion. In full flexion the lumbar rotation is virtually zero. The shoulders and thoracic spine can still rotate. As long as both feet are on the ground, the hips will not permit the pelvis to rotate 90 degrees, as is the case with the baseball pitcher, who throws with only one foot on the ground. In the golfer the pelvis can rotate only about 30 degrees. Thus to obtain the maximum rotation of the shoulders, with both feet on the ground and with the lumbar spine in extension, the pelvis and spine must rotate to achieve about 80 to 90 degrees of rotation at the shoulders.

Another factor to be taken into account to achieve the desired result is flexion/derotation. The golfer must get from the extended lumbar spine—with a rotation of the pelvis, spine, and shoulders—to the flexed lumbar spine with the shoulders and pelvis in the same frontal plane at the time of ball contact, when the movement of the club head is accelerated at the bottom of the swing. There is therefore a strong contraction of the abdominal muscles to flex and derotate the spine. The arms can accelerate the movement of the club until the crucial contact with the ball. At this same instant, the spine must be fully flexed to the λ_0-degree position. The key controlling influence is the contraction of the abdominal muscles. When the movement is well coordinated, the rate of flexion should keep pace with the rotation of the shoulders because, as stated earlier, the flexed spine can support a greater torsional load.

Golf instructors are very careful to explain to a beginner the importance of keeping the knees slightly bent and loose. This ensures that the abdominal muscles are tensed, maintaining the pelvic upward rotation. Failure to coordinate the extension/flexion motion with derotation of the spine results in a duffed ball or, more seriously, if the action is stopped too precipitously, the player may suffer a low back injury.

As a person grows older, the lumbar spine tends to lose some of its flexibility because of attrition of disc thickness. Therefore the golfer can attain the λ_0-degree position with a diminished degree of flexion. The older player does not have to flex as much as the younger person to attain maximum effort. Everything else being equal, the velocity of the club head at ball contact depends on the length of the lever arm (i.e., on the length of the club handle). It would appear reasonable that the older player should choose a club more adapted to the changed λ_0-degree position. This would have the effect of protecting the player's back, as well as preserving the player's skill.

In using the irons, the golfer may not rotate the spine as much. This is automatically corrected for by the length of the clubs and by the stance of the player. Should the player swing with an iron in exactly the same manner as the player swings with a driver, both the extension and the rotation of the spine will be off, unless the player can adjust these two factors while using a shorter club. Thus using the irons, rather than the drivers, is more likely to result in back problems. Furthermore, a player is more likely to apply asymmetric loading to the spine on the fairways and rough than on a driving tee.

American Football

Apart from external causes usually present in the impact sport of American football, certain linemen—the defensive line backers—are particularly prone to lumbar spine injury. These players are discouraged from tackling below the waist and must await the oncoming player in an upright position. Therefore they must resist considerable force from in front.

To exert sufficient counterforce requires that the lumbar spine be fully flexed. Contraction of the abdominal muscles is necessary for maximum effort. The player, even though standing upright, has his spine in full flexion, not in extension, as has been claimed by others.

The least asymmetric effort will produce a torsional effect on the lower lumbar vertebrae, and with sufficient asymmetric effort, the player may develop spondylolysis. Traumatic spondylolysis, on the other hand, often results from a forced hyperextension of the spine. Force delivered in this position causes a fracture of the lamina at its attachment to the pedicle, usually taking a portion of the pedicle.

The offensive quarterback, who throws the ball, is subject to uncoordinated twisting, just like the baseball pitcher, and falls victim to the same type of low back torsional injury.

PREVENTION OF BACK INJURIES

With all sports that involve twisting, there must be emphasis on two requirements. The first is excellent coordination of the flexion/extension motion. In men this excellent coordination is seen to occur naturally up to the age of 25 to 30. At this age the individual may be in good shape, but in most men there is already a loss of coordination, which particularly affects the abdominal muscles. In women this coordination is often lost at a much earlier age—at age 15 to 20. This is partly because of the mother's insistence that the daughter pull her stomach in, in the mistaken belief that this action improves the figure. In actual fact, if the instruction were to harden the abdominal muscles, besides improving the figure, the daughter would preserve her flexion/extension coordination.

It is interesting that coordination begins to fall off almost immediately as growth is completed. Once the athlete reaches the age of 30, the vast majority are no longer able to compete.

The second requirement that must be emphasized is the stamina necessary to maintain coordination. Floor exercises to develop coordination are almost useless. The exercise that is needed is a natural movement that cannot be done without an abdominal contraction. A good example of this sort of exercise is skipping rope, like boxers do, with a tight rope and a minimal jump. Another example is rowing a boat, where virtually all muscles are involved in a coordinated movement, and where one of the principal movements is flexion/extension of the spine.

An antitorsional brace that can be used to protect the low back against torsional overload has also been used successfully in cases of back injury and has been used by some amateur golfers who claim an improvement in their game.

REFERENCES

1. Farfan HF: Muscular mechanism of the lumbar spine and the position of power and efficiency, *Orthop Clin North Am* 6:135, 1975.
2. Farfan HF: Reorientation in the surgical approach to degenerative lumbar intervertebral joint disease, *Orthop Clin North Am* 8:9, 1977.
3. Farfan HF, Baldwin J: Tired neck syndrome: chronic postural strain. In Walciman E, editor: *Trends in ergonomics/human factors,* vol 3, North Holland, 1986, Elsevier Science.
4. Farfan HF, Gracovetsky S: The optimum spine, *Spine* 6:543, 1986.
5. Farfan HF, Gracovetsky S, Lamy C: Mechanism of the lumbar spine, *Spine* 6:249, 1981.
6. Farfan HF, et al: The instantaneous center of rotation of the third lumbar intervertebral joint, *J Biomech* 4:149, 1971.
7. Lamy C, et al: The strength of the neural arch and the etiology of spondylolysis, *Orthop Clin North Am* 6:215, 1975.

Section Two

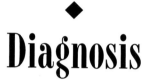

Diagnosis

Chapter Three

◆

Radiology of the Spine

R. Scott Kingston

As enthusiasm for sports and physical fitness increases, the potential for sports-related spinal injuries rises. These may range from minor musculoskeletal strains to more serious fractures and dislocations resulting in temporary or permanent neurologic deficits. Contact sports, such as football, soccer, hockey, and rugby, and highly competitive sports, including gymnastics, dancing, weight lifting, and diving, can result in a wide array of complex spinal injuries; however, common underlying factors are responsible for the basic types of injury. The incidence of spinal cord injury or vertebral instability leading to neurologic impairment following major trauma approaches 60% when vertebral body and posterior element fractures with subluxations are present. Therefore a complete radiologic investigation often requires a combination of diagnostic imaging methods. This chapter reviews the main radiologic imaging procedures and their applications in injuries and disorders of the spine related to sports. Specific mechanisms of injury, related spinal conditions, and how the various imaging modalities are applied in the cervical and thoracolumbar spine are then discussed.

Imaging Modalities

PLAIN FILM ROENTGENOGRAPHY

Examining the spine with plain radiography constitutes the mainstay in evaluating an injured patient. This examination can be performed with relative ease, requiring little or no movement. Once the basic views are obtained, thereby excluding catastrophic injury to the spine, supplemental views may be ordered to evaluate any clinical conditions not visualized on the initial set of films.

In dealing with the cervical spine, the minimum set of films includes the anteroposterior (AP), lateral, and open-mouth or odontoid views. The exact technique in radiographic positioning and filming is not discussed here; the reader is referred to standard radiologic positioning textbooks.

C7 must be visualized on the lateral projection when the cervical spine is being examined because many fracture dislocations occur in the lower cervical spine or at the cervicothoracic junction (Fig. 3-1). Because the muscle bulk of the neck and shoulders in professional athletes lies in the way of the x-ray beam, visualization of the lowermost cervical vertebrae often becomes difficult. It may be necessary to obtain a swimmer's view, with one arm extended above the head and the other by the patient's side for proper visualization of this area. Another excellent technique is the application of passive stretch traction straps (Boger straps) applied to the patient's wrists and wrapped around the feet. With increasing extension of the lower extremities, the patient's shoulders are slowly depressed caudally, allowing improved inspection of the lower cervical spine.

Often the patient is in such severe pain with spasm that placement to obtain the neutral lateral view that could show true ligamentous injuries is not possible. Therefore flexion and extension views are necessary to disclose cases of any occult instability.

A number of imaginary radiographic lines are used in evaluating cervical spine alignment (Fig. 3-2). The three major ones are two smooth convex lines connecting the anterior and posterior vertebral body margins and a third line connecting the junction of the cervical lamina and spinous processes (spinolaminar line). Significant disruption of any of these lines may indicate underlying ligamentous injury, resulting in instability.

The open-mouth view is vital in assessing the normal articulation of the lateral masses of the atlas (C-1) with those of the axis (C-2), especially when one is dealing with a Jefferson burst fracture with disruption of the normal neural ring of C-1 causing lateral displacement of its lateral masses. The bilateral offset of the lateral masses of C-1 with a widened space between the medial margin and the odontoid process of C-2 indicates this type of fracture.

Of equal importance is the articulation between the anterior arch of C-1 and the odontoid process of C-2 on the lateral projection. Either laxity or disruption of the transverse ligament may result in an unstable atlanto-axial joint (Fig. 3-3). This may have grave consequences in cases of flexion, where there is widening of this joint beyond the normal 2.5 mm in the adult, resulting in compression by the odontoid process on the cervicomedullary junction of the spinal cord.

Oblique views of the cervical spine aid in evaluating the neural foramina, as well as the posterior elements (Fig. 3-4). The pillar view is another special view. Using 20 to 30 degrees of caudal angulation of the x-ray beam enables a more precise inspection of the lateral masses when pillar fractures and facet dislocations are suspected in hyperextension and rotational injuries.

Most injuries to the thoracic and lumbar spine can be evaluated with simple AP and lateral radiographs. Many

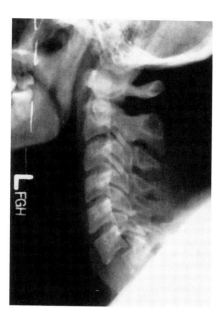

Fig. 3-1. Lateral x-ray film showing significant anterior subluxation of C6 on C7 with depression of the shoulders.

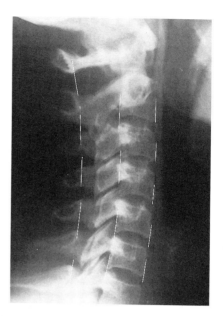

Fig. 3-2. Normal imaginary lines used in evaluating cervical spine alignment.

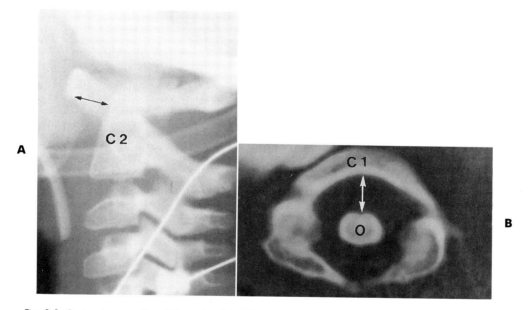

Fig. 3-3. Lateral x-ray film **(A)** and axial CT scan **(B)** demonstrating widening between the anterior arch of C1 and odontoid process *(O)* of C2.

of the same alignment criteria used in evaluating cervical spine fractures are employed elsewhere in the spinal column.

Oblique views of the lumbar spine are particularly helpful in assessing for injuries of the pars interarticularis (the portion of the vertebral posterior arch at the junction of the pedicle with the lamina). Old nonhealed spondylolytic defects of the pars are readily identified by radiolucent gaps or osseous defects with smooth scle-

rotic margins. These generally do not cause pain unless there is compression of the thecal sac or adjacent nerve root caused by hypertrophy of the fibrocartilaginous mass, often associated with the pars defect. Sclerosis or hypertrophy on the contralateral side may indicate compensatory changes or a new fatigue stress fracture with an attempt at healing.

When a spondylolysis exists, the lateral view is used to determine if a spondylolisthesis, or slippage of the

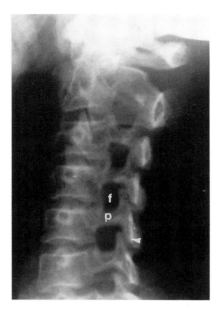

Fig. 3-4. Oblique x-ray film of the cervical spine showing patent normal neural foramina *(f)* bounded by the pedicles *(p)* above and below from the vertebral bodies and disc spaces anteriorly and from the superior facet *(small arrowhead)* and inferior facet *(large arrowhead)* posteriorly.

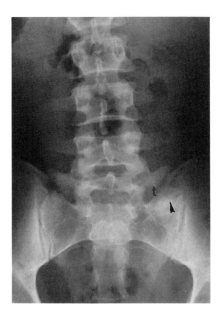

Fig. 3-5. AP x-ray film showing a large transverse process *(t)* of L5 articulating with the sacrum *(arrowhead)*. The L5-S1 disc segment is therefore a transitional segment with little chance of disc degeneration or herniation.

affected vertebral body on the lower one, is present. This may be associated with disc degeneration and a mechanical instability causing pain or may contribute to various forms of lateral or foraminal stenosis resulting in a radiculopathy.

The concept of spinal instability is critical in evaluating the spine-injured patient or someone with back pain. In general, spinal instability refers to the body's inability to maintain its normal anatomic relationships, producing a strong potential for spinal cord or neural damage resulting from any progressive skeletal deformity of the vertebral column. One simple method used to evaluate for lumbar spine instability is the lateral Knuttsen bending view. This is obtained with the patient sitting in the flexed position and then standing in a hyperextended position, which places normal physiologic axial loading stresses on the vertebral column. When there is abnormal angulation or horizontal displacement of one vertebra on another by more than 2.5 mm in flexion or by more than 3 mm in extension, the affected disc segment can be considered unstable.

In the athlete or active individual, disc degeneration results in loss of the normal disc height. Normally the intervertebral discs increase in height from L1 to the sacrum, with the anterior portion being wider than the posterior portion. With the loss in height, biochemical changes occur with degeneration, resulting in hypertrophic osteoarthritic changes. Traction spurs at the attachment of the peripheral annular fibers (Sharpey's fibers) onto the posterior vertebral body cortex, as well

as inflammatory changes occurring in the paraspinal ligaments, result in bony overgrowth with subsequent osteophyte formation. These findings, as well as gas collections forming in the intervertebral disc, are the hallmarks of disc degeneration and are easily evaluated on lateral radiographs.

Caution is advised with regard to lumbosacral transitional vertebrae. A rather large proportion of the general population do not have the typical 12 thoracic vertebrae with their respective ribs and lowermost 5 presacral lumbar vertebrae. Normal congenital variations include atretic twelfth ribs with or without a transitional lumbosacral segment. There is a wide range of the lowest lumbar segment articulation with the sacrum, including large transverse processes with or without fusion to the sacrum (Fig. 3-5). Regardless of the type of the transitional vertebra, the last-formed intervertebral disc segment is usually rudimentary and contributes little to no significant motion to the rest of the vertebral column. Therefore the possibility of a disc herniation or significant degeneration at this formed but nonmobile segment is quite remote. With a transitional intervertebral disc segment, proper nomenclature must be used consistently should the patient require surgery.

NUCLEAR MEDICINE BONE SCAN

The patient who has sustained recent trauma to the neck or back must be evaluated clinically to rule out the possibility of any serious injury that may result in spinal cord trauma with neurologic sequelae. The vast majority of injuries are due to sprains or strains involving the paraspinal ligaments and supporting muscles. Those involving the bony vertebral column may go undetected on the plain radiograph if no obvious subluxation or fracture is present. In addition, isolating the vertebral level of the patient's source of pain may be difficult. Performing a nuclear medicine bone scan not only documents bone or joint pathology, but also helps in pinpointing the level of concern so that a more definitive examination concentrating on that specific area may be undertaken.

In the past, radiopharmaceuticals employing strontium-85, strontium-87m, and fluorine-18 were used, but these have been entirely replaced by newer technetium compounds because the former isotopes had undesirable energy characteristics and long half-lives. Technetium-99m has a low energy of 140 keV, which is ideal for the gamma camera. Its short half-life of 6 hours also makes it quite attractive for use in the proper setting. Currently, technetium can be labeled with a phosphate compound simply and quickly in any nuclear "hot lab." Although the particular phosphate used in our institution is methylenediphosphonate (MDP), a number of different pharmaceuticals are used in today's practice. They differ mainly by their rate of excretion from the body. As a general rule, approximately 50% of the labeled isotope is excreted through the genitourinary system within the first 24 hours. The patient should drink six to eight glasses of fluid after being intravenously injected with the isotope and should empty the bladder immediately before being scanned. This promotes renal excretion, thereby enhancing bone to soft tissue background activity, and lowers the patient's radiation exposure.

With a usual adult dose of 15 to 20 mCi, gonadal and total-body radiation exposures are on the order of 0.2 rad. The skeletal system receives the highest dose: approximately 1 rad.

Patients are scanned 2 to 3 hours after they have been injected with the radioisotope. Whole-body imaging can be obtained in the anterior and posterior projections using the moving scintillation camera with the patient in the supine position. A low-energy, high-resolution parallel-hole collimator is used. For smaller areas, camera spot views may be obtained using converging or pinhole collimators, thereby increasing the spatial resolution of the images. As with all nuclear medicine imaging with technetium, a 20% window is usually centered on its 140 keV photopeak.

At our institution posterior oblique views of the lumbar spine are obtained in addition to the routine anterior and posterior views. This further localizes foci of abnormal uptake in the vertebral body or posterior arch. Newer, more sophisticated imaging may be accomplished with single photon emission computed tomography (SPECT). This allows the image data to be reformatted in any plane, similar to computed tomography (CT). This method is employed for patients with

suspected pars defects or other stress fractures that are not displayed as well with more conventional planar imaging. SPECT imaging also aids in interpreting scans wherein excessive kyphosis or lordosis results in either false-positive or false-negative scans. This occurs when a bone being imaged is closer to the camera and thus appears hotter than a bone farther away from the camera. The scan demonstrates areas of increased activity throughout the lumbar spine in the anterior projection and areas of decreased activity in the posterior projection in patients with increased lordosis.

The technetium phosphate compound becomes incorporated into the calcium hydroxyapatite crystal, depending on the integrity of the skeletal vascular system. This unique feature reflects the physiologic or functional nature of the bone's metabolic state at the time of scanning. The higher sensitivity in detecting abnormalities over plain radiography provides a simple technique for evaluating the osseous system days to weeks before any radiographic changes are detected visually.

Since the bone scan may be thought of as a dynamic physiologic scan, it is often employed in attempts to distinguish active pathologic conditions from inactive ones. Not infrequently, compression fractures of the spine or spondylolytic defects are recognized on plain radiographs. Determining the appropriate treatment and final outcome depends on whether these fractures or defects are the result of acute or prior trauma. By evaluating the bone scan's intensity of activity corresponding to the radiographic abnormality, one may distinguish between old and recent trauma.

One major caveat in interpreting bone scans is the disparity between the scan's specificity and sensitivity in detecting disease. Any pathologic process resulting in an increased blood supply to an affected area will result in positive findings on the bone scan because of the larger amount of delivered isotope available for chemiabsorption into the hydroxyapatite crystal. This is often the case in inflammatory conditions with vasodilation and subsequent hyperemia. Fractures, hypertrophic degenerative changes with osteophytes, degenerative disc disease, cases of discitis, and local inflammatory conditions resulting in myositis ossificans or dystrophic calcifications are some of the many other causes of positive findings.

Careful scrutiny with other diagnostic imaging tests such as x-ray films, CT, or magnetic resonance imaging (MRI) is often required to avoid false-positive bone scan interpretations. Fortunately, these correlative tests demonstrate higher spatial resolution; thus precise diagnoses can usually be achieved without difficulty.

MYELOGRAPHY

Plain film myelography currently uses water-soluble contrast agents with different iodine concentrations in evaluating spinal disorders. In the past, oil-based agents such as iophendylate (Pantopaque) were used but were frequently associated with undesirable side effects and complications, including the late development of epidural fibrosis and arachnoid adhesions when the medium was mixed with blood within the subarachnoid space. Because of its high viscosity and immiscibility with the cerebrospinal fluid, it was customary to withdraw as much as possible on completion of the examination. This attempt required using a larger-bore needle, which often culminated in a postmyelographic headache, presumably caused by spinal fluid leakage at the puncture site.

Newer agents have gained wide popularity because of their lower incidence of adverse effects. Because they are water soluble, they are freely miscible with the cerebrospinal fluid, providing improved radiographic contrast compared with the previous, denser oily agents. The individual intrathecal nerve roots, as well as the spinal cord and conus, are displayed exceptionally well (Fig. 3-6). As these newer agents are absorbed by the bloodstream and excreted by the kidneys, there is no longer any need for aspiration at the close of the procedure. For this reason, as well as because of their lower viscosity, smaller-gauge needles (20 to 22 gauge) are routinely used, thereby minimizing the risk of a postmyelographic headache. The first-generation nonionic water-soluble agent used was metrizamide (Amipaque), but it has largely been replaced with the newer, less toxic iohexol (Omnipaque).

Metrizamide and iohexol are comparable in their sensitivity in detecting disease; however, extensive investigative work has revealed differences in their neu-

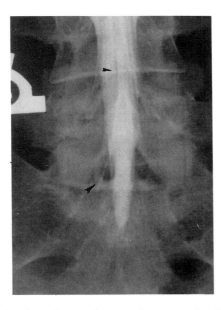

Fig. 3-6. AP view of a myelogram demonstrating intrathecal nerve roots *(small arrowhead)* with filling of the normal nerve root sheath *(large arrowhead).*

rotoxicity. Metrizamide is supplied as a powder that must first be dissolved using the specially prepared diluent. This theoretically could result in unequal concentrations when the mixture is injected intrathecally. Iohexol, on the other hand, is already in aqueous form and is ready for use directly from the vial.

In the work by Kieffer et al.,[10] 350 myelograms using both contrast agents were analyzed with regard to their side effects. Postmyelographic headaches were the most frequent side effect and were nearly twice as common in studies employing metrizamide (38%) than in those employing iohexol (21%). The headaches occurred a mean of approximately 10 hours after the myelogram for metrizamide and 7 hours for iohexol. Nausea was the next most frequent side effect, occurring in 17% of cases using metrizamide versus 10% of cases using iohexol. Vomiting was next in frequency, occurring 8% of the time in the metrizamide group versus 3% of the time in the iohexol group.

Of more significance was the appearance of certain psychobehavioral disturbances, such as confusion, disorientation, aphasia, and auditory, as well as visual, hallucinations. These were noted in 3% of the patients undergoing metrizamide myelography but were not present in those who had iohexol as the contrast medium. The most likely explanation was that metrizamide is chemically related to glucose, which is heavily used by the brain. Not infrequently, a CT scan of the brain performed the day after myelography showed definite cortical enhancement as a result of the diffusion of the metrizamide into the parenchymal extracellular spaces. Also, bathing the frontal cortex with metrizamide results in unusual spike activity on the electroencephalogram (EEG) in nearly 50% of cases. These findings most likely accounted for the more serious complication of convulsions. However, because of the different molecular structure of iohexol, these untoward side effects have not generally been associated with this particular contrast medium.

Myelography of the spine has been used to evaluate patients with a wide array of disorders. In acutely injured patients the most likely reason for performing the myelogram is to look for a disc protrusion that might account for the patient's radiculopathy or compression of the spinal cord in the presence of vertebral fractures. Although myelography has the distinct advantages of demonstrating wider areas of the spinal canal, providing greater spatial resolution than CT reformations, and revealing more obvious changes on the thecal sac and nerve roots because of disc protrusions in the vertical position, it lacks the specificity shared by CT and MRI.

In a prospective study by Modic et al.[15] evaluating cervical radiculopathy using surface coil MRI, CT, and plain film myelography, the surgical confirmation of the predicted findings was 74% for MRI, 85% for CT, and 67% for myelography. Using MRI and CT together led to an improvement of 90%; this increased to 92% when both CT and myelography were employed.

Plain film myelography alone is often inadequate in dealing with the spine-injured patient. More commonly, CT is performed after the intrathecal injection of contrast material for a more accurate inspection of the spinal canal contents. It has been suggested that the optimum time for CT scanning is within 4 hours after the injection. Immediately before scanning, the patient should be positioned so that the contrast pools into the area of clinical concern. This also allows a more even mixing between the spinal fluid and contrast medium and minimizes any layering that might occur during a lengthy time interval between the injection and the CT scan.

Low-dose myelography has been shown to be a safe and practical procedure that can also be performed on an outpatient basis. Using as little as 4 to 5 ml of isotonic contrast medium (180 mg iodine/ml) immediately followed by CT examination has met with wide acceptance and satisfaction. The improved visibility of lesions after the intrathecal administration of contrast medium is more apparent within the cervical and thoracic regions, where there is less fat within the spinal canal surrounding the dural sac and nerve roots. Also, CT affords the detection of more laterally placed disc protrusions that would not indent the thecal sac or proximal nerve root sheaths within the spinal canal.

As an alternative to the routine lumbar puncture, a lateral C1-2 puncture is sometimes used for cervical myelography or when evaluating the cephalad extent in patients with more caudal subarachnoid blocks discovered on lumbar myelography. Although this procedure is considered safe and reliable, certain precautions and considerations should be borne in mind. Since these examinations are usually performed with the patient in the prone position, the neck is usually hyperextended to prevent spillage of contrast medium into the posterior fossa. Therefore patients with spinal stenosis (either congenital or acquired), atlantoaxial disorders, or spinal instability should be carefully examined to prevent any excessive extension, which might predispose them to spinal cord injury.

Since a wider subarachnoid space is posterior to the spinal cord, the needle is usually directed into the posterior third of the spinal canal. The unfortunate complication of developing spinal and intracranial subdural hematomas from anomalous vertebral arteries is thus avoided when inserting the spinal needle posteriorly, since most of these anomalous arteries occur within the anterior two thirds of the spinal canal. Despite the abundance of normal epidural venous channels in the cervical region, there have been no reports of symptomatic venous hemorrhages developing while cervical myelography is being performed.

One major complication in performing a C1-2 puncture for cervical myelography is the potential for puncturing the cervical spinal cord itself. The patient invariably complains of pain on inadvertent cord puncture. Careful fluoroscopic monitoring is therefore needed to prevent such occurrences when cervical punctures are being performed. Slow injection of the contrast medium should then be carried out, observing the medium easily flowing away from the needle tip as it mixes with the cerebrospinal fluid. The persistent collection of contrast medium at the needle tip or visualization of linear collections within the middle of the spinal canal suggests the injection of contrast medium within the substance of the spinal cord. In the four reported cases by Nakstad and Kjartansson,[17] Servo and Laasonen,[18] and Johansen, Orrison, and Amundsen,[9] two of the four patients with cord injections had persistent paresis whereas the other two recovered entirely in a short time. In any event, the myelographer should be wary of such potential complications and should terminate the procedure in the presence of persistent pain, the return of arterial blood flow through the needle, or when contrast material is not localized within the subarachnoid space on injection.

COMPUTED TOMOGRAPHY

Although myelography has been in existence longer than CT, and MR is widely used as the screening test in patients who have sustained trauma or complain of back pain, CT is still considered by many as the method of choice in evaluating patients with spinal disorders. There is no doubt that CT has had an enormous impact on the number of myelograms performed today. However, all three procedures aid in the decision-making process and should be considered complementary rather than competitive studies.

Unless specifically designed to evaluate a designated area identified by either plain film radiography or nuclear medicine bone scanning, a CT scan of the lumbar region should consist of multiple contiguous or overlapping axial cuts parallel to the intervertebral disc spaces from L3 caudal to the sacrum. This is performed routinely, since 90% to 95% of most lumbar disc herniations occur in the lower lumbar region. If there is excessive lordosis at the lumbosacral segment, then the gantry is tilted and additional scans are obtained through the last disc segment. Performing scans through only the disc spaces incurs the potential risk of missing an extruded disc fragment or other space-occupying mass mimicking disc herniation. Reformations are then obtained in at least the sagittal if not both the sagittal and coronal planes. Single-slice reformations through the neural foramina are not sufficient, and thin slices must be obtained throughout the entire length of the foramina (Fig. 3-7) to ensure that any lateral spurs impinging on the exiting spinal nerve are not missed. Once the data have been acquired, then the set of images should be

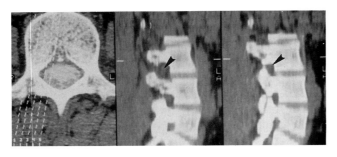

Fig. 3-7. Sagittal CT reformations through neural foramina of the lumbar spine. *Arrowheads,* Exiting nerves surrounded by fat.

photographed at both soft tissue and bone windows.

With the aid of high-resolution thin slices (1 to 3 mm) through the cervical spine, the problem of partial-volume averaging inherent in CT scanning is minimized. The result is a marked improvement in lesion visibility.

Multiplanar three-dimensional reformations may be used to gain a different perspective; however, the acquisition can be time consuming and generally does not add information not readily apparent on conventional axial images (Fig. 3-8).

CT remains unsurpassed in the evaluation of fine bony detail because of its extraordinary sensitivity in detecting calcium. Subtle fractures, small bony spurs, or hypertrophic changes associated with degenerating intervertebral disc and facet disease resulting in spinal stenosis are better delineated on CT than on any other diagnostic examination.

Bubbles of gas within the intervertebral disc (vacuum phenomenon), a radiographic hallmark for disc degeneration, are readily detected by CT. Occasionally gas may be present within the facet joints as well and is usually associated with hypertrophy of the articular processes and ligamentum flavum, subchondral sclerosis, or cyst formation.

Synovial cysts arising from degenerated or inflamed facet joints may be detected. These present little difficulty in diagnosis, since the cysts are located posterolaterally within the spinal canal and are in the immediate proximity of the degenerated joint. The density of the cyst may vary considerably, depending on whether there is internal hemorrhage, synovial fluid, hypertrophy, or collections of gas that might have escaped from the joint into the cyst.

Distinguishing between the various structures within the lumbar spinal canal is facilitated by the higher abundance of epidural fat than is present elsewhere in the cervical and thoracic regions. Caution is advised to avoid misinterpreting the normal lumbar epidural venous plexus for herniated disc material. These veins can become quite prominent, especially in younger individuals. At the exit of the basivertebral venous plexus

from the midpoint of the posterior vertebral body cortex, a small fleck of bone or calcification is frequently observed. The normal intravertebral vascular channels are not surrounded with sclerotic margins and therefore should not be confused with traumatic fractures.

On CT the nonenhanced dural sac is of lower attenuation than the disc itself but higher than the epidural fat. Similar attenuation or density is also noted among the dural sac and the emerging nerve roots, spinal ganglion, spinal nerves, and epidural veins.

Careful analysis of congenitally conjoined nerve roots is necessary because such anomalies may be misinterpreted as disc fragments by an inexperienced observer. The budding sheath encasing both spinal nerves typically occurs midway between both contralateral nerve root sheaths. The caudal anomalous nerve root is frequently already seen within the lateral recess of the subjacent vertebra on the consecutive axial scan after the cephalad nerve takes off and exits through the nerve root canal at a more acute angle than is normally expected. If uncertainty exists, then either contrast-enhanced CT or MRI with sagittal imaging usually suffices in establishing the diagnosis.

Other soft tissue masses that sometimes pose a dilemma in the diagnosis are the so-called perineural cysts. These represent outpouchings of the dural sheath surrounding the spinal nerve and are sometimes referred to as root sleeve diverticula or Tarlov's cysts. They frequently occur in the lower lumbar and sacral regions, and when they approach a substantial size may cause benign erosive changes of the sacral neural foramina. Since it is necessary to exclude the possibility of a neuroma, either myelography or contrast-enhanced CT may be required for proper diagnosis. Because many of these become quite large, there is often dilution of the intrathecal contrast medium, and close inspection is required to observe slight alterations in attenuation or layering of contrast medium.

When CT is performed after routine myelography, often only a small amount of intrathecal contrast medium must be injected into the subarachnoid space for adequate enhancement. At our institution approximately 4 to 5 ml of isotonic (180 mg of iodine per milliliter) water-soluble contrast medium is injected into the lumbar subarachnoid space. The patient is then instructed to roll over to allow proper mixing of contrast medium with the cerebrospinal fluid. Scanning is then performed at the appropriate level of interest. When the thoracic or cervical region is involved, a larger volume of contrast medium at a stronger concentration (240 to 300 mg/ml) may be needed because of the dilution that results as the table is turned in the head-down position to allow the contrast medium to pool in the area of concern. In acutely injured patients with high cervical trauma, a C1-2 puncture with the patient in the supine position may be required.

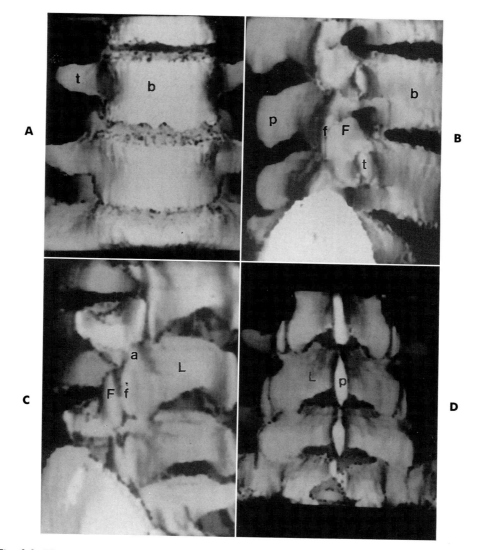

Fig. 3-8. Three-dimensional CT images of the lumbar spine in anterior (**A**), lateral (**B**), posterior oblique (**C**), and posterior (**D**) positions. *b,* Vertebral body; *p,* spinous process; *t,* transverse process; *F, superior facet; f,* inferior facet; *a,* pars interarticularis; *L,* lamina.

Although spondylolytic defects of the pars interarticularis can normally be visualized on MRI, both CT and bone scans are optimal in evaluating for these subtle stress fractures that occur before true isthmic defects develop.

One of CT's major limitations in diagnosing disc disease rests in the fact that only the peripheral disc contour is visualized on the axial images. Normally the disc–thecal sac interface forms a gentle concavity in the lower lumbar region (Fig. 3-9). An exception is at the L5-S1 level, where either a straight or a small gentle convexity is frequently encountered (Fig. 3-10). Focal areas of asymmetry with obliteration of the epidural fat should be regarded as suspicious for subtle disc herniations. More obvious findings include the presence of a focal soft tissue mass having attenuation similar to that of the parent disc and causing displacement of the adjacent nerve root with or without deformity of the dural sac (Fig. 3-11).

In some patients with massive disc extrusions, the axial CT images may actually appear normal. However, the density within the central canal thought to represent the thecal sac really consists of the herniated disc fragment itself. On further inspection, the thecal sac is usually severely compressed against the bony wall of the spinal canal. This unfortunate pitfall can be avoided with sagittal reformations or with the use of intrathecal contrast medium (Fig. 3-12).

Identifying the location of the herniated disc is of extreme importance. Most disc herniations occur posterolaterally within the spinal canal (Fig. 3-13), with central posterior herniations occurring next in fre-

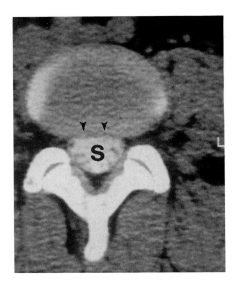

Fig. 3-9. Axial contrast-enhanced CT scan through the L4-5 disc space. Note normal concavity *(arrowheads)* at the disc–thecal sac *(S)* interface.

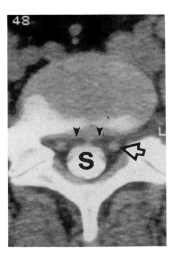

Fig. 3-10. Smooth, gentle convexity *(arrowheads)* seen at the lumbosacral disc segment. *Open arrow,* Left S1 nerve root. *S,* Thecal sac.

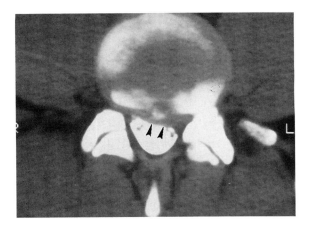

Fig. 3-11. Axial contrast-enhanced CT scan demonstrating a central, posterior, and left-sided broad-based soft tissue mass (herniation, *arrowheads*) indenting on the thecal sac.

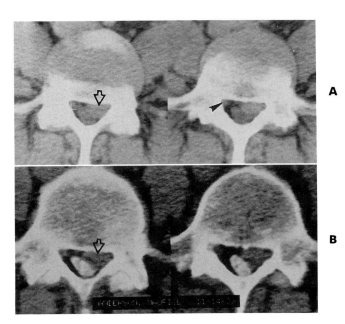

Fig. 3-12. Axial noncontrast **(A)** and contrast-enhanced **(B)** CT scans identifying a large disc herniation *(arrow)* compressing the opacified thecal sac. *Black arrowhead,* Contralateral nerve within lateral recess.

quency. One major advantage of CT over myelography involves its ability to disclose the rarer lateral disc protrusions within or far lateral to the neural foramen, which may go completely undetected on the myelogram (Fig. 3-14). The recognition of these lateral herniations becomes critical to the surgeon, since an entirely different approach is required to reach them.

DISCOGRAPHY

In evaluating the patient with back pain or sciatica, the physical findings must be correlated with imaging

results. Use of a combination of diagnostic imaging tests may be needed when the findings are equivocal or the patient's symptoms remain unexplained after examination. The fact that the patient's pain may be multifactorial further complicates the situation.

Although patients with back pain and/or sciatica are routinely evaluated with CT, myelography, and MRI, serious limitations are inherent in each type of examination. CT is an excellent modality in portraying cross-sectional anatomy in the axial plane, which may then be reformatted in the coronal or sagittal plane.

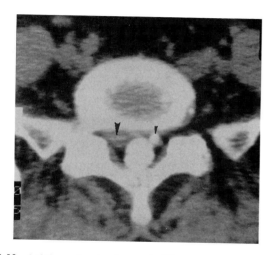

Fig. 3-13. Axial contrast-enhanced CT scan showing a small right posterolateral disc extrusion *(large arrowhead)* preventing opacification of the right S1 nerve root sheath. *Small arrowhead,* Normal contralateral nerve root sheath.

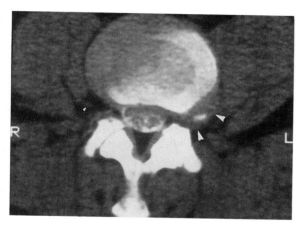

Fig. 3-14. Axial contrast-enhanced CT scan with a large left lateral disc herniation with central calcification *(large arrowheads). Small arrowhead,* Normal contralateral exiting nerve.

Unfortunately, with respect to the intervertebral discs, only the disc's gross morphology or outer contour is displayed. The CT image gives no information concerning the disc's internal architecture or structural changes associated with degeneration. The myelogram is also limited by requiring any disc lesion, whether soft tissue or bone, to directly compress the dural sac or nerve root sleeves for identification.

In Jackson et al.'s prospective study of 124 patients,[8] nonenhanced CT demonstrated an accuracy rate of 74% for disc herniations, CT myelography a 77% rate, and plain myelography a disappointing 70% rate. Foristall, Marsh, and Pay[4] demonstrated an overall accuracy of 88% to 90% for MRI. Although MRI compares favorably with CT myelography, the increased false-positive rate for symptomatic disc herniation and degeneration is well known. In a study of asymptomatic patients by Boden et al.,[1] nearly 35% of those between the ages of 30 and 39 were noted to have evidence of disc degeneration, and in individuals between 20 and 59 years of age, 20% were found to have herniated discs. Although MRI may demonstrate the degenerating disc's signal changes, it still is unable to reveal subtle structural changes occurring within the disc and cannot distinguish between symptomatic and asymptomatic levels, especially in cases of multilevel disc degeneration. Discography, on the other hand, is the only imaging modality that not only delineates the precise internal architecture or degenerative processes occurring within the intervertebral disc but also is able to localize and more accurately define the symptomatic level.

The value of discography remains controversial. Holt[7] and others have questioned its validity because of false-positive pain responses; however, Walsh et al.[19] have shown 17% of the discs in normal subjects to be abnormal at discography with no reproducible symptoms at any of these levels, corresponding to a specificity of 100%.

In a retrospective study performed at our institution, 46 patients, or 122 different lumbar disc levels, were studied using CT, myelography, and discography.[11] Twenty-eight percent of the levels showed no demonstrable abnormalities on myelography but had abnormal findings on discography. Although most of these levels were asymptomatic at discography, nine patients did have a positive pain response identical to their clinical pain. Eighty-three percent had surgical proof of herniated discs causing their sciatica.

In that study, of all the discs interpreted as abnormal on CT, 85% were also abnormal on discography. On examination, however, only a third of these discs reproduced the patient's clinical pain. Of more significance is the fact that 25% of the levels found to be abnormal on discography (which were normal on CT) corresponded to the patient's symptoms.

The diffuse annular disc bulge often encountered on CT presents a problem to the diagnostician. Since only gross morphologic changes of the annulus can be analyzed on CT, significant internal disc pathology not infrequently becomes evident on discography. In our study 30% of all studied levels consisted of diffuse symmetric disc bulges on CT. Of these, 30% experienced a reproduction of their clinical pain at discography. Of the five patients who underwent surgery for sciatica, all had herniated discs confirmed.

The implication of these studies is that discography is seldom required in patients whose clinical examinations and diagnostic tests unequivocally point to a specific etiology for the patient's pain. However, in a substantial number of patients no explanation for the pain is ever found. These patients, as well as those with multilevel disease, may benefit from discography.

In the absence of any detectable disc herniation, a patient may have low back pain with or without sciatica. After exclusion of the facet joints as a possible source of pain, evaluation of the disc with discography may reveal internal annular disruption with tears involving the peripherally innervated annulus and paraspinal longitudinal ligaments. It has been postulated that irritation and inflammation within the abnormal annulus may account for the patient's symptoms. It therefore becomes increasingly important to define the structural nature of the symptomatic and adjacent discs when surgical fusion is being contemplated.

The actual discogram procedure can be accomplished with a modicum of morbidity and may be performed on an outpatient basis. The rate of complicating infection has been reported to be less than 1% and has been less than 0.1% at our institution. The radiologist wears full surgical attire to minimize infection. The patient is premedicated with a sedative before arriving at the radiology department.

All patients are placed on a bolster in the prone, semioblique position to aid in entering the disc space. A modified posterolateral approach is used, thus avoiding penetration of the dural sac and any subsequent headache or nausea, which are frequently encountered during myelography. To minimize any confusion, the patient's side opposite the sciatica is elevated away from the table.

After sterile preparation of the skin with povidone-iodine (Betadine), the patient is covered with a sterile drape, and under fluoroscopic control the Scotty dog appearance of the vertebral posterior bony arch is identified. An 18-gauge spinal needle is then passed down to the mid-disc level just ventral to the superior articular facet of the lower lumbar vertebra relative to the disc (Fig. 3-15). The angle of the needle should remain parallel to the angle of the fluoroscopic image intensifier or C-arm used. The disc spaces must be continuously visualized en face by appropriately angling the image intensifier. If a spinal nerve is encountered, the patient will undoubtedly relate this to the radiologist; after repositioning of the needle, the pain almost immediately disappears.

Once the needle is apposed to the annulus of the disc (this may be visually confirmed by turning the patient to the complete prone position), a 22-gauge (20-cm) Chiba needle is passed coaxially through the larger needle until the beveled tip is centrally located within the disc space. The final location is also confirmed by turning the patient to the prone and lateral positions (Fig. 3-16). Often it is necessary to gently bend the last several centimeters of the Chiba needle in a smooth arc between the thumb and forefinger to facilitate passing the needle into the central nucleus of the disc. It is also important to use the bevel of the needle tip to successfully guide the needle to its desired location, bearing in mind that as the needle is advanced into the disc, the propensity is for the needle to move away from the bevel in the direction of the smooth arc.

Once the needle is in place, iodinated contrast medium is injected under fluoroscopy while the patient's pain pattern response is monitored. All notations of the patient's symptoms are recorded by the x-ray technologist for each injected disc level. The injection is carried

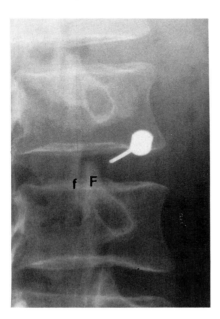

Fig. 3-15. Oblique x-ray film of the lumbar spine demonstrating needle placement for discography. *F,* Superior articular facet; *f,* inferior articular facet.

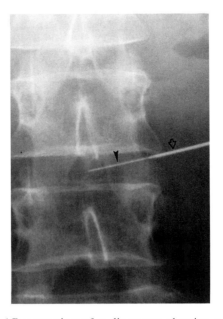

Fig. 3-16. AP x-ray view of a discogram showing a 22-gauge needle *(large arrowhead)* passing through an 18-gauge needle sheath *(open arrow)* with the tip in the center of the disc space.

out until either there is increased resistance in the presence of a normal disc, the patient's symptomatic complaints are reproduced, or there is free extravasation of contrast medium. Typically, the normal disc accommodates 0.5 to 1 ml of medium, and the patient experiences no pain. Degenerated discs often accept up to 5 ml of contrast material and may or may not be associated with back or leg pain.

When an endpoint has been reached, the patient is turned to the lateral and prone positions for lateral and AP radiographs, respectively. Both films are obtained on a 10- by 12-inch cassette with two-on-one programing. Finally, before all the needles are removed, 0.5 to 1 ml of 1% lidocaine (Xylocaine) is injected into the symptomatic discs to abolish pain reproduction, which is almost immediate and makes the remainder of the examination more tolerable for the patient, and to eliminate any potentially confusing pain responses from subsequent injections.

Discographic patterns range from the normal unilocular or bilocular nucleus with its horizontally oriented intranuclear cleft to focal protrusions extending beyond the confines of the normal annulus. Degenerated discs are recognized by the fact that contrast medium is evenly distributed throughout the entire disc and no separate identifiable nucleus pulposus is present (Fig.

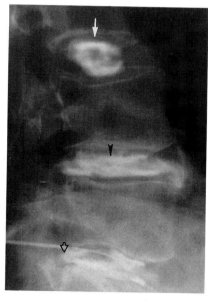

Fig. 3-17. Lateral x-ray view of a discogram showing a normal bilocular nucleus *(white arrow)*, degenerated disc *(black arrowhead)*, and contained posterior disc protrusion *(open black arrow)*.

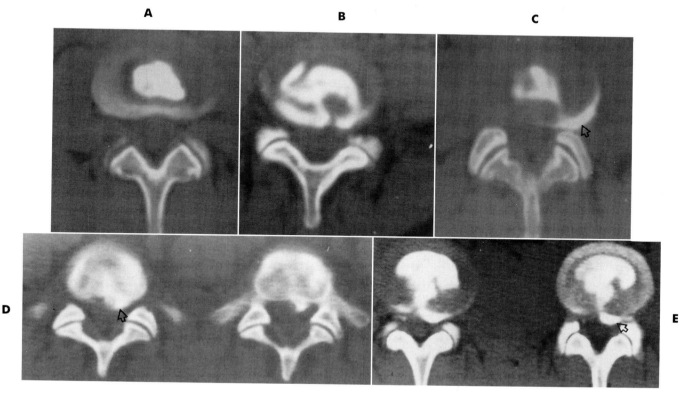

Fig. 3-18. Axial CT discograms. **A,** Normal disc. **B,** Circumferential annular fissures. **C,** Left posterolateral fissure extending into the neural foramen *(arrow)*. **D,** Degenerated disc with focal left posterolateral herniation *(arrow)*. **E,** Left posterolateral disc protrusion *(arrow)*.

3-17). Ruptures through the longitudinal ligaments may result in free extravasation in the paraspinal or epidural spaces.

The discogram is usually complemented with a CT discogram, with several CT scans obtained through the injected disc levels. Various CT configurations of the degenerating disc demonstrate circumferential to radial annular tears (Fig. 3-18). These CT discogram images must then be correlated with either the axial images from a nonenhanced CT scan or an MRI examination. This is essential because the presence of contrast medium outside the normal confines of the disc on the CT discogram may simply represent the extravasation of contrast medium through the posterior longitudinal ligament at discography. The plain scans must show the presence of any space-occupying mass that conforms to the enhancing structure on the CT discogram before the diagnosis of a disc herniation can be made. In the correlative study by Jackson et al.,[8] CT followed by discography was the most accurate (87%) procedure for evaluating disc herniations.

MAGNETIC RESONANCE IMAGING

Since its first clinical use in the early 1980s, MRI has gained recognition based on its high soft tissue contrast, lack of ionizing radiation, and direct multiplanar acquisition (Fig. 3-19). In many institutions it has become the most widely used screening method for evaluating the spine. The underlying physics involved in MRI is beyond the scope of this chapter; however, certain basic concepts are covered.

Each scanning sequence must take into consideration such factors as the field of view, matrix size, repetition time of the radiofrequency pulse (TR), sampling time of the echo (TE), number of excitations, and flip angle used. Selecting the proper surface coil for the desired anatomic site to be examined improves the signal/noise ratio. Combining a smaller surface coil with a smaller field of view generally produces higher-resolution images, although the anatomic coverage is restricted. Although a wide variety of specialized surface coils have been produced, the two most popular ones used in imaging the spine are the rectangular license plate and the 5-inch round coils. With each of these, either the entire cervical, lumbar, or most of the thoracic spine may be imaged in one acquisition. Improvements in coil technology consisting of phased-array coils have allowed imaging of most of the spinal column in one acquisition with no additional scanning time (Fig. 3-20).

Normally, both T1- and T2-weighted images are obtained using a combination of short TR and TE values (TR 500 to 800 msec, TE 20 to 40 msec) for T1-weighted images and long TR and TE values (TR 1600 to 2500 msec, TE 80 to 100 msec) for T2-weighted images. In general, T1-weighted images are best in defining the anatomy but are least sensitive in highlighting pathology. The T2-weighted images are often obtained with two or more TEs (dual-echo imaging), with the longer TE images (second-echo images) being more heavily T2-weighted. T2-weighted images are more sensitive in detecting pathologic conditions. The observed signal intensity is therefore altered according to whether the scan is more T1 or T2 biased. For instance, simple fluid, which has a long T1 and T2, will appear quite dark, or hypointense, on heavily T1-weighted images and will turn white, or become hyperintense, on the more

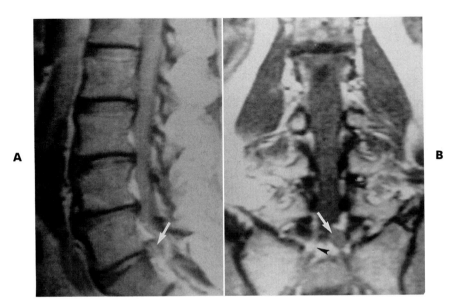

Fig. 3-19. Sagittal (**A**) and coronal (**B**) MRI scans demonstrating a large extruded disc herniation *(white arrow)* posterolaterally within the spinal canal. *Black arrowhead,* Contralateral exiting nerve.

T2-weighted images. Fat, on the other hand, having a short T1, appears quite bright, or hyperintense, on T1-weighted images. This explains why cancellous bone, having an abundance of fat, appears white on T1-weighted images. Compact or cortical bone, with few hydrogen protons to emit signal, remains black on both T1- and T2-weighted images. In general, muscle and cartilage, as well as other soft tissues, have an intermediate or gray signal on T1-weighted images but behave differently on T2-weighted images.

All the aforementioned signal characteristics are typically seen on the conventional spin-echo sequences routinely used. Unfortunately, time is sacrificed when T2-weighted images are obtained, which places a burden on the patient while in the scanner and allows normal physiologic motion (gross bodily motion, swallowing, cerebrospinal fluid pulsations, respiratory and cardiac motion) to degrade image quality. Recent advances in fast scanning or gradient-reversal echoes have significantly reduced scanning time and, thereby, motion artifact considerably. Such techniques go by different acronyms, such as GRASS, FLASH, or FISP, depending on the scanner's manufacturer. These newer techniques allow T2-weighted myelographic images of the spine to be obtained by using smaller flip angles than the typical 90 degrees of conventional spin-echo imaging.

The downside to these newer techniques is that they have inherent undesirable qualities, including higher susceptibility to local magnetic field inhomogeneities. The paramagnetic effect of iron stores within the cancellous bone marrow results in a strong inhomogeneity and negates the normal high signal from fat, resulting in a blackened appearance on gradient-echo

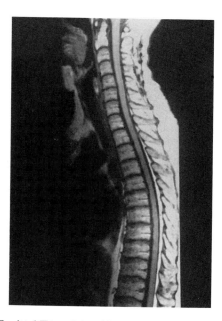

Fig. 3-20. Sagittal T1-weighted image of the entire cervical and thoracic spine using phased-array surface coils.

images. Other artifacts from motion and chemical shift are also common to such gradient-recalled images. By using the shortest TE possible and manipulating other parameters, many of these undesirable side effects can be minimized. Additional techniques, including presaturation radiofrequency pulses, cardiac gating, and first-order gradient-moment nulling (flow compensation), can be used to reduce any flow or pulsatile motion artifact.

Finally, the use of intravenously injected paramagnetic agents has had a tremendous impact on spinal imaging. The MRI contrast medium, gadolinium diethylene triamine pentoacetic acid (gadolinium-DTPA, Magnevist, Berlex), alters the local tissues' magnetic properties, thereby enhancing them on T1-weighted images. In addition to the normal enhancement of the epidural venous plexus and nerve root ganglia, fibrovascular granulation tissue enveloping a herniated disc or in association with annular tears in the unoperated patient is noted to enhance, while the relatively avascular disc does not. This phenomenon has therefore made it easier to distinguish recurrent or residual disc herniation from epidural scarring in patients postoperatively.

At our institution we employ a 1.5-Tesla imager and routinely acquire coronal and sagittal T1-weighted images of the cervical spine in addition to sagittal and axial gradient-reversal echo images (Fig. 3-21). The thoracic spine is studied with T1-weighted and either T2-weighted or gradient images in the sagittal plane (Fig. 3-22). The lumbar spine is examined with coronal T1-weighted images in conjunction with a dual-echo T2-weighted scan in the sagittal and axial planes (Fig. 3-23). Each study is individually tailored to the clinical need. Slice thicknesses range from 3 to 5 mm, with interslice gaps of 1 to 2.5 mm. One must keep in mind that if higher resolution is desired by using a thinner slice, less signal will be emitted from that slice volume and a lower signal/noise ratio will be achieved. To compensate for this reduction, an increase in the number of excitations, prolongation of the TR, or a change in the field of view must be performed. Each technique alteration has the disadvantage of either lengthening the scanning time or changing the anatomic coverage, thereby decreasing spatial resolution. Newer, three-dimensional scanning is gaining popularity with its contiguous, no interslice gap slice (1.5 to 2 mm), high-resolution images that may be reformatted in any plane once the data have been acquired.

Despite the complexity in performing the MRI study, valuable information regarding spinal cord pathology is easily obtained. Although gradient-echo imaging has demonstrated a higher conspicuity for extradural disease, conventional spin-echo imaging is still preferable for evaluating intramedullary pathology. In the work by Goldberg et al.,[5] MR signal intensity patterns corresponding to cord edema and/or hemorrhage have been

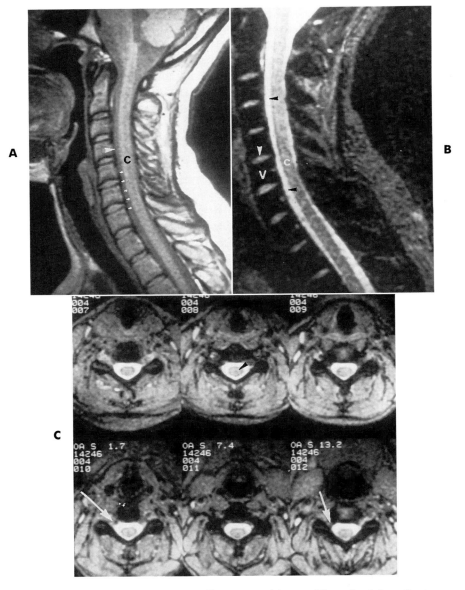

Fig. 3-21. Sagittal proton-density (**A**), gradient-reversal image (**B**), and axial gradient-reversal images (**C**) of the cervical spine. **A** and **B:** *C,* Spinal cord; *large white and black arrowheads,* cerebrospinal fluid; *small white arrowheads,* posterior longitudinal ligament blending in with the posterior vertebral body cortex. **C:** *Black arrowhead,* Cord; *white arrow,* neural foramen.

correlated with the degree of severity of neurologic damage in the spine-injured patient. Focal areas of cord edema as manifested by high-signal intensity on T2-weighted images were found in those patients with the least neurologic sequalae. In contrast, individuals with intramedullary foci of hemorrhage (high signal intensity on T1-weighted images with low signal intensity on T2-weighted images due to the blood breakdown products of deoxyhemoglobin and methemoglobin with surrounding edema) demonstrated the most severe injuries with little or no recovery. Posttraumatic cysts of the cord appear as focal intramedullary areas of hy-

pointensity on T1-weighted images and as hyperintense areas on T2-weighted images (Fig. 3-24). In the early stages of cord contusion, this may be difficult to distinguish from cord edema and myelomalacia, but with time the latter two entities may resolve, with normal cord intensity noted on T1-weighted images.

With respect to degenerative changes occurring within the spinal column, MRI is well known for its ability to detect alterations in disc signal presumed to reflect biochemical changes that occur with normal aging. The normal adult intervertebral disc is composed of a well-hydrated gelatinous matrix of glycosaminogly-

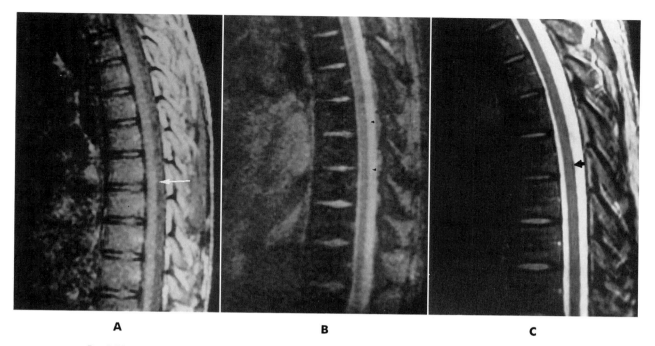

Fig. 3-22. Sagittal T1-weighted **(A),** gradient-reversal **(B),** and heavily T2-weighted **(C)** images of the thoracic spine. *Large white arrow* **(A),** *black arrow* **(C),** Spinal cord; *black arrowheads* **(B),** cerebrospinal fluid.

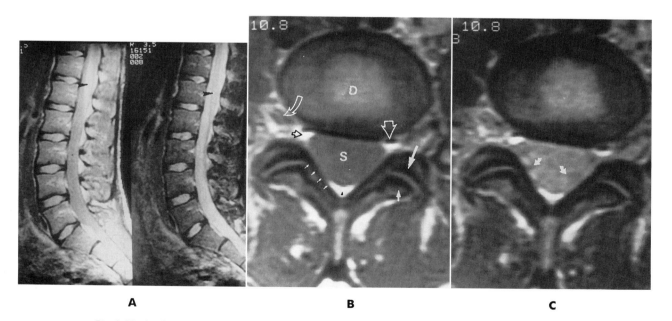

Fig. 3-23. Sagittal T2-weighted **(A),** axial T1-weighted **(B),** and axial T2-weighted **(C)** images of the lumbar spine. *D,* Disc; *S,* sac; *small white arrows,* ligamentum flavum; *large solid white arrow,* cortex of superior articular facet; *small solid white arrow,* inferior articular facet; *curved open white arrow,* exiting nerve; *straight open white arrow,* epidural vein; *open black arrow, small black arrowhead,* epidural fat; *small curved solid arrows,* intrathecal nerve roots.

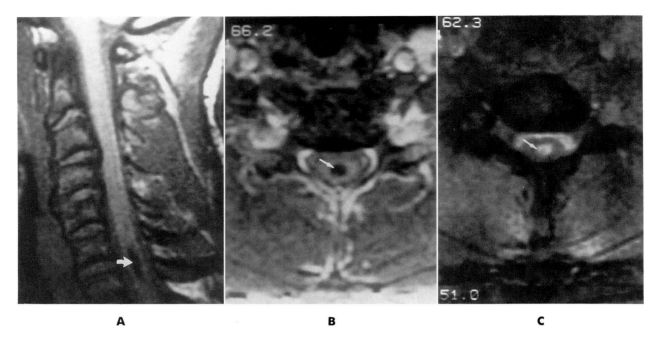

A   **B**   **C**

Fig. 3-24. Sagittal T1-weighted **(A),** axial T1-weighted **(B),** and axial gradient-recalled **(C)** images of the cervical cord revealing a central cavitation within the substance of the spinal cord from hyperextension injury. The posttraumatic cyst *(arrow)* appears hypointense on the T1-weighted images and becomes hyperintense on the T2-weighted image.

cans in the nucleus pulposus surrounded by the loose fibrocartilaginous inner annulus fibrosus. Both of these regions are indistinguishable on MRI and appear hyperintense on T2-weighted images. There is often a normal intranuclear cleft of a more fibrous nature within the central nucleus. Surrounding the nucleus and inner annulus is the dense fibrocartilaginous outer annulus, which appears intermediate in signal on T1-weighted images and considerably less intense than the nucleus on T2-weighted images because of its lower hydration state.

With aging there is a gradual loss of water content from 88% to 70% within the nucleus of the disc. With further desiccation, circumferential annular tears occur and may progress to radial tears. Nuclear material may then be expelled through these annular tears as the disc is subjected to further axial loading. Further degeneration of the disc results in continued loss of signal and height. Nuclear herniations may dissect beneath the peripherally bulging annulus or rupture through the outer annulus still being contained by the posterior longitudinal ligament. If the disc herniation ruptures through the posterior longitudinal ligament, migration away from the disc level results in a sequestered or free fragment.

A grading scale of disc degeneration has been devised at our facility (see box at right). It portrays the ongoing natural occurrences in disc degeneration (Fig. 3-25). However, it should not be misinterpreted to imply symptomatic levels. As stated before, Boden et al.[1] have demonstrated that 30% of asymptomatic individuals had evidence of either disc degeneration or herniation, necessitating a correlation between the patient's clinical symptoms and imaging findings.

Although CT is generally regarded as demonstrating bony detail more accurately than MRI, congenital and acquired spinal stenoses of the central type resulting in a trefoil canal appearance or of the lateral type affecting the nerve root canals can be demonstrated equally well on MRI. Cortical spurs or osteophytes appear markedly hypointense, and subchondral sclerosis appears as decreased signal within the normal bone marrow. High signal from bone marrow may be seen within enlarging osteophytes.

Extruded nuclear disc material may produce various MRI signal intensities, depending on the degree of disc degeneration and chronicity of the herniation. A well-recognized feature is that of a free disc fragment

---

Magnetic Resonance Grading Scale of Degenerating Discs

Grade 1: Normal disc height, normal signal
Grade 2: Normal disc height, slight loss of signal
Grade 3: Normal disc height, moderate loss of signal
Grade 4: Mild to moderate loss in disc height, moderate loss of signal
Grade 5: Complete loss of disc height, severe loss of signal

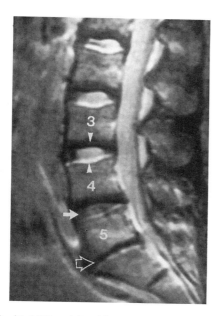

Fig. 3-25. Sagittal T2-weighted image of the lumbar spine. Note grade 4 degenerative changes at the L4-5 disc space *(solid arrow)* with grade 5 degeneration of the L5-S1 disc space *(open arrow)*. Chemical shift artifacts *(arrowheads)* are normal on sagittal MR images and do not reflect abnormalities in adjacent bone marrow.

Cervical Spine Radiographic Measurements

Predental space:
  5 mm in child
  2.5 to 3 mm in adult
Prevertebral soft tissues at C3: less than one half of sagittal diameter of C3 body (usually 4 mm)
Prevertebral soft tissues at C5: less than or equal to sagittal diameter of C5 vertebral body
Prevertebral soft tissues at C6:
  14 mm in child
  22 mm in adult

---

appearing more hyperintense than its parent disc. Routinely acquired T2-weighted images in the axial plane depict the intrathecal nerve roots, allowing for evaluation of nerve root displacement, adhesive arachnoiditis, and perineural cysts.

The relatively few individuals who cannot be scanned with MRI include those with cardiac pacemakers or other electronically implanted devices, intracranial aneurysm clips, or small metallic foreign bodies in vital structures such as the eyes. Even patients with shrapnel, metallic prostheses, most heart valves, or surgical hardware may be scanned, although image quality may be sacrificed.

With newer technologic achievements resulting in faster scanning times and higher spatial resolution, MRI will clearly remain in the forefront in imaging of the spine.

Applications

CERVICAL SPINE

A quick and accurate diagnosis in the traumatized spinal patient is essential. It is vital to assess whether the injury is stable or unstable. Since 5% to 10% of spinal cord injuries occur in the postinjury period because of patient mishandling, any cervical spine motion should be limited until proper examination is performed to exclude any catastrophic fracture. This is usually accomplished with plain film radiography in the AP, lateral, and open-mouth projections. Since there may be spasm or voluntary guarding due to pain, significant ligamentous injury may be masked on the initial x-ray films, thereby necessitating further evaluation with flexion and extension views.

Subtle vertebral body cortical offsets resulting in interruption of the normal imaginary lines may indicate significant underlying ligamentous injury. Other radiographic signs include alteration of the normal parallelism of the interfacet joint spaces, widening or "fanning" of the interspinous process spaces, prevertebral soft tissue swelling, and widening of either the anterior or posterior portions of the intervertebral discs.

Cervical spine instability may be further documented by vertical compression with loss of more than 25% of the vertebral body height, focal angulation of the injured vertebra to either adjacent vertebral level by more than 11 degrees, or slippage (anterolisthesis) of more than 3.5 mm of one vertebra on the subjacent vertebra. Caution is advised when interpreting radiographic findings of the cervical spine in young children, since one may observe up to 2 to 3 mm of subluxation at the C2-3 disc level with the neck in flexion. This pseudosubluxation should not be misconstrued as to imply significant ligamentous damage. A number of other important prevertebral soft tissue measurements of the cervical spine are listed in the box above.

Flexion Injuries

An acute flexion injury may result in a fracture of the dens with the ligament remaining intact (Fig. 3-26). Although AP and lateral radiographs are normally sufficient in demonstrating this fracture, there may be confusion with overlying shadows of the anterior arch of C1 or from the upper front incisor teeth artifactually simulating such a fracture in the normal setting. This can usually be excluded by lack of prevertebral soft tissue swelling on the lateral x-ray film. CT and MRI can easily demonstrate the fracture on images in the coronal projection.

Flexion fractures occur typically at the C5-6 interver-

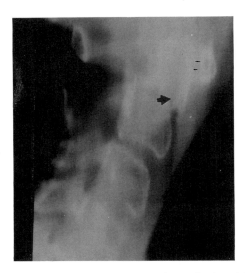

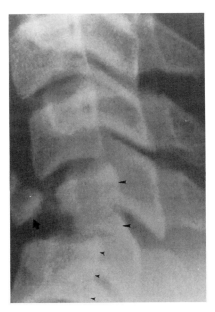

Fig. 3-26. Lateral x-ray film of C1-2 showing a displaced fracture *(arrow)* at the base of the odontoid process with a normal atlantoaxial space *(black lines)*, suggesting integrity of the transverse ligament.

Fig. 3-27. Lateral view of a cervical "teardrop" fracture with posterior displacement *(large arrowheads)* of the remaining body into the spinal canal. *Black arrow,* Displaced anterior vertebral body fracture fragment; *small black arrowheads,* subjacent vertebral body cortex.

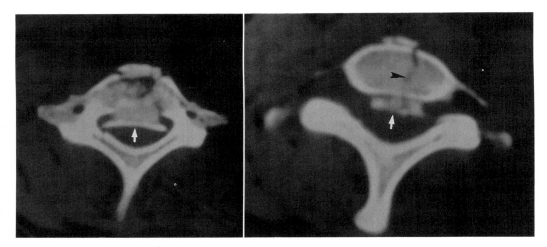

Fig. 3-28. Axial CT images demonstrating the posteriorly displaced bony fragments *(white arrow),* as well as a sagittal cleavage fracture *(black arrowhead)* through the vertebral body.

tebral disc level, the most mobile segment of the cervical spine. The common "teardrop" fracture refers to a triangular piece of bone from the anterosuperior endplate of the compressed vertebral body. With more significant force, the posterior ligamentous complex may be disrupted, resulting in complete bony failure with severe compression and comminution of the vertebral body. This "burst" type of fracture usually involves a sagittal component of the vertebral body, as well as fractures of the posterior arch. Bony fragments are often displaced posteriorly into the spinal canal, resulting in

spinal cord compression and causing severe neurologic damage (Fig. 3-27). CT is excellent in demonstrating any retropulsed bony fragments within the spinal canal (Fig. 3-28). There may be localized kyphosis on the lateral radiograph with fanning of the interspinous space, attesting to the posterior ligamentous damage. MRI, however, remains the procedure of choice in depicting compressive cord changes (hematomyelia, edema, posttraumatic cyst development, or cord transection).

Isolated stable fractures involving the spinous processes are called "clay shoveler's fractures" and occur

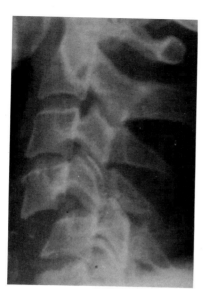

Fig. 3-29. Lateral view of the cervical spine demonstrating a bilateral facet dislocation with significant anterior subluxation.

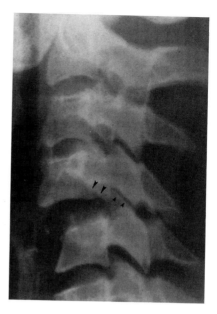

Fig. 3-30. Lateral view of the cervical spine demonstrating a unilateral facet dislocation with rotation of the vertebral bodies. Note the inferior facet *(large arrowheads)* lying anterior to the superior facet *(small arrowheads).*

primarily in the lower cervical spine at the C6 or C7 level. These have been associated with flexion or extension and result from violent traction on the interspinous and supraspinous ligaments. These fractures are easily detected on lateral x-ray films but may also be evident on AP radiographs when two spinous processes are associated with one vertebral body.

When one vertebra is severely subluxed on the subjacent vertebra, bilateral facet dislocations frequently occur (Fig. 3-29). The lateral radiograph shows the inferior articular processes of the subluxed vertebra located anterior to the superior articular processes of the lower vertebra and implies complete disruption of the posterior ligamentous complex, the intervertebral disc, and damage to the anterior longitudinal ligament.

With the head in flexion and slightly rotated, unilateral facet dislocations may occur, but these do not carry the same significance or imply the same degree of damage as does the bilateral facet dislocation. An abrupt difference is seen in the lateral projection of the involved vertebrae as they become obliquely oriented, with the involved inferior articular process lying in front of the superior articular process of the subjacent vertebra (Fig. 3-30). This results in a "bow tie" configuration of the articular processes. On the frontal radiograph the spinous process of the rotated vertebra is deviated toward the side of the locked facet joint, with disruption of the posterior ligaments on that side. CT shows any associated articular process fractures, as well as demonstrating the locked facet joint on the sagittal reformations.

Extension Injuries

With hyperextension, the posterior arch of C1 is compressed between the occiput and posterior arch of C2, resulting in stable vertical fractures of the C1 arch. This is best delineated on either lateral plain radiographs or on axial CT images. Odontoid fractures with or without posterior displacement may also be associated with hyperextension injuries (Fig. 3-31).

The corollary to the flexion "teardrop" fracture is the extension "teardrop" injury wherein the anterior longitudinal ligament avulses a triangular piece of bone from the anteroinferior end-plate, usually from the C2 vertebral body. Localized prevertebral soft tissue swelling prevails; however, the posterior elements and ligaments appear intact (Fig. 3-32).

The "hangman's" fracture occurs through the posterior elements, usually the pedicles, with subsequent anterior spondylolisthesis of C2 (Fig. 3-33). With increasing deformity, the fracture has been classified as either type I (demonstrating minimal displacement), type II (revealing more displacement with abnormal posterior widening of the intervertebral disc), or type III (showing bilateral facet dislocation and anterior subluxation with significant angulation of the body of C2).

The pillar fracture is another stable injury to the cervical spine in extension with the head slightly rotated. The lateral articular mass abuts the adjacent vertebral body. This fracture is suggested on the plain radiograph by overlapping bony shadows and tilting of the involved pillar; CT demonstrates the extent of fracture of the posterior elements with better detail (Fig. 3-34).

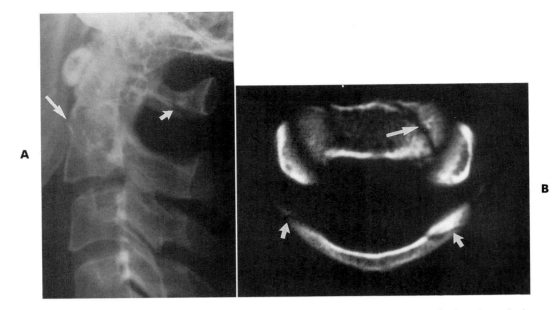

Fig. 3-31. Lateral x-ray **(A)** and axial CT scan **(B)** showing simple, nondisplaced vertical fractures through the posterior arch of C1 *(small arrows),* as well as a type III odontoid fracture *(large arrows).*

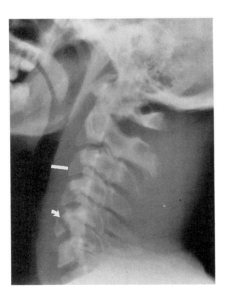

Fig. 3-32. Lateral view of the cervical spine revealing widening of prevertebral soft tissues *(thick white line)* from bleeding due to rupture of the anterior longitudinal ligament with extension "teardrop" fracture of C5 *(arrow).*

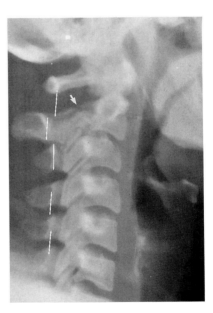

Fig. 3-33. "Hangman's" fracture *(arrow)* through the pedicle of C2. Note the widened spinal canal with slight anterior displacement of the C2 vertebral body and disruption of the spinal laminar line posteriorly *(dashed white line).*

When this mechanism is coupled with axial loading forces applied to the head, a wide combination of hyperextension fracture dislocations may ensue. Fractures through the posterior elements with severe ligamentous damage coupled with rupture of the anterior longitudinal ligament and intervertebral disc occur with rotation and anterior subluxation of the vertebral body.

Again, CT delineates the extent of these fractures to best advantage (Fig. 3-35). Oblique radiographs may show deformity of displaced bony fragments lying within the neural foramina, often resulting in a radiculopathy at the involved level.

A pure hyperextension cervical injury may have serious neurologic effects despite the lack of any

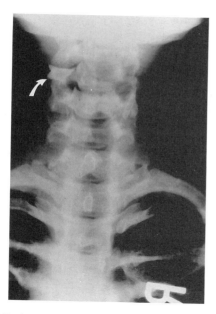

Fig. 3-34. AP view of the cervical spine demonstrating a tilted and asymmetric pillar due to fracture through the lateral mass.

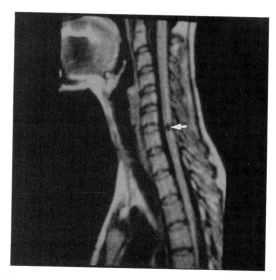

Fig. 3-36. Sagittal T1-weighted image revealing a small central posttraumatic cord cyst from an acute hyperextension injury leaving the patient a quadriplegic.

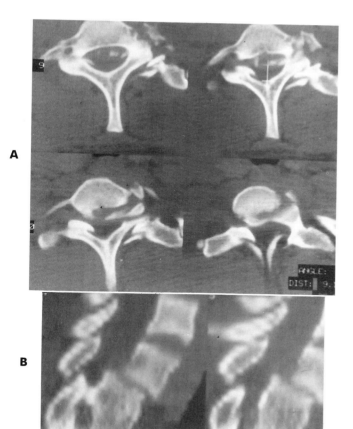

Fig. 3-35. Axial (**A**) and sagittal reformations (**B**) of the lower cervical spine demonstrating severe comminution of the vertebral body and posterior arch with anterior subluxation.

significant bony abnormalities on x-ray examination. A central cord syndrome may result from cord compression due to marked transient narrowing of the spinal canal in extension with the ligamentum flavum compressing the cord from behind (Fig. 3-36). There is usually disruption of the intervertebral disc and anterior longitudinal ligament. Such cord contusions become even more significant in athletes with congenital spinal stenosis or cervical instability. Symptoms of cervical cord neurapraxia ranging from temporary quadriplegia to burning, tingling, and weakness in the upper or lower extremities may occur. These injuries are more typically seen in contact sports, such as football, ice hockey, and boxing, where excessive impact and collision occur. Both CT and MRI are helpful in excluding any bony trauma and spinal cord pathology, respectively. Athletes whose spinal diameter is significantly diminished (less than 80% of the sagittal diameter of the respective vertebral body) or who demonstrate signs of cervical instability and have experienced such episodes should not be permitted to engage in contact sports.

Compression Injuries

As the head is slightly flexed, any significant axial compression on the vertex may result in a wedge deformity or simple compression fracture of the vertebral body. With greater magnitude and strength of the vertically applied forces to the skull, axial compression on the cervical vertebral column culminates in a variety of "burst" fractures.

In the upper cervical spine the Jefferson burst fracture occurs as a result of the occipital condyles transmitting all their energy onto the lateral masses of C1. As the weakened anterior and posterior neural

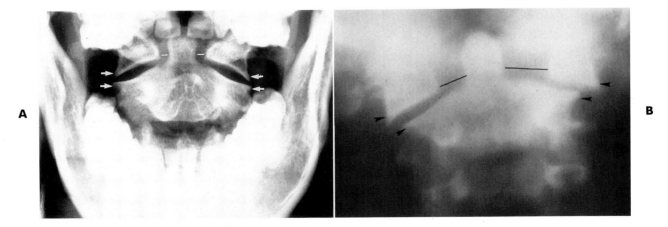

Fig. 3-37. A, Open-mouth view of C1-2 demonstrating normal alignment of lateral masses of the axis with those of the atlas *(arrows),* as well as normal distance between the lateral masses of C1 and the odontoid process. **B,** Bilateral spreading of C1 lateral masses resulting in cortical offset *(arrowheads)* and widening between the odontoid process and medial border of the C1 lateral mass due to a burst fracture of the C1 ring.

arches of C1 fail and fracture, outward displacement of the lateral masses occurs and becomes evident on frontal radiographs as the lateral masses overhang the articular processes of C2 (Fig. 3-37). The open-mouth view is essential in clearly portraying the bilateral spreading of the lateral masses of C1 in relation to those of C2. CT pictorially demonstrates in the axial plane the widened spinal canal produced with this type of injury, accounting for the relative lack of significant neurologic deficit.

Burst fractures in the lower cervical spine typically result in narrowing of the intervertebral disc immediately above the fracture, since the nucleus pulposus is driven into the subjacent vertebra and causes explosive comminution of the lower vertebral body. Retropulsed bony fragments within the spinal canal can produce significant neurologic damage and are best demonstrated on axial CT scanning. As with other types of injuries compressing the cord, MRI is the preferred method of evaluation in this regard.

Cervical Disc Disease

Certain biochemical changes occur in the degenerating intervertebral disc with gross morphologic structural alterations within the annulus fibrosus and nucleus pulposus. Annular fissures or rents may develop in the degenerating disc and may coalesce, thereby allowing avenues for nuclear material to extrude when the disc is subjected to increased axial loading. As the extruded nucleus forms a broad-based extension of the disc beyond the peripheral confines of the vertebral endplate, the disc is said to be bulging. When focal asymmetric nuclear material extends beyond the endplate but is still contained by the posterior longitudinal ligament, a disc protrusion is said to exist. With further expulsion of nuclear material, a disc extrusion occurs

and a free or sequestered disc fragment may migrate away from the parent disc level. The nuclear material may then press on the thecal sac anteriorly, on the cord and cervical nerve root anterolaterally, or on the exiting nerve root if the herniation lies far enough laterally within the foramen (Fig. 3-38).

Whether one is dealing with acute disc herniation or chronic degenerative disc disease with or without herniation, plain radiography falls far short of CT, myelography, MR, and contrast-enhanced CT with respect to distinguishing between nerve root or spinal cord compression. Myelography has the advantage of displaying the entire thecal sac and normal nerve root sheaths (Fig. 3-39) but is often limited by requiring subsequent CT to clarify the diagnosis. Plain CT also is limited because of the paucity of epidural fat in the cervical area and often requires the intrathecal injection of contrast medium to detect subtle soft tissue masses deforming the dural sac or nerve root sheaths (Fig. 3-40). One major disadvantage with CT is frequently encountered in imaging the cervical-thoracic junction. Multiple dark streaks appear as a result of the x-ray attenuation by the individual's shoulders (beam hardening artifact). In addition, patients with subarachnoid block from extradural disease may require the injection of contrast medium above and below the level of the block to adequately evaluate the extent of disease. Despite these limitations, CT has the distinct advantage of obtaining ultrathin axial sections, thus minimizing partial-volume artifact and allowing differentiation between osteophytic spurs and herniated disc material.

Some patients have focal soft tissue masses ventral to the dural sac on CT or MRI scans that disappear on follow-up diagnostic examinations after conservative treatment or that are absent at subsequent surgery (Fig.

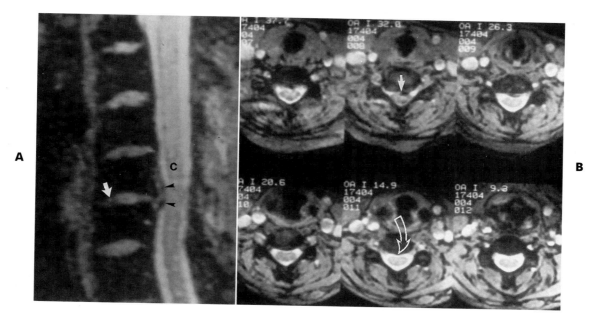

Fig. 3-38. Sagittal **(A)** and axial gradient-recalled **(B)** MRI scans of the cervical spine showing central disc extrusion *(black arrowheads)* effacing ventral subarachnoid space *(small white arrow)* in contrast to normal subarachnoid space *(open curved white arrow)*. *C,* Spinal cord.

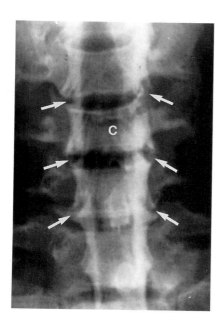

Fig. 3-39. AP view from a cervical myelogram showing normal cervical nerves *(arrows)* outlined with contrast in nerve root sheaths. *C,* Spinal cord.

3-41). The mass may represent a transient epidural hematoma related to minor degrees of trauma resulting from tearing of one of the small epidural veins. (In this case the MRI signal characteristics may vary, depending on the age of the clot, but almost always resolve in time. Alternately, these masses may represent true disc herniations that incite a reactive granulation tissue

response, resulting in the enzymatic digestion of the mass over time. The body tends to react to the normally occurring degenerative processes of the intervertebral disc by the ingrowth and proliferation of vascular granulation tissue in an attempt to repair damage. Modic et al.[15,16] have demonstrated this phenomenon within the lumbar spine with histologic correlation of surgical disc specimens with MRI scans after the intravenous administration of gadolinium-DTPA. The observed enhancing granulation tissue in the postoperative patient has proved helpful in distinguishing recurrent disc herniation (which does not enhance) from normal fibrosis or scar tissue (which does enhance). It has also been observed in nonoperated patients with granulation tissue in association with extruded disc material (Fig. 3-42).

Although MRI is generally regarded as being equal or superior to both CT and myelography in evaluating the traumatized cord, cervical radiculopathy is difficult to evaluate with the thicker axial slices used in MRI. Poor spatial resolution results from MRI partial-volume artifact. However, improvements with surface coil technology and gradient-echo three-dimensional thin-section imaging have improved the overall image quality to such an extent that these imaging techniques are now used routinely in many institutions as the method of choice for evaluating cervical radiculopathy.

THORACOLUMBAR SPINE

Fractures that occur in the thoracolumbar region usually arise from flexion injuries due to axial compres-

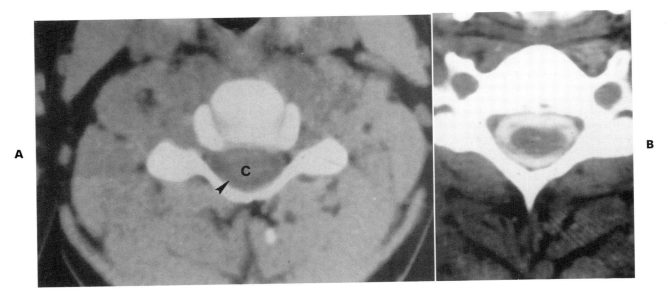

Fig. 3-40. A, Axial noncontrast CT scan demonstrating poor soft tissue contrast due to insufficient epidural fat in the cervical area. *C,* Cord; *arrowhead,* cerebrospinal fluid. **B,** Contrast-enhanced CT scan showing normal configuration of the thecal sac and spinal cord with emerging nerve roots.

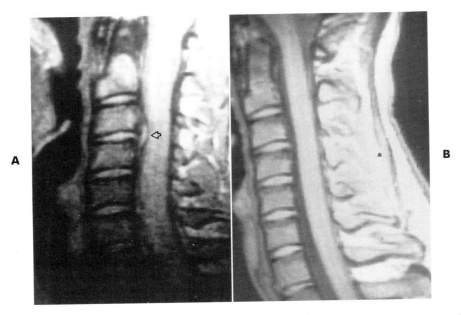

Fig. 3-41. Sagittal T1-weighted images at presentation **(A)** and at follow-up 6 months later **(B).** Disappearance of ventral soft tissue *(arrow)* in the absence of surgery was thought to represent resolving epidural hematoma or disc herniation.

sive loading on the anterior vertebral column. The vast majority of these fractures occur between T12 and L2, although it is not uncommon to have multiple, noncontiguous areas of injury.[2] When one level of injury is detected, the entire spine should be examined with at least frontal and lateral radiographs to exclude this possibility.

The location of the traumatized vertebral body is easily identified on plain x-ray films, although it is sometimes difficult to assess whether the compression fracture is recent or old. The intensity of activity on the radionuclide bone scan often helps in this distinction, since simple vertebral compression fractures should revert back to normal activity after 6 to 12 months. Unless the compression exceeds more than 50% of height or multiple compression fractures are seen that

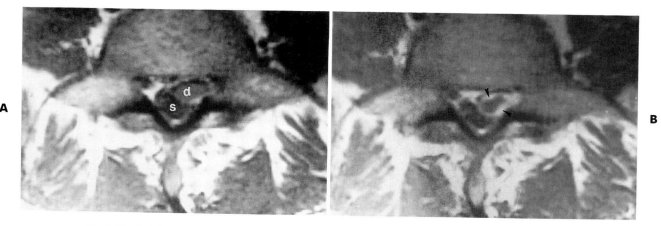

Fig. 3-42. Axial precontrast T1-weighted image **(A)** and postcontrast image **(B)** of the lumbar spine demonstrating rim enhancement *(arrowheads)* representing fibrovascular granulation tissue surrounding a herniated disc fragment *(d)* adjacent to the thecal sac *(s).* There was no history of surgery.

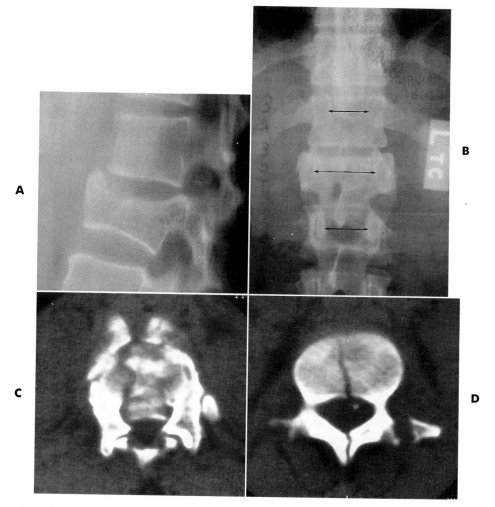

Fig. 3-43. Lateral x-ray film **(A)**, AP x-ray film **(B)**, and axial CT scans **(C** and **D)** of comminuted burst fractures. Note the significant loss of vertebral body height, posterior angulation, and widened interpediculate distance *(arrows)* compared with the adjacent vertebrae, and the comminution of bony fragments with retropulsion into the spinal canal with concomitant sagittal cleavage fracture of the vertebral body.

may result in progressive kyphotic deformity, the posterior spinal column usually remains intact.

As the axial loading vector is increased on the flexed spine, the intervertebral disc is driven into the caudal vertebra, resulting in a comminuted burst fracture (Fig. 3-43), possibly accompanied by disruption of the posterior vertebral column. These injuries are more likely to demonstrate posteriorly displaced bony fragments that

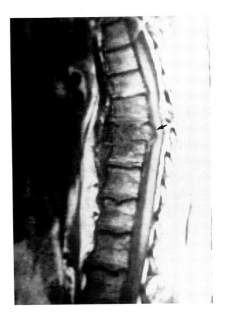

Fig. 3-44. Sagittal T1-weighted MRI scan of a thoracic burst fracture showing retropulsed bony fragments *(arrow)* impinging on the spinal cord. Decreased signal within the vertebral body is secondary to acute hemorrhage and edema.

may press on the spinal cord. MRI's superb soft tissue characterization makes it the preferred modality for demonstrating posttraumatic changes of the cord, such as hematomyelia or cyst formation (Fig. 3-44).

Flexion-distraction injuries occur when the fulcrum of force is located anterior to the anterior longitudinal ligament. Posterior column tension results in either bony or ligamentous disruption with compression of the anterior spinal column. Horizontal cleavage fractures (Chance's fracture) extending through the posterior bony neural arch and vertebral body create the visible linear radiolucent clefts seen on plain radiographs (Fig. 3-45). Since these fractures typically run parallel to the scanning plane on CT, they may be overlooked on the axial images and often require sagittal reformations for detection.

Flexion-rotation injury is one of the most severe thoracolumbar fractures, nearly always producing neurologic sequelae. This three-column injury often leads to subluxation, with extensive oblique fractures through the vertebral body and associated posterior arch fractures, as well as marked ligamentous or disc disruption. Distortion of the vertebral body is readily identified on x-ray films (Fig. 3-46), although CT often displays more subtle fractures and rotational deformity to better detail.

In young adolescents competing in weight-lifting or gymnastics, small bony avulsions off the lumbar apophyseal ring may be produced. This circular mound fuses onto the superior and inferior vertebral body end-plates at about 17 years of age and provides attachment of the major paraspinal ligaments. With repetitive axial loading and frequent hyperextension of the trunk, vertebral end-plate failure and fracture of this ring may occur with

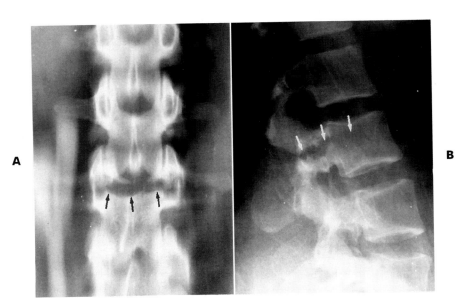

Fig. 3-45. A distraction fracture demonstrated on an AP tomogram **(A)** as a horizontal cleft *(black arrows)* through the pedicles and posterior arch extending through the vertebral body *(white arrows)* on the lateral view **(B).**

posterior displacement into the spinal canal. Diagnosis is usually not difficult and may be easily made either with plain radiography, CT, or MRI.

Although not truly designated as a fracture, there is often irregularity involving the anterosuperior aspect of one or more of the mid-lumbar vertebrae (limbus vertebra) (Fig. 3-47). This represents herniation of the disc's nucleus pulposus anteriorly beneath the unfused ring apophysis in early adolescence. It is usually of no

clinical significance but should not be inadvertently mistaken for vertebral fracture on conventional radiographs.

Spondylolysis

Young athletes with a history of trauma or persistent low back pain often show a bony defect in the pars interarticularis between the superior and inferior articular processes on lateral radiographs of the lower lumbar spine. This spondylolysis almost always occurs at the L4 or L5 level. A bone scan is frequently used in evaluating for spondylolysis when an athlete complains of low back pain. Increased uptake on the symptomatic side in the presence of normal x-ray findings indicates bony microfractures with attempts at healing. Faint sclerosis about the stress line may be visible either on x-ray films or high-resolution CT (Fig. 3-48). However, old healed pars defects may appear quite sclerotic, with a "hockey stick" deformity, on the x-ray but will not be hot on the bone scan. Instead, there may be contralateral activity on the radionuclide bone scan, suggesting increased stress bearing or impending fracture on that side (Fig. 3-49).

When spondylolysis is present bilaterally, a fibrous mass with hypertrophic bony spurring is often associated with the pars defect. Lateral constriction of the dural sac may be noted on myelography (Fig. 3-50). Spondylolisthesis, or slippage of the affected vertebral body on the caudal vertebra, can ensue with underlying degenerative disc disease.

Degenerative Disc Disease

Both biochemical and structural changes occur within the intervertebral disc in degenerative disc disease.

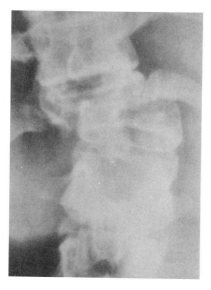

Fig. 3-46. The distorted vertebral body configuration on this AP view attests to the significant trauma to the vertebral column in flexion-rotation injuries resulting in severe spinal cord damage with paraplegia.

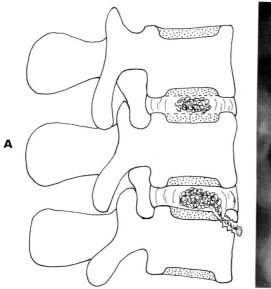
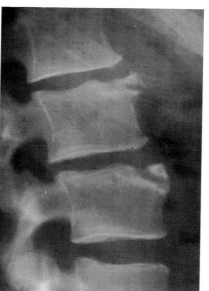

Fig. 3-47. Schematic drawing (**A**) of herniation of nuclear material beneath an unfused anterior apophyseal vertebral ring with subsequent radiographic evidence (**B**), forming the limbus vertebra.

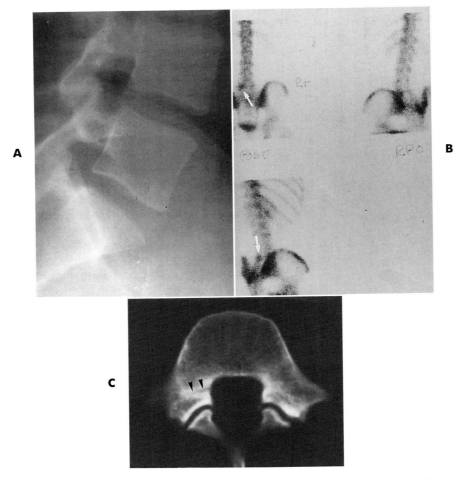

Fig. 3-48. Acute stress fracture in a young athlete complaining of left low back pain with normal x-ray findings (**A**) and abnormal bone scan findings (**B**), signifying the acute nature of the trauma *(arrows)*. **C,** Axial CT scan demonstrating the stress fracture *(arrowheads)* surrounded by faint sclerosis that could not be detected on the plain radiograph.

Farfan[3] and Kirkaldy-Willis et al.[12,13] have stressed that repeated axial loading with rotation leads to desiccation of the normally hydrated disc, causing circumferential annular rents or tears. The coalescence of these tears through the weaker posterolateral regions of the disc produces radial tears, herniated nuclear material from the disc's center, and further degeneration of the disc. The radiographic findings include progressive disc space narrowing, vertebral end-plate sclerosis, marginal hypertrophic spurs or osteophytes, and the appearance of intradiscal gas (vacuum phenomenon). All of these findings can be portrayed on plain radiographs, CT, and MRI; however, MRI has the advantage of demonstrating the signal intensity changes occurring within the disc and bone marrow adjacent to the vertebral end-plates as the degenerative process evolves (see box on p. 39).

MRI of the sagittal spine reveals the hyperintense hydrated nucleus pulposus and inner annulus fibrosus on T2-weighted images surrounded by the dense, hy-pointense fibrous outer annulus. The peripheral annulus blends with the posterior longitudinal ligament and posterior vertebral body cortex to produce the signal void or black line on sagittal images. This is usually interrupted at the mid–vertebral body level where the basivertebral venous plexus resides. This landmark is easily recognized because of the surrounding fat and slow flow of blood within the vessels, which produce its bright signal (Fig. 3-51).

Changes occur in cancellous bone marrow with normal aging. From birth into early adulthood, the central axial skeleton is composed primarily of red or hematopoietic marrow for erythropoiesis. This type of marrow produces the intermediate signal seen within the vertebral bodies on T1-weighted and proton density images and the decreased signal on T2-weighted images on MRI.

As degenerative disc disease progresses, one sees an alteration in the bone marrow signal intensity adjacent to

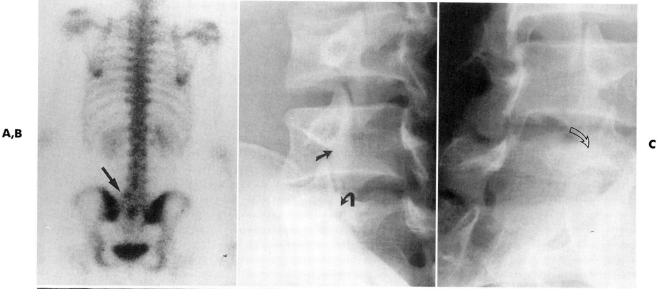

A,B

C

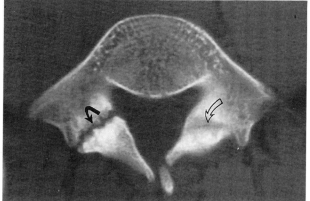

D

Fig. 3-49. A, Abnormal bone scan findings *(arrow)* in the lower lumbar spine (left side) in a young basketball player with a recent history of back trauma, now complaining of left low back pain. **B,** Posterior oblique view of the right pars interarticularis, showing an intact pars *(straight arrow)* at L4 with a complete pars defect at L5 *(curved arrow)*. **C,** Opposite side from symptomatic side, demonstrating a thickened and sclerotic pars *(open arrow)* at L5. **D,** Axial CT scan through L5 disclosing the old, nonhealed pars defect on the right *(solid arrow)* that is cold on the bone scan while a new healing stress fracture *(open arrow)* is noted on the left side, accounting for the bone scan finding.

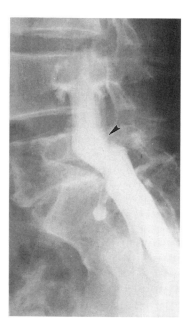

Fig. 3-50. Posterolateral impression *(arrowhead)* on a myelogram due to the fibrous soft tissue associated with a pars defect.

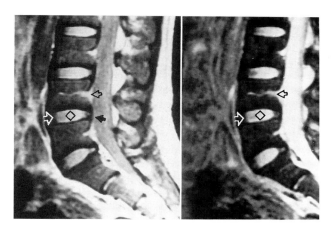

Fig. 3-51. Sagittal proton-density and T2-weighted MRI scans of the lumbar spine demonstrating a basivertebral venous plexus *(open black arrow)* with adjacent fat noted midway posterior to each vertebral body. The central hydrated nucleus pulposus and inner annulus *(open diamond)* are surrounded by the less-hydrated outer fibrous annulus *(open white arrow)*. *Solid black arrow,* Thick posterior longitudinal ligament blending in with the peripheral annulus.

the vertebral end-plates. As discussed by Heithoff,[6] the strong bone marrow signal noted in these areas is thought to reflect inflammatory changes (Modic type I) resulting from the diffusion of inflammatory agents from the abnormal, degenerating disc through damaged vertebral end-plates. This theory accounts for the T2-weighted sagittal spinal images demonstrating hyperintensity within the bone marrow on either side of the disc space primarily as a result of the higher water content within vascular granulation tissue. As the inflammatory granulation tissue is replaced with fat, the marrow signal behaves similarly to that of fat seen elsewhere in the body on MRI (Fig. 3-52). At this stage, one observes the increased signal in the bone marrow adjacent to the vertebral end-plates on the T1-weighted images. This variable appearance of the peridiscal bone marrow correlates well with histologic sectioning of bone

marrow specimens obtained at surgery. There has been some correlation between the presence of these inflammatory changes seen on MRI and the occurrence of back pain.

In the past the patient with intractable low back pain or sciatica underwent various diagnostic tests such as myelography or CT after conservative management failed to alleviate the symptoms within a given time frame. The presumptive diagnosis of a herniated disc was made on the myelogram when an anterior extradural defect was present at the disc space level either with or without amputation of the adjacent nerve root sheath (Fig. 3-53). Fortunately, CT can complement the myelogram, often disclosing different findings accounting for the myelographic defects. However, despite CT's improved sensitivity over myelography in detecting disc disease, it, too, has drawbacks.

As previously mentioned, the diagnosis of disc herniation on CT is based on the gross morphologic appearance of the disc-thecal sac interface and symmetry of the neural tissues within the spinal canal. The bulging, protruding, or extruding disc may indent the thecal sac, obliterate the normal epidural fat, or displace the budding or traversing nerve roots (Fig. 3-54). Sequestered or free fragments that have migrated away from the parent disc may involve a spinal nerve at a different level, thus confusing the clinical presentation. Anomalous conjoined nerve root sheaths may be distinguished from disc fragments by observing their typical course and position within the neural foramina on the parasagittal MRI scans (Fig. 3-55).

The presence of a massive disc herniation nearly occupying the entire spinal canal may appear deceptively normal at first glance. The administration of intrathecal contrast medium followed by CT myelography clearly

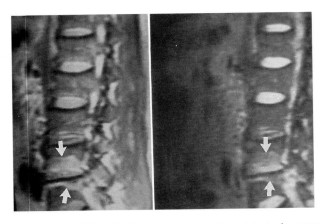

Fig. 3-52. Fat within the bone marrow adjacent to a degenerated disc appearing bright on T1-weighted sagittal image (*arrows*) and losing signal intensity on the T2-weighted image.

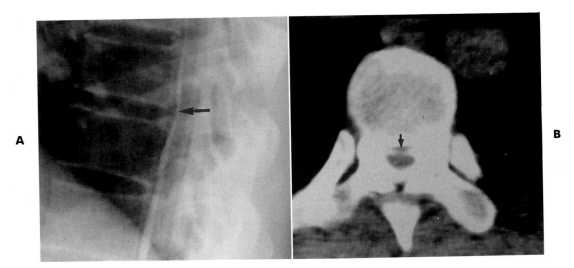

A   B

Fig. 3-53. Lateral myelogram (**A**) and axial contrast-enhanced CT scan (**B**) showing a small ventral extradural defect consistent with a small disc herniation (*arrow*) imprinting on the thecal sac.

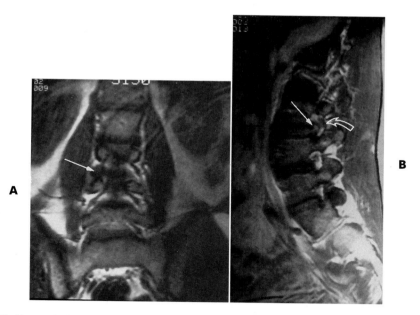

Fig. 3-54. Coronal (**A**) and sagittal (**B**) T1-weighted images demonstrating a large lateral disc extrusion *(thin arrow)* within the neural foramen, displacing the exiting nerve *(open arrow).*

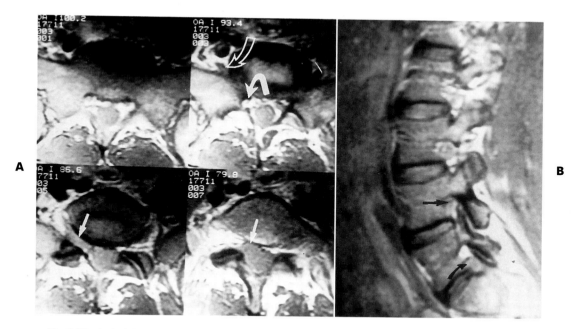

Fig. 3-55. A, Axial MRI scan demonstrating L5 and S1 conjoined nerve roots *(straight solid white arrow)* budding off late from the thecal sac and dividing into the L5 nerve *(open curved white arrow)* and S1 nerve root *(solid curved white arrow)* already within the lateral recess. **B,** Sagittal image showing a normal nerve root *(straight black arrow)* within the cephalad portion of the neural foramen while the conjoined nerves below *(curved black arrow)* bud off the thecal sac at a lower point and exit through the foramen in the caudal portion of the foramen.

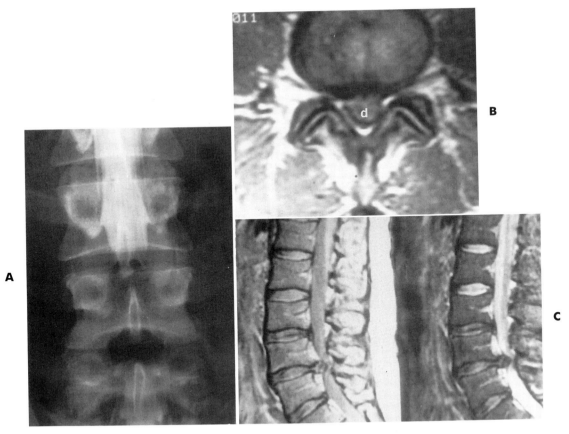

Fig. 3-56. Complete subarachnoid block noted on the myelogram (**A**) may go undetected on the axial MRI scan (**B**) if the sagittal images (**C**) are not inspected, revealing a massive disc extrusion *(d)* that mimics the thecal sac on the axial image.

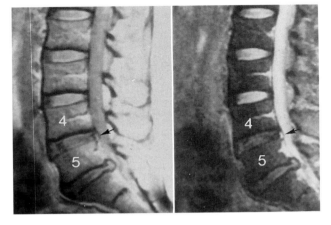

Fig. 3-57. Sagittal MRI scans demonstrating a large disc herniation at L5-S1. Within the peripherally bulging L4-5 annulus is a hyperintense focus *(arrow)* representing either fluid or inflammatory granulation tissue in an annular tear.

demonstrates the compressed dural sac and distinguishes it from the herniated nucleus. This mistake can also be obviated by employing both T1- and T2-weighted images on MRI (Fig. 3-56).

Modic et al.'s revelation of the body's attempt to heal itself by forming hypervascular granulation tissue[14-16] has provided strong support for disc inflammation as the origin of low back pain and sciatica. The peripheral annulus is well known to be innervated with sensory pain fibers and often contains radially oriented fissures or rents that enhance after the intravenous injection of gadolinium-DTPA. Similarly, they appear as small hyperintense foci in the peripheral annulus on sagittal T2-weighted images on MRI (Fig. 3-57). It is therefore conceivable that the presence of inflammation associated with these annular rents might relate to the patient's symptoms.

Despite MRI's ability to portray the changes associated with degenerative disc disease, it cannot provide information regarding the symptomatology of each disc. The discogram, on the other hand, has been instrumental in resolving these cases by discriminating between symptomatic and asymptomatic discs when multiple

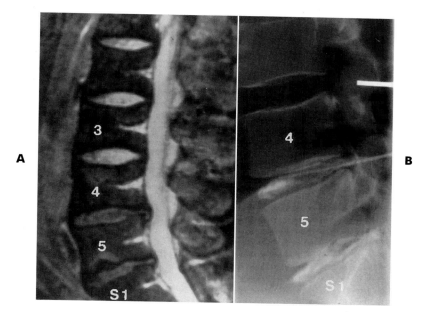

Fig. 3-58. A, Sagittal T2-weighted image showing grade 4 degenerative changes occurring at both the L4-5 and L5-S1 levels with small disc protrusions. **B,** The corresponding discogram revealed that the patient's pain originated from the L4-5 disc, and no pain response was elicited from the L5-S1 disc level.

levels of abnormality are demonstrated on the MRI scan. Not infrequently, what may have initially appeared to represent a symptomatic degenerated or herniated disc by conventional imaging has appeared entirely asymptomatic on the discogram, thereby altering the patient's treatment (Fig. 3-58).

Degenerative Facet Disease

The posterior lumbar facet joints are true synovial joints innervated by sensory branches of the primary dorsal ramus of the spinal nerve. As with any joint, local irritation and inflammation may occur, and the athlete or active individual may subsequently complain of low back pain with or without referred leg pain. Any underlying degenerative disc disease eventually results in loss of disc height and settling of the vertebral bodies, which can exert additional abnormal biomechanical forces on the facet joints and predispose them to early degeneration. This manifests as bony and ligamentous hypertrophy in an attempt to stabilize any potential subluxation. As the inflammation progresses and the stabilizing capsular and ligamentous attachments become lax, degenerative spondylolistheses may occur, further contributing to the patient's back pain.

Large synovial cysts (Fig. 3-59) associated with deranged facet joints present as soft tissue masses projecting posterolaterally into the spinal canal, an unusual location for free disc fragments. Recognizing the cyst's base centered over the joint space within the posterolateral portion of the spinal canal facilitates

arriving at the proper diagnosis. Intracystic hemorrhage, fluid, gas, or hypertrophied synovium accounts for the variable signal characteristics noted on MRI. Either diagnostic or therapeutic injection of the abnormal facet joint under fluoroscopic or CT guidance with bupivacaine and steroids has been advocated by some in helping to reduce any inflammation occurring in and around the facet joint once a diagnosis has been established.

Stenosis

CT and MRI have generally been regarded as the preferred imaging modalities in evaluating the spinal canal and neural foramina for stenosis. Individuals with a congenitally narrowed spinal canal and a significant disc bulge or herniation are at higher risk of developing symptoms than those with a larger canal. In general, CT and MRI correlate well in evaluating spinal stenosis (Fig. 3-60) despite CT's improved capability for displaying fine bony detail.

Both the axial and sagittal planes are needed when inspecting for central spinal canal stenosis (Fig. 3-61). The central stenosis may be congenital, resulting from short pedicles with reduced AP canal dimension, or acquired, caused by the development of hypertrophy of the ligamentum flavum and facet joints in conjunction with disc pathology (Fig. 3-62). The "trefoil"-appearing canal created by hypertrophy of the superior articular processes and lamina may result in stenosis of the spinal recess or subarticular gutter, which is where the spinal

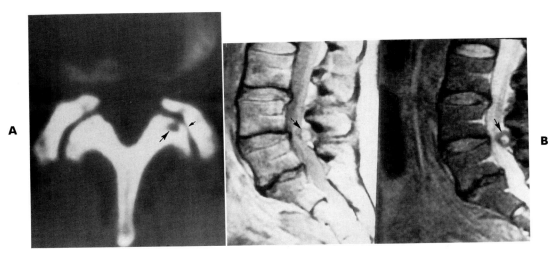

Fig. 3-59. A, Axial CT scan showing a degenerated left facet joint with narrowing *(small arrow)* and subchondral cyst formation *(large arrow).* **B,** Sagittal MRI scans portray a rounded soft tissue mass *(arrow)* posterolaterally within the spinal canal, representing a synovial cyst associated with the degenerated facet joint. The heterogeneous internal signal represents hemorrhage, synovium, and fluid surrounded by a thick fibrous capsule.

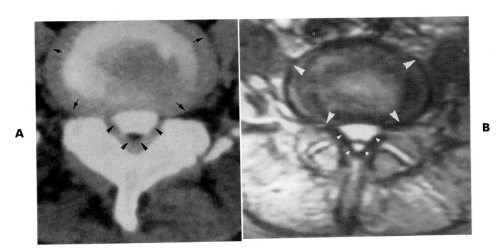

Fig. 3-60. Good correlation between an axial CT scan **(A)** and MRI scans **(B)** in demonstrating central canal stenosis due to a diffusely bulging disc *(arrows)* and hypertrophy of the ligamentum flavum *(arrowheads).*

nerve root passes in a downward-sloping course as it enters the more lateral recess before passing beneath the pedicle and exiting through the foramen.

Other forms of central stenosis may be noted in patients with calcification of the posterior longitudinal ligament encroaching on the spinal canal (Fig. 3-63). This can occur in the cervical and thoracic regions, where there is less epidural fat than in the lumbar region. As the calcification enlarges in the presence of underlying disc disease, anterior cord compression may progress to ischemic changes, leading to cord atrophy, myelomalacia, and eventually central cavitation. More laterally

located calcifications or spurs within the neural foramina may contribute to a radiculopathy of a thoracic intercostal nerve. Because of the small size of the offending spur, high-resolution axial CT scanning through the region of interest is needed for identification, although the larger calcifications within the spinal canal may be easily recognized on plain x-ray films and MRI.

Lateral stenosis in the lumbar spine helps explain why a number of patients who undergo surgical laminectomy for back or leg pain do not experience alleviation of symptoms (failed back syndrome). Osseous spurs may originate from the lumbar uncinate processes, analogs to

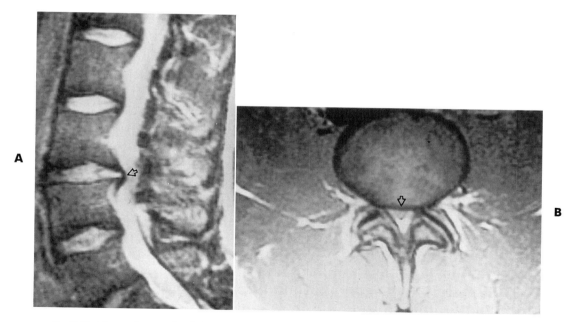

Fig. 3-61. Central stenosis of the spinal canal primarily due to a posteriorly bulging disc *(arrow)* on sagittal **(A)** and axial **(B)** MRI scans.

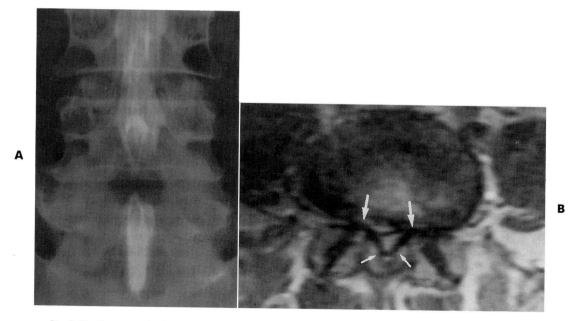

Fig. 3-62. Severe spinal stenosis at the L4-5 disc level on the myelogram **(A)** corroborated the axial MR image **(B)** because of the diffusely bulging disc *(large arrows)* and posterior ligamentous hypertrophy *(small arrows)*.

the small bony ridges seen posterolaterally in the cervical spine (Fig. 3-64). Since these localized osteophytes tend to protrude in a cephalad direction, they may be overlooked if only axial images are examined. Thus sagittal reformations through the entire nerve root canal should be performed. This type of stenosis has been

called "up-down" stenosis because of the craniocaudal compromise of the nerve root canal, as opposed to the more widely recognized "front-back" stenosis where there is hypertrophy of either the superior articular process or the ligamentum flavum in conjunction with a posteriorly bulging disc or osteophyte that causes

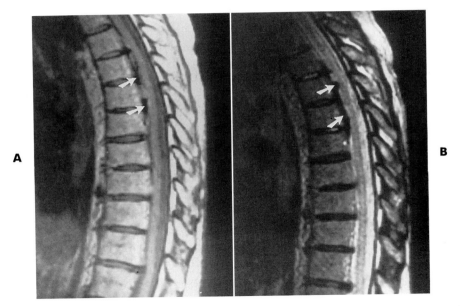

Fig. 3-63. Sagittal proton-density **(A)** and T2-weighted **(B)** MRI scans of the thoracic spine demonstrating dense calcification of the posterior longitudinal ligament represented by signal void structures *(arrows)* in anterior epidural spaces.

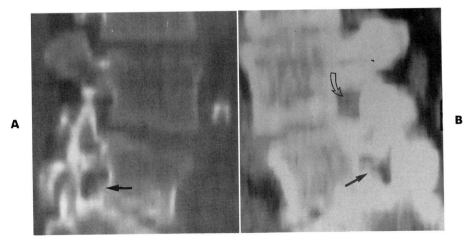

Fig. 3-64. Sagittal CT reformations photographed at bone **(A)** and soft tissue windows **(B)** revealing bony spurs projecting from the uncinate processes of L5 *(solid arrows),* encroaching on the neural foramina. Note the normally patent foramen at the L4-5 level with fat *(curved open arrow)* surrounding the exiting nerve.

narrowing anteroposteriorly. In severe cases compression of the dorsal root ganglion may produce an enlarged edematous ganglion simulating a soft tissue mass that might be mistaken for lateral disc herniation.

In patients with isthmic spondylolisthesis, the nerve may become trapped within the narrowed nerve root canal as the normal vertically oriented foramen assumes a horizontal orientation as a result of vertebral body slippage. The floor of the nerve root canal becomes the intervertebral disc (Fig. 3-65) rather than the pedicle of the subjacent vertebra, and any disc bulge or herniation compresses the exiting nerve from below against the pars defect from above. Because of the traversing nerve's immobility resulting from the tiny extradural ligaments extending from it to the posterior margin of the disc space and vertebral body as it exits the foramen, it is

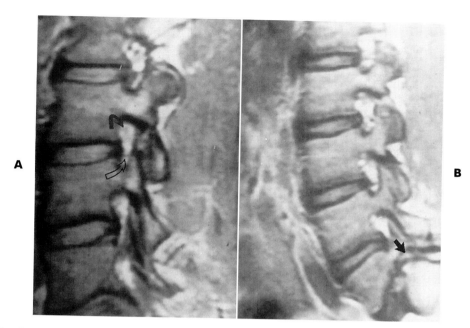

Fig. 3-65. A, Normal neural foramen showing an exiting nerve *(solid curved arrow)* in the cephalad portion of the foramen with vascular structures *(open curved arrow)* in the caudal portion of the foramen. There is ample epidural fat surrounding the neurovascular structures. **B,** Sagittal MRI scan at the level of an isthmic spondylolisthesis demonstrating severe narrowing of the distorted neural foramen, with the floor of the neural foramen consisting of the intervertebral disc rather than the pedicle of the subjacent vertebral body. There is compression of the exiting nerve *(solid arrow)*, resulting in radiculopathy at the involved disc segment.

securely anchored within the ventral and cephalad compartment of the nerve root canal as it passes downward and beneath the pedicle. This predisposes the nerve to compression from the spondylolisthesis, adjacent osteophyte, or lateral disc herniation at the level of the slip. These preoperative findings are critical to the surgeon, since a routine decompressive laminectomy and medial facetectomy may not alleviate the situation and a false sense of security may be established by probing a patent posterior compartment of the nerve root canal in checking for stenosis.

REFERENCES

1. Boden SD et al: Abnormal magnetic resonance scans of the lumbar spine in asymptomatic subjects, *J Bone Joint Surg* 72A:403, 1990.
2. Calenoff L et al: Multiple level spinal injuries: importance in early recognition, *AJR* 130:665, 1978.
3. Farfan HF: The pathological anatomy of degenerative spondylolisthesis: a cadaver study, *Spine* 5:412, 1980.
4. Foristall RM, Marsh HD, Pay NT: Magnetic resonance imaging and contrast CT of the lumbar spine: comparison of diagnostic methods and correlation with surgical findings, *Spine* 13:1049, 1988.
5. Goldberg AL et al: The impact of magnetic resonance on the diagnostic evaluation of acute cervicothoracic spinal trauma, *Skeletal Radiol* 17:89, 1988.
6. Heithoff KB, Amster JL: The spine. In Mink JH, Deutsch AL, editors: *MRI of the musculoskeletal system: a teaching file,* New York, 1990, Raven Press.
7. Holt AP: The question of lumbar discography, *J Bone Joint Surg* 50B:720, 1968.
8. Jackson RP et al: The neuroradiographic diagnosis of lumbar herniated nucleus pulposis. I. A comparison of computed tomography (CT), myelography, CT myelography, discography, and CT discography, *Spine* 14:1356, 1989.
9. Johansen JG, Orrison WW, Amundsen P: Lateral C1-2 puncture for cervical myelography. I. Report of a complication, *Radiology* 146:391, 1983.
10. Kieffer A et al: Lumbar myelography with iohexol and metrizamide: a comparative multicenter prospective study, *Radiology* 151:665, 1984.
11. Kingston S, Schneiderman G: Comparative use of myelography, computed tomography, and disc discography. In Watkins RG, Collis JS, editors: *Lumbar discectomy and laminectomy,* Rockville, Md, 1987, Aspen.
12. Kirkaldy-Willis WH et al: Lumbar spinal stenosis, *Clin Orthop* 99:30, 1974.
13. Kirkaldy-Willis WH et al: Pathology and pathogenesis of lumbar spondylosis and stenosis, *Spine* 3:319, 1978.
14. Modic MT, Masaryk TJ, Paushter DM: Magnetic resonance imaging of the spine, *Radiol Clin North Am* 24:229, 1986.
15. Modic MT et al: Cervical radiculopathy: prospective evaluation with surface coil MR imaging, *Radiology* 161:753, 1986.
16. Modic MT et al: Magnetic resonance imaging of intervertebral disc disease: clinical pulse and sequence considerations, *Radiology* 152:103, 1984.
17. Nakstad PH, Kjartansson O: Accidental spinal cord injection of contrast material during cervical myelography with lateral C1-C2 puncture, *Am J Neuroradiol* 9:410, 1988.
18. Servo A, Laasonen EM: Accidental introduction of contrast

medium into the cervical spinal cord: a case report, *Neuroradiology* 27:80, 1985.

19. Walsh TR et al: Lumbar discography in normal subjects, *J Bone Joint Surg* 72:1081, 1990.

SUGGESTED READINGS

Afsbani E, Kuhn J: Common causes of low back pain in children, *Radiographics* 11:269, 1991.

Antti-Poika I et al: Clinical relevance of diskography combined with CT scanning: a study of 100 patients, *J Bone Joint Surg* 72B:480, 1990.

Becker E, Griffiths HJ: Radiologic diagnosis of pain in the athlete, *Clin Sports Med* 6:699, 1987.

Beers GJ et al: MR imaging in acute cervical spine trauma, *J Comput Assist Tomogr* 12:755, 1988.

Bellah RD et al: Low back pain in adolescent athletes: detection of stress injury to the pars interarticularis with SPECT, *Radiology* 180:509, 1991.

Browne TD, Yost RP, McCarron RF: Lumbar ring apophyseal fracture in an adolescent weight lifter, *Am J Sports Med* 18:533, 1990.

Cacayorin ED, Hochhauser L, Petro GR: Lumbar and thoracic spine pain in the athlete: radiographic evaluation, *Clin Sports Med* 6:767, 1987.

Crawford AH: Operative treatment of spine fractures in children, *Orthop Clin North Am* 21:325, 1990.

Daffner RH: Thoracic and lumbar vertebral trauma, *Orthop Clin North Am* 21:463, 1990.

Duchesneau PM: Myelography. In Watkins RG, Collis JS, editors: *Lumbar discectomy and laminectomy,* Rockville, Md, 1987, Aspen.

Elster AD: Bertlotti's syndrome revisited: transitional vertebrae of the lumbar spine, *Spine* 14:1373, 1989.

Enzmann DR, Rubin JB: Cervical spine: MR imaging with a partial flip angle, gradient-refocused pulse sequence. I. General considerations and disk disease, *Radiology* 166:467, 1988.

Enzmann DR, Rubin JB: Cervical spine: MR imaging with a partial flip angle, gradient-refocused pulse sequence. II. Spinal cord disease, *Radiology* 166:473, 1988.

Flannigan B: Magnetic resonance imaging of the lumbar spine. In Watkins RG, Collis JS, editors: *Lumbar discectomy and laminectomy,* Rockville, Md, 1987, Aspen.

Flaunders AE et al: Acute cervical spine trauma in correlation of MR imaging findings with degree of neurologic deficit, *Radiology* 177:25, 1990.

Grenier N et al: Normal and degenerative posterior spinal structures: MR imaging, *Radiology* 165:517, 1987.

Haughton VM: MR imaging of the spine, *Radiology* 166:297, 1988.

Heithoff K, Ray CD: CT of lateral spinal stenosis. In Watkins RG, Collis JS, editors: *Lumbar discectomy and laminectomy,* Rockville, Md, 1977, Aspen.

Karnaze MG et al: Comparison of MR and CT myelography in imaging the cervical and thoracic spine, *AJR* 150:397, 1988.

Kaye JJ, Nance EP: Cervical spine trauma, *Orthop Clin North Am* 21:449, 1990.

Kaye JJ, Nance EP: Thoracic and lumbar spine trauma, *Radiol Clin North Am* 28:361, 1990.

Keene JS: Thoracolumbar fractures in winter sports, *Clin Orthop* 216:39, 1987.

Kingston S: Contrast-enhanced computed tomographic scanning. In Watkins RG, Collis JS, editors: *Lumbar discectomy and laminectomy,* Rockville, Md, 1987, Aspen.

Kricun R, Kricun ME, Dalinka MK: Advances in spinal imaging, *Radiol Clin North Am* 28:321, 1990.

Kronberg M: Diskography and magnetic resonance imaging in the diagnosis of lumbar disk disruption, *Spine* 14:1368, 1989.

Letts M et al: Fracture of the pars interarticularis in adolescent athletes: a clinical biomechanical analysis, *J Pediatr Orthop* 6(1):40, 1986.

Maly P: Sex and age related differences in postmyelographic adverse reactions: a prospective study of 1765 myelographies, *Neuroradiology* 31:331, 1989.

Martine JR: The role of nuclear medicine bone scan in evaluating pain in athletic injuries, *Clin Sports Med* 6:713, 1987.

Murphy MD, Batnitzky S, Bramble JM: Diagnostic imaging of spinal trauma, *Radiol Clin North Am* 27:855, 1989.

Paley D, Gillespie R: Chronic repetitive unrecognized flexion injury of the cervical spine (high jumper's neck), *Am J Sports Med* 14:92, 1986.

Pavlov H, Torg JS: Roentgen examination of cervical spine injuries in the athlete, *Clin Sports Med* 6:751, 1987.

Robertson HJ, Smith RD: Cervical myelography: survey of modes of practice and major complications, *Radiology* 174:79, 1990.

Ross JS, Modic MT, Masaryk TJ: Tears of the annulus fibrosus: assessment with Gd-DTPA enhanced MR imaging, *AJR* 154:159, 1990.

Rothman SL: Computed tomography of the spine in older children and teenagers, *Clin Sports Med* 5:247, 1986.

Rothman SLG, Glenn WV: Multiplanar CT in the diagnosis of disc herniation. In Watkins RG, Collis JS, editors: *Lumbar discectomy and laminectomy,* Rockville, Md, 1987, Aspen.

Sand T et al: Side effects after lumbar iohexol myelography: relation to radiological diagnosis, sex, and age, *Neuroradiology* 31:523, 1989.

Schiebler ML et al: Normal and degenerated intervertebral disk: in vivo and in vitro MR imaging with histopathologic correlation, *AJR* 157:93, 1991.

Schneiderman G et al: Magnetic resonance imaging in the diagnosis of disc degeneration: correlation with discography, *Spine* 12:276, 1987.

Thomas JC: Plain roentgenograms of the spine in the injured athlete, *Clin Sports Med* 5:353, 1986.

Thomas JC: Plain X-rays in lumbar disc disease. In Watkins RG, Collis JS, editors: *Lumbar discectomy and laminectomy,* Rockville, Md, 1987, Aspen.

Torg JS et al: Neuropraxia of the cervical spinal cord with transient quadriplegia, *J Bone Joint Surg* 68A:1354, 1986.

Tsuruda JS et al: Three dimensional gradient-recalled MR imaging as a screening tool for the diagnosis of cervical radiculopathy, *AJR* 154:375, 1990.

Vezina JL, Fontaine S, Laperriere J: Outpatient myelography with fine-needle technique: an appraisal, *AJR* 153:383, 1989.

Watkins RG: Neck injuries in football players, *Clin Sports Med* 5:215, 1986.

Wilcox PG, Spencer CW: Dorsolumbar kyphosis or Scheuermann's disease, *Clin Sports Med* 5:343, 1986.

Chapter Four

◆

Electrodiagnostic Evaluation of Spinal Problems

Joel M. Press
Jeffrey L. Young
Stanley A. Herring

Electrodiagnostic studies, such as electromyelography (EMG), are an extension of the clinical examination and should be guided by pertinent information gathered in the history, physical examination, and anatomic or radiologic data.[2] Furthermore, any resultant electrophysiologic information must be interpreted in light of the complete clinical picture. The electrodiagnostic examination evaluates the physiology of the nerves and muscles studied *at that time.* Some abnormalities might not yet have appeared; others may have resolved, leaving no detectable residual deficit. Therefore the electrodiagnostic impression must be based on the entire clinical picture. A lack of electrophysiologic abnormality does not necessarily mean that nerve damage has not occurred. Conversely, lack of nerve damage does not mean that the patient is free of pathologic conditions.

This chapter describes the electrophysiologic events that occur with nerve injuries, the usefulness and limitations of various electrophysiologic tests, the sensitivity and specificity of these tests, common clinical presentations of cervical and lumbar radiculopathies, and indications and limitations of electrodiagnostic studies in the evaluation of athletes with spinal problems.

NEUROLOGIC ANATOMY

The spinal nerves are composed of dorsal and ventral roots (Fig. 4-1). The axons of the ventral root originate primarily from cells in the anterior and lateral gray columns of the cord, whereas those of the dorsal roots originate in the dorsal root ganglia. The dorsal root ganglia are usually situated within the entrance of the bony intervertebral foramen.[21,22] This is situated along the distal portion of the dorsal root near the area where the dorsal and ventral roots join to form the spinal nerves. The spinal nerve is formed at about the level of the intervertebral foramen. Disruption of the nerve root by a herniated disc occurs before the exit at the intervertebral foramen and therefore proximal to the dorsal root ganglia.[67] As a result, the sensory fibers to the periphery are not affected. However, the afferent fibers from the dorsal root ganglia to the spinal cord can be affected, therefore explaining why hypesthesia can be present despite normal sensory study results.

Nearly all muscles are innervated by more than one root level, except the rhomboids, which are believed to be exclusively C5 in origin.[72] The specific nerve root supplies of some muscles have yet to be determined, and there is natural variability in muscle innervation, which adds further confusion.[72] Thus when EMG studies are performed, several muscles with overlapping innervations must be studied to obtain a clear picture of which nerve root is the one most likely affected. Sensory dermatomes overlap extensively. Because of overlap, myofascial pain syndromes, and nonneural causes that simulate radicular pain, it is difficult to adequately assess sensory symptoms with standard nerve conduction studies.[63,67]

PATHOPHYSIOLOGIC PATTERNS

Compression of nerve tissues can induce structural damage to the nerve fibers, impairment of intraneural blood flow, and the formation of intraneural edema, as well as axonal transport block.[52] Some electrodiagnostic changes occur from the onset of irritation or damage to a nerve. If the initial injury is mild, a focal conduction slowing or block occurs, which can be transient (neurapraxia) or, if more persistent, can result in focal demyelination.[17-20,51] With mild injury the sensory or motor deficit may last only hours to days. Spontaneous single muscle fiber discharges (e.g., positive waves and fibrillation potentials or changes in the parameters of the motor unit action potential [MUAP]) never occur because no axonal loss has taken place. Clinically apparent weakness may, however, be recognized electrophysiologically as a reduced recruitment pattern on maximal contraction.[31,32] On the other hand, if weakness is minimal, the recruitment pattern may not be identified as reduced. Then, with minimal contraction, a reduced recruitment interval can be seen because there are fewer motor units available and the first unit fires more rapidly when the second unit is recruited.

Other electrodiagnostic changes detectable from the onset of nerve injury are alterations in the H-reflex latency and amplitude of the compound muscle action potential (CMAP). In S1 radiculopathies the H-reflex latency is prolonged from the onset.[67] Opinions about

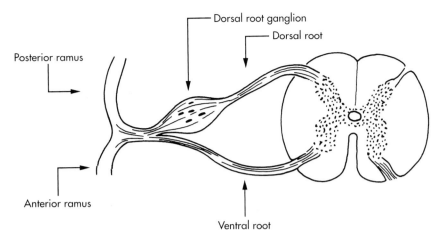

Fig. 4-1. Spinal nerve root anatomy. Note that the spinal nerves terminate by dividing into anterior and posterior rami.

what constitutes significant differences in H-reflex latency from side to side in unilateral radiculopathies vary among authors from 1 to 2 msec.[30,58,56] The reduced amplitude of the CMAP over the appropriate muscle group can also be seen soon after nerve injury.[31,32]

With more severe injuries, axonal loss occurs, so that sensory abnormalities are prominent, muscle stretch reflexes are reduced or lost, and denervation occurs in the muscles of that myotome.[69] The electrophysiologic hallmark of axonal degeneration is the spontaneous single muscle fiber discharges called positive sharp waves and fibrillation potentials. Positive sharp waves are first noticed in paraspinal muscles (posterior primary ramus distribution) within 7 to 10 days after loss of axon function.[31,32] By 14 to 18 days, positive sharp waves can appear in the limb muscles, beginning proximally and quickly becoming evident throughout the involved myotome. Soon the positive waves are accompanied by fibrillation potentials.[31,32,34,42] By 18 to 21 days, all muscles in the involved myotome have abnormalities, including positive sharp waves and fibrillation potentials. Positive sharp waves start out as large-amplitude waves of approximately 200 μV that gradually drop over many weeks to about 100 to 150 μV.[30,53,54] Fibrillation potentials follow a similar course. With time, if reinnervation of muscle fibers remains incomplete, both positive sharp waves and fibrillation potentials decrease to 20 and 50 μV. As the nerve root disorder resolves, paraspinal muscles, which are the first muscles to show abnormalities on EMG, are also the first muscles to reinnervate and cease fibrillating. Thereafter, proximal limb muscles and later the more distal muscles follow suit.

Most radiculopathies will not demonstrate positive waves and fibrillations within the first 3 weeks of symptoms, so electrodiagnostic studies are not immediately pursued. If, however, the athlete has had previous episodes of radicular symptoms or prior spinal surgery, it may be useful from both a diagnostic and a medical-legal standpoint to perform initial electrodiagnostic studies as soon as possible after new symptoms appear.[59] If positive waves are seen within 1 or 2 weeks, they can be assumed to have been present before the onset of symptoms. Different EMG abnormalities seen 4 to 6 weeks later can be assumed to represent new findings.

In chronic radiculopathies, fibrillation potentials typically are seen only in distal muscles. If the radiculopathy resolves (does not become chronic), the spontaneous single muscle fiber discharges (positive sharp waves and fibrillation potentials) begin to diminish in 5 to 6 weeks and then disappear in 6 months or less unless the root lesion was severe. Evidence of reinnervation (long-duration, large-amplitude polyphasic MUAP) may be found several weeks after the onset of symptoms, but this is not readily apparent unless the radiculopathy was severe. Absence of positive waves (i.e., absence of denervation) even though weakness is present portends a good prognosis, assuming sufficient time has passed since the onset of nerve compromise for them to develop.[42]

SPECIFIC ELECTRODIAGNOSTIC STUDIES

Many specific steps constitute a comprehensive electrodiagnostic evaluation. Each is discussed separately to delineate its usefulness and limitations in evaluating patients with back pain. Specific procedural details of each of these studies are not discussed in this chapter because they are explained fully in standard electrodiagnostic texts.[31,32,38]

Nerve Conduction Studies

Results of distal peripheral motor and sensory nerve conduction studies are often normal in a single-level radiculopathy. They may, however, be useful to evaluate the possibility of nerve entrapment or peripheral neuropathy, which may mimic symptoms of radiculopathy. In radiculopathy, if the root lesion is purely demyelinative, no change occurs in the CMAP amplitude after stimulation distal to the lesion. If axonal degeneration occurs at one root level, the CMAP amplitude may still be relatively preserved, as a result of either reinnervation of the muscles by fibers from the other uninvolved roots or the relatively small contribution of the injured root to that muscle compared with the uninvolved levels. Also, root compromise is nearly always incomplete; only rarely do most motor fibers degenerate. When considerable axon degeneration does occur, the CMAP amplitude may be reduced. Maximum reduction is reached 7 days after injury[72] and is easily recognized in the peroneal muscle groups in L5 radiculopathy and in the tibial groups when S1 is involved. A reduction of the CMAP of a specific muscle of more than 50% compared with the uninvolved side probably is significant. In general, the CMAP is likely to be significantly reduced only when considerable axonal degeneration has occurred or multiple nerve roots are acutely involved. In clinical situations in which the muscle is very weak, yet the CMAP is large, the prognosis for recovery is good. Chronic nerve root compression, such as occurs with central lumbar stenosis, tends not to cause axonal degeneration until later.

Sensory nerve action potentials and conduction velocities are often normal in radiculopathies. Because the lesion in a herniated disc is almost always proximal to the dorsal root ganglion, degeneration of peripheral sensory fibers does not occur.[6,11,12,72] However, in a far lateral lumbar disc herniation, particularly at the L5-S1 level, the dorsal root ganglion may be injured and cause abnormal sensory study findings. In the cervical spine, a disc that herniates into the intervertebral foramen and impinges on the posteriorly located dorsal root ganglion causes sensory symptoms and shows positive electrophysiologic findings on sensory studies. In the cervical spine, rarely does a herniated disc impinge only on the anterior roots, cause no sensory deficits, and show a normal sensory nerve action potential with only motor weakness as evidence of the radiculopathy.

H-Reflex

The H-reflex is the electrophysiologic analog to the ankle muscle stretch reflex. It measures afferent and efferent conduction along mainly the S1 nerve root and is used in localizing nerve root compromise at that level.* Authors differ as to which component, the distal latency or the amplitude of the response, is more important in determining S1 root abnormalities. Comparing side-to-side latency differences is even more critical in tall athletes with long limbs (and therefore longer nerves) inasmuch as absolute distal latencies may be prolonged on the sole basis of nerve length. A latency difference of

* References 1, 5, 8, 13, 41, 62.

at least 1 to 2 msec is significant. H-reflex latency shows a high correlation with S1 nerve root pain production, as demonstrated by selective nerve root blocks.[53,54] Amplitude differences of less than 25% to 50% compared with the uninvolved side or less than 1 mV also are significant.[13,71,72] However, the amplitude of this reflex is sensitive to contraction of the plantar flexor muscles; thus caution is recommended about accepting a significant finding based solely on amplitude changes.

Several advantages are seen in performing H-reflex studies as part of the electrodiagnostic evaluation of athletes with spinal problems. H-reflex parameters can become abnormal as soon as root injury occurs and therefore are detectable much earlier than with the use of standard EMG.[23] Because the H-reflex allows a view of both afferent and efferent pathways, it can give information about the status of sensory fibers that is not available with standard EMG, which evaluates only motor nerve fibers. H-reflexes are also helpful in distinguishing S1 from L5 radiculopathies. Because these two levels are involved in more than 90% of lumbar radiculopathies, H-reflex studies may help construct a clear clinical picture. If surgery is contemplated, H-reflexes may assist in localizing the involved level and help guide the surgical approach.

H-reflexes in the forearm, recorded from the flexor carpi radialis (FCR), are found in an overwhelming number of normal subjects.[13] As with the physiologically similar phasic myotatic reflexes, however, symmetrically absent H-reflexes are not necessarily abnormal and the percentage of absent responses increases in elderly persons.[70] Nevertheless, FCR H-reflexes may be abnormal with C6 or C7 root injury.[55] Upper limits of normal for side-to-side latency differences is 1 msec for FCR H-reflexes.[28,31,32,47]

Certain limitations must be understood in performing H-reflex studies.[13] These studies provide direct information only about the segmental level being studied (i.e., S1), although by inference they also provide information about L5.[23,56] The H-reflex sometimes is normal in persons with proven S1 radiculopathies, presumably because of incomplete root involvement and sparing of the fibers over which the reflex is mediated.[72] H-reflex studies give no information about chronic versus acute radiculopathies, nor do they correlate with the severity of the radiculopathy. Once inelicitable, the H-reflex may remain so indefinitely.[72] H-reflex studies reveal nothing about the cause of the S1 root abnormality, and, in fact, do not even specifically localize the lesion to the root because findings also can be abnormal in peripheral neuropathies (often bilaterally), tibial or sciatic nerve injuries, and disorders of the lumbosacral plexus, spinal cord, and even central nervous system. Therefore evaluation of other peripheral nerves by means of standard nerve conduction studies may be helpful if the clinical situation warrants it. Furthermore, patient relaxation is important because mild muscle contraction of the antagonist muscles inhibits the H-reflex.[23,34]

In conclusion, the H-reflex may be part of an electrodiagnostic study in athletes with low back and leg complaints in whom the clinician suspects an S1 nerve injury or in a patient with arm pain who is suspected of having a C6 or C7 root injury. When EMG abnormalities on needle examination are limited to the paraspinal muscles, a prolonged H-reflex suggests an S1 or a C6 or C7 radiculopathy. H-reflex studies are especially important when EMG abnormalities are inconclusive. They may be helpful in making a diagnosis early in the course of nerve irritation in an athlete with radicular symptoms before needle EMG findings are present.

F Wave

The F wave is a late muscle potential that results from the backfiring of antidromically and supramaximally activated anterior horn cells.[13,45,53,54,73-75] F wave studies have been shown by some to be useful in the diagnosis of lumbar nerve root lesions when the side-to-side minimal latency is greater than 2 msec.[16,62] Like H-reflexes, F wave abnormalities occur immediately after injury to a nerve root. In one study, F wave abnormalities were found to be the only abnormality in up to 15% of patients with radiculopathy.[15] Other studies have found that the F waves, which most often are abnormal when other abnormalities are also present, are rarely the only abnormality noted.[62,72] Unlike the H-reflex, the F wave can be elicited at many spinal levels and from any muscle.

The use of the F wave in evaluating athletes with spinal problems is affected by several limitations. First, F wave studies, like needle EMG, assess only motor fibers, not sensory fibers.[23] Second, only a small population of all the fibers of an axon is evaluated, and if these fibers are not involved, study results will be normal. Third, F wave studies, like the H-reflex, view the entire pathway of the nerve, and small, focal abnormalities tend to be obscured by the longer segments. Fourth, because the F wave is elicited by stimulating the nerve of the muscle studied and all muscles receive more than one nerve root innervation, it is not specific for a given nerve root level. Fifth, like the H-reflex, the F wave cannot distinguish between acute and chronic changes. Sixth, because there is a range of latencies, 10 to 20 stimuli are required for each nerve studied to determine the shortest and longest latencies. Finally, as with H-reflexes, various conditions can injure the nerve pathways at sites other than the nerve root and result in abnormal F waves. In conclusion, F wave studies can be useful in evaluating radiculopathies and should be employed as clinical indications dictate.

Needle Examination

The chronology of electrophysiologic changes that occur with nerve injury has been discussed, and the steps in performing a proper needle examination study are well documented.[31,32] Needle EMG is probably the single most useful electrodiagnostic study in evaluating athletes with low back and neck complaints for evidence of nerve injury. Despite the fact that EMG evaluates only motor fibers, the diagnostic yield is considerably higher than with other techniques.[3,71,72] Although the needle examination is an excellent way to evaluate limb symptoms associated with neck and back pain, study findings are not always abnormal even though true nerve injury exists. Some of the reasons for this discrepancy are based on electrophysiologic factors. First, a normal finding on needle examination can result from weakness caused by neurapraxia or conduction block (e.g., the nerve is not conducting normally but no axonal injury has occurred). Second, if only a few axons degenerate, the lesion could be missed by random sampling of the muscles.[72] Third, the timing of the needle examination is important. If the examination is performed more than 4 to 6 months after symptoms have occurred, reinnervation by collateral sprouting has probably halted the occurrence of spontaneous single muscle fiber discharges (positive waves and fibrillations). If the examination is performed less than 2 to 3 weeks after onset, spontaneous single muscle fiber discharges have not yet appeared. Therefore the needle examination performed too early (i.e., in less than 2 to 3 weeks) or too late (i.e., after more than 4 to 6 months) does not reveal the abnormalities that may be prominent between these time limits.

The needle study is particularly useful in localizing a nerve injury to a specific root level. Sampling is done on various muscles in a multisegmental distribution that are innervated by different peripheral nerves. Then if the abnormalities are confined within a single myotome but fall outside the distribution of a single peripheral nerve, the evidence strongly favors a radiculopathy. However, individual variations in muscle innervation occur, sometimes making exact localization less precise.[74] Clinical experience has shown that certain muscles have higher yields for positive needle examination findings in specific nerve root injuries[42] (Table 4-1).

The needle examination can help differentiate acute from chronic denervation. In an acute radiculopathy, positive waves, fibrillation potentials, and fasciculations are usually present in the affected muscle at rest. Chronic radiculopathy without significant ongoing denervation shows large or giant motor unit potentials with polyphasia and often very small fibrillation potentials or positive waves.

Needle examination of paraspinal muscles in suspected radiculopathies or nerve injury is essential. Paraspinal fibrillation potentials indicate that the lesion is proximal to the posterior primary ramus, eliminating the concern of a possible plexopathy.[12,34,72] Chronologically, paraspinal muscles also are the first muscles to

Table 4-1. Findings in Radiculopathy

Area of Radiculopathy	Clinical Findings	Electrodiagnostic Findings (PSW)	Comments (DD)
L3	P/D in groin, medial thigh, weak hip flexion	Adductors, iliopsoas	Psoas and adductor strain
L4	P/D in hip to groin and anterior thigh to medial leg and foot; decreased knee MSR; weak knee extensors, ankle dorsiflexors	Anterior tibialis quadriceps	Saphenous nerve entrapment, anterior compartment syndrome
L5	P/D in back of thigh and anterior tibial region to first web space on dorsum of foot; weak ankle dorsiflexor, great toe extension; diminished medial hamstring MSR; SLR positive	Anterior tibialis hamstrings, hip abductors, TFL, medial gastrocnemius; peroneal F wave may be abnormal	Peroneal neuropathy at the fibular head or anterior compartment syndrome
S1	P/D from hip to posterior thigh and calf to lateral aspect of foot; weak plantar flexors and ankle eversion; diminished ankle MSR; SLR positive	Gluteus maximus, medial hamstrings, lateral gastrocnemius; ± sural SNAP	Deep posterior compartment syndrome, ACL injury with posterior tibial translation, plantar fasciitis; "chronic" hamstring strain; persistent "tennis leg"
C5	P/D over lateral deltoid, weak deltoid; ±biceps weakness; decreased biceps MSR	Rhomboids (C5 only), supraspinatus, infraspinatus biceps, deltoid	Rotator cuff abnormality, acromioclavicular joint, suprascapular nerve, axillary nerve, "stinger," brachial neuritis
C6	P/D over shoulder to lateral forearm and thumb; weak biceps, wrist extensors; decreased biceps and pronator MSR	Pronator teres, ECR, brachioradialis biceps; NL deltoids supraspinatus, infraspinatus	Carpal tunnel syndrome, "stinger," musculocutaneous nerve entrapment, brachial neuritis
Thoracic level	P/D in bandlike distribution	Local paraspinals, possibly intercostal muscles	Herpes zoster
C7	P/D in index and long fingers; decreased triceps MSR; weak elbow extension, wrist flexion	Triceps, pronator teres, FCR, EDC, ECR, ECU; median FCR H-reflex may be abnormal	Carpal tunnel syndrome, proximal median nerve entrapment
C8/	P/D radiating to ulnar aspect of arm into fourth and fifth digits; weak intrinsics of hand	EDC, first digit, APB; prolonged median and ulnar F waves	Ulnar entrapments at elbow or Guyon's canal; TOS

PSW, positive sharp waves and/or fibrillation potentials; *DD,* differential diagnosis; *P/D,* paresthesias and/or dysesthesias; *MSR,* muscle strength reflex; *SLR,* straight leg raising; *TFL,* tensor fascia lata; *SNAP,* sensory nerve action potential; *ACL,* anterior cruciate ligament; *ECR,* extensor carpi radialis; *NL,* normal; *FCR,* flexor carpi radialis; *EDC,* extensor digitorum communis; *ECU,* extensor carpi ulnaris; *APB,* abductor pollicis brevis; *TOS,* thoracic outlet syndrome.

show fibrillation after the onset of radiculopathies in patients with low back or neck pain. They are the first to stop showing fibrillations as the athlete recovers.[53,54] Of all patients with positive EMG findings 3 weeks or longer after the onset of symptoms, about 70% have abnormalities in the distribution of the posterior primary rami (paraspinal muscles) and 90% will have abnormalities in the anterior rami distribution.[42] Of all cases of lumbar radiculopathy, 10% to 30% have EMG abnormalities only in the distribution of the posterior primary rami.[34,42] Thus an evaluation of the paraspinal muscles as part of the needle examination is important.

Certain limitations apply to the needle examination of the paraspinal muscles. First, fibrillation potentials are present in the paraspinal muscles for up to 3 days after lumbar myelography.[65] Similar findings have been noted in the paraspinal muscles after lumbar epidural injections, as well as lumbar selective nerve root blocks in which abnormalities may last as long as 4 weeks.[53,54] Second, inasmuch as paraspinals are the first muscles to reinnervate, needle EMG findings may not be noted because reinnervation has already occurred. Furthermore, incomplete root involvement that does not affect the posterior ramus may exist.[72] Like other aspects of electrodiagnostically confirmed abnormalities, positive sharp waves and fibrillation potentials in paraspinal muscles only indicate very proximal nerve or muscle abnormalities and are not diagnostic for radiculopathy. Although not common in the athletic population, other causes for these changes include metastatic disease that affects the proximal nerve roots, anterior horn cell disease, inflammatory myopathies (e.g., polymyositis), and particularly diabetes mellitus, which can cause widespread fibrillation potentials throughout the paraspinal muscles.[71] Because of overlapping innervation, questions have been raised about the localizing value of paraspinal EMG findings. The specificity of this information is probably enhanced if care is taken to examine the main muscles of the deeper group of intrinsic back muscles, the multifidi.[15] Anatomic data indicate relatively localized innervation by dorsal rami in these muscles.[36] It is prudent to try to correlate findings in peripheral muscles with paraspinal muscle findings for precise localization of nerve root injuries. Because it can be difficult to achieve complete relaxation of the athlete's paraspinal muscles, reaction of distant motor units can be misinterpreted as positive waves. Also, nonreproducible trains or bursts of positive waves in the paraspinal muscles are usually normal and are generated by the needle passing through an end-plate zone.[58,66,67]

Positive sharp waves and fibrillations in the paraspinal muscles of athletes who have undergone lumbar surgery or other invasive procedures, such as recent injections or even recent electrodiagnostic studies, should not be used also to diagnose radiculopathies.[12,31-34,57] These findings should be correlated with the clinical history, physical findings, and anatomic studies.

Although the presence of positive waves and fibrillation potentials confined to a single myotome is the most reliable EMG evidence of acute radiculopathy, analysis of motor unit potentials and their recruitment patterns plays a role in evaluating patients with subacute, chronic, and old resolved radicular syndromes. Abnormal motor unit recruitment occurs almost immediately after the onset of any nerve injury in which interrupted conduction of nerve impulses takes place.[11,31,32,38] The use of abnormal recruitment intervals or frequencies to evaluate radiculopathy has been described, and it is believed to possibly be of particular benefit early in the course of the nerve injury before positive sharp waves and fibrillation potentials occur.[11] Johnson[32,35] suggested that in early and mild L5 radiculopathy a recruitment interval of 70 to 90 msec in the extensor digitorum longus as compared with the normal interval of 100 to 120 msec was significant. Motor unit recruitment abnormalities are unlikely to be recognized, however, unless muscle weakness is easily detectable clinically. Mild weakness is accompanied by only minimal alterations in recruitment intervals, which can be difficult to detect, even for the experienced electromyographer. Although the recruit-

ment pattern at maximal contraction is believed to indicate the number of active motor unit potentials, Johnson[30,32] showed this parameter to be less sensitive in patients with radiculopathy than are positive sharp waves and fibrillations.

Changes in motor unit size and configuration are seen in patients after the acute phase of radiculopathy. They are due to reinnervation of denervated muscle fibers and include polyphasic potentials, often of long duration and sometimes of large amplitude, but such changes by themselves cannot be considered evidence of ongoing, active nerve degeneration. In radiculopathy, reinnervation occurs by intramuscular collateral sprouting from the distal portions of the remaining viable nerves. Many viable nerves supply any given muscle in monoradiculopathy because muscles are innervated by more than one nerve root. As viable nerves sprout, they begin to reinnervate the denervated muscle fibers. Then, when the nerve discharges, it activates both its own muscle fibers and some of those belonging to an adjacent denervated nerve fiber. The recorded motor unit potential under such conditions is larger and wider than normal and may be polyphasic. Polyphasicity has long been recognized as an electrophysiologic abnormality found in radiculopathy.[27,39,53,54,71]

When a muscle fiber is reinnervated, it stops fibrillating. Therefore persistent fibrillations indicate ongoing nerve degeneration, reflecting chronic radiculopathy. Although it is not uncommon for pain to persist chronically after acute radiculopathy, it is relatively uncommon to find evidence of progressive nerve degeneration. Such findings are more often seen in the chronic, progressive narrow spinal canal syndromes.[42]

In conclusion, the needle examination appears to be the most reliable aspect of the electrodiagnostic examination in athletes with neck and low back complaints and reveals the highest yield of abnormalities in radiculopathy.[3,50,67] Nerve conduction studies and late responses also reveal useful information, which, when taken within the entire context of the athlete's complaints, physical findings, and anatomic studies, aid in diagnosing nerve injuries in the back and upper and lower extremities.

Single-Fiber Electromyography

Single-fiber electromyography (SFEMG) is not used in routine electrodiagnostic studies of patients being evaluated for low back or neck pain because many electromyographers lack the expertise to perform these studies, these tests are lengthy, and the value of additional information gained can be questioned. SFEMG can be helpful in evaluating athletes with low back complaints, particularly when it is used to evaluate recurrent radiculopathy and to assess the onset and process of reinnervation. The electrophysiologic changes that occur and how the parameter of blocking and jitter are affected are well described elsewhere.[67] Useful information is obtainable only if serial studies are performed and compared or the study is completed very soon after a new nerve injury occurs. Depending on the timing of the examination and the availability of comparative SFEMG studies, these types of examinations may allow differentiation of an acute injury from a chronic one; however, they are rarely used in clinical practice.

ACCURACY OF ELECTRODIAGNOSTIC STUDIES

For decades, clinical investigators have compared EMG results, which reveal the electrophysiologic properties of nerve and muscle, with imaging studies, which delineate anatomic configuration of the tissues.[37,40,73] Comparisons between surgically "proven" nerve root compromise and EMG findings have also been made.[15,41,75] The misconception that the two can be compared with accuracy comes from the observed high coincidence of nerve root abnormality at the site of, and often caused by, disc protrusion and other anatomic distortions. Although distorted spinal architecture can damage a nerve root, a nerve root problem can be demonstrated in the absence of macroanatomic abnormality.[43,54] Furthermore, disc protrusion can be seen at postmortem examination in the spine of almost all patients older than 40 years of age, most of whom were asymptomatic for radiculopathy.[46]

The EMG supplies the following information. First, it reveals the presence and to some degree the extent of motor nerve degeneration. This information is provided neither by imaging studies nor by direct observation of the tissues during surgery. In radiculopathy, during the acute or subacute phase of muscle fiber denervation, the observation of fibrillation (i.e., the sensitivity of the test) approaches 100% accuracy: there either has been nerve degeneration (fibrillation is present) or there has not. By the time muscle fibers have been reinnervated, EMG must rely on findings that are sometimes less obvious than fibrillation potentials, but the presence of such findings indicates that nerve degeneration has led to reinnervation of muscle fibers. The specificity for radiculopathy, based on the findings of positive waves and fibrillation potentials, is not known; however, it greatly increases when the distribution of the abnormalities is clearly segmental. Second, the EMG also allows recognition of the segmental level involved as long as the abnormality is distributed to at least three or four muscles within a single myotome.[14] Detection of anatomic abnormality at another level does not alter the location of nerve root damage.

Some studies have attempted to compare findings on physical examination with those on EMG.[24,40] This is also improper. The EMG is an extension of the physical examination; one does not supplant the other. The presence or absence of EMG abnormalities always adds information. At times the EMG reveals abnormality when no neurologic deficits can be found on physical examination. This is particularly true in chronic radiculopathy such as with spinal stenosis.[24,29,58]

CLINICAL AND ELECTROPHYSIOLOGIC PRESENTATIONS OF RADICULOPATHIES

The most common referral to an electrophysiology laboratory for arm pain, leg pain, or back pain is to obtain an evaluation for potential radiculopathy. Athletes often manifest symptoms of numbness, tingling, dysesthesias, or weakness in various distributions. Although radiculopathy is most commonly due to a herniated disc or degenerative foraminal stenosis, electrophysiologic studies reveal only the presence of nerve root irritation, not the cause of the radiculopathy. Table 4-1 shows some common signs, symptoms, and electrophysiologic findings in common cervical, thoracic, and lumbar radiculopathies, as well as clinical points to consider when the clinician evaluates patients for potential radiculopathy. Included in this table are common entrapment neuropathies and other common clinical conditions that mimic spinal problems in athletes.

Details of all the potential peripheral nerve entrapments that can mimic radiculopathy are beyond the scope of this text, but the confusion is well documented.* Some peripheral nerve entrapments may present with symptoms similar to those of radiculopathy (see Table 4-1). All athletes who report numbness, tingling, or pain in an extremity must not be assumed to have only radiculopathy. Although the condition is not common, concomitant cervical radiculopathy and rotator cuff tear, or plantar fasciitis and an S1 radiculopathy are seen in clinical practice. Furthermore, the "double crush" syndrome is well documented, wherein a nerve can be injured in more than one place, possibly as a result of the first injury making the nerve more susceptible to injury in a second location.[61] An example is carpal tunnel syndrome with a C6 radiculopathy. Understanding the anatomy of peripheral nerves and their dermatomal distributions can lead to more effective electrophysiologic evaluation of athletes with suspected spinal problems.

STINGERS

Electrophysiologic studies may have a place in evaluating athletes with a "stinger," or "burner," described as a nerve injury to many different components of the proximal nerve root/brachial plexus complex.† Bergfeld, Hershman, and Wilbourn[7] have stated that electrophysiologic studies may be quite limited in evaluating athletes with stingers, noting that 80% of follow-up study results on patients with stingers were abnormal 3 years later. However, the most abnormalities they describe are those

---

* References 25, 26, 34, 38, 48, 60.
† References 4, 7, 9, 10, 25, 44, 49, 64, 68, 69.

of MUAP changes, which may be abnormal indefinitely after any type of nerve injury. Of greater significance would be the presence or absence of active nerve irritation (e.g., positive waves and fibrillation potentials). Electrophysiologic studies, especially EMG, in an athlete with persistent motor weakness, may pinpoint where the injury occurred, as well as the presence of acute denervation. It may also help to distinguish stingers from acute radiculopathy.

INDICATIONS FOR ELECTROPHYSIOLOGIC TESTING

The utility of electrodiagnostic testing in a given athlete may be evaluated after a thorough history and physical examination, a review of supplemental information (i.e., imaging studies), and an appreciation of the chronology of electrophysiologic changes that occur following nerve injury. Some helpful generalizations as to the indications and limitations of electrodiagnostic studies are worthy of review:

1. *To establish and/or confirm a clinical diagnosis.* Pain in the upper or lower extremities and back is often referred from pain-sensitive structures other than nerve tissue. This pain may even appear to follow a dermatomal pattern. If there is no electrophysiologic abnormality, the studies give the physician confidence that this is the case, which may help in patient management and reassurance. With nerve injury, however, a properly timed EMG can show evidence of the nature, location, and severity of the injury. A thorough electrophysiologic examination may alert the examiner to the possibility of an unsuspected pathologic condition (e.g., concomitant peripheral neuropathy with radiculopathy, an active common peroneal nerve entrapment superimposed on a chronic L5 radiculopathy, or carpal tunnel syndrome concomitant with a C6 radiculopathy). In a small percentage of patients the diagnosis of radiculopathy is established by EMG when the diagnosis on clinical grounds seems unlikely.[42]

2. *To localize nerve lesions.* Signs or symptoms of nerve injuries in the extremities can result from a number of causes, including root lesions (radiculopathy), brachial or lumbosacral plexus or root lesions (e.g., stingers, metastasis, retroperitoneal hematoma), or peripheral nerve injuries (e.g., carpal tunnel syndrome, ulnar lesions at the elbow, meralgia paraesthetica, saphenous nerve entrapment, tarsal tunnel syndrome). Various conduction studies and EMG can specifically localize the lesion and provide an evaluation of many of these nerve segments. Occasionally what may appear clinically as a single-level radiculopathy may in fact be multilevel or, in the case of spinal stenosis, bilateral. Frequently, clinical assessment predicts only a uniradicular lesion, but EMG may reveal involvement of two roots. This has importance in planning an operative approach.[73]

3. *To determine the extent of nerve injury.* A properly timed EMG can differentiate neurapraxic injury (conduction block) from active axonal degeneration. It can also semiquantitatively assess the degree of reversible motor axon damage and the severity of the neuronal deficit. This information may have a significant impact on the aggressiveness of treatment for a lumbar radiculopathy. The acuteness or chronicity of the lesion may also be obtained.

4. *To correlate findings on anatomic studies.* The existence of nerve root dysfunction cannot be determined or even assumed from diagnostic procedures that determine structural abnormalities.[23] EMG can show if physiologic nerve injury has occurred or is ongoing and if these findings correlate with the symptoms and results of radiologic studies. This information may have significant importance as to what type of treatment is instituted (surgical versus nonsurgical). Furthermore, to plan the most appropriate approach and level in presurgical candidates, it is useful to know which nerve root levels are most involved. Selective nerve blocks can complement EMG studies in localization of abnormalities.

5. *To assist in prognosis.* With proper timing of the examination, the paucity of positive sharp waves and fibrillation potentials in acute radiculopathy portends an excellent prognosis for return of muscle strength. A comparison of the compound muscle action potential of a very weak muscle with that of the same muscle on the asymptomatic side provides an idea of the extent of neurapraxia and of potential recovery. A side-to-side amplitude difference of greater than 50% is probably significant. Recovery is prolonged and less complete when more than one root is involved, which may be determined at times only by EMG.[6,73]

LIMITATIONS OF ELECTROPHYSIOLOGIC TESTS

The EMG is not a perfect test and should not be used for every athlete referred for evaluation of spinal problems. The following limitations of electrophysiologic testing provide a guide and present situations in which EMG may not be necessary:

1. *In the first 2 to 4 weeks after onset of symptoms.* In most cases if the clinical situation and examination strongly suggest radiculopathy, treatment can be instituted without EMG. Many findings may not be seen if the examination is performed too early. If the patient has progressive neurologic deficits, the results of EMG will not be important inasmuch as the patient will require emergent care. If a patient is not improving to the extent that is anticipated for

that level of care, then EMG may be useful, but not in the very acute situation.

2. *In unequivocal radiculopathy.* When the clinical history and the motor, sensory, and reflex changes are consistent, EMG adds little information and generally is not necessary. It may still be required, however, if the patient is not improving with treatment.

3. *When the history and examination are highly inconsistent with acute radiculopathy.* If the clinical situation is not clear, some important points need to be considered. When a patient with back or neck pain is being evaluated, acute radiculopathy is unlikely if the pain is confined to the axial skeleton, if it involves both upper or lower limbs, or if it occurs intermittently. If, in addition, there is no detectable neurologic deficit on physical examination, acute radiculopathy is highly improbable and electrodiagnostic studies may not be needed.

4. *When no change has occurred in a previously studied patient's clinical situation.* Many patients have had multiple EMG studies in an attempt to determine a causative factor for nonsegmental, nondermatomal complaints. When multiple studies of high quality have been completed, with no change in the clinical signs or symptoms, very little information will be gained with further studies.

5. *If the results will not change medical or surgical management.* For whatever reasons (e.g., extreme illness, patient refusing surgery), if the results of the studies will in no way change the treatment plan, EMG should probably be avoided.

6. *If barriers to acquiring sufficient information are present.* If a patient cannot be moved from a prone to a supine position (or vice versa), or if dressings, casts, or stabilizing devices cannot be repositioned or temporarily removed, the information from performing the electrodiagnostic studies may be limited.

ELECTROPHYSIOLOGIC REPORT

The electrophysiologic report should include a variety of important data for the referring physician. First, the electrophysiologic findings should be correlated with any physical findings noted or discrepancies identified. Inconsistencies may have as much importance in the clinical management of the patient as consistent results, if not more. Second, the degree of certainty or "hardness" of the finding needs to be conveyed to the referring physician. A diagnosis of an S1 radiculopathy by H-reflex changes will carry different weight only if compared with abundant spontaneous discharges in an S1 myotomal distribution. Third, the diagnoses that have been excluded can be as important as those confirmed. Fourth, information should be noted about potential diagnoses that are suggested by the clinical examination but not

supported by results of the electrophysiologic study. Fifth, a significant concomitant pathologic condition (e.g., carpal tunnel syndrome superimposed on a cervical radiculopathy) should be mentioned. Sixth, any change from previous studies may be useful information. Seventh, the degree of acuteness or chronicity of the lesions identified needs to be stated. Finally, prognosis, when possible, is critical information for managing patients. This is particularly important when the EMG shows only neurapraxic changes in contrast to significant axonal degeneration.

REFERENCES

1. Aiello I, et al: The diagnostic value of H-index in S1 root compression, *J Neurol Neurosurg Psychiatry* 44:171, 1981.
2. American Association of Electrodiagnostic Medicine: Guidelines in electrodiagnostic medicine, *Muscle Nerve* 15:229, 1992.
3. Aminoff MJ, et al: Electrophysiologic evaluation of lumbosacral radiculopathies: electromyography, late responses, and somatosensory evoked potentials, *Neurology* 35:1514, 1985.
4. Archambault JL: Brachial plexus stretch injury, *J Am Coll Health* 31:256, 1983.
5. Baylan SP, Yu J, Grant AE: H-reflex latency in relation to ankle jerk, electromyographic, myelographic, and surgical findings in back pain patients, *Electromyogr Clin Neurophysiol* 21:201, 1981.
6. Benecke R, Conrad B: The distal sensory nerve action potential as a diagnostic tool for the differentiation of lesions in dorsal roots and peripheral nerves, *J Neurol* 223:231, 1989.
7. Bergfeld JA, Hershman EB, Wilbourn AJ: Brachial plexus injury in sports: a five year follow up, *Orthop Trans* 12:743, 1988.
8. Braddom RL, Johnson EW: Standardization of H-reflex and diagnostic use in S1 radiculopathy, *Arch Phys Med Rehabil* 55:161, 1974.
9. Chrisman OD, et al: Lateral flexion neck injuries in athletic competition, *JAMA* 192:613, 1965.
10. Clancy WG: Brachial plexus and upper extremity peripheral nerve injuries. In Torg JS, editor: *Athletic injuries to head, neck and face,* Philadelphia, 1982, Lea & Febiger.
11. Eisen A: Electrodiagnosis of radiculopathy. In Aminott MJ, editor: Symposium on electrodiagnosis, *Neurol Clin* 3:495, 1985.
12. Eisen A, Schamer D, Melmed C: An electrophysiological method for examining lumbosacral root compression, *Can J Neurol Sci* 2:117, 1977.
13. Fisher MA: AAEM minimonograph No 13: H reflexes and F waves physiology and clinical indications, *Muscle Nerve* 15:1223, 1992.
14. Fisher MA, Kaur D, Houchins J: Electrodiagnostic examination, back pain and entrapment of posterior rami, *Electromyogr Clin Neurophysiol* 25:183, 1985.
15. Fisher MA, et al: Clinical and electrophysiological appraisal of the significance of radicular injury in back pain, *J Neurol Neurosurg Psychiatry* 41:303, 1978.
16. Fisher MA, et al: The F-response: a clinically useful physiological parameter for the evaluation of radicular injury, *Electromyogr Clin Neurophysiol* 19:65, 1979.
17. Fowler T, Danta G, Gilliatt R: Recovery of nerve conduction after a pneumatic tourniquet: observations on the hind limb of the baboon, *J Neurol Neurosurg Psychiatry* 35:638, 1972.
18. Gilliatt RW: Acute compression block. In Sumner AJ, editor: *The pathophysiology of peripheral nerve disease,* Philadelphia, 1980, WB Saunders.
19. Gilliatt RW: Chronic nerve compression and entrapment. In Sumner AJ, editor: *The physiology of peripheral nerve disease,* Philadelphia, 1980, WB Saunders.
20. Gilliatt RW: Recent advances in the pathophysiology of nerve

conduction. In Desmedt J, editor: *Developments in electromyography and clinical neurophysiology,* vol 2, Basel, 1983, Kargar.

21. Glantz RH, Haldeman S: Other diagnostic studies: electrodiagnosis. In Frymoyer JW, editor: *The adult spine: principles and practice,* New York, 1991, Raven Press.
22. Goss CM, editor: *Gray's anatomy of the human body,* ed 29, Philadelphia, 1973, Lea & Febiger.
23. Haldeman S: The electrodiagnostic evaluation at nerve root function, *Spine* 9:41, 1984.
24. Hall S et al: Clinical features, diagnostic procedures and results of surgical treatment in 68 patients, *Ann Intern Med* 103:271, 1985.
25. Herring SA, Weinstein SM: Electrodiagnosis in sports medicine, *Phys Med Rehabil State Art Rev* 3:809, 1989.
26. Hirasawa Y, Sakakida K: Sports and peripheral nerve injury, *Am J Sports Med* 11:420, 1983.
27. Hoover BB, et al: Value of polyphasic potentials in diagnosis of lumbar root lesions, *Arch Phys Med Rehabil* 51:546, 1970.
28. Jabre JF: Surface recording of the H-reflex of the flexor carpi radialis, *Muscle Nerve* 4:435, 1981.
29. Jacobson RE: Lumbar stenosis: an electromyographic evaluation, *Clin Orthop* 115:68, 1976.
30. Johnson EW: Electrodiagnosis of radiculopathy: advanced concepts in evaluation of focal neuropathy. Text of training workshop, American Association of Electromyography and Electrodiagnosis, Las Vegas, 1985.
31. Johnson EW: Electrodiagnosis of radiculopathy. In Johnson EW, editor: *Practical electromyography,* Baltimore, 1988, Williams & Wilkins.
32. Johnson EW: The EMG examination. In Johnson EW, editor: *Practical electromyography,* Baltimore, 1988, Williams & Wilkins.
33. Johnson EW, Burkhart JA, Earl WC: Electromyography in postlaminectomy patients, *Arch Phys Med Rehabil* 53:407, 1972.
34. Johnson EW, Melvin JL: Value of electromyography in lumbar radiculopathy, *Arch Phys Med Rehabil* 52:239, 1971.
35. Johnson EW, Stocklin R, LaBan MM: Use of electrodiagnostic examination in a university hospital, *Arch Phys Med Rehabil* 46:573, 1965.
36. Jonsson B: Morphology, innervation, and electromyographic study of the erector spinae, *Arch Phys Med Rehabil* 50:638, 1969.
37. Khatri BO, Barvah J, McQuillen MP: Correlation of electromyography with computed tomography in evaluation of lower back pain, *Arch Neurol* 41:594, 1984.
38. Kimura J: *Electrodiagnosis in diseases of muscle and nerve,* Philadelphia, 1985, FA Davis.
39. Lajoie WJ: Nerve root compression: correlation of electromyographic, myelographic and surgical findings, *Arch Phys Med Rehabil* 53:390, 1972.
40. Lane ME, Tamhankar MN, Demopoulos JJ: Discogenic radiculopathy: use of electromyography in multidisciplinary management, *NY State J Med* 32:432, 1978.
41. Leyshon A, Kirwan EOG, Wynn PCG: Electrical studies in the diagnosis of compression at the lumbar root, *J Bone Joint Surg* 63B:71, 1981.
42. MacLean IC: Acute radiculopathy. Paper presented at the meeting of the American Association of Electromyography and Neurophysiology: *a high-intensity review,* Chicago, April 6, 1989.
43. Marshall LL, Trethewie ER, Curtain CC: Chemical radiculitis: a clinical, physiological and immunological study, *Clin Orthop* 129:61, 1987.
44. Marshall TM: Nerve pinch injuries in football, *J Med Assoc* 14:648, 1970.
45. Mayladeny JW, McDougall DB: Electrophysiological studies of nerve and reflex activity in normal man: identification of certain reflexes in EMG and conduction velocity of peripheral nerve function, *Bull Johns Hopkins Hosp* 86:265, 1950.
46. McCrae DL: Asymptomatic intervertebral disc protrusions, *Acta Radiol* 46:9, 1956.
47. Ongerboer de Visser BW, Schimsheimer RJ, Hart AAM: The

H-reflex of the flexor carpi radialis muscle: a study in controls and radiation-induced brachial plexus lesions, *J Neurol Neurosurg Psychiatry* 47:1098, 1984.
48. Pease WS: Entrapment neuropathies, *Phys Med Rehabil State Art Rev* 3:741, 1989.
49. Robertson WC, Eichman PL, Clancy WG: Upper trunk brachial plexopathy in football players, *JAMA* 241:1480, 1979.
50. Rodriguez AA, et al: Somatosensory evoked potentials from dermatomal stimulation as an indicator of L5 and S1 radiculopathy, *Arch Phys Med Rehabil* 68:366, 1987.
51. Rudge P, Ochoa J, Gilliatt R: Acute peripheral nerve compression in the baboon, *J Neurol Sci* 23:403, 1974.
52. Rydevik B, Braun MD, Lundborg G: Pathoanatomy and pathophysiology of nerve root compression, *Spine* 9:7, 1984.
53. Saal JA: Electrophysiologic evaluation of lumbar pain: establishing the rationale for therapeutic management, *Spine* 1:21, 1986.
54. Saal JS: The role of inflammation in lumbar pain, *Phys Med Rehabil State Art Rev* 4:191, 1990.
55. Schimsheimer RJ, et al: The flexor carpi radialis H-reflex in lesions of the sixth and seventh cervical nerve roots, *J Neurol Neurosurg Psychiatry* 48:445, 1985.
56. Schuchmann JA: H-reflex latency in radiculopathy, *Arch Phys Med Rehabil* 59:185, 1978.
57. See DH, Kraft GH: Electromyography in paraspinal muscles following surgery for root compression, *Arch Phys Med Rehabil* 56:80, 1975.
58. Seppalainen AM, Alaranta H, Solni J: Electromyography in the diagnosis of lumbar spinal stenosis, *Electromyogr Clin Neurophysiol* 21:55, 1981.
59. Spindler HA, Felsenthal G: Electrodiagnostic evaluation of acute and chronic radiculopathy, *Phys Med Rehabil Clin North Am* 1:53, 1990.
60. Takazawa H, et al: Statistical observation of nerve injuries in athletes, *Brain Nerve Injuries* 3:11, 1971.
61. Thomas JE, Lambert EH, Czevz KA: Electrodiagnostic aspects of the carpal tunnel syndrome, *Arch Neurol* 16:635, 1967.
62. Tonzola RF et al: Usefulness of electrophysiological studies in the diagnosis of lumbosacral root disease, *Ann Neurol* 9:305, 1981.
63. Travell JG, Simons DG: *Myofascial pain and dysfunction: the trigger point manual,* Baltimore, 1983, Williams & Wilkins.
64. Watkins RG: Nerve injuries in football players, *Clin Sports Med* 5:215, 1986.
65. Weber RJ, Weingarden SI: EMG abnormalities following myelography, *Arch Neurol* 36:588, 1979.
66. Weichers DO: Electromyographic insertional activity in normal limb muscles, *Arch Phys Med Rehabil* 60:359, 1979.
67. Weichers DO: Radiculopathies, *Phys Med Rehabil State Art Rev* 3:713, 1989.
68. Wiens JJ, Saal JA: Rehabilitation of cervical spine and brachial plexus injuries, *Phys Med Rehabil State Art Rev* 1:583, 1987.
69. Weinstein SM, Herring SA: Nerve problems and compartment syndrome in the hand, wrist and forearm, *Clin Sports Med* 11:161, 1992.
70. Weintraub JR et al: Achilles tendon reflex and the H response, *Muscle Nerve* 11:972, 1988.
71. Wilbourne AT: The value and limitations of electromyographic examination in the diagnosis of lumbosacral radiculopathy. In Hary RW, editor: *Lumbar disc disease,* New York, 1982, Raven Press.
72. Wilbourne AJ, Aminoff MJ: The electrophysiologic examination in patients with radiculopathies and nerve, *Muscle Nerve* 11:1099, 1988.
73. Young A, Wynn PCB: The assessment and management of the failed back, part I, *Int Disabil Stud* 9:21, 1987.
74. Young A et al: Variations in the pattern of muscle innervation by the L5 and S1 nerve roots, *Spine* 8:616, 1983.
75. Young RR, Shahani BJ: Clinical value and limitation of F-nerve determination, *Muscle Nerve* 13:248, 1978.

Chapter Five

◆

History, Physical Examination, and Diagnostic Tests for Neck and Upper Extremity Problems

James P. Bradley
James E. Tibone
Robert G. Watkins

HISTORY

The history is critical in determining the diagnostic plan (see Appendix). The history and physical examination proceed as follows:

1. Quantitate the morbidity.
2. Delineate the psychosocial factors.
3. Eliminate tumors and infections.
4. Identify the clinical syndrome.

The standardized history form is used to obtain the necessary information, starting with:

1. What is the problem?
2. What caused the problem?
3. When did the problem begin, and how long have you had it?
4. What makes the problem better or worse?

The location of the pain, weakness, or numbness; the exact mechanical maneuvers that reproduce the pain; the time of day the pain is worse; and the activities of daily living or occupation that are restricted by the pain are important parts of the history. At the Kerlan-Jobe Orthopaedic Clinic the history is checked by the nurse, the fellow, and the physician. Certainly, the physician must identify the difference between a spinal tumor, cervical radiculopathy, cervical myelopathy, postural cervical strain, and psychosomatic reaction.

The physician should review the history before seeing the patient and then listen to the patient's description of the symptoms and how they affect the patient. This is critical for establishing the physician-patient relationship; no form can take the place of hearing patients' own words as they describe their symptoms. Patients must feel that all of their symptoms and concerns have been fully expressed and their questions answered by the end of the interview.

PHYSICAL EXAMINATION

The examination for neck and arm pain is initiated with the patient seated on the end of the table and the physician on a movable stool with rollers, seated lower than the patient. First, reflexes—patellar, Achilles tendon, crossed adductor and posterior tibial, Chaddock's, Oppenheim's, and Babinski's—are evaluated. Sensation—pinprick, light touch, and vibratory sense—

and motor function—foot dorsiflexion, plantar flexion, inversion, eversion, toe dorsiflexion, plantar flexion, and knee flexion and extension—are noted.

Neck Pain

The examination of the patient with neck pain begins at the feet to diagnose any lower extremity spasticity present and then proceeds to the upper extremities with the patient seated. The physician checks the biceps, triceps, brachial radialis, Hoffmann's sign, bilateral upper extremity pulses, and motor and sensory function, and then checks Tinel's sign at the wrist and elbows, performs Phalen's maneuver, and notes any signs or symptoms of peripheral entrapment syndrome. The physician also reviews the cranial nerve examination; checks for extraocular muscular function and the presence of nystagmus; checks the pupillary reflex, corneal reflex, gag reflex, and shoulder shrug; and asks questions concerning numbness in the face or head and concerning hearing or vision changes.

The upper extremity examination starts with the shoulder abduction test. The examiner places a hand on the head and asks the patient if that relieves the symptoms of radiating arm pain. A rotator cuff test and Adson's maneuver are performed, and then cervical range-of-motion testing is begun by telling the patient to touch the chin to the chest, extend the head back and rotate left and right, and then do a lateral tilt right and left. The range of motion (ROM) and any pain are recorded. Spurling's maneuver (Fig. 5-1) is then done, first with head compression in the neutral position. (If that reproduces radicular symptoms, one does not need to check the full maneuver.) Next, the head is extended. (If that reproduces the symptoms, one may stop there.) Then the patient is told to extend the head and look toward the painful arm. Finally, the patient extends the head and looks toward the painful arm while head compression is applied.

At the Kerlan-Jobe Orthopaedic Clinic the patient generally stands and is examined from behind for shoulder heights, pelvic height, and scoliosis. The history and physical examination combined allow identification of the clinical syndrome.

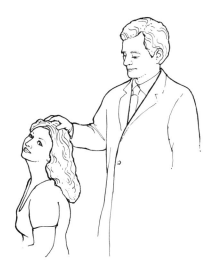

Fig. 5-1. Spurling's maneuver.

The clinical syndromes to be identified are nonmechanical neck pain and mechanical neck and/or arm pain. Nonmechanical neck pain is pain that is not particularly affected by mechanical activity in the neck. More unrelenting, severe pain is possibly worse at night. The pain can be worse with certain positions but generally is unaffected by position.

As with lumbar disease, an important distinction to be made under the category of mechanical neck and/or arm pain is whether the pain is true radiculopathy or referred cervical pain. Cervical intervertebral discs and neuro-motion segments do produce referred pain. A more typical pattern is into the cephalad medial tip of the scapula, across the brim of the scapula, or down the medial border of the scapula to the tip of the scapula. Referred shoulder pain or cervical radiculopathy may produce shoulder joint dysfunction as a result of compensating for the referred pain. Trigger points may exist that are very tender, especially in the trapezius area. Deep palpation of these very tender trigger points can reproduce radiating arm and/or neck pain. The distinction should be made in terms of the intensity or percentage of pain in the neck versus that in the arm. The arm in this instance starts at the acromioclavicular joint and lateral shoulder tip. We do not consider scapular pain arm pain. These areas are so commonly part of a referred pain pattern that to attribute this pain solely to radicular pain might lead to a wrong recommendation. Scapular pain may certainly be accompanied by radicular pain, but the distinction should be made in terms of the intensity of the pain. Paresthesias, muscle dysfunction, and sensory changes are all very important, but so is the percentage or intensity of the pain in the neck and scapula versus that in the arm. The head compression test, Spurling's maneuver, and other techniques can produce neck and referred scapular pain.

Cervical rotation may produce a significant amount of neck pain.

Shoulder Pain

Ideally the examination of an athlete with shoulder pain begins with the inspection of both shoulders, using the uninjured shoulder as a basis for comparison. Watching the patient remove clothing can frequently reveal more information about shoulder function than a detailed examination;[18] attitude, muscle features (atrophy), deformities, asymmetry (swelling), and skin manifestations are noted. The presence of a short neck, low hairline, and neck webbing are all associated with Klippel-Feil syndrome. A high-riding scapula should alert the examiner to the possibility of Sprengel's deformity. The abnormal posture of the entire upper extremity in Klumpke's or Erb's palsy is obvious. More subtle conditions such as a posterior dislocation, sternoclavicular joint pathology, or early atrophy of the supraspinatus muscle may be much more challenging. Prominence of the scapular spine is indicative of supraspinatus and/or infraspinatus atrophy, which is a classic sign of a rotator cuff tear or, more rarely, of a suprascapular nerve lesion.[4,19] Throwers, particularly volleyball players, classically induce traction injuries of the suprascapular nerve at the scapular spine, causing only atrophy of the infraspinatus. Deltoid atrophy, indicated by prominence of the acromion and squaring off of the injured shoulder, is often noted in axillary nerve lesions from fractures, dislocations, or a direct blow; it is also seen in the rare quadrilateral space syndrome. Fullness of the trapezius and paracervical muscles, indicating spasm, may be seen with cervical spine anomalies. It should be remembered that relative hypertrophy of the dominant extremity in throwers is normal.

Palpation identifies tenderness, crepitation, deformity, and temperature. All four joints of the shoulder complex (glenohumeral, acromioclavicular, sternoclavicular, and scapulothoracic), should be addressed. Tenderness at the coracoid is of little value in diagnosis because it is common in normal shoulders.[2] Although palpation of the biceps tendon is rarely possible, localized tenderness about the intertubercular groove may indicate biceps tendinitis.

Tenderness of the acromioclavicular joint is significant and usually represents degeneration of the joint with or without associated impingement. Anterior acromial tenderness associated with crepitation about the acromion suggests impingement. Specific palpation for trigger points of pain around the scapula (rhomboids, levator scapulae insertions) may indicate muscle spasm from cervical spine (C5-6) origins. Temperature differences, especially coolness, may be the first finding of thoracic outlet syndrome.

ROM, including total range (active, passive), rhythm,

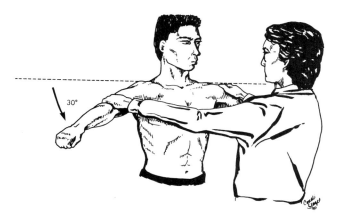

Fig. 5-2. Supraspinatus testing.

Table 5-1. Shoulder Innvervation

Muscle	Nerve	Root Level
Deltoid	Axillary	Posterior cord C5-6
Teres minor	Axillary	Posterior cord C5-6
Supraspinatus	Suprascapular	C5-6
Infraspinatus	Suprascapular	C5-6
Subscapularis	Subscapular	Posterior cord C5-6
Teres major (C6)	Subscapular (lower)	Posterior cord C5-6
Biceps (C7)	Musculocutaneous	Lateral cord C5-6
Coracobrachialis	Musculocutaneous	C5 to C7
Rhomboid major	Dorsal scapular	C5
Rhomboid minor	Dorsal scapular	C5
Trapezius	Spinal accessory XI	C3-4
Pectoralis major	Lateral pectoral	C5-6
Levator scapula	Scapular	C3-4
Serratus anterior	Long thoracic	C5-6 (C7)
Latissimus dorsi	Thoracodorsal	C6-7 (C8)

Table 5-2. Sensory and Reflex Levels in the Upper Extremity

Level	Sensory	Reflex
C5	Lateral deltoid	Biceps
C6	Thumb	Bracioradialis
C7	Middle finger	Triceps
C8	Ulnar border of little finger	—
T1	Medial side of proximal arm	—

scapulohumeral synchrony, and pain hindering or at the limits of motion should be evaluated. The normal glenohumeral/scapulothoracic motion ratio during the first 30 degrees is 4.3:1. From 30 degrees to maximum abduction, it decreases to 1.25:1.[15] Controversy exists over this point: various reports state that the ratio between glenohumeral and scapulothoracic motion varies from 2:1 to 5:4, with the scapulothoracic motion decreasing with elevation.[5,15] Adhesive capsulitis and osteoarthritis restrict glenohumeral motion, producing a relative increase in the scapulothoracic segment.[2] Conversely, rotator cuff tears or labral problems produce a catching pain with a resultant jerky, hesitant glenohumeral rhythm.[2] Active and passive ROM for maximum total elevation, internal rotation, external rotation, and extension should be done. Maximum elevation occurs in a plane between the coronal and sagittal planes. ("Scaption" is the term coined to describe this motion.[14]) Discrepancies between passive and active ROM are usually noted with rotator cuff tears, with passive ROM showing greater values. In delineating rotation it should be remembered that skilled overhand throwers may have an excess of external rotation, often 15 to 20 degrees greater than in the nondominant side.[18] Commonly this increase in external rotation is at the expense of internal rotation.

Muscle strength testing of the shoulder allows the orthopaedist to appraise the competency of the musculotendinous units, as well as the neurologic elements. Special attention is given to discriminating between peripheral innervation and root innervation of the muscle groups as they relate to the aches of shoulder motion. Strength testing should include forward flexion, abduction, and external and internal rotation. The anterior portion of the deltoid muscle (C5-6, axillary nerve) is the chief flexor of the shoulder. Assistance is provided by the pectoralis major muscle (C5-6, lateral pectoral nerve), biceps, and coracobrachialis muscle (C5 to C7, musculocutaneous nerve). Abduction is achieved mainly by the middle deltoid muscle (C5-6, axillary nerve) and supraspinatus muscle (C5, suprascapular nerve). Enhanced testing of the supraspinatus is accomplished by abducting the arm to 90 degrees, placing the arm 30 degrees forward in the coronal plane with the forearm maximally pronated[8] (Fig. 5-2). External rotation is provided by the infraspinatus muscle (C5, suprascapular nerve) and the teres minor muscle (C5-6, axillary nerve); the posterior portion of the deltoid is an accessory muscle (C5-6, axillary nerve). Selective testing of the scapular rotators (trapezius C3-4, spinal accessory XI, serratus anterior C5-6, long thoracic nerve) may uncover deficiencies in the scapular rotators of throwing athletes.[6] Serratus anterior weakness can be demonstrated by having the patient lean against the wall and do a "push-up." If the findings are positive, scapular winging will be apparent.

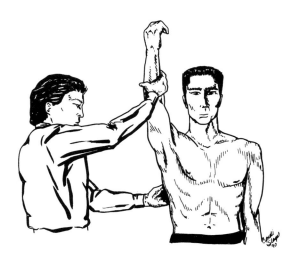

Fig. 5-3. Neer's impingement sign.

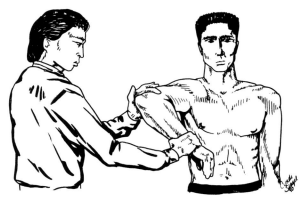

Fig. 5-4. Hawkins' impingement test.

The neurologic examination of the upper extremity should include muscle testing to elicit radicular or peripheral nerve function, a sensory examination, reflex testing, and evaluation of the sympathetic chain. The magnitude of the examination is determined by the patient's clinical presentation. A summary of the neurologic levels is presented in Tables 5-1 and 5-2.

DIAGNOSTIC TESTS
Specific Tests

Impingement tests. Clinical signs of impingement include pain localized to the anterior acromion or greater tuberosity, a painful arch of from 60 to 100 degrees of abduction, and a positive impingement sign. Impingement signs have been well documented by Hawkins and Kennedy,[3] Jobe and Jobe,[7] and Neer and Welsh.[11] The principle is to forcibly elevate the arm, causing the critical segment of the supraspinatus tendon to be impinged against the anterior inferior acromion. In Neer's method the shoulder is forcibly forward flexed and internally rotated, causing the greater tuberosity to be jammed against the anterior interior acromion (Fig. 5-3). Hawkins' test involves positioning the arm at approximately 90 degrees of forward flexion, followed by forcibly internally rotating the shoulder, impaling the supraspinatus tendon against the anterior inferior acromion and coracoacromial ligament (Fig. 5-4). Pain relief may be demonstrated on the impingement test by injecting 10 ml of 1% lidocaine (Xylocaine) beneath the acromion and then repeating the impingement signs; however, this does not distinguish between pure impingement and anterior subluxation causing impingement.

Biceps tests. Examination of the biceps should begin with palpation over the bicipital groove. Direct palpation of the tendon is usually not possible, and firm pressure over the area almost invariably causes discomfort (even

in those without pathology). Pain with palpation, therefore, is not a very specific sign of biceps tendinitis. The best-known stress tests to help identify bicipital pathology are Speed's test and Yergason's test. Speed's test is performed by having patients flex their shoulder against resistance while the elbow is extended and the forearm supinated. The findings are positive when pain is localized to the bicipital groove.[1] Yergason's test findings are positive if pain is present in the bicipital groove when the elbow is flexed 90 degrees and the wrist is supinated against resistance.[17] The most useful test in daily practice is Speed's test. Although tests for subluxating biceps tendons that involve palpating the tendon have been described,[12] the validity of such maneuvers is questionable. In the athletic patient with questionable biceps subluxation, true anterior glenohumeral instability should be suspected. Dimpling over the proximal biceps with fullness of the lower half of the muscle on the lateral side is indicative of a proximal biceps rupture.

Tests for rotator cuff tears. The salient tests for rotator cuff tears include the supraspinatus test and the drop arm test.[7,16] The supraspinatus test is mentioned earlier under strength testing. In the drop arm test, the examiner abducts the shoulder to 90 degrees and then asks the patient to lower the arm to the side slowly in the same arc. Severe pain or inability to lower the arm smoothly and slowly constitutes a positive finding. Positive drop arm test findings rarely, if ever, occur in young athletes and usually are reserved for an older population with large degenerative tears.

Stability tests. When stability is being tested, two primary concerns should be addressed: (1) the amount and direction of passive translation of the shoulder and (2) the ability to reproduce apprehension and subluxation. Passive translation of the humerus in relation to the glenoid is best accomplished by first grasping the humeral head, making sure it is reduced in the glenoid. Once the humeral head is reduced, directional stresses may be applied. The physician is seated behind the patient, and one hand is used to stabilize the shoulder

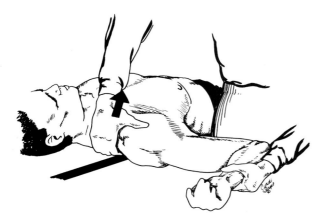

Fig. 5-5. Anterior subluxation test.

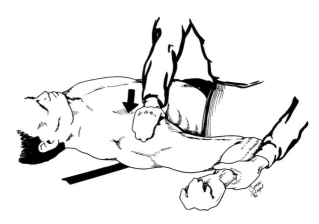

Fig. 5-6. Relocation test.

while the outer hand grasps the humeral head and selectively applies anterior, posterior, and inferior stress. The humeral head may be felt to translate to the glenoid rim and sometimes over it. Hawkins and Bokor[2] have found a combination of a percentage and grading system to be helpful. Generally, up to 10% anterior translation and up to 50% posterior translation are considered normal. Next, an inferior stress is applied to the arm, pulling on the elbow; the area of the skin just inferior to the acromion is observed for dimpling (sulcus sign).[9]

Once the degree of glenohumeral translation is documented, it is important to correlate these findings with the patient's complaints. Subluxation and apprehension tests try to reproduce the symptom complex of instability (subluxation, dislocation). In young overhand athletes the incidence of anterior subluxation with secondary impingement signs is more common than previously thought. Experience and sensitive fingers are the tools to uncovering this silent subluxation. The best test for discovering this shoulder instability is the anterior subluxation test, performed with the patient supine and the arm off the table at 90 degrees of abduction and external rotation. The examiner grasps the humeral head with the fingers and pushes the humeral head anteriorly (Fig. 5-5). Any anterior subluxation is considered pathologic; typically the patient complains of pain, not apprehension. Then the relocation test is performed; the humeral head is pushed posteriorly, and if the pain is relieved, the findings are considered positive (Fig. 5-6). The most common site of subluxation in overhand athletes is the anteroinferior quadrant. During the anterior subluxation maneuver, it is important to discern whether the patient's complaint is pain or apprehension. Pain during the anterior subluxation test relieved by the posteriorly directed relocation test implies anterior subluxation with secondary impingement. Apprehension during the anterior subluxation test conversely indicates a prior episode of dislocation, and a history of gross dislocation should be

investigated. The subjective feeling of apprehension is common for anterior instability; however, it is not as reliable for posterior instability. Often the athlete does not realize that the shoulder is posteriorly subluxed but complains of pain with forward flexion of the arm. A snapping sensation of the shoulder with extension and positive posterior subluxation or dislocation during stability testing helps clarify the diagnosis.

One of the most commonly overlooked conditions is the athlete with multidirectional instability. These patients demonstrate anterior, posterior, and inferior laxity as described in the preceding tests. The hallmark, however, is abnormal inferior laxity in the absence of labral detachments.[10] In addition to the sulcus sign, inferior apprehension can be illustrated by abducting the shoulder and pushing the humeral head inferiorly.[9] Generally, the athlete (throwers, weight lifters, swimmers) complains of vague aching or recurrent slipping of the shoulder with an associated decrease in performance. Intermittent pain and paresthesias, sometimes radiating distally to the elbow, may be present. However, the neurologic examination is normal.[13] Every examination should include testing of the thumb, fingers, elbows, and knees for generalized ligamentous laxity. Multidirectional shoulder instability is more common in patients with some degree of generalized laxity.[9]

Acromioclavicular joint tests. Acromioclavicular joint pathology is primarily suggested by pain with direct superior palpation of the acromioclavicular joint. Provocative tests include pain on flexing the arm to 90 degrees and forcibly adducting and internally rotating the arm across the chest, thus jamming the anterior acromioclavicular joint together (Fig. 5-7). A variation involves abducting the shoulder to 90 degrees and horizontally extending the arm to compress the posterior aspect of the acromioclavicular joint[16] (Fig. 5-8).

Thoracic outlet syndrome tests. Three specific tests are useful in identifying thoracic outlet problems: Adson's maneuver, the costoclavicular maneuver, and the hy-

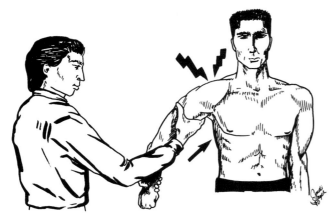

Fig. 5-7. Anterior provocative acromioclavicular test.

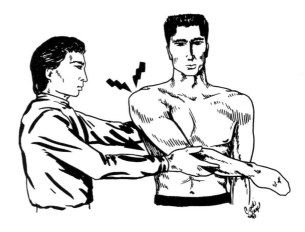

Fig. 5-8. Posterior provocative acromioclavicular test.

Table 5-3. Distribution of Typical Anatomic Findings With Each of the Cervical Nerve Roots

Root	Disc	Muscle	Reflex	Sensation	Myelogram/CT/MRI Deficit
C5	C4-5	Deltoid Biceps	Biceps	Lateral arm Deltoid area Axillary nerve	C4-5
C6	C5-6	Biceps Wrist extensors	Brachioradialis	Thumb, index, ring fingers Lateral forearm Musculocutaneous nerve	C5-6
C7	C6-7	Triceps Wrist flexors Finger extensors	Triceps	Middle finger and/or ring finger	C6-7
C8	C7-T1	Hand intrinsics Finger flexors		Ring and fifth fingers Medial forearm Medial anterior brachial cutaneous nerve	C7-T1
T1	T1-2	Hand intrinsics		Medial arm Medial brachial cutaneous nerve	

perabduction maneuver. Adson's maneuver is performed while the patient is seated, with the head extended and turned to the involved side. With deep inspiration there is a diminution or total loss of the radial pulse. The costoclavicular maneuver involves drawing downward and backward in the shoulder after the patient takes a deep breath (head and neck in neutral position). Thoracic outlet compression is suspected if this maneuver reproduces symptoms or obliterates the radial pulse. The hyperabduction test is performed while the patient is standing with the head extended; the shoulder is manually hyperabducted, and the patient is asked to take a deep breath. Thoracic outlet compres-

sion is indicated if the radial pulse is diminished or if this reproduces symptoms. Thoracic outlet syndrome is a diagnosis of exclusion; the work-up is troublesome, and the condition is very rare in athletes.

Cervical spine tests

Cervical radiculopathy. Cervical radiculopathy is certainly a more common syndrome than cervical myelopathy. It consists of pain and neurologic dysfunction produced by irritation or injury to a spinal nerve. This injury may be caused by a herniated cervical disc, cervical foraminal stenosis, tumors, fractures, or dislocations. The hallmark of cervical radiculopathy is pain in the distribution of a radicular nerve. Neurologic loss (i.e., muscle weakness, sensory changes, and/or reflex changes) may help localize the problem for the clinician. Table 5-3 shows the distribution of typical anatomic findings with each of the cervical nerve roots. To summarize this table, in patients with a C4-5 cervical disc herniation or C4-5 foraminal stenosis, we would expect a pathologic condition related to the C5 nerve root: pain radiating to the deltoid area, decreased biceps reflex, and decreased strength in the deltoid shoulder elevation muscles and possibly the biceps. The sensory loss would follow the distribution of the pain to the lateral deltoid area. For a C5-6 posterolateral disc herniation or C5-6 foraminal stenosis, we would expect upper arm pain radiating to the lateral epicondylar area, to the dorsolateral surface of the forearm, and to the thumb, index, and middle fingers. Distribution to the thumb is a critical distinguishing factor for the C6 nerve root. There may be weakness of wrist extension and some abduction in extension, a decreased brachial radialis reflex, and a sensory pattern in the distribution of the pain. For a C6-7 disc herniation or C6-7 foraminal stenosis, one might expect pain radiating to the posterior upper arm, to the dorsal surface of the arm, and to the ring and middle fingers; weakness in the triceps; and decreased triceps reflex. For a C8 disc herniation there may be pain radiating to the posterior arm, to the medial forearm, and to the ring and little fingers; and weakness in hand and finger abduction and in the intrinsic muscles of the hand.

The neuromechanical test for cervical spine disease is of great importance. To summarize, the neuromechanical signs of the cervical spine are as follows:

1. *Spurling's maneuver* (see Fig. 5-1) — Spurling's maneuver begins with simple neck extension. If neck extension reproduces radicular symptoms — pain not just in the neck but radiating to the arm — then the findings are positive. It is of more significance when the maneuver produces pain in the exact dermatomal distribution of a radicular nerve; it is of minimal significance when the maneuver produces neck pain only. When the maneuver produces neck pain only, the findings should be considered negative. If the findings are positive with head extension only, there is no reason to carry the test any further.

   The second stage of Spurling's maneuver is rotation of the extended head toward the symptomatic arm. If this produces pain in a radicular dermatomal pattern or arm pain, the findings are considered positive.

   The last stage of Spurling's maneuver is head extension, rotation toward the symptomatic side, and compression on the forehead.

2. *Head compression test* — Radicular arm pain on head compression constitutes a positive finding, which indicates cervical radiculopathy.

3. *Shoulder abduction test* (Fig. 5-9) — If abducting the

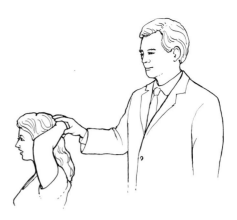

Fig. 5-9. Shoulder abduction test.

arm, putting the hand behind the head, produces relief of arm pain, it is an excellent sign that relief of tension in the nerve root has relieved the arm pain and the findings are positive, indicating cervical radiculopathy.

   If elevating the shoulder and placing the hand behind the head produces a severe increase in shoulder pain, shoulder pathology is present.

4. *Rotator cuff test* (Fig. 5-10) — The upper arm is held in 90 degrees of abduction and neutral, out from the body; with the arm maximally internally rotated and the elbow at 90 degrees of flexion, downward pressure is put on the elbow, thereby producing resistive abduction. Pain in the shoulder indicates shoulder joint pathology (Fig. 5-10, *A*).

   The arm is flexed 90 degrees, and the elbow is flexed to 90 degrees with the hand in the salute position across the chest. Downward pressure on the hand producing shoulder pain indicates shoulder pathology (Fig. 5-10, *B*).

   With the arm extended, the thumb is pointed toward the ground, and downward pressure is resisted (Fig. 5-10, *C*). Tenderness on the point of the shoulder and the bicipital groove with signs of impingement can indicate shoulder pathology.

5. *Lhermitte's sign* — Flexion of the neck producing bilateral upper and/or lower extremity paresthesias or paresis constitutes a positive finding. This can occasionally be seen with extension and is indicative of cervical cord pathology.

6. *Adson's maneuver* (Fig. 5-11) — This maneuver consists of abduction of the arm to 90 degrees at the elbow, with external rotation of the arm. The patient looks toward the abducted arm. If this maneuver reproduces symptoms, the cause is more likely the cervical root. Then the patient looks away from the arm, and the pulse is felt. If the pulse decreases and arm numbness or pain is reproduced, the findings are considered positive

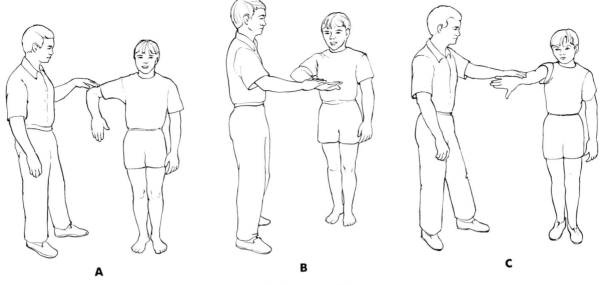

Fig. 5-10. Rotator cuff test.

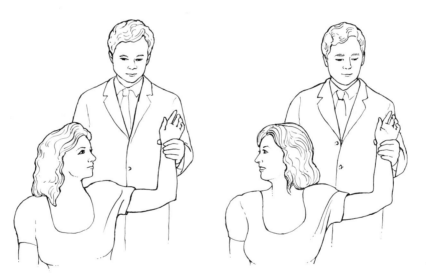

Fig. 5-11. Adson's maneuver.

for thoracic outlet obstruction. Sometimes a deep breath will further exacerbate the symptoms.

These neuromechanical signs are similar to straight leg raising, the Cram test, neck flexion, foot dorsiflexion, and other tests in the lumbar spine that indicate nerve root tension. In the cervical spine the pathomechanics are different. Maneuvers that extend and rotate the cervical spine produce narrowing of the spinal canal and intervertebral foramina. The phenomenon that reproduces the pain is more of a compressive one with these maneuvers. The pathologic condition may be a disc herniation or intervertebral foraminal stenosis, but what exactly is causing the pain is not necessarily as significant as distinguishing between radicular symptoms that are reproduced with maneuvers of the neck as opposed to neck pain without radicular symptoms or arm pain that is not related to the cervical spine. The last-mentioned category brings up a whole series of peripheral nerve entrapment and peripheral nerve injury categories that are obviously common in athletes. A peripheral nerve trapped or irritated anywhere along its course can hurt anywhere along its course. Carpal tunnel syndrome can present with shoulder and neck pain. Brachial plexus pathology can present with neck pain radiating to the hand. It is important to determine whether the pain is caused by radiculopathy. If the problem is radiculitis, it is important to determine how severe the radicular pain is.

Cervical myelopathy. Cervical myelopathy is a syndrome of symptoms resulting from spinal cord injury caused by cervical spine pathology, such as spondylitic spurs, central disc herniation, tumors, and dislocations of the cervical spine.

Initially, the feet are examined. Checking for cervical myelopathy is of paramount importance in evaluating every patient with a spinal problem. Key historical and physical examination factors should be noted. During the history, every patient should be asked about a gait disturbance (i.e., "Have you had any difficulty walking? Maintaining your balance? Knowing where your feet are in the dark? Any stumbling? Loss of balance or control? Feet further apart when you walk? Lack of agility? Lack of ability to stand on one foot?"). Often, questioning patients about their sports activity (such as golf) can review the key aspects of loss of balance and control, potentially pointing to cervical myelopathy. Asking family members and friends if they have noticed any change in the patient's gait pattern can be helpful. Questions concerning inability to stop walking when one wants to stop, an inability to get going when one is trying to get up from a seated position, and various tremor activity is approached at this time. Questions concerning numbness and tingling in the legs, numbness in the hands, loss of agility in the hands, inability to fasten small buttons, deterioration in handwriting, loss of ability to stand on one foot, and a decrease in bowel, bladder, or sexual function should be asked of every patient with spinal pain and certainly of every patient with cervical pain.

When the history and physical examination suggest the presence of cervical myelopathy, the appropriate diagnostic tests with indications of abnormality are magnetic resonance imaging (MRI) or a contrast computed tomography (CT) scan of the cervical spine. With significant neurologic symptoms, an electromyelogram (EMG) and nerve conduction study can also be ordered to rule out radiculopathy, a medical evaluation can be made for diabetes, and a neurologic evaluation can be done for demyelinating disease or cerebral abnormalities. Any abnormality of the cranial nerves with gait disturbance immediately points toward a more systemic neurologic dysfunction—either cerebral or neurologic disease. Diabetes and peripheral neuropathy may explain the gait disorder. Parkinsonism should be diagnosed on the initial history and physical examination by the typical characteristics of dyskinesia.

Tests to Determine Treatment

The morbidity found on the history and physical examination determines the aggressiveness of the diagnostic plan (see box above, right). The diagnostic tests ordered in the presence of cervical and arm pain can be

---

Morbidity Classification

Pain

1. No pain to mild pain, minimal discomfort with activity
2. Moderate pain, may take nonnarcotic medication
3. Constant low-grade or severe intermittent pain; intermittent narcotic use; may interfere with sleep
4. Constant severe pain; regular narcotic use; minimal to no relief of pain

Function

1. No impairment
2. Impairment of function (no sports)
3. Ineffective community ambulator
4. Ineffective household ambulator

Occupation

1. Full-time work
2. Part-time work
3. Changed jobs
4. Unemployed

---

divided into nonoperative and preoperative. Nonoperative tests allow the physician to pursue nonoperative care. The history and physical examination alone may allow the physician to proceed without diagnostic tests, but tests ordered should reflect (1) factors in the history and physical evaluation and (2) the severity of the patient's problems. Tests should be ordered when the results will change the recommended treatment or are necessary for an accurate diagnosis or prognosis.

Nonmechanical inflammatory neck and arm pain

Nonoperative tests. Tests include a bone scan, MRI, protein electrophoresis, complete blood count (CBC), sedimentation rate, SMA12, bone marrow aspiration, rheumatoid work-up, chest x-ray study, and electrocardiogram (ECG).

Operative tests. Tests include MRI, myelography, a contrast CT scan, needle aspiration, and Craig needle biopsy or open-incision biopsy.

Mechanical axial neck pain, with or without arm pain. This is predominantly a mechanical neck problem.

Nonoperative tests. Tests include MRI and a bone scan. MRI diagnoses levels of disc degeneration, tumors, infections, disc herniations, and cervical stenosis. A bone scan may help identify localized areas of arthritis and inflamed facet joints amenable to interarticular cortisone injections.

Operative tests

Myelography and contrast CT. Full examination of the spinal canal and spinal cord and subarachnoid space is imperative to properly diagnose disc herniations, cervical stenosis, intraforaminal tumors, foraminal stenosis, extruded disc fragments, and certain congenital anomalies. In the cervical spine, determining whether the nerve roots fill, how far out the foramina fill, and the exact bony contours of the intervertebral foramina is best done with a contrast CT scan. Measuring central canal diameters, volume, and intrathecal volume versus cord volume versus canal volume are all best done with a contrast CT scan.

MRI. The quality of most MRI scans available, as well as the interpretation available, does not equal that of the contrast CT scan in determining the exact anatomy of the foramina, the nerve roots, the spinal canal, and its contents. Still, MRI can accurately show causes of cervical neck and arm pain, cervical radiculopathy, and cervical myelopathy. MRI is a noninvasive study and is very accurate in ruling out intrathecal tumors and infections.

Discography. Cervical discography is both a subjective and an objective test. It is designed to reproduce pain from intervertebral discs by injecting the disc with water-soluble dye. It may reproduce pain from a painful neuromotion segment or from a herniated cervical disc. Some have considered it imperative in the diagnostic work-up for cervical neck and arm pain. However, at the Kerlan-Jobe Orthopaedic Clinic very little cervical discography is used, certainly much less than lumbar discography. Cervical discography requires a certain technique in which the discographer's finger presses down on the spine to push the esophagus off the spine. This requires x-ray exposure of the finger. Also, the incidence of esophageal perforation and probably higher incidence of infection, although undocumented, mitigate against its use. As in lumbar stenosis, cervical stenosis is less likely to reproduce symptoms from injection of the disc because the disc plays less of a role in the pathomechanics, so discography can be less useful. For cervical radiculopathy due to cervical stenosis, discography plays a greater role.

Cervical radiculopathy and cervical radiculitis. Radiculopathy implies neurologic deficit, and radiculitis is pain in the dermatomal distribution of a radicular nerve.

Nonoperative tests. A primary screening test, MRI diagnoses disc herniations, intrathecal tumors, spinal column tumors, and disc degeneration.

Operative tests. The contrast CT scan allows better visualization of nerve root filling and its relation to the bony architecture of the foramina.

Cervical myelopathy

Nonoperative tests. MRI can accurately diagnose cervical stenosis and the levels involved in patients with myelopathy, as well as cervical cord tumors.

Operative tests. A myelogram and contrast CT scan may allow a more exact measurement of the canal and can add information, but both MRI and the contrast CT scan can diagnose cervical myelopathy well. Intrathecal tumors and other conditions accompanying myelopathy

are diagnosed well with both MRI and CT. MRI shows changes in the cord, such as cervical edema, cervical injury, and syrinx, with excellent accuracy. The signs and symptoms of cervical myelopathy are a major medical problem. Using two different testing methods that demonstrate possibly the same thing is certainly indicated with a critical problem such as cervical myelopathy. The MRI scan identifies areas of cord pathology possibly not appreciated on the contrast CT scan, and the contrast CT scan allows better measurements to be made on the canal and cord.

A third group of tests involve functional testing. Dynamic MRI is a newer treatment technique that can demonstrate areas of cord impingement not seen on a standard MRI scan, or at least these areas can be better appreciated with dynamic MRI. Cineradiography studies show motion abnormalities, probably with greater emphasis than standard flexion/extension films, and extension motion studies are important in cervical myelopathy to demonstrate dynamic problems. These tests should be used with great care and under the proper circumstances. EMG testing can be important in patients with symptoms similar to or compatible with cervical myelopathy, demonstrating demyelination or other neurologic diseases that present with gait abnormalities, and should be part of the patient's work-up when cervical myelopathy is suspected. Additional testing for myelopathy should involve a gamut of tests from muscle biopsy to blood work for pernicious anemia to a long differential diagnosis for gait abnormality.

All the factors of morbidity determine the aggressiveness of the diagnostic plan. Determining psychosocial factors, eliminating tumors, and eliminating neurologic catastrophes all have the same importance here as they do in lumbar disease. The percentage of neck and arm pain plays a vital role in determining the clinical syndrome.

OUTCOME

The diagnostic plan must answer three questions: (1) what level, (2) what nerve, and (3) what pathologic condition. The distribution of pain and neurologic dysfunction may follow a distinct radicular pattern, allowing the surgeon to determine which nerve is involved. An EMG can, at times, determine which nerve when the EMG can identify a pathologic condition in the anterior primary ramus. Posterior primary ramus pathology, as in the lumbar spine, is not of great localizing significance. The EMG and nerve conduction study allow the clinician to diagnose peripheral nerve entrapment syndromes and peripheral neuropathy. This is vitally important in the upper extremity because carpal tunnel, thoracic outlet syndrome, and brachial plexus injuries are very common. What level of the spine is involved and what the pathologic condition is can be determined by changes on anatomic studies such as the myelogram, contrast CT scan, and MRI. As in lumbar spine disease, there is a very high incidence of false-positive findings, meaning that anatomic findings are not producing symptoms. The incidence of significantly pathologic structures in the cervical spine of athletes that are not causing any symptoms may run as high as 30% to 50% of studies.

The conclusion—and the most important aspect of the diagnostic plan—is that the x-ray studies must match the clinical syndrome to determine their true significance.

REFERENCES

1. Crenshaw AH, Kilgore WE: Surgical treatment of bicipital tenosynovitis, *J Bone Joint Surg* 48A:1496, 1966.
2. Hawkins RJ, Bokor DJ: Clinical evaluation of shoulder problems. In *The shoulder,* Philadelphia, 1990, WB Saunders.
3. Hawkins RJ, Kennedy JC: Impingement syndrome in athletes, *Am J Sports Med* 8:151, 1980.
4. Howell SM et al: Clarification of the role of supraspinatus muscle in shoulder function, *J Bone Joint Surg* 68A:398, 1986.
5. Inman VT, Saunders JB, Abbott LC: Observation of the function of the shoulder joint, *J Bone Joint Surg* 26A:1, 1944.
6. Jobe FW, Bradley JP: The diagnosis and nonoperative treatment of shoulder injuries in athletes, *Clin Sports Med* 8:419, 1989.
7. Jobe FW, Jobe CM: Painful athletic injuries of the shoulder, *Clin Orthop* 173:117, 1983.
8. Jobe FW, Moynes DR, Brewster CE: Rehabilitation of shoulder joint instabilities, *Orthop Clin North Am* 18:473, 1987.
9. Neer CS: Involuntary inferior and multidirectional instability of the shoulder: etiology, recognition and treatment. In *AAOS Instructional Course Lectures,* vol 34, St Louis, 1985, Mosby.
10. Neer CS II, Foster CR: Inferior capsular shift for involuntary inferior and multidirectional instability of the shoulder, *J Bone Joint Surg* 62A:897, 1980.
11. Neer CS II, Welsh RP: The shoulder in sports, *Orthop Clin North Am* 9:583, 1977.
12. Neviaser RJ: Anatomic considerations and examination of the shoulder, *Orthop Clin North Am* 11:187, 1980.
13. Norris TR: History and physical examination of the shoulder. In Nicholas JA, Hershman EB: *The upper extremity in sports medicine,* ed 2, St Louis, 1995, Mosby.
14. Perry J: Personal communication, 1989.
15. Poppen NK, Walker PS: Normal and abnormal motion of the shoulder, *J Bone Joint Surg* 58A:195, 1976.
16. Shields CL, Glousman RE: Open management of rotator cuff tears, *Adv Sports Med Fitness* 2:223, 1989.
17. Yergason RM: Supraspinatus sign, *J Bone Joint Surg* 13:60, 1931.
18. Yocum LA: Assessing the shoulder: history, physical examination, differential diagnosis, and special tests used, *Clin Sports Med* 2:281, 1983.
19. Zarins B, Andrews J, Carson W: *Injuries to the throwing arm,* Philadelphia, 1985, WB Saunders.

Chapter Six

♦

Differential Diagnosis of Upper Extremity Problems

Norman P. Zemel
James P. Bradley
James E. Tibone

Upper Extremity Injuries

Various injuries can occur in the upper extremity during athletic competition. Injury to the cervical spine, spinal nerves, and brachial plexus can produce symptoms of burning, weakness, pain, and loss of function. However, similar complaints can occur from neurovascular or musculotendinous lesions originating within the upper extremity. In addition, a "double-crush" syndrome[40,71] can occur that involves both the cervical spine and the peripheral nerves of the upper extremity.

Neurovascular problems in the upper extremity can occur anywhere along the pathway of the nerve or vessel. The peripheral nerves and vessels pass beneath muscles or fascial tunnels in their course from the neck to the tip of the digits. Certain anatomic sites are more prone to injury, usually by compression, and knowledge of the anatomy of the area helps in localizing, evaluating, and diagnosing these injuries (see Chapter 1 and box at right). A detailed medical examination and various diagnostic modalities assist the clinician in determining the proper diagnosis and treatment.

Stress placed on the hand, wrist, forearm, and elbow of athletes as a result of repeated blunt trauma, sustained forceful gripping, and stretching because of the various postures of the extremity while playing (e.g., the elbow in throwing sports) can lead to several neurovascular disorders. However, neurovascular disorders in the upper extremity of athletes are less common than musculoskeletal lesions. These disorders are predominately closed injuries.

Upper extremity pain, weakness, tingling, numbness, and burning causing an inability to compete in a particular athletic activity must be accurately diagnosed and treated to allow the athlete to return to full athletic activity. It is extremely important to differentiate between recurring cervical spine injuries leading to "burners" ("stingers"),[62,75] brachial plexus injury,[25] thoracic outlet syndrome,[12] peripheral nerve and vascular disorders, and musculotendinous abnormalities. This part of the chapter discusses the various peripheral nerve disorders, vascular conditions, and musculotendinous abnormalities in the upper extremity that can arise from

---

Muscle Innervations in the Upper Extremity

Musculocutaneous Nerve

Coracobrachialis
Biceps
Brachialis

Radial Nerve

Triceps
Anconeus
Brachioradialis
Extensor carpi radialis longus
Extensor carpi radialis brevis

Posterior Interosseous Nerve

Supinator
Extensor carpi ulnaris
Extensor digitorum
Extensor digiti quinti
Extensor pollicis longus
Extensor indicis proprius
Abductor pollicis longus
Extensor pollicis brevis

Ulnar Nerve

Flexor carpi ulnaris
Flexor profundus (ring finger, little finger)
Hypothenar muscles
Adductor pollicis
Interosseous muscles
Lumbrical muscles (ring finger, little finger)

Median Nerve

Pronator teres
Flexor carpi radialis
Palmaris longus
Flexor superficialis (all fingers)
Abductor pollicis brevis
Opponens pollicis
Flexor pollicis brevis
Lumbrical muscles (index finger, middle finger)

Anterior Interosseous Nerve

Flexor pollicis longus
Flexor profundus (index finger, middle finger)
Pronator quadratus

athletic activity. Many of these conditions can cause symptoms similar to more proximal disorders or can be associated with symptoms that radiate proximally to the shoulder or neck.

NEUROLOGIC DISORDERS

When neurologic injuries occur in the upper extremities, they generally result from blunt trauma, repetitive overuse, stretching, or extended forced gripping. These injuries are rarely due to open wounds.[41]

The most common nerve injury in the upper extremity is a compressive neuropathy or entrapment syndrome. Usually the injury is a neurapraxia (Seddon classification), or first-degree nerve injury (Sunderland classification)[47] (Table 6-1). Neurapraxia is the least severe type of injury and is characterized by transient loss of nerve function but no disruption of the integrity of the nerve fibers or sheath.

The exact pathophysiologic changes associated with compressive neuropathies have yet to be elucidated. Theories of nerve compression include (1) anoxia caused by venous obstruction within the nerve and (2) a mechanical lesion that produces local structural changes to the myelin sheath.[52] If left untreated, these lesions cause progressive damage to the nerve. The peripheral fibers tend to be involved initially, whereas the central fibers are preserved, unless the compression continues.[64] Depending on the forces involved, the nerve injury can be a combination of first-, second-, and third-degree changes.

Systemic diseases, such as thyroid disorders and diabetes mellitus, should be considered in the overall evaluation of the athlete with upper extremity injury.[36]

Peripheral Nerve Disorders

Lacerations of a nerve in the upper extremity rarely occur during sporting activities. Injury to the nerve usually occurs from blunt trauma, repeated stretching, or compression.

Musculocutaneous Nerve

The musculocutaneous nerve is rarely injured. Bassett and Nunley[2] reported a series of patients with compression of the sensory portion of this nerve (lateral antebrachial cutaneous) by the biceps aponeurosis and the biceps tendon. A compression force can be exerted on the nerve as it pierces the brachial fascia lateral to the biceps tendon. The compression force occurs with elbow extension and can be exaggerated with forearm pronation. These patients have pain on the anterolateral aspect of the elbow and burning dysesthesias along the volar radial aspect of the forearm.

The musculocutaneous nerve can be injured with activities causing forceful repetitive forearm pronation with elbow extension, direct trauma, or a muscular hypertrophy. These injuries occur in swimmers and racquetball or tennis players. Compressive injury must be differentiated from lateral epicondylitis, proximal median nerve compression, cervical radiculitis, or injury to the biceps tendon.

Radial Nerve

In the arm, radial nerve injury is usually associated with direct contusion or is secondary to a fracture of the humerus.[27] In addition to the obvious bony injury, the patient may be unable to extend the wrist, fingers, or thumb. The nerve can also be compressed as a result of repeated strenuous muscular activities such as weight lifting.[39]

Radial tunnel syndrome. The radial tunnel, which is about 5 cm long, begins where the radial nerve passes anterior to the humeroradial joint and ends where the posterior interosseous nerve passes beneath the proximal edge of the superficial part of the supinator muscle (arcade of Frohse). (Fig. 6-1.) In the tunnel the radial nerve lies on the anterior capsule of the humeroradial joint, 1 cm lateral to the biceps tendon. Four potential

Table 6-1. Classification of Nerve Injury

Seddon	Sunderland
Neurapraxia	First-degree nerve injury
Axonotmesis	Second-degree nerve injury Third-degree nerve injury
Neurotmesis	Fourth-degree nerve injury Fifth-degree nerve injury

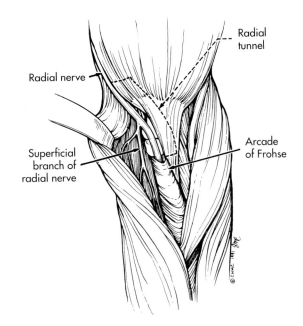

Fig. 6-1. The course of the radial nerve within the radial tunnel is outlined by the dotted line. The posterior interosseous nerve then passes beneath the arcade of Frohse.

causes of radial tunnel syndrome are (1) fibrous bands anterior to the radial head, (2) a fan-shaped leash of vessels lying across the radial nerve (leash of Henry), (3) the tendinous margin of the extensor carpi radialis brevis, and (4) the arcade of Frohse.[38,55]

Patients with radial tunnel syndrome complain primarily of pain and aching in the dorsum of the proximal forearm distal to the elbow. Activity often causes the pain to increase. The pain can radiate to the distal arm and to the distal forearm. Paresthesias along the superficial radial nerve distribution can also occur.

Examination shows tenderness three to four finger-breadths distal to the lateral epicondyle at or distal to the head of the radius, pain on resisted supination of the extended forearm, and pain with resisted extension of the middle finger with the elbow extended. If the radial nerve is compressed above its bifurcation, both motor and sensory findings will be noted on physical examination. Electrodiagnostic studies are not very helpful unless denervation of the muscle is noted on the electromyogram.

Lateral epicondylitis. The primary differential diagnosis with radial tunnel syndrome is lateral epicondylitis,[43] although more proximal lesions must also be considered. The distinction between lateral epicondylitis and radial tunnel syndrome is often difficult. Pain with lateral epicondylitis is usually sharp and is found with pressure over the ridge of the lateral epicondyle.

Compression injuries. The deep branch of the radial nerve is the posterior interosseous nerve. Spinner[63] reported on his study of a fibrous arch, originally described by Frohse, at the most proximal point of the supinator muscle. The arcade of Frohse can compress the posterior interosseous nerve as the nerve passes beneath its fibrous edge (see Fig. 6-1). At this site the nerve can be compressed by any inflammatory swelling, blunt trauma, or repeated pronation and supination of the forearm. If the arcade is narrow, the nerve can be tethered by hyperextending the elbow.

Compression of the posterior interosseous nerve results in weakness or loss of motor function without any loss of sensibility. Active wrist extension is present, but the wrist deviates radially because of weakness of the extensor carpi ulnaris muscle. The long extensors to the fingers and thumb are affected. A partial compression of the nerve can occur, affecting only one or two fingers. Electrodiagnostic studies may be helpful in diagnosing this condition.

Verhaar and Spaans,[72] in a study of 16 patients, indicated that the data did not support the concept of compression of the posterior interosseous nerve as the cause of the complaints reported in radial tunnel syndrome.

Entrapment injury. An isolated entrapment of the superficial radial nerve (cheiralgia paresthetica, Wartenberg's syndrome) can occur in the distal third of the forearm as the nerve emerges from beneath the brachio-radialis tendon (Fig. 6-2). In athletes this is usually caused by blunt trauma or repeated rotation of the forearm. Burning or pain is present in the distribution of the superficial radial nerve, and the nerve is tender in the distal third of the forearm.[14,16] This condition must be differentiated from a lesion of the more proximal radial nerve or from de Quervain's tenosynovitis.

Ulnar Nerve

The ulnar nerve is injured or compressed at the elbow or wrist, with the former site being the more common. The nerve is partially protected, but its superficial location at the elbow makes it susceptible to injury. Direct trauma to the nerve can occur in contact sports, whereas indirect trauma can occur in weight lifting, gymnastics, and throwing sports.[21] Ulnar nerve symptoms in the throwing athlete occur secondary to direct trauma, repeated traction of the ulnar nerve, cubital tunnel compression, bony changes secondary to fracture or arthritis on the medial aspect of the elbow, recurrent dislocations or subluxations of the nerve out of its groove, congenital soft tissue abnormalities, and inflammatory conditions. The athlete is susceptible to any of these conditions because of the biomechanical forces involved in throwing and the vigorous and repeated

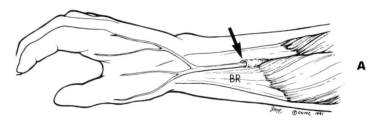

A

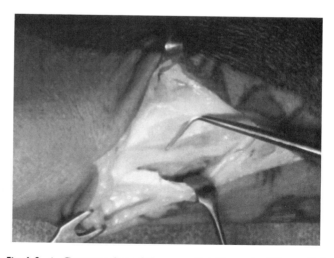

B

Fig. 6-2. A, Compression of the superficial branch of the radial nerve (Wartenberg's syndrome) occurs in the distal forearm *(arrow).* The nerve emerges from beneath the tendon of the brachioradialis muscle *(BR).* **B,** The nerve has been decompressed by incising the tight fascia.

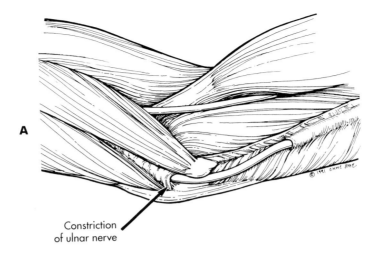

Constriction
of ulnar nerve

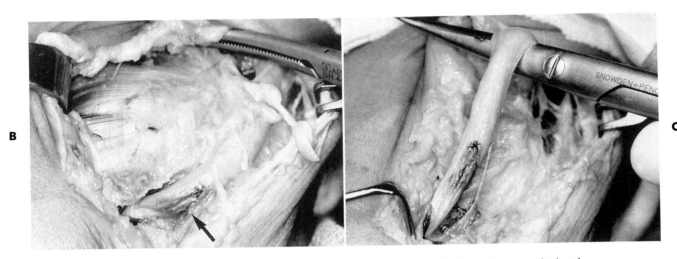

Fig. 6-3. A and **B,** The ulnar nerve is often compressed as it enters the hiatus between the heads of the flexor carpi ulnaris muscle just distal to the ulnar groove at the elbow *(arrow).* **B,** The localized site of compression of the nerve is hemorrhagic. **C,** Beyond the site of compression, the nerve seems to be normal.

tensile stresses on the medial aspect of the elbow. The nerve is usually mechanically compressed (Fig. 6-3) as a result of traction or friction.[79] The term *cubital tunnel syndrome* was first used by Feindel and Strafford.[18]

Complaints are most likely to be reported by the athlete who uses an overhand throwing motion (e.g., in baseball, football, javelin throwing, and tennis). Numbness, tingling, or burning in the ring and little fingers can be early complaints, usually preceding any muscle weakness or atrophy. Sometimes the person complains of a clumsy or heavy feeling in the hand. Symptoms can subside with rest, but they recur with activity and tend to increase in frequency. A painful pop or snap may be felt at the elbow when the ulnar nerve subluxes or dislocates. Then a burning or tingling feeling can radiate into the fingers.

Examination shows tenderness of the ulnar nerve at the elbow and Tinel's sign; the nerve may be felt to move

out of the ulnar groove. Abnormal sensitivity to pinprick or two-point discrimination is present in the ring and little fingers and possibly also over the dorsal ulnar aspect of the hand. Mild intrinsic weakness may be noted early, but often the long flexor tendons to the ring and little fingers are functioning. This may be related to the configuration of the nerve bundles within the ulnar nerve at the elbow. The fibers to the flexor carpi ulnaris and flexor digitorum profundus muscles lie deep within the nerve, whereas the fibers to the intrinsic muscles are more superficial. Thus it is usually late in the compression curve of the nerve that weakness of the flexor carpi ulnaris and flexion of the digitorum profundus muscles are found. The elbow flexion test described by Wadsworth[74] is useful in diagnosing compression of the ulnar nerve at the elbow. The test is performed by acutely flexing both elbows with the forearm in supination to determine if the patient's complaints can be reproduced.

The differential diagnosis includes cervical nerve root compression, cervical rib with pressure on C8 and T1 nerve roots, scalenus anticus syndrome, and compression of the ulnar nerve at the wrist.

Roentgenograms of the elbow, including a cubital tunnel view, should be part of a routine evaluation. Electromyogram and nerve conduction studies should also be done; however, in the early stages of injury and compression, these test results may be negative. It is then important to evaluate and treat the patient on a clinical basis.

The ulnar nerve can also be injured or compressed at the wrist. This occurs most commonly at or within Guyon's canal. Shea and McClain[60] described three types of ulnar nerve compression syndromes at the wrist. Type I occurs proximal to or in Guyon's canal and produces both sensory and motor symptoms. Type II is an isolated compression of the deep (motor) branch of the nerve at the hook of the hamate. Type III also can occur at the hook of the hamate, but it involves only the superficial (sensory) branch. Thus a type II lesion produces only motor abnormalities—weakness or atrophy of the ulnarly innervated intrinsic muscles of the hand—and a type III lesion produces only loss of sensibility in the ring and little fingers. Lesions of the ulnar nerve at the wrist spare the dorsal sensory branch of the ulnar nerve and do not affect the profundus tendons to the ring and little fingers. In addition to the compression within Guyon's canal, the ulnar nerve at the wrist may be injured by direct trauma, fractures of the hook of the hamate,[66] injuries of the pisiform, or repeated power grip. These injuries occur most commonly in baseball, tennis, golf, racquetball, and gymnastics. The hyperextended wrist and constant pressure on the hypothenar muscles by the handlebars of a bicycle can result in compression of the ulnar nerve known as *handlebar palsy*.[1]

Roentgenograms of the wrist should include a carpal tunnel view and supinated oblique view to show the hook of the hamate and pisitriquetral joints. If necessary, a computed tomography (CT) scan of these areas should be obtained. Electrodiagnostic studies help differentiate ulnar nerve lesions at the wrist and elbow from the more proximal lesions of the brachial plexus and cervical spine.

Median Nerve

Disorders of the median nerve in the athlete usually occur from repetitive motion. This activity can cause compression of the nerve by hypertrophy of normal or abnormal muscles, by fascial thickening, or by flexor tenosynovitis. Two common sites of compression of the median nerve are the proximal forearm and the wrist.

Compression at the wrist. Although compression of the median nerve at the wrist (carpal tunnel syndrome) is fairly common in the general population, it is uncommon

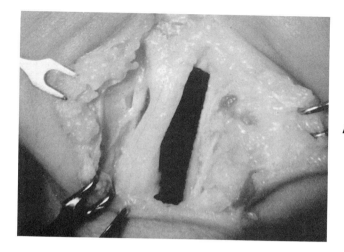

A

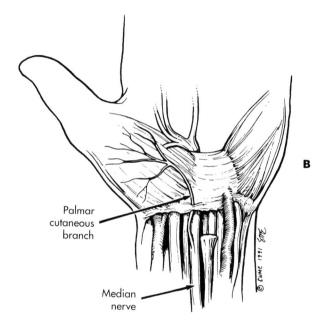

B

Palmar cutaneous branch

Median nerve

Fig. 6-4. A, Significant constriction of the median nerve at the wrist from a sports injury is unusual. **B,** The palmar cutaneous branch of the median nerve can be injured by direct trauma or compressed as it passes through the transverse carpal ligament.

as a sports-related injury (Fig. 6-4). In athletic activities carpal tunnel syndrome occurs from forced gripping, throwing, or any activity involving repetitive flexion and extension of the wrist.[34,41] Gelberman, Hergenroeder, and Hargeus[20] showed that the pressure within the carpal canal in normal subjects rose tenfold with acute flexion and extension of the wrist. In patients with carpal tunnel syndrome, the pressure increased to three times greater than when the measurements were taken with the wrist at neutral.

Typical complaints are numbness and tingling in the thumb, index finger, and middle and radial half of the ring finger and/or night pain or numbness in the wrist and fingers. These complaints are aggravated or initiated by exertional activity. Occasionally pain is referred proximally to the shoulder.[33]

Percussing the median nerve at the wrist (Tinel's sign) and Phalen's test (wrist flexion test) provide important physical findings that indicate that the compression of the median nerve is at the wrist.[50] Thenar atrophy is a late finding on physical examination. Routine roentgenograms should include a carpal tunnel view to rule out any bony abnormality in the carpal canal. Magnetic resonance imaging (MRI) of the wrist may also provide useful information about the median nerve or flexor tendons.

Findings obtained from an electromyogram and nerve conduction velocity tests are extremely valuable in verifying the diagnosis of carpal tunnel syndrome. Although there is a 10% incidence of false-negative findings in these tests, especially during the early stages of nerve compression,[77] this can be overcome by stressing the upper extremity to recreate the symptoms and then retesting the patient.

The differential diagnosis should include compression of the median nerve in the proximal forearm, brachial plexus injury, and cervical radiculopathy. Coexistence of carpal tunnel syndrome and cervical radiculopathy, usually at the C6 or C7 level, as well as brachial plexus lesions, also has been reported.[1,40]

Compression in the forearm. Compression of the median nerve in the proximal forearm is uncommon in sports-related activities. Repetitive upper extremity exertion, particularly in throwing sports, can result in proximal nerve compression. This presents as either a pronator teres syndrome or an anterior interosseous nerve syndrome.

Pronator teres syndrome can result from athletic activities requiring forced gripping, repetitive forearm pronation, or direct trauma. Throwing sports, racquet sports, weight lifting, and gymnastics are activities that may produce this particular nerve compression.[9] The sites of compression are the lacertus fibrosus, between the superficial and deep heads of the pronator teres muscle, and the proximal edge of the flexor superficialis muscle (Fig. 6-5).

Complaints are predominantly sensory and often vague. They consist of numbness and tingling in all or part of the median nerve distribution. These complaints frequently occur after exertion and are relieved with rest. There may be tenderness in the proximal forearm, and motor weakness sometimes occurs. Johnson, Spinner, and Shrewsbury[32] described specific diagnostic maneuvers that are useful in diagnosing entrapment of the median nerve in the proximal forearm. The stress tests, which provoke paresthesia, include (1) flexion of the elbow with supination of the forearm against resistance (lacertus fibrosus), (2) pronation of a flexed forearm against resistance and increased paresthesia when the forearm is extended (pronator teres), and (3) independent flexion of the middle finger against resis-

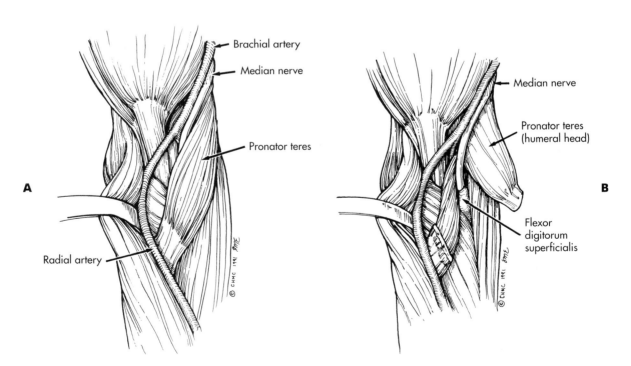

Fig. 6-5. A, The median nerve passes under the lacertus fibrosus (not shown) and then between the two heads of the pronator teres muscles. **B,** It continues beneath the fibrous arch of the flexor superficialis muscles.

tance (flexor digitorum superficialis). In these patients, Phalan's test results will be negative.

Only 15% to 20% of the patients have positive findings on electrodiagnostic studies, but even some of these are not specific.[64] A high index of suspicion regarding pronator teres syndrome is important. Postexertional electrodiagnostic testing may be useful in making this difficult diagnosis.

Anterior Interosseous Nerve

Compression of the anterior interosseous nerve is rare (Fig. 6-6). Patients complain of vague discomfort in the proximal forearm and of motor weakness. The anterior interosseous nerve is a motor nerve that innervates the flexor pollicis longus, the flexor digitorum profundus to the index and occasionally the middle finger, and the pronator quadratus muscle. Thus the injured person demonstrates a weak pinch with loss of active flexion at the distal joints of the thumb and index finger. An incomplete compression of this nerve has also been reported.[26]

VASCULAR DISORDERS

Vascular disorders in the upper extremity in athletes are uncommon. They tend to occur in athletes who have a significant energy absorption in the hands, either from a single traumatic event or repeated trauma.[8,46,51,54,68] Allen's test (Fig. 6-7) is a useful diagnostic test that can be performed in the office. Both the radial and ulnar arteries are compressed at the wrist while the patient rapidly flexes and extends the fingers. Each vessel is then released to test its patency. Allen's test can also be used

to test the patency of the vessels to the individual digits. Doppler testing of the vessels also provides useful information.

MUSCULOTENDINOUS DISORDERS

Abnormalities of the musculotendinous system must be included as part of the differential diagnosis of upper extremity disorders in the athlete. Various muscle overuse problems and ligament and tendon inflammatory conditions arise as a result of vigorous training and stressful use of the extremity during various sporting events. In particular, medial and lateral epicondylitis, de Quervain's syndrome, tenosynovitis, intersection syndrome, dorsal tenosynovitis, tendinitis of the flexor carpi ulnaris and flexor carpi radialis tendons, and tenosynovitis of the flexor tendons must be carefully evaluated as causes of pain and decreased function in the upper extremity.[9,15,67,77]

Various upper extremity disorders in the athlete have been described that must be differentiated from abnormalities of the cervical spine and brachial plexus. This can be accomplished with a detailed history and physical examination of the upper extremity, in conjunction with electrodiagnostic studies and various imaging techniques.

Shoulder Pain

Athletes who engage in overhand sports frequently sustain injuries localized to the rotator cuff or ligamentous shoulder capsule and occasionally to the neurologic elements. Chronic stress initiated by the repetitive high-velocity nature of these overhand throwing activities often predisposes the shoulder to impingement syndrome and rotator cuff abnormalities. The activities most commonly implicated include baseball (especially pitching), tennis (serve, overhead smash), football (quarterbacks), swimming (especially backstroke), gymnastics, and javelin throwing.

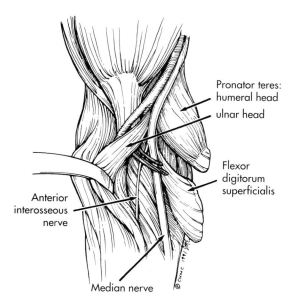

Fig. 6-6. A variety of structures can compress the anterior interosseous nerve after it originates from the ulnar side of the median nerve. A group of vessels is shown in the diagram.

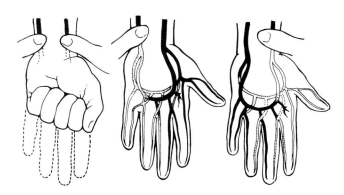

Fig. 6-7. The patency of the radial and ulnar arteries is determined by Allen's test. A negative test result indicates the vessels are patent. A positive test result indicates some obstruction of the vessel.

In treating shoulder problems in athletes it is useful to divide them into two separate categories: the older population and the younger population. The problem in the older population (over 35 years of age) is commonly secondary to a degenerative process that is hallmarked by subacromial spur formation, compromise of the subacromial space, and decreased vascular supply. This group has a propensity for pure subacromial impingement with its associated rotator cuff tear. Concomitant or isolated cervical spine disorders with symptomatic overlap is common in this group. In contrast, the most common cause of shoulder dysfunction in young athletes (ages 18 to 35 years) is anterior instability (a result of inherent increased range of motion with anterior capsular attenuation), causing secondary impingement. Associated cervical spine problems are uncommon in this group and thus present less of a problem in the differential diagnosis.

When presented with an athlete with shoulder pain, it is paramount to delineate whether the problem is one of labral, capsular, rotator cuff, or coracoacromial arch abnormality, secondary to neurovascular problems or distant referred conditions. Generally, shoulder pain in athletes can be divided into one of five groups: (1) posttraumatic, (2) degenerative, (3) instability, (4) neuromuscular, or (5) referred. Once the structures involved are determined and an accurate diagnosis is established, conservative modalities usually alleviate the problem. Occasionally surgery is indicated if conservative measures fail.

SIGNS AND SYMPTOMS

Occasionally the patient complains of instability ("my arm goes out" or "my arm goes dead").[56,59] Pain occurring simultaneously with a specific phase of throwing (i.e., cocking or acceleration) may be due to underlying instability causing anterior capsular pain and eventually impingement symptoms.[28] Pain during cocking and acceleration that is suddenly alleviated at follow-through and localized to the inferomedial angle of the scapula usually represents scapulothoracic bursitis.[61] Nocturnal pain and pain at rest are classic symptoms of a rotator cuff tear, whereas persons with rotator cuff tendinitis develop pain with progressive shoulder activity, particularly overhand elevation. Albeit rare in athletes, nocturnal pain may be a harbinger to an insidious neoplastic process, which should always be considered, especially when the examination is uncharacteristic of common shoulder maladies. A burning or vague ache centered about the posterior lateral shoulder (with subtle atrophy of the infraspinatus) that is sometimes referred to the arm or neck during or after throwing may indicate suprascapular nerve syndrome. Although rare, complaints of activity-related fatigue that is associated with aching, subtle fullness, and swelling of the arm should arouse suspicions of effort thrombosis.[73] There should be a high index of suspicion of pain related to specific circumstances (e.g., a competitive swimmer having pain when training with paddles but being pain free during routine swimming or a young pitcher having pain on a 2- to 3-day pitching rotation but being pain free on a 5-day rotation). Simple overuse with improper rest may be the only underlying cause under these circumstances.

The duration of the pain (acute versus chronic) is revealing. Adhesive capsulitis is usually more common after a long, protracted course of shoulder pain. Prolonged immobilization for fractures, or convalescence in bed in a postoperative situation, may be a setup for adhesive capsulitis. Calcific bursitis is characterized by a long course of intermittent mild to moderate shoulder pain that may, during the resorptive phase, become extremely painful. Rotator cuff tears can be acute or chronic, but an extended period of shoulder problems is the norm.

The character of the pain may often lead the orthopaedist to the diagnosis. The dull, toothachelike night pain of a rotator cuff tear obviously differs from the burning pain of an acute calcific bursitis.[78] A deep burning pain in the posterior shoulder extending down the arm to the fingers, associated with paresthesias in the digits and less frequently in the forearm, is characteristic of a protrusion of a cervical disc. Generally, crepitation and discomfort with passive shoulder motion can be attributed to inflammation disorders of bursal structures. Pain associated with pseudolocking is indicative of possible loose bodies or labral tears, particularly in the throwing shoulder.[22]

Shoulder pain does not always equate to primary shoulder pathology, because it is often the site of referred pain, most commonly from the cervical spine (C5-6). Intradural, preforaminal, and postforaminal lesions of the neck can all induce shoulder pain.[3] Ruptured intervertebral discs (preforaminal) remain the most common source of pain. The type of pain may often help differentiate a pathologic condition of the cervical spine from primary shoulder problems. Cervical spine pain is characterized by a deep, burning discomfort usually located in the middle of the upper neck and sometimes the suboccipital region along the distribution of the greater occipital nerves. Frequently the discomfort spreads across the shoulders, where it may localize to the supermedial angle of the scapula at the insertion of the levator scapulae and rhomboids. Not uncommonly, the discomfort presents in the shoulder, elbow, or hand without cervical spine symptoms. It is helpful when the radiation of pain is into the fingers with associated paresthesias in the digits, alerting the physician to evaluate the cervical spine. Sometimes patients are more comfortable with the shoulder abducted, allowing the forearm to rest on the top of the head. This maneuver presumably decreases some of the tension on the involved cervical roots.[69] A good guideline is to ask the patient to indicate the site of maximal pain. Pain localized distal to the lateral acromion usually repre-

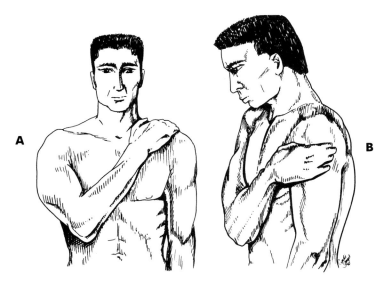

Fig. 6-8. **A,** Pain localized to the top of the shoulder is common with cervical spine pathology. **B,** Pain isolated distal to the acromion about the deltoid insertion is common with primary shoulder pathology.

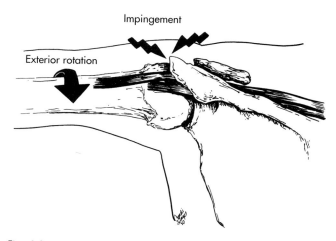

Fig. 6-9. Impingement pathology. The supraspinatus, biceps tendon, subacromial bursa, and sometimes the acromioclavicular joint are anatomically involved in the impingement process.

sents a primary pathologic condition of the shoulder. However, pain localized to the top of the shoulder should alert the physician to possible cervical spine abnormalities. Patients with cervical spine–referred pain commonly cup their hand over the top of the shoulder and supermedial angle of the scapula (Fig. 6-8).

Less frequent causes of referred shoulder pain include cardiac, visceral (gastric, pancreatic), diaphragmatic (gallbladder, hepatic disorders mediated through the phrenic nerve), and pleural etiologies. An especially noteworthy cause is Pancoast's tumor residing in the apex of the lung. Coincident Horner's syndrome (ptosis, miosis, anidrosis, and enophthalmos) may sometimes present first because of an apical tumor. A plethora of symptom complexes, some with subtle variations, may be evident when one is evaluating athletes with shoulder pain; therefore all shoulder pain in an athlete should not automatically be considered to originate from the shoulder.

Finally, a review of the past medical history and any recent medical work-ups or surgical procedures should be completed. Inquiry is made regarding any history of diabetes, gout, chondrocalcinosis, rheumatoid arthritis, physiologic anomalies, metabolic disorders, infections, or spinal or neuromuscular disorders. Although rare in this population, symptoms of neoplastic disease, both primary and metastatic, should be addressed.

COMMON SHOULDER CONDITIONS IN ATHLETES
Subacromial Impingement Syndrome

The shoulder's functional arc in both athletes and the general population is forward, not lateral, and impingement of the rotator cuff, biceps tendon, and subacromial

bursa occurs against the anterior edge of the acromion, coracoacromial ligament, and undersurface of the acromioclavicular joint.[44] It is important to understand that the supraspinatus tendon, long head of the biceps, subacromial bursa, and sometimes the acromioclavicular joint are involved in the impingement process.[45] (Fig. 6-9) The space available for the rotator cuff to pass beneath the coracoacromial arch is limited. Therefore any processes that increase the volume of structures that pass beneath the coracoacromial arch or decrease the space available for the supraspinatus and biceps tendons will result in irritation of the cuff, biceps tendon, and subacromial bursa, leading to impingement. In athletes the usual mechanism is an increase in volume by (1) hypertrophy of the musculotendinous structures or (2) a local inflammatory response, incited by microtrauma, that causes edema and thickening of the cuff and subacromial bursa. Throwing, by virtue of its force, velocity, and repetition, predisposes the shoulder to impingement by either of the aforementioned mechanisms. In the older athlete, a diminution of the size of the subacromial space is more common. Anterior acromial osteophytes, enlargement of the greater tuberosity, inferior distal clavicular spurs, proximal migration of the humeral head, and rotator cuff degeneration can be coconspirators in exacerbating the impingement process.

Impingement is described in three progressive stages: stage I, edema and hemorrhage; stage II, fibrosis and tendinitis; and stage III, bone spurs and tendon ruptures.[45] Jobe modified this classification into four stages, with stage III divided into cuff tears of less than 1 cm and stage IV consisting of cuff tears of greater than 1 cm.[31]

Stage I impingement. Overuse from throwing sports causes microtrauma that produces supraspinatus and bursal edema and hemorrhage. This stage is prevalent in young athletes (younger than 25 years of age) and responds well to activity modification and conservative treatment (reversible lesion).

Stage II impingement. Several bouts of repeated mechanical irritation and inflammation (stage I impingement) may cause the subacromial bursa to become fibrotic and thicken. This and supraspinatus and/or biceps tendinitis are the prominent features of stage II. This stage is common in an older age group (25 to 40 years of age) and is usually responsive to conservative measures.

Stage III impingement. Typically, this stage presents in persons over 40 years of age with a past history of multiple episodes of subacromial impingement symptoms. The hallmark of this stage is the presence of a rotator cuff tear and associated anterior acromion osteophytes, greater tuberosity enlargement, and, sometimes, inferior distal clavicular spurs. It is thought that repeated traction from the deltoid and supraspinatus muscles cause the anomalies of the anterior acromion and greater tuberosity. Conservative treatment of stage III lesions can be rewarding in the elderly patient; however, in athletes it usually fails, and surgical management is generally indicated.

Stage IV impingement. A stage IV impingement lesion has a rotator cuff tear that is larger than 1 cm. In athletes, surgical management is necessary.

Anterior Instability With Secondary Impingement

Anterior instability producing secondary impingement is unique to groups of young (ages 18 to 35 years), throwing athletes, especially pitchers. Most throwing problems commonly seen during training are related to overuse of the rotator cuff (pure impingement). However, in a select group, unrecognized anterior instability, or silent subluxation, is becoming more apparent as our index of suspicion and diagnostic ability improve. A delicate balance exists between mobility and stability, which makes the shoulder susceptible to injury when stressed by high athletic stresses. A pathologic condition will ensue when (1) chronic overuse causes the physiologic healing response to lag behind the repetitive microtrauma, (2) prolonged throwing causes increased external rotation with subsequent attenuation of the anterior capsule and associated subluxation, or (3) an imbalance in the shoulder's four-joint complex causes altered throwing mechanics and added anterior strain.[28]

The concept to understand in young overhand athletes is one of a progressive continuum of shoulder pathology: overuse leads to microtrauma, which leads to instability, which leads to subluxation, which leads to impingement, which finally terminates in a rotator cuff tear. This cascade is known as the instability complex.[6,29,30]

The typical presentation is a young high-caliber overhand athlete with long-standing insidious shoulder pain that has increased in intensity, resulting in an alteration in performance. The pain may be anterior or (sometimes) posterior and is maximal during the late-cocking or acceleration phase of throwing. Physical examination demonstrates positive anteroinferior subluxation and relocation tests, impingement signs, and symptoms that are usually overshadowed by the patient's cognizant feeling of subluxation.

On the basis of the history, physical, and arthroscopic findings, the athletes can be divided into one of four groups. Group I consists of those with pure and isolated impingement and no instability; typically these are older athletes. In group II are those with impingement findings with concurrent instability resulting from labral and capsular repetitive microtrauma; this is the most common group. Group III consists of those who have impingement findings and associated instability caused by hyperelasticity and a lax joint. In group IV are those with isolated instability without impingement findings. Treatment in all four groups initially requires a specific supervised rehabilitation program as described by Jobe and Bradley.[28,29]

Rotator Cuff Tension Failure Without Impingement

Distinguishing rotator cuff (supraspinatus) tension failure from incomplete rotator cuff tears secondary to progressive impingement is extremely difficult in throwing athletes. In both situations the athletes have impingement symptoms, one or more positive impingement signs, and, commonly, a positive impingement test result (subacromial lidocaine injection). No conclusive evidence by either history or physical examination has proved to be diagnostic. Arthroscopy has proved to be very beneficial in the diagnosis of this problem; diagnostic arthroscopy has revealed a small linear, incomplete undersurface tear of the supraspinatus muscle, paralleling the greater tuberosity at or near its insertion. The subacromial space has no signs of an inflammatory process typical of subacromial impingement. The appropriate treatment is not yet known, but we advocate conservative management.

Acromioclavicular Problems

Acute traumatic acromioclavicular injuries are usually easily apparent to the examiner by the history, physical findings, and radiographic findings. Treatment is dependent on the type of injury, but for most types of acute acromioclavicular injuries, conservative management is generally advocated in athletes.

Repetitive impact loading may cause idiopathic osteolysis of the clavicle. This syndrome is associated especially with weight lifters and is sometimes difficult to diagnose in its early stages.[7,10]

Degenerative problems and spurring within the acromioclavicular joint can be more troublesome and can mimic several shoulder maladies (Fig. 6-10). Clinically, degenerative acromioclavicular problems usually localize to the joint itself; however, they may cause mechani-

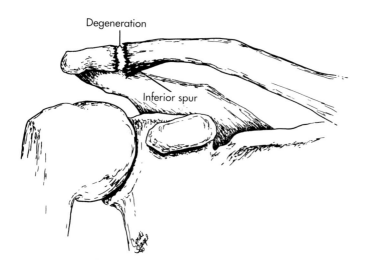

Fig. 6-10. Acromioclavicular joint degeneration—the great impersonator.

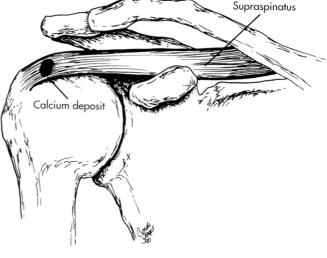

Fig. 6-11. Typical location of calcific (bursitis) tendonitis.

cal pain radiating toward the lateral border of the acromion or into the neck and trapezius.[4,49] Three maneuvers help to isolate this process: (1) direct palpation, (2) an anterior provocative test, and (3) a posterior provocative test as described in the physical examination section of this chapter. A local injection of 1 to 2 ml of lidocaine may help to verify the diagnosis by temporarily eliminating the pain during these maneuvers.

In the event that clinical and radiographic evidence of acromioclavicular degeneration is present and unresponsive to conservative measures, a Mumford's procedure can produce rewarding results (resection of the distal 1 to 2 cm of the clavicle).

Biceps Tendinitis

Anterior shoulder pain associated with Speed's sign and/or Yergason's sign directs attention to the biceps tendon as a possible source for the patient's pain. Although inflammation may be localized to the biceps tendon, the problem is far more commonly one of impingement, with biceps tendinitis constituting only a small component of a greater problem. Ruptures of the long head of the biceps, at the top of the bicipital groove, are commonly associated with impingement in middle-aged athletes. Conversely, in very young athletes tears at the musculotendinous junction have been reported.[5,35] Treatment should be directed toward alleviating the impingement process as described earlier. We do not believe that primary biceps tenodesis should be performed in athletes.[69]

Frozen Shoulder (Adhesive Capsulitis)

The etiology of frozen shoulder is not well understood; however, any stage of impingement syndrome may produce this process. Therefore it is important to ex-

clude the many other causes of frozen shoulder before implying that it is secondary to a primary pathologic condition of the shoulder. These other conditions include cervical spine lesions, diabetes, autoimmune disease, cerebrovascular accident (CVA), immobilization, myocardial infarction, calcific tendinitis, and thyroid disorders.[22,24,58] Most cases will resolve with physical therapy and attention to the underlying cause; however, patients with diabetes seem to have a prolonged course of recovery.

Calcific Bursitis

Clinical findings of chronic calcific bursitis are analogous to impingement findings, and a distinction based on the history and physical findings alone is difficult. Conversely, acute calcific bursitis produces a lancinating shoulder pain that is quite characteristic, paralleled only by gout, pseudogout, and nerve injuries of the shoulder. Many investigators believe that a metabolic rather than local rotator cuff degenerative process may be the etiologic factor.[23,53] In support of this is the finding that calcification is rarely observed in association with degenerative rotator cuff disease.[24] Radiographic findings show calcification of the supraspinatus and/or infraspinatus tendons (Fig. 6-11). No correlation has been found between the size of the deposit and the symptoms.[76] Many other conditions may produce periarticular calcifications, including gout, hypervitaminosis D, hyperparathyroidism, renal osteodystrophy, collagen vascular disease, pseudogout, and humeral calcinosis.[57] The natural history progresses from a precalcific stage (fibrocartilage metaplasia) to a calcific phase (calcium deposition and stabilization), followed by a postcalcific stage (resorption and reconstitution).[70] Treatment is conservative, and a subacromial steroid injection is sometimes helpful during an acute flare.

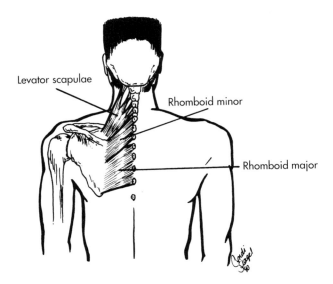

Fig. 6-12. Anatomy of superior medial scapula.

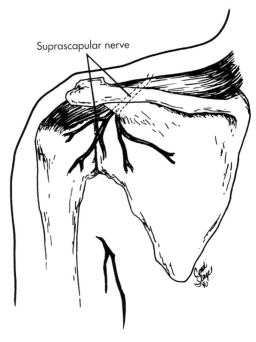

Fig. 6-13. Suprascapular nerve anatomy.

Levator Scapulae Syndrome

Characteristically, levator scapulae syndrome is a local tendinitis of the insertion of the levator scapulae localized to the superior medial scapula (Fig. 6-12). The pain is deep, and the athlete usually cannot isolate the primary site of pain. When the symptoms localize to the scapular border, a neck evaluation is helpful to rule out referred pain from the cervical spine. Golf, swimming, boxing, wrestling, gymnastics, karate, and weight lifting have all been implicated.[17] An acute or chronic overload of the insertion of the levator is thought to be the mechanism of injury. Physical examination helps to segregate the maximal tenderness to the area of the insertion of the levator scapulae in the posterior shoulder. Typically, the patient's symptoms abate with a specific course of physical therapy and a steroid injection at the levator insertion.

Scapulothoracic Bursitis

Situated at the inferomedial angle of the scapula, the scapulothoracic bursa can become inflamed, especially in baseball pitchers. This condition is secondary to repetitive, high-velocity microtrauma applied to the anterior surface of the scapula, the underlying musculature, and the rib cage.[61] Classically, the pain is localized to the inferior angle of the scapula during the cocking and acceleration stages of pitching and is alleviated at follow-through. Sometimes a mass can be palpated at the intermedial angle of the scapula. Commonly, elevation to 60 degrees and forward flexion to 30 degrees enhances the examiner's ability to palpate the bursal sac. Range of motion is not usually affected. An association with impingement and/or anterior instability has been shown. Treatment is conservative; however, in recalcitrant cases a steroid injection into the bursa has been beneficial; rarely, excision of the bursa is necessary.

NEUROLOGIC PROBLEMS
Suprascapular Nerve Entrapment

Generally, suprascapular nerve entrapment (C5-6) occurs in the suprascapular notch; however, in the throwing athlete, the nerve is commonly compressed distally as it journeys around the base of the scapular spine to innervate the infraspinatus muscle (Fig. 6-13). Volleyball spikers seem to have an increased incidence of isolated distal palsies.[19] The pain pattern is varied and is commonly diagnosed as an impingement process. Careful physical examination will show atrophy and weakness of the infraspinatus, but a normal-functioning supraspinatus. Because of this weakness, a secondary impingement syndrome may occur concomitantly. Surgical decompression of this lesion has not proved to be beneficial in athletes. Treatment is centered on maximizing the residual infraspinatus muscle function while concurrently strengthening the remaining of the rotator cuff. The pain will typically decrease with this exercise program, and the athletes commonly are able to resume full competition.[69]

Long Thoracic Nerve Injury

Tension injuries to the long thoracic nerve (C5 to C7) produces winging of the scapula. Prolonged use of a backpack or falling with a backpack has been associated with this lesion. Overhead weight lifters also have an increased incidence of this palsy.[65] The diagnosis is made by having the patient do a wall push-up and observing the scapula being separated from the rib cage. The associated serratus anterior muscle weakness causes a dysfunction of scapular protraction with shoulder

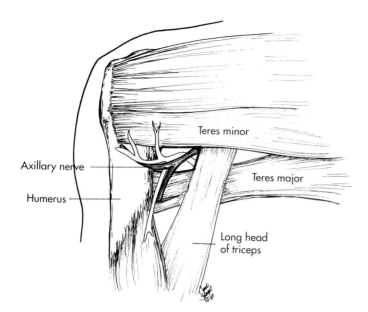

Fig. 6-14. Quadrilateral space.

elevation. Scapulothoracic and glenohumeral asynchrony ensues, initiated by poor protraction of the scapula and, therefore, inadequate elevation of the acromion, causing a decrease in the available clearance for the cuff tendons. This asynchrony predisposes the athlete to impingement syndrome, which can be very resistant. Treatment entails a physical therapy program to strengthen the scapular rotators, specifically the serratus anterior.

Quadrilateral Space Syndrome

Quadrilateral space syndrome is caused by compression of the axillary nerve and posterior humeral circumflex artery in the quadrilateral space (Fig. 6-14). The symptomatology is insidious, consisting of periodic pain and paresthesias in the upper extremity.[13] Aggravation of the symptoms is caused by forward flexion and/or abduction and external rotation of the humerus. Throwing athletes, especially pitchers, seem most susceptible.[48] The pain is poorly localized to the anterior and/or lateral shoulder, and paresthesias are sometimes experienced in a nondermatomal pattern.[11,48] Direct palpation about the quadrilateral space causes pain, and hyperabduction and external rotation cause the pain to increase after several minutes. A subclavian arthrogram can be diagnostic by demonstrating a patent posterior humeral circumflex artery while the arm is at the side and occlusion of the artery with the humerus hyperabducted and externally rotated.[11,13,42,48] Occlusion of the artery indirectly indicates compression of the axillary nerve by fibrous bands that tether the quadrilateral space.[11,48] Initially, conservative treatment is indicated; failure may require a surgical decompression of the quadrilateral space.[11,13,42,48]

Referred Pain

It is extremely important to remember that all shoulder pain does not indicate a primary pathologic condition of the shoulder. A meticulous history and examination will often uncover symptoms and/or signs that are not consistent with primary shoulder pathology.

The character of the pain may guide the orthopaedist to the site of pathology. Cervical spine pain is the most common referred pain in the shoulder. It is characterized by a deep burning or aching pain localized to the insertion of the levator scapula or rhomboids. Radicular pain or paresthesias in the fingers or, less frequently, the forearm support the diagnosis. A pathologic condition of the cervical spine may occur concomitantly with shoulder pathology. Usually, primary shoulder pathology will not present with pain extending below the elbow. Distinction between the two entities is often troublesome and may require further testing. A good guideline is to ask the patient to localize the site of maximal pain; if the patient cups the hand over the top of the shoulder, proximal to the lateral acromion, then a cervical spine abnormality should be investigated. Conversely, if the patient localizes the pain about or distal to the lateral acromion, a primary shoulder problem should first be considered. Spurling's, Valsalva's, and distraction tests, which are described earlier, have proved to be helpful in our hands to differentiate between the entities. To help clarify a diagnostic dilemma, additional radiographs, arthrography, electromyographic studies, computed tomography (CT) scans, and magnetic resonance imaging (MRI) have all proved to be beneficial.

Cervical pathologic conditions that present as shoulder pain include (1) cervical arthrosis, (2) spondylosis, (3) foraminal osteophytes, (4) herniated discs, and (5) syringomyelia.

A C5-6 disc herniation presents in much the same way as either a suprascapular nerve entrapment or a rotator cuff tear. Each presents with atrophy and weakness of the spinalis muscles in external rotation; an arthrogram, electromyogram (EMG), and nerve conduction studies or MRI may be helpful in these cases.

Although rare, pain referred from the pleural cavity can present a diagnostic problem. Horner's syndrome (ptosis, miosis, anhidrosis, and enophthalmos) may sometimes be the first clue to a superior sulcus tumor. Routine radiographs should always include the ipsilateral lung field to assess possible pulmonary lesions, especially Pancoast's tumor. Pulmonary infarction causes shoulder pain (mediated by the phrenic nerve) secondary to diaphragmatic irritation.

Thoracic outlet syndrome (TOS) is caused by compression of the neurovascular bundle at or near the thoracic outlet. A multitude of symptoms such as pain, paresthesias, dysesthesias, numbness, weakness, atrophy, and temperature changes have been described.[29] Women of childbearing age have a much higher incidence of TOS.[37] Adson's, costoclavicular, and hyperabduction maneuvers can aid in making this difficult diagnosis.

Gastric, pancreatic, cardiac, gallbladder, and hepatic referred shoulder pain have been described.[29] Gastric and pancreatic diseases tend to refer pain to the interscapular region, whereas gallbladder and hepatic problems refer pain over the top of the shoulder with concomitant tenderness and scapular pain.[22] Cardiac ischemic pain usually radiates to the neck in the clavicular region, through the shoulder, and down the medial border of the left arm.[22] Because of the large variation in presentation and symptom patterns, it is prudent not to assume that all shoulder pain in the athlete is always indicative of a pathologic condition of the shoulder.

REFERENCES

1. Aulicino PL: Neurovascular injuries in the hands of athletes, *Hand Clin* 6:455, 1990.
2. Bassett FH, Nunley JA: Compression of the musculocutaneous nerve at the elbow, *J Bone Joint Surg* 64A:1050, 1982.
3. Bateman JE: Neurologic painful conditions affecting the shoulder, *Clin Orthop* 173:55, 1983.
4. Bergfeld JA, Andrish JT, Clancy WG: Evaluation of the acromioclavicular joint following first- and second-degree sprains, *Am J Sports Med* 6:153, 1978.
5. Bosworth DM: The supraspinatus syndrome: symptomatology, pathology, and repair, *JAMA* 116:2477, 1941.
6. Bradley JP, Perry J, Jobe FW: The biomechanics of the throwing shoulder, *Perspect Orthop* (in press).
7. Brunet ME et al: Atraumatic osteolysis of the distal clavicle: histologic evidence of synovial pathogenesis, *Orthopedics* 9:557, 1986.
8. Buckhont BC, Warner MA: Digital perfusion of handball players: effects of repeated ball impact on structures of the hand, *Am J Sports Med* 8:206, 1980.
9. Cabrera JM, McCue FC III: Nonosseous athletic injuries of the elbow, forearm and hand, *Clin Sports Med* 5:681, 1986.
10. Cahill BR: Osteolysis of the distal part of the clavicle in male athletes, *J Bone Joint Surg* 64A:1053, 1982.
11. Cahill BR, Palmer RE: Quadrilateral space syndrome, *J Hand Surg* 8A:65, 1983.
12. Carroll RE, Hurst LC: The relationship of thoracic outlet syndrome and carpal tunnel syndrome, *Clin Orthop* 164:149, 1982.
13. Cormier PJ, Matalon TAS, Wolin PM: Quadrilateral space syndrome: a rare cause of shoulder pain, *Radiology* 167:797, 1988.
14. Dellon AL, Mackinnon SE: Radial sensory nerve entrapment in the forearm, *J Hand Surg* 11A:199, 1986.
15. Dobyns JH, Sim FH, Linscheid RL: Sports stress syndromes of the hand and wrist, *Am J Sports Med* 6:236, 1978.
16. Ehrlich W, Dellon AL, Mackinnon SE: Cheiralgia paraesthetica (entrapment of the radial sensory nerve), *J Hand Surg* 11A:196, 1986.
17. Estwanik JJ: Levator scapulae syndrome, *Physician Sportsmed* 17(10):57, 1989.
18. Feindel W, Strafford J: The role of the cubital tunnel in tardy ulnar palsy, *Can J Surg* 1:287, 1958.
19. Ferretti A, Cerullo G, Russo G: Suprascapular neuropathy in volleyball players, *J Bone Joint Surg* 69A:260, 1987.
20. Gelberman RH, Hergenroeder PT, Hargeus AR: The carpal tunnel syndrome: a study of carpal canal pressures, *J Bone Joint Surg* 63A:380, 1981.

21. Glousman RE: Ulnar nerve problems in the athlete's elbow, *Clin Sports Med* 9:365, 1990.
22. Hawkins RJ, Bokor DJ: Clinical evaluation of shoulder problems. In Matsen R: *The shoulder,* Philadelphia, 1990, WB Saunders.
23. Hawkins RJ, Hobeika PE: Impingement syndrome in the athletic shoulder, *Clin Sports Med* 2:391, 1983.
24. Hawkins RJ, Kennedy JC: Impingement syndrome in athletes, *Am J Sports Med* 8:151, 1980.
25. Hershman EB, Wilbourn AS, Bergenfeld JA: Acute brachial neuropathy in athletes, *Am J Sports Med* 17:655, 1989.
26. Hill NA, Howard FM, Huffer BR: The incomplete anterior interosseous nerve syndrome, *J Hand Surg* 10A:4, 1985.
27. Hiraswa Y, Sakakida K: Sports and peripheral nerve injury, *Am J Sports Med* 11:420, 1983.
28. Jobe FW, Bradley JP: Rotator cuff injuries in baseball: prevention and rehabilitation, *Sports Med* 6:377, 1988.
29. Jobe FW, Bradley JP: The diagnosis and nonoperative treatment of shoulder injuries in athletes, *Clin Sports Med* 8:419, 1989.
30. Jobe FW, Bradley JP: The treatment of impingement syndrome in overhand athletes. I. A philosophical basis, *Surg Rounds Orthop* 4:19, 1990.
31. Jobe FW, Jobe CM: Painful athletic injuries of the shoulder, *Clin Orthop* 173:117, 1983.
32. Johnson RK, Spinner M, Shrewsbury MM: Median nerve entrapment syndrome in the proximal forearm, *J Hand Surg* 4A:48, 1979.
33. Kummel BM, Zazanis GA: Shoulder pain as the presenting complaint in carpal tunnel syndrome, *Clin Orthop* 92:227, 1973.
34. Layfer LF, Jones JV: Hand paresthesias after racquetball, *Ill Med J* 190:191, 1977.
35. Leach RE, Schepsis AA: Shoulder pain, *Clin Sports Med* 2:123, 1983.
36. Leffert RD: Diabetes mellitus initially presenting as peripheral neuropathy in the upper limb, *J Bone Joint Surg* 51A:1005, 1969.
37. Leffert RD, Gumley G: The relationship between dead arm syndrome and thoracic outlet syndrome, *Clin Orthop* 223:20, 1987.
38. Lister GD, Belsole RB, Kleinert HE: The radial tunnel syndrome, *J Hand Surg* 4A:52, 1979.
39. Lotem M et al: Radial palsy following muscular effort: a nerve compression syndrome possibly related to a fibrous arch of the lateral band of the triceps, *J Bone Joint Surg* 53B:500, 1971.
40. Massey EW, Riley T, Pleet AB: Coexistent carpal tunnel syndrome and cervical radiculopathy (double crush syndrome), *South Med J* 74:957, 1981.
41. McCue FC et al: Hand and wrist injuries in the athlete, *Am J Sports Med* 7:275, 1979.
42. McKowen JC, Voorhies RM: Axillary nerve entrapment in the quadrilateral space: case report, *J Neurosurg* 66:932, 1987.
43. Moss SH, Switzer HE: Radial tunnel syndrome: a spectrum of clinical presentations, *J Hand Surg* 8A:414, 1983.
44. Neer CS II: Anterior acromioplasty for the chronic impingement syndrome in the shoulder, *J Bone Joint Surg* 54A:41, 1972.
45. Neer CS II, Welsh RP: The shoulder in sports, *Orthop Clin North Am* 9:583, 1977.
46. Nuber GW et al: Arterial abnormalities of the hand in athletes, *Am J Sports Med* 18:520, 1990.
47. Omer GE, Spinner M: *Management of peripheral nerve problems,* Philadelphia, 1980, WB Saunders.
48. Pedler MR, Ruland LJ III, McCue FC III: Quadrilateral space syndrome in a throwing athlete, *Am J Sports Med* 14:511, 1986.
49. Penny JN, Welsh RP: Shoulder impingement syndromes in athletes and their surgical management, *Am J Sports Med* 9:11, 1981.
50. Phalen GS: The carpal tunnel syndrome: clinical evaluation of 598 hands, *Clin Orthop* 83:29, 1972.
51. Porubsky GL, Brown SI, Urbaniak JR: Ulnar artery thrombosis: a sports related injury, *Am J Sports Med* 14:170, 1986.

52. Posner MA: Compressive neuropathies of the median and radial nerves at the elbow, *Clin Sports Med* 9:343, 1990.

53. Resnick CS, Resnick D: Crystal deposition disease, *Semin Arthritis Rheum* 2(4):39B, 1983.

54. Rettig AC: Neurovascular injuries in the wrists and hands of athletes, *Clin Sports Med* 9:389, 1990.

55. Roles NC, Maudsley RH: Radial tunnel syndrome: resistant tennis elbow as a nerve entrapment, *J Bone Joint Surg* 54B:499, 1972.

56. Rowe CR: Recurrent transient anterior subluxation of the shoulder: the "dead arm" syndrome, *Clin Orthop* 223:11, 1987.

57. Rowe CR: Tendinitis, bursitis, impingement "snapping scapula and calcific bursitis." In Rowe CR: *The shoulder,* New York, 1988, Churchill Livingstone.

58. Rowe CR, Leffert RD: Idiopathic chronic adhesive capsulitis ("frozen shoulder"). In Rowe CR: *The shoulder,* New York, 1988, Churchill Livingstone.

59. Rowe CR, Zarins B: Recurrent transient subluxation of the shoulder, *J Bone Joint Surg* 63A:863, 1981.

60. Shea JD, McClain EJ: Ulnar nerve compression syndromes at and below the wrist, *J Bone Joint Surg* 51A:1095, 1969.

61. Sisto DJ, Jobe FW: The operative treatment of scapulothoracic bursitis in professional pitchers, *Am J Sports Med* 14:192, 1986.

62. Speer KP, Bassett FH: The prolonged burner syndrome, *Am J Sports Med* 18:591, 1990.

63. Spinner M: The arcade of Frohse and its relationship to posterior interosseous nerve paralysis, *J Bone Joint Surg* 50B:809, 1968.

64. Spinner M: *Injuries to the major branches of peripheral nerves of the forearm,* 2 ed, Philadelphia, 1978, WB Saunders.

65. Stanish WD, Lamb H: Isolated paralysis of the serratus anterior muscle: a weight training injury, *Am J Sports Med* 6:385, 1978.

66. Stark HH et al: Fracture of the hook of the hamate, *J Bone Joint Surg* 71A:1202, 1989.

67. Stern PJ: Tendinitis, overuse, syndrome and tendon injuries, *Hand Clin* 6:467, 1990.

68. Suguwara M et al: Digital ischemia in baseball players, *Am J Sports Med* 14:329, 1986.

69. Tibone JE, Bradley JP: Management of resistant subacromial impingement lesions in competitive athletes, Unpublished manuscript, 1990.

70. Unthoff HK, Sarkar K: Calcifying tendonitis. In Rockwood M: *The shoulder,* Philadelphia, 1990, WB Saunders.

71. Upton RM, McComas AJ: The double crush in nerve-entrapment syndromes, *Lancet* ii:359, 1973.

72. Verhaar J, Spaans F: Radial tunnel syndrome: an investigation of compression neuropathy as a possible cause, *J Bone Joint Surg* 73A:539, 1991.

73. Vogel CM, Jensen JE: "Effort" thrombosis of the subclavian vein in competitive swimmer, *Am J Sports Med* 13:269, 1985.

74. Wadsworth TG: The external compression syndrome of the ulnar nerve at the cubital tunnel, *Clin Orthop* 124:189, 1977.

75. Watkins RG: Neck injuries in football players, *Clin Sports Med* 5:215, 1986.

76. Weiss J: The painful shoulder. In Kelly WN et al, editors: *Textbook of rheumatology,* Philadelphia, 1981, WB Saunders.

77. Wood MB, Dobyns JH: Sports related extra-articular wrist syndromes, *Clin Orthop* 202:93, 1986.

78. Yocum LA: Assessing the shoulder: history, physical examination, differential diagnosis, and special tests used, *Clin Sports Med* 2:281, 1983.

79. Zemel NP, Jobe FW, Yocum LA: Submuscular transposition/ulnar nerve decompression in athletes. In Gelberman RH, editor: *Operative nerve repair and reconstruction,* Philadelphia, 1991, JB Lippincott.

Chapter Seven

◆

History, Physical Examination, and Diagnostic Tests for Back and Lower Extremity Problems

Robert G. Watkins

Along with an understanding of the morphologic changes in the spine and the potential sources of pain, the history and physical examination are the key to relating the science of spinal pain to the patient. The commonly used diagnostic tests, such as plain x-ray films, computed tomography (CT) scans, and myelograms, demonstrate the morphology of the spine. These tests can show pathologic anatomy capable of producing pain. Surgery should be directly correlated to the anatomic pathologic changes and the patient's complaints and findings, as well as limited to the areas of morbidity. These limits are set during the history, physical examination, and testing.

To obtain a proper history and perform an appropriate physical examination, the examiner should follow a standardized form that focuses on the following objectives (see Appendix):

I. Quantitate the morbidity. Use a value scale to quantify the pain, function, and occupation in order to understand how sick the patient is (see box on p. 79). Converse in detail with the patient to detect the patient's inflections and manner as he or she describes the pain.

II. Delineate the psychosocial factors. Know what psychologic effect the pain has had on the patient. Understand the social, economic, and legal ramifications of the patient's disability. Be aware of what can be gained by the patient's being sick or healthy. Determine what role these factors play in the patient's complaints. At the Kerlan-Jobe Orthopaedic Clinic we use the Oswestry pain-rating scale. Each patient completes a pain drawing using the rating system, which distinguishes organic from psychologic pain fairly well. The pain drawing helps to accomplish the goals of the physical examination and localizes the symptoms for future reference.[9,14]

III. Eliminate the possibility of tumors, infections, and neurologic crisis. These diseases require immediate attention according to a therapeutic regimen very different from that for disc disease.

IV. Diagnose the clinical syndrome. Note the following definitions:

A. *Nonmechanical back or neck pain* — Inflammatory, constant pain, minimally affected by activity, usually worse at night or early morning

B. *Mechanical back or neck and/or leg or arm pain* — Made worse by activity and relieved by rest

1. *Sciatica* — Predominantly radicular leg pain, positive stretch signs, with or without neurologic deficit

2. *Cervical radiculopathy* — Predominantly arm pain in a dermatomal distribution made worse by neck extension and rotation and relieved by putting the arm behind the head

3. *Neurogenic claudication* — Radiating leg pain or calf pain made worse with ambulation; negative stretch signs, made worse with spinal extension and relieved with flexion

4. *Cervical myelopathy* — Wide-based gait, loss of agility, stumbling, hand numbness, loss of finger function or bowel and bladder control

The other important determinations to be made are as follows:

1. What level or neuromotion segment is involved?
2. What nerve is involved?
3. What pathologic condition is involved? What is the exact structure or disease process in that neuromotion segment that is causing the pain?

The history and physical examination are the first steps to take in determining the clinical syndrome and determining appropriate treatment.

CAUSES OF SPINAL PAIN

Spinal pain usually results from injury or from noxious stimuli to the spinal nerve or the joints of the spine. The usual source of such stimuli lies in the structure and biomechanics of the intervertebral disc and its neuromotion segment. A neuromotion segment is defined as an intervertebral disc, its adjacent vertebral body endplates, two facet joints, and the nerves, vessels, ligaments, and muscles functioning in conjunction with those structures.

Motion and Function

Every spinal motion segment undergoes certain morphologic changes as a result of acute or chronic injury or age.[2] Nociceptors present in the spine translate pathophysiologic and biomechanical abnormalities related to these morphologic changes into pain.[3] Critical for the transition from morphology to pain is function. Function is expressed by motion and activity in a living human. Function studied scientifically is the biomechanics of spinal motion. From a person bending over, to straight leg raising, to abnormal motion present in a damaged disc, these functional biomechanics are what connects morphology to pain. Current understanding of the normal motion and stress in a living spinal motion segment is rudimentary. The concepts of dysfunction, instability, and restabilization form a reasonable view of the sequence of events that translate morphology into pain,[7] but a biomechanical definition of dysfunction, instability, and stabilization is vague.

Spinal Instability

Spinal instability in spinal injuries is best defined as the inability of the structural integrity of the spinal column to prevent neurologic deficit.[7] This instability is usually caused by one major injury. It represents a defect in the biomechanical functioning of a neuromotion segment that results in pain. The segmental motion present in spinal instability is not necessarily excessive motion but rather abnormal motion. This biomechanical abnormality in the intervertebral disc and its neuromotion segment can be caused by a single, acute injury; repeated, multiple traumas; or wear and tear over time.

Disc damage. An intervertebral disc may be damaged by various combined stresses and loads.[15] Rotational loading and axial loading are common mechanisms of injury to an intervertebral disc. The resulting damage may be a circumferential or radial tear in the annulus fibrosus, fractures in the vertebral body end-plate, or avulsion of the annulus from the end-plate. A single high-strain rate rotation of 15 to 20 degrees of body motion or 3 degrees of forced axial rotation in the neuromotion segment can produce annular injury in the lumbar disc.[4] The disc transforms compression into radially directed tensile forces in the annulus. Torsion, bending, and forced rotation can produce disc rupture and nuclear extrusion. The posterolateral corner is probably more vulnerable because of the shape of the disc, the axis of rotation, and the resultant force vectors. This is the usual location for the earliest changes of disc degenerations that result from repeated small annular tears and for eventual disc herniations.

Change in disc morphology changes joint kinematics.[1,5,11] A damaged disc does not exhibit the same mechanical behavior that it did before it was injured and the degenerative process began. A degenerative disc has less viscoelasticity, so it distributes stress less evenly.

Motion, such as twisting or bending, may produce an axis change and an abnormal rotational pattern in the damaged neuromotion segment. That abnormal motion produces friction. Friction increases inflammation, producing pain from pain fibers in the annulus and the facet joints. In a similar fashion, a torn shoulder rotator cuff produces mechanical dysfunction, inflammation, and pain.

The total amount of motion is irrelevant to this pain-producing process. The micromotion of the neuromotion segment is altered, producing a mechanical dysfunction. Most investigators have found the correlation between disc degeneration and a specific amount of spinal motion to be poor.[10,12] As in a knee pyarthrosis, an inflamed joint moves very little, but what motion there is produces an extreme amount of pain. In cases of an acute isolated disc resorption or an infected disc, it is the stiff, poorly moving segment that is painful, not the hypermobile joints above that may be moving more to compensate for the inflamed joint. Measuring the total amount of flexion/extension in a damaged spinal segment may correlate little with the origin of the patient's pain. Abnormal motion may be only a change in the axis of rotation, not an increase in the flexion/extension range of motion.

There is no good way to measure pain-producing micromotion. A logical sequence is that damage produces abnormal motion, leading to inflammation, which leads to pain with any motion in the segment. Pain with any motion leads to reflex muscle spasm and joint stiffness. Abnormal motion resulting from damaged articular structures produces posttraumatic scar, stiffness, and osteophytic changes of localized degenerative arthritis. The eventual loss of range of motion accompanying the osteophytic changes allows the painful motion to dissipate and the neuromotion segment to stabilize. The concept of dysfunction, instability, and stabilization as a chronologic sequence applies very well to this sequence of events.[8]

Disc degeneration. Disc degeneration is associated with biomechanical changes in the tissue of the disc, vascular changes in the subchondral bone of the vertebral end-plate, and changes in the type of mechanical stresses endured by that motion segment. There is difficulty in relating disc degeneration to any one specific injury, any certain testable mechanical alteration, and any specific amount of pain.

Understanding the relation of morphologic changes, such as disc degeneration, to pain is limited by our means of diagnosing disc degeneration. A degenerated disc may or may not demonstrate bulging on a CT scan.[15] Many of the discs that demonstrate bulging on CT scans are asymptomatic. Disc narrowing and osteopathic changes are generally accepted as changes of disc degeneration and may result from injury.[8] However, many degenerated discs are not narrowed,[11] and 53% of a group of pain-free persons showed degeneration on x-ray examination.[6]

The nerve root sleeves, the dural sac, the annulus of the disc, the posterior longitudinal ligament, and the facet joint capsules are richly innervated with sensory nerves. The biomechanical environment of the spinal column (i.e., the discs, bone, joints, and ligaments) is a major determinant of whether there will be spinal pain. Biomechanical stresses on the neurologic structure, such as the dural sac and nerve roots, also determine a major component of spinal pain.[13] This is especially true with the increase in leg pain associated with sciatica. Nerve root inflammation may result from compression, tension, or other noxious stimuli. The sudden appearance of a disc herniation into the spinal canal initially compresses and contuses the nerve root. The herniation becomes a space-occupying lesion around which the nerve root is stretched. The root and dural root sleeve are under tension: stretching the nerve—putting it under more tension by straight leg raises, foot dorsiflexion, or neck flexion—increases the pain from the inflamed, tense lumbar nerve. Lumbar extension produces radicular pain from foraminal stenosis or disc herniations that narrow the canal and foramina.

Spinal column extension produces smaller spinal canal and intervertebral foraminal diameters. The disc bulges posteriorly or in the direction of the motion, but the neurologic structures, the dura, and the nerve roots slacken and experience less tension on extension. Disc space collapse is usually accompanied by an annular bulge into the canal, but this can relieve root tension. Spinal column flexion has the opposite effect, causing larger canal diameters but greater root tension. With flexion, intradiscal pressure increases, but the disc bulges anteriorly.

If neurogenic claudication is caused by microvascular shunting from compressed nerve roots, the enlargement of canal and foraminal diameters with flexion may help explain why flexion relieves neurogenic claudication from spinal stenosis. The relief of root tension may explain why sciatica caused by acute disc herniation is alleviated by extension exercises that are done correctly. The criterion for a successful intraoperative decompression is relief of root tension that is tested by retractability. Understanding the biomechanical functioning of the neurologic column is critical to understanding the diagnosis and treatment of back and leg pain.[13]

HISTORY

Some key factors to be explored in the history are the percentage of back versus leg pain; a comparison of pain levels during walking, sitting, standing, and lying; the effects of Valsalva's maneuver, coughing, and sneezing on the pain; the type of injury and duration of the problem; and the time of day when the pain is worse. By means of the history, the examiner can determine whether the pain is caused by an axial (back or neck) or extremity (arm or leg) problem.

The classic history given for radiculopathy resulting from disc herniation is back or neck pain that progresses to predominantly leg or arm pain. It is made worse by increases in intraspinal pressure, such as occur with coughing, sneezing, and sitting. Extremity pain predominates over spinal pain, and mechanical factors increase the pain.

PHYSICAL EXAMINATION

The same questions that the history seeks to answer serve as the basis for the physical examination. The examination begins with the patient in the seated position and the physician seated on a low, movable stool in front of the patient (Fig. 7-1). Final aspects of the history are reviewed, a rapport is established with the patient, and a brief explanation of the examination is given. The physician checks the patellar, Achilles tendon, posterior tibia, and crossed adductor reflexes, followed by pinwheel, light touch, and vibratory sensation. The posterior tibia and dorsalis pedis pulses are checked, as well as motor function, foot dorsiflexion, toe dorsiflexion, foot inversion and eversion, Chaddock's reflex, Oppenheim's reflex, Babinski's reflex, and clonus with the knee flexed and extended. The physician then helps the patient extend each knee individually, the painless leg first. With the knee fully extended and the foot dorsiflexed, the Cram test is applied, and the patient is asked to slowly flex the chin to the chest (Fig. 7-2). The Cram test involves the examiner pushing on the sciatic nerve just medial to the lateral hamstring tendon. The

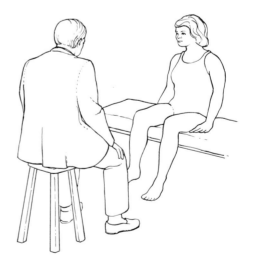

Fig. 7-1. The physician begins the examination sitting on a low stool to examine the feet of the patient. This is for both neck and low back pain. The examination begins with the assessment of the patellar and Achilles reflexes, sensation in the lower extremities, pulses in the lower extremities, straight leg raising, foot dorsiflexion, and motor function of the lower extremity below the knee.

patient is then asked to stand, and from a position behind the patient, the physician examines the bare back while the patient points directly to the source of the pain and to other tender areas. The physician palpates each of these tender areas and determines whether most tenderness is in the midline of the spine, in the paralumbar region, or in the sacroiliac joint, sacral notch, buttock, or costovertebral angle. Tender areas on the ribs and thoracic spine are evaluated.

Next the patient is evaluated for scoliosis and decompensation of T1 or the occiput to the gluteal cleft. Pelvic heights are evaluated for leg length differences. Chest expansion is checked when necessary. The gown is held together at the sacrum, and the patient is asked to bend forward, to the left, and to the right.

After the range of motion of the spine is evaluated, the patient is asked to place his or her hands against the wall and do repetitive toe raises, first bilaterally, then the right foot only, then the left foot only, to check for gastrocnemius weakness. Pain and restriction of range of motion are noted. The physician then clasps the patient's knees between the physician's knees, holds the pelvis, and asks the patient to extend the back, and the same notations are made.

Next the patient lies on a table with the head on a pillow and an additional sheet placed between the legs. This part of the examination begins with the hip flexed, the knee flexed, and the foot flat on the table (Fig. 7-3). The hip is slowly brought up to 90 degrees, and the knee is extended to 90 degrees; the patient is now in the hip 90-degree/knee 90-degree supine position. This is done first with the contralateral leg and then with the ipsilateral leg. The patient is checked for hip internal and external rotation, and pain with range of motion is noted. Patrick's (faber) test (Fig. 7-4) is then performed; this involves abduction and external rotation of the hip while the ankle is placed on the opposite knee. The lateral malleolus of the examined leg is placed on the opposite knee, and pressure is applied toward the table. Pain in the anterior hip joint area indicates a positive finding. Then the leg is returned to the 90-degree/90-degree position, and the knee is extended on the flexed hip. A notation is made as to whether this reproduces radicular pain. Then the foot is dorsiflexed, and the Cram test is performed (Fig. 7-5). Next the leg is brought down to the full knee-extended/hip-extended position, and straight leg raising is applied (Fig. 7-6). Again with foot dorsiflexion (Fig. 7-7), the Cram test and internal rotation are performed, and the presence or absence of radicular pain is noted.

Back pain may be reproduced with any of these straight leg raising maneuvers. Back pain absent in the sitting position and present in the supine position may be the result of rotation of the spine from straight leg raising in the supine position. The same process is then repeated with the ipsilateral, or painful, leg.

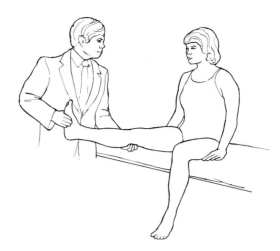

Fig. 7-2. With the patient in the sitting position, straight leg raising is checked; the patient is asked to flex the neck, and the physician dorsiflexes the foot, pushing on the lateral popliteal space on the sciatic nerve, which may or may not reproduce sciatica.

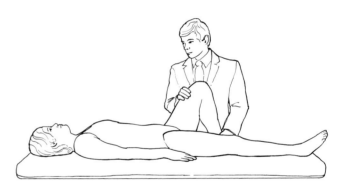

Fig. 7-3. After examination of the back with the patient standing, in which range of motion is checked and tender areas are evaluated, the patient is asked to lie supine on the table. The hip and knee are flexed initially, and the examination begins from this position.

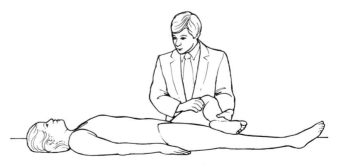

Fig. 7-4. Patrick's (faber) test involves flexion, abduction, and external rotation of the hip while the ankle is placed on the opposite knee. Groin pain reproduced with this maneuver indicates a pathologic condition of the hip joint. Back pain with the maneuver is not a positive finding.

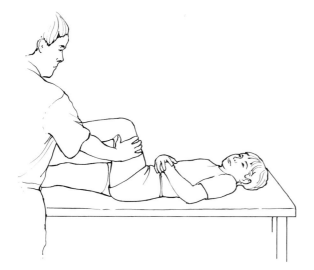

Fig. 7-5. With the hip and knee in the 90/90 position, range of motion in the hip is checked; then straight leg raising and the Laségue's test are performed. Extension of the knee on a flexed hip producing radiating leg pain constitutes a positive finding. The Cram test is a further check for pain by applying pressure on the sciatic nerve in the popliteal fossa just medial to the lateral hamstring tendon.

The patient is then asked to lie first on the right and then on the left side. The hip is extended to just past neutral with the knee extended (Fig. 7-8). The knee is flexed in that position to reproduce anterior thigh pain with a positive femoral stretch (Fig. 7-9). If there is a question, the patient is rolled prone, and with the knee flexed at 90 degrees, the hip is further extended past 90 degrees in an attempt to elicit anterior thigh pain of a positive femoral stretch.

Sensory examination of the buttocks and posterior area is performed. A rectal examination is performed when necessary. The rectal examination, when done for motor and sensory function, consists of evaluation first for sensation in the perianal and perineum area. Then the examiner checks for an anal wink reflex. Stroking beside the anus produces a puckering of the anus. The rectal digital examination begins by the physician inserting a lubricated, gloved finger and testing the resting tone; then the examiner asks the patient to squeeze the finger to test for voluntary control, cephalad, caudad, medially, and laterally. Next the bulbocavernosus reflex is checked by applying pressure on the glans, producing a reflex contraction of the anal musculature and asking

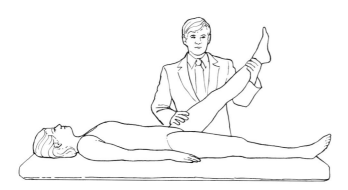

Fig. 7-6. Laségue's test is carried out; radiating pain produced with extension of the knee on the flexed hip is a positive finding, indicative of radiculitis.

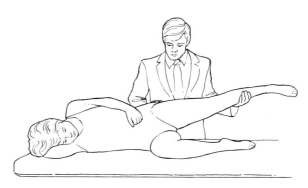

Fig. 7-8. Femoral stretch test. The patient is positioned on the side, and the hip is extended; then the knee is flexed on the extended hip. If this maneuver reproduces anterior thigh pain or radiating pain typical of the patient's femoral neuritis, then it is indicative of an upper lumbar root radiculitis.

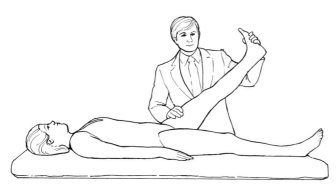

Fig. 7-7. Foot dorsiflexion from the straight leg position may further accentuate the problem.

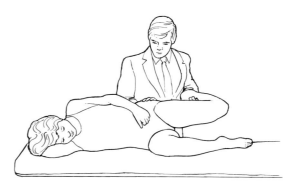

Fig. 7-9. Flexion of the knee on the extended hip.

if the patient can feel the finger. Finally, the patient is returned to the supine position, and an anterior sensory examination is carried out.

Stethoscopic evaluation for abdominal and femoral bruits, and femoral and popliteal pulses are carried out at this time, or an abdominal examination is performed when necessary. Additional evaluations for spasticity may be completed with the patient in the supine position and Chaddock's, Oppenheim's, Babinski's, and Clonus reflexes checked. The patient is then asked to sit, and the x-ray findings are discussed. Other tests may be included or excluded according to the patient's specific complaints.

In summary, the physical examination should address:
1. The presence of sciatic stretch signs or cervical radicular signs
2. The neurologic deficit
3. Neck or back and extremity stiffness and loss of range of motion
4. The exact location of tenderness and radiation of pain or paresthesias
5. Maneuvers during the examination that reproduce the pain

In the categories of back and leg pain, one must distinguish between referred pain and radicular pain. Pain in the disc, facet joint, or other structure of the neuromotion segment can be referred to the hip, buttock, or leg. The most common referred pain pattern from discogenic disease is from the paraspinous area to the sacroiliac joint across the posterior ilium to the trochanteric area. Pain may be referred to the leg, and facet blocks have relieved pain referred to the lower leg area. All leg pain is not true radiculopathy. In determining the percentage of back and leg pain, one considers the leg to include the muscle of the buttock and/or the thigh, lower leg, and foot. The percentage is based on the intensity and consistency of the pain. Dysesthesia in the leg is important, but one should concentrate on the percentage of the intensity of the pain—back versus leg.

Classic radiculopathy causes radicular pain radiating in a specific dermatomal pattern, with paresis, loss of sensation, and reflex loss. The radicular pattern of the pain and neurologic examination determine the nerve involved.

Physical examination also shows positive nerve mechanical signs. In lumbar disease, leg pain in a dermatomal distribution that is made worse by straight leg raising with the patient sitting or supine, foot-dorsal flexion, neck flexion, jugular compression, and direct palpation of the popliteal nerve or sciatic notch is characteristic of radiculopathy. A source of radicular pain not found in this description is that caused by spinal stenosis. Spinal stenosis usually lacks positive stretch signs but has the characteristic history of neurogenic claudication (i.e., leg and calf pain produced by ambu-

lation). Pain that does not go away immediately on stopping is made worse with spinal extension and is relieved by flexion. The pain progresses from proximal to distal.

DIAGNOSTIC TESTS

After the four objectives of the history and physical examination have been achieved (see box below), a succinct summary should be prepared delineating what nerve is affected, what level is involved, and what pathologic condition is present. Then the diagnostic studies can be used to pinpoint the specific origins of the clinical syndrome. The spinal pain/extremity pain ratio is an important factor in determining which diagnostic tests are indicated. The clinical syndrome should be divided into predominantly mechanical pain, nonmechanical pain, axial pain, and extremity pain.

The level of involvement can be evaluated by a discogram or magnetic resonance imaging (MRI). Almost every nerve can be injured or irritated by pathologic conditions at different levels. For example, an L5 radiculopathy is produced by an L4-5 posterolateral herniation, an L5-S1 lateral foraminal herniation, or, theoretically, a central herniation at L3-4. A central disc herniation of L4-5 may produce S1 symptoms; a posterolateral herniation may produce an L5 radiculopathy, and a foraminal herniation of L4-L5 may produce an L4 radiculopathy.

Tests are also used to direct treatment. The operative procedure may differ for different pathologic conditions at the same level and producing the same root symptoms. Table 7-1 demonstrates the typical radicular dysfunctions associated with each nerve root; see Fig. 19-3, *B*, for a demonstration of the location of potential noxious stimuli to each individual nerve.

Tests to Determine Treatment

The morbidity found on the history and physical examination determine the aggressiveness of the diagnostic plan. As with diagnostic tests for upper extremity problems, the diagnostic tests can be divided into nonoperative and operative (see Chapter 5). As with upper extremity problems, tests should be ordered when their results will change recommended treatment or are mandatory for an accurate diagnosis or prognosis.

Four Objectives of the History and Physical Examination

1. To quantitate the morbidity of the patient
2. To delineate psychosocial factors
3. To diagnose tumors, infections, and neurologic disasters
4. To diagnose the clinical syndrome

Table 7-1. Typical Pattern of Dysfunction Seen With Specific Radiculopathies

Nerve	HNP	Foramen	Muscle	Reflex	Sensation
T10					Umbilicus
T12					Pubis
L1	T12-L1	L1-2			Upper anterior thigh
L2	L1-2	L2-3			Mid–anterior thigh
L3	L2-3	L3-4	Quadratus		Lower anterior thigh
L4	L3-4	L4-5	Quadratus Anterior tibial	Patella	Anterior thigh Medial leg Foot (occasionally)
L5	L4-5	L5-S1	Anterior tibial EHL	Posterior tibial	Lateral leg Dorsum of foot Big toe
S1	L5-S1		Toe raise Peroneal	Achilles tendon	Posterior leg Sole of foot Lateral foot Little toe

Nonmechanical inflammatory back and/or leg pain

Nonoperative tests. Tests include a bone scan, MRI, protein electrophoresis, a complete blood count (CBC), SMA 12, an erythrocyte sedimentation rate (ESR), a bone marrow aspiration, and a rheumatoid work-up.

Operative tests. Tests include MRI, a myelogram, a contrast CT scan, spinal needle aspiration, and a Craig needle biopsy or open excisional biopsy.

Mechanical axial back pain with or without leg pain. This is predominantly a mechanical back pain problem.

Nonoperative tests. MRI diagnoses levels of disc degeneration, disc herniations, spinal stenosis, and spondylolisthesis and eliminates neurologic intradural tumors. A plain CT scan can diagnose spondylolysis, arthritic change in the spine, and significant disc bulges. A CT scan and MRI aid in interabdominal and retroperitoneal causes of back pain. The bone scan diagnoses active stress fractures and localizes areas of arthritis. MRI is preferable to a CT scan for initial diagnostic screening in this category of pain. MRI can reveal a large posterior lateral herniation in patients with all of the history and physical examination findings of a disc herniation but with predominantly back pain. This can lead to surgery in certain circumstances.

Operative tests

Myelography and contrast CT scan. Full examination of the spinal canal and dural contents is imperative to diagnose disc herniations, stenosis, intrafocal tumors, arachnoiditis, and congenital anomalies. Myelography and CT scanning in cases of minimal leg signs and symptoms cannot be expected to yield valuable information in regard to the etiology of the pain and can be dangerously misleading when one is contemplating fusion or decompression.

Discography. Discography is both a subjective and an objective test. It is designed to reproduce pain from an intervertebral disc by injection pressure and irritation of the dye. In this category of pain, discography is of paramount importance.

CT-enhanced discography. CT-enhanced discography has shown a number of patterns of discographic dye. The dye frequently outlines extruded disc fragments from inside the disc to the outside, through the annulus. An annular tear with dye flowing through a radial laceration in the annulus can often be demonstrated. CT discography can demonstrate a herniated disc with sublaminar or extruded nuclear fragments. There are also subannular collections of dye that are indistinguishable from annular nuclear material on the discogram. Some cases of subannular dye collection show a meniscus of dye in an intraannular fissure on CT discography that looks like a herniation on the discogram.

The symptomatology aspect of discography involves pain reproduction of a clinical pain pattern. The patient draws the pain pattern at the time of the initial visit. The radiologist does the discography and either draws the pain pattern or comments very specifically as to its intensity, character, and location. The radiologist determines if the pain pattern reproduced was similar to prior pain experienced by the patient. Some patients are unable to participate in this symptom reproduction portion of the study. Some are hysterically oriented toward pain, either everywhere or nowhere. These human factors must be kept in mind in evaluating the symptomatologic reproduction of pain. It is best not to discuss with patients which levels of the spinal column are being evaluated, not to allow them to watch the monitor, and not to inform them when the dye is being injected. The accuracy of discography is dependent on the skill and experience of the discographer.

Operative care for predominantly back pain is controversial. If a surgeon does not do fusions for back pain, discography is less important. This is a preoperative invasive diagnostic study only. Fusion for the instability stage of disc degeneration may relieve a patient of symptoms for a socioeconomically very important 10 years. Discography is critically important in determining which levels to fuse for back pain.

If a normal morphology discogram fails to reproduce the patient's pain pattern, the chance of success in fusing that disc is poor. An exception may be an acute posterior element fracture. The chance of clinical success in fusion for back pain is decreased if discography demonstrates multiple symptomatic levels. The ideal candidate for selective fusion for predominantly back pain is one in which discography exactly reproduces the pain at one level only; additional intradiscal anesthetic injection at that level totally blocks the pain, and adjacent levels are totally normal and asymptomatic.

Operative care of patients without radiculopathy includes care of individuals with spondylolisthesis. It is critically important to examine, with discography and/or MRI, levels adjacent to a spondylolisthetic level. Fusion of a spondylolisthetic level, when pain is from an annular disruption at an adjacent level, will be met with clinical failure.

In patients with a higher percentage of back pain than leg pain or fifty-fifty back and leg pain, discography can be helpful in determining which level is the origin of the pain. MRI is becoming increasing effective in screening the adjacent levels. In a review of discography and MRI cases, Schneiderman et al.[13] found a 99% correlation between degeneration on the MRI and degeneration on discography. They concluded that the MRI can be used to screen for levels of degeneration. If degeneration is present, discography is helpful in determining whether it is symptomatic in the patient.

Sciatica. The history and physical examination point to a discogenic origin for sciatica, with or without neurologic deficit.

Nonoperative tests. MRI is the primary outpatient screening test. It diagnoses disc herniations, intradural tumors, and disc degeneration. The second preference is the CT scan, which pinpoints more exactly the diagnosis, the location of disc fragments in the canal, and the presence of stenosis and arthritic spurs. In young people it is preferable to use the MRI as a screening test, since it accomplishes the objectives of a working diagnosis for nonoperative care. In a young person with predominant leg pain from probable disc herniation, the MRI is performed with a CT scan as the second test. In older patients, where stenosis is a more likely diagnosis, the CT scan is used.

Operative tests. The contrast CT scan with cuts through the conus medullaris is preferred. This allows a better interpretation of spinal stenosis, whether the stenosis is central, lateral recess, foraminal, or extraforaminal. A determination of the exact size and location of a disc

herniation and extruded disc fragment is possible. A full myelogram is not mandatory preparation for operative care in this category of pain. Electromyography (EMG), sensory-evoked potentials, and selective nerve root blocks, along with the clinical examination, are used to distinguish which nerve root is responsible for the patient's pain and to eliminate other neurologic diagnoses. The CT scan, myelogram, and discography help determine which level and the pathologic condition at that level. Discography may be of benefit in patients with predominantly leg pain of a discogenic source, but it is not routinely indicated. If there is a question as to the differential diagnosis of a major canal-obstructing lesion, discography with CT can clearly outline a fragment from the intervertebral disc.

A primary benefit of discography may lie in a negative discogram. An asymptomatic, well-contained nucleus should not be the source of true radicular pain from that neuromotion segment. Discography is this case helps rule out possible diagnoses. In cases in which there are bulges and protrusions of intervertebral discs at levels adjacent to a herniation that could be producing radicular symptoms, discography may be helpful. Under these circumstances, discography may very clearly reproduce that patient's exact pain pattern, giving greater indication that this is the spinal column level with the problem. The definitive test is usually a contrast CT scan, but MRI can give an exact diagnosis. The other tests are more supportive. The more tests that point to the same level, same nerve, and same pathologic condition, the more exact the diagnosis and successful the surgery.

Older patients with predominantly claudicatory leg pain and no sciatic signs

Nonoperative tests

Vascular evaluation. Evaluation includes Doppler studies, a bicycle test, and evaluation by a vascular surgeon.

Plain CT scan. The plain CT scan eliminates bone tumors and metastatic tumors, which are reasonably common in the older age group, and shows spinal stenosis. The levels for the CT scan are determined by the plain films.

MRI. MRI eliminates tumors and diagnoses stenosis.

Operative care. The myelographic patterns of spinal stenosis give a good indication of which levels to decompress. A contrast CT scan follows the myelogram. CT demonstrates foraminal and extraforaminal stenosis. The morbidity of the myelogram is higher in older persons, and nausea, vomiting, or mental changes may last several days. The contrast CT scan may soon eliminate the full myelogram. Discography plays little role in evaluation of these patients. Patients in this class are in the stabilization phase of degenerative disease, not the instability stage. Soft disc herniations are less frequent in older patients with stenosis. The decision to fuse is primarily based on flexion/extension films demonstrating dynamic instability, not discography. Fusions are to prevent further destabilization from the decompression, leading to a return of radicular symptoms; they are not for back pain.

Positive and Negative Aspects of the Tests

The comparative use of myelography, CT scanning, and discography with regard to accuracy depends on the condition being diagnosed. The following lists the optimum diagnostic categories for each test based on symptoms:

1. *Discography*—Mechanical back and leg pain
2. *MRI*—Mechanical back and leg pain
3. *CT scan*—Radicular pain, claudicatory pain
4. *Myelography*—Radicular pain, claudicatory pain

To make a clinical decision in a specific case, the facts in the case are weighed according to the patient's symptoms. The more facts pointing to a specific area, the better the ultimate result of treatment.

REFERENCES

1. Brown T, Hanson R, Yorra A: Some mechanical tests on the lumbosacral spine with particular reference to the intervertebral disc, *J Bone Joint Surg* 39A:1135, 1957.
2. DuPuis P: The natural history of degenerative changes in the lumbar spine. In Watkins RG, editor: *Lumbar discectomy and laminectomy,* Rockville, Md, 1987, Aspen.
3. Dyck P: Sciatic pain. In Watkins RG, editor: *Lumbar discectomy and laminectomy,* Rockville, Md, 1987, Aspen.
4. Farfan H: *Mechanical disorders of the low back,* Philadelphia, 1973, Lea & Febiger.
5. Hirsch C: The reaction of intervertebral discs to compression forces, *J Bone Joint Surg* 37A:1188, 1955.
6. Hult E: Cervical, dorsal, and lumbar spinal syndromes, *Acta Orthop Scand Suppl* 17:5, 1954.
7. Kiraldy-Willis WH, editor: *Pathology and pathogenics of low back pain in managing low back pain,* New York, 1983, Churchill Livingstone.
8. McNab I: *Backache,* Baltimore, 1977, Williams & Wilkins.
9. Mooney V, Cairns D, Robertson J: A system for evaluating and treating chronic back disability, *West J Med* 124:370, 1976.
10. Nachemson A, Schultz A, Berkson M: Mechanical properties of human lumbar spine motion segment: influence of age, sex, disc level, and degeneration, *Spine* 4:1, 1979.
11. Pennal GF et al: Motion studies of the lumbar spine, *J Bone Joint Surg* 54B: 442, 1972.
12. Posner I et al: A biomechanical analysis of clinical stability of the lumbar and lumbo-sacral spine, *Spine* (in press).
13. Schneiverman et al. In Brieg A, editor: *Adverse mechanical tension in the central nervous system,* New York, 1978, John Wiley & Sons.
14. Watkins R et al: Comparison of preoperative and postoperative MMPI data in chronic back patients, *Spine* 11:385, 1986.
15. White AA, Panjabi MM: *Clinical biomechanics of the spine,* Philadelphia, 1978, JB Lippincott.

Chapter Eight

◆

Differential Diagnosis of Back and Lower Extremity Problems

Michael F. Mellman
Edward J. McPherson
Lawrence D. Dorr
Philip Kwong

Backache

The differential diagnosis of backache extends through all regions and organ systems of the body. Backache that originates in the dorsal spine is usually mechanical in nature. Atypical pain patterns or presentations should trigger suspicion regarding a systemic cause, one not exclusively mechanical or of isolated nerve root origin. Factors to be noted in history taking relevant to backache include unexplained weight loss, night sweats, fever, nocturnal pain unrelated to position changes during sleep, pain that does not limit activity, and pain that is not improved by recumbency.[14] Also of note is any history of infection, malignancy, rheumatologic problems, or metabolic disorders.

Any low back pain seemingly of systemic origin must be evaluated fully. Normal findings on lumbosacral spine radiographs are rare in individuals with back pain who are older than 35 years of age. When radiographs of matched populations with and without low back pain were compared, the prevalence of degenerative and congenital deformities was similar.[12] Thus only a normal radiographic finding is helpful in evaluating low back pain because it rules out a primary spinal condition as causing the pain.

One approach to patients with backache is to consider, first, the region of pain, with the intent of defining a possible anatomic pathologic association, and, second, the systemic disease states that may further define etiologic factors.

REGIONS OF PAIN

The anatomic regions most commonly associated with referred spinal pain include the thorax and the abdomen. Intrathoracic structures tend to project pain in the region of the neck, thorax, and abdomen. Abdominal abnormalities rarely refer pain above the shoulder.

Upper Torso

Neck. Esophageal conditions refer pain to ventral structures, most typically to the sternum and the epigastrium. Occasional dorsal midline spine discomfort is also noted. Usually some relationship to swallowing and, in some instances, to position is noted. Food tends to stick in the midsternal region, regurgitation occurs, or a bitter taste is present when the person bends at the waist, all of which are consistent with reflux of gastric contents into the esophagus. The person notes similar symptoms in assuming a supine posture or on wearing garments that are tight across the abdomen. These last two positional manifestations usually are associated with an improperly functioning gastroesophageal sphincter and/or hiatal hernia. Often food associations are noted that worsen the pain. Typical esophageal problems include esophagitis, esophageal spasms, Zenker's diverticulum, esophageal webs, and esophageal strictures.

Lung. Lung conditions can be associated with thoracic pain. Shortness of breath and cough are cardinal symptoms. Shortness of breath may be due not only to a pulmonary parenchymal abnormality but also to limited bellows function as a result of pain during chest wall motion. Pleuritic chest pain that is described as worsening with deep inspiration, cough, or sneeze usually suggests involvement of the pleura. Chest wall pain of spinal origin, however, may have a pleuritic component. Chest wall symptoms as a result of rib or intercostal muscle injury caused by cough may suggest a thoracic spine problem. Sputum production likewise has a nonspinal origin and suggests sinus, airway, or pulmonary parenchymal involvement. Typical pulmonary disorders include pneumonia, pleurisy, pneumothorax, and pulmonary embolization.

Chest

Chest wall. Pain originating from the chest wall can be confused with intercostal nerve injury secondary to a pathologic condition of the thoracic spine and the resultant radiculopathy. Most chest wall problems have a component of pleuritic pain. Chest compression, however, in either the anteroposterior (AP) or the left/right orientation, localizes the region of the rib abnormality, which is identical to the region of maximum pain on compression. Costochondral joint involvement is manifested by point tenderness over the involved joint and simply needs to be identified. Intercostal muscle pain as a result of local injury from trauma or muscle strain, usually from cough, also is a cause of localized tenderness.

Pulmonary embolization. Pulmonary embolization is a special consideration, not only because it can be life-threatening but also because it frequently is a complication of a dorsal spine condition. Pulmonary embolization results from deep venous thrombosis, typically involving the larger veins of the lower extremities and, less frequently, the pelvic and intraabdominal venous structures. Deep venous thrombosis is a result of venous stasis, as noted, with immobility. Causes of immobility can include surgery and/or bed rest for a dorsal spine condition. Additional risk factors for pulmonary embolization include a prior history of deep vein thrombosis, venous trauma, and, much more rarely, the hypercoagulable state.

Heart. The heart, its surrounding pericardium, and great vessels must be included in a differential diagnosis of pain of thoracic origin. As with pulmonary embolization, a missed diagnosis in these situations can prove to be fatal. Pericardial pain is described typically as sharp and peristernal, and it can radiate to the dorsal spine. It is unique in that the pain lessens when the patient leans forward. Thus this pain can be positional, but unlike coronary artery disease, it is not exertional.

Heart vessels. Coronary artery disease and its cardinal symptom, angina pectoris, is classically exertional and is associated with the risk factors of hypertension, hypercholesterolemia, diabetes mellitus, and cigarette smoking. In its more severe forms, angina may occur at rest. It is not positional. Classic anginal pain is retrosternal, with radiation to the shoulder or jaw, and is associated with palpitations, shortness of breath, nausea, vomiting, or diaphoresis. The pain itself is dull and described as deep. It is usually pressurelike and is often demonstrated by the patient placing a fist over the chest—like a Roman soldier saluting. Symptomatic myocardial infarction is simply an extreme of anginal pain that is longer lasting and that may have a pericardial component.

Pain emanating from the great vessels is far more difficult to distinguish from spinal pain than is pain of cardiac or pericardial origin. Dissection of, or direct pressure from, an aortic aneurysm may actually cause symptoms localized to the back. Aortic dissection classically causes a tearing type of back pain, especially when the transverse or descending aorta is involved. This may be associated with the pain of myocardial infarction when proximal dissection occurs with involvement of the coronary cusps of the aortic valve. Arm and/or shoulder pain may occur with dissection of the ascending aorta. Aortic dissection represents a surgical emergency. Signs include the onset of an aortic insufficiency murmur, change in contour of the carotid pulses, asymmetric radial pulses, or a change in the timing of radial versus femoral pulses, with the radial pulse arriving sooner on simultaneous examination than the femoral pulse. One may also see a widening of the aortic arch on sequential chest radiographs.

Marfan's Syndrome

Marfan's syndrome is a special concern in athletes. No specific characteristic verifies the diagnosis. It is believed to be an inborn error of metabolism that involves connective tissue and results in alterations of collagen or elastin.[11] Physical characteristics include mild joint laxity; chest deformity; long, thin fingers (arachnodactyly); limbs disproportionately long compared with the trunk; aortic aneurysm and valvular dysfunction; and displacement of the lens in the eye. In less than extreme forms, the long limbs may make a person unusually tall and thus especially well equipped for certain sporting endeavors. The most worrisome involvement includes that of the aorta. Often, aortic dilation and subsequent aortic valve regurgitation or dissection can be a late finding that goes unnoticed on an early chest radiograph because the initial dilation occurs within that portion of the aorta that is within the cardiovascular silhouette.[10] The diagnosis is obtained from an echocardiogram. Not only is there aortic root involvement, but prolapse of the mitral valve occurs in approximately 80% of persons with Marfan's syndrome. Scoliosis, which may occur along the thoracolumbar spine, is most noticeable during the adolescent growth spurt. Even at its least evident presentation, straightening of the thoracic kyphosis occurs to some degree. Finally, inguinal hernias can occur and recur with unexpected frequency after surgical correction. Pulmonary manifestations can include changes caused by chest wall abnormalities or—even in those with normal chest wall architecture—a forced vital capacity that is less than predicted.

Lower Torso: Abdomen and Pelvis

Abdominal and pelvic abnormalities may mimic symptoms and diseases of the mid to lower thoracic, or sacral, spine.

Peptic ulcer disease. Peptic ulcer disease, especially with posterior penetration, leads to lower thoracic or upper lumbar spine symptoms. These symptoms are usually associated with fasting. Peptic ulcer disease often is linked to the use of nonsteroidal antiinflammatory drugs, which are frequently prescribed to treat athletic injuries.

Pancreatitis. Pancreatitis usually causes epigastric or intrascapular pain. The quality of pain varies from dull to sharp and may be worsened by oral intake. Factors contributing to pancreatic pain include concomitant cholelithiasis, peptic ulcer disease with posterior penetration, malignant disease, trauma, alcohol, and other drugs.

Cholelithiasis. Cholelithiasis leads to a colicky pain

Table 8-1. Systemic Diseases Producing Backache

Disorder	Description	Effects
Metabolic Syndromes		
Diabetes mellitus	Common disease; produces polyneuropathy; affects vasa nervorum of nerve	Dorsal spine disease, manifested by rapid onset of pain, weakness in distribution of one or two nerves of leg (usually femoral or sciatic); mimics herniated nucleus pulposus
Guillain-Barré syndrome	Acute idiopathic polyneuritis; autoimmune, demyelinating disorder usually associated with antecedent event of gastrointestinal or respiratory origin within 8 weeks of onset	Produces ascending motor weakness, and in half of cases patients have bulbar involvement, some needing ventilatory support to sustain life; polyneuropathy; paresthesia in glove-and-stocking distribution; elevated level of cerebrospinal fluid with minimal cellular response
Porphyria	Group of inborn errors of metabolism sharing a disorder of heme synthesis; hepatic and erythropoietic forms exist; latency common; death can occur when condition is unrecognized or treated inappropriately; autosomal dominant inheritance	Pain, weakness, and paresthesia in the paraspinous musculature and extremities; depression, deep tendon reflex suppression, cranial nerve abnormalities, extremity weakness, either single or multiple; sensory changes include hypoesthesia and anesthesia; neurodiagnostic studies may be altered
Gout and pseudogout (chondrocalcinosis)	Rare causes of back pain; diagnosed by aspiration of crystals from articular joints	Concomitant, acute, peripheral, crystal-induced articular pain and spinal pain
Ochronosis	Rare autosomal recessive disorder in tyrosine metabolism; alkaptonuria, blue-black connective tissue	Usually affects knees and includes globally stiff spine; acquired weakening of annulus fibrosis may mimic herniated nucleus pulposus
Osteoporosis	Loss of bone mineral content beyond what is expected for age and sex-matched controls	Causes back pain due to compression fractures of thoracic and lumbar vertebrae with secondary impingement of neural structures, as well as primary bone pain; marked kyphosis; correction of primary spinal disorder without treating osteoporosis will result in therapeutic failure
Paget's disease	Localized alteration of bone metabolism and architecture; greater radiographic appearance than symptomatology; immobility leads to hypercalcemia; elevated serum alkaline phosphatase and 24-hour urinary hydroxyproline levels common; usually in patients over 40 years of age	Low back pain without radiculopathy; spine involved frequently; diagnosis of exclusion
Malignant Conditions	Usually metastatic from breast, prostate, thyroid, or lung tumors; multiple myeloma (a disorder of plasma cells) displaces normal bone marrow, causing anemia and affecting the spine in particular; suggested by presence of anemia and albumin/globulin ratio near unity; perineoplastic syndrome represents distant effects of malignancy	Malignant tissue replaces bony structures or occurs indirectly as a result of hormonal factors
		Perineoplastic syndrome produces pure sensory and sensorimotor neuropathy, primarily in elderly patients and secondary to carcinoma of lung, ovary, breast, stomach, and colon

Continued.

Table 8-1. Systemic Diseases Producing Backache — cont'd

Disorder	Description	Effects
Infectious Diseases		Rarely involve spine; spinal epidural abscess causes symptoms localized to area of spinal involvement; increased incidence of infections in diabetic patients; disc space infections can result from investigatve processes, vertebral osteomyelitis, or Pott's disease; varicella zoster remains sequestered in paraspinal ganglia after childhood infection and produces dermatomal vesicular eruptions
Inflammatory Disorders		
Nonarticular rheumatism	Vague collection of symptoms that emanate from muscles and tendons as opposed to bones and joints; primary complaints are pain and stiffness; often multiple areas of localized tenderness of skeletal muscles	Myofascial pain syndrome; fibromyalgia involving the axial skeleton and proximal extremities
Myofascial pain syndromes	Characterized by painful muscle groups with associated trigger points	Pain is produced distal to site of stimulation but within same muscle group
Seronegative spondylo-arthropathies	Inflammatory rheumatologic disorders, including ankylosing spondylitis, Reiter's syndrome, psoriatic arthritis, inflammatory bowel disease (enteropathic arthropathy), juvenile chronic arthropathy, Behçet's syndrome, and Whipple's disease	Enthesis, secondary infections, sacroiliitis; men are more likely to have progressive spinal disease; women show peripheral joint manifestations; low back pain with morning stiffness common, improves with exercise; diminished mobility of spine in both AP and lateral planes Spondyloarthropathy
Reiter's syndrome	Occurs in patients with HLA-B27 positivity, especially after infection, such as *Shigella flexneri;* psoriatic arthritis typical; joint changes in apparent absence of skin changes; diagnosed as a triad of urethritis, conjunctivitis, and arthritis	Causes inflammatory oligoarthropathy in young male patients; sacroiliitis, ascending spinal sacroiliitis disease; may occur with acquired immunodeficiency syndrome (AIDS)
Inflammatory bowel disease (Crohn's disease and ulcerative colitis)		Sacroiliitis that progresses to ankylosing spondylitis; may precede bowel disease

involving the right subcostal region and is precipitated by oral intake of solids or liquids. This pain may radiate around the right costal margin. Icterus may be a late finding, as can lightening of fecal and darkening of urine color. Contributing factors include obesity, prior family history, and recent limitation of caloric consumption. Limited caloric consumption is often associated with sports that divide competitors into categories by weight. It is more common in females than in males.

Perforated viscus. A perforated viscus resulting from appendicitis, diverticulitis, or peptic ulcer disease rarely brings on localized pain in the dorsal spine. Free air in the abdominal cavity in a subdiaphragmatic position, however, can be associated with shoulder pain, suggesting a cervical or thoracic spine abnormality. Usually the intraabdominal catastrophe is apparent; however, this may not be so in a person treated with glucocorticoids.

Renal disease. A renal disease, such as nephrolithiasis or pyelonephritis, may refer pain to the costovertebral angle region, thus also suggesting thoracic or lumbar spine disease. Pain of kidney origin is usually manifested in the ipsilateral costovertebral angle or subcostal region. Renal colic from nephrolithiasis follows the course of the ureter, is intense, and causes restlessness. Hematuria is a cardinal signal but may also be seen with prolonged marching or running. Patients with pyelonephritis show evidence of systemic infection, as well as gastrointestinal symptoms that include nausea and vomiting.

Pelvic disease. Pelvic abnormalities can be associated with lumbar or sacral discomfort. Pelvic inflammatory disease, which is chronic and recurrent, is associated with systemic manifestations of infection and may include a vaginal discharge and diarrhea. Endometriosis in its early stages may manifest symptoms that parallel hormonal variation in the menstruating female patient. However, this condition is just as likely to become chronic and noncyclic over time as the ectopic sites of endometrial tissue deposition scar and show chronic irritation. Prostatitis and prostate carcinoma with metastases to the regional lymph nodes and ultimately the lumbosacral spine must always be considered in the male patient with low back pain. On rare occasions, ovarian and testicular abnormalities may refer pain to the lumbodorsal spine.

SYSTEMIC DISEASE

A number of systemic diseases involve bones, soft tissue, and joints at all levels and thus cannot be categorized by regional or anatomic associations. These processes may be metabolic, inflammatory, infectious, malignant, or idiopathic and can involve any spinal segment. Although symptoms are defined by the region of spinal involvement, the etiologic factors are not. A brief description of these systemic diseases and their effects, particularly on the back, is presented in Table 8-1.[1-9,13,15]

Hip Pain

Injuries to the hip and pelvic area in athletes may be classified as soft tissue or skeletal injuries. The following factors must be considered in evaluating the type of injury and presenting symptoms:
1. Skeletal and physiologic age of the athlete
2. Sport in which the athlete is participating
3. Severity of the trauma
4. Athlete's physiologic condition

Either macrotrauma or repetitive microtrauma may be causing the hip pain. Skeletal trauma can be epiphyseal, diaphyseal, or apophyseal, depending on the patient's age, the sport involved, and the velocity of the injury. Soft tissue injuries include acute strains, sprains, and repetitive overuse syndromes. In skeletally immature athletes, growth plate injuries are more common than ligamentous or musculotendinous injuries. Nonmusculoskeletal conditions can also present with symptoms similar to those of hip or pelvic injury. In addition, pathologic conditions can mimic orthopaedic injury in some cases. A complete list of the conditions to be considered in the differential diagnosis of hip pain in athletes is given in the box at right.

REFERRED PAIN

Hip joint pain may be perceived in various locations — medial, lateral, anterior, or posterior — because of its multiple sensory innervations. In general, hip pain is felt in the groin or in the anterior or medial aspect of the proximal thigh, but knee pain can be a predominant feature (i.e., referred pain from the obturator nerve).

Conditions of the Hip and Pelvis Presenting With Hip Pain in Athletes

Soft Tissue Injuries
A. Contusions
  1. Hip pointer
  2. Myositis ossificans
B. Muscle strains
C. Musculotendinous strains
  1. Osteotitis pubis
  2. Iliac apophysitis
D. Sprains
E. Hip snaps, clicks, and pops
  1. Iliopsoas snap
  2. Proximal iliotibial band snap
  3. Acetabular labral tears
F. Bursitis
  1. Trochanteric
  2. Ischiogluteal
  3. Iliopectineal
G. Neuritis
  1. Sciatic
  2. Piriformis syndrome
  3. Meralgia paresthetica

Skeletal Injuries
A. Apophyseal avulsion fractures
  1. Anterosuperior iliac spine (sartorius)
  2. Ischium (hamstring)
  3. Lesser trochanter (iliopsoas)
  4. Anteroinferior iliac spine (rectus femoris)
  5. Iliac crest (abdominal musculature)
B. Nonphyseal fractures
  1. Pelvic fractures
    a. Unstable pelvic ring
    b. Acetabular
    c. Stable pelvic: iliac wing
  2. Femoral neck fractures
    a. Transphyseal
    b. Subcapital
    c. Transcervical
    d. Cervicotrochanteric
    e. Intertrochanteric
  3. Subtrochanteric fractures
C. Stress fractures
  1. Pelvis
  2. Femoral neck
  3. Subtrochanteric
D. Growth plate injuries
  1. Salter-Harris physeal fractures
  2. Slipped capital femoral epiphysis
E. Avascular necrosis of femoral head
  1. Legg-Calvé-Perthes disease
  2. Adult
F. Traumatic dislocation of hip

Structural Abnormalities
A. Femoral anteversion
B. Leg length discrepancy
  1. Congenital leg length discrepancy
  2. Functional leg length discrepancy

Inflammatory Disorders
A. Transient synovitis
B. Septic arthritis
C. Osteoarthritis

Pathologic Conditions
A. Benign and malignant lesions of bone
B. Metastatic tumors
C. Synovial tumors
D. Endocrinopathies

Medical Conditions
A. Urologic disorders
B. Pelvic inflammatory conditions

Pain caused by a pathologic condition in the spine or pelvis is often referred to the hip. Hip pain referred from the lower lumbar vertebrae and sacrum is usually felt in the gluteal region, often radiating down the back or outer side of the thigh. In contrast, lesions from the upper lumbar vertebrae often refer pain to the proximal anterior hip and thigh region. Intrapelvic or lower abdominal conditions often refer pain to the groin and proximal part of the thigh.

TESTS FOR HIP PAIN

Because most hip joint pain results from capsular irritation, tests used to identify hip joint dysfunction involve provoking the hip joint capsule. Exact or similar reproduction of hip pain implicates the hip joint as the area of dysfunction, whereas dissimilar symptoms or lack of pain clears the hip. Three tests are used to provoke hip pain, and positive findings in at least two indicate hip joint dysfunction. Both the involved hip and the uninvolved hip are tested.

Faber (Patrick's) Test

With the athlete lying supine, the examiner flexes, abducts, and externally rotates the hip. In each position the examiner places one hand on the contralateral anterosuperior iliac spine and the other hand on the medial side of the knee. A complaint of hip pain when both hands are pressed down simultaneously is a positive result. This test can also detect sacroiliac joint pain.

Passive Abduction Test

With the athlete lying supine, the examiner passively abducts the hip to its end range. A complaint of hip pain with passive abduction is a positive result.

Internal Rotation of the Femur With the Hip Flexed

With the athlete lying supine, the examiner flexes the hip to 90 degrees and then maximally internally rotates it. A complaint of hip pain with this movement is a positive result.

CONDITIONS PRODUCING HIP PAIN IN ATHLETES
Contusions

Contusions are probably the most common injury in contact sports, although they are usually not referred to a sports medicine facility. Contusions cause hemorrhaging from blood vessel ruptures in the skin, subcutaneous fat, muscle, and even bone. Soft tissue damage and disruption of underlying muscle fibers are common. Occasionally contusions cause significant muscular hemorrhage, producing prolonged muscle spasm, disuse atrophy, and decreased range of motion.

Common sites of deep contusions about the hip that can result in significant disability are the anterior and lateral aspects of the proximal thigh. The force and duration of the blow determine the degree of soft tissue

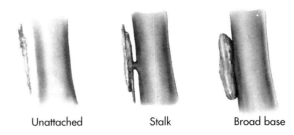

Unattached   Stalk   Broad base

Fig. 8-1. Various forms of myositis ossificans involving the femur. Initial radiographs after a thigh contusion will show only a soft tissue mass. After 2 weeks, calcific flocculations can be identified that evolve into one of three types of bone formation: (1) the unattached type that has no direct communication to bone, (2) the stalk type that is connected to the adjacent femur, and (3) the broad-based periosteal type that is broadly connected to the femur. (From Kulund DN: *The injured athlete,* Philadelphia, 1982, JB Lippincott.)

injury. The severity of a thigh contusion can be judged by its effect on knee flexion after the immediate, acute pain has subsided. With the athlete lying prone, the knee is flexed to the point of discomfort. If 90 degrees or less of flexion is achieved, the injury is severe; if more than 120 degrees of flexion is achieved, the injury is minor.

Because of its superficial location, the greater trochanter can suffer significant contusion, possibly leading to trochanteric bursitis with persistent pain and tenderness. A blow to the ischial tuberosity in a fall on the buttocks can cause a painful contusion. The ascending ramus of the ischium or descending ramus of the pubis may be contused by a direct blow, such as a fall across a bar or a blow from the saddle while horseback riding.

The most disabling contusion in the pelvis is the hip pointer. This contusion is caused by a driving blow to the iliac crest by a helmeted head, which is common in football and hockey. The overlying muscle is contused, and a subperiosteal hematoma forms. Over the 24-hour period following the injury, the athlete develops appreciable edema, pain, and ecchymosis, with motion of the abdominal muscles, hip abductors, and flexor muscles aggravating the condition. If the athlete develops post-traumatic periostitis of the iliac crest, the crest will remain painful and tender.

Severe contusion can lead to myositis ossificans, wherein a hematoma develops secondary to trauma. In approximately 2 weeks calcific flocculations develop, which then mature into heterotopic bone about 8 weeks after the injury (Figs. 8-1 and 8-2). Adjacent hip motion may be lost as a result of restricted muscle function.

Muscle Strains

The most commonly strained muscles around the hip are the hamstrings, adductor longus, iliopsoas, and rectus femoris. Muscle strains result from excessive tension (stretching) of the muscle, which results from

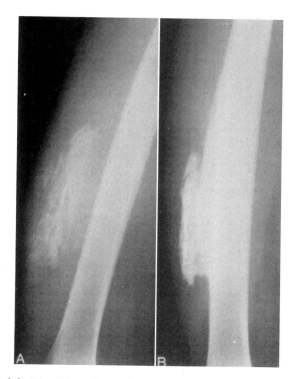

Fig. 8-2. Myositis ossificans in an 11-year-old boy who fell from the stairs of a swimming pool. Lateral radiographs of the femur 1 month (**A**) and 5 months (**B**) after the injury show maturation of the ossifying process. Initially separated from the bone, the heterotopic ossification subsequently merged with the anterior surface of the femur. (From Resnick D, Niwayama G: *Diagnosis of bone and joint disorders,* ed 2, Philadelphia, 1988, WB Saunders.)

both external and internal mechanisms. External factors include activities that stretch the muscle beyond its limit, such as extralong strides to catch a ball; internal factors that predispose to muscle strain are short muscles, weak muscles, muscle imbalance, or an anteriorly or posteriorly tilted pelvis.

If the injury is on the tendinous side of the musculotendinous junction, it is usually painless and involves minimal hemorrhage. If the muscle portion is involved, hemorrhage is always present. Usually the athlete perceives pain immediately at the time of injury and complains of tenderness on palpation.

Musculotendinous Strains

Osteitis pubis. Osteitis pubis is most commonly seen in soccer players, race walkers, and long-distance runners, although it is an unusual injury. While its cause is not clear, evidence favors repeated minor trauma from excessive or repetitive biomechanical stresses to the symphysis pubis, resulting in shear forces transmitted to the symphysis. There is a gradual onset of localized pain around the pubis and entending to the groin, lower abdomen, and occasionally the hip. Movements such as pivoting on one leg, kicking a ball, sprinting, jumping,

climbing stairs, suddenly changing direction, or stretching aggravate the pain. Pain may become intense; when the condition is severe, adductor spasm develops, resulting in a waddling gait. The disorder seems to be self-limiting.

Iliac apophysitis. Iliac apophysitis primarily affects adolescent long-distance runners. The process of long-distance running induces an inflammatory response to a subclinical stress fracture of the iliac apophysis through repeated contractions of the tensor fascia lata, gluteus medius, and oblique abdominal muscles. Usually an intensive training program or a recent escalation of a training regimen precedes the development of iliac apophysitis. Generally, nonspecific pain occurs along the anterior iliac crest and increases during running, especially with crossover arm swings. This condition is self-limiting, responding to rest and antiinflammatory medication.

Sprains

The stability of the hip joint depends primarily on ligaments of the joint and the hip's bony anatomic configuration. Ligamentous sprains are rare but should be suspected when there has been a violent injury to the hip, placing it in a position of extreme abduction, flexion, and external rotation, or in a position of extreme adduction, flexion, and internal rotation.

Hip Snaps, Clicks, and Pops

Snaps, clicks, and pops around the hip joint are noted mostly in dancers and gymnasts, but they can also be seen in various other athletes.

Iliopsoas snap. Iliopsoas snap syndrome occurs when the hip is at about 45 degrees of flexion, coming into extension. The click or snap is palpable anteriorly and is caused by the iliopsoas tendon snapping across a bony prominence on the anterior acetabulum (Fig. 8-3). Occasionally there is pain or a slight jerk. Usually the condition resolves without invasive treatment.

Proximal iliotibial band snap. In "snapping hip" syndrome a tight iliotibial band causes irritation of the greater trochanteric bursa during hip flexion and extension, especially with internal rotation (Fig. 8-4). A sensation like that of hip dislocation may be associated with an audible snap or pop. Iliotibial band tightness can be demonstrated by Ober's test.

Acetabular labral tears. Although little has been written regarding acetabular labral tears, this injury is analogous to glenoid labral tears. The athlete complains of a sharp, catching pain localized to the groin and anterior aspect of the thigh. Pivoting movements cause catching, along with a sharp pain in the groin and anterior hip area; residual soreness may persist. Passive maneuvers produce an audible and palpable click as the extended hip is moved into positions of adduction and external rotation.

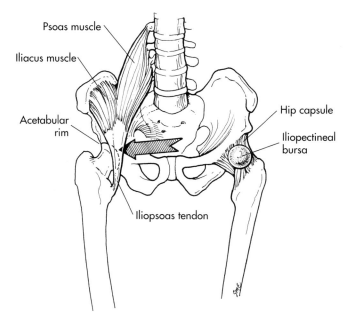

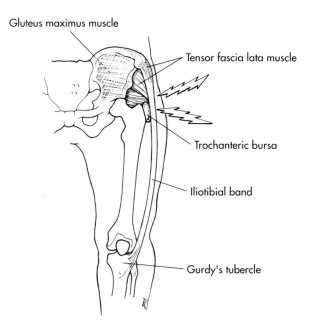

Fig. 8-3. Diagram of the anterior pelvis and hips demonstrating the etiology of iliopsoas sna p syndrome. The left hip shows the hip capsule with an overlying iliopectineal bursa. The right hip shows the iliopsoas tendon as it crosses over the iliopectineal bursa and anterior acetabular edge. If repetitive snapping of this tendon occurs over a prominent acetabular edge, then iliopsoas tendonitis or iliopectineal bursitis may develop.

Fig. 8-4. Proximal iliotibial band snap. This condition is a result of a tight iliotibial band that causes irritation of the greater trochanteric bursa as the hip is brought between flexion and extension. The athlete frequently describes a sensation of the "hip dislocating" as the iliotibial band snaps anteriorly or posteriorly over the trochanter.

Bursitis

Numerous synovial lined sacs called bursae overlie bony prominences or separate tendons from muscles in the hip area. These can become inflamed and cause significant disability.

Greater trochanteric bursitis. Bursitis of the greater trochanter is the most common form in this area and is caused essentially by increased stress in the iliotibial band over the bursa. Frequently the cause is abnormal running mechanics, such as feet crossing over the midline, thereby increasing the adduction angle and increasing friction between the trochanter and overlying iliotibial band; imbalance between the adductor and abductor muscles in female athletes who have a broad pelvis and increased Q angle; or excessive posterolateral heel wear on the shoe or running on a banked surface. Trochanteric bursitis produces pain over the lateral aspect of the hip and thigh that may radiate down to the knee or proximally to the posterolateral buttocks. Usually the athlete notices an insidious onset of pain while participating in sports and later notes pain with walking, when attempting to cross the legs when seated, or when lying on either side. Palpation reveals an area of warmth and tenderness over the greater trochanter; on internal and external rotation of the hip, there is guarding, with pain localized over the greater trochanter. Ober's test findings are usually positive, with significant tenderness over the greater trochanter.

Ischiogluteal bursitis. The ischiogluteal bursa lies between the tuberosity of the ischium and the gluteus maximus. It can become inflamed after a direct blow to the ischial tuberosity, as in a fall on the buttocks, or can develop insidiously during activities requiring prolonged sitting, especially with the legs crossed or on a hard surface. It has been referred to as "bench warmer's bursitis." The athlete reports pain with walking, climbing stairs, and flexion of the hip or trunk, with tenderness localized over the ischial tuberosity, which is easily palpated with the patient in the side-lying position with the hip flexed, or in the prone position with the involved leg in the frog-leg position. Pain often radiates to the hamstrings but can also be referred to the hip region.

Iliopectineal bursitis. The iliopectineal bursa lies deep to the tendon of the iliopsoas muscle and on top of the anterior acetabular wall and hip capsule. It can communicate with the hip joint and lies next to the femoral nerve, often irritating it. A common cause of iliopectineal bursitis in athletes is a sudden increase in performance requirements, such as competing in tournaments or trying new dance steps. Acute hemorrhage into the iliopsoas bursa can occur, usually in association with an overlying iliopsoas muscle strain, with the typical history of resisted violent flexion of the hip. Clinical findings include pain on tensing of the iliopsoas muscle against resisted flexion of the hip or passive stretching of the iliopsoas in full extension. Tenderness is noted on

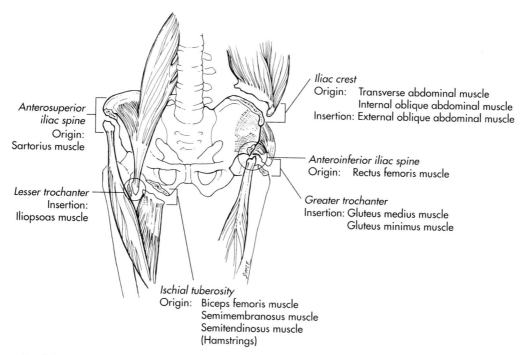

Anterosuperior
iliac spine
Origin:
Sartorius muscle

Iliac crest
Origin: Transverse abdominal muscle
            Internal oblique abdominal muscle
Insertion: External oblique abdominal muscle

Anteroinferior iliac spine
Origin: Rectus femoris muscle

Lesser trochanter
Insertion:
Iliopsoas muscle

Greater trochanter
Insertion: Gluteus medius muscle
            Gluteus minimus muscle

Ischial tuberosity
Origin: Biceps femoris muscle
           Semimembranosus muscle
           Semitendinosus muscle
           (Hamstrings)

Fig. 8-5. Muscle insertions and origins relevant to avulsion fractures of the pelvis and hips.

palpation in the inguinal region. Pain can be referred to the anterior thigh, hip, or knee as a result of adjacent irritation of the femoral nerve.

Neuritis

Sciatic neuritis. Sciatic neuritis can occur in athletes who have little adipose tissue, placing the sciatic nerve at risk as it exits the greater sciatic notch into the posterior buttocks. The sciatic nerve is traumatized in a fall as the buttocks strike the floor and the nerve receives a direct blow. Sciatic neuritis may also occur as a chronic injury caused by repetitive stretching of the nerve over the posterior acetabular region. The athlete usually complains of pain in the posterior buttocks and hip. Palpation of the sciatic nerve elicits localized pain with radiation to the hip and posterior thigh, associated with paresthesias. Treatment consists of rest and antiinflammatory medication. Occasionally convalescence may take as long as 6 to 8 weeks.

Piriformis syndrome. Piriformis syndrome is irritation of the sciatic nerve as it passes through the piriformis muscle. Usually the sciatic nerve passes entirely under the muscle, but in 15% of the population the nerve cuts through it. The syndrome is caused by compression of the nerve by a tight piriformis muscle. It occurs six times as often in females as in males. Significant to its diagnosis is the fact that pain occurs both with active external rotation with resistance and with passive stretch into internal rotation. Direct palpation over the piriformis elicits localized tenderness and paresthesias. Treatment

is conservative, employing passive stretching of the piriformis muscle once inflammation has subsided.

Meralgia paresthetica. Meralgia paresthetica is an inflammation of the lateral femoral cutaneous nerve, which is a direct branch of the lumbar plexus, which is formed by the posterior branches of the second and third lumbar nerves. The nerve becomes superficial as it passes just medial to the anterosuperior iliac spine into the proximal thigh and is susceptible to direct injury. In athletes it can be injured by a direct blow to the anterior hip (e.g., from a helmet or fall onto a hard surface). Symptoms include dysesthesias or paresthesias along the distribution of the lateral femoral cutaneous nerve, which affects the area of the lateral thigh down to the knee. If a neuroma is present, Tinel's sign may be elicited.

Avulsion Fractures

Avulsion fractures of the hip and pelvis are caused by either a sudden violent muscular contraction or an excessive amount of muscle stretch across an open apophysis. Often no external trauma is present. The injury usually occurs in adolescent athletes, with similar mechanisms producing muscle strains in adults. Avulsion injuries are more common in males and occur most frequently in the anterosuperior iliac spine (the origin of the sartorius muscle), the ischium (hamstrings), the lesser trochanter (iliopsoas), the anteroinferior iliac spine (rectus femoris), and the iliac crest (abdominal muscles) (Fig. 8-5). Rarely, avulsion of the greater trochanter occurs by the insertion of the abductors. These fractures can be seen in competitive athletes in the course of exerting extreme effort, but they generally occur in sprinters, jumpers, and soccer and football players. Pain may be intense.

Nonphyseal Fractures

Unstable pelvic ring and acetabular fractures. High-energy, violent trauma produces significant or displaced fractures of the pelvic ring and acetabulum. Generally, auto and motorcycle racing, hang gliding, or snowmobiling is involved. Because other life-threatening injuries are usually present, these injuries are most often managed at trauma centers.

Stable pelvic fractures. Generally, stable pelvic fractures cause only minimal impairment to the athlete. The iliac wing fracture, which occurs after a direct blow to the lateral aspect of the iliac wing (usually during horseback riding), is associated with pain, swelling, and tenderness over the iliac wing. Weight bearing is difficult because of the discomfort associated with contraction of the pelvic muscles used in locomotion.

Femoral neck fractures. With femoral neck fractures the athlete is disabled and complains of excruciating pain in the hip region. Any attempt to move through the range of motion causes severe pain.

Subtrochanteric femur fractures. As with femoral neck fractures, subtrochanteric femur fractures result from violent injury to the athlete. The clinical picture resembles that in a patient with an intertrochanteric or femoral neck fracture in that the athlete is in extreme pain and unable to move the affected leg. Usually the iliopsoas, gluteus musculature, and hip external rotators are attached to the proximal fragment, which pulls this fragment into the characteristic position of flexion, abduction, and external rotation. The proximal thigh is markedly swollen and shortened.

Stress Fractures

The athlete with a stress fracture almost always has a history of high training intensity and frequently reports a recent increase in the training regimen. Sharp, persistent, progressive pain or a deep, persistent, dull ache located over the bone are the most common symptoms of stress fracture. Impact activities aggravate the symptoms. The most specific diagnostic sign is point tenderness over the bony surface. Common sites are the pubic ramus, femoral neck, and subtrochanteric regions.

Pubic ramus stress fractures. Pubic ramus stress fractures occur typically in female joggers, long-distance and marathon runners, and military recruits. The fracture produces pain in the groin, buttock, or thigh. It is nondisplaced, occurs at a single site on the pubic ring, and is very occult radiographically before healing callus and resorption are present along the fracture margins.

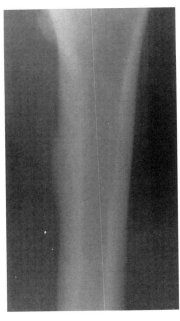

Fig. 8-6. AP radiograph of the proximal left femur demonstrating the typical location and appearance of a subtrochanteric stress reaction/fracture. Note the stress reaction evidenced by localized periosteal and endosteal thickening along the medical cortex without a radiolucent fracture line. (From Butler JE, Brown SL, McConnell BG: *Am J Sports Med* 10:228, 1982.)

Augmented isotope uptake in the inferior pubic arch confirms the diagnosis.

Femoral neck stress fractures. Runners, soccer players, and military recruits are the most common victims of femoral neck stress fractures. They are associated with vague, poorly localized pain, and the athlete may have thigh or knee pain. The discomfort is more noticeable in the morning, and walking affords some relief. Continued activity and impact activities exacerbate the pain. Clinical examination may reveal an antalgic gait, limitation of flexion and internal rotation, and localized pain with palpation over the anterior hip. Radionuclide bone scanning can be used to detect the fracture before radiographs are able to do so.

Subtrochanteric stress fractures. Subtrochanteric stress fractures are seen at the origin of the vastus medialis muscle and at the insertion site of the adductor brevis and may represent a traction avulsion phenomenon (Fig. 8-6). Causes include a change in running surface, increased intensity of workouts, and repetitive jumping with and without weights. The athlete notes medial thigh or groin pain that may extend anteriorly over the hip. Radiographs reveal a localized area of periosteal reaction along the medial femoral cortex that, with continued participation in athletic activities, causes a localized area of periosteal and endosteal irregularity and cortical hypertrophy. AP tomograms may demonstrate a fracture line in the area of cortical hyperostosis.

Growth Plate Injuries

Salter-Harris physeal fractures. Although children may sustain typical adult injuries, including sprains, strains, contusions, and fractures, they are also susceptible to growth plate and epiphyseal injuries. In the hip, Salter Harris fractures of the proximal femur and acetabulum are rare in sports but, when identified, indicate severe trauma or an associated disease process.

Slipped capital femoral epiphysis. Slipped capital femoral epiphysis (SCFE) is a well-recognized condition affecting children and adolescents and should be considered in any athlete who complains of pain in the hip, thigh, or groin. It is usually seen in males between the ages of 10 and 17 years and in females between 8 and 15 years of age. It tends to occur in individuals who are large, obese, and sexually immature and among those who are tall and thin. Contributing factors include the adolescent growth spurt, a deficiency of sex hormones relative to growth hormones, excess weight, and strenuous physical activity. Usually the patient complains of pain in the groin region, which is often referred to the anteromedial aspect of the thigh and knee; sometimes knee pain is the only presenting complaint. The athlete will have an antalgic gait and holds the extremity in an externally rotated position. Hip motion, especially internal rotation and abduction, is limited. A hip flexion contracture may be present. Extension of the hip may be increased consistent with the amount of slip. An acute slip may occur after an injury, such as a fall, tackle, or collision, and presents with sudden pain in the hip and groin with associated muscle spasm. Preexisting gradual slipping is often associated with an acute slip. Radiographs are essential to the diagnosis of SCFE (Fig. 8-7). Both AP and frog lateral projections are needed. The characteristic deformity described is posteroinferior displacement of the capital epiphysis on the femoral neck.

Avascular Necrosis of the Femoral Head

Legg-Calvé-Perthes disease. Legg-Calvé-Perthes disease affects children 3 to 12 years of age, with a peak incidence at 6 years. Males are affected five times more frequently than females. It must be considered in any child athlete who has a persistent limp and symptoms of hip, groin, or thigh pain. Clinical findings include gradual onset of intermittent hip pain, involving the groin, anterior thigh, and knee; development of an antalgic gait; spasm of the adductor muscles and iliopsoas on the affected side; atrophy of the thigh and buttocks muscles; limited hip motion, particularly abduction, internal rotation, flexion, and extension; and flexion contracture. Radiographs are diagnostic, showing capsular swelling, a diminutive femoral head ossific nucleus, lateral displace-

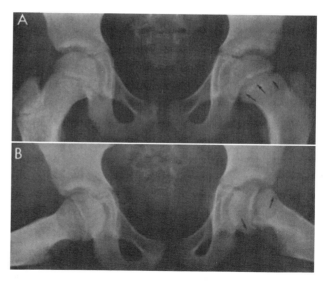

Fig. 8-7. Slipped capital femoral epiphysis in a 10-year-old boy. This patient complained of progressive left groin pain and anterior thigh pain over a 6-month period, with development of a limp several weeks before these radiographs were taken. **A,** In this AP radiograph with the hips in adduction, the physeal plate of the left femur is widened. Also note the minimal inferior displacement of the epiphysis. **B,** In this frog lateral radiograph, the amount of slip is more dramatic, emphasizing the importance of lateral radiographs. The epiphysis of the left femur maintains its normal relationship with the acetabulum, but it has slipped inferiorly and posteriorly in relation to the femoral neck. (From Caffey J: *Pediatric x-ray diagnosis,* St Louis, 1972, Mosby.)

Clinical Conditions Predisposing to Avascular Necrosis of the Femoral Head

Traumatic disruption of blood supply
  Femoral head dislocation
  Femoral neck fracture
Exogenous steroid therapy
  Corticosteroids
  Anabolic steroids
Alcoholism
Dysbaric disorders
  Deep sea diving
Hemoglobinopathies
  Sickle cell disease
  Sickle cell trait
  Sickle cell thalassemia
Lipid storage disease
  Gaucher's disease
Cushing's disease
Pregnancy
Radiation therapy
Idiopathic (Chandler's disease)

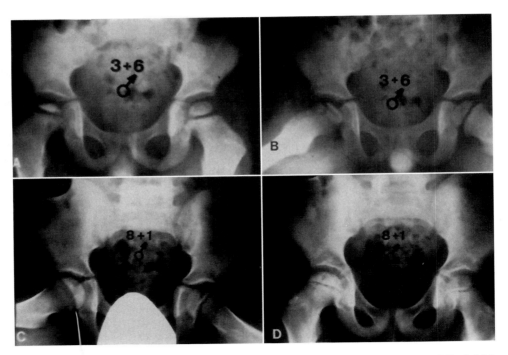

Fig. 8-8. Radiographs of a young child with Legg-Calvé-Perthes disease. **A** and **B,** Initial radiographs demonstrating complete head involvement of the right capital femoral epiphysis (Catterall classification, group IV). **C** and **D,** Minimal deformity is present after treatment; the child regained full range of motion. (From Lovell WW, Winter RB, editors: *Pediatric orthopaedics,* ed 2, Philadelphia, 1986, JB Lippincott.)

ment of the femoral ossification center, fissuring and fracture of the femoral ossific nucleus, flattening and sclerosis of the femoral ossification, metaphyseal cysts, and widening and shortening of the femoral neck as the disease progresses (Fig. 8-8). Further disorders may develop, including degenerative arthritis.

Ischemic necrosis of the femoral head in adult athletes. These patients have recalcitrant hip pain and a limp. The basic lesion is mechanical interruption of the blood supply to the femoral head. Causes include exogenous steroid consumption, alcoholism, and posttraumatic injury to the hip (see box on p. 117).

Traumatic Dislocation of the Hip

Traumatic dislocation of the hip in athletes represents a severe disruption in the mechanical integrity of the hip joint. This injury is seen in such sports as skiing, football, rugby, soccer, and hockey. Acute hip dislocation is one of the few orthopaedic emergencies encountered in sports. At best, femoral head circulation is compromised, with the hip in the dislocated position. Early reduction is of paramount importance to prevent the complication of avascular necrosis.

Structural Abnormalities

Structural abnormalities of the hip can predispose to overuse problems and cause hip pain. Conditions to be evaluated include femoral anteversion and leg length discrepancy.

Femoral anteversion. Fig. 8-9 illustrates the femoral condyle alignment in mature and immature skeletal systems. Femoral anteversion declines with age in the growing child, as follows:

1 year	40 degrees
2 years	30 degrees
3 to 9 years	Decline of 1 to 2 degrees every 2 years
10 years	Average 24 degrees
14 to 16 years	Average 15 degrees

In athletes with increased femoral anteversion, the head of the femur is uncovered anteriorly if the patella and knee point straight forward. To bear weight adequately, the leg must be internally rotated to cover the femoral head completely (Fig. 8-10). The patella points medially when walking, and the gait is noticeably intoed. Significant concern over this condition is seen particularly in ballet dancers and gymnasts. Young athletes who participate in these activities and develop chronic hip pain should be evaluated for femoral anteversion.

Leg length discrepancy. Pelvic obliquity resulting from a true or apparent leg length discrepancy produces an altered resting position of the hip joint, which changes the way the acetabulum articulates with the femoral head, causing hip dysfunction and pain. In children a

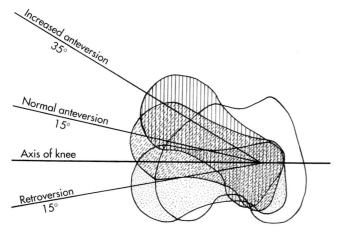

Fig. 8-9. Version of the neck of the femur evaluated by looking down on the hip and knee joint with the femoral head and neck superimposed over the femoral condyles. Version of the femoral neck is the angle made between the coronal axis of the knee and the axis of the femoral neck. When the axis of the femoral neck is anterior to the axis of the knee, this is referred to as anteversion. Likewise, if the axis of the femoral neck is posterior to the axis of the knee, this is referred to as retroversion.

careful appraisal of both the anatomic and the functional leg lengths should be carried out, since the occurrence of a discrepancy is most apparent between the ages of 6 and 14 years. In anatomic leg length discrepancy the legs are actually different lengths. In functional leg length discrepancy, or apparent leg length discrepancy, the anatomic leg lengths are equal, with the discrepancy resulting from an abnormal pelvic tilt.

Athletes with a congenitally short leg have anatomic leg length discrepancy, and the athlete may have developed compensatory scoliosis, hip abduction contracture on the affected leg, and adduction contracture on the contralateral leg.

Athletes with functional leg length discrepancy must be evaluated for primary scoliosis, hip adduction and abduction contractures, and an uneven medial longitudinal arch.

Inflammatory Disorders

Transient synovitis. Acute transient synovitis of the hip is a nonspecific inflammatory and self-limited condition that affects males more often than females in a ratio of 3:2. It occurs mainly in early childhood (peak age 3 to 6

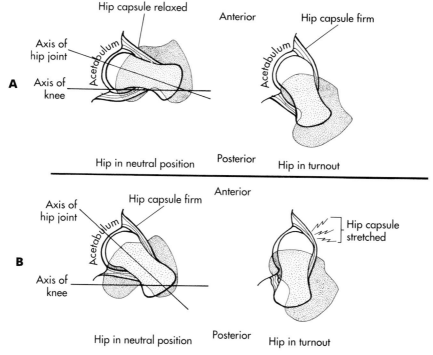

Fig. 8-10. Demonstration of the effect of femoral anteversion in turnout (external rotation). **A,** The femoral neck has normal anteversion. In the neutral position, the anterior and posterior capsular structures are relaxed, and the femoral head is centered within the acetabulum. With hip turnout, the femoral head stretches the anterior capsule within its normal limits. **B,** The femoral neck is excessively anteverted. In the neutral position (with the knee pointing straight forward), the anterior aspect of the femoral head is partly uncovered, and the anterior hip capsule is taut. With hip turnout, the athlete must force the anteverted femoral head against the already-taut anterior capsule, causing microscopic ruptures of collagen fibers. If turnout exercises are not performed in a controlled and gradual manner, significant pain and disability may result.

years) but can be seen in early adolescence and is more prevalent in spring and summer months. It is almost always unilateral, and its cause is unknown, although trauma, infection, and allergy have been suggested. Clinically the young athlete may report gradual or acute onset of symptoms, such as pain in the groin and anterormedial thigh, antalgic gait, and painful, restricted hip motion, with the hip "grabbing" on logrolling of the leg. Palpation reveals tenderness over the anterior hip. Any fever present is usually less than 101° F. Radiographs reveal capsular swelling with no bony changes, and laboratory tests show a near-normal white blood cell count and slightly elevated erythrocyte sedimentation rate.

Septic arthritis. Acute septic arthritis is a true orthopaedic emergency that primarily affects the neonate and young child, although it may occur at any age. The inflammation of the hip is caused by pus-forming organisms. Generally, a history of recent injury or infection, such as otitis media or skin infection, is given, with the hip symptoms developing and becoming excruciating over a very short period of time. Most patients are unable to bear weight on the affected leg because of the severe pain. These individuals are apprehensive, irritable, anorectic, and feverish, with the temperature reaching as high as 104° to 105° F. The hip is held in a position of minimum articular pressure (30 to 65 degrees of flexion, 15 degrees of abduction, and 10 to 15 degrees of external rotation). Radiographs demonstrate significant capsular swelling and surrounding soft tissue edema. Because of the increased intracapsular pressure, the femoral head may be displaced laterally or even subluxed (Fig. 8-11).

Osteoarthritis. Osteoarthritis is a common painful affliction affecting the hip joint and can cause significant disability in senior athletes. The pain and decreased range of motion limit athletic pursuits. This disorder affects 20% of people over the age of 55, with a female/male ratio of 3:2. Osteoarthritis is characterized by progressive degenerative changes in the articular cartilage and bones of the affected joint. The sequence of degeneration, inflammation, and destruction results in the eventual loss of the normal joint congruity. Synovial inflammation develops as a result of resorbing cartilaginous fragments from within the joint. Continued synovitis leads to capsular fibrosis and restricted motion.

Many of the clinical manifestations of osteoarthritis are related to capsular fibrosis, which causes shortening and deformity into flexion, adduction, and external rotation, exposing the capsule to painful stretching. This in turn elicits a reflex guarding by the muscles supplied by the motor branches of the sensory nerves to the hip capsule.

The predominant symptom is progressive pain, described as an aching sensation that is exacerbated by movement and relieved with rest. Stiffness occurs after

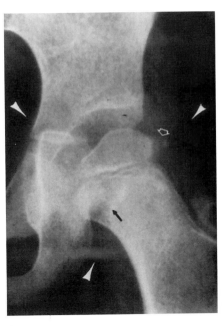

Fig. 8-11. Septic arthritis of the hip in a young child, complicated by metaphyseal osteomyelitis. Observe osseous destruction (*solid arrow*), soft tissue swelling with displacement of fat planes (*arrowheads*), widening of the joint space due to lateral subluxation of the femoral head, and periarticular calcification (*open arrow*). (From Resnick D, Niwayama G: *Diagnosis of bone and joint disorders,* ed 2, Philadelphia, 1988, WB Saunders.)

rest and then disappears with movement. The patient is easily fatigued with walking, has night pain (which may be a prominent feature), and has tenderness over the anterior and posterior regions of the hip. Active and passive range of motion is restricted, and flexion, abduction, and external rotation contractures may be present. Crepitation, often both audible and palpable, is usually elicited. The patient has an antalgic gait, with a Trendelenburg component late in the disease, which indicates abductor weakness. The affected leg may be shortened.

Radiographs show both sides of the joint narrowing or obliteration of the joint space, sclerotic subchondral bone on beginning in the superolateral weight-bearing portion and expanding, and osteophytes at the joint margins. As the disease progresses, the neck of the femur may become distorted, and superior erosion of the acetabulum may occur (Fig. 8-12).

Pathologic Conditions

Pathologic fractures occur through abnormal bone, causing the severity of the injury to exceed the severity of the trauma producing the injury. Pathologic conditions present either with an acute fracture through a lesion or with complaints of persistent, activity-related pain similar to that of an overuse injury. Radiographs are

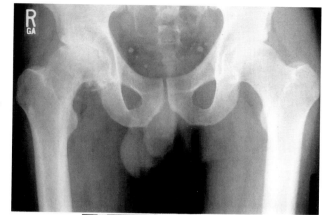

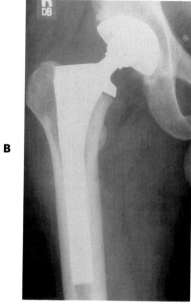

Fig. 8-12. Forty-six-year-old retired professional football lineman with osteoarthritis of the hips. **A,** AP radiograph of both hips. Observe on the right hip the nearly complete obliteration of the joint space, the femoral head and acetabular subchondral sclerosis, and marginal osteophytes. Also note loss of the superior femoral head. These degenerative changes are also evident to a lesser extent in the left hip. **B,** Because of this patient's recalcitrant pain and progressive dysfunction, he was treated with a right total hip replacement using an uncemented APR-IIT prosthesis (Intermedics Orthopaedics, Austin, Tex.)

needed for definitive diagnosis. Not uncommonly, athletes with pathologic lesions are initially treated at a sports facility for a sprain or strain and then later develop the pathologic fracture.

Benign bone lesions include osteoid osteoma, osteochondroma, enchondroma, unicameral bone cyst, giant cell tumor, and fibrous dysplasia. Malignant bone lesions include osteogenic sarcoma, chondrosarcoma, Ewing's sarcoma, and multiple myeloma. Metastatic lesions to the hip are more common in older patients and include those from carcinoma of the breast, lung, kidney, thyroid,

prostate, and colon. Tumors of synovium that can affect the hip include pigmented villonodular synovitis and synovial chondromatosis. Endocrinopathies may affect the quality of bone within the hip and predispose to fracture. Examples include hyperthyroidism, Paget's disease, osteomalacia, and osteoporosis.

Medical Conditions

Pain of urologic origin, including a ureteral stone, cystitis, or urethritis, may be referred to the hip. The pain is often referred to the respective lower abdominal quadrant, groin, or medial thigh, as well as the testicle. Symptoms may appear to be those of an adductor or hamstring strain. Cystitis is common in young female athletes, and a history of nocturia, polyuria, or dysuria in addition to the hip pain is helpful in making the diagnosis. Appropriate laboratory tests confirm the diagnosis. Gynecologic problems must also be considered, such as pelvic inflammatory disease (vaginitis, endometriosis, salpingitis, and ovarian cyst disease). A pap smear and appropriate cultures should be used to assist in the diagnosis. With acute lower quadrant abdominal pain and hip pain, ectopic pregnancy is a possibility.

In males prostatitis, epididymitis, and orchitis often present symptoms of groin and medial thigh pain. Again, a physical examination and appropriate laboratory tests differentiate these conditions. Other diseases, such as proctitis and perirectal abscess, cannot be overlooked.

Foot and Ankle Problems

NERVE ENTRAPMENT NEUROPATHIES

Several nerve entrapment neuropathies have been recognized clinically in the foot and ankle. Entrapment exists when an anatomic configuration creates constriction of a nerve; at these points there is little latitude for dimensional change allowing for unrestricted physical passage of the nerve. Common foot and ankle compression syndromes affect the interdigital nerve (Morton's neuroma), lateral plantar nerve (medial calcaneal nerve entrapment), posterior tibial nerve (tarsal tunnel syndrome), medial plantar nerve (jogger's foot), superficial peroneal nerve, and deep peroneal nerve (anterior tarsal tunnel syndrome).

Although nerve compression relates to a mechanical basis, other causes exist. Inflammatory arthritides such as rheumatoid arthritis, Reiter's syndrome, ankylosing spondylitis, and gout are known to be associated; even a case of tarsal tunnel syndrome was reported in a patient with seronegative spondyloarthropathy. Metabolic abnormalities (diabetes mellitus in particular), electrolyte imbalance, and alcoholism are conditions often exhibiting peripheral neuropathies.

While most local nerve compression exists independently in the foot, the possibility of a second and concurrent proximal nerve entrapment site in the leg or back must be considered. The "double-crush" phenomenon exists when a more proximal nerve injury (perhaps subclinical) impairs the axoplasmotic activity and decreases the nerve's tolerance to compression at a second and more distal site. Examination of common proximal sites for compressive conditions include the lumbar sacral spine (involving nerve roots), the greater sciatic notch (involving the sciatic nerve), and around the proximal fibula (involving the peroneal nerve). Chronic or acute compartment syndromes involving posterior, anterior, or lateral spaces in the lower leg can create compressive neuropathies by constricting along a greater length of the nerve rather than at a discrete point; this diffuse-type nerve compression is less frequently encountered than point-specific entrapment.

MODIFICATION OF FUNCTIONAL BODY MECHANICS USING FOOT ORTHOTICS

Modification of functional body mechanics by foot orthotics has implications for the spine and lower extremity. The center of mass (CM) in the human body is located within the pelvis. While standing, a person's weight-bearing line projected from the CM to the floor in the sagittal plane passes through the hip joint, anterior to the knee, and in front of the ankle; knee stability depends 70% on passive structures and 30% on muscle activity; ankle stability is provided by continuous calf muscle activity, especially the soleus. Similarly, the line projected proximally passes behind the cervical vertebrae, in front of the thoracic spinal segments, and behind most lumbar vertebral bodies; the center of gravity line then passes through the fifth lumbar vertebrae and anterior to the sacrum. Because the center of gravity intersects the transitional vertebral bodies T9 to L1 and L4 to S1, these spinal segments are subject to the greatest mechanical stress. Consequently, they experience the greatest movement and are more unstable when compared with other vertebrae; these characteristics of transitional segments correlate to areas of greatest incidence of surgical pseudarthrosis. The L5-S1 area is particularly vulnerable to mechanical shear, not only because of its transitional position but also because of its abrupt directional change; spondylolisthesis results when a deficiency in the laminae is present. The lumbar vertebrae cannot rotate but do ventroflex, extend, and laterally flex. Net spinal mobility is due to the summation of limited movement between vertebral segments supported by muscles and ligaments and occurs with compression of the intervertebral disc and gliding of facet joints.

A slight positive lift (8 mm) built into an orthotic device elevates and reorients the heel, resulting in reduced duration of pronation and maximum excursion. Patients with low back mechanical dysfunction may not tolerate the added stress at the vulnerable L5-S1 junction created by the heel lift; chronically inflamed ligaments and muscles are easily aggravated while attempting to stabilize the transitional vertebrae under greater shear forces. In such cases little or no heel lift effect is preferred, and an orthotic of soft, low-density material cushions loading impact and lessens the shock transmitted to the spine. A longer break-in period is better tolerated; occasionally, foot orthotic use is discontinued when the aggravated back discomfort persists.

Foot orthotic devices are frequently prescribed for excessive pronation deformity. Although data are inconclusive, some evidence indicates that foot appliances can successfully modify selected pathomechanical pronatory effects at the hip, knee, and foot. Orthotics have been observed to reduce both the duration and the severity of pronation. Foot appliances that contact and support the longitudinal arch may limit excessive motion at the subtalar-midtarsal complex and also reduce femur-tibia internal rotation. Appropriate correction of an excessive pronatory deformity can reduce hip bursitis, relieve anterior knee pain, and minimize foot strain. Because pronation is a necessary functional mechanism, overcorrection can create new problems, since the stress must be absorbed by other mechanisms in the foot, leg, and spine. In addition, the effectiveness of controlling excessive pronation depends on both the foot orthotic device and the mediolateral stability of the shoe used.

REFERENCES

1. Altman RD, Brown M, Gargano F: Low back pain in Paget's disease of bone, *Clin Orthop* 217:152, 1987.
2. Asbury AK: Diagnostic considerations in Guillain-Barré syndrome, *Ann Neurol* 9(supp):1, 1981.
3. Benson DR: The back: thoracic and lumbar spine. In D'Ambrosia RD, editor: *Musculoskeletal disorders, regional examination and differential diagnosis*, ed 2, Philadelphia, 1986, JB Lippincott.
4. Brown MJ, Asbury AKL: Diabetic neuropathy, *Ann Neurol* 15:2, 1984.
5. Clague JE, MacMillan RR: Backache and the Guillain-Barré syndrome: a diagnostic problem, *Br Med J* 293:325, 1986.
6. Flugel KA, Druschky KF: Electromyogram and nerve conduction in patients with acute intermittent porphyria, *J Neurol* 214:267, 1977.
7. Fox R et al: The chronicity of symptoms and disability in Reiter's syndrome: an analysis of 131 consecutive patients, *Ann Intern Med* 91:190, 1979.
8. Gran JT, Ostensen M, Husby G: A clinical comparison between males and females with ankylosing spondylitis, *J Rheumatol* 12:126, 1985.
9. Lewis GW: Zoster sine herpete, *Br Med J* 2:418, 1958.
10. Pyeritz RE, McKusick VA: The Marfan syndrome: diagnosis and management, *N Engl J Med* 300:772, 1979.
11. Pyeritz RE, McKusick VA: Basic defects in the Marfan syndrome, *N Engl J Med* 305:1011, 1981 (Editorial).
12. Reuler JB: Low back pain, *West J Med* 143:259, 1985.
13. Stein JA, Tschudy DP: Acute intermittent porphyria: a clinical and biochemical study of 46 patients, *Medicine* 49:1, 1970.
14. Waddel G: An approach to backache, *Br J Hosp Med* 28:187, 1982.
15. Waldenstrom J: The porphyrias as inborn errors of metabolism, *Am J Med* 22:758, 1957.

SUGGESTED READINGS

Berquist TH, Coventry MB: The pelvis and hips. In Berquist TH, editor: *Imaging of orthopaedic trauma and surgery,* Philadelphia, 1986, WB Saunders.

Birrer RB, Brecher DB: *Common sports injuries in youngsters: trauma to the hip, thigh, knee and leg,* Oradell, NJ, 1987, Medical Economics.

Bray TJ, Templeman DC: Fractures of the femoral neck. In Chapman MW, Madison M, editors: *Operative orthopaedics,* Philadelphia, 1988, JB Lippincott.

Chapman MW, Zickel RE: Subtrochanteric fractures of the femur. In Chapman MW, Madison M, editors: *Operative orthopaedics,* Philadelphia, 1988, WB Saunders.

Cibulka MT: Rehabilitation of the pelvis, hip, and thigh, *Clin Sports Med* 8:777, 1989.

Cohen JL, Bindelglass DF, Dorr LD: Total hip replacement using the APR II System, *Techniques Orthop* 6:40, 1991.

D'Ambrosia RD: Musculoskeletal disorders: regional examination and differential diagnosis. In *The hip,* ed 2, Philadelphia, 1986, JB Lippincott.

Goldberg B: Pre-sport participation. In Nudel DB, editor: *Pediatric sports medicine,* New York, 1989, PMA.

Kulund DN: *The injured athlete,* ed 2, Philadelphia, 1988, JB Lippincott.

Meyer CM: Muscle strains and contusions. In Smith NJ, editor: *Common problems in pediatric sports medicine,* St Louis, 1989, Mosby.

Micheli LJ: Sites of overuse injury. In Lovell W, Winter W, editors: *Pediatric orthopaedics,* Philadelphia, 1986, JB Lippincott.

Micheli LJ, Smith AD: Injury recognition and evaluation: lower extremity. In Cantu RC, Micheli LJ, editors: *ACSM'S guidelines for the team physician,* Philadelphia, 1991, Lea & Febiger.

O'Neill DB, Micheli LJ: Overuse injuries in the young athlete, *Clin Sports Med* 7:591, 1988.

Pavlov H: Roentgen examination of groin and hip pain in the athlete, *Clin Sports Med* 6:829, 1987.

Reilly JP, Nicholas JA: The chronically inflamed bursa, *Clin Sports Med* 6:345, 1987.

Resnick D, Niwayama G: Degenerative disease of extraspinal locations. In Resnick D, Niwayama G, editors: *Diagnosis of bone and joint disorders,* Philadelphia, 1988, WB Saunders.

Sim FH, Rock MG, Scott SG: Pelvis and hip injuries in athletes: anatomy and function. In Nicholas JA, Hershman EB, editors: *The lower extremity and spine in sports medicine,* ed 2, St Louis, 1995, Mosby.

Sweet DE, Madewell JE: Pathogenesis of osteonecrosis. In Resnick D, Niwayama G, editors: *Diagnosis of bone and joint disorders,* Philadelphia, 1988, WB Saunders.

Wojtys EM: Sports injuries in the immature athlete, *Orthop Clin North Am* 18:689, 1987.

Section Three

◆

Common Spinal Problems and Syndromes

Chapter Nine

Cervical Spine Injuries

Robert G. Watkins

In many of today's sports, particularly contact sports (Fig. 9-1), the neck is at risk for injury because of an inability to pad, brace, or protect the cervical spine while maintaining its function. The cervical spine must be flexible enough to allow the head and eyes to move to the right place at the right time. The spine also serves as a conduit for the central nervous system, with the spinal cord and the cervical nerve roots passing through it, making injury to the neck a potentially catastrophic event. Mueller and Cantu[13] evaluated injuries and fatalities occurring in high school and college sports from the fall of 1982 to the spring of 1988 (Tables 9-1 to 9-3). In this study fatalities were described as either direct (resulting directly from participation in the sport) or indirect (caused by systemic failure as a result of exertion while participating in the sport). The injuries were classified as catastrophic when they resulted in permanent, severe neurologic dysfunction and as serious when symptoms were serious but transient and did not result in permanent neurologic disability.

Clark[5] has reported that 54% of all spinal cord injuries in high school and college athletics are sports related. Torg et al.[25] have reported on the findings of the National Football Head and Neck Injury Registry, which was established to document the incidence and nature of severe intracranial and cervical spine injuries resulting from tackle football. The criteria for inclusion in the registry are that injuries require hospitalization for at least 72 hours, involve fracture subluxation or dislocation, involve intracranial hemorrhage, or be associated with quadriplegia or death. In the period from 1971 to 1984, 1412 cervical spine injuries met these criteria. The prevention of cervical spine and spinal cord injuries is of paramount importance, and the responsibility for educating athletes in methods to prevent neck injury is most important in those sports carrying the highest risk of trauma to the cervical spine. Contact sports, such as football, rugby, and wrestling, have been identified as being particularly high risk activities for cervical trauma.[16] The use of the head as an offensive weapon to block and tackle makes football a significant source of cervical injuries. Even noncontact sports, such as diving, water skiing, surfing, water polo, and body surfing, can be responsible for traumatic spinal injuries.[4] The prevention of neck injuries in athletes involves the education of players, trainers, and physicians. Prevention of these injuries must incorporate appropriate rule changes for high-risk sports.

Jackson and Lohr[8] reviewed a broad spectrum of cervical injuries occurring in athletes. Herniation in the cervical intervertebral disc is not uncommon in athletes, even though an epidemiologic study of acute prolapse of the cervical intervertebral disc shows that the majority of persons affected are in the fourth decade of life and men outnumber women by 1.4 to 1. Statistically significant associated factors include the heavy lifting of objects on the job, smoking, and frequent diving from a board; operating vibrating equipment and time spent in motor vehicles are borderline statistically significant factors. Variables not affecting the risk for a herniated cervical disc include participation in certain sports other than diving.[9] Although fractures with spinal cord injuries are common, fractures without neurologic deficits are more common in athletes[14,24] (Figs. 9-2 and 9-3).

There are several specific activities within certain sports that have led to a high incidence of cervical spine injuries. The following are a few examples:

Rugby—Injuries occur in the tackle as well as in the scrum, although collapsing the scrum has been identified as a significant source of fracture dislocations in quadriplegia.[7,18] In the long term, rugby players have significant increases in degenerative

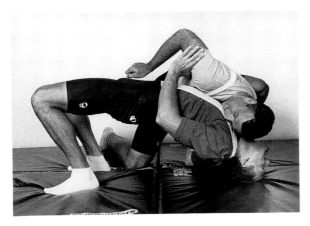

Fig. 9-1. "Bridging" is a wrestling move that places large hyperextension forces on the cervical spine. (From Vessa PP: Wrestling. In White AH, Schofferman JA, editors: *Spine care*, vol 1, *Diagnosis and conservative treatment*, St Louis, 1995, Mosby.)

Table 9-1. Fall Sports Injuries: Fall 1982 to Spring 1988

Sport	Fatalities		Catastrophic Injuries	Serious Injuries	Total
	Direct	Indirect			
Cross country					
High school	0	5	1	0	6
College	0	1	0	0	1
Football					
High school	33	27	53	74	187
College	3	10	8	29	50
Soccer					
High school	1	4	0	2	7
College	0	0	0	1	1
TOTAL	37	47	62	106	252

Table 9-2. Winter Sports Injuries: Fall 1982 to Spring 1988

Sport	Fatalities		Catastrophic Injuries	Serious Injuries	Total
	Direct	Indirect			
Basketball					
High school	0	18	1	1	20
College	0	8	0	1	9
Gymnastics					
High school	1	0	3	3	7
College	0	0	2	1	3
Ice hockey					
High school	0	0	3	2	5
College	0	1	0	1	2
Swimming					
High school	0	2	1	3	6
College	0	1	1	0	2
Wrestling					
High school	2	8	7	6	23
College	0	0	0	0	0
TOTAL	3	38	18	18	77

Table 9-3. Spring Sports Injuries: Fall 1982 to Spring 1988

Sport	Fatalities		Catastrophic Injuries	Serious Injuries	Total
	Direct	Indirect			
Baseball					
High school	2	2	3	5	12
College	1	1	0	0	2
Lacrosse					
High school	0	1	0	0	1
College	0	0	1	2	3
Track					
High school	5	7	2	4	18
College	0	1	1	1	3
Tennis					
High school	0	1	0	0	1
College	0	2	0	0	2
TOTAL	8	15	7	12	42

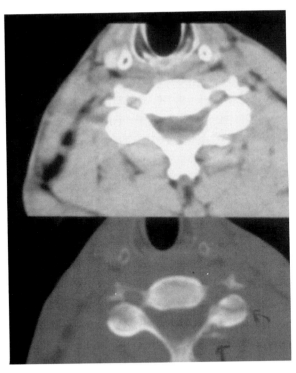

Fig. 9-2. A fractured lamina and facet of this kind can occur with head trauma. Positive head compression tenderness and decreased range of motion are key features.

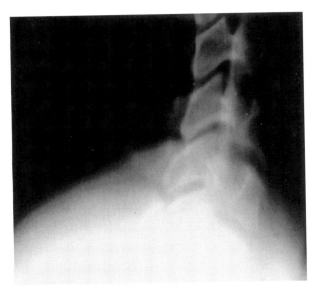

Fig. 9-3. A facet fracture in a 24-year-old downhill skiing racer healed with nonoperative care and produced a stiff but stable segment. The racer was cleared to return to racing in a mild-risk category. Facet fractures depend significantly on the type of residual deformity in the presence of instability.

arthritis of the cervical spine as compared with the rest of the population.[17]

High jumping—A high jumper's neck is subject to chronic, repetitive, unrecognized flexion injury.

Hockey—The most common cause of injury is a push or a check from behind that causes the player to be catapulted headfirst into the boards.[20,21]

Weight training—Injuries vary from neck strain, lumbar strain, and cervical disc herniation to the more rare posttraumatic syringomyelia.[1,3]

Wrestling—Takedown techniques in which the head is smashed into the neck lead to the potential for neck injuries, and the training needed to prevent neck injuries produces chronic degenerative changes.[30]

Other injuries associated with specific sports are outlined in the chapters on those sports (see Section Six, Specific Sports).

CLINICAL ANATOMY AND SIGNS AND SYMPTOMS OF INJURY

The cervical spinal cord is housed under the rigid, intercalated spinal motion units. Protection against direct blows, as well as against axial loading, flexion, extension, and torsional injuries, is afforded by the lamina, spinous processes, facet joints, and vertebral bodies of the cervical spine. However, when axial loading and bending surpass the bony element's biomechanical capability and strength, fractures and/or dislocations

may result. This failure of the bony elements of the spine may cause injury to the spinal cord or cervical nerve roots. The same may occur when the mechanical limits of the ligamentous and muscular support of the neck are exceeded in traumatic situations.

In the neck the cervical spinal cord produces the cervical nerve roots, which exit above the corresponding cervical vertebrae via the neural foramina. This relationship between spinal level and root level has important diagnostic and prognostic implications when an athlete sustains a spinal cord injury. From a surgical viewpoint, the precise anatomic level corresponding to nerve tissue damage is critical in ensuring that any surgical intervention is performed at the correct level. Prognostically, the potential for functional independence in a quadriplegic patient increases dramatically with each functioning root level below the fourth cervical nerve root. Clinically, the difference between C5-level quadriplegia and C7-level quadriplegia is dramatic. In fact, the recovery of a single additional cervical nerve root level in a quadriplegic patient can mean the difference between a completely dependent existence and a completely independent and functional life.

Cervical spine or spinal cord injury has a more favorable prognosis when the injury is identified before the injured patient is moved any further. An unstable fracture or dislocation without neurologic injury can have catastrophic sequelae if improper transportation techniques are used. The athlete with an unstable cervical spine injury may not be aware of the magnitude of the injury because of the minimal amount of pain felt at the time of injury. However, once the injury has been identified as a spinal cord injury, the level of injury can be quickly assessed by simple pinprick sensation testing along the cervical dermatomes and by manual muscle strength testing. The fifth cervical nerve root supplies sensation to the deltoid region in the lateral brachium distally to the elbow. The sixth cervical nerve root supplies skin sensation to the lateral forearm from the elbow distally to include the thumb and index finger. The seventh cervical nerve root supplies the sensation to the upper extremity and the dermatomal region that includes the midpalm, as well as the long finger. The eighth cervical nerve root supplies the dermatomal region that includes the ulnar border of the forearm, as well as the ring and small fingers. The first thoracic nerve root supplies the dermatomal region medially at the elbow and proximally up toward the middle part of the arm. It is not unusual for there to be some overlap of adjacent dermatomes.

EXAMINATION AND DIAGNOSIS

The motor deficits identifiable in cervical spinal cord injury are categorized according to which motor groups are spared. It should be remembered that the third cervical root exists at the level of the second and third cervical discs. Schneider[15] has summarized the injury levels as follows:

C3-4 level — Injury may result in complete paralysis of the trunk and extremities, with complete loss of all normal, unassisted respirations as a result of paralysis of the diaphragm, as well as of the thoracic musculature. Loss of pinprick sensation to a point just below the clavicle, including the upper extremities, may be seen.

C4-5 level — The athlete can only shrug the shoulders, indicating trapezius innervation via the second and third cervical nerve roots to the motor branch of the spinal accessory nerve. There is no movement of the arms, lower extremities, and trunk, and the toes point outward. Only abdominal breathing is present, and if only one more segment toward the head is involved, spontaneous respirations cease. Spinal cord swelling or hemorrhage progresses, especially if inappropriate immobilization techniques are used. The motor fibers extending to the diaphragm via the phrenic nerve from the C3 and C4 nerve cell bodies exit from the spinal cord with the upper portion of the C5 root. Pain sensation is absent to the level of the outer border of the upper extremity between the shoulder and the elbow.

C5-6 level — The player can bend the arms at the elbows, and they will tend to remain flexed in that position unless they fall downward with the pull of gravity. Attempted movements of the hands result in hyperextension at the wrists with inability to

voluntarily close the fingers. Extension of the arms is markedly impaired. Loss of pinprick sensation may occur over the region of the thumb and index finger of the hand.

C6-7 level — The athlete can close the hands very weakly and grasp with the fingers. The arms can be flexed and extended weakly at the elbows. The athlete may be unable to strongly spread the fingers apart because of loss of innervation of the intrinsic musculature of the hands. Pinprick sensation is intact over the thumb and index finger but is usually lost over the middle and radial half of the ring finger.

C7-T1 level and below — Muscle function of the upper extremities may be completely spared, with only lower extremity paraplegia. Trunk control, including control of the rectus abdominis, internal and external oblique, and spinal extensor muscles, is, however, affected by the level of the thoracic spinal cord injury. With more caudal thoracic spinal cord injury, the patient is more able to adapt to activities requiring controlled and coordinated trunk muscle activity. Pinprick sensation is impaired from the dermatomal level corresponding to the level of injury. Fracture dislocations of the thoracic or lumbar spine are much less common in athletes, partly because of protective equipment, such as shoulder pads, covering the area. Also, the thoracic rib cage imparts significant structural support to the thoracic spine.

It should be noted that these are fairly simple tests and are meant only as a quick method of determining the level of neurologic impairment while the player is still on the playing field. Even if the player's complaints include only vague neck stiffness or pain, the examiner should proceed as if a true spinal cord injury is present until it is proved otherwise.

Examination of the player on the sidelines usually reveals the mechanism of injury by careful questioning concerning purely radicular symptoms. Spurling's maneuver reproduces the symptoms. The shoulder abduction test, in which the hand is placed palm down on the top of the head, may alleviate the symptoms somewhat.[28] Davidson, Dunn, and Metzmaker[6] observed a series of patients with cervical myeloradiculopathies due to extradural compressive disease in whom clinical signs included relief of radicular pain with abduction of the shoulder. The mechanism by which shoulder abduction may relieve pain from cervical root impingement at the level of the neural foramen is thought to be the shorter distance that the nerve root must traverse (and thus be under less tension) when the shoulder is abducted. Davidson, Dunn, and Metzmaker's study included two patients who had myelographically proven extradural impingement of the cervical root. Sixty-eight percent of their patients noted relief of pain with abduction of the affected shoulder. On the field the player with a "stinger," or "burner," classically maintains a head-forward and flexed posture and complains of a stiff neck. The arm is too weak to elevate. Attempts to elicit Spurling's sign are generally met with pain. Occasionally, head compression will reproduce the symptoms. It should be remembered that persistent neck pain with head compression is considered evidence of a fracture or disc herniation until it is proved otherwise.

Radiologic Evaluation

Once x-ray films are available, it is mandatory to obtain adequate visualization of the cervicothoracic junction at C7-T1, as well as an x-ray film of adequate quality that can be safely interpreted. Generally, the lateral x-ray film is obtained first and should be interpreted and evaluated before proceeding with the remainder of the radiographic evaluation. Thomas[23] has reported the appropriate sequence of radiographs that should be obtained in the neck-injured player; these include the anteroposterior projection, the lateral x-ray film and the neutral position, the open-mouth view of the atlantoaxial articulation, and each oblique position. Not until the initial sequence of cervical spine films has been reviewed and evaluated for any potential instability, fracture, or dislocation, should subsequent flexion-extension radiographs be considered (Fig. 9-4). If such instability, fracture, or dislocation is identified, the next appropriate step is to continue cervical spine immobilization and proceed with definitive treatment or further diagnostic studies, including a computed tomography

(CT) scan or magnetic resonance imaging (MRI), as indicated by the nature of the lesion. When the basic radiographic evaluation indicates spinal instability, fracture, or dislocation, then the lateral flexion-extension films may be contraindicated and unsafe.

The x-ray films should be evaluated for obvious vertebral body fracture or malalignment, and the anterior retropharyngeal space should also be evaluated. At the anterior aspect of the body at C3, there should be no more than 4 mm of space between the posterior pharynx and the anterior vertebral body. An increased retropharyngeal space indicates soft tissue swelling and may indicate cervical spine injury. The posterior margins of the vertebral bodies and the spinal laminar lines should

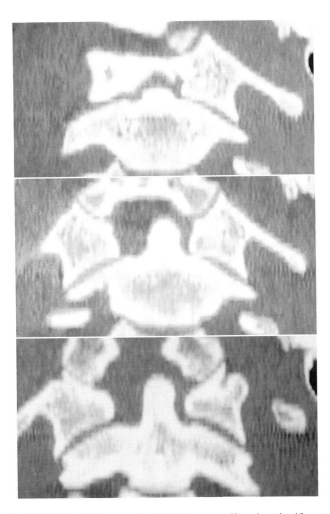

Fig. 9-5. This adolescent football player suffered a significant neck injury with residual torticollis. The C1-2 evaluation revealed no fracture, but the patient had a residual rotatory subluxation of C1-2. Since chronic rotatory subluxation with torticollis presents a considerable risk to an adolescent athlete, the recommendations were to avoid football, work hard in an upper body–strengthening and conditioning program, and hopefully return to noncontact sports.

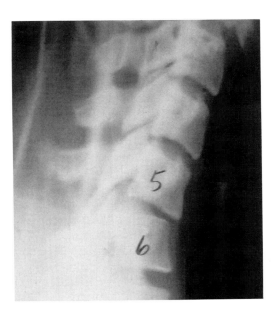

Fig. 9-4. A lateral x-ray film under emergency conditions should allow the diagnosis of a unilateral facet dislocation or facet fracture.

be evaluated for a symmetric and smooth contour. The facet joints should be evaluated for symmetry and congruity. Changes in the rotational position of the spinal column from one motion segment to the next may indicate facet subluxation or dislocation. The criteria of White et al.,[29] including subluxation of 3.5 mm or more and kyphotic angulation of the injured level that is 11 degrees or more greater than an adjacent level, are generally considered evidence of cervical spine instability (Fig. 9-5). These criteria pertain to any lateral cervical spine view, including a flexion view.

The evaluation of C1 through T1 is imperative and can be facilitated by using downward traction on the player's hand by an assistant or by the use of Boger straps. At the Kerlan-Jobe Orthopaedic Clinic we prefer the Boger straps, which are passive-action Velcro straps connected to the wrists and passed around the bottoms of the feet. They are tightened with the knees flexed. As the knees are pushed down to straighten them out, the straps tighten and pull the arms down. A sandbag can be placed on the knees in an unconscious patient, thereby maintaining traction on the arms. We have never had a patient in which C7 was not visualized using the Boger straps. Occasionally traction on an arm with cervical radiculopathy produces too much pain to pull for a long time. If Boger straps are not available, the "swimmer's view" can be used, which is a special radiographic view obtained by centering the beam on the lateral projection at C7. The patient's arm closest to the source of the radiographic beam is left at the patient's side while the opposite arm, which is adjacent to the radiographic plate, is fully abducted over the patient's head. If adequate visualization of the cervicothoracic junction remains a problem after the "swimmer's view" is obtained, a CT scan is done of that region. We will not clear a patient's cervical spine film unless the full cervical spine is visualized. Also important on the lateral view is the atlantodens interval. An atlantodens interval greater than 2 to 3 mm may be considered indicative of cervical spine instability at the atlantoaxial articulation, particularly if this atlantodens interval markedly increases on flexion films.

One difficult aspect of the radiographic evaluation is to determine if there is an acute injury, an old injury, or an asymptomatic finding. A complicating factor is the presence of a hypermobile segment over a stiff, arthritic segment. Many athletes who do neck-strengthening exercises regularly, especially those starting at a young age, have relative osteoarthritic changes in the lower cervical spine region. The biomechanical stiffness of these levels may produce a relative increase in mobility through a compensatory mechanism at the levels just above these less mobile lower segments. To find an asymptomatic, never-injured level that exceeds the White-Punjabi criteria would be rare.[29]

Adequate identification of an area of ligamentous instability may be particularly difficult in acute situations secondary to associated muscle spasm from the injury.

A compression fracture noted in the lateral film must be interpreted with caution because it may include an injury with associated cervical spine instability. A review of 27 patients with cervical compression fractures revealed that 6 of these patients were later noted to have associated cervical spine instability.[12] When doubt continues as to the stability of a cervical spine injury, such as when there is too much spasm to obtain flexion extension views, immobilization with a cervical orthosis is continued until additional radiographic evaluation is obtained in subsequent days with flexion-extension views. Once a fracture has been identified on a plain film or CT scan, it should be classified according to the standard classification system used today, depending on the spinal level affected and the fracture configuration.

Often important in the radiologic evaluation is the determination of whether a radiographic finding is an acute injury, on old injury, or an asymptomatic degenerative change. Boden et al.[2] identified the incidence of asymptomatic degenerative changes occurring in the cervical spine in a group of volunteers who underwent MRI of the cervical spine while being asymptomatic for problems related to the neck. They were able to identify a 14% to 35% incidence of herniated cervical discs, osteophytes, or degenerative disc disease in these asymptomatic individuals, which underscores the importance of clinical correlation between the radiographic findings and the history and physical examination findings in individuals being evaluated for cervical injuries.

In-Depth Studies

The logical answer to the question of when should in-depth studies be done is "when they are needed to make the diagnosis" or "when the results would change the treatment." As a practical measure, studies are obtained on players with severe, persistent, or recurring problems. For a stiff, painful neck due to a recent injury, a bone scan may identify an acute fracture. MRI and plain CT scans are helpful, and a contrast CT scan helps identify disc herniations and fractures (Fig. 9-6). An electromyogram (EMG) with nerve conduction study can help distinguish a peripheral nerve problem from a cervical nerve root problem but is not as helpful in detecting progression in a case. Making liberal use of whatever tests are taken to diagnose the problem is the way to proper treatment and prognosis.

MANAGEMENT

Managing neck injuries sustained by athletes often centers on what risks are involved in returning to play either on that day or later.[10,11,26] Risk can include permanent injury or recurrent symptoms. The diagnosis,

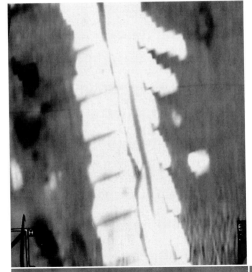

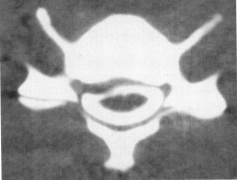

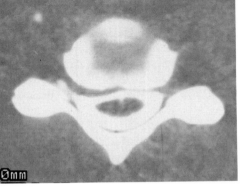

Fig. 9-6. This 20-year-old major league outfielder had intense radicular right arm pain. He had radiation into the thumb and index finger and signs of C6 radiculopathy. The patient was treated nonoperatively in the last 2 months of the season but continued to have problems throwing the ball. His shoulder joint was developing some strain, and he was advised not to throw the ball; he was told that he could return to base running and hitting as long as he developed no pain. If symptoms continued, the recommendation was to have an anterior cervical fusion during the off season. **A,** Parasagittal view. **B,** Transverse view. **C,** Transverse view showing some nerve root filling but considerable herniation.

prognosis, and risk factors for future injury must be weighed. The physician must be trained in evaluating, diagnosing, and treating neck injuries and have a thorough understanding of the mechanics involved in the particular sport, as well as an understanding of the effects of game stresses on the particular injury that the player has received. Factors to be considered include the mechanism of the player's injury, any prior history of neck injury, the findings on physical examination immediately after injury, and the results of diagnostic studies. Factors to be avoided are contract provisions, disability contracts, the player's desire to play, and the desires of others (e.g., spouse, coach, team owner, parents). The physician should state the medical facts of the case and provide the same information to all concerned about the known risk factors. If there is a history of prior neck injury, it must include the frequency of occurrence of such incidents as stingers, transient neuropraxia, and neck stiffness, as well as the length of duration of these episodes. The type of treatments that the player has received and the player's response to these treatments are also important considerations, along with published clinical scientific information related to the specific neck

injury and the physician's personal experience in diagnosing and treating neck injuries in athletes.

Immobilization and Transportation

When confronted with an individual on the playing field who complains of symptoms of neck pain or stiffness, or who has any upper or lower extremity neurologic manifestations, the trainer or team physician should initially ensure prompt and adequate immobilization of the cervical spine and establish an airway. In an emergency setting, the helmet should not be removed from a player suspected of having sustained cervical spine injury. In a player with neck injury and respiratory compromise, either the face mask must be removable or large bolt cutters capable of transecting the metallic face mask must be available. If the player is unconscious and respiratory effort is inadequate, the airway may be opened by grasping the angle of the mandible with both hands and thrusting the jaw forward. Hyperextension of the head to obtain an open airway is usually not necessary when cervical spine injury is a possibility. It is only after cervical spine immobilization has been provided that the individual may be transported to the

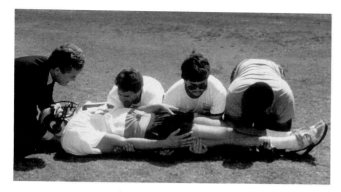

Fig. 9-7. Multiman carry. The team chief immobilizes the head and neck and calls the signals. Three men on each side of the body (the three on the near side are not pictured) join hands and lift. The spine board is brought in underneath.

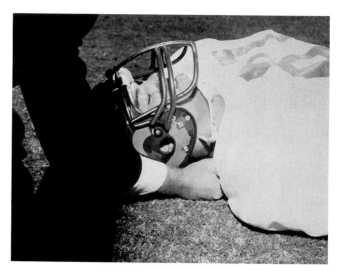

Fig. 9-8. Method of immobilizing the head to the trunk. The team chief holds the trapezius-clavicle-scapula area with his hands and holds the head between his forearms.

sidelines, the locker room, or the emergency room. When there is doubt concerning the necessity for neck immobilization and player transportation, the recommendation is to consider the player a victim of spinal injury until further evaluation is possible. The precise and safe implementation of cervical spine immobilization and transportation require proper instruction of the coach and trainer by the team physician, as well as practice in the transportation techniques by those involved. The team trainer, as well as rescue personnel, must have available and be comfortable with the application of standard cervical immobilization collars. Those commonly in use are the Nek-Loc and the Philadelphia collar. When appropriate, the collar can be applied to the player before transportation.

The transport technique should be standardized and practiced by the trainer, coach, and team physician before the start of the playing season; five to six people are needed to move the player safely (Fig. 9-7). One person controls the head and shoulders (Fig. 9-8). As the person in charge of the timing of transportation, this individual should grab the trapezius, clavicle, and scapular area with his hands while cradling the helmeted head of the player between his forearms. The person in charge, or transportation team chief, should not be responsible for any of the weight of the transfer. The other members of the transportation team include one person who holds the player's shoulders and upper torso and two persons who hold the player's trunk and upper thighs on each side. Two more members are responsible for lifting and turning the legs. The person holding the head announces each move in the transportation process. When practicing these maneuvers, the team chief may try holding only the head in an awake, uninjured volunteer and proceed through the turning maneuvers. The awake volunteer should then be asked how much neck movement was felt during the turning procedure.

Generally, a significant amount of neck motion can be felt, reinforcing the need of the team chief to maintain a firm grasp on the shoulders and the head, thus ensuring adequate immobilization of a potentially unstable cervical spine. The team chief can grasp both the trapezius inside and a shoulder pad outside, but this is not quite as stable as the preceding method. Another person may be used to squeeze the team chief's forearms to the head, thus further increasing the stability of the team chief's grasp on the player's shoulders and head.

Once all individuals are in place on each side of the body, they join hands in an Indian-grip fashion, with the palm placed against the forearm of the individual directly across, underneath the player. On the team chief's signal, the assistants gently elevate the player off the ground while a rigid backboard is slid directly under the player.

If the player is face down on the field, the team chief rotates his arms and grasps the player's head and shoulders in a similar fashion (Fig. 9-9). An assistant must grasp the team chief's arms and squeeze them against the head to increase the hold on the player's shoulders and head. Safely turning the prone player to the supine position requires several assistants to gently roll the player over while the team chief maintains the alignment of the head with the shoulders during the turn. Once the player is turned, the standard transportation protocol is used.

Once the player is on the backboard, the player can be safely transported off the field to the appropriate health care facility while the team chief maintains his grasp on the player's shoulders and head. If an appropriate cervical orthosis is available, the team chief may

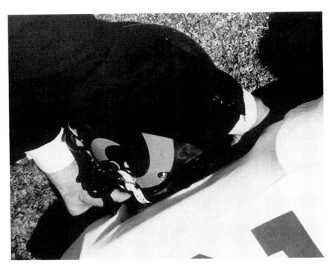

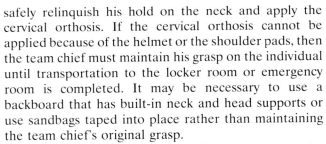

Fig. 9-9. If the player is face down on the field, the team chief rotates his arms and grasps the player's head and shoulders in a similar fashion. In this situation it is mandatory that an assistant grasp the team chief's arms and squeeze them against the head to increase the hold on the player's shoulders and head. Safely turning the prone player to the supine position requires several assistants to gently roll the player over while the team chief maintains the alignment of the head with the shoulders during the turn. Once the player is turned, then the standard transportation protocol is used.

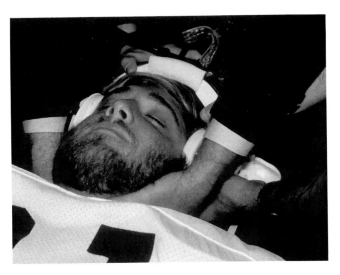

Fig. 9-10. To remove the helmet, the surgeon should stand with hands grasping both the occiput and the base of the neck in order to allow the assistants to remove the helmet. The face mask should be removed to allow proper elasticity in the helmet to enable it to be removed. Several assistants should help remove the helmet while the surgeon steadies the head and neck.

safely relinquish his hold on the neck and apply the cervical orthosis. If the cervical orthosis cannot be applied because of the helmet or the shoulder pads, then the team chief must maintain his grasp on the individual until transportation to the locker room or emergency room is completed. It may be necessary to use a backboard that has built-in neck and head supports or use sandbags taped into place rather than maintaining the team chief's original grasp.

Once the player is in a controlled environment, the helmet should be removed in a safe fashion. First, the face mask is removed (Fig. 9-10). The appropriate hand position of the team chief for helmet removal includes grasping the base of the occiput and the base of the neck with open palms and fingers. An assistant may first spread the sides of the helmet and then gently slide the helmet in a cephalad direction off the player while neck control is maintained by the team chief. Absolutely no cervical flexion should be allowed during this maneuver. If the shoulder pads do not allow for adequate physical examination and radiography of the cervical spine, they should be removed at this time, in a similar fashion while cervical immobilization is maintained and cervical or head flexion is prevented.

REHABILITATION PRINCIPLES

A number of different modalities and techniques are used for rehabilitation of cervical spine injuries.[19,22,27]

Certainly, in the athlete who is expecting to return to contact sports, it is imperative to regain a full, pain-free range of motion of the cervical spine.

We recommend a progressive isometric trunk-strengthening exercise program aimed at placing the neck in a biomechanically sound position with the shoulders, back, and chest in a posturally correct position. This exercise program concentrates on trunk strengthening and trunk mobility. Throughout the program the patient is instructed in postural modifications that place the patient in a chest-out posture, which effectively normalizes the lumbar lordosis while bringing the shoulders backward and bringing the head and neck back over the shoulders (see Upper Extremity Postural Exercises in Chapter 27). In this position, which is quite similar to the military position of attention, the cervical lordosis is normalized while the neural foramina are opened. Athletes involved in the use of the upper extremities require a rigid cylinder of strength in their torso in order to transfer torque from their legs to their upper extremities. Trunk and leg strength generate the strength of the upper extremity activity, whereas the arms and hands generally provide the fine control. Fatigue in the trunk or legs can reduce the fine control available in the upper extremities for overhead activities, such as in racquet sports and throwing sports. With loss of rigid trunk cylinder strength, loss of synchrony between the arms and legs results. There is a similar linkage between the legs, trunk, neck, and head in regard to the fine control.

Our trunk-conditioning program is aimed at developing power in the torsional strength of the trunk musculature, including the trapezius muscles; the spinal erector musculature; the latissimus dorsi; the internal and external oblique muscles; the transversus abdomins; the rectus abdomins sheath of muscle; the gluteal musculature; the hip flexors, extensors, abductors, and adductors; and the thigh musculature. Trunk-strengthening exercises are designed not only to enhance performance, but also to prevent subsequent injury to the back, the neck, and the arms.

When an individual trainer or physician treats an athlete with neck or back pain after an injury, the full clinical details of that patient must be incorporated into a rehabilitation and exercise protocol that is designed specifically for that individual and for that individual's injuries. The isometric trunk-conditioning program can be effective in preventing back injuries and is useful in treating many individuals with neck or back pain. Any trunk–strengthening and conditioning program places a biomechanical strain on the spine and can exacerbate any underlying inflammatory or degenerative condition that is symptomatic. Implementation of this isometric trunk-strengthening and posture correction program proceeds progressively from less vigorous activity to more vigorous activity as the patient's symptoms diminish.

The key to safe strengthening of the back and neck is an ability to maintain the spine in a safe, neutral position during the strengthening exercises. For upper body strengthening, the spine must be well aligned with a chest-out posture. Isometric trunk exercises and upper body exercises that emphasize this chest-out posture also strengthen the supporting structures for the cervical spine, strengthen the postural muscles necessary for maintaining proper body alignment, and ultimately are useful measures to prevent neck pain during athletic activity. In individuals other than football players, we do not recommend specific neck-strengthening exercises except for modest isometric exercises that can be performed manually only. There are certainly exceptions; in sports such as wrestling, rugby, and other contact sports the individual neck-strengthening exercises must be tailored appropriately.

Every exercise in this program could be done by any reasonably conditioned athlete with no training whatsoever, but the key is doing the exercises correctly. The program starts with the athlete learning to obtain and maintain a neutral, pain-free position for the trunk and being able to hold the trunk muscles, including the buttocks, the paraspinous musculature, the abdominal oblique musculature, the rectus abdomins musculature, and the thigh musculature, in a tight, rigidly controlled neutral trunk position. These exercises teach a balanced and coordinated muscle-firing sequence of adequate strength to protect the spine during the sport activity. Being able to do 5000 sit-ups may protect one's back

while doing the sit-ups, but not while throwing a football, throwing a baseball, or tackling another player. The key to the exercises is the first step: being able to isolate the trunk musculature, provide a tight contraction, and hold the spine in a neutral, pain-free position. The therapist and trainer initially assist the individual in learning where the neutral, pain-free position is and how to use the muscles to maintain that position.

This exercise program is helpful in the postoperative recovery of patients after neck and back surgery. After neck surgery an appropriate period of spinal immobilization with an orthotic device is required. Then the patient may initiate this series of exercises with the assistance of the physical therapist.

Generally, within 3 to 6 weeks after neck or back surgery that does not require bony healing or bony fusion to take place, we initiate our isometric trunk stabilization program if the wound is well healed and the patient is able to safely take part in a water rehabilitation program. We allow patients to enter into a gentle water rehabilitation program at 3 weeks, doing exercises in a swimming pool by running in the water while wearing a wet vest. By 6 weeks postoperatively, the patient is usually able to advance to dry-land exercises that include progressive walking for aerobic conditioning.

Further details of the exercise program recommended for cervical spine injuries are offered elsewhere in this text.

REFERENCES

1. Balmaseda MT Jr et al: Post-traumatic syringomyelia associated with heavy weightlifting exercises, *Arch Phys Med Rehabil* 69:970, 1988.
2. Boden SD et al: Abnormal magnetic resonance scans of the cervical spine in asymptomatic subjects: a prospective investigation, *J Bone Joint Surg* 72A:1178, 1990.
3. Brady TA, Cahill BR, Bodnar LM: Weight training–related injuries in the high school athlete, *Am J Sports Med* 10:1, 1982.
4. Burke DC: Spinal cord injuries from water sports, *Med J Aust* 2:1190, 1972.
5. Clark KS: The survey of sports related spinal cord injuries in schools and colleges: 1973-1975, *J Safety Res* 9:140, 1977.
6. Davidson RI, Dunn EJ, Metzmaker JN: The shoulder abduction test, *Spine*. 6:441, 1981.
7. Hoskins TW: Prevention of neck injuries playing rugby, *Public Health Engl* 101:351, 1987.
8. Jackson DW, Lohr FP: Cervical spine injuries, *Clin Sports Med* 5:373, 1986.
9. Kelsey JL: An epidemiological study of acute prolapsed cervical intervertebral disc, *J Bone Joint Surg* 66A:907, 1984.
10. Marks MR, Bell GR, Boumphrey FR: Cervical spine fractures in athletes, *Clin Sports Med* 9:13, 1990.
11. Mashala LJ: Sports following spinal injury in the young athlete, *Clin Orthop* 198:152, 1985.
12. Mazur JW, Stauffer ES: Unrecognized spinal instability associated with seemingly simple cervical compression fractures, *Spine* 8:687, 1983.
13. Mueller FO, Cantu R: Catastrophic injuries and fatalities in high school and college sports, *Med Sci Sports Exerc* 22:737, 1990.
14. Neuber GW, Schafer MF: Clay shovelers injury report of two injuries sustained from football, *Am J Sports Med* 15:182, 1987.
15. Schneider RC: The treatment of the athlete with neck, cervical spine and spinal cord trauma. In Schneider RC, editor: *Sports*

injuries: mechanisms, prevention and treatment, ed 1, Baltimore, 1985, Williams & Wilkins.

16. Schneider RC: Serious and fatal neurosurgical football injuries, *Clin Neurosurg* 12:226, 1966.

17. Sher AT: Premature onset of degenerative disease in cervical spine rugby players, *S Afr Med J* 77:577, 1990.

18. Sovio OM, Van Peteghem PK, Schweigel JF: Cervical spine injuries in rugby players, *Can Med J* 130:735, March 1984.

19. Tan JC, Nordin M: The role of physical therapy in the treatment of cervical disc disease, *Orthop Clin North Am* 23:435, 1992.

20. Tator CH, Edmonds VE: National survey of spinal injuries in hockey players, *Can Med Assoc J* 130:185, 1984.

21. Tator CH, Edmonds VE, Lapezak L: Spinal injuries in ice hockey players, 1966-1987, *Can J Surg* 34:63, 1991.

22. Teitz CC, Cook DM: Rehabilitation of neck and low back injuries, *Clin Sports Med* 4:455, 1985.

23. Thomas JC: Plain roentgenograms of the spine in the injured athlete, *Clin Sports Med* 5:353, 1990.

24. Torg JS, Senate B, Vegso JJ: Spinal injury at the level of the 3rd and 4th cervical vertebrae resulting from axial loading and analysis of classification, *Clin Sports Med* 6:159, 1987.

25. Torg JS, et al: The National Football Head and Neck Injury Registry: 14 year report on cervical quadriplegia, 1971-1984, *JAMA* 254:3439, 1985.

26. Vegso JJ, Lehman RC: Field evaluation and management of head and neck injuries, *Clin Sports Med* 6:1, 1987.

27. Vegso JJ, Torg JS: Rehabilitation of cervical spine, brachial plexus, and peripheral nerve injuries, *Clin Sports Med* 6:135, 1987.

28. Watkins RG: Neck injuries in football players, *Clin Sports Med* 5:215, 1986.

29. White AA III et al: Biomechanical analysis of clinical stability in the cervical spine, *Clin Orthop* 109:89, 1975.

30. Wroble RR, Albright JP: Neck and low back injuries in wrestling, *Clin Sports Med* 5:295, 1986.

Chapter Ten

♦

Lumbar Spine Injuries

Robert G. Watkins

The lumbar spine is a highly vulnerable area for injury in a number of different sports. The incidence varies from 27%[11] to 7%[6] or 13%.[12] While the incidence is significant and the time lost may be significant, probably the most important problems are related to the fear of spinal injuries and the need for a therapeutic plan. Lumbar pain is significant in many sports, but an organized diagnostic and therapeutic plan can prevent permanent injury, allowing full function and maximum performance.

Among the sports most often associated with lumbar spine injury are the following:

Gymnastics — The motions and activities of gymnastics produce tremendous strains on the lumbar spine. The hyperlordotic position used with certain maneuvers, such as back walk-overs, requires extreme flexibility, and the lumbar flexion/extension used during flips and vaulting dismounts requires great strength to support the spine during these extremes of flexibility. It is believed that the vigorous lumbar motion in hyperextension in gymnastics produces a fatigue fracture, resulting in spondylolysis. There is also a hereditary predisposition to the stress fracture of spondylolysis, and finding occult spina bifida in some of these gymnasts reveals a possible weakness.

Ballet — Many of the motions used in ballet resemble those in gymnastics, particularly the arabesque position, which requires both extension and rotation of the lumbar spine. Ballet also involves lifting of dancers, especially in awkward positions. Off-balance bending and lifting are hallmarks of back problems in industrial workers and, yet, ballet, while balanced, is often designed to produce extremely difficult lifts. Resulting spondylolysis and spondylolisthesis often produce severe mechanical back dysfunction.

Water sports — In addition to injuries to the wrist and cervical spine, in diving the lumbar spine is subjected to added strain, both in rapid flexion/extension changes and in severe back arching after entering the water. Although swimming and water exercises form a major component of back rehabilitation programs, certain kicks, such as the butterfly, produce vigorous flexion/extension of the lumbar spine, especially in young swimmers. The swimmer must attain good abdominal tone and strength to protect the back during vigorous kicking motions.

Weight lifting — The incidence of lower back pain and problems in weight lifters is estimated to be 40%.[1] The tremendous forces exerted on the lumbar spine by lifting weights over the head produce extreme lever-arm effects and compressive injury to the spine. Extension forces of the lumbar spine naturally lead to increased risks of spondylolysis and spondylolisthesis.[7] Many newer training techniques in weight lifting emphasize the role of general body conditioning, flexibility, aerobic conditioning, speed, and cross-training in addition to the ability to lift weight.

Running — Low back pain is commonly reported in runners. In achieving the aerobic conditioning that running provides, the runner often must experience stiffness, contractures, and selected areas of muscle weakness. Runners also have a natural tendency to develop isolated abdominal weakness, frequently producing a significant imbalance between flexor and extensor muscles, both in the legs and in the trunk.

Golfing — Golfers have the highest incidence of back injury of all professional athletes. Lumbar spine pain in golfers results from torsional stress on the lumbar spine.

Baseball — Torsional problems develop in both pitchers and hitters. Pitchers require a rigid cylinder of strength in order to transfer torque from their legs to their throwing arm. Fatigue reduces the control of the pitching motion and ball location. As the abdominal musculature weakens because of fatigue, lumbar lordosis increases and the back arches. Attempts to compensate for loss of trunk strength and a "slow arm" increase the use of the arm musculature and predispose the shoulder to injury. Hitters initiate a violent lumbar rotation based on instantaneous ocular information. Therefore the head position and maintenance of that position are as critical as acuity and eye focus. Delayed recognition of the ball produces a rotation with the hips too far in front of the shoulders, a loss of parallelism of the shoulders and hips, and increased torsional strain of the lumbar spine.

In summary, the keys to proper management of lumbar spine problems in athletes include the following:

1. Comprehensive diagnosis
2. Aggressive, effective nonoperative care
3. Pinpointing operations that do as little damage as possible to normal tissue but correct the pathologic lesion

CLINICAL ANATOMY AND BIOMECHANICS OF THE LUMBAR SPINE

Understanding the basic biomechanics of the lumbar spine begins with an understanding of the forces and stresses applied to the spine in relation to the normal curvatures of the spine. Because of the lordotic shape of the spine, vectorial forces on the spine are usually made up of two vertical axial loading compressive forces—one perpendicular to the surface of the disc and one horizontal to the disc—producing a shear strain. The combination of these two forces produces both tensile stress in the annulus fibrosis and a shear force on the neural arch.[4] The center of gravity of body weight is anterior to the spine. This weight times the distance back to the spine produces a lever-arm effect of the weight of the body. This is resisted by the erector spinae muscles, the abdominal musculature, the lumbodorsal fascia, and the gluteus maximus.[4] When abnormal stresses are applied, the result may be annular tears of the intervertebral discs or stress fractures on the neural arch as a result of the excessive resistive force. The most common place for stress fractures is the pars interarticularis.

The basic mechanism of injury is a combined vector of force that may be difficult to analyze in a force diagram.[5]

Three common mechanisms of injury to consider are:
1. Compression or weight loading to the spine
2. Torque or rotation (may result in various shear forces in a more horizontal plane)
3. Tensile stress produced through excessive motion on the spine

The compressive type of stress is more common in sports that require high body weight and massive strengthening, such as football and weight lifting. Torsional stresses occur in athletes participating in sports such as javelin throwing, baseball, and golf. Motion sports that put tremendous tensile stresses on the spine include gymnastics, ballet, dance, pole vaulting, and high jumping.

Some injuries result from direct blows. In sports such as football there can be muscle contusions, muscle stretches, and tears of fascia, ligaments, and occasionally muscle.

Lumbar fractures can occur from direct blows to the back with fracture of the spinous process or twisting injuries that avulse the transverse process. Vertebral body end-plate fractures from axial compression loading on the disc is a relatively common source of compressive disc injury. Whereas the annulus is more likely to be injured in rotation, the end-plate is more vulnerable to compression than the annulus. Axial loading compression injuries can result from jarring injuries in motor sports or boating. Flexion rotation fracture dislocations of the cervical and lumbar spine are possible. In any sport in which one athlete falls on another, an athlete can suffer an asymmetric loading, rotational injury to the thoracolumbar spine. Any time equipment is involved, such as a motorcycle, board, or automobile, direct translational blows can produce a fracture dislocation.

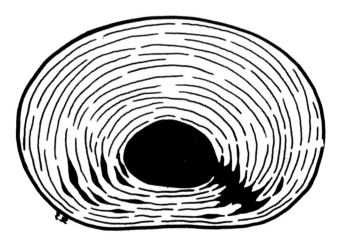

Fig. 10-1. The disc is a multilayered, woven basket, with round, concentric rings of tough, ligamentous structure, that develops first circumferential tears and then radial tears and should be treated as any other ligament tear, such as a sprained ankle or a torn knee ligament. The pain resulting from the annular disruption produces abnormal motion, inflammation, and pain. The outer layers of the annulus are richly innervated, as is the granulation tissue that grows into the injury. Discogenic pain produces excruciating back and referred leg pain and should be treated as one would most other significant joint injuries.

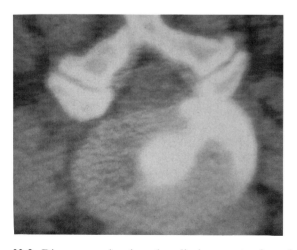

Fig. 10-2. Discogram showing the displacement of nuclear material into the tear in the annulus that may produce a bulge that may contribute to the nerve root irritation and is part of the scenario of an annular tear leading to progressive herniation.

The intervertebral disc is injured predominantly through rotation and shear, producing circumferential tears and radial tears (Figs. 10-1 and 10-2). Initially the layers may actually separate, or the inner layers may break. As the inner layers weaken and are torn, additional stress is placed on the outer layers. This can produce a radial tear of the intervertebral disc. With the outer layers torn, the inner layers of annulus break off and, along with portions of the nucleus, are forced with axial loading to the place of least resistance, the weak area in the annulus. The outer areas of annulus are richly innervated, producing tremendous pain and reflex spasm when the annulus tears. The nuclear material can produce a chemical neuritis and inflammation. The spasm and pain are mediated through the sinovertebral nerve with anastomosis through the spinal nerve and the posterior primary ramus. As the herniated annular fragment extrudes, producing pain from the traversing or exiting nerve root itself, the patient may develop sciatica or radiculopathy. Intradiscal infiltration of the granulation tissue adds increased potential for painful sensation in the annulus. The annulus, with time, can heal. Although the healing annulus will not retain the same biomechanical function capability as the original intervertebral disc, it can be completely compatible with pain-free function.

Biomechanical functioning of the spinal column and its relationship to the biomechanics of nerve tissue involve several basic concepts:

1. In the spine, flexion of the lumbar spine increases the size of the intervertebral canal and the intervertebral foramina.[10]
2. Extension decreases the size of the intervertebral canal and the intervertebral foramina.[10]
3. Flexion increases dural sac and nerve root tension.[9]
4. Extension decreases dural sac and nerve root tension.[9]
5. Front flexion, axial loading, and an upright posture increase intradiscal pressure.
6. With flexion the annulus bulges anteriorly.[14]
7. With extension the annulus bulges posteriorly.[14]
8. Nuclear shift in an injured disc is poorly documented, but the disc probably shifts in the direction of the annular bulge.[10]
9. Rotation and torsion produce annular tears and disc herniations.[2]

These facts indicate that motion does have an effect on the nerves and the neuromotion segments of an injured area. For example, if there is a spinal obstructive problem such as spinal stenosis, extension exercises can further compress the neurologic structures and make them worse; if there is a nerve root tension problem, such as disc herniation, then flexion can produce increased tension in an already-tense nerve and increase symptoms.

HISTORY AND PHYSICAL EXAMINATION

The key to a proper history and physical examination is to have a standardized form that accomplishes the needed specific objectives:

1. Quantitate the morbidity. Use a value scale of pain, function, and occupation to determine how sick the patient is. Converse with the patient and listen to the inflections and manner of pain description. Detail the time of disability and the time of origin of the pain. We use the Oswestry scale and the disability rating. The severity of the morbidity often determines the aggressiveness of the diagnostic and therapeutic plan.
2. Delineate the psychosocial factors. Know what psychologic effect the pain has had on the patient. Know the social, economic, and legal results of the patient's disability. We use the pain drawing on the initial visit and a detailed psychologic report in certain instances. Understand what can be gained by the patient's being sick or well. Derive an understanding of what role these factors are playing in the patient's complaints.
3. Eliminate the possibility of tumors, infections, and neurologic crisis—these conditions have a certain urgency that requires immediate attention and a diagnostic therapeutic regimen that is very different from that required for disc disease. Constant, unrelenting pain more at night than during the day is an indication of tumor or infection. Ask about bowel, bladder, and sexual dysfunction and do a thorough examination.
4. Diagnose the clinical syndrome:
   a. *Nonmechanical back and/or leg pain*—Inflammatory, constant pain; minimally affected by activity; usually worse at night or in early morning
   b. *Mechanical back and/or leg pain*—Made worse by activity; relieved by rest
   c. *Sciatica*—Predominantly radicular pain; positive stretch signs, with or without neurologic deficit
   d. *Neurogenic claudication*—Radiating leg or calf pain; negative stretch signs; made worse with ambulation and spinal extension; relieved by flexion

Pinpoint the pathophysiology causing the syndrome. Three important determinations are:

1. What level? Which neuromotion segment?
2. What nerve (especially in radiculopathy)?
3. What pathology? What is the exact structure or disease process in that neuromotion segment that is causing the pain?

Some key factors in the history and physical examination are:

1. What caused the injury
2. The time of day when the pain is worse

3. A comparison of pain levels during walking, sitting, and standing
4. The effects of Valsalva's maneuver, coughing, and sneezing on pain
5. The type of injury and duration of the problem
6. The percentage of back versus leg pain (We insist on getting an accurate estimate of the relative amount of discomfort in the back versus that in the legs. These two numbers must add up to 100%.)

The physical examination should address:

1. Maneuvers during the examination that reproduce the pain
2. The presence of sciatic stretch signs
3. The neurologic deficit
4. Back and lower extremity stiffness and loss of range of motion
5. The exact location of tenderness and radiation of pain or paresthesias

Most athletic injuries to the lumbar spine fall under the category of mechanical, axial, back, or leg pain. Within this categorization several different syndromes exist:

Annular tear of the intervertebral disc — Usually a loaded compressive rotatory injury to the lumbar spine producing severe, disabling back spasm and pain. The pain is usually worse on flexion with coughing, sneezing, straining, an upright posture, sitting, and any other situations that increase intradiscal pressure. There may be referred leg pain, low back pain with straight leg raising, and anterior spinal tenderness. Annular tears can be produced with as little as 3 degrees of high-torque rotation.[3] Facet joint alignment that protects the disc from rotatory forces may lead to facet joint injuries as the annulus fails in rotation.

Facet joint syndrome — More typically occurring in extension with rotation, reproduced with extension and rotation during the examination. This syndrome may present with pain on rising from flexion, with a lateral shift in the extension motion. Point tenderness may occur in the paraspinous area over the facet joint in association with referred leg pain. The facets and the disc are all part of the same joint — three joints of a one-joint complex. If the facet joint injury causes pain and is accompanied by an annular tear of the intervertebral disc, it is the entire joint that is injured.

Tears of the lumbodorsal fascia, as well as muscle injuries and contusions — Present with muscle spasm, stiffness, and many of the characteristics of facet joint syndrome or annular tears.

Sacroiliac joint pain and pain in the posterior superior iliac spine — The most common area of pain referred from the annulus in the intervertebral disc and the neuromotion segment of the spine. Sciatic pain can occur in the sciatic joint area, as well as in

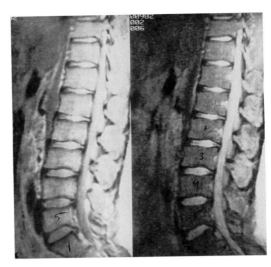

Fig. 10-3. This 22-year-old professional basketball player had significant back and bilateral radiating leg pain. His nonoperative treatment included an aggressive trunk stabilization program that enabled him to return to full activity and play.

the sciatic notch and buttocks. Although injuries can occur to the sacroiliac joint, the vast majority of syndromes presenting with sacroiliac joint pain are believed to be a result of referred pain from a neuromotion segment in the spine.

Herniated nucleus pulposus — The annulus tears, and a fragment of the inner layers of the annulus breaks off and extrudes out of the tear and into the spinal canal (Figs. 10-3 and 10-4). Disc herniations should be viewed as a continuum of injuries to the annulus of the intervertebral disc. The intervertebral disc is a multilayered, woven basket with layers of annulus that are injured first with circumferential tears and then with radial tears. These circumferential and radial tears produce inflammation and mechanical back pain. The outer layers of the annulus are richly innervated and become inflamed. As the structure progressively deteriorates, a complete radial tear results in herniation in which the inner layers of the annulus break off and extrude out the rent in the disc material, producing injury and pain to the radicular nerves coursing posterior to the disc. Severe back mechanical irritative pain progresses to predominant leg pain, often without back pain. The leg pain may course in the distribution of a radicular nerve, causing radiculitis, with or without neurologic deficit and radiculopathy.

MANAGEMENT AND REHABILITATION PRINCIPLES
Nonoperative Care

The objective of the rehabilitation program is to safely return the patient to whatever level of function the patient wants, and to allow the patient to safely test the

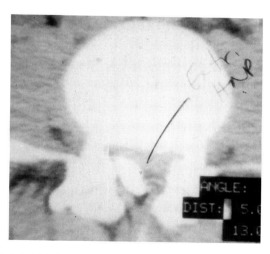

Fig. 10-4. This 28-year-old professional basketball player had an extruded fragment of the intervertebral disc that was removed through a microscopic lumbar discectomy. He returned to play 3 months later after an intensive trunk stabilization program.

limits of future performance. Patients who are better at a sport (having the proper muscle coordination patterns to perform the sport) find it easier to return to the sport without injury. When and whether patients can return to a sport (except for a few conditions) are usually based on their ability to perform the rehabilitation program and to apply the program to their sport.

The nonoperative treatment plan consists of several basic steps:
1. Stop the inflammation.
2. Restore strength.
3. Restore flexibility.
4. Restore aerobic conditioning.
5. Restore balance and coordination.
6. Adapt the rehabilitation program to sport-specific training and exercises.
7. Start back into the sport slowly.
8. Return to full function.

Stopping inflammation of the spine in an injured athlete often requires rest and immobilization. We try to limit the rest and immobilization to a minimum. Bed rest produces stiffness and weakness, which prolong the pain. Every day of rest and immobilization may necessitate weeks of rehabilitation before the athlete can return to performance. As in the treatment of lower extremity injuries (i.e., fracture bracing and postoperative continuous motion machines), rapid rehabilitation of lumbar injuries in athletes requires effective means of mobilizing the patient. Rapid mobilization requires strong antiinflammatory medications, ranging from epidural steroids, oral methylprednisolone (Medrol Dosepak), and indomethacin (Indocin SR) to other nonsteroidal antiinflammatory agents and aspirin. Lots of ice, a transcuta-

neous electrical nerve stimulation (TENS) unit, and mobilization with casts, corsets, and braces are required. Strengthening techniques are started when the brace is applied so that the brace can be removed as soon as possible, since braces cause stiffness and weakness. As a general rule, our patients with acute disc herniations are treated with up to 3 days of bed rest; physical therapy within 1 to 5 days; a corset to be worn for no more than 10 to 14 days; and indomethacin, occasionally methylprednisolone, and epidural injections. The therapist begins the neutral-position, isometric trunk-strengthening program and, depending on the response of the patient, evolves into resistive strengthening, motion, and aerobic conditioning as tolerated.

Concern has been raised about the risk of increasing neurologic deficit or producing a neurologic deficit through nonoperative care. As a result, nonoperative care for neurologic deficit has consisted of no care. Today, a short period of bed rest is the usual, initial stage of treatment of the athlete with a disc herniation and neurologic deficit. It is believed that bed rest protects the patient from increasing injury to the spine and therefore increasing neurologic deficit. However, bed rest can actually increase the risk of injury, and other methods should be used, depending on the goal. If the purpose of bed rest is to decrease inflammation, the logical substitute is aggressive antiinflammatory medication. If the objective of bed rest is to prevent motion, braces and casts can be substituted. If the objective of bed rest is to prevent abnormal motion that could injure the spine, it is with the understanding that certain mechanical functions must take place, such as getting on and off bed pans, getting up to go to the bathroom, rolling over in bed, coughing, sneezing, and eventually walking. An exercise program should prevent abnormal motion while restoring strength and flexibility in a biomechanically sound fashion to protect the spine from abnormal motions that produce injury and to enhance healing.

Lumbar spine injuries in athletes demand prevention of atrophy and stiffness and restoration to maximum function as early as possible. The key to the nonoperative program lies in safety and effectiveness. Rehabilitation begins with the concept of neutral-position isometric strengthening for the spine, emphasizing trunk isometric control and strength, followed by extremity strengthening, extremity stretching, and, finally, trunk mobility. Neck and upper extremity strengthening can be added after trunk stability for neck problems.

Trunk stabilization rehabilitation program. The principles for the trunk stabilization rehabilitation program outlined here are derived from work by the Folsom Physical Therapy Office, Jeff Saal, M.D., Arthur White, M.D., and others, including Celeste Randolph, Ann Robinson, Clive Brewster, and others at the Kerlan-Jobe Orthopaedic Clinic.[8,13] The exercise program concentrates on trunk strength, balance, coordination, flexibility, and aerobic conditioning. It is a practical application of the use of trunk strengthening in back treatment, injury prevention, and improved performance in athletes.

The role of muscle coordination in athletic function cannot be underestimated. Coordinated muscle activity produces the athletic activity necessary for a sport. In our study of the dynamic electromyographic (EMG) analysis of the trunk muscles in professional baseball pitchers, we demonstrated three significant facts: (1) the opposite side of the abdominal oblique muscle is probably the most important muscle in the throwing athlete; (2) trunk strength is important in any torsional athlete (power must be transferred from the legs and hips and through the trunk to the fine control of the arms); and (3) it is coordinated trunk muscle activity that distinguishes higher performance, more effective performance, and pain-free performance.

In an EMG study of professional baseball hitters, the role of coordinated trunk activity was demonstrated clearly, and based on discussions with Ben Hines, hitting coach for the Dodgers, and a number of other sources on baseball hitting, it can be concluded that the general trunk activity of a baseball hitter consists of a coiling-up mechanism followed by uncoiling in which the hips rotate quickly toward the pitcher; getting the hips through the swing quickly is necessary for proper bat speed. This maneuver is followed by a tightly controlled derotation of the upper body that demands a synchrony of upper body and lower body function to transmit the power of the thighs and hips through the end of the bat. The ratio of upper body derotation to lower body derotation is controlled through coordinated muscle function of the trunk. Any adjustment in the speed of derotation of the upper body must involve rapid, coordinated trunk muscle function and occurs in less than a second.

Another important aspect of muscle coordination is the role of eye function and muscle coordination. Eye focus on the ball is necessary for coordinated muscle function. For example, the tightrope walker is not looking around at the audience or walking the rope with the eyes closed. This performer focuses on a point, and it is this focus that produces maximum muscle coordination. Although seeing the ball clearly in maximum focus is certainly important for seeing the rotation on the ball and other aspects, it also produces maximum muscle coordination.

At the heart of the trunk stabilization rehabilitation program is coordinated trunk strength. Therefore an ideal muscle-strengthening program begins trunk muscle coordination exercises as early as possible. All the trunk strengthening is done in response to proprioceptive stimulation and incorporates balance and coordination into the trunk-strengthening exercises. This is why, with the trunk stabilization rehabilitation program, we would rather have a participant do 50 sit-ups while balancing on a green exercise ball than 500 sit-ups on the floor. The program teaches trunk control while teaching trunk strength.

The neutral, pain-free position is used because it is the same position a normal lumbar spine assumes when a person walks a tightrope, balances on a slideboard, or attempts to lift 150 pounds at waist level. It is the position of power—the position of balance. It is not an exaggerated flat-back position. In a patient with back pain, it may involve a slight degree of flexion or extension, depending on the painful structures, but as the pain resolves, this position of power and balance becomes the neutral position for the strengthening exercises. In patients with back pain, this has the added advantage of the patient's finding and maintaining a pain-free position and thus being able to make faster progress in reestablishing isometric muscle control.

The program has the added benefit of producing back strength without having to use unprotected back motion; back motion without fine muscle control and without the proper strength in coordinated trunk muscle function can produce injury to joints whose vector forces are distributed across the joint surface without proper muscle control. Injury to joints is more likely to occur when trunk motion is used for trunk strengthening than when a neutral, pain-free position is used for trunk strengthening.

What role does the neutral position play in the actual performance of a sport? Using baseball as an example, when a shortstop sprints for a ball and bends over to catch it, his trunk muscles fire to protect his back because they have been trained to do so in response to off-balance peripheral septal stimuli and in response to extremity motion. When the shortstop puts his arm out for the ball, the trunk muscles almost return the spine to the neutral position of balance and power.

A program of this type differs from one wherein back strengthening is done with a back-strengthening machine. The ability to bend forward or backward against increasing resistance can be beneficial (it is better than no strength), and it is a factor that can be measured objectively. The disadvantages of using a back-strengthening machine are that (1) back motion is used for back strength (abnormal forces are more likely to be transmitted through injured joints with resisted back motion than with maintenance of the neutral, pain-free position), and (2) the ability to perform the function on the machine may not translate to the proper muscle coordination necessary to perform the tasks the athlete must perform. For example, the ability to bend forward against resistance on the back machine is not the ability needed to throw a javelin. If coordinated muscle strength can be taught from day one in the program, we believe the program will be more comprehensive and effective.

The rehabilitation program in a patient with an injured lumbar spine, with or without neurologic deficit, begins with the patient finding a neutral, pain-free position with isometric muscle control; lying supine on the ground with the knees flexed and the feet on the ground is the position generally used. This is as atraumatic a beginning to rehabilitation as possible. Also, it forms the basis of an important concept, not only in athletic function but also in activities of daily living for everyone. We retrain muscles to work to support the spine while the patient is using the arms and legs. This is not only theoretically ideal but also practically possible. Teaching muscle control with tight, rigid contraction of the trunk muscles and controlling the spine through muscle control of the lumbodorsal fascia not only results in protection of the lumbar spine but also can improve athletic performance. The power and strength of any throwing athlete come from his trunk. Lifting weight requires functioning of the muscles attached to the lumbodorsal fascia.

Trunk strength is an important treatment method for back pain and can prevent back injuries. While treatment plans for symptomatic patients with back pain may include similar exercises, each treatment plan should be designed to match the examination findings and the symptoms. Any trunk-strengthening plan puts strain on the spine and can produce back pain due to overload. Therefore it should be conducted in a controlled, progressive manner.

The key to safe strengthening is the ability to maintain the spine in a safe, neutral position during the strengthening exercises. For upper body strengthening, the spine must be well aligned, with the chest-out posture. Doing isometric trunk exercises and upper body exercises emphasizing this chest-out posture strengthens the support for the cervical spine, builds up the postural muscles needed for maintaining proper body alignment, and prevents neck pain due to bad postural alignment.

The neutral pain-free position obtained in the stability program is one of relative flexion. The patient learns to tighten muscles around that position. Just as a patient who has had knee surgery starts with the first quadriceps set, the patient feels and learns the proprioception for trunk muscles from this position. The patient, feeling (sometimes for the first time) the abdominal oblique muscles, the gluteal muscles, and other muscles contracting, squeezes to hold that position. The program progresses through a series of balancing and resistive exercises while the patient maintains that position. The muscles are strengthened during balancing. They are trained to maintain or restore that position while attempts are made through resistive maneuvers to move that position. There is an actual time in which the spine is "loaded in position" or moving under maximum muscle control that not only delivers the maximum torque transfer and performance but also delivers maximum protection from overload injuries to the spine.

The specific program is outlined in Chapter 27.

Aerobic conditioning. Numerous methods are available for aerobic conditioning. Chapter 25 discusses this topic in detail.

Restoration of balance and coordination. Restoration of balance and coordination is vital to an effective return to full activity and sports. Incorporation of balancing techniques into the strengthening program, as is done in the spinal stabilization and rehabilitation program, begins the process of retraining muscles to fire at the right time with the proper strength. Balance and coordination are the key to friction-free performance, which is safer and more effective. Coordination is the key to swinging the golf club, throwing a baseball, or even lifting weights. Using the Swiss exercise ball, balance beam, standing positions for resistive exercises, exercises bands, and such techniques as one-legged squats while resisting an exercise band pulling on the waist are methods that use balance with strengthening. Balance and coordination need to be incorporated into all the strengthening, stretching, and aerobic conditioning aspects of a rehabilitation program.

Sport-specific exercise. The physical therapist, trainer, physician, and coach all come together in the rehabilitation program in relation to the sport-specific exercise. After relief of inflammation and pain, and restoration of strength, flexibility, conditioning, and coordination from doing the rehabilitation exercises, these techniques must be incorporated into the sport. Much will be lost and injury is likely to recur if this does not take place properly. New exercises in addition to the old ones are added that more closely simulate the sport. Proprioceptive neuromuscular facilitation-type techniques of resistive rotation and other techniques blend in with the old techniques and are done by the athlete to prepare for the sport. The coach may be able to change certain techniques, such as using a slight external rotation of the lead foot in golf or a different foot plant in baseball. Sport-specific training incorporates certain things that coaches have taught for years. One should be innovative. Being able to understand the sport and design ways to simulate that sport's activity in the rehabilitation program will facilitate transfer of the principles of the rehabilitation program to the sport.

The athlete should *start slowly back into the sport,* taking time to test out the new techniques, the new awareness of trunk muscle function, and body alignment. Too fast a return means returning too quickly to the same old rut that often led to the injury. One should build up to the maximum performance.

Operative Care

The chief indications for surgery in the athlete are the indications for surgery in any patient. The basic principles of dealing with any patient are also of major importance in the athlete:

1. Sufficient morbidity to warrant surgery

2. Failure of conservative care
3. An anatomic lesion that can be corrected with a safe, effective operation
4. A proper, fully developed postoperative rehabilitation program

Not enough emphasis can be placed on the last-mentioned principle: a proper postoperative rehabilitation program. Failure to do postoperative spinal rehabilitation would be equivalent to failure to do postoperative knee strengthening after reconstruction of the knee or failure to do postoperative strengthening and range-of-motion exercises after surgery on a shoulder. The patient wants restoration of function. The surgeon should be able to guide the patient through the restoration process. The morbidity of the patient, amount of pain, loss of function, and occupation are the critical factors.

Spinal operations to enhance performance rather than relieve disabling pain are a part of managing the care of athletes, a part that requires a great deal of experience, not only in spinal surgery but also in dealing with athletes.

There are numerous factors to consider. One must always keep in mind the longevity of the patient. Young players can stay out a year after significant spinal surgery and still return to play. Older players are less likely to return to play after a major spinal reconstructive operation.

What the player will be like after retiring from the sport—the condition of the spine at that time—should be of major importance in decision making early in the player's career.

A major factor involves calculating the odds of the operation being successful. In many sports, after a spinal fusion for example, or a major resection of a supporting structure in a decompression, the chance of returning to the sport may be no greater with the operation than without it.

A surgeon must carefully question the use of surgery if the surgeon does not have a proper alternative to the surgery in good, effective nonoperative care. If all one knows is the surgical technique, and if one does not have a proper understanding of and delivery system for a rehabilitation program, then that person should not

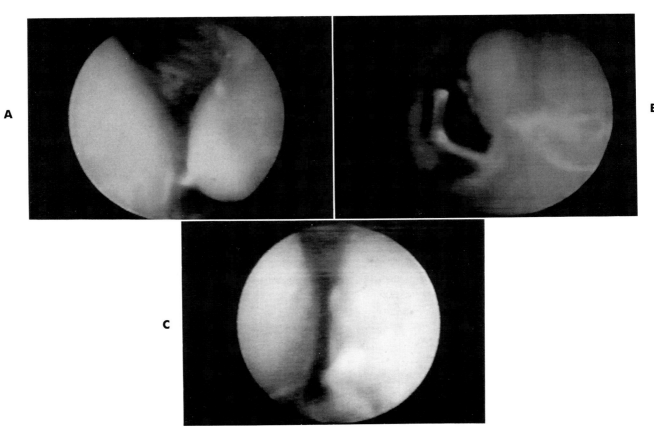

Fig. 10-5. A, Spinalscopic view showing a disc herniation in a cadaveric specimen with the probe coming through the tip of the herniation and the nerve root above. **B,** Spinalscopic view showing instrument inserted through the disc herniation through a working portal, removing the disc fragment. **C,** Spinalscopic view with the fragment removed, showing the annulus and the nerve root in place.

advise surgery for the athlete. An appropriate team approach among specialists in rehabilitation and specialists in operative care can be worked out so that the decision for surgery is well founded, but the surgeon must understand and participate in all aspects of the decision-making process. The surgeon must understand spinal rehabilitation in order to understand whether the patient has had a sufficient nonoperative treatment program and whether there is a proper postoperative plan for return to full function.

The anatomic lesion is critical to the decision. A simple extruded disc herniation, of course, can be very amenable to a single-level microscopic lumbar discectomy, but an annular tear of the intervertebral disc with mild nerve root irritation will not be made better by a decompressive laminectomy and usually will be made worse because of abnormal motion in the injured disc (segmental instability), now with a nerve root that is scarred to the back of the annulus.

A surgical procedure must be designed to do as little damage as possible to normal tissue. The spinalscope is both a diagnostic and a therapeutic tool. New developments in technique and technology are allowing us to diagnose with intracanal spinoscopy, to treat contained herniations with intradiscal spinoscopy, and to remove extruded fragments percutaneously from the spinal canal with a working canal spinalscope (Fig. 10-5). Percutaneous surgery techniques, such as neucleotomy, may be effective for contained disc herniations.

The microscopic discectomy is our standard treatment at this time for removing an extruded disc fragment. A small skin incision is used because that is all that is needed with a microscope. The subcutaneous tissue is gently opened to find the fascia. The fascia is opened just off the spinous process to allow a tight fascial closure. Muscle is gently elevated and protected. The ligamentum flavum is detached, and only the minimum necessary for exposing the fragment and nerve is resected. The microscope, proper positioning, and relative hypotensive anesthesia may allow the surgeon to avoid bleeding and having to use the bipolar electric cautery and cottonoids. The annulus should be handled with care to enhance healing. A blunt puncture with a No. 4 micro-Penfield dissector, expanding the hole with a regular Penfield dissector and a micropituitary rongeur, produces less annular damage than a cruciate incision, which is better than a square incision. Every operation is not necessarily done exactly this way, but an important principle in surgery on athletes is to protect the normal tissue. Tissue-handling techniques should be designed to enhance postoperative healing with a minimum of scar formation. Obviously, this is a proper mandate for all surgery. The extent of the surgery is also determined by the need to fully correct the pathologic condition. The skill is in being able to fully correct the pathologic condition with a minimum of surgery.

In spondylolisthesis the obvious solution may be a spinal fusion, as it is in the majority of the patients facing surgery for spondylolisthesis. Some athletes can return to their sport after a successful spinal fusion, and some cannot. Part of the danger lies in curing the x-ray results, and not the patient. Another possibility is to cure the patient with a successful operation and leave the player without a job. As with everyone, an absolute indication for surgery for lumbar disc disease is progressive cauda equina syndrome or progressive neurologic deficit. Relative indications include static significant neurologic deficit, unrelenting night pain, major loss of functional capability, and inability to play the sport because of spinal pain. There will always be patients who could live the way they are but who cannot perform the way they are. This is a relative indication for surgery, but it must be a frequent consideration in lumbar spine injuries in athletes. A simple question often asked is, how long does one "wait" before doing surgery for a disc herniation? The key word is "wait." A vulture "waits" until the victim quits moving. A spinal surgeon is not "waiting"; the surgeon is aggressively treating the patient, judging the response to treatment, listening to the patient's expectation of the sport and of life outside of the sport, understanding the patient's concern about timing or surgery relative to the start of spring training, and understanding the patient's fears concerning the sport and the patient's life. The number one factor in *when* or *whether* to recommend surgery is *what* is in the patient's best interest.

REFERENCES

1. Aggrawal ND et al: A study of changes in weight lifters and other athletes, *Br J Sports Med* 13:58, 1979.
2. Farfan HF: *Mechanical disorders of the low back,* Philadelphia, 1973, Lea & Febiger.
3. Farfan HF: Muscular mechanism of the lumbar spine and the position of power and efficiency, *Orthop Clin North Am* 6:135, 1975.
4. Farfan HF: The biomechanical advantage of lordosis and hip extension for upright activity, *Spine* 3:336, 1978.
5. Keene JS: Drummond DS: Mechanical back in the athlete, *Comp Ther* 11:7, 1985.
6. Keene JS et al: Back injuries in college athletes, *J Spinal Dis* 2:190, 1986.
7. Kotani PT et al: Studies of spondylolisthesis found among weight lifters, *Br J Sports Med* 9:4, 1981.
8. Saal JA: Common American football injuries, *Sports Med* 24:42, Aug 1991.
9. Schnebel BE, Watkins RG, Willin WH: The role of spinal flexion and extension in changing nerve root compression in disc herniations, *Spine* 14:835, 1989.
10. Schnebel BE et al: A digitizing technique for the study of movement of intradiscal dye in response to flexion and extension of the lumbar spine, *Spine* 12:309, 1988.
11. Sieman RL, Spangler D: The significance of lumbar spondylolysis in college football players, *Spine* 6:174, 1981.
12. Spencer CW, Jackson DW: Back injuries in the athlete, *Clin Sports Med* 2:191, 1983.
13. Watkins RG: *Trunk stretching and strengthening program.* Pamphlet prepared for the Professional Baseball Athletic Trainers Society (PBATS), 1987; revised 1989, 1991, 1993.
14. White AA, Panjabi MM: *Clinical biomechanics of the spine,* Philadelphia, 1978, JB Lippincott.

◆

Chapter Eleven

Muscle Imbalance Patterns Associated With Low Back Syndromes

Michael B. Schlink

Treatment of vertebrogenic pain appears to follow the inverse knowledge syndrome: the less known, the more answers. Pathogenesis of low back pain is obscure and full of controversies or even myths. This explains why so many types of treatment claim to be the panacea, but hard evidence is lacking for all.

Part of the problem is that vertebrogenic pain presents as a multifactorial problem. The presence of a specific pathologic condition will certainly inform the physical therapist of contraindications regarding treatment and in broad terms define the parameters of treatment. However, it cannot be relied on to clearly determine the therapeutic approach.[50] This is illustrated by the McKenzie approach to disc derangement syndromes. McKenzie[41] developed seven clinical categories under the same medical diagnosis. Treatment of each category is approached differently. In this manner pathologic conditions can be viewed as the manifestation of compensatory factors that developed to create the symptoms and that continue to precipitate the symptoms. It would seem prudent to base treatment on the interdependence of all mechanisms involved in the control and production of abnormal movement behavior relating to patients' symptoms rather than focusing treatment on one structure or motion segment. Failure to recognize the multifactorial nature of vertebrogenic pain not only may lead to poor therapeutic results but can contribute to "late-onset" sequelae.[30,31]

The role of the physical therapist is to interpret through communication, observation, and manual techniques the mechanical components responsible for the patient's symptoms and dysfunction. Treatment then must be approached in a stepwise manner with development of a plan from which predicted outcomes are realized and reassessed. This chapter focuses on muscle imbalance patterns that are believed to develop in a predictable manner. These patterns can begin to develop in the acute condition or, conversely, may be the cause of the acute episode. If not corrected, these muscle imbalance patterns can precipitate exacerbations resulting in a chronic condition and preventing the athlete's unrestricted return to function.

FUNCTIONAL PATHOLOGY OF THE MOTOR SYSTEM

The evaluation and treatment of joint and soft tissue dysfunction has been well documented in the field of manual therapy.* Working rules have been developed that allow the therapist to approach the evaluation and treatment in a methodic manner, yielding predictable results and clarifying the morass of signs and symptoms. Much has been written about the aspects of individual muscles and their response to exercise, fatigue, and pain.† However, much less is known and understood about muscle function and its role in the pathogenesis of many syndromes, including low back pain. We lack a system to understand muscle function and dysfunction as it applies to the entire organism.

The term *functional pathology of the motor system* was introduced by Lewit in 1974.[22,35] This was an attempt to define functional changes in the motor system that play a role in the pathogenesis of various conditions, including low back pain. These functional changes, or "functional lesions," relate to abnormal movement behaviors that can occur because of a painful stimulus, through poor postural habits, through repetitive motions, or perhaps independently because of predetermined poor central nervous system control. Each functional lesion can lead to other lesions in a compensatory manner and if left untreated can eventually develop into a chronic condition that responds only temporarily to treatment and is never fully resolved.

Seasoned physical therapists have encountered conditions resistant to treatment. Only after reassessment has a far-distant dysfunction been identified as the perpetuator of symptoms. One example is headache symptoms that have been determined through testing to originate at the occipital atlantal complex (OAA) complex. Appropriate treatment results in excellent symptom relief and normal motion, but the carryover is negligible and the symptoms persist. Only after evaluation and treatment of dysfunction of the pelvis are symptoms resolved. Another example is low-grade chronic low back pain that persists until an abnormal foot-to-ground orientation is corrected.

One can think of any musculoskeletal condition as having a cause, compensations, and perhaps complications. The cause is the pain generator, that structure from which the noxious stimulus arises. The compensations relate to how the musculoskeletal system has

---

* References 6, 8, 15, 16, 37, 43.
† References 1-5, 9-11, 17, 18, 33, 34, 39, 42, 46-48, 52-54.

responded to the symptoms and/or how it may be perpetuating the symptoms. Complications cannot be changed (e.g., a pathologic condition or a postural abnormality that has become fixed). Appropriate treatment must be directed not only to relieving the noxious stimulus but to addressing all compensatory factors that may perpetuate it. Complications must be taken into consideration when the clinician determines the final prognosis—will those complications affect the motor system to the extent that certain compensations cannot be resolved, resulting in the eventual return of symptoms?[2] The term *compensation* in this discussion is another way to describe the *functional lesion*.

MUSCLE IMBALANCE PATTERNS

The literature reports observed such muscle reactions as strength deficits, abnormal motor-unit activity, susceptibility to fatigue, and apparent or real muscle shortening.* Results vary greatly. The state of our knowledge of trunk muscle performance can perhaps be summed up by Beimborn and Morrissey's review of the literature.[3] The most outstanding finding of their review is the great need for further research in the area of trunk and muscle performance and for increased specificity regarding pathology. Part of the confusion may come from the premise of studying low back dysfunction and disability as the primary effect of one structure or motion segment rather than as a multifactorial problem. Nevertheless, the wide range of results makes it difficult for the clinician to determine how to approach observed muscle reactions such as weakness, poor firing patterns, and tightness. Does the confusion indicate that muscle reactions occur in a random and independent manner, or are these changes part of a general muscle reaction that presents in typical patterns? Do muscles become tight because biomechanically some muscles are strong and others weak? Does imbalance between muscles develop as a mechanical response to faulty posture or to reflex relationships among various muscles in the pattern? Is there a difference between innervation of the two systems?

Janda believes that there are predictable patterns of muscle imbalance and dysfunction. His clinical and electromyographic observations and analysis indicate that there are two functional divisions of muscles: postural and phasic. The muscle system with predominantly tonic or postural function has a tendency to develop tightness, hypertonia, shortening, or contractures. These muscles are readily activated in most movement patterns and even dominate when certain conditions, such as fatigue or working out new movement patterns, are present. The postural muscle system is less fragile and less likely to atrophy; these muscles primarily cross two joints and are associated with flexor

---

Functional Divisions of Muscle Groups

Muscles Prone to Tightness

Gastrocsoleus
Tibialis posterior
Short hip adductors
Hamstrings
Rectus femoris
Iliopsoas
Tensor fasciae latae
Piriformis
Erector spinae (especially lumbar, thoracolumbar, and cervical portions)
Quadratus lumborum
Pectoralis major
Upper portion of trapezius
Levator scapulae
Sternocleidomastoid
Scalenes
Flexors of the upper limb

Muscles Prone to Weakness

Peroneal
Tibialis anterior
Vastus medialis and lateralis
Gluteus maximus, medius, and minimus
Rectus abdominus
Serratus anterior
Rhomboids
Lower portion of trapezius
Short cervical flexors
Extensors of the upper limb

From Jull G, Janda V: Muscles and motor control in low back pain. In Twomey LT, Taylor JR, editors: *Physical therapy for the low back: clinics in physical therapy,* New York, 1987, Churchill Livingstone.

---

reflexes. The other system has a predominantly phasic function, with a tendency to develop hypotonia, to be inhibited, and therefore to develop weakness. It is less activated in most movement patterns and tends to become fatigued more easily and to a greater extent. The phasic muscles primarily cross only one joint and are associated with extensor reflexes.[20-24,26,27,29,32] The box above lists the muscles prone to tightness and those prone to weakness, and the box on p. 148 lists the characteristics of muscles prone to tightness and those prone to weakness.

Despite the consistency of these clinical and electromyographic observations and analyses, no histologic, histochemical, nor physiologic studies explain these different functional roles of muscles.[22,32] As electromyographic studies indicate, muscles prone to tightness are readily activated with movement (i.e., these muscles have a shorter chronaxie). The explanation of functional differences may lie in the central nervous system control over each of these muscle systems. Janda[20,22,27,32]

---

* References 1-5, 9-11, 17, 18, 33, 34, 39, 42, 46-48, 52-54.

Characteristics of Divisions of Muscle Groups

Muscles Prone to Tightness

Predominantly postural function
Associated with flexor reflexes
Primarily two-joint muscles
Readily activated with movement (shorter chronaxy)
Tendency to tightness, hypertonia, shortening, or contractures
Resistance to atrophy

Muscles Prone to Weakness

Primarily phasic function
Associated with extensor reflexes
Primarily one-joint muscles
Not readily activated with movement (longer chronaxy)
Tendency to hypotonia, inhibition or weakness
Atrophies easily

From Jull G, Janda V: Muscles and motor control in low back pain. In Twomey LT, Taylor JR, editors: *Physical therapy for the low back: clinics in physical therapy,* New York, 1987, Churchill Livingstone.

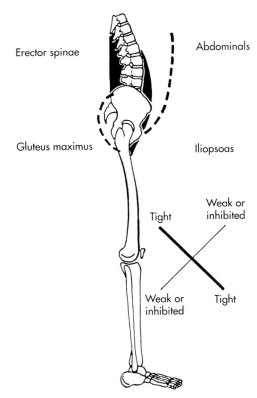

Fig. 11-1. Pelvic crossed syndrome. (From Jull G, Janda V: Muscles and motor control in low back pain. In Twomey LT, Taylor JR, editors: *Physical therapy for the low back: clinics in physical therapy,* New York, 1987, Churchill Livingstone.)

studied a group of 100 chronic low back pain sufferers who were unexpectedly resistant to treatment. A thorough neurologic examination indicated that 80% of this group exhibited a slight but definite minimal cerebral dysfunction, which implicated central nervous system dysfunction. Others believe that the same abnormal patterns of muscular dysfunction can be attributed to repetitive activity in which the actual path of instantaneous center of rotation of a movement is not consistent with the standard kinesiologic axis of motion.[19,51] Muscle imbalance patterns in this sense are learned, and this scenario applies to the athlete. This repetitive activity can lead to a painful syndrome or exacerbate a preexisting condition. Sahrmann[51] believes that biased recruitment of the more tonic or postural muscles may be related to (1) a less available range of the muscle and therefore less slack and a tendency to shorten earlier, and/or (2) greater afferent input via stretch receptors to the spinal cord, thereby creating a bias of the motoneuron pool of the short muscle that results in earlier recruitment.

A region of the body where this pattern of muscle imbalance is more evident and from which other levels of imbalance emanate is in the lumbar-pelvic-hip complex. Janda[20,22,23,26,32] refers to this as the pelvic crossed syndrome, which is characterized by the imbalance between short and tight hip flexors and lumbar erector spinae and weakened gluteal and abdominal muscles (Fig. 11-1). This imbalance can affect both the static and dynamic function of the lumbar-pelvic-hip region. This imbalance pattern promotes a forward pelvic tilt, increased lumbar lordosis, and hip flexion contractures.

Weakness of the gluteal muscles results in compensatory increased activity of the thoracolumbar erector spinae and hamstrings to provide hip extension. Weakness of the posterior fibers of the gluteus medius results in compensatory increased activity of the ipsilateral quadratus lumborum and tensor fascia latae/iliotibial band to provide lateral lumbopelvic stabilization. Weakness of the abdominals results in compensatory increased activity of the iliopsoas muscle to provide trunk flexion. Hamstring tightness could be present to lessen the anterior pelvic tilt.

The significance of this syndrome is that it demonstrates the strength or weakness of one muscle group that in itself does not have specific bearing on low back dysfunction, but rather forms a series of muscles acting as prime movers, stabilizers, and synergists that act together to produce movement whether or not that movement is appropriate. The sequence of the firing pattern of muscles is more important than the actual weakness tested. In an imbalanced state the phasic muscle action is delayed, so that the order in which the individual muscles are activated changes to the more postural muscles and their synergists. Whether the tight overactive muscle inhibits its antagonist as described by Sherrington's law of reciprocal innervation or as a response to general reprogramming of the motor systems is not known. Regardless of the mechanism, this pattern of muscle imbalance is self-sustaining, as evidenced in an electromyographic (EMG) study indicating that when a weakened muscle is resisted in a motion designed to elicit a maximal contraction, its activity tends to decrease rather than increase.[20,22-24,32] In one study, a woman whose low back condition was resistant to treatment had EMG electrodes attached to the rectus abdominis and lumbar extensors. She was asked to perform a curl-up exercise—designed to contract the abdominals. The abdominals showed little to no activity, whereas the extensors exhibited marked activity. After stretching of the extensors, the reverse was true. It is the tight postural groups that are activated first in conditions of muscle imbalance. Therefore a therapeutic approach to strengthening—no matter how specific the method of strengthening is—only reinforces the muscle imbalance pattern, making it worse, and is more likely to increase symptoms. However, if the tight and hypertonic muscle is stretched or relaxed to its normal length and tone, an immediate and spontaneous activation of the previously weakened muscle occurs and the previously abnormal EMG activity is normalized. The general implication here is that emphasis in therapy programs should be directed at regaining normal length and tone of the tight postural groups so that strengthening can then commence. Also indicated is the importance of inadequate proprioceptive control and sensorimotor integration in the pathogenesis of low back pain.

EVALUATION

The medical diagnosis sets the parameters of the evaluation and treatment, not the direction. A thorough mechanical examination must be performed to indicate the type and sequence of treatment.[50] An excellent format for mechanical evaluation was developed by Maitland.[37] This stepwise approach includes effective questioning, history taking, observation, and manual techniques to determine the presence, nature, and stage of dysfunction. Proper evaluation looks at all systems that may affect the patient's dysfunction. This chapter deals with the assessment of muscle dysfunction, which rarely takes place during the acute stage. The level of irritability of symptoms is too high to effectively evaluate muscle imbalance patterns. The effects of pain and/or active pathology on movement behaviors would invalidate testing. After the acute episode has passed or with more chronic problems, the movements involved with the evaluation of muscle imbalance can commence without an exacerbation of symptoms.

Assessment of muscle dysfunction is accomplished in three stages: evaluation in standing and gait, examination of movement patterns, and examination of muscle tightness and tone. The evaluation is a stepwise process in which the information gained at one level determines

further tests to be done, resulting in an efficient use of time and movement.

Standing and During Gait

Although the therapist's observations begin as the patient walks to the treatment room, the first step of a detailed examination of muscle imbalance patterns begins with observation of the patient standing still. The need to look at the entire patient and not just one region needs to be emphasized. It is important to view the patient from the front, back, and sides to gain a full appreciation of the effects of muscle dysfunction on static positions.

A basic appreciation of architectural design is achieved by identification of the position of some key bony landmarks. Abnormal pelvic girdle position will commonly reflect abnormalities of the lumbar spine, sacroiliac joint (SIJ), and hip. These abnormalities present as excessive sagittal curves of the lumbar spine, lateral shift of the lumbar spine, pelvic rotations, and/or iliac torsions or flares. The pelvic crossed pattern is often recognized by an anteverted pelvis and increased lordosis of the lumbar spine. Unilateral weakness of posterior fibers of the gluteus medius with concurrent overactivity of the ipsilateral quadratus lumborum and iliotibial band (ITB)/tensor fascia latae (TFL) can result in a contralateral shift. Rotation of the pelvis is often associated with tightness of the piriformis, whereas iliac torsions are often associated with tightness of the piriformis and iliopsoas.

The shape of muscles can reveal the presence of muscle imbalances. A distinct groove along the iliotibial band strongly suggests increased tone of the TFL and quadratus lumborum compensating as lateral pelvic stabilizers for weak posterior fibers of the gluteus medius. Sagging gluteal and abdominal muscles associated with predominance of the thoracolumbar erector spinae and hamstrings may confirm their part in the pelvic crossed syndrome. As this pattern progresses cephalad, further compensation of weak lower scapular stabilizers and tight cervical erector spinae, upper trapezius, and levator scapulae occurs. Janda[32] calls this the layer syndrome and considers it to be a more established muscle imbalance pattern and an indication of marked impairment of the central nervous system's motor regulation. (Fig. 11-2). The layer syndrome reflects hyperactivity of the postural groups and hypoactivity of the phasic groups that extend beyond the pelvic girdle.

Effects of more distal dysfunction on the lumbopelvic complex cannot be ignored. Foot-to-ground orientation can have profound effects on both static and dynamic function of the lumbar spine. For example, excessive pronation can give rise to a series of muscle imbalances throughout the lower extremity, pelvis, and lumbar spine. These may include tightness of the gastrocsoleus,

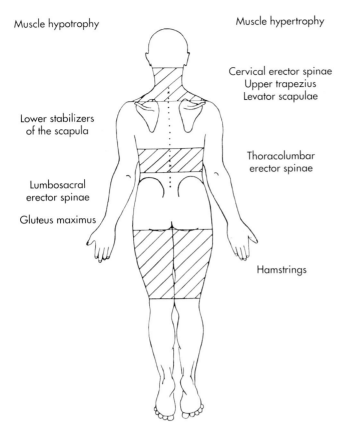

Muscle hypotrophy

Muscle hypertrophy

Cervical erector spinae
Upper trapezius
Levator scapulae

Lower stabilizers
of the scapula

Thoracolumbar
erector spinae

Lumbosacral
erector spinae

Gluteus maximus

Hamstrings

Fig. 11-2. Layer syndrome. (From Jull G, Janda V: Muscles and motor control in low back pain. In Twomey LT, Taylor JR, editors: *Physical therapy for the low back: clinics in physical therapy,* New York, 1987, Churchill Livingstone.)

internal rotation of the tibia, abnormal patellar femoral dysfunction with overactivity of the vastus lateralis and rectus femoris, and atrophy of the vastus medialis oblique (VMO). Increased tone of the ipsilateral short hip adductors and ITB/TFL will occur in an attempt to balance the pelvis over the pronated foot. This abnormal tone of the short adductors may have an effect on the pubic symphysis, resulting in possible sacroiliac and lower lumbar spine dysfunction. This is an example of how muscle imbalance patterns can proliferate to involve far-distant structures.

Observation of the static position in standing sets the outer parameter of recognizing muscle imbalance patterns. Observed bony abnormalities and aberrations of muscle shape and tone alone do not implicate muscle imbalance patterns—there are many other possible causes for these distinctions. It provides a basis from which to direct further investigation.

Gait is the dynamic manifestation of the static standing position. Gait is best observed with the use of a treadmill and videotape. Inasmuch as that is not possible in most clinics, my focus is on the more obvious

but still pertinent aspects of gait in relation to muscle imbalance patterns.

Poor lateral stability on heel strike and midstance positions noted with Trendelenburg's or antalgic positions can be associated with tightness and increased tone of the ITB, TFL, and quadratus lumborum to compensate for weakness of the posterior fibers of the gluteus medius. An anteverted pelvis that is accentuated at toe-off can implicate a poor firing pattern of the gluteal muscles and associated tightness of the iliopsoas and rectus femoris. Excessive and prolonged foot pronation can lead to tightness and hypertonicity of a series of muscles previously discussed. It is during gait that the therapist can begin to note the dynamic aspect of abnormal muscle firing patterns. One should focus on the manner in which the lumbopelvic region compensates. Excessive sacral, iliac, and lumbar motion gives rise to abnormal stresses on these joints occurring with each step. One should appreciate how many lumbopelvic syndromes are the result of repetitive mechanical stress.

Movement Patterns

Classical manual muscle testing, while serving a purpose in the determination of specific muscle weakness, does not give information about poor motor control. It is this poor quality of movement and substitution or compensatory patterns that will depict the presence of muscle imbalance patterns and better direct treatment.

Observation of the patient's gait pattern will commonly indicate the dynamics of muscle imbalance patterns. However, for the novice and even the more experienced therapist it is difficult to observe gait efficiently and be able to pick out all abnormal movement patterns. Some of the more common abnormal patterns have been discussed. There is a need to develop specific and more simple movement patterns that will clearly exhibit the presence of subsets of muscle imbalance patterns. A few such movement patterns are offered here for illustration.

Movement of the upper and lower extremities in the four-point position provides the opportunity to examine the manner in which the patient achieves hip extension. Fig. 11-3, *A*, depicts an abnormal movement pattern with alternate upper extremity and lower extremity extension. Here hip extension is achieved primarily through the hamstrings and back extensors. The hip extensors fire only at the end of movement once an abnormal lumbopelvic position of an anteverted pelvis and hyperlordotic lumbar spine has been achieved. There is poor stabilization of the abdominals. Fig. 11-3, *B*, depicts a more normal firing pattern in which better gluteal contraction is clearly visible and the lumbopelvic complex is stable in a more neutral lordotic position. The abnormal pattern depicts early and excessive firing of the postural groups—the lumbothoracic back extensors and

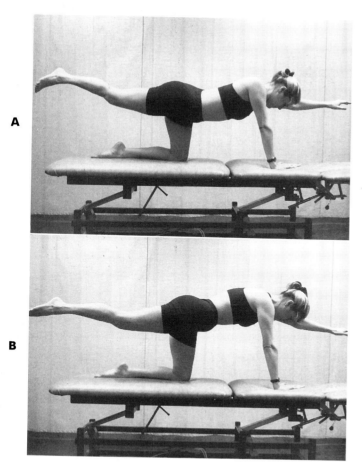

Fig. 11-3. A, Abnormal movement pattern. Hip extension is achieved through the hamstrings and back extensors. The gluteals fire only at end range. **B,** Normal movement pattern. Appropriate firing of the gluteals occurs on a stable pelvis and lumbar spine.

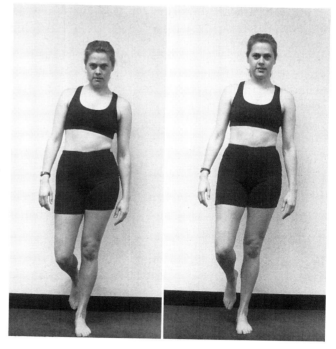

Fig. 11-4. A, Compensated single-limb stance. The antalgic position is secondary to poor firing of the posterior fibers of the gluteus medius. **B,** Normal single-limb stance. Lateral pelvic stability is provided by appropriate firing of the posterior fibers of the gluteus medius.

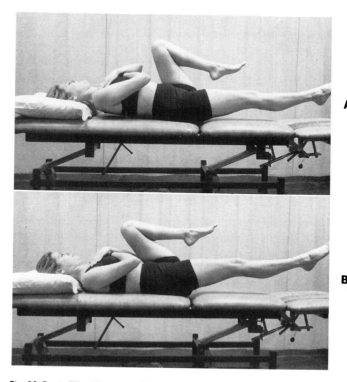

Fig. 11-5. A, The iliopsoas fires earlier and incorrectly to achieve right hip flexion on an unstable lumbopelvic complex. **B,** Normal firing pattern. Appropriate abdominal contraction stabilizes the lumbopelvic complex as the iliopsoas provides hip flexion.

hamstrings—with inhibition of the phasic muscle groups—the abdominal and gluteal muscles.

Single-limb stance is an effective way to determine lateral lumbopelvic stability. Fig. 11-4 depicts poor and good movement patterns in this position. The key weakness here is of the posterior fibers of the gluteus medius. The patient compensates with either an antalgic position as shown in Fig. 11-4, *A,* or Trendelenburg's position. Abnormal tone and/or shortness of the TFL and quadratus lumborum occur in a compensatory fashion. The evolution of a further developing compensatory pattern can be seen in Fig. 11-4, *A.* Here compensation of knee valgus and foot pronation occurs, leading to a progression of muscle imbalance patterns distally.

Hypertonicity of the iliopsoas is a common finding in many lumbopelvic syndromes. In the absence of good abdominal tone a hypertonic iliopsoas will produce abnormal stresses on the low lumbar spine. Fig. 11-5 shows a high-level abdominal exercise in the supine position. Abnormal and earlier firing of the iliopsoas results in abnormal extension of the lumbar spine and anteversion of the pelvis. With normalized iliopsoas tone and concurrent appropriate firing of the abdominals, the lumbo/pelvic junction is stabilized and the motion of the right lower extremity occurs through the hip alone.

These serve only as examples of testing positions to determine the presence of muscle imbalance patterns. Evaluation of abnormal movement patterns is a continuing process as the athlete is returned to full function. These examples demonstrate that predictable patterns of abnormal movement do occur and define the interplay between dysfunctional postural and phasic muscle groups. One also appreciates the self-sustaining nature of these movement patterns in which the tight and hypertonic groups have an inhibitory effect on the weak groups. This pattern is self-sustaining unless specific measures are taken to break this cycle.

Muscle Length and Tone

The next step in the objective examination of muscle imbalance patterns is to assess abnormal muscle length and or tone. Observations made in the static standing position, during gait, and with specific movement patterns will determine which muscles the therapist believes needs closer inspection. Initially it is wise to look at all the muscles that have a tendency to become tight (see box on p. 147). This knowledge gives the therapist a clear idea of the degree of muscle imbalance compensation that has developed. Usually the more compensations, the more resistant the condition will be to treatment and the more likely it is that distal structures are involved. This provides an index of prognosis for both the patient and the therapist.

Descriptions of muscle length testing can vary with the author and/or course presenter. Janda[25] published a full description of muscle length tests. There is always the question of how much force one should apply in determining tightness. The purpose of muscle length testing is to determine if the length of the muscle will have an abnormal effect on the joints to which it is attached. It is important to ensure that the limb or trunk position achieved with testing will be in the plane of normal motion. End range of testing is determined when either the joint to which the muscle is attached begins to move and/or the soft tissue slack is taken up. Attempts to take the limb beyond this point will result in compensatory movement that will not reflect the functional length of that muscle.

Straight leg raising is a typical test for hamstring tightness. However, tight neuromeningeal structures may confound this test, giving a false-positive result.[8] Even if one palpates the anterior superior iliac spine (ASIS) and notes when it first moves, that movement might be due to restriction of the neuromeningeal tissue

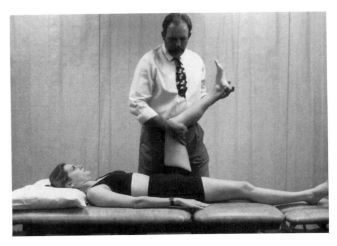

Fig. 11-6. Testing of hamstring length.

versus the hamstrings. I believe a more functional test is depicted in Fig. 11-6. Here the hip is flexed to 90 degrees. The therapist palpates the distal tendons of the hamstring as the knee is moved into extension. The time that soft tissue restriction is palpated in the hamstrings reflects its functional range. Although specific ranges are determined by age, premorbid status, and comparisons with the opposite limb, normal ranges vary from negative 25 to 35 degrees of knee extension.

Testing of gastrocnemius length may be confounded by abnormalities of the subtalar joint. It is important to maintain the subtalar joint in its neutral position when one tests restriction into dorsiflexion. Fig. 11-7 depicts the mechanics of this testing procedure. It is only after the talus is in the neutral position that testing begins. The point at which soft tissue restriction is encountered without movement of the talus denotes the end of functional range. Without this precise positioning one may push harder only to achieve more pronation of the subtalar joint, which is indeed one of the compensations often seen with tight calf musculature. It is not surprising to find that many patients with low back syndromes cannot even achieve a plantargrade position with this test. One can imagine how they must compensate just to stand.

The Thomas position is often used to simultaneously test the iliacus, psoas, rectus femoris, TFL, and one-joint hip adductors. I believe this is a good screening test but that it could be followed up with more precise testing that would better direct subsequent treatment. Alternate tests to distinguish between tightness of the iliacus and psoas is indicated in Fig. 11-8. In the prone position, hip extension is performed while the examiner palpates the ASIS and observes the lumbar spine. Thus the therapist either encounters movement of the ASIS, which indicates iliacus end range, or sees increased lumbar lordosis, which indicates psoas end range. This distinction may direct the sequence of treatment. For

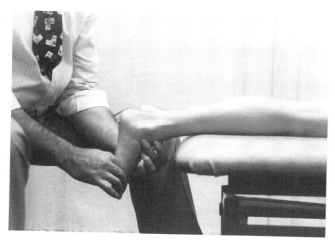

Fig. 11-7. Testing of gastrocnemius length.

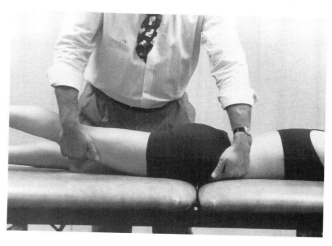

Fig. 11-8. Testing of iliacus and psoas length.

patients with hyperlordotic postures in the supine position, a pillow should be used to normalize the lordotic curve.

Abnormal muscle shortening is not always reflected by adaptive shortening or a true decrease in the muscle length. Often, abnormal muscle tone is responsible for muscle shortening. This hypertonicity is evidence of the speculation by Janda that muscle imbalance patterns are driven by impaired motor regulation of the central nervous system.[22,24] Increased afferent input via the muscle spindle to the spinal cord can bias the motoneuron pool and result in a higher level of resting tone.

Palpation of the muscle bellies and simple inspection may give some indication of hypertonicity. However, this level of observation and palpation is too cursory to be effective other than as an initial screening. Travell and Simons[55] clearly define trigger points associated with myofascial pain and dysfunction. The question is how much pressure should the therapist apply to determine a positive response. On a clinical basis, I have found that enough pressure to blanch the finger or thumb pad is sufficient. If this much pressure elicits a painful response, one may assume that abnormal tone is present. In addition, it has been my clinical experience that pressure applied at the insertion of muscles and the trigger points is an excellent index of hypertonicity of that muscle.

Testing of muscle length and tone should be as specific as possible and provide a methodology that is reproducible. Muscle length should be determined at the point that the appropriate joint moves or at the beginning of soft tissue restriction. Muscle tone can be effectively determined by a painful response attained with enough pressure to blanch the finger or thumb pad at the appropriate trigger or insertion point. Specific tests of muscles confirm the clinician's suspicions of muscle imbalance patterns observed in stance, gait, and movement patterns.

TREATMENT

Treatment of muscle imbalance patterns, as with evaluation, takes place after the acute period has ended—when symptoms and the pathologic condition are under control. The treatment philosophy is based on good balance between muscle groups in terms of length and strength with coordinated and controlled motion. Achieving this balance of postural and phasic groups will result in better motor programing and eliminate adverse mechanical stresses that could result in future sequelae of symptoms.

Janda* describes three stages of treatment: (1) restoring normal muscle length and tone of involved postural muscles, (2) strengthening the phasic muscles that have been inhibited and are weak, and (3) establishing optimal motor patterns that protect the spine and encourage normal muscle balance patterns.

The initial goal of treatment is to resolve abnormal tone or length of postural muscles. If normal length is not achieved, the muscle imbalance pattern will be perpetuated. Attempts to strengthen first tend only to increase the activity of the tight postural groups inasmuch as they have a shorter chronaxie and are likely to activate before the phasic muscles. Abnormal length can be due to adaptive shortening or to abnormal tone. If abnormal length is due to true shortening, aggressive stretching will be required. Hold or contract-relax techniques are effective. Stretching should be performed in a manner to focus on one muscle group while keeping the spine in a "neutral" position. One such method is illustrated in Fig. 11-9.[13,14] Here the iliopsoas group is being stretched. Near-maximum contraction activates the maximum number of motor units and is followed by an aggressive stretch. This aggressive stretching is usually needed with more chronic and long-standing low back syndromes. It is essential to follow up with home

*References 20, 22, 24, 26, 30, 32.

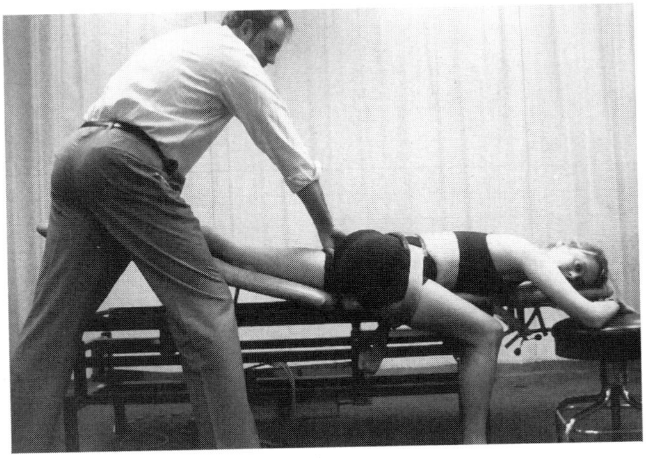

Fig. 11-9. Stretching of the iliopsoas with the spine in a "neutral" position.

stretching. The phrase "little bits often" applies.[40] The patient should stretch many times a day for 30 to 60 seconds.

Often the cause of abnormal muscle length of tight postural groups is abnormal tone. This results in greater afferent input via stretch receptors to the spinal cord, biasing the motoneuron pool and causing earlier recruitment. Aggressive stretching here would result only in increased tone by activating the stretch reflex and should be avoided. There are a variety of techniques to effectively decrease tone. All should be gentle to encourage relaxation of the muscle. Muscle energy and postisometric relaxation techniques are gentle forms of contract-relax exercises that are effective when hypertonicity is present.[36,43] Other manual techniques include myofascial release, trigger point release, and "pump tacking." With these techniques the therapist can feel the muscle tone release and direct the degree of pressure accordingly. A newer and very effective technique is the use of microcurrent electrical nerve stimulation. This form of treatment applied to the origin and insertion and through the muscle belly of the involved hypertonic muscle is thought to increase the adenosine triphosphate (ATP) available to the muscle and thus result in less resting tone.[38,56] The advantage of this technique is that it can be used on patients who cannot tolerate even light[1] palpation. Once tone is normalized, the therapist can proceed with more aggressive muscle stretching techniques if adaptive shortening is also present.

Whatever the technique used, the result should achieve normal tone and/or length of the involved postural muscle. Concurrently, once the inhibitory effect of tight muscles has been removed, there should be an immediate improvement in motor patterns. Movement patterns should always be reassessed after treatment.

The next step is to strengthen muscles that have been inhibited and therefore weakened. This is a delicate procedure. Strengthening must be approached slowly and quite specifically. Aggressive strengthening tends to fire the hypertonic postural groups. Even after abnormal muscle length has been achieved, the patient still tends to substitute and use old and abnormal movement patterns. The exercises must be designed so that the correct muscle is activated. Janda[28] believes that this reeducation program is divided into two stages: first conscious control, then subcortical and postural reflex control. Emphasis is placed on gaining appropriate control of lumbopelvic movement. Practice and repetition of the exercises are essential to the learning process and ultimately to spontaneous and correct use of the muscle groups during function.

An effective approach has been developed to achieve functional training for low back injuries and for trunk stabilization.[44,45,49] The underlying philosophy is based on the view that low back syndromes involve a movement disorder either resulting in or perpetuated by low back dysfunction. The exercises are designed to include planned, repetitive, and quality movement that breaks abnormal movement patterns and establishes new ones. The exercises are meant to simultaneously achieve coordination, strength, endurance, and mobility.

The basic tenant of this training is to keep the lumbar spine in the most symptom-free position for the task at hand—the functional position. The training follows a progression of exercises. The first exercises train the patient to find the functional position and maintain that position with appropriate isometric contraction. Mass body movements are introduced that will reinforce the functional position. This becomes more difficult when the same mass body movements are made with head and limb movement away from positions of reinforcement. Next the patient is asked to perform superimposed and independent movement of the extremities while automatically maintaining the proper functional position of the lumbar spine. This training eventually leads to the specific athletic performance.

This training program follows the levels of achieving motor control as defined by Brooks.[7] First strength is achieved—in this case through isometric contraction. Coordinated movement occurs when appropriate muscles are selected and stimulated at the right time with proper inhibition of antagonists. Skill is achieved through practice to achieve coordinated movement that is well organized and efficient. When the patient develops the skills to achieve a predetermined set of neural commands, motor programs are then introduced. The movement becomes automatic—it has been learned. In the early stages of training, feedback is required for the patient to achieve coordinated movement. As a motor skill is programmed, the muscles become set to perform a movement that requires no feedback if the need arises. This learned muscle behavior is a feed-forward or open-loop system. There is mounting evidence that motor learning depends on patterning of inhibition in motor neurons. With increased skill there is a marked reduction of activity in the auxiliary muscles, whereas the prime movers neither gain or lose.[12]

The training itself serves as an invaluable evaluative tool. The functional position becomes the index for proper movement behaviors. If the athlete is unable to maintain that position, the therapist must decide how the patient is compensating and correct the "functional lesion." In this manner. techniques are guided by the compensations seen in attempts to maintain the functional position with higher-level skill.

REFERENCES

1. Addison R, Schultz A: Trunk strengths in patients seeking hospitalization for chronic low-back disorders, *Spine* 5:539, 1980.
2. Alston W et al: A quantitative study of muscle factors in the chronic low back syndrome, *J Am Geriatr Soc* 14:1041, 1966.
3. Beimborn DS, Morrissey MC: A review of the literature related to trunk muscle performance, *Spine* 13:655, 1988.
4. Berkson M et al: Voluntary strength of male adults with acute low back syndromes, *Clin Orthop* 129:84, 1977.
5. Biering-Sorensen F: Physical measurements as risk indicators for low-back trouble over a one-year period, *Spine* 9:106, 1984.
6. Bourdillon JF: *Spinal manipulation,* London, 1982, W Heinemann.
7. Brooks V: Motor control, *Phys Ther* 63:664, 1983.
8. Butler DS: *Mobilisation of the nervous system,* Melbourne, 1991, Churchill Livingstone.
9. Davies GJ, Gould JA: Trunk testing using a prototype Cybex II dynamometer stabilization system, *J Orthop Sports Phys Ther* 3:164, 1982.
10. de Vries HA: Quantitative electromyographic investigation of the spasm theory of muscle pain, *Am J Phys Med* 45:119, 1966.
11. de Vries HA: EMG fatigue curves in postural muscles: a possible etiology for idiopathic low back pain, *Am J Phys Med* 47:175, 1968.
12. Engelhorn R: Agonist and antagonist muscle EMG activity pattern changes with skill acquisition, *Res Q Exerc Sport* 54:315, 1983.
13. Evjenth O, Hamberg J: *Muscle stretching in manual therapy: a clinical manual—the extremities,* vol 1, Alfta, Sweden, 1984, Alfta Rehab Forlag.
14. Evjenth O, Hamberg J: *Muscle stretching in manual therapy: a clinical manual—the spinal column and the TM joint,* vol 2, Alfta, Sweden, 1984, Alfta Rehab Forlag.
15. Grieve GP: *Common vertebral joint problems,* Edinburgh, 1981, Churchill Livingstone.
16. Grieve GP: *Mobilisation of the spine,* London, 1984, Churchill Livingstone.
17. Hasue M, Fujiwara M, Kikuchi S: A new method of quantitative measurement of abdominal and back muscle strength, *Spine* 5:143, 1980.
18. Hemborg B, Moritz U: Intra-abdominal pressure and trunk muscle activity during lifting, *Scand J Rehabil Med* 17:5, 1985.
19. Jackson R: *Functional relationships of the lower half,* course notes, San Francisco, 1992, San Francisco Spine Center.
20. Janda V: Postural and phasic muscles in the pathogenesis of low back pain. In *Proceedings of the Eleventh Congress Rehabilitation International,* Dublin, 1969.
21. Janda V: Muscle and joint correlations: proceedings of the Fourth Congress FIMM, *Rehabilitacia* (suppl 10-11):154, 1975.
22. Janda V: Muscles, central nervous motor regulation and back problems. In Korr IM, editor: *The neurobiologic mechanisms in manipulative therapy,* New York, 1978, Plenum Press.
23. Janda V: Muscles as a pathogenic factor in back pain. In *Proceedings, Fourth Conference IFOMT,* Christ Church, New Zealand, 1980.
24. Janda V: Introduction to functional pathology of the motor system. In Bullock MI, editor: *Proceedings of the Seventh Commonwealth International Conference,* vol 3, Brisbane, Australia, 1982.
25. Janda V: *Muscle function testing,* London, 1983, Butterworth.
26. Janda V: On the concept of postural muscles and posture in man, *Aust J Physiother* 29:83, 1983.
27. Janda V: Pain in the locomotor system: a broad approach. In Glasgow EW, editor: *Progress in manipulative therapy,* Edinburgh, 1985, Churchill Livingstone.
28. Janda V: Rational therapeutic approach to chronic back pain syndromes. In *Proceedings of the symposium "Chronic back pain, rehabilitation and self help,"* 1985.
29. Janda V: Muscle weakness and inhibition (psuedoparesis) in back pain syndromes. In Grieve GP, editor: *Modern manual therapy of the vertebral column,* Edinburgh, 1986, Churchill Livingstone.
30. Janda V: Muscles and cervicogenic pain syndromes. In Grant R, editor: *Physical therapy of the cervical and thoracic spine: clinics in physical therapy,* New York, 1988, Churchill Livingstone.
31. Janda V: Prevention of injuries and their late sequelae. In *A collection of articles by Vladimir Janda, MD,* Visiting scholars program at Los Angeles College of Chiropractic, 1988.
32. Jull G, Janda V: Muscles and motor control in low back pain. In Twomey LT, Taylor JR, editors: *Physical therapy for the low back: clinics in physical therapy,* New York, 1987, Churchill Livingstone.
33. Kravitz E, Moore ME, Glaros A: Paralumbar muscle activity in chronic low back pain, *Arch Phys Med Rehabil* 62:172, 1981.
34. Langrana NA et al: Quantitative assessment of back strength using isokinetic testing, *Spine* 9:287, 1984.
35. Lewit K: Functional pathology of the motor system: proceedings of the Fourth Congress FIMM, *Rehabilitacia* (suppl 10-11), 1975.
36. Lewit K: *Manipulative therapy in rehabilitation of the locomotor system,* London, 1988, Butterworth.
37. Maitland GD: *Vertebral manipulation,* ed 5, London, 1986, Butterworth.
38. Manley LW: *Microcurrent electrical neuromuscular stimulator,* Anaheim Hills, Calif, 1989, Linda W Manley (instruction manual).
39. Mayer TG et al: Use of non-invasive techniques for quantification of spinal range-of-motion in normal subjects and chronic low-back dysfunction patients, *Spine* 9:588, 1984.
40. McConnell J: *McConnell advanced patellofemoral course notes,* 1992.
41. McKenzie RA: *The lumbar spine: mechanical diagnosis and therapy,* New Zealand, 1981, Spinal Publications.
42. McNeil T et al: Trunk strengths in attempted flexion, extension and lateral bending in healthy subjects and patients with low-back disorders, *Spine* 5:529, 1980.
43. Mitchell FL, Moran PS, Pruzzo NA: *An evaluation and treatment manual of osteopathic muscle energy procedures,* Valley Park, Mo, 1979, Mitchell, Moran & Pruzzo.
44. Moore M et al: *Training the patient with low back dysfunction,* course notes, Folsom, Calif, 1987, 1990, Folsom Physical Therapy.
45. Morgan D: Concepts in functional training and postural stabilization for the low-back-injured, *Top Acute Care Trauma Rehabil* 2(4):8, 1988.
46. Nachemson A: Measurement of abdominal and back muscle strength with and without low back pain, *Scand J Rehabil Med* 1:60, 1969.
47. Parianpour M et al: The triaxial coupling of torque generation of trunk muscles during isometric exertions and the effect of fatiguing isoinertial movements of the motor output and movement patterns, *Spine* 13:982, 1988.
48. Pederson OF, Petersen R, Staffeldt ES: Back pain and isometric back muscle strength of workers in a Danish factory, *Scand J Rehabil Med* 7:125, 1975.

49. Saal JA, Saal JS: Nonoperative treatment of herniated lumbar intervertebral disc with radiculopathy: an outcome study, *Spine* 14:431, 1989.

50. Sahrmann S: Diagnosis by the physical therapist—a prerequisite for treatment: a special communication, *Phys Ther* 68:1703, 1988.

51. Sahrmann S: *Diagnosis and treatment of muscle imbalances associated with regional pain syndromes*—level 1, course notes, St Louis, 1992, Washington University.

52. Smidt G et al: Assessment of abdominal and back extensor function: a quantitative approach and results for chronic low-back patients, *Spine* 8:211, 1983.

53. Suzuki N, Endo S: A quantitative study of trunk muscle strength and fatigability in the low back pain syndrome, *Spine* 8:69, 1983.

54. Thortensson A, Arvidsson A: Trunk muscle strength and low back pain, *Scand J Rehabil Med* 14:69, 1982.

55. Travell JG, Simons DG: *Myofascial pain and dysfunction: the trigger point manual,* Baltimore, 1983, Williams & Wilkins.

56. Wallace LA: *M.E.N.S. therapy,* vols 3 and 4, Cincinnati, 1989, Lynn Wallace.

Chapter Twelve

◆

Spondylolisthesis

Mark F. Hambly
Leon L. Wiltse
Richard D. Peek

Over the past two decades the number of young people engaging in highly competitive individual and team sports has skyrocketed. In 1979 it was reported that 50% of all boys and 25% of all girls between the ages of 14 and 17 participated in some organized competitive team sport,[38] and it is safe to assume that these numbers continue to grow. Serious practice and rigorous training methods are begun at an early age so that athletes can successfully compete on an international level.

The number of complaints of low back pain in this highly motivated population is increasing. Persistent low back pain without nerve root tension signs should signal the possibility of a stress reaction or fracture of the pars interarticularis.[26] An increased incidence of spondylolisthesis has been documented in athletes involved in sports requiring repetitive twisting, hyperextension, and/or hyperflexion movements.

This chapter describes the etiology, incidence, typical clinical presentation, and work-up of the athlete with spondylolisthesis.

INCIDENCE

An increased incidence of spondylolysis has been associated with numerous sporting activities, ranging from pole vaulting to crew (Table 12-1). The four sports most frequently associated with a significantly increased incidence are diving, gymnastics, wrestling, and weight lifting.[33] The incidence of pars interarticularis defects in female gymnasts is four times that of the general female Caucasian population.

The incidence of pars interarticularis defects in the Caucasian population is very low in preschool children but increases to about 4.5% during the first year in school. It is twice as common in males as in females; however, high-grade olisthesis is twice as common in females.[9] It is half as common in blacks as in whites.[31] There is a definite familial predisposition to pars defects in cases appearing at age 6 or 7, but no studies have determined if there is such a predisposition in cases that develop in the young athlete, except that an increased incidence of spina bifida occulta (a hereditary condition) has been noted in young athletes who have spondylolysis at the L5 level.[18] Progression of the slip is most likely to occur between the ages of 9 and 12 in girls and 10 and 14 in boys.[22]

An additional 0.8% of patients previously negative for pars defects develop fatigue fractures between the ages of 10 and 20.[4] Those individuals who develop fractures of the pars after age 12 engage in very strenuous athletics. A prospective study of incoming freshman football players at the University of Indiana demonstrated a 2.4% incidence of acquired spondylolysis during their 4-year career.[25]

ETIOLOGY

Spondylolysis appearing between ages 6 and 7 is due to a fatigue fracture of the pars interarticularis and is very seldom caused by one acute, traumatic event. When spondylolysis is due to one event, it is secondary to major trauma and there are virtually always other fractures in the vertebrae besides the pars. Stress fractures of the pars differ from other fatigue fractures associated with athletics in that they occur at an earlier age. We have been unable to determine if there is a hereditary element in the pars fractures occurring in the adolescent super

Table 12-1. Incidence of Spondylolisthesis

Researchers	Incidence (%)
Judo	
Rubens-Duval et al.[36]	12
Gymnastics	
Rossi[33]	32.8
Jackson et al.[19]	11
Wrestling	
Rossi[33]	33.3
Granhead and Morelli[13]	12
Weight Lifting	
Kotani et al.[21]	30.7
Rossi[33]	36.2
Granhead and Morelli[13]	15
Football	
Simon and Spenger[40]	21
McCarroll, Miller, and Ritter[25]	15.2
Diving	
Rossi[33]	63.3

athlete, but there is an increased incidence of spina bifida that is hereditary.

It has been demonstrated experimentally that while the pars interarticularis has great inherent tensile and shear strength, cyclic loading may produce a fatigue fracture at lesser loads.[17]

It is likely that all motions contribute to the development of the condition if they are repeated often enough. This being the case, it is easy to see why there is an increased incidence in gymnasts,[4,6,18] interior linemen,[25,40] weight lifters, Little League pitchers,[16] and the like.* Those athletes who develop pars fractures and participate in sports that do not require these repetitive movements may use training techniques, such as weight lifting, that involve these movements, thus increasing their risk.

There are several biomechanical reasons why athletes may be predisposed to developing spondylolysis at L5.[1] There is an abrupt change in stiffness at the lumbosacral junction where the flexible spinal column joins the fixed pelvis.[17] This, coupled with the viscoelasticity of a healthy young disc, allows significant stresses to be transmitted across the pars.[7,8] Extension of the lumbosacral junction closes the joint of the vertebral arch. Any rotational forces while in extension are directly transmitted to the pars, thus stressing it.[37] Against this view, a significant number of athletes develop defects higher up in the lumbar spine, even up to L1.

High-caliber Swedish athletes with spondylosis have been noted to have a slightly increased sacrohorizontal angle when compared with unaffected athletes and nonathletic controls.[43] This leads to conversion of vertical compression forces to shear forces at the lumbosacral junction, which may predispose the pars to fracture.

It is not known why pars fractures that have probably been present and quiescent for years suddenly become painful. Intuitively, one surmises that the fracture is the source of the pain. Indeed, in the young athlete just developing or recently having developed a pars fracture, it is. However, in athletes with an established pars defect, tension on the posterior longitudinal ligament and the annulus fibrosis may be the source of the pain. Tension on the disc itself may also generate pain. The pain is most probably the result of abnormal mechanical stresses coupled with a change in the local chemical environment, causing an irritation of the primary sensory neurons.[44] Also, the disc itself may be undergoing internal disc disruption, which is often painful.

CLINICAL FINDINGS

Typically, patients with an impending or existing pars fracture complain of low back pain. Young athletes often report that they had been playing a sport even though they had a backache and some spasm, and that they then

*References 11, 13, 20, 23, 24, 33, 41, 42.

noted a sudden worsening of symptoms after a specific traumatic episode. They believe this episode to be the cause of their pain. Most probably, these athletes were developing a fatigue fracture, and the severe episode was actually the completion of the stress fracture. It is at this point that medical attention is usually sought.

Affected athletes commonly complain of chronic, dull, aching, and/or cramping pain in the low back.[18] The pain may be unilateral or bilateral, usually "along the belt line."[19] The ache is usually constant and made worse with rotation and/or hyperextension of the low back. There are usually no radicular findings or true sciatic tension signs present. The range of motion, although painful, is usually full. There may be palpable paraspinal spasm and hamstring tightness. Commonly, having the patient stand on one leg and bend backward (the one-legged lumbar extension maneuver) reproduces and accentuates the pain if a fatigue fracture is present (Fig. 12-1). In the presence of a unilateral defect, hyperextension while standing on the ipsilateral leg will worsen the pain on the side of the defect.

Radiographic examination should include appropriate shielding of the gonads.[5] An anteroposterior (AP) spot lateral view (with the patient standing) of the lumbosacral junction and, if necessary, oblique projections should be taken. If a significant slip is present, Ferguson's view may be helpful. If the 45-degree oblique

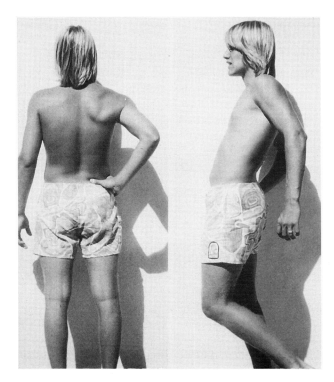

Fig. 12-1. Jackson's one-legged hyperextension test. The patient stands on one leg and hyperextends the back. Back pain will be reproduced on the symptomatic side if there is an impending pars fracture. (Courtesy Douglas Jackson, M.D.)

views suggest a pars defect but are not definitive, oblique projections taken at 30 degrees and 60 degrees may afford better visualization of the fracture.

If a frank defect is present on one side, bony sclerosis of the pars and, rarely, the pedicle may be seen on the other side. This is a reaction to the contralateral pars defect and heralds the presence of extra stress on the as-yet-not-fractured pars. This sclerosis must be differentiated from an osteoid osteoma, which has a predilection for the pedicle or pars.[39] Rothman[35] believed that the sclerosis of the opposite pedicle so often reported in association with a unilateral pars defect is in most cases actually sclerosis of the proximal part of the pars and not of the pedicle. When the radiographic examination fails to provide useful information, a technetium pyrophosphate bone scan should be performed. Scintigraphy has repeatedly been shown to reliably detect early stress fractures or areas of increased bone turnover in both the spine and the extremities.* The pars is commonly "hot" in this "subradiologic" phase.[10] During this phase plain radiographs usually show normal results.

Bone scanning is also invaluable in the evaluation of the relative acuteness of the defect. The combination of a plain radiograph and bone scan assists in forming a treatment plan and is discussed further in the following section.

On rare occasions, even though an early stress reaction is present, the radiographic examination and the bone scan are normal. This may occur if the bone scan is ordered too soon after the stress reaction has started or if it is misinterpreted.[35] In this case computed tomography (CT) scanning with sagittal reconstruction may be appropriate (Fig. 12-2). Because of the lack of radiation exposure, magnetic resonance imaging (MRI)

* References 10, 12, 17, 29, 30, 32.

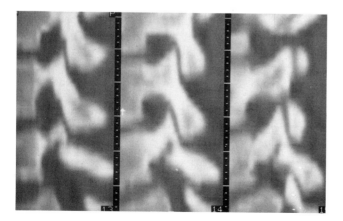

Fig. 12-2. Sagittal reformation demonstrating an incomplete fracture of the pars interarticularis. (Courtesy Stephen Rothman, M.D.)

would be preferred for this evaluation, especially in young people. Unfortunately, it is more difficult to appreciate pars defects on MRI scans than it is with CT scanning. Thus, as of this writing, a CT scan is the examination of choice.[14]

TREATMENT

The treatment of spondylolysis in the athlete must be individualized. The goals of treatment are to relieve pain and to possibly heal the defect. Consideration should be given to the age, physical maturity, and relative athletic talent of the child. The impact of both the disease and the treatment must be considered. Obviously, the treatment of the "weekend warrior" or casual competitor should be more conservative. These individuals can usually be treated with activity modification alone. The discontinuation of athletics in the high-caliber athlete may cause great emotional stress and/or even financial loss. It is with this in mind that the following treatment recommendations are offered.

Treatment of any patient with low back pain should begin with a careful history and physical examination. All of the potential sources of low back pain, such as tumor, infection, or spondyloarthropathy, should be ruled out. It is important to keep in mind that the majority of people with spondylolysis are asymptomatic. Automatically assuming that the spondylolytic defect is the source of the pain may lead one astray.

As previously mentioned, the young athlete with a history of low back pain that suddenly worsened probably was already developing the fracture, and a moment of slight extra stress merely completed it. Plain x-rays films may reveal a crack in the pars without a slip, and there may or may not be evidence of periosteal reaction at the pars. The technetium pyrophosphate bone scan is very helpful in assessing both the relative acuteness of the fracture and its healing potential. If there is significant uptake at the pars with radiographic evidence of fracture, there is good potential for healing the defect.

Studies have shown defect healing either with an antilordotic orthosis, such as the Boston brace,[26,27] or with a lumbosacral corset. The corset is significantly less expensive, which may actually be a negative factor, since the expense of the brace may cause some parents to insist that it be worn. The corset is less restrictive, less cumbersome, and esthetically more appealing. We recommend that the corset be removed after the patient is in bed and put back on while the patient is still in bed. This is done to avoid leaving the corset off for long periods before retiring and after getting up. During this period, the athlete should be participating in a gentle stabilization exercise program, along with cardiopulmonary training to avoid deconditioning. The corset is also removed for showering.

Once the symptoms have improved, practice is al-

Table 12-2. Diagnosis and Treatment of Spondylolysis

X-Ray Study	Bone Scan	Treatment	Repeat X-Ray Study	Repeat Bone Scan	Likelihood of Pars Healing	Length of Immobilization	Time off Athletics
Negative	Unilateral pars uptake	Off athletics Wear corset	3 months	6 months	Nearly 100%	Until bone scan shows significant healing	Until bone scan shows significant healing Probably 6 months
Possible unilateral pars fracture	Bilateral pars uptake	Off athletics Wear corset	3 months	6 months	Nearly 100%	Until bone scan shows significant healing	Until bone scan shows significant healing Probably 6-9 months
Possible bilateral pars fracture	Bilateral pars uptake	Off athletics Wear corset	3 months	6 months	Fair	Until plain x-ray films and bone scans show pars healing or else it is clear that healing will not take place	Until plain x-ray films and bone scans show pars healing or else it is clear that healing will not take place
Definite bilateral pars fracture appearing fresh	Still very "hot"	Off athletics Wear corset	3 months	6 months	Poor	Until plain x-ray films and bone scans show pars healing or else it is clear that healing will not take place	Until plain x-ray films and bone scans show pars healing or else it is clear that healing will not take place
Fracture appears old	Negative or only mildly positive	Treat symptomatically, posterior fusion or pars repair			Poor, nearly nonexistent	May choose not to use a corset	Only until symptoms allow return

lowed while wearing the corset and avoiding stressful maneuvers. An oblique x-ray film is taken 3 months later to assess whether the defect is showing signs of healing. Treatment is continued and the x-ray study is repeated 3 months later. Nine months after injury, if the patient is asymptomatic, he or she may return to full athletics, regardless of whether the defect has healed. The assumption is that if the defect was ever going to heal, it would have by then. If symptoms are still present at this time, the patient is asked if he or she can compete in spite of the pain. If the answer is yes, an attempt to compete is allowed. If this fails, or if the answer is no, a decision must be made to either discontinue strenuous athletics or undergo surgical treatment.

If an acute defect is discovered before the age of 15 but does not heal and surgery is not elected, the patient

is followed radiographically with a single spot lateral view of the lumbosacral junction (with the patient standing) every 4 months until the patient is asymptomatic and then semiannually until the age of 16. This is important only in those athletes in whom the defect fails to heal, because if a slip is going to occur, it will usually do so between the ages of 9 and 15. Girls are twice as likely to develop a high-grade slip as are boys.

If a slip of less than 50% is noted incidentally in an asymptomatic athlete, no restrictions are necessary. However, until the age of 16, radiographic follow-up is recommended. If a slip of 50% or more is present, the patient is advised not to compete in high-risk sports and is examined semiannually until growth stops. These patients are more likely to require fusion. It is unlikely that the physician will be faced with making this decision, because patients with a high-grade slip generally are not able to compete in any of the sports requiring great physical activity.

Athletes may present with complaints of low back pain but have normal radiographic findings. In this situation, if the scan demonstrates uptake in the region of the pars but the x-ray findings are negative, the fracture is in the "subradiologic"[10] phase. Athletics are stopped, and a corset is worn. If the x-ray findings suggest a fracture, oblique x-ray films are taken at 30, 45,

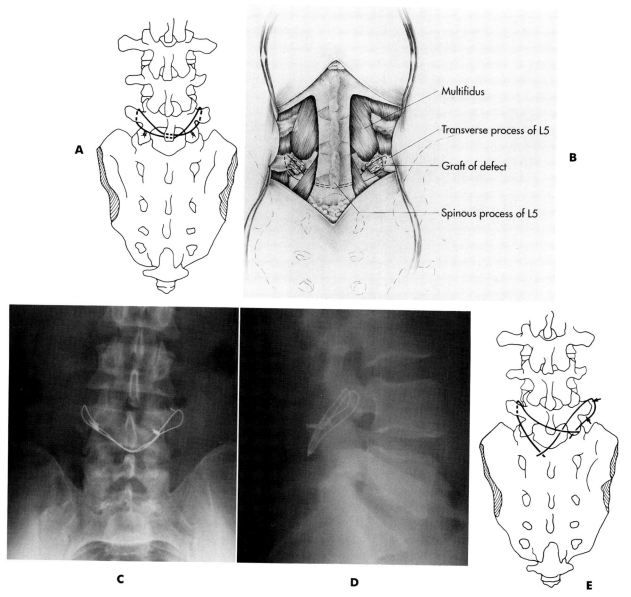

Fig. 12-3. A, Hambly's modification of Nicol and Scott's technique for tension band wiring and bone grafting. With two wires and two knots, a more even tension can be obtained. Also, the knots are very accessible through the paraspinal approach. To get the wire through the midline soft tissue when the paraspinal approach is used, a long hemostat is passed through just caudal to the L5 spinous process and the wire is passed through. **B,** Hambly's modification showing the paraspinal approach with the bone grafts and wires in place. **C,** AP x-ray film of a patient in whom the double-wire and double-knot technique is being used. **D,** Lateral x-ray film of the same patient as in **C. E,** Getting the wire around the transverse process can be difficult. We go around from the caudal side of the process; we clear the soft tissue off with a Cloward ligamentum flavum dissector and then bend the wire as in passing a wire around the lamina in a Luque spinal fixation. If too much difficulty is encountered in passing the wire, it is permissible to cut the ligament from the tip of the process and simply loop the wire around as on the right side.

and 60 degrees, or a sagittally reconstructed CT scan may demonstrate the fracture. If there still is no evidence of fracture, all sports are discontinued and a corset is prescribed. Bed rest is generally not helpful and only leads to deconditioning. At 6 weeks the x-ray studies are repeated to determine if a fracture is now present. At 4 months the bone scan is repeated, and if it shows decreased uptake with respect to the previous scan and symptoms have resolved, activities may be resumed. These patients have excellent healing potential.

Low back pain in the athlete with the combination of a radiographic pars defect and a "cold" bone scan is not likely to resolve. The absence of uptake indicates that the defect is probably chronic and may not be the source of the pain. Relief of pain with injection of the pars with local anesthetic using radiologic localization would implicate the pars as the source of the pain. If the pain does not resolve on pars injection, a disc is probably responsible.

A T2-weighted MRI scan may demonstrate the presence of disc degeneration or disc herniation. Discography may localize the painful disc. If patients become asymptomatic or can compete with the help of activity modifications or antiinflammatory medications, they are cleared to do so even though they have pars defects. Appropriately ordered and monitored epidural steroid injections may be beneficial in breaking the pain cycle in the skeletally mature athlete but should not be used more than three or four times a year.

Surgical intervention is obviously the last resort in athletes. It is impossible to assure those competing at international levels that their "fine edge" will not be lost after surgery. However, surgery is occasionally necessary in the athlete who either refuses to stop competing or who has stopped and is still symptomatic. However, the exact source of the pain must be localized if surgery is to help.

In those with long-standing spondylolisthesis, the likelihood is that the pain is discogenic. An MRI scan may reveal disc degeneration, and in the skeletally mature patient discography may be helpful in diagnosing the source of the pain. If one is convinced that the pain is discogenic, a bilateral fusion of just the involved level is performed. Autologous bone graft is used. Special care must be taken in the athlete when harvesting bone graft for fusion, since this is a significant source of morbidity.[44] To minimize muscle stripping, cancellous graft is harvested from between the inner and outer tables of the ilium. A paraspinal approach is preferred because it allows one to address the pathologic condition directly, affords excellent exposure, and, most important, preserves the midline ligamentous structures. If there is significant degeneration at the L4-5 level (when the pars defect is in L5) and it is very painful on discography, this level may need to be included in the fusion. However, every effort should be made to treat these patients nonoperatively.

Direct Repair of the Pars Fracture

In cases of a minimal slip, if injection of the pars defect with local anesthetic gives significant short-term relief, the pars is presumed to be the source of the pain, and direct repair of the defect may be indicated. The advantages of this technique are that only the pathologic condition is addressed, and a motion segment is not lost, which might be crucial in an athlete. There must be only a minimal slip present and no more than mild evidence of disc degeneration. There are several techniques for repairing the defect. In our experience, a paraspinal approach is preferable.

The first direct pars repair was described by Buck[3] in 1970. In this technique, a screw is passed across the pars defect, and bone graft taken from the iliac crest is packed into the freshened defect. Morscher, Gerber, and Frasel[28] described a technique using a hook screw device to apply compression across the defect.

Perhaps the simplest and least challenging technique is a combination of tension band wiring and bone grafting, which was originally described by Nicol and Scott.[29] A significant rate of defect healing has been achieved with this technique.[2,13] Nicol and Scott's technique can be performed using a paraspinal approach that leaves the important midline ligamentous structures undisturbed. Also, we find it easier to work through this lateral approach. A modification of this technique that we find makes the operation easier was designed by one of us (M.F.H.).[15] In this technique, two tension band wires are used, and thus two knots are made (Fig. 12-3). This works especially well with the paraspinal approach.

REFERENCES

1. Alexander MJI: Biomechanical aspect of lumbar spine injuries in athletes: a review, *Can J Appl Sports Sci* 10:1, 1985.
2. Bradford D, Iza J: Repair of the defect in spondylolysis or minimal degrees of spondylolisthesis by segmental wire fixation and bone grafting, *Spine* 10:673, 1985.
3. Buck J: Direct repair of the defect in spondylolisthesis: preliminary report, *J Bone Joint Surg* 52B:432, 1970.
4. Cahill BR: Chronic orthopedic problems in the young athlete, *J Sports Med* 3:36, 1973.
5. Commandre FA et al: Spondylolysis and spondylolisthesis in young athletes: 28 cases, *J Sports Med Phys Fitness* 28:104, 1988.
6. Cuillo JV, Jackson DW: Pars interarticularis stress reaction, spondylolysis and spondylolisthesis in gymnasts, *Clin Sports Med* 4:95, 1985.
7. Cyron BM, Hutton WC, Troup JD: Spondylolytic fractures, *J Bone Joint Surg* 58B:462, 1976.
8. Cyron BM, Hutton WC: The fatigue strength of the lumbar neural arch in spondylolysis, *J Bone Joint Surg* 60B:234, 1978.
9. Dandy DJ, Shannon MJ: Lumbo-sacral subluxation (group 1 spondylolisthesis), *J Bone Joint Surg* 53B:578, 1971.
10. Elliot S, Hutson MA, Wastie ML: Bone scintigraphy in the assessment of spondylolysis in patients attending a sports injury clinic, *Clin Radiol* 39:269, 1988.
11. Gainor B, Hagen RJ, Allen WC: Biomechanics of the spine in the pole vaulters as related to spondylolysis, *Am J Sports Med* 11:53, 1983.
12. Gelfand MJ, Strife JL, Kerelakes JG: Radionuclide bone imaging in spondylolysis of the lumbar spine in children, *Radiology* 140:191, 1981.

13. Granhead H, Morelli B: Low back pain in athletes, *Physician Sportsmed* 10:77, 1982.
14. Grogan JP et al: Spondylolysis studied with computerized tomography, *Radiology* 145:737, 1987.
15. Hambly MF et al: Tension band wiring—bone grafting for spondylolysis and spondylolisthesis: a clinical biomechanical study, *Spine* 14:455, 1989.
16. Hoshima H: Spondylolysis in athletes, *Physician Sportsmed* 8:75, 1980.
17. Hutton WC, Stott JRR, Cryon BM: Is spondylolysis a fatigue fracture? *Spine* 2:202, 1977.
18. Jackson DW, Wiltse LL, Cirincione RJ: Spondylolysis in the female gymnast, *Clin Orthop* 117:68, 1976.
19. Jackson DW et al: Stress reactions involving the pars interarticularis in young athletes, *Am J Sports Med* 9:304, 1981.
20. Keene JS, Alkert MJ, Ritter MA: Back injuries in college athletes, *J Spinal Dis* 2:190, 1989.
21. Kotani PT et al: Studies of spondylolysis found among weight lifters, *Br J Sports Med* 6:4, 1971.
22. Lament LE, Einola S: Spondylolisthesis in children and adolescents, *Acta Orthop Scand* 82:45, 1961.
23. Leach R: Disc disease, spondylolysis, and spondylolisthesis, *Athletic Training* 12(1), 1977.
24. Letts M et al: Fracture of the pars interarticularis in adolescent athletes: a clinical biomechanical analysis, *J Pediatr Orthop* 6:40, 1980.
25. McCarroll JR, Miller JM, Ritter MA: Lumbar spondylolysis and spondylolisthesis in college football players, *Am J Sports Med* 14:404, 1986.
26. Micheli LJ: Back injuries in gymnastics, *Clin Sports Med* 4:85, 1985.
27. Micheli LJ, Hare JE, Miller ME: Use of modified Boston brace for back injuries in athletes, *Am J Sports Med* 8:351, 1980.
28. Morscher E, Gerber B, Frasel J: Surgical treatment of spondylolisthesis by bone grafting and direct stabilization of spondylolysis by means of hook screw, *Acta Orthop Trauma Surg* 103:175, 1984.
29. Nicol R, Scott J: Lytic spondylolysis repair by wiring, *Spine* 11:1027, 1986.
30. Papanicola N et al: Bone scintigraphy and radiography in young athletes with low back pain, *AJR* 145:1039, 1985.
31. Reference deleted in proofs.
32. Rosen PR, Micheli LJ, Treves S: Early scintigraphic diagnosis of bone stress and fractures in athletic adolescents, *Pediatrics* 70:11, 1982.
33. Rossi F: Spondylolysis, spondylolisthesis and sports, *J Sports Med Phys Fitness* 18:317, 1978.
34. Rothman SLG: Computed tomography of the spine in older children and teenagers, *Clin Sports Med* 5:247, 1986.
35. Rothman SLG: Personal communication, 1989.
36. Rubens-Duval A et al: Le rachis de ceintures noines de judo, *Rev Rheum* 27:233, 1960.
37. Schultz KP, Niethard FU: Strain on the interarticular stress distribution, *Arch Orthop Trauma Surg* 96:197, 1980.
38. Shaffer RE. In Smith NJ, editor: *Sports medicine for children and youth: report of the tenth Ross roundtable on critical approaches to common pediatric problems,* Columbus, Ohio, 1979, Ross Laboratories.
39. Sherman FC, Wilkinson RH, Hall JE: Reactive sclerosis of a pedicle and spondylolysis in the lumbar spine, *J Bone Joint Surg* 59A:49, 1977.
40. Simon RL, Spenger D: Significance of lumbar spondylolisthesis in college football players, *Spine* 6:172, 1981.
41. Stallard MC: Backache in oarsmen, *Br J Sports Med* 14:105, 1980.
42. Stanitski CL: Low back pain in athletes, *Physician Sportsmed* 10:77, 1982.
43. Swaid L et al: Spondylolysis and the sacrohorizontal angle in athletes, *Acta Radiol* 30:359, 1989.
44. Weinstein J, Rydevic B: The pain of spondylolisthesis, *Semin Spine Surg* 1:100, 1989.

Chapter Thirteen

◆

Degenerative Disorders of the Cervical Spine

James M. Odor
William H. Dillin
Robert G. Watkins

NECK PAIN

Intelligent decision making in the evaluation and treatment of patients with neck complaints requires an understanding of the anatomic mechanisms responsible for pain, a complete history and physical examination, and compilation of a differential diagnosis for use in further evaluation and treatment.

In 1949 Kellgren[86] stated, "The phenomenon of pain belongs to that borderland between the body and the soul about which it is so delightful to speculate from the comfort of an armchair, but which offers such formidable obstacles to scientific inquiry." Over the past 40 years scientific attempts to hurdle these obstacles have shed some light on pain pathogenesis. Rather than discussing the entire spectrum of neurophysiologic and biochemical events and pathways, this chapter summarizes known anatomic events leading to pain production.

In the intervertebral disc, known physiologic, age-related changes begin in the third decade but are expressed as disease-related processes only at a later time. Accompanying the aging process is a gradual increase in collagen and decrease in mucoprotein in the intervertebral disc, with a consequent lowering of water content.[172] The subsequent changes lead to a loss of disc space height. As this occurs, the bony prominences formed by the neurocentral joints approach each other. With further disc degeneration these processes are pressed together and osteophytic excrescences form.[59,95]

This process may not necessarily be painful, as evidenced by the fact that these findings are found in a high percentage of x-ray films of asymptomatic persons.[65] The midcervical region is the most common site for disc degeneration, with C5-6 being the most frequently involved segment.[37]

Cervical disc degeneration may cause local or referred pain as a result of inflammation, annular nerve fiber stimulation, or posterior joint strains caused by instability of the neuromotion segment.[8] In 1988 histologic studies of cervical discs by Bogduk et al.[11] showed that nerve fibers occur as deeply as the outer third of the annulus fibrosus. They found that the cervical sinovertebral nerves follow an upward course in the vertebral canal, supplying the disc at their level of entry, as well as the disc above. Branches of the vertebral nerves supply the lateral aspects of the cervical discs.[11]

In addition to local and referred pain, the neurocentral osteophyte formation and foraminal narrowing may produce nerve root irritation or impairment of root conduction, causing a radicular-type pain in the distribution of that nerve root. If an osteophyte extends laterally, encroaching on the vertebral artery foramen, vertebral artery occlusion symptoms may result, including dizziness, tinnitus, intermittent blurring of vision, and retroocular pain.[106] Severely diminished flow in one vertebral artery may lead to occlusion of the posteroinferior cerebellar artery on that side, resulting in a lateral medullary infarction (Wallenberg's syndrome). This syndrome is associated with the following symptom complex[106]:

1. Dysphagia, ipsilateral palatal weakness, and vocal cord paralysis caused by involvement of the nucleus ambiguous of the vagus nerve
2. Impairment of sensation to pain and temperature on the same side of the face caused by involvement of the descending root and nucleus of the fifth nerve
3. Horner's syndrome in the homolateral eye caused by involvement of the descending sympathetic fibers
4. Nystagmus caused by involvement of the vestibular nuclei

In addition to discogenic pain, nerve root pain, inflammation, and symptoms related to vascular occlusion, cervical disc degeneration may lead to central canal stenosis from posterior osteophytes or bars that cause spinal cord compression and vascular impairment of the radicular arteries, leading to cervical spondylotic myelopathy.[71] The manifestations of this disorder are discussed later in this chapter.

The syndrome of cervical disc degeneration encompasses many potential pathologic culprits responsible for pain. However, a differential diagnosis must be entertained even with seemingly obvious causes for the symptoms. Other offending lesions can be classified as either intraspinal or extraspinal.[33] Intraspinal lesions may present with various patterns of pain and neurologic changes. Intramedullary tumors or hydromyelia usually cause a pattern of diffuse deep pain. Extramedullary tumors, such as schwannoma or neurofibroma, may present with radicular pain of the nerve root involved.[33]

164

Oblique views of the cervical spine may show foraminal widening created by tumor expansion. Anterior horn cell disease, such as the early stages of acute poliomyelitis, may present with neck and upper extremity pain.[33] If associated predominant motor weakness, fasciculations, widespread denervation seen on electromyography (EMG) or debilitating prodromal symptoms are present, they aid in the diagnosis of this gray matter disease of the spinal cord.

Disseminated white matter abnormalities, as seen in the demyelinating diseases, may occasionally be associated with neck pain.[33] When suspected, cerebrospinal fluid (CSF) counts, biochemical analysis (myelin basic protein, oligoclonal bands, IGG, and IGG complex), and magnetic resonance imaging (MRI) should be ordered. MRI shows demyelinating white plaques if present.[33]

Pain of brachial plexus origin due to brachial neuritis is a well-defined clinical entity and was described by Parsonage and Turner[125] in 1948. Shoulder pain at the onset appears as a primary symptom of brachial neuritis, with referred pain to the neck and upper extremity. It is important to distinguish this disorder because of its dramatic symptoms and relatively good prognosis.[41] The pain is usually short lived, but as it is subsiding, weakness generally ensues, most frequently involving the deltoid, spinati, serratus anterior, biceps, and triceps. A hallmark of this process is that EMG studies usually show changes indicating combined nerve root and peripheral nerve involvement.[41] The cause of brachial neuritis is still under debate, but one theory relates its onset to a systemic or local infection, presumably of viral origin. In as many as 25% of patients in large reported series,[100,177] an infection immediately preceded the syndrome's onset.

Other phenomena causing brachial plexus neuropathy must also be considered when evaluating patients with cervical, shoulder, and upper extremity symptoms. Compression by vascular and skeletal structures,[65] fibrous bands, and tumors are included.[171] The brachial plexus closely approximates the subclavian artery and vein as these elements pass through a triangle formed by the anterior and middle scalene muscles and the first rib.[171]

Compromise of the space in this triangle may result from a cervical rib, an elongated seventh cervical transverse process, an abnormality of the scalene muscles, or narrowing of the space between the first rib and the clavicle when the arm is abducted.[111,137] The abnormal compromise of this space may create symptoms often referred to as thoracic outlet syndrome, first described in 1821 by Sir Astley Cooper.[175] The vast majority of symptomatic patients with the syndrome have symptoms resulting from direct compression of the brachial plexus.[137] Symptoms are generally those of aching pain in the neck, shoulder, or medial arm, frequently radiating along the distribution of the ulnar nerve to involve the hypothenar palm and fourth and fifth digits. Numbness and tingling may be present, and discomfort is often worse after the arm is used, rather than during use, and may be worse at night.[35,123] The principal differential diagnosis includes cervical disc disease and more distal compressive neuropathies. Less frequent entities include costoclavicular syndrome, pectoralis minor syndrome, posttraumatic sympathetic dystrophy, and superior sulcus carcinoma of the lung (Pancoast's tumor).[137]

Apical carcinomas of the lung where the neurovascular bundle is close to the parietal pleura may occur.[21] Symptoms can be caused by irritation of the parietal pleura itself or by tumor invasion of adjacent structures, including the vertebrae, ribs, brachial plexus, or stellate ganglion. When brachial plexus involvement occurs, the C8-T1 nerve roots are most commonly affected, since they are the most medial in the brachial plexus.[21] The diagnosis is usually suggested by a mass at the apex of the lung, seen on apical lordotic chest x-ray examination.[21,33]

Diaphragmatic irritation, whether on pleural or peritoneal surfaces, can refer pain to the ipsilateral shoulder via stimulation of the roots from which the phrenic nerve originates (i.e., the third, fourth, and fifth cervical nerves). Since these nerves innervate the skin of the neck, the supraclavicular area, and the shoulder, pain is felt in these areas.[21] Pneumonia, pulmonary infarction, empyema, neoplasm, hepatobiliary disease, subphrenic abcess, splenic injury, or a pseudocyst of the pancreas are processes that may irritate the diaphragm, producing a painful neck and shoulder.[21]

Primary disorders of the shoulder may occasionally masquerade as cervical pathology, but a careful physical examination generally shows signs localized to the shoulder. Patients with adhesive capsulitis have limited glenohumeral range of motion. Those with subacromial bursitis with impingement syndrome have localized tenderness in the subacromial area and over the coracoacromial ligament with forward flexion and internal rotation through the impingement arc. When patients with suspected cervical pathology are being evaluated, a careful examination of the shoulder itself should always be carried out.

Finally, angina pectoris may present with varying forms of left shoulder and upper extremity symptoms. This is usually described as a deep aching or crushing pain, exacerbated by exertion, and usually associated with a chest pain component and absence of exacerbation with cervical spine movement. Angina pectoris is occasionally misinterpreted as cervical radiculopathy, but more commonly the opposite occurs.[33] In 1927 Phillips[131] was perhaps the first to point out that anginoid precordial pain can occur as a result of cervical root compression. Since then, it has been suggested that the referred pain in cervical angina most likely results from compression or irritation of the ventral nerve root, creating pain along the myotome innervated by the motor nerves of that level.[15]

In summary, a multitude of entities can masquerade as problems originating from the cervical spine, and unusual presentations of cervical spine pathology may occur. However, careful attention to the history, physical examination, EMG abnormalities, and radiographic findings usually allows the differentiation of these disorders, as well as appropriate localization of the process.

RADIOLOGIC EVALUATION

A complete cervical spine series should consist of anteroposterior (AP), lateral, flexion/extension lateral, oblique, and open-mouth odontoid views. This series screens for osseous pathology, although a more subtle expression of pathologic conditions cannot be ruled out. Osseous conditions identifiable by plain radiography include cervical spondylosis, sagittal spinal canal dimensions, calculation of canal/body ratios, measurement of intervertebral disc space height, congenital abnormalities, basilar impression, and destructive lesions from infection, tumor, or other causes. Oblique views allow a general assessment of osseous foraminal patency, and flexion/extension lateral views evaluate stability.

Cervical spondylosis is a common x-ray finding in asymptomatic persons.[50,59,65] Gore et al.,[65] in a study of cervical spine x-ray findings in 200 asymptomatic persons, found that by age 60 to 65, 95% of men and 70% of women had at least one degenerative change detectable radiographically. The same study also found that 9% of the 200 patients had kyphotic deformities. The findings seen on screening radiographs must be correlated with the clinical history and physical findings.

See Chapter 3 for further discussion of radiologic evaluation of the cervical spine.*

RADICULOPATHY

Cervical radiculopathy is defined as pain in the distribution of a cervical nerve root caused by nerve root compression.[42] It is not uncommon; Hult[81] estimated that 51% of the adult population has neck and arm pain at some point.[46] An epidemiologic study by Kelsey et al.[87] has shown that cervical disc herniations are most common in the fourth decade of life and occur in a male/female ratio of 1.4:1; risk factors are frequent lifting, cigarette smoking, and diving from a board. This section focuses on the pathogenesis, clinical presentation, differential diagnosis, natural history, and treatment alternatives in cervical radiculopathy.

Pathogenesis

Nerve root irritation may be secondary to compression by either hard or soft disc herniations.[156,169] A "hard

disc" refers to the presence of cervical spondylosis with osteophytes originating from the degenerative neuro-central joints and protruding into the nerve root foramina. A "soft disc" refers to the more acute stage of disc herniation with prolapse of the nucleus pulposus through the annulus.[95,152,169] Nuclear prolapse may occur intraforaminally, ventrolaterally, or in the midline.[169] Of these, intraforaminal extrusions are the most common, producing pain in the neck and shoulder that radiates down a specific nerve root distribution. The C5-6 level is most commonly involved, followed by C6-7, C4-5, C3-4, and C7-T1.[72,99] Regardless of the acute versus chronic presentation, nerve root irritation caused by mechanical compression is a denominator in producing symptoms of cervical radiculopathy.

Clinical Presentation

Patients with acute cervical disc herniation complain of a sudden onset of severe pain leading to voluntary neck immobilization. Pain usually radiates to the dermatome of the involved nerve root and may also occur in the suboccipital region along the greater occipital nerve distribution, giving some patients the complaint of "headaches." Pain is usually aggravated by neck motion, especially extension, and may be relieved by rest and immobilization. The onset may be associated with heavy lifting, trauma, or, commonly, awakening in the morning. Although the pathologic changes of spondylosis occur over time, either acute or chronic presentations may occur.

Although the classic presentations are usual, variations may be encountered. Anatomic variations may result from anastomoses between posterior cervical roots, variations of root contribution, and anastomoses within the brachial plexus and the peripheral nerves.[9] Benini's excellent analysis of 119 single–nerve root syndromes caused by single-level disc herniation[9] points to the variation in clinical presentation for cervical nerve roots C5 through C8. Reasons offered as anatomic explanation include:

1. Differences between Foerster's and Keegan's dermatomal charts from single–nerve root loss
2. Anastomoses between adjacent posterior cervical nerve roots but limited to adjacent segments and reputedly never three-segment involvement
3. Brachial plexus variations such as C7 contribution of the medial cord in 39%, bridging of the ulnar nerve and lateral cord in 18%, and medial cord and lateral cord involvement in 12.5%
4. Connection between the median and ulnar nerves in the forearm

In addition, nerve root involvement associated with cervical spondylosis may be unilateral or bilateral and may present with multiple ipsilateral nerve root irritation, with variable degrees of involvement at each level.

Various physical examination tests have been cited to increase the pain radiation in cervical radiculopathy

---

* See also references 3, 28, 29, 34, 39, 40, 58, 77, 78, 82, 90, 92, 102, 103, 105, 107, 151, 152, 166, 173, 186, 191.

through provocative means. Valsalva's maneuver, which increases intrathecal pressure, and the cervical compression test have been used to elicit pain, whereas the cervical distraction test theoretically releases cervical nerve root compression, thus transiently relieving pain.[79] Spurling's sign reproduces arm pain by hyperextension and lateral cervical rotation.[167] The shoulder abduction test, which relieves arm pain, is an excellent indication of cervical radiculopathy caused by extradural compression.[36] In Davidson, Dunn, and Metzmaker's series[36] 68% of those with cervical radiculopathy demonstrated this sign, and it correlated with parasthesis in 73%, weakness in 100%, and positive myelography for extradural compression. This test was found to have a significant correlation with surgical success. The most likely reason for symptom relief was reduced nerve root tension.

How often are "the classic" presentations of specific nerve root involvement encountered in patients with cervical radiculopathy? In Henderson and Hennessy's retrospective analysis of 846 consecutive operative cases for cervical radiculopathy,[72] only 53.9% had pain and/or parasthesia in a dermatomal pattern, whereas in 45.5% the pattern was nondermatomal. In addition, 79.7% had neck pain, 52.5% had scapular pain, 17.8% had anterior chest pain, and 9.7% had headaches. Lunsford et al.'s retrospective series of 295 patients with cervical radiculopathy due to either a hard or soft disc herniation[99] did not demonstrate significant differences between the two conditions for neck pain, arm pain, chest pain (rare), interscapular pain, or unilateral or bilateral presentations. In their series patients with hard disc herniations had headaches and shoulder pain. Patients with soft disc herniations predominantly experienced mechanical signs such as cervical tenderness, restricted movement, Spurling's sign, and cervical spasm. Sensory deficits involving multiple dermatomes were more common with hard disc herniations, whereas deficits in a single dermatome were more common with soft disc herniations. A motor deficit involving a single myotome was more common with soft disc herniations, whereas the opposite was true with multiple myotomes and hard disc herniations. Atrophy was rare in both cases. Specific reflex loss was more common with soft disc herniations.

In a study of 43 patients looking at the validity of clinical tests in the diagnosis of root compression in cervical disc disease, Spurling's test,[167] the axial manual traction test,[180] and the shoulder abduction test[36] were performed.[181] All of these tests were highly specific for nerve root compression. However, the sensitivity ranged from 26% to 50% for the three single validity parameters in roots C6 through C8, and from 40% to 64% for combined neurologic and radiologic signs. It was concluded that despite low sensitivity these tests are a valuable aid in the clinical examination of a patient with neck and arm pain.[181] Finally, cervical nerve root compression can coexist with peripheral nerve root compression in a double-crush phenomenon,[119] whose symptoms may be those of a cervical nerve and the peripheral nerve, thus potentially confusing the "radicular" clinical picture.

Differential Diagnosis

Nerve root pain may result from other pathologic conditions, and other pathologic conditions can masquerade as nerve root pain. These include disc compression, posterior fossa tumors, spinal canal tumors, trauma, degenerative disorders, inflammatory diseases, brachial neuritis, toxic and allergic conditions, hemorrhage, congenital defects, compression neuropathies, thoracic outlet syndrome, chest and shoulder pathology, and phrenic nerve stimulation from diaphragmatic irritation.*

The more commonly encountered differential diagnoses involve compressive neuropathies of the upper extremity.[16,46] EMG and nerve conduction velocity tests can confirm the presence of these neuropathies.[88] Various compression neuropathies in the upper extremity are identifiable, such as those involving the median nerve in the carpal tunnel syndrome, the anterior interosseous syndrome, and the pronator teres syndrome; and at the supracondylar process and in the infraclavicular course of the nerve.[16,46,88] Other entrapment syndromes to be considered involve the axillary nerve, the suprascapular nerve, the musculocutaneous nerve, the dorsal scapular nerve, and the radial and ulnar nerves.[16,46,88] Thoracic outlet syndrome, superior sulcus tumors, shoulder pathology, and other problems have already been discussed.

Natural History

It is a generally held opinion that most patients with cervical radiculopathy will get better with the passage of time. Lees and Turner[94] studied the natural history of cervical radiculopathy. They found that although it rarely progressed to a myelopathic state, two thirds of the patients who were not operated on manifested persistent symptoms. The natural history of cervical disc degeneration was evaluated by Rothman and Simeone.[153] Of 68 patients treated conservatively, 69% had neck and radicular pain at a 5-year follow-up, and 31% had neck pain only. At the 5-year follow-up of patients treated nonoperatively, 45% were considered to have satisfactory results, 55% were considered to have unsatisfactory results, and 23% of these were completely disabled. Patients with hyperextension injuries and litigation tended to do more poorly than the group as a whole. When the surgical results were reviewed in the context of this nonoperative group, there was no statistical difference at the 5-year follow-up period between the surgical group and the control group. The implication from this study is that in dealing with

---

* References 16, 46, 50, 88, 91, 132, 147.

predominant neck pain in the absence of neurologic deficit and discrete radicular symptomatology, the results of surgery do not significantly alter the natural course of the disease.[42]

Although these studies suggest that persistent symptomatology is not an exceptional condition, the majority of patients with cervical radiculopathy do not require surgical intervention. It should be noted that in the diagnosis of cervical radiculopathy the goal of the evaluation process is the determination of nerve root compression and the elimination of other diagnoses. EMG and nerve conduction velocities, MRI, myelography, and contrast CT scanning all assist the history and physical examination in meeting this goal.

Treatment

Nonsurgical management. The primary treatment of cervical radiculopathy is supportive and includes rest, immobilization, antiinflammatory medication, patient education, and frequent reevaluation. Relative immobilization of the neck may be accomplished by educating the patient and limiting his or her activities. A soft cervical collar in slight flexion helps act as a reminder. Cervical manipulation has been shown to have no value in the treatment of neck pain or cervical radiculopathy.[97,165] In a double-blind prospective study of the influence of a single manipulation done with the patient under diazepam sedation, there was no difference in the outcome of the study group from that of a control group.[165] In a clinical study by Livingston,[97] it was found that up to 7% of patients receiving spinal manipulation sustained significant injuries, including joint injury, nerve and spinal cord damage, vascular injury, and fracture-dislocation. Intermittent cervical traction, ultrasound, acupuncture transcutaneous electrical nerve stimulation, and other therapy modalities have been used in the treatment of cervical radiculopathy, but the long-term benefit of these methods remains controversial.[67,83,153]

Surgical management. Those patients who have cervical radiculopathy unresponsive to conservative therapy and who have intractable pain lasting for an intolerable period of time may be candidates for surgical intervention. This is assuming that other pathologic entities have been excluded and that the criteria for the establishment of a diagnosis of cervical radiculopathy have been met, including the documentation of a nerve compression lesion by radiographic study (either by MRI, myelogram, or contrast CT scan), as well as a root distribution neurologic deficit and radicular arm pain.[42] Although they are uncommon, in cases of patients with a progressive motor weakness, a general philosophy employed is aggressive decompression of these nerve roots. The natural history of motor function as a result of decompressive surgery is excellent.[72] In Henderson and Hennessy's series[72] 98% returned to full function, and excellent results have been cited in most series for recovery of motor function after cervical disc surgery.

Once the lesion is localized and surgical intervention is planned, the ongoing controversy is encountered and centers on the questions of anterior versus posterior decompression for cervical radiculopathy and of fusion versus no fusion in anterior approaches. Support can be found in the orthopedic and neurosurgical literature for the use of anterior and posterior approaches. In most studies there is no significant statistical difference in results between anterior and posterior approaches for the management of cervical radiculopathy. This has been demonstrated by multiple authors in large series.*

Anterior approach with fusion. The anterior cervical fusion was initially described by Robinson and Smith[143] in 1955. A follow-up study in 1958 presenting the first 14 cases by the same authors was the first reported series in the orthopaedic literature using this approach.[144] The benefits proposed by Smith and Robinson for using the anterior discectomy and fusion were:

1. Spur formation would stop.
2. Spurs that were already present would regress because of the stability of the fusion.
3. By disc space distraction the neuroforamen would be enlarged, aiding in nerve root decompression.[144]

Since this introduction of anterior cervical discectomy and fusion, modifications and various graft configurations have been introduced.[7,27,84,164] However, biomechanical studies looking at various graft configurations have shown the Robinson iliac crest horseshoe graft to have the strongest load-bearing capacity.[183]

Since its original description in 1955,[143] numerous reports reviewing large series of anterior cervical fusions have been published.† Reported results range from 63% to 98% good and excellent. Many series combined patients with cervical spondylosis without significant radicular components with those having pure radiculopathy. In one review looking at the results of eight large series with a total of 784 cases, the overall improvement rate was 91%.[185]

It appears from reviewing these studies that the best results are obtained in treating patients with an identifiable level correlating with primarily root radiculopathy.[138,184] In a recent review of 146 patients with radiculopathy from degenerated or protruded discs who underwent anterior cervical discectomy and fusion without an attempt to remove osteophytes, pain relief was total in 78% and partial in 18%, with a fusion rate of 97%.[64] In this study it was also found that patients with pain only in the arm, forearm, and hand are the

---

* References 5, 6, 8, 14, 15, 23, 26, 27, 31, 35, 43, 51, 53, 54, 64, 68, 69, 72, 74, 75, 99, 101, 104, 109, 110, 116, 128, 129, 133, 136, 138-140, 142, 145, 148, 155, 158, 159, 164, 168, 170, 179, 184, 187-189.
† References 5-8, 14, 15, 26, 27, 31, 38, 43, 45, 85, 99, 101, 104, 138, 139, 145, 148, 150, 153, 164, 170, 184, 187.

most likely to obtain complete pain relief after surgery. This is in agreement with other studies.[138,184,187]

Potential complications of anterior cervical discectomy and fusion do exist. These can be divided into those occurring at the neck and those occurring at the graft donor site. In a review of 11 different series of anterior cervical fusions totaling 1244 cases, there was a 0.2% incidence of complications related to the neck and a 20% incidence related to the donor site.[185] Those at the neck included hoarseness, dysphagia, graft displacement, spinal cord or nerve root injury, visceral perforation, and others.[185] Those at the graft donor site included persistent drainage, hematoma formation, superficial or deep wound infection with osteomyelitis, hernia, and injury to the lateral femoral cutaneous nerve.[185]

Reports of pseudarthrosis rates in large series of anterior cervical fusions vary from 0% to 37%.* Pseudarthrosis rates are higher in multiple-level fusions.[31,73,184] Whether pseudarthrosis affects the ultimate surgical outcome is controversial. There are those who report no correlation;† however, in Riley, Robinson, and Johnson's series[139] better results were present when fusion was achieved. In their series symptoms in patients who had pseudarthrosis were improved after the patients underwent posterior fusion at the involved level.[15]

Posterior surgery for cervical radiculopathy. Posterior procedures that have been used for treatment of cervical radiculopathy include laminectomy, laminoplasty, and foraminotomy.‡ An advantage of the posterior approach includes better visualization of the neural structures, allowing generous decompression.[161] As noted earlier, when patients with multiple-level radiculopathy were treated, anterior surgery produced better results than laminectomy and laminoplasty in one series.[73] However, many reports using the posterolateral foraminotomy technique with or without use of the microscope have yielded successful results in high numbers of patients with cervical radiculopathy.§ In Henderson and Hennessy's series[72] 736 patients underwent 846 posterolateral foraminotomies for simple cervical radiculopathy. Ninety-one percent of patients reported good or excellent results, and 98% of patients with preoperative motor deficit had full motor return postoperatively. In another series 235 patients with 585 symptomatic cervical nerve roots underwent simple posterolateral foraminotomy using microsurgical technique, with excellent results reported.[188] There is no statistical difference between the results of posterolateral foraminotomy for soft or hard disc herniations.[68,72,116,153,158] This was also confirmed by Lunsford et al.[99] in an analysis of 295 patients with anterocervical discectomy. There was no difference between hard disc and soft disc statistical

results. Therefore the hard versus soft disc issue should not play a role in determining the surgical approach in these patients.

Potential complications of posterior surgery also exist. In the sitting position, air embolism has been reported.[153] Problems with instability and late kyphosis with late swan-neck deformity have been associated with laminectomy.[93,141,149,160] This seems to be related to mechanical loss of posterior cervical support after laminectomy.[98,99] Bilateral resection of more than 50% of a facet joint has been shown to compromise the shear strength of a cervical spine motion segment.[135] In Henderson and Hennessy's series of posterolateral foraminotomies,[72] complications included wound infection in 1.2% and wound breakdown in 0.3%. In Williams' series[188] 10.1% of the operations were accompanied by complications, the most frequent being transient symptoms lasting less than 6 days. Prolonged postsurgical paresis was present in 2% of cases.

◆ ◆ ◆

In summary, cervical radiculopathy is a relatively common specific diagnostic entity requiring specific diagnostic criteria. The majority of patients will respond to conservative nonoperative treatment. Exclusion of other pathologic processes that can masquerade as cervical radiculopathy is required. When surgical intervention is necessary, the approach should be selected on the basis of the location of the lesion, surgical goals, and the experience and confidence of the surgeon.

CERVICAL MYELOPATHY

Cervical spondylotic myelopathy is a neurologic disorder consisting of a spectrum of features related to pathologic attack of the cervical spinal cord. It is the most common cause of spinal cord dysfunction in patients over the age of 55, but despite advanced current diagnostic technology, cervical spondylotic myelopathy has probably been understudied, underdiagnosed, and undertreated.[182]

Cervical spondylotic myelopathy is probably multifactorial in origin with multiple influencing factors, including congenital or developmental narrowing of the cervical spinal canal, progressive cervical spondylosis, direct spinal cord compression, and alterations of the blood supply to the spinal cord.[13,18,25]

Pathophysiology

Canal size. Lindgren,[96] in 1937, pointed out the importance of the sagittal diameter in the cervical region. Since then, the importance of canal size in relation to the existence of cervical spondylotic myelopathy has been well documented.* Wolfe, Khilnani, and Malis[190] in

* References 6, 30, 31, 38, 73, 139, 145, 164, 170, 184, 187.
† References 6, 31, 38, 73, 145, 184.
‡ References 53, 54, 72, 153, 158, 159, 161, 189.
§ References 53, 61, 153, 158, 159, 188.

* References 1, 4, 22, 48, 52, 76, 108, 117, 120, 122, 125, 127, 128, 146, 176, 189.

1956, established the currently accepted normal values of the sagittal diameters of the cervical spine. In their study 200 random asymptomatic subjects underwent lateral cervical spine radiographs at a fixed target-film distance of 72 inches. AP diameters were measured from the posterior aspects of the vertebral bodies to the most anterior point on the spinolaminar line. For C1 the average AP diameter was 22 mm. For C2 the average was 20 mm. From C3 to C7 inclusively, the most frequent measurement was 17 mm. In addition to knowing the average diameter of the cervical spinal canal, it is important to know the average diameter of the cervical spinal cord. Most authors agree that there is little variation in the sagittal diameter of the spinal cord from C1 to C7, the average cord diameter being 10 mm.[146] Therefore if a spinal canal sagittal diameter approaches 10 mm, ischemia and cord compression are predictable, the effects of multisegmental disease additive, and the risk of myelopathy very high.[76]

Thus it is clear that canal size is an important determinant of the pathologic condition that leads to the expression of cervical myelopathy. But the cervical spine is indeed a dynamic mobile system, and static canal measurements and pathology do not define the full spectrum of etiologies responsible for cervical myelopathy.

Dynamic factors. In 1956 O'Connell[115] suggested that repeated cord trauma may be a more important factor than compression in patients in whom spondylotic protrusions were not severe. The amount of motion present in the cervical spine is important. Increased cervical spine movements are seen with myelopathy or radiculopathy; also, results of laminectomy were poorer in myelopathy patients with a high range of motion.[1]

It has been shown that changes in head position can cause intermittent spinal subarachnoid block in patients with spondylotic cord compression.[85] Indeed, the functional diameter of the cervical spine may be reduced to a critical level with hyperextension, as well as flexion.[52,108,127] In extension the posteroinferior margin of the superior vertebral body approximates the arch of the adjacent vertebrae and protrudes slightly into the canal, reducing the sagittal diameter of the canal by 1 to 2 mm.[55] Penning[127] has suggested that the canal diameter is 2 to 3 mm smaller in extension than in flexion, and it has been shown that the spinal cord thickens in extension, which further reduces its available space.[19] Hyperextension also produces buckling of the ligamentum flavum posteriorly, with or without disc protrusion into the canal anteriorly.[112,157,174] In flexion the cervical spine increases in length up to 2.8 cm as compared with maximal extension, with a maximal change at C5.[19,20] Thus, in flexion, axial tension on the cord decreases, deforming the lateral and anterior columns.[19,20] In a study looking at the radiographic changes of the cervical spine in relation to aging, it was shown that both static and dynamic AP canal diameters decrease with age.[71] In the same study it was shown that the dynamic canal

became much narrower than the static canal. Bohlman,[12] in 1977, pointed out the dynamic problem of pathologic compensatory subluxation in the upper cervical spine above stiff spondolytic segments producing severe cord compression and myelopathy. Hypermobility of a segment adjacent to a congenital blocked vertebra can cause cord compression.

Soft disc herniation presenting as acute myelopathy represents a group requiring acute surgical intervention.[134] Acute disc herniations should be suspected in patients with myelopathy who have normal findings on plain radiographs that show congenital or spontaneous fusion and in patients with a previous history of cervical injury.[118]

Ischemic factors. Interruption of the blood supply to the spinal cord can occur and may play a significant role in the etiology and pathophysiology of myelopathy. Criteria for inclusion in this group include the acute nature of the event, absence of obstruction on myelography, lack of pain, and failure to respond to surgery.[55]

Usually, single anterior spinal artery branches originate from each distal intracranial vertebral artery and join to form a single artery that descends in a midline anterior position to supply the rostral cervical spinal cord.[17,70] The cervical portion of the vertebral arteries gives off radicular arteries that accompany the anterior and posterior roots and feed into the anterior spinal artery system.[55]

Compression of the radicular spinal arteries at some point in their course or in the anterior spinal axis itself, by disc protrusion or bars, can produce ischemia of the spinal cord with characteristics of cervical myelopathy.[124,154]

Clinically the anterior spinal artery syndrome may have a variety of etiologic factors but usually presents with sudden quadriparesis, dissociation of sensory loss with preservation of vibration, position, and touch.[10] Sensory and motor recovery from the anterior spinal artery syndrome after sprains of the cervical spine has been observed.[56,57] Perhaps the vulnerability to this syndrome is more prominant in those whose blood supply to the anterior two-thirds of the spinal cord is derived from only one anterior radicular artery, as was demonstrated in 7 of 36 cadavers studied.[44] Recovery from cord contusion or the anterior cord syndrome may vary, ranging from complete recovery from a transitory vascular compromise to no recovery from an injury to the vascular supply of the cord.

Thus it is evident that multiple factors can play a role in the production of myelopathy. These factors may occur independently or in conjunction. Together the effects are additive; separately each has less profound effects on neurologic function than when combined.[63,94]

Clinical Presentation

The initial presenting complaints of patients with cervical myelopathy vary, ranging from those with minimal spinal cord involvement and normal gait to those with profound neural involvement and inability to walk. The course of presentation is, in general, slow and progressive, occurring frequently in stepwise deterioration.[113,162]

The gait pattern of myelopathy is well known.[162] Although variable in its severity, it is characteristically stooped, wide based, and somewhat jerky. Weakness and atrophy of the upper extremities can occur, with loss of hand dexterity. This may be compounded by progressive sensory deficits. Long-tract signs with spasticity, hyperreflexia, and extension plantar responses are characteristically present.[24]

Sympathetic chain involvement may be responsible for some of the vague and indefinite symptoms, such as dizziness, diplopia, tinnitus, and a feeling of separation from the environment or constriction of the neck.[24]

Typically, motor findings include lower and upper motor neuron signs. Lower motor neuron signs usually occur at the level of the lesion, and upper motor neuron signs occur below this level.[24] Sensory findings may be confusing, since compression of sensory pathways may occur at three anatomic locations.[162] With spinothalamic tract involvement, contralateral pain and temperature sensation is affected. If posterior column involvement is present, ipsilateral position and vibration sense may be altered. Finally, dorsal nerve root compression will lead to dermatomal sensory changes.[162]

Reflexes will typically be diminished at the level of the lesion, reflecting lower motor neuron involvement, and hyperactive below the lesion, reflecting upper motor neuron involvement.[162] Extensor plantar reflexes (Babinski's reflex) usually occur late in the clinical course.[24] Hoffman's reflex, ankle clonus, and Lhermitte's sign, the feeling of generalized electrical shock sensation with neck flexion, may be present.[24]

The gait abnormality associated with myelopathy constituted one of the major clinical effects of the disease.[162] Gorter[66] reviewed the world literature and concluded that cervical myelopathy usually presents initially as a subtle gait disturbance with gradual deterioration. He emphasized that spasticity and paretic dysfunction occur first, followed in the upper extremities by numbness and loss of fine motor movements. Nurick[113,114] used gait as a major basis for his classification of cervical spondylotic myelopathy into five grades. Grade 0 patients have root symptoms only. Grade 1 patients have cord symptoms with normal gait. Grade 2 patients have gait abnormalities but are able to be employed. Grade 3 patients have gait problems preventing employment and the performance of activities of daily living. Grade 4 patients walk only with assistance, and Grade 5 patients are confined to a chair or are bedridden.[80]

The severity of symptoms has been found to correlate with the degree of spinal cord deformity.[191] Ferguson and Caplan[55] delineated four intermingled but defined clinical syndromes on the basis of neurologic malfunction due to spondylosis. The "lateral," or radicular, syndrome is essentially an expression of nerve root compressive pathology, with absence of spinal cord dysfunction. The "medial," or spinal, syndrome is a manifestation of spinal cord abnormality. The combined "medial and lateral" syndrome presents with evidence of both spinal cord and spinal nerve root symptomatology. This is the most common presenting syndrome.[55] This group demonstrates an even greater heterogeneity of clinical symptoms and signs due to the frequent root dysfunction in the upper extremities in conjunction with "upper motor neuron" findings in the lower extremities on clinical examination. The "vascular" syndrome comprises a group of patients with acute-onset myelopathy in association with spondylosis where no other clear mechanism for the acute deterioration appears plausible.[55]

Ferguson and Caplan[55] identified this category of patients with sudden, painless myelopathy in the absence of trauma, frequently in association with unimpressive myelographic findings in relationship to symptoms, and in whom the surgical results have been unrewarding. Fortunately, this is the rarest of the syndromes.

Crandall and Batzdorf[32] classified patients into five groups based on dominant cord syndromes: Patients with transverse lesions with involvement of the appropriate neurologic tracts (corticospinal, spinothalamic, posterior columns) had severe spasticity and frequent sphincter involvement, and a third of these patients exhibited Lhermitte's sign. Patients with motor system lesions (anterior horn cells, corticospinal tract) showed spasticity but relatively innocuous or absent sensory disturbance.[32] Patients with central cord syndrome were characterized by severe motor and sensory disturbances with greater expression in the upper extremities. Patients with Brown-Séquard syndrome were characterized by contralateral sensory deficits and ipsilateral motor deficits. Patients with brachialgia and cord syndrome demonstrated lower motor neuron upper extremity involvement and upper motor neuron lower extremity involvement.[32,99]

Hand involvement in myelopathy continues to draw attention. "Myelopathy hand," coined by Ono et al.,[121] is defined as "loss of power of adduction and extension of the ulnar two or three fingers, and an inability to grip and release rapidly with these fingers." The finger escape sign, which shows the deficiency of adduction and/or extension, can be distinguished from other causes (motor neuron disease or peripheral nerve entrapment syndrome) by normal active range of motion of the wrist.[121] Ono et al. found that myelopathy hand was associated with spasticity in the lower extremities, and their grading system correlated with the performance of hand function.

Good, Couch, and Wacaser[62] reported a series of patients with cervical myelopathy with compression between C3 and C5 in whom the main attribute was numbness in the hands. In this group decreased vibratory and position sense, stereoanesthesia, and diminished fine motion were present in the hands. Although hyperreflexia was present in the upper extremities, only one half of the patients were noted to have gait disorders and Babinski's reflex on examination.

Ebara et al.[47] associated myelopathy hand with muscle wasting—the "amyotrophic type." Clinical features in this group of patients included hand muscle wasting and weakness, minimal sensory changes, and no gait disorders. The emphasis of this information is that the hand, by symptom and physical examination, may be conceptualized as the potential distal expression of the cervical spinal cord.

Proximal upper extremity involvement has been focused upon by Phillips,[130] who identified a subgroup of patients with cervical myelopathy associated with shoulder wasting and weakness. The scapular and deltoid muscles were involved, with 32 of the 40 cases being due to myelopathies associated at the C3-4 level.

In the lower extremities spasticity has been shown to be a common finding; however, one must remember that other coexistent pathology may present a confusing clinical picture. In addition to the classic upper motor neuron changes, there may be lower motor neuron findings, as evidenced by absent or diminished ankle jerks.[49] Concomitant lumbar stenosis or neuropathy may mask upper motor neuron signs in the lower extremities or present a mixed upper and lower motor neuron picture.

From this review it is evident that because of the global nature of the myelopathic process, the heterogeneity of clinical presentations, and the variable clinical signs dependent on the anatomic location of the pathologic lesion, it is difficult to make the diagnosis of "early myelopathy." Yet these patients are precisely the ones in whom treatment is more efficacious.[13] Since no single neurologic exponent is unique to cervical myelopathy, the diagnosis must be established by the affirmation of the associated clinical signs and symptoms and the exclusion of those clinical entities that may mimic the same. This leads us to the differential diagnosis of cervical myelopathy.

In a patient with the classic signs and symptoms, with appropriate correlative radiographic findings, the diagnosis of cervical myelopathy is less difficult to make. However, since cervical spondylosis is so common in patients over the age of 50, strict correlation is necessary to establish that an observed myelopathy is due to the degenerative process and not to some other pathologic event.[23]

In a group of 102 cases of cervical myelopathy followed over a 10-year period, 23 additional cases of myelopathy associated with cervical spondylosis graphically depicted other diagnoses associated with my-

elopathy: "Disseminated sclerosis, motor neuron disease, subacute combined degeneration, syringomyelia, Arnold-Chiari malformation, vertebrobasilar ischemia, peripheral neuritis, astrocytoma of the spinal cord, and cysts of the spinal cord" were examples. In a series reported by Veidlinger et al.[179] other diagnoses considered included cerebral hemisphere disease, motor neuron disease, multiple sclerosis, poliomyelitis, Guillain-Barré syndrome, peripheral neuropathy, and arthritis.[178]

To discuss each syndrome that could be confused with cervical spondylotic myelopathy is beyond the scope of this chapter; however, the following outline gives one a good basis on which to consider other diagnostic entities. For an indepth review of each of these processes, one is referred to a neurology text, from which this outline was derived.[2]

I. Spinal cord injury
   A. Posttraumatic
   B. Postradiation
II. Inflammatory diseases of the spinal cord (myelitis)
   A. Viral
   B. Bacterial, fungal, parasitic, tubercular
   C. Unknown etiology
      1. Postinfectious, postvaccinal
      2. Acute and chronic relapsing multiple sclerosis
      3. Neurotic or degenerative
III. Vascular diseases of the spinal cord
   A. Infarction (myelomalacia)
   B. Hemorrhage (hematomyelia) into the spinal cord
   C. Hemorrhage into the spinal canal (hematorrhachis)
   D. Vascular malformations
   E. Caisson's disease
   F. Fibrocartilaginous embolism
IV. Syndrome of subacute or chronic spinal ataxia with paraparesis
   A. Hereditary spinal (Friedreich's) ataxia and spastic paraparesis
   B. Multiple sclerosis (demyelinative diseases)
   C. Syphilitic meningomyelitis
   D. Subacute combined degeneration of the spinal cord
   E. Combined-system disease of nonpernicious anemia type
   F. Spinal arachnoiditis
V. Other spinal abnormalities (besides spondylosis) with myelopathy
   A. Anomalies of the craniocervical junction
   B. Platybasia and basilar invagination
   C. Odontoid process abnormalities—atlantoaxial instability—rheumatoid arthritis
VI. Intraspinal tumors
   A. Extramedullary

B. Intramedullary
VII. Foramen magnum tumors
VIII. Syringomyelic syndrome
  A. Syringomyelia
IX. Multiple sclerosis and allied demyelinative diseases
  A. Multiple sclerosis
  B. Diffuse cerebral sclerosis
  C. Acute disseminated encephalomyelitis
  D. Acute and subacute necrotizing hemorrhagic encephalitis
X. Metabolic diseases of the nervous system
  A. Inherited
  B. Nutritional
  C. Acquired
XI. Degenerative diseases of the nervous system
  A. Huntington's chorea
  B. Parkinson's disease
  C. Friedreich's ataxia
  D. Amyotrophic lateral sclerosis
  E. Progressive spinal muscular atrophy
  F. Charcot-Marie-Tooth disease
  G. Dystonia musculorum deformans (torsion spasm)

REFERENCES

1. Adams CBT, Logue V: Studies in cervical spondylotic myelopathy. II. The movement and contour of the spine in relation to the neural complications of cervical spondylosis, *Brain* 94:569, 1971.
2. Adams RD, Victor M: *Principles of neurology*, ed 3, New York, 1985, McGraw-Hill.
3. Alker G: Neuroradiology of cervical spondylotic myelopathy, *Spine* 13:850, 1988.
4. Arnold JG Jr: The clinical manifestations of spondylochondrosis (spondylosis) of the cervical spine, *Ann Surg* 141:872, 1955.
5. Aronson N: The management of soft cervical disc protrusions using the Smith-Robinson approach, *Clin Neurosurg* 20:253, 1973.
6. Aronson N, Filtzer D, Bagan M: Anterior cervical fusion by the Smith-Robinson approach, *J Neurosurg* 29:397, 1968.
7. Bailey R, Badgley C: Stabilization of the cervical spine by anterior fusion, *J Bone Joint Surg* 42A:565, 1960.
8. Bailey R et al: *The cervical spine*, Philadelphia, 1983, JB Lippincott.
9. Benini A: Clinical features of cervical root compression C5-C8 and their variations, *Neuro-Orthopedics* 4:74, 1987.
10. Blennow G: Anterior spinal artery syndrome, *Pediatr Neurosci* 13:32, 1987.
11. Bogduk N et al: The innervation of the cervical intervertebral discs, *Spine* 13:2, 1988.
12. Bohlman HH: Cervical spondylosis with moderate to severe myelopathy: a report of seventeen cases treated by Robinson anterior cervical discectomy and fusion, *Spine* 2:151, 1977.
13. Bohlman H, Emery S: The pathophysiology of cervical spondylosis and myelopathy, *Spine* 13:843, 1988.
14. Bohlman H, Goodfellow D: The treatment of cervical disc disease with Robinson anterior cervical discectomy and fusion: a review of 103 consecutive cases with long-term follow-up. Paper presented at the annual meeting of the Cervical Spine Research Society, New York, Dec 1982.
15. Bollati A et al: Microsurgical anterior cervical disk removal without interbody fusion, *Surg Neurol* 19:329, 1983.
16. Bora F, Osterman A: Compression neuropathy, *Clin Orthop* 163:23, 1982.
17. Brain WR, Knight GC, Bull JWD: Discussion on rupture of the intervertebral disc in the cervical region, *Proc R Soc Med* 41:509, 1948.
18. Brain WR, Northfield DW, Wilkinson M: The neurologic manifestations of cervical spondylosis, *Brain* 75:187, 1952.
19. Brieg A: *Biomechanics of the central nervous system*, Stockholm, 1960, Almquist & Wiksel.
20. Brieg A: *Adverse tension in the central nervous system*, New York, 1978, John Wiley & Sons.
21. Brown C: Compressive, invasive referred pain to the shoulder, *Clin Orthop* 173:55, 1983.
22. Burrows HR: The sagittal diameter of the spinal canal in cervical spondylosis, *Clin Radiol* 14:77, 1963.
23. Campbell AMG, Phillips DG: Cervical disc lesions with neurological disorder, *Br Med J* 47:481, 1960.
24. Clark CR: Cervical spondylotic myelopathy: history and physical findings, *Spine* 13:847, 1980.
25. Clarke E, Robinson PK: Cervical myelopathy: a complication of cervical spondylosis, *Brain* 79:483, 1956.
26. Cloward RB: Treatment of ruptured intervertebral discs: observations on their formation and treatment, *Am J Surg* 84:151, 1952.
27. Cloward R: The anterior approach for removal of ruptured cervical disks, *J Neurol* 15:602, 1958.
28. Cloward RB: Cervical discography: a contribution to the etiology and mechanism of neck, shoulder, and arm pain, *Ann Surg* 150:1052, 1959.
29. Cloward RB: Cervical discography, *Acta Radiol* 1:675, 1963.
30. Cloward RB: Lesion of the intervertebral discs and their treatment by interbody fusion methods, *Clin Orthop* 27:51, 1963.
31. Connolly E, Seymour R, Adams J: Clinical evaluation of anterior fusion for degenerative cervical disc disease, *J Neurosurg* 23:431, 1965.
32. Crandall PH, Batzdorf U: Cervical spondylotic myelopathy, *J Neurosurg* 25:57, 1966.
33. Cusick JF: *The cervical spine*, Philadelphia, 1989, JB Lippincott.
34. Czervionke LF, Daniels DL: Imaging in neuroradiology. II. Cervical spine anatomy and pathologic processes: applications of new MR imaging techniques, *Radiol Clin North Am* 26:921, 1957.
35. Dale WA, Lewis MR: Management of thoracic outlet syndrome, *Ann Surg* 181:575, 1975.
36. Davidson R, Dunn E, Metzmaker J: The shoulder abduction test in the diagnosis of radicular pain in cervical extradural compressive monoradiculopathesis, *Spine* 6:441, 1981.
37. DePalma AF, Rothman RH: *The intervertebral disc*, Philadelphia, 1970, WB Saunders.
38. DePalma A et al: Anterior interbody fusion for severe cervical disc degeneration, *Surg Gynecol Obstet* 134:755, 1972.
39. DiChiro G et al: Tumors and arteriovenous malformations of the spinal cord: assessment using MR, *Radiology* 156:689, 1985.
40. DiChiro G, Schellinger D: Computed tomography of spinal cord after lumbar intrathecal introduction of metrizamide (computer-assisted myelography), *Radiology* 120:101, 1976.
41. Dillin L, Hoaglund FT, Scheck M: Brachial neuritis, *J Bone Joint Surg* 67A:878, 1985.
42. Dillin W et al: Cervical radiculopathy: a review, *Spine* 11:988, 1986.
43. Dohn D: Anterior interbody fusion for treatment of cervical-disk conditions, *JAMA* 197:175, 1966.
44. Dommisse GF: *The arteries and veins of the lumbar spinal cord from birth*, Edinburgh, UK, 1975, Churchill-Livingstone.
45. Dunsker S: Anterior cervical discectomy with and without fusion, *Clin Neurosurg* 24:516, 1977.
46. Dyck P et al: *Peripheral neuropathy*, vols 1 and 2, Philadelphia, 1984, WB Saunders.
47. Ebara S et al: Myelopathy hand characterized by muscle wasting, *Spine* 13:785, 1988.
48. Edwards WC, LaRocca H: The developmental segmental sagittal

diameter of the cervical spinal canal in patients with cervical spondylosis, *Spine* 8:20, 1983.

49. Edwards W, LaRocca H: The developmental segmental sagittal diameter in combined cervical and lumbar spondylosis, *Spine* 10:42, 1985.

50. Elias F: Roentgen findings in the asymptomatic cervical spine, *NY State J Med* 58:3300, 1958.

51. Epstein J, Carras R, Lavine LS: The importance of removing osteophytes as part of the surgical treatment of myeloradiculopathy in cervical spondylosis, *J Neurosurg* 30:219, 1969.

52. Epstein JA et al: Cervical myelopathy caused by developmental stenosis of the spinal canal, *J Neurosurg* 51:362, 1979.

53. Fager C: Management of cervical disc lesions and spondylosis by posterior approaches, *Clin Neurol* 24:48, 1977.

54. Fager C: Posterior surgical tactics for the neurological syndromes of cervical disc and spondylotic lesions, *Clin Neurol* 25:218, 1978.

55. Ferguson RJL, Caplan LR: Cervical spondylotic myelopathy, *Neurol Clin* 3:373, 1985.

56. Foo D, Rossier A: Anterior spinal artery syndrome and its natural history, *Paraplegia* 21:1, 1983.

57. Foo D, Rossier A, Cochran T: Complete sensory and motor recovery from anterior spinal artery syndrome after sprain of the cervical spine, *Eur Neurol* 23:119, 1984.

58. Fox AJ, Vinuela F, Debrun G. Computed myelography with metrizamide, *AJNR* 2:79, 1983.

59. Freidenberg ZB, Miller WT: Degenerative disc disease of the cervical spine: a comparative study of asymptomatic and symptomatic patients, *J Bone Joint Surg* 45A:1171, 1963.

60. Glassenberg M: The thoracic outlet syndrome: an assessment of 20 cases with regards to new clinical and electromyographic findings, *Angiology* 32:180, 1981.

61. Glover J et al: Evoked responses in the diagnosis of thoracic outlet syndrome, *Surgery* 89:87, 1981.

62. Good D, Couch J, Wacaser L: "Numb, clumsy hands" and high cervical spondylosis, *Surg Neurol* 22:285, 1984.

63. Gooding MR, Wilson CB, Hoff JT: Experimental cervical myelopathy: effects of ischemia and compression of the canine cervical spinal cord, *J Neurosurg* 43:9, 1975.

64. Gore D, Sepic S: Anterior cervical fusion for degenerated or protruded discs, *Spine* 9:667, 1984.

65. Gore DR et al: Roentgenographic findings of the cervical spine in asymptomatic people, *Spine* 11:521, 1986.

66. Gorter K: Influence of laminectomy on the course of cervical myelopathy, *Acta Neurochir* 33:265, 1976.

67. Grieve GP: Neck traction, *Physiotherapy* 68:260, 1982.

68. Haft H, Shenkin H: Surgical end results of cervical ridge and disk problems, *JAMA* 186:312, 1963.

69. Hankinson H, Wilson C: Use of the operating microscope in anterior cervical discectomy without fusion, *J Neurosurg* 43:452, 1975.

70. Hassler O: Blood supply to human spinal cord: a microangiographic study, *Arch Neurol* 15:302, 1966.

71. Hayashi H et al: Etiologic factors of myelopathy: a radiographic evaluation of the aging changes in the cervical spine, *Clin Orthop* 214:200, 1987.

72. Henderson C, Hennessy R: Posterolateral foraminotomy as an exclusive operative technique for cervical radiculopathy: a review of 846 consecutively operated cases, *Neurosurgery* 13:504, 1983.

73. Herkowitz HN: A comparison of anterior cervical fusion, cervical laminectomy, and cervical laminoplasty for the surgical management of multiple level spondylotic radiculopathy, *Spine* 13:774, 1988.

74. Hirsch C: Cervical disk rupture: diagnosis and therapy, *Acta Orthop Scand* 30:172, 1960.

75. Hirsch C et al: Cervical-disc resection, *J Bone Joint Surg* 46A:1811, 1964.

76. Hoff J et al: The role of ischemia in the pathogenesis of cervical spondylotic myelopathy, *Spine* 2:100, 1977.

77. Holt EP: Fallacy of cervical discography, *JAMA* 188:799, 1964.

78. Holt EP: Further reflections on cervical discography, *JAMA* 231:613, 1975.

79. Hoppenfeld S: *Orthopedic neurology* Philadelphia, 1977, JB Lippincott.

80. Hukuda S et al: Operations for cervical spondylotic myelopathy, *J Bone Joint Surg* 67B:609, 1985.

81. Hult L: The Munkfors investigation, *Acta Orthop Scand Suppl* 16:1, 1959.

82. Hyman RA et al: 0.6 T MR imaging of the cervical spine: multislice and multiecho techniques, *AJNR* 6:229, 1985.

83. Jette DU, Fulkel JE, Trombley C: Effect of intermittent, supine cervical traction on the myoelectric activity of the upper trapezius muscle in subjects with neck pain, *Phys Ther* 65:1173, 1985.

84. Kambin P: Anterior cervical fusion using vertical self-locking T-graft, *Clin Orthop* 153:132, 1980.

85. Kaplan L, Kennedy F: The effect of head posture on the manometrics of cerebrospinal fluid in cervical lesions: a new diagnostic test, *Brain* 73:337, 1950.

86. Kellgren JH: Deep pain sensibility, *Lancet* 1:943, 1949.

87. Kelsey J et al: An epidemiological study of acute prolapsed cervical intervertebral disc, *J Bone Joint Surg* 66A:907, 1984.

88. Kimura J: *Electrodiagnosis in diseases of nerve and muscle: principles and practice* Philadelphia, 1983, FA Davis.

89. Kirschner P, Simon M: Radioisotopic evaluation of skeletal disease, *J Bone Joint Surg* 63A:4, 673, 1981.

90. Klafta LA: The diagnostic inaccuracy of the pain response in cervical discography, *Cleve Clin Q* 36:35, 1969.

91. Kofoed H: Thoracic outlet syndrome, *Clin Orthop* 156:145, 1981.

92. LaMasters DL et al: Multiplanar metrizamide enhanced CT imaging of the foramen magnum, *AJNR* 3:485, 1982.

93. Laoire S, Thomas D: Spinal cord compression due to prolapse of cervical intervertebral disc: treatment of 26 cases by discectomy without interbody bone graft, *J Neurosurg* 59:847, 1983.

94. Lees F, Turner J: Natural history and prognosis of cervical spondylosis, *Br Med J* 2:1607, 1963.

95. Lestini WF, Wiesel SW: The pathogenesis of cervical spondylosis, *Clin Orthop* 239, 69, 1989.

96. Lindgren E: The importance of the sagittal diameter of the spinal cord in the cervical region, *Nevenartz* 10:240, 1937.

97. Livingston M: Spinal manipulation causing injury, *Clin Orthop* 81:82, 1971.

98. Longstein J: *Post-laminectomy kyphosis spinal deformities and neurologic dysfunction,* New York, 1978, Raven Press.

99. Lunsford L et al: Anterior surgery for cervical disc disease, *J Neurosurg* 53:1, 1980.

100. Magee KR, DeJong RN: Paralytic brachial neuritis: discussion of clinical features with review of 23 cases, *JAMA* 174:1258, 1960.

101. Martins A: Anterior cervical discectomy with and without interbody bone graft, *J Neurosurg* 44:290, 1976.

102. Masaryk TJ et al: Cervical myelopathy: a comparison of magnetic resonance and myelography, *J Comput Assist Tomogr* 10:184, 1986.

103. Massacre C, Bard M, Tristant H: Cervical discography: speculation on technique and indications from our own experience, *J Radiol* 55:395, 1974.

104. Mayfield F: Cervical spondylosis: a comparison of the anterior and posterior approaches, *Clin Neurosurg* 13:181, 1965.

105. McAfee PC et al: Comparison of nuclear magnetic resonance imaging and computed tomography in the diagnosis of upper cervical spinal cord compression, *Spine* 11:295, 1986.

106. McNab I: *The cervical spine* Philadelphia, 1989, JB Lippincott.

107. Meyer RR: Cervical discography: a help or hindrance in evaluating neck, shoulder, arm pain, *AJR* 90:1208, 1963.

108. Murone I: The importance of the sagittal diameters of the cervical spinal canal in relation to spondylosis and myelopathy, *J Bone Joint Surgery* 56B:30, 1974.

109. Murphey F, Simmons J, Brunson B: Surgical treatment of laterally ruptured cervical disc, *J Neurosurg* 38:679, 1973.

110. Murphy M, Gado M: Anterior cervical discectomy without interbody bone graft, *J Neurosurg* 37:71, 1972.
111. Nichols HM: Anatomic structures of the thoracic outlet, *Clin Orthop* 207:13, 1986.
112. Nugent GR: Clinico-pathologic correlations in cervical spondylosis, *Neurology* 9:273, 1959.
113. Nurick S: The natural history and results of surgical treatment of the spinal disorder associated with cervical spondylosis, *Brain* 95:101, 1972.
114. Nurick S: The pathogenesis of the spinal cord disorder associated with cervical spondylosis, *Brain* 95:87, 1972.
115. O'Connell JEA: Discussion on cervical spondylosis, *Proc R Soc Med,* 49:202, 1956.
116. Odom G, Finney W, Woodhall B: Cervical disk lesions, *JAMA* 166:23, 1957.
117. Ogino H et al: Canal diameter: anteroposterior compression ratio, and spondylotic myelopathy of the cervical spine, *Spine* 8:1, 1983.
118. O'Laoire S, Thomas D: Spinal cord compression due to prolapse of cervical intervertebral disc, *J Neurosurg* 59:847, 1983.
119. Omer G, Spinner M: *Management of peripheral nerve problems,* Philadelphia, 1980, WB Saunders.
120. Ono K et al: Cervical myelopathy secondary to multiple spondylotic protrusions: a clinicopathologic study, *Spine* 2:109, 1977.
121. Ono K et al: Myelopathy hand, *J Bone Joint Surg* 69B:215, 1987.
122. Pallis C, Jones AM, Spillane JD: Cervical spondylosis, incidence and implications, *Brain* 77:274, 1954.
123. Pang D, Wessel HB: Thoracic outlet syndrome, *Neurosurgery* 22:105, 1988 (review article).
124. Parke W: Correlative anatomy of cervical spondylotic myelopathy, *Spine* 13:831, 1988.
125. Parsonage MJ, Turner JWA: Neuralgic amyotrophy: shoulder girdle syndrome, *Lancet* 254:973, 1948.
126. Pavlov H et al: Cervical spinal stenosis: determination with vertebral body ratio method, *Radiology* 164:771, 1987.
127. Penning L: *Functional pathology of the cervical spine* Baltimore, 1968, Williams & Wilkins.
128. Penning L, Van der Fwagg P: Biomechanical aspects of spondylotic myelopathy, *Acta Radiol* 5:1090, 1966.
129. Phillips D: Upper limb involvement in cervical spondylosis, *J Neurol Neurosurg Psychiatry* 38:386, 1975.
130. Phillips D: The shoulder girdle disc, *J Neurol Neurosurg Psychiatry* 39:817, 1976.
131. Phillips J: The importance of examination of the spine in the presence of intrathoracic or abdominal pain, *Proc Interest Postgrad MA North Am* 3:70, 1927.
132. Pollok E: Surgical anatomy of the thoracic outlet syndrome, *Surg Gynecol Obstet* 150:97, 1980.
133. Raaf J: Surgical treatment of patients with cervical disk lesions, *J Trauma* 9:327, 1969.
134. Raynor R: Cervical cord compression secondary to acute disc protrusion in trauma, *Spine* 2:39, 1977.
135. Raynor R, Pugh J, Shapiro I: Cervical facetectomy and its effect on spine strength, *J Neurosurg* 63:278, 1985.
136. Rhoton A, Henderson E: Cervical disk disease with neural compression, *Minn Med* 998, 1972.
137. Riddell DH, Smith BM: Thoracic and vascular aspects of thoracic outlet syndrome—1986 update, *Clin Orthop* 207:31, 1986.
138. Riley L: Anterior cervical spine surgery. In *AAOS Instructional Course Lectures* vol 27, St Louis, 1978, Mosby.
139. Riley L, Robinson R, Johnson K: The results of anterior interbody fusion of the cervical spine, *J Neurosurg* 30:126, 1969.
140. Robertson JT: Anterior removal of cervical disc without fusion, *Clin Neurosurg* 20:259, 1973.
141. Robertson JT: Anterior cervical discectomy without fusion: long-term results, *Clin Neurosurg* 27:440, 1980.
142. Robertson JT: Anterior operations for herniated cervical disc and for myelopathy, *Clin Neurosurg* 25:245, 1978.
143. Robinson RA, Smith GW: Anterolateral cervical disc removal and interbody fusion for cervical disc syndrome, *Bull Johns Hopkins Hosp* 96:223, 1955.
144. Robinson RA, Smith GW: The treatment of certain cervical spine disorders by anterior removal of the intervertebral disc and interbody fusion, *J Bone Joint Surg* 40A:607, 1958.
145. Robinson R et al: The results of anterior interbody fusion of the cervical spine, *J Bone Joint Surg* 44A:1569, 1962.
146. Robinson RA et al: Cervical spondylotic myelopathy: etiology and treatment concepts, *Spine* 2:89, 1977.
147. Roos D: The place for scalenectomy and first-rib resection in thoracic outlet syndrome, *Surgery* 92:1077, 1982.
148. Rosen RNJ, Hansen E, Rosenhorn M: Anterior cervical discectomy with and without fusion, *J Neurosurg* 59:252, 1983.
149. Rosenorn J, Hansen E, Rosenorn M: Anterior cervical discectomy with and without fusion, *J Neurosurg* 59:252, 1983.
150. Rosonoff H, Rossman F: Treatment of cervical spondylosis by anterior cervical discectomy and fusion, *Arch Neurol* 14:392, 1966.
151. Roth DA: Cervical analgesic discography: a new test for the definitive diagnosis of the painful disc syndrome, *JAMA* 235:1713, 1976.
152. Rothman RH, Marvel JP: The acute cervical disk, *Clin Orthop* 109:59, 1975.
153. Rothman RH, Simeone S: *The spine,* Philadelphia, 1982, WB Saunders.
154. Rovira M, Torrant O, Ruscalleda J: Some aspects of the spinal cord circulation in cervical myelopathy, *Neurology* 9:209, 1975.
155. Saunders R, Wilson D: The surgery of cervical disk disease: new perspectives, *Clin Orthop* 146:119, 1980.
156. Schmidelz HH: Cervical spondylosis, *AFT* 33:89, 1986.
157. Schneider RC: The syndrome of acute anterior spinal cord injury, *J Neurosurg* 12:95, 1955.
158. Scoville WB, Dohrmann GJ, Corkill G: Late results of cervical disc surgery, *J Neurosurg* 45:203, 1976.
159. Scoville WB, Whitcomb B: Lateral rupture of cervical intervertebral disks, *Postgrad Med* 39:174, 1966.
160. Sim FH et al: Swan neck deformity following extensive cervical laminectomy, *J Bone Joint Surg* 56A:564, 1974.
161. Simeone F, Dillin W: Treatment of cervical disc disease: selection of operative approach, *Contemp Neurosurg* 8 (14):1, 1986.
162. Simeone FA, Rothman RH: Cervical disc disease. In Rothman RH, Simeone FA: *The spine,* Philadelphia, 1982, WB Saunders.
163. Simmons EH: An evaluation of discography in the localization of symptomatic levels in discogenic diseases of the spine, *Clin Orthop* 108:57, 1975.
164. Simmons EH, Abhalla S: Anterior cervical discectomy and fusion, *J Bone Joint Surg* 51B:225, 1969.
165. Sloop PR et al: Manipulation for chronic neck pain: a double-blind controlled study, *Spine* 7:532, 1982.
166. Smith GW, Nichols P Jr: The technique of cervical disgography, *Radiology* 68:718, 1957.
167. Spurling RG, Scoville WB: Lateral rupture of the cervical intervertebral discs, *Surg Gynecol Obstet* 78:350, 1944.
168. Spetzler R, Roski R, Selman W: The microscope in anterior cervical surgery, *Clin Orthop* 168:17, 1982.
169. Stookey B: Compression of spinal cord and nerve roots by herniation of nucleus pulposus in cervical region, *Arch Surg* 40:417, 1940.
170. Stuck R: Anterior cervical disc excision and fusion, *Rocky Mt Med J* 60:25, 1963.
171. Swash M: Diagnosis of brachial root and plexus lesions, *J Neurol* 233:131, 1986.
172. Sylven B: On the biology of nucleus pulposis, *Acta Orthop Scand* 20:275, 1951.
173. Taveras J: Is discography a useful diagnostic procedure? *J Can Assoc Radiol* 18:294, 1967.
174. Taylor AR: The mechanism of injury to the spinal cord in the

neck without damage to the vertebral column, *J Bone Joint Surg* 33B:543, 1951.

175. Tilney NL, Griffins HJG, Edwards EA: Natural history of major venous thrombosis of the upper extremity, *Arch Surg* 101:792, 1970.

176. Torg J, Pavlov H, Genuario S: Neuropraxia of the cervical spinal cord with transient quadriplegia, *J Bone Joint Surg* 68A:1354, 1986.

177. Tsairis P, Dych PJ, Mulder DW: Natural history of brachial plexus neuropathy: report of 99 patients, *Arch Neurol* 27:109, 1972.

178. Veidlinger OF et al: Cervical myelopathy and its relationship to cervical stenosis, *Spine* 6:550, 1981.

179. Verbiest H, Paz Y, Geuse H: Anterolateral surgery for cervical spondylosis in cases of myelopathy or nerve-root compression, *J Neurosurg* 25:601, 1966.

180. Viikari-Juntura E: Interexaminer reliability of observations in physical examinations of the neck, *Phys Ther* 67:1526, 1987.

181. Viikari-Juntura E, Porras M, Laasonen EM: Validity of clinical tests in the diagnosis of root compression in cervical disk disease, *Spine* 14:253, 1989.

182. White AA: Symposium on cervical spondylotic myelopathy, *Spine* 13:829, 1988.

183. White A, Hirsch C: An experimental study of the immediate load capacity of some commonly used iliac bone grafts, *Acta Orthop Scand* 42:482, 1971.

184. White A, Southwick W, Deponte RJ: Relief of pain by anterior cervical spine fusion for spondylosis, *J Bone Joint Surg* 55A:525, 1973.

185. Whitecloud TS: Complications of anterior cervical fusion. In *AAOS Instructional Course Lectures,* vol 27, St Louis, 1978, Mosby.

186. Whitecloud TS, Seago RA: Cervical discogenic syndrome: results of operative intervention in patients with positive discography, *Spine* 12:313, 1987.

187. Williams J, Allen M, Harkess J: Late results of cervical discectomy and interbody fusions: some factors influencing the results, *J Bone Joint Surg* 50A:227, 1968.

188. Williams R: Microcervical foraminotomy, *Spine* 8:711, 1983.

189. Wilson D, Campbell D: Anterior cervical discectomy without bone graft, *J Neurosurg* 47:551, 1977.

190. Wolf BS, Khilnani M, Malis L: The sagittal diameter of the bony cervical spinal cord and its significance in cervical spondylosis, *J Mt Sinai Hosp* 23:283, 1956.

191. Yu YL et al: Computer-assisted myelography in cervical spondylotic myelopathy and radiculopathy, *Brain* 109:259, 1986.

Chapter Fourteen

◆

Thoracic Pain Syndromes

Robert G. Watkins

Thoracic pain can be a perplexing and difficult area in terms of both diagnosis and treatment. Thoracic pain is commonly seen in athletes whose throwing actions cause excessive torsional stress. The most commonly involved area is the thoracolumbar junction. Interscapular pain and high thoracic pain of the T1 to T7 area usually are more typically associated with upper extremity function, whereas thoracolumbar junction problems are more commonly associated with lower extremity function and torsional activities. There are more radiologic abnormalities in the thoracolumbar spine of athletes than in the thoracolumbar spine of nonathletes and more back pain than other injuries in athletes. Localized tenderness and pain of the T4 spinous process is a common clinical syndrome, and is referred to as the T4 syndrome. It results from chronic postural strain of both shoulder elevators and oppressors, their combined muscle function producing a significant tendinous strain and localized inflammation over the proximal T4 spinous process. Treatment of the T4 syndrome involves trunk stabilization, upper body–strengthening exercise, and local therapy in that area, as well as techniques to take strain off the shoulders and elbows (such as adding arms to the working chair and to the seat in the car), and other methods to take the chronic pull and strain off this interscapular area.

The thoracolumbar spine is a transitional zone between the coronally oriented facets of the thoracic spine and the more sagittally oriented facets of the upper lumbar spine. The rib cage produces a stabilizing effect on the thoracic spine. Twisting motion occurs in the lower lumbar spine, and the transitional zone between this very mobile lower lumbar segment and the rigidly fixed thoracic segment is the thoracolumbar junction. Flexion/rotation fracture dislocations that occur in the thoracolumbar junction area are less commonly seen in other parts of the thoracic spine. Therefore this area receives a certain degree of torsional stress and strain, especially in certain sports. At the Kerlan-Jobe Orthopaedic Clinic we also see, at times, a compressive load applied disproportionately at the thoracolumbar junction. Problems of disc degeneration and other discogenic changes in the thoracolumbar junction occur more frequently in certain elite athletes, such as gymnasts, than in the average population.[16]

Pain in the interscapular area is commonly associated with fatigue problems in the upper extremity and with postural abnormalities of the cervical spine and upper thoracic lumbar spine. There may be tenderness on the spinous process. There is very little radiation to the pain, which is paraspinous and is also located at the medial scapular border and tips of the spinous processes. A typical work-up includes any test used for mechanical or nonmechanical axial pain. A bone scan and/or magnetic resonance imaging (MRI) scan are obtained when indicated. Constant pain, unrelenting in nature, is more likely to require MRI and a bone scan than a clearly fatigue-related postural pain.

Treatment for muscle strains in this area typically consists of therapy for cervical strains: trunk stabilization, joint mobilization, chest-out posturing exercises, local modalities, and shoulder-strengthening exercises. Posture correction is the key to curing interscapular pain, whether it is of a referred cervical or a thoracic muscle insertion origin. Operations for resection of the costovertebral joint and costotransverse joint have been performed with success by certain surgeons, but it is highly unusual to use this surgery for a high-performance athlete.

NONOPERATIVE CARE

Midthoracic or thoracolumbar junction problems in the torsionally stressed athlete typically occur unilaterally—on the opposite side from the throwing arm—and definitely are related to rotation in the lower thoracic area. Because of the necessary pull of the lateral oblique musculature on the opposite side from the throwing arm, costocartilage and rib injuries in this area are common.[17] This area undergoes severe stress; thus injuries to the opposite side of the chest wall in throwing athletes can produce a major disability. Another common differential diagnosis of thoracic and thoracolumbar junction problems is injury to the ribs, soft tissue, and cartilage of the rib cage. Although selective blocks of these specific structures can be of some benefit, they do not necessarily exclude thoracic radicular pain as a causative factor. Bone scans can reveal rib injuries. Costocartilage crepitus and relief through local injection can better demonstrate costocartilage injury such as at the tip of the eleventh and twelfth ribs.

Stress fractures of the ribs, very typically on the opposite side of the throwing arm, are not uncommon in throwing athletes and can be diagnosed with a bone scan. Also, spondylitic defects, especially in the immature athlete, can occur in the thoracic spine and produce radiating intercostal pain. Again, the bone scan is the key to the diagnosis of stress fractures in this area.

Probably the most important diagnosis to make in thoracic and thoracic-radiating pain is that of a thoracic disc herniation. The incidence of thoracic disc herniation is one in a million.[6] Surgery on the thoracic disc is employed in 0.15% to 0.80% of all disc herniations, and thoracic disc herniations can involve the spinal cord or the thoracic nerve. Pressure on the exiting thoracic nerve at that level produces pain in the chest and back. Pressure on or damage to the spinal cord carries the grave risk of permanent cord injury.[7] A thoracic disc herniation can result in paraplegia, with weakness and numbness in the legs and complete loss of bowel, bladder, sexual, and leg function. At some centers up to 50% of patients with thoracic disc herniation have significant spinal cord injury.[3,7]

It is important to realize that thoracic disc herniations can and do occur. There is a risk of neurologic injury in this area, but a complete history and physical examination according to the guidelines noted elsewhere in this text will usually reveal whether radicular pain exists. Radicular pain in the thoracic area follows a basic dermatomal pattern that extends laterally and anteriorly on the chest or abdominal wall. Each patient whose thoracic spine is evaluated must undergo examination for myelopathy. Often, subtle findings and changes in myelopathy are not obvious to the patient. If myelopathy is present, then a myelogram and contrast computed tomography (CT) scan should be done. If no myelopathy is present and the patient has radiating thoracic pain in a dermatomal pattern, MRI or a myelogram and contrast CT scan still constitute the preferred test. Although MRI may demonstrate a thoracic disc herniation, the intervertebral foramina of the thoracic spine probably are best evaluated by a contrast CT scan. A foraminal spur that produces radicular symptoms in a throwing athlete is not uncommon. Nonradicular pain of the thoracic spine can come from the same sources as in the lumbar spine—intervertebral disc and facet joints. The additional structures in the thoracic spine involve the costotransverse and costovertebral joints. Costovertebral joint pain is an enigma. Certainly, these joints can be blocked with provocative selective blocks. Because of cross-innervation of different levels, it still is very difficult to localize the specific level of the problem when the symptoms involve axial pain only.

Thoracic disc herniations may present with a great variety of symptoms. In the lower thoracic spine a flaccid neurologic loss may occur rather than the spastic presentation of an upper thoracic disc herniation, and often it mimics lumbar spine disease.[2,9] Lower herniated thoracic discs may present with the signs and symptoms of neurogenic claudication or sciatica.[11] High thoracic disc herniations at T1-2 or T2-3 may present as a cervical spine problem, with pain radiating to the medial aspect

of the arm, hand, and shoulder, with possible intrinsic hand weakness and/or Horner's syndrome.[1] The nonoperative treatment of radicular pain is similar to that for lumbar pain and starts with a proper trunk stabilization program.

The indications for surgery in thoracic disc herniation are significant progressive myelopathy and unrelenting radiculopathy. Intermittent thoracic radiculopathy is a relative indication for surgery and depends on the degree of morbidity. A large asymptomatic thoracic disc herniation can be a relative indication for surgery; if it expands, it could produce myelopathy under heavy loading situations, which certainly can be anticipated in an athlete. There is still significant room and indication for proper nonoperative care in thoracic disc herniations with minimal or absent symptoms. The presence of the herniation alone does not necessitate surgery. In the review article by Brown et al.,[4] the cases of 55 patients with 72 thoracic disc herniations were reviewed to determine the natural history of the disease. Although 27% of these patients eventually required surgery, most did not and continued to perform activities of everyday living, even participating in sports activities such as skiing, without any paraneurologic deficit. Herniated thoracic discs do not always lead to major neurologic compromise, and appropriate rehabilitation and careful observation certainly are possible.

Athletes may experience a much higher incidence of thoracic disc herniations than one would think, and many of the rib injuries and radicular chest pain injuries that are seen intermittently in athletes may be due to thoracic disc herniation that heals quite well nonoperatively. Certainly, any return to function without surgery should come only after a detailed, comprehensive, and intense nonoperative rehabilitation program, with a slow return to the sport, that would place significant strain on

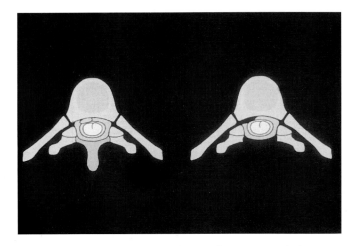

Fig. 14-1. The standard posterior laminectomy technique requires manipulation of the cord to get to an extruded lumbar calcified or soft disc fragment.

the area to verify whether the person has a chronically asymptomatic lesion.

SURGICAL CARE

Of the surgical approaches available for excision of a thoracic disc herniation, one is a standard thoracic laminectomy through a posterior approach (Fig. 14-1). However, standard posterior thoracic laminectomy has been shown to result in a high incidence of neurologic deficit.[10] A posterior approach requires at least some degree of spinal cord manipulation. In one study[12] thoracic disc herniation through the posterior approach demonstrated some element of neurologic loss in all 23 patients.[12] Certainly laminectomy by the posterior approach has poorer results and a higher rate of neurologic complication.[3,8,15] In a review of posterior approaches by Perot and Monroe in 1969,[13] 40 of 91 patients were not improved and 16 were permanently paralyzed by the operation. Thus the posterior approach is considered unacceptable for the treatment of thoracic disc herniation because of complications and poor results.[15]

The preferred approaches involve posterior lateral foraminotomy with pedicle resection and anterior discectomy. Evolution of the posterolateral or lateral rachiotomy approach occurred in the treatment of tuberculosis.[5] An approach from the intervertebral foramina to the anterior half of the body may give access to the thoracic disc prolapse under scrutiny without retraction of the dura (Fig. 14-2). Different techniques for the costotransversectomy approach include use of the last section of the rib and the costovertebral articulation or resection of these structures plus the transverse process and portion of the pedicle (Fig. 14-3). Good results have been obtained with this lateral costotransversectomy approach (Figs. 14-4 and 14-5). Proper positioning of the patient on the table in a prone, oblique position to allow the lateral view is important. In addition, use of the microscope to better visualize structures has improved the technique for costotransversectomy by means of the posterolateral approach. The anterolateral transthoracic approach to the intervertebral disc described by Ransohoff et al.[14] has proved to be a safe, effective method of resecting thoracic disc herniation.

Although a posterolateral costotransversectomy approach can be effective, most spinal surgeons recommend a thoracotomy and an anterior disc excision, with

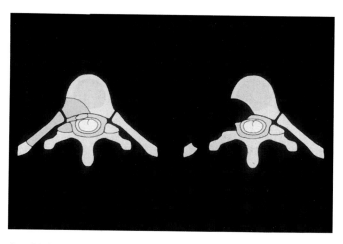

Fig. 14-3. The more expansive and more lateral rachiotomy approach involves resection of the costovertebral articulation and/or pedicle and exposure through the intervertebral foramen of the floor of the spinal canal.

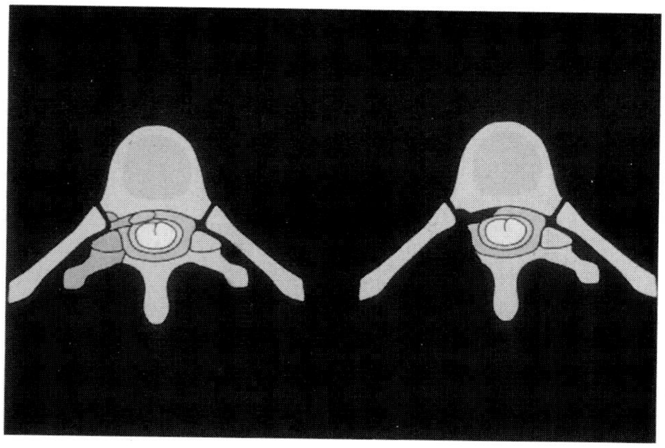

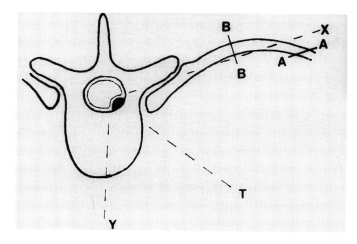

Fig. 14-2. The lateral rachiotomy approach may involve only resection of the pedicle. It may also include resection of the transverse process. Done through the microscope, this approach can produce excellent visualization of the floor of the spinal canal.

Fig. 14-4. Approach line of the lateral and anterior approaches: *Y* is midline; *X* is the posterolateral line; *T* is the approach for anterior thoracotomy; *B* is the osteotomy site for a proximal costotransverse joint resection; *A* is the osteotomy site for a more expansive posterolateral rhachotomy approach.

or without fusion[3] (Fig. 14-6). The anterior approach varies from surgeon to surgeon; it may be extrapleural[12] and sometimes involves an interbody fusion. The recommendation at our clinic is anterior thoracotomy with resection of the rib head of the involved rib (Figs. 14-7 and 14-8). For example, for T6-7 disc herniation, a transpleural approach is made by following the seventh rib and resecting its rib head to expose the T6-7 disc. Ribs articulate with the disc space above; therefore the seventh rib leads to the T6-7 disc space.

Our surgical treatment of herniated thoracic discs usually involves a transthoracic approach. We do not use the costotransversectomy approach or transpedicular approach except under the most unusual circumstances. The transthoracic approach follows the rib head to the disc involved; the key is to use the costovertebral articulation to find the disc and to resect a portion of the disc anterolaterally from the canal. We use the arthroscope or microscope to resect the disc herniation and fuse the disc (Figs. 14-9 to 14-11). The arthroscopic technique is becoming our standard operation. Isolated foraminal spurs that produce radicular pain can

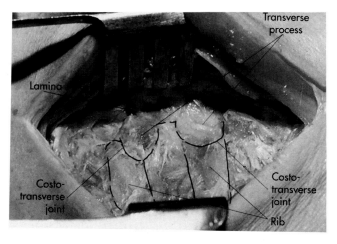

Fig. 14-5. Curvilinear paraspinous (posterolateral Kapner-type) approach with visualization of the rib and the costotransverse joint. (From Watkins RG: *Surgical approaches to the spine,* New York, 1983, Springer-Verlag.)

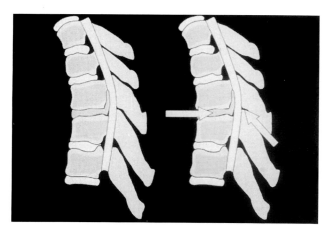

Fig. 14-6. Example of the differences between the anterior approach and the posterolateral approach. The anterolateral approach goes through the herniated portion of the disc, and the posterolateral approach invariably approaches the nerve and dural sac before approaching disc herniation.

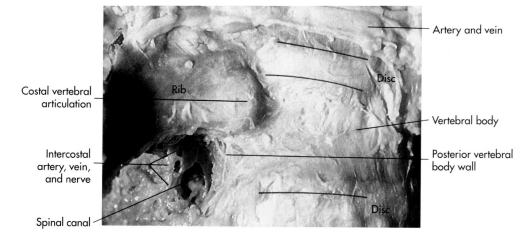

Fig. 14-7. The rib articulates with the cephalad half of its appropriately numbered vertebral body and with the disc space above. Therefore the 10th rib articulates at T9-10. Removal of the head of the rib and its articulation allows excellent exposure of the posterolateral aspect of the intervertebral disc. After removal of the rib head and disc, the intercostal nerve, dural sac, posterior vertebral body wall, and spinal canal are identified. (From Watkins RG: *Surgical approaches to the spine,* New York, 1983, Springer-Verlag.)

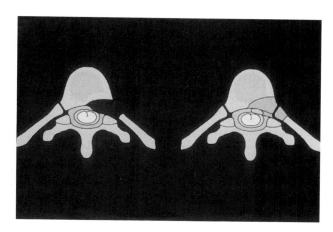

Fig. 14-8. Anterior resection of the costovertebral joint for entry into the disc space.

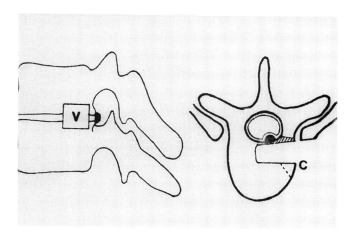

Fig. 14-9. Path of the anterior excision as it approaches under the extruded fragment of the disc, allowing easy manipulation of the fragment into the space available for the fragment.

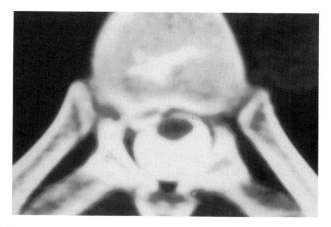

Fig. 14-10. Clinical example of a lateral disc fragment and the approach through the costovertebral articulation under the fragment; this is a very safe approach to the disc fragment.

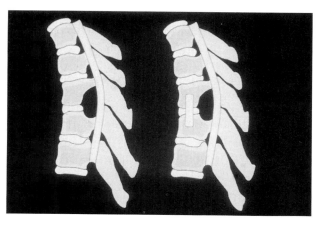

Fig. 14-11. Very large resection of a lesion in the spinal canal from the anterior approach and the resulting fusion when this large resection is necessary.

be resected through a posterolateral foraminal approach. The surgeon identifies the nerve, follows the nerve into the spine, and performs the foraminotomy using the microscope or arthroscope. Lateral disc herniations can be resected through a modified costotransversectomy approach. With this approach a transverse incision is made along the rib, the transverse process is resected, approximately 4 to 5 inches of rib is resected, the rib head is followed again to the disc space, the rib head is resected, and the disc space is exposed. This approach is easier with soft tissue fragments than with calcified fragments. We use the microscopic wound retractors and the microscope for the procedure.

Pain in the thoracic spine is relatively common, and the initial work-up is much like that for the cervical spine. The examiner must determine whether the condition is a radiculopathy, a myelopathy, or a musculoskeletal joint complaint and whether the problem is cervical pain, a posterior penetrating duodenal ulcer, renal colic, or some other internal medicine problem. The key is to use a standardized history and physical form that provides enough detail for an adequate review of systems, as well as an extensive neurologic examination. The examiner must be alert to signs and symptoms of neurologic dysfunction, particularly because thoracic disc herniations can cause permanent paraplegia. Every effort must be directed toward making this diagnosis when symptoms suggest such a pathologic condition. The use of diagnostic tests depends on the results of the history and physical examination. If there is a suggestion of a neurologic dysfunction, MRI of the thoracic spine can provide sufficient detail and quality to diagnose a thoracic disc herniation. If there are questions, then a thoracic myelogram and contrast CT scan may add additional information. Thoracic radiculopathy, radiating pain, or intercostal pain, with or without associated sensory loss, can be diagnosed with MRI, but for the greatest detail of the thoracic intervertebral foramina, a thoracic contrast CT scan may be necessary. For musculoskeletal joint problems of the thoracic spine, a bone scan can be helpful if it reveals sufficient detail to identify a stress fracture, an inflamed arthritic joint, or even a bone tumor of the thoracic spine.

In summary, the key to the treatment of thoracic area pain is as follows:

1. Identify postural strain syndromes and use posture-correcting techniques.
2. Identify radicular syndromes or the appropriate diagnostic tests, and institute as aggressive a therapeutic technique as possible to prevent potential cord or nerve injury to the patient.
3. Always check for myelopathy.
4. Initiate a prompt diagnostic and therapeutic plan when thoracic myelopathy is suspected or diagnosed.

CASE ILLUSTRATIONS

Figs. 14-12 to 14-16 illustrate cases of thoracic pain syndrome encountered in athletes.

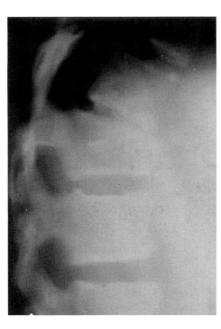

Fig. 14-12. This 14-year-old athlete was involved in a motorcycle accident and sustained a compression fracture of T12. He was neurologically intact. He underwent open reduction and internal fixation for stability and fusion.

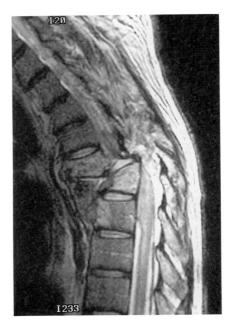

Fig. 14-13. Original MRI scan of a thoracolumbar fracture dislocation in a 32-year-old professional motorcycle racer. The dislocation produced bilateral hemopneumothoraces and complete T6 paraplegia. An operative open-reduction internal fixation was carried out for spinal alignment, stability, and fusion.

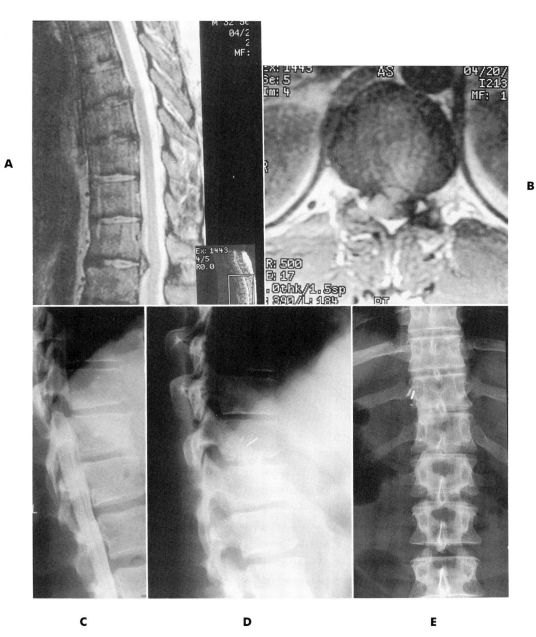

Fig. 14-14. **A** to **C,** This 32-year-old recreational athlete was injured while lifting, which caused severe back and thoracolumbar junction pain radiating into the groin. He had definite but vague and ill-defined bilateral leg weakness that was worse with activity. There was slight hyperreflexia in the lower extremities. **D** and **E,** Postoperative views showing a satisfactory rib graft in place after an extrapleural eleventh rib approach, disc excision, and grafting. The patient's postoperative recovery was satisfactory, with return of neurologic function.

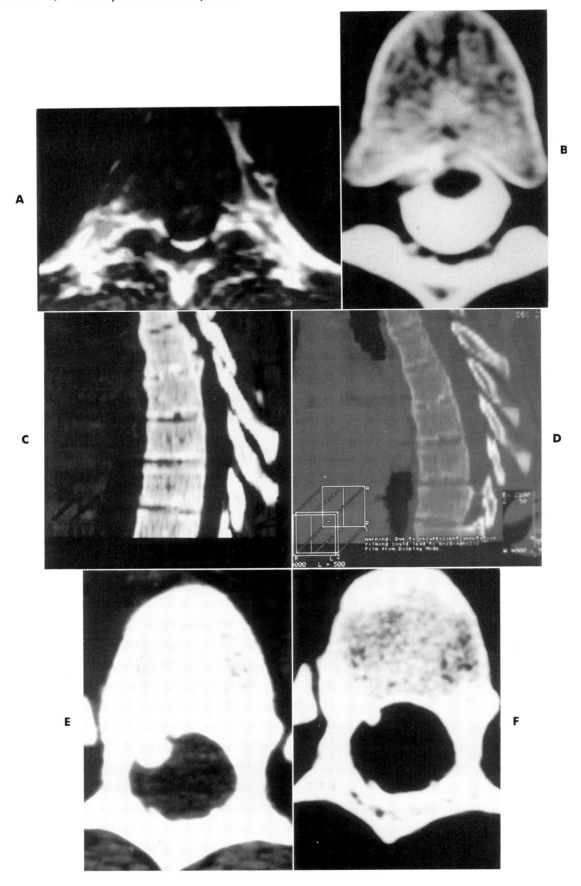

Fig. 14-15. For legend see opposite page.

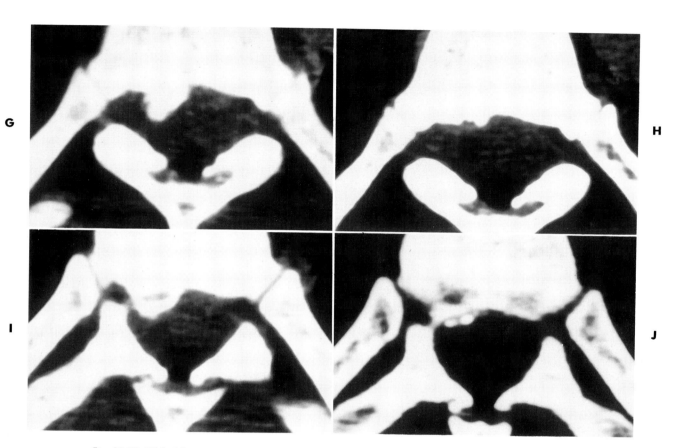

Fig. 14-15. This 32-year-old professional athlete had thoracic radiculopathy but no thoracic myelopathy. The radiculopathy began with a blow from behind during a professional sports activity, which produced intense radiculopathy unresponsive to nonoperative care over a considerable period of time. **A,** MRI scan showing extruded fragment of a herniated disc. **B,** Contrast CT scan showing a calcified extruded fragment of the intervertebral disc. **C,** Parasagittal section of the plain CT scan showing a calcified extruded fragment from the T6-7 disc space, extruding up behind the body of T6. **D,** Parasagittal section 90 days from the time of the intense radiculopathy. The intense radiculopathy slowly resolved. The patient was maintained on a regimen of aggressive trunk stabilization, chest-out posture correction, and a body-reconditioning program. He was able to return to his sport 90 days after the original onset of symptoms and performed at full function for the rest of the professional season. **E,** Transverse section of the CT scan at the time of intense radiculopathy. **F,** Appearance 90 days later. **G,** Large, calcified, extruded fragment. **H,** Resolution of the fragment. **I,** Another section of the extruded fragment. **J,** Resolution in that approximate area. This herniation was an extrusion of an intradiscal calcification that was resorbed by a combination of pulsations of the thoracic cord and healing of the injured area.

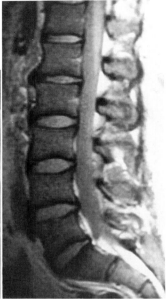

Fig. 14-16. This 27-year-old professional defensive lineman experienced an acute lifting episode that caused severe thoracolumbar junction pain. The pain was worse with rotation. There was some radiation around the flank into the abdomen and severe pain with coughing, sneezing, and deep breathing, as well as an acute inflammatory reaction. X-ray films revealed an anterior herniation and degeneration of the L1-2 disc. Time, rest, physical therapy, and rehabilitation allowed a satisfactory return to play without future complications.

REFERENCES

1. Alberico A et al: High thoracic disc herniation, *Neurosurgery* 19:449, 1986.
2. Balague F et al: Unusual presentation of thoracic disc herniation, *Clin Rheumatol* 8:269, 1989.
3. Bohlman H, Zdeblick T: Anterior excision of herniated thoracic discs, *J Bone Joint Surg* 70A:1038, 1988.
4. Brown CW et al: The natural history of thoracic disc herniation, *Spine* 17:597, 1992.
5. Capener N: The evolution of lateral rhachotomy, *J Bone Joint Surg* 36B:173, 1954.
6. Carson J, Gumpert J, Jefferson A: Diagnosis and treatment of thoracic intervertebral disc protrusion, *J Neurol Neurosurg Psychiatry* 34:68, 1971.
7. Dommisse GF: The arteries, arterioles and capillaries of the spinal cord: surgical guidelines in the prevention of postoperative paraplegia, *Coll Surg Engl* 62:369, 1980.
8. Fidler MW, Goedhart ZD: Excision of prolapse of thoracic intervertebral disc: a transthoracic technique, *J Bone Joint Surg* 66B:518, 1984.
9. Hamilton MG, Thomas HG: Intradural herniation of a thoracic disc presenting as flaccid paraplegia: case report, *Neurosurgery* 27:482, 1990.
10. Hedge S, Staas WE: Thoracic disc herniation and spinal cord injury, *Am J Phys Med Rehabil* 228, 1988.
11. Morgenlander J, Massey EW: Neurogenic claudication with positionally dependent weakness from a thoracic disc herniation, *Neurology* 39:1133, 1989.
12. Otani K et al: Thoracic disc herniation: surgical treatment in 23 patients, *Spine* 13:1262, 1988.
13. Perot PL Jr, Munro DD: Transthoracic removal of midline thoracic disc protrusions causing spinal cord compression, *J Neurosurg* 31:452, 1969.
14. Ransohoff J et al: Case reports and technical notes: transthoracic removal of thoracic disc—report of three cases, *J Neurosurg* 31:459, 1969.
15. Stillerman C, Weiss M: Management of thoracic disc disease, *Clin Neurosurg* 38:325, 1992.
16. Sward L et al: Disc degeneration and associated abnormalities of the spine in elite gymnasts: a magnetic resonance imaging study, *Spine* 16:437, 1991.
17. Watkins R et al: Dynamic EMG evaluation of trunk musculature in professional baseball players, *Spine* 14:404, 1989.

Section Four

◆

Surgery

Chapter Fifteen

◆

Anesthetic Care of the Spine-Injured Athlete

Irv Klein

Anesthesia, whether by general or regional technique, facilitates the performance of surgical procedures. Just as surgical techniques have evolved to optimize clinical results, so have anesthesiologists attempted to hone their skills to best assist the surgical team in performing the task at hand. This chapter focuses on current anesthetic practices often used to facilitate surgery of the spine-injured athlete.

PREPARATION FOR SURGERY

The anesthesiologist should have a thorough understanding of the patient's medical history and condition before transport of the patient to the operating room suite. During the preoperative period, volume status and coexisting medical conditions, such as asthma, hypertension, and electrolyte imbalance, should be optimized with the assistance of internal medicine consultants. Prophylaxis with medications that are useful in minimizing gastric acid secretion may be helpful in preventing peptic symptoms, especially in those patients who may be receiving supplemental glucocorticoid therapy. For those elective procedures that may require perioperative blood transfusion, autologous blood donation should be performed during the preoperative period. Patients receiving salicylates or nonsteroidal antiinflammatory medications should have these withheld preoperatively to allow the template bleeding time to return to normal before surgical intervention. Although well conditioned, the spine-injured athlete may manifest a sinus bradycardia during the perioperative period. This does not require treatment unless the medications administered, including narcotic analgesics, further reduce the heart rate to alarmingly low levels.

HYPOTENSIVE ANESTHESIA

During most surgical spinal procedures the anesthesiologist may best assist the surgeon by attempting to minimize blood loss in the operative field. This may be accomplished best by the vigorous use of hypotensive anesthetic techniques. We routinely attempt to maintain the systolic blood pressure between 75 and 85 mm Hg during the period from skin incision to closure of the superficial skin layers. Hypotensive anesthesia is best accomplished through a combination of patient positioning and judicious use of volatile anesthetics and intravenous medications, including fentanyl, labetalol, and hydralazine. Rarely do we find it necessary to use sodium nitroprusside for its hypotensive effect. This avoids the possibility of cyanide toxicity during prolonged surgical procedures. Continuous intraarterial blood pressure monitoring, usually via cannulation of the nondominant radial artery, is often used during cervical, thoracic, and prolonged lumbosacral procedures. Central venous pressure monitoring, usually by cannulation of the right internal jugular vein, is employed during cases in which prominent fluid shifts may occur during the perioperative period. Body temperature is maintained at normothermic levels by use of warming irrigation, intravenous fluids, and humidified breathing circuits.

BLOOD LEVELS

Perioperative nonautologous blood transfusions are a rarity in caring for the spine-injured athlete. This is accomplished through the combination of hypotensive anesthetic techniques, vigilant scavenging of blood from the operative field via the cell saver, and its subsequent transfusion after appropriate processing, as well as perioperative transfusion of preoperatively collected autologous blood. When it is indicated, patients orally receive iron-containing medications to hasten the return of hemoglobin levels to the normal range.

PATIENT POSITIONING

Optimal patient positioning facilitates good surgical results and minimizes pressure on bony prominences. For those spinal procedures performed in the prone or prone-kneeling position, particular attention is paid to avoid or at least minimize pressure on both ulnar nerves as they traverse their respective ulnar grooves. In positioning the patient on the Andrews frame for lumbosacral procedures, the arms are kept at a maximum of 90 degrees from the major axis of the body. The forearms are maintained on padded armrests somewhat inferior in plane to the major body axis. The face is carefully positioned on a slotted head-positioner cushion to avoid pressure on the eyeballs, ears, nasal tip, chin, and lips. The neck should not be subject to extremes of flexion or extension. The abdominal cavity is dependent without encroachment from the operating room table or its attachments.

For patients undergoing cervical spine procedures, the degree of stability of the bony axis must be communicated to the anesthesiologist preoperatively. In instances of instability, preoperative application of a halo vest may make intubation by conventional methods impossible. Fiberoptic intubation techniques are usually mandated in such instances. In such cases, evoked potential monitoring is often used during positioning to ensure optimal neurologic status.

Complex thoracic spine procedures occasionally require a transthoracic approach facilitated by rib resection. In these cases the anesthesiologist can greatly facilitate exposure to the ventral surface of the thoracic spine by providing single-lung anesthesia via the use of a double-lumen endotracheal tube or retractable bronchial blocker. Deflating the nondependent lung on those thoracic procedures performed in the lateral position allows the surgeon maximal maneuverability to perform the surgical procedure in an expeditious manner.

PREOPERATIVE AND POSTOPERATIVE CARE

Preoperatively, athletes, whether professional or amateur, often have considerable anxiety relating to both their clinical condition and their ultimate status on recovery. This anxiety may best be alleviated by giving the patient a detailed explanation of the expected sequence of events on the day of surgery and by ordering anxiolytic premedication, such as midazolam. Postoperatively, pain is often best minimized through the use of patient-controlled analgesia with morphine or meperidine (Demerol).

◆

Chapter Sixteen

Anterior Cervical Spine Surgery

Robert G. Watkins

The most common operation for cervical radiculopathy is anterior cervical fusion.

CERVICAL ANATOMY
Muscles and Arteries

The hyoid bone is situated at approximately the C3 level and serves as a dividing area for the musculature of the anterior neck. The suprahyoid region is covered by the suprahyoid portion of the external investing fascia. The musculature includes the digastric muscle, which lies inferior to the mandible and extends from the mastoid process to the symphysis mandibularis. The sling around the tendinous midportion of the digastric muscle separates the posterior belly from the anterior belly. It holds the midportion of the muscle to the greater cornu of the hyoid bone. The digastric muscle helps form the carotid triangle, which is bordered superiorly by the posterior belly of the digastric muscle, inferiorly by the omohyoid muscle, and posteriorly by the sternocleidomastoid muscle. It is essentially through this triangle that the approach is made.

The stylohyoid muscle lies anterior and superior to the posterior of the digastric and rises from the styloid process, passing to the hyoid bone. The stylohyoid ligament is a ligamentous band that passes with the stylohyoid muscle from the styloid process to the hyoid bone. The mylohyoid and sternohyoid muscles run from the mandible to the hyoid bone. Structures coursing from the mastoid to the hyoid and from the mandible to the hyoid must be either retracted in a cephalad direction or severed.

The sequential branches of the external carotid from caudad to cephalad are the superior thyroid artery, the facial artery, and the lingual artery. The external carotid artery continues coursing through the parotid gland and terminates just in front of the ear and the maxillary artery, which crosses anteriorly through the parotid gland. The occipital artery arises from the posterior aspect of the carotid artery at the level of the facial artery. It crosses under the posterior belly of the digastric and stylohyoid muscles through a loop of the hypoglossal nerve and ascends in the interval between the transverse process of C1-2 and the mastoid process.

Nerves and Bony Structures

In addition to the hypoglossal nerve, the superior laryngeal nerve also arises from the inferior ganglion of the vagus and crosses caudally and medially under the internal carotid artery to the superior border of the thyroid cartilage, where it joins the superior thyroid artery. The superior laryngeal nerve has external and internal branches; the external branch crosses at the more caudad level. The recurrent laryngeal nerve on the right side loops under the subclavian artery, passing dorsomedial to it to the side of the trachea and esophagus. It is vulnerable to damage as it passes from the subclavian artery to the right tracheoesophageal groove.

On the left side the recurrent laryngeal nerve loops under the arch of the aorta and is much more protected in the left tracheoesophageal groove. Both recurrent laryngeal nerves enter the larynx through the cricothyroid membrane, as does the inferior thyroid artery, and therefore should not be present in more cephalad exposures. The seventh cranial nerve (facial nerve) emerges from the stylomastoid foramen and crosses anteriorly into the parotid gland across the external carotid artery. Although this is a very superior position in the dissection, care must be taken to avoid the facial nerve with any cephalad retraction.

Important bony landmarks are the mastoid process and the smaller, more pointed styloid process, which projects off the temporal bone just medial to the mastoid process. The styloid process is the origin of the stylohyoid muscle and ligament. The stylohyoid foramen is just medial to the styloid process and serves as the exit for the facial nerve. The jugular foramen lies between the occipital bone and the temporal bone and is the exit for the glossopharyngeal, vagus, and accessory nerves. The hypoglossal canal in the occipital bone is the exit foramen for the hypoglossal nerve.

POSITIONING FOR ANTERIOR APPROACHES

The head must be extended enough to allow exposure of the spine. Patients vary from fixed kyphotic deformity to short neck to no neck. The amount of extension possible is affected by the stiffness of the neck and the type of abnormality (care should be taken in hyperextending a patient with myelopathy because this condition further closes the spinal canal). The surgeon holds the head, taking spinal cord precautions, and places a rolled towel under the patient's shoulders, allowing the head to extend gently to find its limit of extension. Then the surgeon flexes to less than this limit and observes the amount of anterior clearance, assessing the distance of the cricoid and thyroid cartilages from the sternal notch.

The amount of extension should be the amount needed to make the approach in terms of the aforementioned precautions. Then a firm flotation pad and towel are placed under the patient's head to establish the amount of extension. Rotation of the head away from the side of the approach may be needed to provide adequate exposure. Remember, extension and rotation close the intervertebral foramina opposite the approach. A small sandbag or inflatable cushion is molded under the neck to provide support for the neck itself. Boger straps are positioned loosely around the patient's wrists to provide traction on the arms when needed during the procedure. At the time that x-ray films are taken, we place these straps around the bottoms of the patient's feet, with the knees flexed, and push down on the knees, extending the legs and pulling down the shoulders: a sandbag is placed on the knees, and x-ray films are obtained without exposure to the operating room personnel. The straps are released after the radiographs are completed.

CHOICE OF APPROACH

To determine whether to approach the spine from the right or the left, the surgeon considers the following. Approaches from the left in the supraclavicular area require caution because of the point of entry of the thoracic duct into the jugular vein–subclavian vein junction (Fig. 16-1). A large, fatty meal the day before surgery in this area is an aid to identifying the duct, but most approaches are well medial to this area and do not require definitive identification. Approaches from the right from C4 and below require identification of the right recurrent laryngeal nerve. This nerve passes from

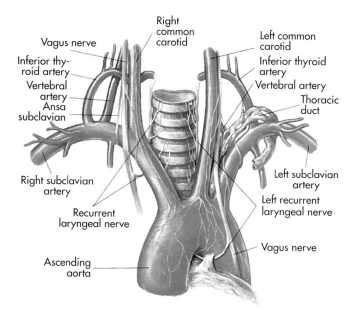

Fig. 16-1. Neurovascular structures of the base of the neck. Both vagus nerves seen here are in the carotid sheath. (From Watkins RG: *Surgical approaches to the spine,* New York, 1983, Springer-Verlag.)

the area of the carotid sheath to the medial musculovisceral column in the C5 to C7 area. The left recurrent laryngeal nerve is in the tracheoesophageal groove throughout the neck. It can be injured by using a sharp, angled retractor in the tracheoesophageal groove. For this reason we use blunt finger dissection from the medial border of the sternocleidomastoid muscle to the midline of the spine. Then the nonlipped, hand-held Cloward retractor is placed directly on the spine, and rigorous retraction into the soft tissue is avoided.

Anatomic Landmarks

The significant anatomic landmarks for differentiating the various approaches to the cervical spine are the sternocleidomastoid muscle, the carotid sheath, and the longus colli muscle. Categorization of the approach is based on the direction of the approach relative to these specific structures. For example, in C1 to C3 an anterior medial approach is medial to the sternocleidomastoid muscle (therefore retracting it laterally) and medial to the carotid sheath (therefore retracting it laterally as well). A lateral approach to the midcervical spine is directed lateral to the sternocleidomastoid muscle and lateral to the carotid sheath. A significant differential feature of these approaches is whether to approach the carotid sheath medially or laterally. Approaching the carotid sheath medially and retracting it laterally often requires sacrifice of vessels coursing from the carotid sheath to the medial musculovisceral column. Nerves running from lateral to medial also must be retracted. Approaching the carotid sheath laterally and retracting it medially, as in the anterolateral approaches, produces a more avascular plane but may also result in a more limited, more lateral exposure. Both the anteromedial and the anterolateral approaches have common points of dissection and anatomy.[2,3] At the Kerlan-Jobe Orthopaedic Clinic we prefer the anteromedial Smith-Robinson, Cloward approach for pathologic conditions in C2 to T1. For T2 abnormalities the approach is usually through a third rib under the arm.

Skin incisions. The skin incision must be cosmetically acceptable but efficient. Superficial landmarks used to place the incision over the appropriate level of the spine are C3-4, which is above the thyroid cartilage, and C5-6, which is at the cricoid cartilage.[5] Alternately, two fingerbreadths above the clavicle can be used for C5-6 and one fingerbreadth for C6-7 (Fig. 16-2). Other superficial landmarks to be identified are the angle of the jaw, the sternocleidomastoid muscle, the hyoid bone, the cricoid cartilage, the superior border of the thyroid cartilage, and the insertion of the sternocleidomastoid to the clavicle. For best cosmesis a 3-cm transverse incision is made in a skin crease from midline to the anterior border of the sternocleidomastoid muscle. A longer transverse incision allows adequate exposure for three vertebral bodies and two disc levels (Fig. 16-3). The exact

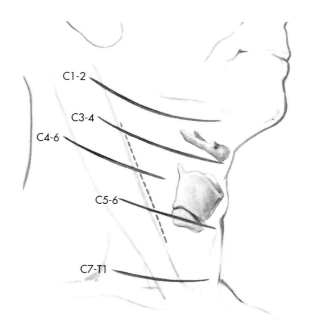

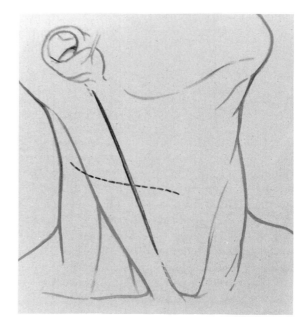

Fig. 16-2. The approximate skin areas for approaches to specific spinal levels are usually indicated by palpable subcutaneous structures. C1-2 lies under the angle of the jaw, C3-4 is a centimeter above the thyroid cartilage in the region of the hyoid bone, C4-6 is at the level of thyroid cartilage, C5-6 is at the cricoid cartilage, and C7-T1 is in the supraclavicular area. For best cosmesis a transverse skin incision is made (see text). A vertical incision along the anterior border of the sternocleidomastoid muscle, as seen on the dotted line, may be used for long exposures of the cervical spine. (From Watkins RG: *Surgical approaches to the spine,* New York, 1983, Springer-Verlag.)

Fig. 16-3. The more cosmetically suitable transverse incision is made at the appropriate level and should allow exposure of up to two discs and three vertebrae. A vertical incision can be used for greater exposure. (From Watkins RG: *Surgical approaches to the spine,* New York, 1983, Springer-Verlag.)

abnormality and the technical demands of the operation determine the size of the exposure and the structures that must be transected rather than retracted.

Platysma muscle. After the skin incision has been made and a well-developed platysma muscle is visible, it is best to open the platysma muscle along the line of its fibers. The platysma muscle should be elevated with Adson forceps and opened carefully to avoid damage to underlying veins and the sternocleidomastoid muscle.[5] (A well-developed platysma muscle may be closed as an individual layer, although usually this layer is not individually closed but allowed to reapproximate itself.) The sternocleidomastoid must be identified as the initial key to the approach: for anteromedial approaches, the medial border of the sternocleidomastoid; for lateral approaches, the lateral border of the sternocleidomastoid. The second landmark, the carotid sheath, is first identified by finger palpation of the carotid pulse. The carotid sheath contains the carotid artery, internal jugular vein, vagus nerve, and elements of the sympathetic plexus.

Longus colli muscle. The third landmark structure is the longus colli muscle, which must be identified under the prevertebral fascia over the spine. The surgeon palpates

for the spine. Often the anterior tubercle of the transverse process is mistaken for the vertebral body. Inadvertent dissection in this more lateral area can damage the sympathetic plexus and cause bleeding from the longus colli. The more avascular area of the spine is the midline. Opening the prevertebral fascia in the midline allows lateral dissection and retraction of the longus colli and causes less bleeding. Special note should be taken of the esophagus in any approach to the anterior cervical spine; it is frequently a flat ribbonlike structure lying over the anterior prevertebral fascia. A nasogastric tube aids in identification of the esophagus. The surgeon uses finger dissection to progress from the medial border of the sternocleidomastoid muscle to the midline of the spine.

Retraction of Neurovascular Structures

Vessels may be either ligated or retracted, usually depending on their size and location. The retraction of nerves and arteries varies, but general guidelines can be used. For more cephalad exposures, the hypoglossal nerve, glossopharyngeal nerve, and digastric muscle cephalad are retracted. The superior laryngeal nerve and superior thyroid artery and vein are often retracted caudad for C1 to C3 approaches and cephalad for C4 to C7 approaches. The middle thyroid vein is ligated when necessary. The inferior thyroid artery and vein are retracted caudally for C7 and above, possibly cephalad

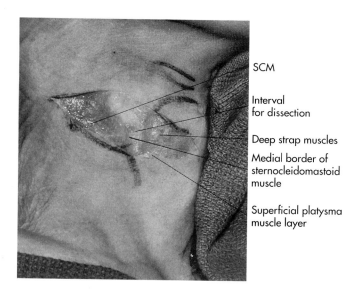

Fig. 16-4. Dissection through subcutaneous tissue to the platysma muscle, which in this specimen is very thin. (From Watkins RG: *Surgical approaches to the spine,* New York, 1983, Springer-Verlag.)

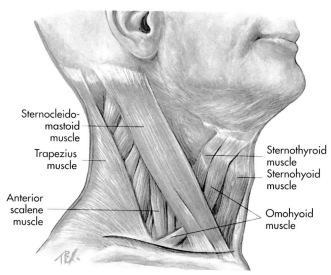

Fig. 16-5. Muscles of the neck. (From Watkins RG: *Surgical approaches to the spine,* New York, 1983, Springer-Verlag.)

for levels distal to T1. In addition, the omohyoid muscle crosses around C6 and is divided or retracted for C6-7 and below.

ANTEROMEDIAL APPROACH TO THE MIDCERVICAL SPINE

Although head-halter traction may be used, we prefer insertion of the Gardner-Wells tongs to allow for cervical distraction during the procedure. A roll is placed under the shoulders. A small, curved sandbag is contoured under the neck to support the spine. The head is positioned in slight extension and rotation. Adhesive towels drape the entire neck. The skin incision level is chosen.

After a transverse skin incision at the appropriate level, the surgeon dissects through the subcutaneous tissue to the platysma muscle and inserts the spring retractors (Fig. 16-4). The platysma muscle is lifted with Adson forceps and opened carefully in line with the fibers. The surgeon takes care to avoid damage to veins and the sternocleidomastoid muscle.[1,5] Under the platysma is the external jugular vein, which courses on the external surface of the sternocleidomastoid muscle, and the anterior jugular vein, which is in a more anteromedial location over the sternocleidomastoid-strap muscle interval or on the lateral aspect of the strap musculature. The anterior and external jugular veins must be divided and ligated only when their presence interferes with the procedure.

The first key to successful exposure is adequate identification of the medial border of the sternocleidomastoid (Fig. 16-5). The superficial cervical fascia is opened, and the medial border of the sternocleidomas-

toid muscle is identified.[7] The posterior cutaneous nerves, when present, are retracted. With identification of this medial border, the surgeon bluntly develops the interval between the sternocleidomastoid muscle and the musculovisceral column.[6] The middle cervical fascia invests the sternocleidomastoid medially. This may be opened with scissors and spread vertically, or the wound can be developed with blunt dissection only.

The sternocleidomastoid is retracted laterally, and the strap musculature is retracted medially (Fig. 16-6). The omohyoid muscle crosses from proximal medial to lateral distal through the middle cervical fascia at around C6-7. The omohyoid is retracted and, when necessary, divided laterally in the tendinous portion, tagged, and later repaired.

Vertical finger dissection spreads the middle cervical fascia just medial to the carotid sheath.[6] The inconstant middle thyroid vein crossing at approximately C5 is identified, ligated, and divided when needed. The anterior surface of the vertebral body is identified with a finger. The blunt, nonlipped Cloward hand-held retractor is then inserted into the wound directly down to the spine. The surgeon holds the retractor on the right longus colli muscle and takes care to avoid entering the tracheo-esophageal groove with the retractor tip (and thereby damaging the left recurrent laryngeal nerve).[4]

The surgeon retracts distally the inferior thyroid artery and vein at the C6-7 level and retracts proximally the superior thyroid artery and vein and the superior laryngeal nerve at C3-4.

The transverse process must not be mistaken for the midline of the vertebral body inasmuch as an incision deep in this area will damage the longus colli muscle, the sympathetic chain, and possibly the vertebral artery. An

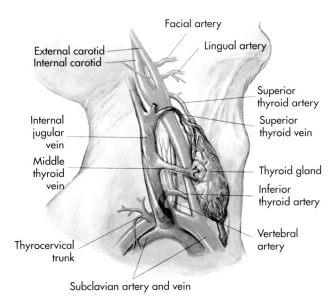

Facial artery
Lingual artery
External carotid
Internal carotid
Superior thyroid artery
Superior thyroid vein
Internal jugular vein
Middle thyroid vein
Thyroid gland
Inferior thyroid artery
Vertebral artery
Thyrocervical trunk
Subclavian artery and vein

Fig. 16-6. Arteriovenous structures of the middle cervical fascial layer. (From Watkins RG: *Surgical approaches to the spine,* New York, 1983, Springer-Verlag.)

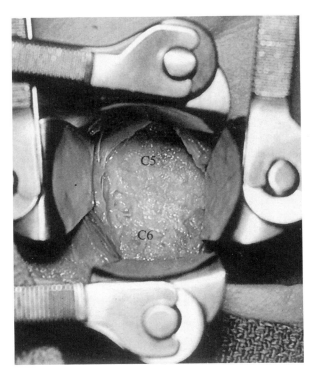

C5
C6

Fig. 16-7. Insertion of the Cloward self-retaining retractor with the clawed blades into the longus colli muscle on both sides of the spine. (From Watkins RG: *Surgical approaches to the spine,* New York, 1983, Springer-Verlag.)

incision into the longus colli muscle produces bleeding. The key to avoiding this is to stay in the midline.

A retractor is inserted. The empty esophagus is only a soft, flat, ribbonlike structure simulating the musculature over the anterior portion of the spine. Either an esophageal stethoscope or a nasogastric tube is used to help identify the esophagus by feel.

The esophagus, trachea, and anterior strap muscles are retracted medially, and the carotid sheath and sternocleidomastoid muscle are retracted laterally.

With the prevertebral fascia opened in the midline and the disc identified, a needle is inserted into a disc for lateral x-ray confirmation of the level.

After the prevertebral area is exposed, a hand-held Cloward, nonlipped retractor is placed on the right longus colli muscle and then held by the assistant. The surgeon then uses the peanut to sweep the prevertebral fascia, exposing the discs and vertebrae, and, with a low setting on the Bovie cautery, cuts the medial edge of the longus colli. Using the bipolar cautery in the right hand and the sucker in the left, the surgeon cauterizes the leading edge of the longus colli muscle for the full width of the self-retaining retractor. Then the assistant takes the sucker, and the surgeon uses a Cloward periosteal elevator in one hand and the bipolar in the other and gently elevates the longus colli muscle; elevating the muscle and using the bipolar cautery are alternated until a flap of longus colli muscle is fashioned on the right side. At this point the lipped, hand-held Cloward retractor is placed underneath the lip of the flap of the longus colli muscle and hemostasis is obtained. By means of this technique, using the bipolar cautery and the curved Cloward periosteal elevator each step of the way, a bloodless

elevation of the longus colli muscle can be carried out. At this point the nonlipped Cloward retractor is used to retract the left side of the spine just to the midportion of the left longus colli muscle. The sucker, the curved Cloward periosteal elevator, and the bipolar cautery are used in the same way to fashion a similar flap of the left longus colli muscle.

Retraction Procedure

The entire operation can be performed by repositioning the hand-held Cloward retractors. The flap of the longus colli muscle can be used, and pressure on the medial and lateral structures can be relaxed as frequently as possible.

If self-retaining retractors are desired, clawed retractors, smooth blades, or serrated-edge retractors can be used. First, the curved Cloward periosteal elevator can be used to hold the flap up while the retractor is placed under the right longus colli muscle and the left-sided retractor is placed. The retractor is opened enough to expose the spine medial to the longus colli muscle. Care is taken not to produce undue stress on soft tissues with the self-retaining retractor (Fig. 16-7).

Distraction

If the Kaspar distractor is used, the Gardner-Wells tongs will not be needed. The Kaspar distractor provides retraction in a cephalad/caudad direction, as well as disc space distraction. The Cloward nonlipped retractor is placed cephalad, and the midportion of the body above is used for the self-tapping Kaspar distractor pin to be placed. The same procedure on the midportion of the caudal body allows the two spikes of the Kaspar distractor to be used.

It is important to align the Kaspar distractor with the disc space, making sure that the two prongs are parallel to each other and aligned with the disc space, because the Kaspar distractor can block easy insertion of the graft if the prongs are not aligned with the disc space. The distractor is placed on the distractor pins. This also applies for a cephalad/caudad retraction. The hand-held Cloward retractor can be used for supplemental retraction in any aspect of the wound if the soft tissue is protruding over the spine.

If attention is turned away from the wound for any reason, we loosen the retractors. In most instances the graft is obtained at the same time as the approach to the cervical spine.

X-Ray Level Identification

The marker film for the disc space is usually taken as soon as the spine is exposed with the hand-held Cloward retractor, and indigo carmine is placed in the disc space after the x-ray film is completed. Before the needle is removed, a spot of indigo carmine is clearly identified on the disc surface before the rest of the exposure. Occasionally the needle and x-ray film may be obtained after insertion of the Cloward retractors, but we prefer to do so before the insertion.

Disc Space Preparation

With the retractors in place and the x-ray film having confirmed the level, a No. 15 blade is used to incise the annulus of the disc. This cutting motion is taken over the rim of the osteophyte to remove the soft tissue, not only at the true disc space level but over the osteophyte as well. From the initial work on the disc space, it is important to remember that the graft may be as wide as 15 mm, and spending an excessive amount of time fashioning too narrow a slot for the graft is a waste of time. After the annulus is incised, a pituitary rongeur is used to remove enough of the disc material to see the articular surface of the disc space. The surgeon should be aligned with the probable angle of the articular surfaces at this point and have a good feel for the direction of the disc space. Attention is turned back to the lip, where straight curettes and a Leksell rongeur are used to remove the osteophytes from the anterior surface of the disc space down to its true bony edge. On identification of the true edge of the disc space and the angles of the articular surface, we remove the cartilaginous surface of the end-plates without removing any subchondral bone at this point.

With the osteophytes removed and the annulus excised, the outer annulus and a portion of the center of the intervertebral disc are removed with a micropituitary rongeur. The Cloward curettes are used to clear enough disc material from the center of the disc to allow the surgeon to see clearly the end-plates of the intervertebral disc.

Using a straight No. 1 Karlin curette, we curette the cartilage off the end-plates. Every attempt is made not to gouge into the soft cancellous bone at the center of the disc space and to concentrate on using a rotating motion laterally and removing the cartilage in the most lateral aspects of the disc space. A common tendency is to fashion too narrow a recipient site when the iliac crest in some patients may be 14 to 15 mm wide.

The objective at this point is to rectangularize the disc space. The joints of Luschka curve laterally, and the posterior osteophytes curve posteriorly in the wound. The disc has a biconcave surface from both an antero-posterior and a lateral view. This biconcave aspect of the end-plates must be considered in fashioning the receptor site for the graft inasmuch as the goal is to rectangularize the biconcave surfaces. After the true plane of the joint is detected, this biconcave surface can be clearly identified. An AM8 drill is used to drill down the right and left sides of the disc space, which are drilled to the height of the center portion of the disc space. Then the drill, paralleling the end-plate, is used to cut into the sloping surface of the posterior end-plate. Additional leveling of the interspace is performed anteriorly as well, to produce the rectangularization of the disc space. This step eliminates the slope from the posterior aspect of the superior and inferior end-plates. It also creates a bony abutment to prevent the graft from going into the spinal canal. We use the disc space measurers that show graduated millimeter heights. Using the smaller spacer, we can slowly pick up the narrow areas and expand those with the drill. This rectangularization of the disc space removes all articular cartilage and certain areas of subchondral bone. The idea is to leave subchondral bleeding bone.

Cutting into the center portion of the body may lead to delays in union because the hard graft pushes into the soft cancellous bone, leaving crushed cancellous bone and areas for fibrous ingrowth. Obviously, leaving cartilage on the end-plate is inappropriate, and many clinicians believe the subchondral bone should be penetrated to allow proper vascularization. We follow the philosophy of erring on the side of leaving proper support for the graft. Measuring the depth of the prepared interspace, which is accomplished with the depth gauge, is very important. The depth gauge usually is set at 1.4 mm, and then the depth of the disc space is evaluated. It is important to measure on the end-plates, not in the center of the disc space. The end-plate is where the graft will be entering and where the graft will

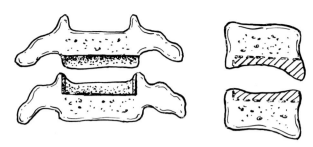

Fig. 16-8. **A,** Resculpturing the disc space requires fashioning a graft from a biconcave surface, with the rounded surfaces cut into a rectangle. **B,** The graft is a rectangle placed into a rectangularized slot in the disc space.

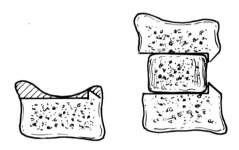

Fig. 16-9. If the bone spurs are to be removed, they are cut cephalad and caudad, leaving a posterior buttress on at least 50% of the back edge of the body.

have contact. Therefore that is where the measurement should be taken. The most common mistake leading to inadequate graft positioning is failure to cut the biconcave sloping surface and rectangularize the disc space. If there is a slope on the surface, then the graft will impinge on the initial foot of the slope, and if the measurement is taken at the depth of the disc space, then the difference in these two figures is how much the graft will be sticking out anteriorly (Figs. 16-8 and 16-9). Therefore rectangularization of the disc space and measurement of the end-plate grafts are vital.

THE GRAFT

The graft, which is usually taken while the end-plate is being prepared, is obtained through a 2-inch incision just below the iliac crest. Dissection is carried directly to the top of the iliac crest, and the oscillating saw removes a 1-cm plug of bone. After periosteal elevation of both inner and outer tables, a 1-cm plug of bone is removed, and the small quarter-inch osteotome is used to cut the inferior surface of the graft. The wound is copiously irrigated, and the fascia is closed. Subcuticular sutures are used.

Microscopic Removal of the Disc Fragment

Before the end-plates are fashioned, which causes some bleeding, visualization of the posterior lipped

surface of the disc space is completed. In cases in which there is an extruded fragment of intervertebral disc, the indigo carmine used to mark the disc space usually colors the extruded fragment a bright blue. After vertebral body spreading, the AM8 drill is used to drill end-plates down to the posterior longitudinal ligament. It is still easy to leave a bony bridge to protect against graft extrusion of the canal by opening up only a portion of the lipped surface to remove an extruded fragment of intervertebral disc. Once the end-plates are drilled down, the operating microscope is used to enter the tear in the posterior longitudinal ligament. The blue hole made by the indigo carmine is seen, and the micro-rongeur Kerrison, the No. 4 micro-Penfield dissector, and the micro–nerve hook are used to open the adjacent portions of the posterior longitudinal ligament. The fragment is manipulated with the No. 4 Penfield and removed with the micro–nerve hook. Use of the microscope allows adequate fragment removal and protection of neurologic tissue.

Osteophyte Removal

In those instances in which it is believed necessary to remove a large osteophyte from a posterolateral corner, the AM8 drill and microscopic curettes can remove this tissue by thinning it, drilling it down to a small thin layer of bone, and gently peeling that out. We do not routinely remove osteophytes from the anterior approach, because in most instances it is unnecessary. Distraction of the disc space, fusion in distraction, and a solid fusion relieve the symptoms of cervical radiculopathy caused by foraminal stenosis with the same success rate as combining these procedures with a joint of Luschka or vertebral body spur removal. Removal of true osteophytes is reserved for instances in which the patient has signs or symptoms of cervical myelopathy. Distraction alone produces an improvement in the central canal diameter. Fusion alone produces a decrease in the signs and symptoms of cervical myelopathy.

When the spur is to be removed, it should be remembered that the base of the spur extends cephalad and caudad a number of millimeters on the back of the vertebral body. Going directly to the center of the disc space and removing 2 to 3 mm of the posterior aspect of bone is rarely adequate, and the tangential cut cephalad and caudad of the lipped posterior surface of the vertebral body removes a considerable portion of bone. It also removes the bony bridge to prevent graft extrusion into the canal. With good carpentry work in the disc space, it is possible to remove these spurs and still allow a slight ridge to protect the graft and allow adequate anterior graft fixation. Removal of large osteophytes, however, carries a greater risk of losing a graft position. If the posterior third or fourth of the end-plate is removed in removing a posterior osteophyte, there is less support for the graft and a greater chance of graft dislodgment.

Graft Preparation

After the graft is obtained, the tangential saw and a small rongeur are used to fashion the graft. The graft is measured carefully in its depth, height, and maximum width in case it rotates, and it is put onto the Kaspar pinned impacter. The distractor provides distraction as the graft is tapped into place. We prefer posterior placement of the cortical surface. It provides more support and is less likely to extrude and break off the surface, but in one case a slight kyphotic deformity occurred because the softer cancellous portion of the graft collapsed while healing. X-ray films are obtained before closure.

The graft is taken through a 2-inch incision over the iliac crest. The area between the muscle layers is carefully dissected down to the fascia, allowing removal of a 6- to 8-mm graft with minimal bleeding and complications. This graft is then rectangularized, just as with the receptor site. The height, width, and depth of the graft are carefully measured. If one wall of the graft is a little higher than the other, it should be the most posterior portion. The cortical portion of the tricortical graft is inserted into the depth of the receptor site. We place the screw-enhanced Kaspar inserter into the cancellous portion, inserting the cortical portion posteriorly in the receptor site. Distraction is done with the Kaspar distractor, or if that is not available, we use the Gardner-Wells tongs. With distraction of the disc space, the graft is tapped into place in a snug fashion. X-rays films are always obtained to confirm the position of the graft. Every attempt is made to avoid using the height of the graft to force open the disc space. This produces fractures of the graft and/or the end-plate and rarely allows a properly seated graft. The disc space is distracted with the Gardner-Wells tongs, and the graft, sized to be 0.5 mm more so that it is snug, will be held in place by the friction of the end-plates when the distraction is removed. After the x-ray film is obtained, the wound is copiously irrigated. Subcutaneous tissue and skin are closed after Hemovac drains have been placed directly in front of the spine.

REFERENCES

1. Bailey RW, Bagley CD: Stabilization of the cervical spine by anterior fusion, *J Bone Joint Surg* 42A:565, 1960.
2. Hodgson AR, Rau ACM: Anterior approach to the spinal column, *Recent Adv Orthop* 9:289, 1969.
3. Nanson EM: The anterior approach to the upper dorsal sympathectomy, *Surg Gynecol Obstet* 104:118, 1957.
4. Perry J: Surgical approaches to the spine. In Pierce D, Nichols V, editors: *The total care of spinal cord injuries,* Boston, 1977, Little, Brown.
5. Riley L: Surgical approaches to the anterior structures of the cervical spine, *Clin Orthop* 91:10, 1973.
6. Robinson RA: *The craft of surgery,* ed 2, Boston, 1971, Little, Brown.
7. Robinson RA, Southwick WO: Surgical approaches to the cervical spine. In *AAOS instructional course lectures,* vol 17, St Louis, 1960, Mosby.

◆

Chapter Seventeen

Microscopic Posterior Foraminotomy for Cervical Radiculopathy

David R. Campbell
William H. Dillin

The clinical features of posterior foraminotomy for the treatment of cervical radiculopathy can be divided into four different groups. Three of the groups are distinguished by differences in the underlying pathologic condition and include cervical radiculopathy from a posterolateral soft disc herniation, cervical radiculopathy from foraminal stenosis due to osteophyte encroachment into the cervical neural foramen, and radiculopathy after a failed anterior cervical disc excision and fusion that has developed a pseudarthrosis. The fourth group includes the athletic patient who has cervical radiculopathy from one of these causes. This fourth group differs not in the underlying pathologic condition but rather in the functional and biomechanical demands placed on the operated cervical spine. Athletes with cervical radiculopathy due to either a soft posterolateral disc herniation or to foraminal stenosis from bony encroachment of the neural foramen require a treatment approach that accommodates the increased demand that has been and will be placed on the cervical spine. Individuals involved in both recreational and competitive athletic activities often have incorporated their commitment to training into their life-style. Dedication to improvement within their chosen sport is generally reflected by long hours of training, trips to competitive events, and sacrifice of other pleasurable activities for the sake of the sport. These individuals expect and demand an excellent result from any surgical treatment aimed at relieving pain, weakness, or numbness in the affected extremity. It is encumbent on the treating orthopaedic surgeon or neurosurgeon to recognize that this group of individuals with cervical radiculopathy differs from other, nonathletic patients with the same spinal disorder. The desired postoperative goals in athletes must include the prompt relief of pain, weakness, or numbness in the extremity; the early return to unencumbered functional activities; a timely return to their premorbid level of conditioning and training; and, perhaps most important, a durable operative outcome with minimal risk of long-term problems, such as advanced degenerative disc disease in adjacent nonoperated levels. A thorough review of the available literature has failed to reveal any published series of posterolateral cervical foraminotomy classified accord-

ing to the athletic demand placed on the operated spine. Therefore we will review the surgical history of the first three groups and discuss our approach at the Kerlan-Jobe Orthopaedic Clinic to the recreational or competitive athlete with isolated cervical radiculopathy, including nonoperative treatment, surgical recommendations, and postoperative rehabilitative protocol and restrictions.

MICROSCOPIC POSTERIOR CERVICAL FORAMINOTOMY

Microscopic posterior cervical foraminotomy, also known as posterolateral microdiscectomy, has been documented extensively in the literature as an effective and safe method of surgical treatment of cervical radiculopathy caused by posterolateral disc herniations and cervical foraminal stenosis. Specific contraindications to the procedure have included cervical myelopathy and central disc herniations with bilateral upper extremity symptoms. However, judging from the larger volume of available literature documenting the similarly safe and effective treatment of cervical radiculopathy with anterior surgical procedures, posterolateral cervical foraminotomy may be underused. The reasons for this underuse may be related to the increased diagnostic demand placed on the surgeon to ensure proper patient selection and excellent clinical outcome.

Posterior cervical foraminotomy has uncontested and distinct advantages over anterior procedures, such as no risk of injury to anterior cervical structures, no donor bone graft site pain, and no stress concentration at adjacent spinal motion units. The potential disadvantages include postoperative neck and muscle discomfort, spinal instability and facet fractures, injury to neural structures, and, possibly, incomplete neural decompression. The disadvantages have been addressed by the microsurgical techniques currently used, which employ a smaller incision and a minimal partial unilateral facetectomy, often with less than 20% of the medial facet joint requiring resection. Inappropriate patient selection for this procedure remains a potential disadvantage and requires careful attention to the details of the physical examination and the diagnostic imaging studies.

Aldrich[1] recently reviewed his surgical experience with posterolateral microdiscectomy for cervical monoradiculopathy caused by posterolateral cervical disc sequestration. Over a 5-year period he identified 53 patients who had acute monoradiculopathy caused by soft cervical disc herniation; 36 were included in this study when they were identified as having a posterolateral soft disc sequestration on computed tomography (CT) myelography. His treatment policy has evolved to include an anterior approach for central disc protrusions, a posterolateral microdiscectomy for posterolateral sequestrations, and either an anterior or a posterior approach for paracentral disc protrusions. He defined a paracentral protrusion as one that compresses both the dura and the nerve root sleeve on CT myelography. (The posterolateral disc herniation only obliterates the cervical nerve root with minimal compression of the spinal dura.) Immediate postoperative pain relief and motor improvement occurred in all patients. Only 7 of 21 patients with preoperative numbness had improvement in the numbness by the time of discharge. At the 26-month mean follow-up, no relapses had occurred, all patients were symptom free, and any neck pain (present in 7 of 8 patients) had resolved.

Herkowitz, Kurz, and Overholt[22] published a prospective report of their results with the surgical management of cervical soft disc herniation. These authors compared anterior cervical discectomy, including autogenous iliac crest bone graft fusion, with posterior laminotomy/foraminotomy. An analysis of the data on the patients in their study showed that the improvement (excellent/good/fair) was slightly better for anterior fusion versus posterior laminotomy in the treatment of posterolateral cervical disc herniations (100% and 93%, respectively). However, they found a wide difference in the percentage of excellent/good results when they compared anterior discectomy and fusion with posterior laminotomy (94% versus 75%, respectively). There remains a substantial volume of orthopaedic and neurosurgical literature that documents a high percentage of good to excellent results with both the anterior and the posterior approach to the neck for cervical radiculopathy.*

Simeone and Dillin[41] commented on their findings in the second group of patients with cervical radiculopathy: those with foraminal stenosis caused by osteophyte encroachment into the neural foramen. They found the results of posterolateral foraminotomy for either soft disc herniations or hard disc herniations (e.g., osteophytes) to be similar. The presence of osteophytes projecting from the adjacent joint of Luschka or bony ridges protruding from the edge of the vertebral body at the disc space level may be associated with more chronic symptoms than the acute soft disc herniation. The possibility for increased periradicular fibrosis in chronic cases suggests that a more cautious approach to the hard disc is indicated. Lunsford et al.[32] mirrored this finding

in patients undergoing anterior cervical discectomy, with no difference in outcome identified between hard or soft disc herniations that were surgically decompressed.

The third group of patients includes those with cervical radiculopathy and a pseudarthrosis of the cervical spine after anterior discectomy and arthrodesis. These patients represent a failure of the original surgical intervention. A recent study of the surgical treatment of these patients included the technique of posterior nerve root decompression with a posterolateral foraminotomy approach, coupled with wire fixation and posterior bone graft arthrodesis. Farey et al.[13] studied 19 patients who had symptomatic pseudarthrosis after a failed anterior cervical arthrodesis. All patients had cervical pain and radiculopathy with pain, paresthesia, hypoesthesia, or muscle weakness present in different combinations. Their operative technique included a standard posterolateral foraminotomy with a Bohlman triple-wire technique[49] spinal fusion with autogenous unicortical iliac crest bone graft. They achieved solid arthrodesis in all patients, and the radiculopathy was relieved in all but one.

The use of posterolateral foraminotomy for cervical radiculopathy in athletes has not been evaluated in any well-controlled clinical trial. At the Kerlan-Jobe Orthopaedic Clinic we have used this operative approach in many of our athletic patients. Several details related to the anterior versus the posterior approach to cervical radiculopathy have contributed to this choice of operative technique in athletes, including decreased rehabilitation time, decreased time to presurgery levels of training, no donor bone graft site pain, no possible meralgia paresthetica, decreased biomechanical alterations of the cervical spine, and an unaltered natural history of cervical spondylosis above or below the operative level.[26,48]

CERVICAL RADICULOPATHY
Natural History

Contemporary surgical treatment, with microscopic technique, for cervical radiculopathy is often recommended after an appropriate but unsuccessful nonoperative treatment regimen. The concern in this group of patients is that failure to surgically relieve the mechanical compression on the affected nerve root will lead to permanent neurologic dysfunction.

Lees and Turner[30] analyzed the natural history of cervical radiculopathy and found that it rarely progresses to a myelopathic state. These two entities are quite separate in their clinical signs and symptoms. However, these authors did find that persistent symptomatology in patients with cervical radiculopathy that was not treated surgically was not an exceptional condition. Two thirds of the patients who were not operated on manifested persistent symptoms.

Rothman and Simeone[40] evaluated the natural his-

* References 1, 10, 11, 21, 22, 28, 32, 45.

tory of cervical disc degeneration in 68 patients treated conservatively for 5 years; 69% had neck and radicular pain, and 31% had only neck pain. At 5-year follow-up, 45% who had not had surgery were considered to have satisfactory results; 55% had unsatisfactory results, and of these, 23% were considered disabled. By comparing their surgical results with those obtained in their unoperated patients, the authors were able to conclude that surgery for neck pain alone, without radiculopathy, does not significantly alter the natural course of the disease.

In his study, Aldrich[1] identified an important subgroup of patients in whom the acute radiculopathy pain cleared after a few weeks, but who had progression of their motor findings despite conservative treatment. He believed that delay in recognizing and surgically treating this group might lead to residual nerve damage.

The basic science literature supports the clinical observation that persistent nerve root compression will lead to residual intrinsic nerve damage. A compressive neuropathy leads to deformation of the intraneural vascular bed, which results in impairment of nutritive blood flow in the nerve roots.[17] Prolonged or repeated vascular compression leads to increased permeability of the blood vessels, resulting in intraneural edema formation.[35] The resultant intraneural edema may adversely affect the nerve impulses and potentially allow for the development of intraneural fibrosis with residual nerve damage. Experimental constriction of the cauda equina in dogs has shown that constriction of 50% or more of the nerve root diameter leads to edema, loss of myelin, venous congestion, blockage of axoplasmic flow, and wallerian degeneration distal to the constriction. This constriction also causes severe arterial narrowing and, ultimately, complete nerve root atrophy.[6]

Incidence

The incidence of cervical radiculopathy in the population can be studied by asking the question "How many individuals develop cervical radiculopathy within a given segment of the population per year?" Hult[25] estimated that 51% of the adult population will experience neck and arm pain at some point. Kondo et al.[28] studied cervical radiculopathy and found it to be a significant health problem commonly causing morbidity in patients during their prime working years: 35 to 54 years of age. The incidence of cervical radiculopathy was found to be 5.5 per 100,000 persons per year. Kelsey et al.[27] analyzed acute cervical disc disease and found a strong predilection among individuals who lift heavy objects or smoke cigarettes and among competitive divers; they noted a borderline increased incidence among those who operate vibrating equipment and ride for prolonged intervals in cars. Boden et al.[2] prospectively studied 63 volunteers with no history of symptoms, using cervical magnetic resonance imaging (MRI). The incidence of abnormal

scans in those asymptomatic volunteers less than 40 years old was 14%. In volunteers older than 40 years, the incidence was 28%. The existence of abnormal radiographic findings in asymptomatic persons has been confirmed in other studies using discography (Holt[24]) and plain roentgenograms (Friedenberg and Miller[15]).

It is also relevant to ask the question "Which cervical levels are likely to be causing symptomatic cervical radiculopathy?" Most studies indicate that cervical disc herniation is most common at the C5-6 level, followed by C6-7, C4-5, C3-4, and C7-T1,[21,32] with the frequency almost zero at more cephaled levels. However, we recently treated a professional baseball player who had unilateral atrophy of the trapezius and sternocleidomastoid muscles. He also had a painful neck and shoulder region but no sensory deficit. He was found to have a posterolateral herniated cervical disc at C2-3. CT myelography revealed compression of the third cervical nerve root. This patient had consulted several orthopaedic surgeons and neurosurgeons about this unusual disorder until an astute neurologist was able to make the diagnosis. The loss of motor contribution of the third cervical nerve root to the spinal accessory nerve was thought to be the underlying compressive neuropathy.

History

The presenting complaints of cervical radiculopathy vary in their chronicity, severity, and dermatomal distribution. The athlete, by virtue of his or her dedication to the sport, may come to the physician after months to years of symptoms, especially when the underlying pathologic condition is more insidious (e.g., caused by foraminal narrowing and degenerative disc disease). The athlete may, however, have an acute disc herniation with profound motor weakness and functional disability before muscle atrophy is readily apparent.

The term *cervical radiculopathy* is commonly used to describe pain in the distribution of a specific cervical nerve root.[9] It also encompasses numbness, paresthesias, dysesthesias, and motor weakness in the dermatomal or myotomal distribution of an affected nerve root. Cervical radiculopathy is distinct from cervical myelopathy in terms of the underlying pathologic compression of neurologic structures. Cervical myelopathy is characterized by compression of the spinal cord, whereas cervical radiculopathy is characterized by compression of cervical nerve roots. Early in the clinical course of cervical myelopathy, the neurologic manifestations of spinal cord compression may be quite subtle. A report of vague symptoms with no objective neurologic findings is not unusual. Subtle changes in the gait pattern or loss of fine manual dexterity of the hands may be the only early sign of myelopathy. Pain is not a helpful symptom in the diagnosis of cervical myelopathy, which is in sharp contrast to the clinical presentation of cervical nerve root compression. Patients with nerve root compression generally complain of pain as their most bothersome symptom. The pain typically begins in the cervical region, radiating into the interscapular region, shoulder region, or distally into the arm, forearm, and fingers. The arm and hand pain of cervical radiculopathy is generally greater than any neck pain that the patient may complain of. However, mild neck pain and restriction in cervical spine flexibility are common. The neck pain may be discogenic and referred to the posterior cervical region or shoulder region, or it may represent a more proximal nerve root compressive neuropathy with true radicular pain in the distribution of the more cephalad nerve roots.[39] Radiating arm pain in cervical radiculopathy follows the distribution of the primary anterior division of the nerve root and may be localized by the patient anywhere in the distribution of that root.[39] The failure of radicular pain to follow an understandable neurologic pattern should raise some suspicion of an alternate diagnosis.[8]

Williams[45] studied 235 patients treated with micro-cervical foraminotomy for intractable radicular pain, the majority of whom had experienced pain for months or years. He found that trauma was stated as the precipitating factor in 27%, 81% of these representing industrial compensation cases. He also found that discogenic neck pain was associated with radicular pain in 40%, with the majority of patients in his series demonstrating objective neurologic deficits. He found radicular pain associated with myelopathy in only 1% of cases. The anatomic distribution of pain, weakness, sensory abnormalities, and reflex changes are specific for each individual nerve root.[41]

The symptoms of cervical radiculopathy generally associated with herniated cervical disc or foraminal stenosis may also be caused by metastatic tumors of the spine, spinal cord or spinal canal, primary neoplasms of the spine, trauma to the spine, inflammatory disorders, nerve root tumors, nerve root entrapment, reflex sympathetic dystrophy, or the thoracic outlet syndrome. The thoracic outlet syndrome or other lesions of the brachial plexus may mimic cervical radiculopathy quite closely. Herpes zoster (shingles) typically affects a single intercostal nerve, causing pain in a specific dermatomal pattern. Inflammation of a cervical root by herpes zoster would be unusual but may cause symptoms of cervical radiculopathy that would be quite difficult to differentiate from other causes. Bilateral or multiple cervical root involvement may result from extensive degenerative disc disease with foraminal stenosis or herniated intervertebral discs at more than one level. The pain associated with cervical radiculopathy may be associated with straining, sneezing, coughing, or performing overhead activites with neck extension. Patients may note that extending their neck or turning the head to the affected side exacerbates their radicular pain, and they may compensate for this loss of functional range of motion by turning their shoulders and torso with their head.

Henderson et al.,[21] in their study of 846 consecutive operative cases for cervical radiculopathy, found that 53% of patients had pain or paresthesias in a dermatomal pattern, whereas 45% had pain that did not follow a dermatomal pattern. In addition, 79% had neck pain, 52% had scapular region pain, 17% had anterior chest pain, and 9% had headaches. Aldrich[1] reported on 36 patients with single-level monoradiculopathy as their chief complaint. Twenty-four of these patients had very minor neck symptoms that caused little discomfort. Twenty-five of these patients related a history of injury or a specific incident as a cause of their symptoms. Aldrich found that the older patients in his group who had preexisting cervical spondylosis more commonly had experienced severe cervical discomfort for variable periods of time in the past than had the younger patients, who had less degenerative disc disease and spondylosis in the cervical spine.

Patients who had cervical radiculopathy associated with pseudarthrosis after anterior cervical discectomy were reported on by Farey et al.[13] These authors found that the symptoms in their patients, including pain, paresthesia, hypoesthesia, or muscle weakness, corresponded to a nerve root distribution and were similar to the preoperative symptoms. However, not all patients who develop pseudarthrosis after attempted anterior cervical fusion have recurrent symptoms, as evidenced by DePalma et al.[7] in their series of 150 patients, of whom 12% developed a pseudarthrosis after attempted anterior cervical fusion. These authors felt that the presence of a pseudarthrosis after anterior cervical discectomy and a bone graft attempt at fusion did not affect the quality of the final result. In our experience, the athlete with cervical radiculopathy is most commonly afflicted by the acute onset of arm pain and motor deficit secondary to an extruded intervertebral disc fragment. There are no well-documented reports that have evaluated athletes separately from nonathletic patients for any differences in their clinical presentation, incidence of disease, etiology of disease, or outcome after treatment for cervical radiculopathy.

Physical Examination

The history, physical examination, and location of the offending pathologic condition on diagnostic imaging studies are the key determinants in deciding on an anterior or a posterior surgical approach to the spine for cervical radiculopathy. The two critical components of the physical examination needed to consider a microscopic posterolateral foraminotomy are a positive hyperextension test (Spurling's maneuver) and a positive shoulder abduction test. Spurling's maneuver was described in 1956 in Spurling's textbook on cervical radiculopathy.[44] This maneuver includes extension coupled with lateral flexion of the head and neck toward the painful side. Reproduction or exacerbation of the pain or paresthesia in the involved nerve root distribution is considered a positive finding. Garfin, Rydevik, and Brown[17] reviewed the biologic response to nerve root mechanical deformation in both normal nerve roots and in nerve roots that had been irritated by a compression lesion, such as a herniated disc or foraminal stenosis. In their review of the experimental literature, including studies by Lundborg et al.,[31] MacNab,[33] Smyth and Wright,[42] Greenbarg et al.,[19] and others, Garfin, Rydevik, and Brown[17] concluded that inflammation of the nerve root tissue is a critical factor that has to be present before mechanical nerve root deformation will give rise to pain.

With Spurling's maneuver, the neural foramina of the cervical spine on the side to which the neck is laterally flexed are narrowed. Mechanical impingement of the nerve root by a herniated disc, osteophyte, or hypertrophic facet joint in an already irritated nerve root will reproduce the patient's pain. A positive response to Spurling's maneuver localizes the mechanical impingement to the level of the neural foramen.

Davidson et al.[5] observed a series of over 200 patients with cervical radiculopathy due to osteophytes and herniated cervical discs in whom clinical signs included marked relief of radicular pain with abduction of the shoulder. The shoulder abduction test is a sign that can be elicited by having the patient position the affected arm overhead with the palm resting on the top of the head and then describe whether the arm pain is relieved. The precise mechanism by which shoulder abduction relieves radicular pain is presumed to be related to the decreased tension placed on the root, by shortening the distance between the brachial plexus and the nerve roots, as well as directly elevating the sensory root cephalad or lateral to the offending osteophyte or herniated disc.

It can be appreciated that multiple root involvement is possible, especially in the patient with significant underlying degenerative cervical disc disease and foraminal stenosis. In persons with multiple root involvement, there may be a confusing overlap of the objective findings that requires close correlation with both diagnostic imaging studies and electrodiagnostic studies. CT, myelography, CT myelography, and MRI are the standard diagnostic imaging studies obtained today for the radiologic evaluation of cervical radiculopathy. The neurodiagnostic studies are also important tools to assist in the precise localization of the offending pathology in patients with multiple cervical levels that appear abnormal on the imaging studies. These neurodiagnostic studies include electromyograms (EMG), nerve conduction velocities (NCV) and evoked potentials (sematosensory [SSEP], dermatosensory [DSEP], and motor [MEP]).

Diagnostic Tests

Magnetic resonance imaging. MRI has become the most common diagnostic imaging method used to study cervical radiculopathy. The quality of MRI has improved in the last few years to the point that the resolution of soft tissue and bony structures on MRI is comparable to the resolution of structures on CT myelography. The use of image-enhancing agents, such as gadolinium, and specialized pulse-sequence techniques used in high-quality powerful MRI machines, certainly has made MRI an excellent imaging technique to study cervical radiculopathy. Wilson, Pezzuti, and Place[46] studied the use of MRI in the preoperative evaluation of cervical radiculopathy and now regard MRI as the initial procedure of choice and usually the only preoperative study necessary. In their retrospective review of 40 cases of cervical radiculopathy, they used effacement of the subarachnoid space in the vicinity of the nerve root as the primary criterion for the interpretation of clinically significant lesions. In their study MRI correctly demonstrated a herniated nucleus pulposus in 84% of cases. They had a 92% success rate in demonstrating a cervical lesion, which included herniated nucleus pulposus and/or spondylosis. Modic et al.[34] studied cervical radiculopathy in a prospective evaluation with surface-coil MRI, contrast CT, and metrizamide myelography. MRI and CT myelography both had a sensitivity of 83% for herniated discs in a study of 28 patients undergoing surgery for cervical radiculopathy. In that same study, MRI was slightly less successful than CT myelography in differentiating herniated discs from osteophytes.

The difficulty in distinguishing osteophytes from herniated discs was lessened by the use of a gradient-echo imaging sequence rather than a spin-echo sequence by Hedberg et al.[20] in 1988. These authors found that with the gradient-echo sequence the sensitivity in differentiating osteophytes from herniated discs in patients evaluated for cervical radiculopathy was 93%. The drawback of gradient-echo sequencing is that the imaging time is increased over the imaging time necessary for spin-echo sequencing techniques.

MRI has a comparable efficacy in the diagnosis of clinically significant spinal pathology in patients with cervical radiculopathy. There have not been any detectable health risks associated with MRI, and the MRI often costs less than a CT myelogram of the cervical spine. Perhaps the one difficulty with MRI has been the patient's intolerance of the confining atmosphere of the MRI unit, and this at times has required the use of sedative-type medications to overcome the claustrophobic tendencies of some patients. The axial images are most helpful in delineating the precise location of pathologic structures impinging on the nerve root. Thus we agree with others[34] that high-quality MRI is the first choice for diagnostic imaging in patients with cervical radiculopathy. However, the difference in quality of images obtained from different MRI units can be striking, and we would caution against accepting poor-quality images that would make the precise interpretation of the film and the precise localization of the pathologic condition more difficult than with high-quality MRI. The sensitivities noted in the published information related to MRI in the diagnosis of cervical radiculopathy have been reported from centers that generally have higher-quality machines and newer software that enables increased resolution.

It is critical that the diagnostic imaging findings, whether MRI, CT, or myelography, correlate precisely with the patient's symptoms, physical findings, and neurologic studies. Investigations with plain radiography, myelography, CT, and MRI have shown the frequent occurrence of degenerative disc disease of the cervical spine in patients without any clinical symptoms. Boden et al.[2] recently defined the incidence of abnormal cervical spine MRI findings in asymptomatic volunteers. They conclusively demonstrated the necessity for correlating all patient data before making a decision to perform surgery.

CT myelography. Before the advent of CT more than a decade ago, oil-soluble myelography was a common diagnostic method used in patients with radiculopathy. With the more recent introduction of safer water-soluble contrast agents for myelography, the use of CT after the introduction of intrathecal contrast media has improved diagnostic capabilities over noncontrast CT or myelography without contrast agents. A recent study by Brown et al.[4] of 34 patients undergoing surgery for cervical radiculopathy and myelopathy found that MRI correctly revealed a herniated disc in 91% of cases. These authors determined the accuracy of imaging methods in detecting all types of lesions responsible for the cervical radiculopathy and myelopathy and found that 88% were detected correctly with MRI, 81% with CT myelography, 58% with myelography, and 50% with CT. The lesions responsible for the radiculopathy or myelopathy included herniated nucleus pulposus, osteophytes, neoplasm, and syrinx.

A study comparing myelography, CT myelography, and MRI for cervical spondylosis and disc degeneration, performed both preoperatively and postoperatively on 26 patients, showed that MRI, CT myelography, and myelography were of comparable accuracy in detecting lesions causing nerve root compression.[29] These authors recommended the replacement of CT myelography with MRI in the preoperative evaluation of patients with cervical radiculopathy. The use of gradient-echo sequencing on the axial MRI scans gives the cerebrospinal fluid an increased signal intensity, the bone a decreased signal intensity, and the disc material an intermediate signal intensity, allowing for images that are similar to CT myelography without the inherent risks and discomfort associated with CT myelography.[46]

CT without intrathecal contrast enhancement for the diagnosis and preoperative evaluation of cervical radiculopathy is not typically used at our institution because of the much more precise information available from MRI or CT myelography. Similarly, plain myelography without CT generally does not provide additional useful information in the preoperative planning of patients with cervical radiculopathy over and above CT myelography or MRI.

Electromyography and nerve conduction velocities. The radicular pattern of pain, paresthesias, and numbness; the pattern of motor weakness; the presence of reflex changes; the presence of sensory abnormalities to light touch and pinprick testing; and the diagnostic imaging findings generally represent a sufficient data base on which a precise operative plan can be formulated. In some cases of cervical radiculopathy, however, there may be several suspected areas of pathologic nerve root impingement within an apparent overlap of clinical findings. Or there may be findings that do not correlate with the normal anatomic radicular patterns that one would expect to find. In these unusual and diagnostically challenging cases, patient evaluation with neurodiagnostic studies, such as electromyography (EMG), nerve conduction velocities (NCVs), or somatosensory-evoked potentials (SSEPs) may be helpful in clarifying a confusing diagnostic picture.

Somatosensory-evoked potentials. The use of SSEPs to assess the adequacy of neural decompression for lumbar nerve root decompressive surgery has been well documented.[18,22] However, there are no well-documented studies of intraoperative SSEPs used for the evaluation of neural decompression during surgery for cervical radiculopathy in order to predict the postoperative clinical outcome. Herron et al.,[23] in a study of the intraoperative use of SSEPs in lumbar stenosis surgery, found that decreases in the latency of the operated side correlated with the surgeon's assessment of the adequacy of decompression. They found the use of SSEPs helpful in assessing the adequacy of neural decompression intraoperatively. Gepstein and Brown[18] published a report on the use of SSEPs to assess the adequacy of lumbar nerve root decompression for spinal stenosis and herniated disc surgery. They also considered intraoperative physiologic testing with SSEPs to be valuable in determining the adequacy of lumbar nerve root decompression and for the prediction of the successful relief of symptoms. In surgery for cervical radiculopathy we occasionally use this method of intraoperative physiologic monitoring. We have been impressed by the consistent improvement seen in both the latency and the amplitude of the evoked potentials after successful decompression of the affected nerve root. Perhaps the most useful aspect of using SSEPs intraoperatively is that the surgeon can feel confident before leaving the operating room that the correct spinal nerve root has been decompressed, as evidenced by marked improvement in the latency and amplitude, and thus decreasing the possibility of surgery at the wrong spinal level.

PREOPERATIVE PREPARATION

The development and implementation of an efficient routine to prepare patients for surgery is critical to the smooth transition of the patient from the office setting to hospital admission and through surgical and postsurgical rehabilitation. An up-to-date review of all diagnostic studies available shortly before the surgery, coupled with a current assessment of the patient's symptoms and physical findings, will avoid wrong-level surgery and inappropriate surgery by correlating the pathology with the symptoms and signs. A careful review of the cervical MRI scan or CT myelogram should rule out the more unusual and unexpected findings that could cause cervical radiculopathy, such as spinal infection, spinal cord tumor, metastic spine tumor, or a more peripheral nerve root or brachial plexus entrapment mimicking cervical radiculopathy. Obtaining operative consent and blood transfusion consent (required in some states) can be addressed in the office setting to allow for a complete discussion with the patient of the proposed procedure so that there is complete understanding of the alternatives to surgery, risks of surgery, and potential benefit of surgery.

Autologous blood donation is offered to all surgical patients, by law, in the State of California. Preoperative medical evaluation and clearance is routinely performed by the patient's internist to assess systemic diseases. The internist, after evaluation of the medical condition of the patient, should make recommendations for preoperative optimization of the patient's medical condition, if necessary, as well as perioperative and postoperative medical recommendations. We believe that each patient should be offered HIV testing preoperatively in accordance with the current local laws and hospital policy.

The cessation of smoking is required of all preoperative patients because of the increased risk of infection[14] and decreased capacity for wound healing in smokers.[38] We recommend that aspirin products and nonsteroidal antiinflammatory medications, narcotics, muscle relaxants, and sleeping pills be stopped before surgery. The patient is asked to shampoo the night before surgery. Compressive lower extremity stockings are applied the morning of surgery.

OPERATIVE PROCEDURE

Loupe magnification or the operating microscope is used throughout the procedure. Additional special instruments include the micro–bipolar electrocautery, high-speed burr, blunt micro–nerve hook, No. 4 micro-Penfield dissector, 45-degree microrongeur, and the microcurette.

The Mayfield three-pin head holder, or the horseshoe

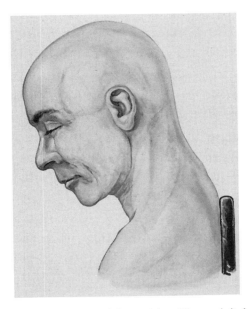

Fig. 17-1. Patient in the upright position. The occipital scalp is sufficiently shaved to tape the head in place and to allow operative preparation of the surgical field. (From Dyck P: Cervical foraminotomy: indications and technique. In Watkins RG, editor: *Surgical approaches to the spine*, New York, 1983, Springer-Verlag.)

head holder, is used to support the head. Skeletal pin fixation remains an option, but the horseshoe headrest is preferred. Use of the seated position depends on preference (Fig. 17-1).[11,45] However, the intraoperative seated position in cervical spine surgery may have an increased risk of intraoperative air embolism, and care must be taken to avoid this. After the patient is positioned prone, on chest bolsters, the knees are bent 90 degrees and secured with a padded upright knee-stop attachment on the operating table. The shoulders are gently retracted with very wide adhesive tape attached from the shoulders to the foot of the operating table. This allows for the lower cervical levels to be properly visualized on the intraoperative radiograph. The eyes, elbows, and knees are particularly protected. The anesthesiologist is asked during the case to recheck the eyes for any malposition of the head holders that may cause pressure to be exerted on the eyes. The pedal pulses should be assessed both before and after positioning. The shoulders are not abducted beyond 90 degrees to avoid brachial plexus neurapraxia. The neck is placed in a neutral position with the chin slightly tucked in toward the chest. This allows the cervical spine to straighten out, widening the neural foramen and enhancing the surgical exposure. In addition, Dyck[10] uses slight lateral flexion contralateral to the painful side to further enlarge the neural foramen.

SSEPs may be used throughout the procedure to monitor both the spinal cord and the specific nerve roots

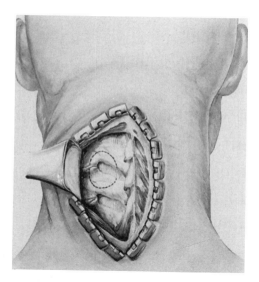

Fig. 17-2. The incision should extend two spinous processes above and two below the desired level. The skin and subcutaneous tissue are opened, the subcutaneous tissue is undercut slightly, and hemostatic Raney clips are applied. After placement of the self-retaining retractor and incision of the trapezius fascia, the muscle mass on either side of the lesion is retracted. Either a periosteal elevator or a cutting electrocautery is used to remove the paraspinous musculature from the spinous process and the lamina of the involved side. (From Dyck P: Cervical foraminotomy: indications and technique. In Watkins RG, editor: *Surgical approaches to the spine,* New York, 1983, Springer-Verlag.)

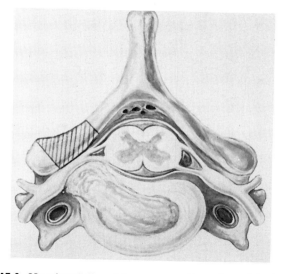

Fig. 17-3. Herniated disc. After x-ray confirmation of the level, the medial two thirds *(shaded area)* of the zygapophyseal joint is exposed. (From Dyck P: Cervical foraminotomy: indications and technique. In Watkins RG, editor: *Surgical approaches to the spine,* New York, 1983, Springer-Verlag.)

to be decompressed. However, evoked potentials are only an adjunct to the surgeon's technical assessment of the adequacy of neural decompression.

General anesthesia with endotracheal intubation is used in 100% of our cases. The skin should be shaved up to the occiput. After positioning, preparation, and draping, a lateral x-ray film with paraspinous needles can better limit the skin incision, and a midline skin incision is made through the superficial dermis. Epinephrine solution, 1:500,000, may be injected into the paraspinal musculature to enhance hemostasis, if desired. It is important to incise the skin before piercing it with the needle to avoid introducing a piece of plastic skin drape deep into the wound. The incision is carried sharply down to the bulbous spinous processes at this point. A self-retaining retractor is placed deep into the wound. The trapezius fascia is then incised, allowing the introduction of a Langenbach elevator to subperiosteally dissect the splenius and semispinalis capita, the lower semispinalis cervicis, and the multifidus muscles off of the spinous processes and lamina of the two adjacent levels (Fig. 17-2).[10] Hemostasis is achieved with electrocautery, with care taken to avoid contacting the ligamentum flavum and particularly any underlying dura, nerve root sleeve, or neural structures. The electrocautery power on both the cutting and coagulation modes should

be turned down to the minimum effective level. This dissection is carried out to the midportion of the cervical zygoapophyseal joint (facet joint), retaining the lateral joint capsule.

An intraoperative lateral radiograph is obtained at this time, with a Kocher clamp attached to each of the adjacent two spinous processes to precisely define the surgical level. A high-speed drill (e.g., Midas Rex AM-3) is used to thin the overlying superior facet, and to a lesser extent, the inferior facet from the underlying neural foramen (Fig. 17-3). From 20% to 50% of the medial facet with its overlying capsule is removed. The posterior cortical shell and the intervening cancellous bone is drilled until only a thin cortical shell remains, covering the nerve (Fig. 17-4). Intermittent irrigation during the drilling keeps the bone cool and protects the underlying neural structures while enhancing exposure. A micro-curette and micro-Kerrison rongeur can then be used to delicately remove the remaining ligamentum flavum and cortical bone. Bone wax is used to control medullary bone bleeding. Williams[45] believes that coagulating instruments should not be used for hemostasis once neural structures are exposed, although we have not identified any complications from the use of the micro–bipolar electrocautery on the extradural veins. The risk of increased scar formation after use of electrocautery about the neural structures is always considered, and, when possible, Gelfoam pads soaked in thrombin and small cotton pledgets are used as hemostatic agents instead of electrocautery.

The three-dimensional path of the nerve root is determined by gentle palpation with a micro–nerve hook

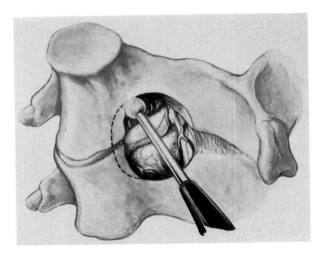

Fig. 17-4. With the burr, the inferolateral lamina of the vertebra above and the superolateral lamina of the vertebra below are cautiously removed. The interposed flavum comes away with the bony removal. (From Dyck P: Cervical foraminotomy: indications and technique. In Watkins RG, editor: *Surgical approaches to the spine,* New York, 1983, Springer-Verlag.)

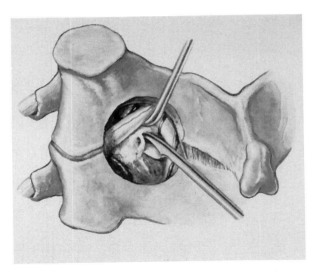

Fig. 17-5. Chisels and curettes may be used to remove osteophytes arising in the vertebral disc space and osteophytes emanating from the joint of Luschka. (From Dyck P: Cervical foraminotomy: indications and technique. In Watkins RG, editor: *Surgical approaches to the spine,* New York, 1983, Springer-Verlag.)

or Woodson dental tool and direct observation. This allows a microcurette to safely enlarge and remove the remaining thinned superior and inferior edges of the neural foramen without putting pressure on the neural elements. Once any tight stenotic lesions have been relieved by the microcurette technique, microrongeurs are used to widely hollow the foraminal walls from the entrance to the outlet.[45] When soft disc protrusion is encountered, it may be an extrusion of a substantial part of the nucleus pulposus, requiring delicate handling of the nerve.[10] All easily accessible extruded fragments are teased free of the neural foramen and removed. No attempt is made to enter the disc space, however. For hard disc protrusions or osteophytes, the curved and straight microcurettes may be used to remove these bony projections, if this can be safely done without undue neural trauma. Both osteophytes arising from the edges of the intervertebral disc space and osteophytes protruding into the nerve root axilla from the joint of Luschka can be removed[10] (Figs. 17-5 to 17-8). In chronic cases, with a long history of symptoms, there may be significant adherence of the nerve root to the foraminal wall by fibrosis. Care must be taken to avoid injury to the neural tissue and to avoid a tear in the nerve root sleeve, with subsequent spinal fluid leak requiring repair.

Aldrich[1] identified only three nerve roots with a periradicular fibrous cuff in a series of 36 patients. All three patients had chronic radicular symptoms. In the remainder of his patients, the nerve and sequestered disc were covered by a thin layer of venous-laden, loose,

fibrous tissue. We incise the venous cuff if the root is not clearly pulsatile after adequate decompression. A final check of the evoked potentials is done at this time.

Wound closure is accomplished over a Hemovac drain after copious irrigation and meticulous hemostasis is achieved. No fat graft or absorbable gelatin is left in the wound. The wound is closed in multiple layers. We use a rigid foam collar for patient comfort postoperatively. Generally, we have the patient begin gentle isometric aquatic exercises at 3 weeks. By 6 weeks a trunk stability program of isometric exercises may be initiated. The chest-out posturing stressed as part of our trunk stabilization program effectively brings the head back over the shoulders, squares off the shoulders, and positions the neck in a more comfortable, biomechanically sound position.

BIOMECHANICS OF POSTERIOR CERVICAL FORAMINOTOMY
Stability

The classic definition of clinical spine instability was given by White, Southwick, and Panjabi[47] in 1976. They defined "instability as the loss of the ability of the spine, under physiologic loads, to maintain relationships between vertebrae in such a way that there is neither damage or subsequent irritation to the spinal cord or nerve roots and, in addition, no development of deformity with excessive pain."

The minimally invasive approach to the posterior cervical spine using microscopic dissection techniques

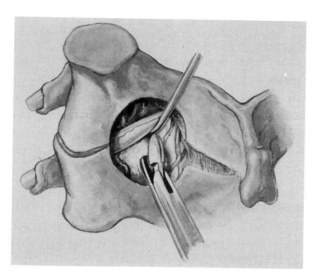

Fig. 17-6. The pituitary rongeur may be used to remove the disc. (From Dyck P: Cervical foraminotomy: indications and technique. In Watkins RG, editor: *Surgical approaches to the spine,* New York, 1983, Springer-Verlag.)

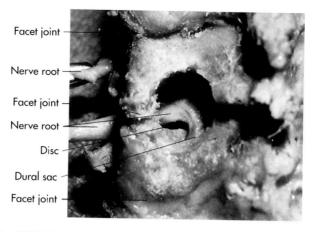

Fig. 17-7. Nerve root and disc space in the intervertebral foramen without the veins. (From Dyck P: Cervical foraminotomy: indications and technique. In Watkins RG, editor: *Surgical approaches to the spine,* New York, 1983, Springer-Verlag.)

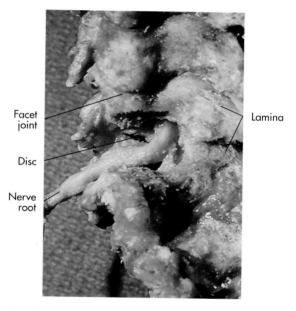

Fig. 17-8. Ventral retraction of the nerve root shows the intervertebral disc. (From Dyck P: Cervical foraminotomy: indications and technique. In Watkins RG, editor: *Surgical approaches to the spine,* New York, 1983, Springer-Verlag.)

and minimal removal of bone and ligament affords protection of the stability of the operated spinal motion unit. Unlike the alternative anterior cervical discectomy with fusion, the posterior foraminotomy approach avoids the potential for alteration of the biomechanical functioning of the adjacent spinal motion units. Unlike anterior discectomy without fusion, the posterior foraminotomy approach avoids the collapse of the intervertebral disc space with subsequent localized kyphosis. The technique of anterior cervical fractional interspace decompression using microscopic techniques for the treatment of cervical radiculopathy has been described by Snyder and Bernhardt.[43] This approach provides adequate neuroforaminal decompressions but avoids segmental collapse, or fusion. These authors found the preservation of spinal biomechanics to be an advantage with that procedure over other anterior procedures.

In performing microscopic posterolateral foraminotomy, the avoidance of excessive bone or ligamentum flavum removal is possible with meticulous surgical technique. As always, adequate decompression of neural elements is the primary objective of the procedure, but minimizing facet joint destruction maximizes the residual stability of the motion unit. This is even more important if multiple unilateral levels are decompressed posteriorly or if a single spinal level is decompressed bilaterally.

There is disagreement in the literature regarding the necessity of removing osteophytes or herniated disc material from beneath the affected nerve root. The controversy is seated in the increased amount of bone

and facet joint necessarily removed when nerve root retraction is to be performed safely, in order to pass instruments anteriorly to remove the offending material.[3,16] Excellent results have been achieved by Epstein et al.[12] by removing osteophytes anteriorly. In a series of patients treated for cervical radiculopathy with a posterolateral foraminotomy, they found that 90% of the patients who had osteophytes removed had good results, whereas only 50% who had simple posterior root decompression without anterior osteophyte removal had good results.

The experimental assessment of cervical facetectomy and its effect on spinal strength has been performed by several authors. Panjabi, White, and Johnson[36] found that complete removal of the facet caused an increase in the horizontal displacement of the spine in flexion. This has direct clinical relevance when facets are fractured or surgically removed. Radiographically, facet fracture or facet removal is evidenced by forward translation of one vertebra with respect to the others.

In a study of 14 fresh-frozen cervical spine motion segments, Raynor, Pugh, and Shapiro[37] found that 3 to 5 mm of nerve root could be exposed with 50% facetectomy and 8 to 10 mm of nerve root could be exposed with 70% facetectomy. In their biomechanical testing, these authors found a significant difference in the spine's ability to withstand shear stress without fracture if only 50% of the facet was excised. They recommended that facet excision not exceed 50%. However, if it becomes necessary to gain greater exposure to adequately decompress the neural elements, which is the primary objective of the procedure, then adding a stabilizing procedure with spinal wiring and spinal fusion to the posterolateral foraminotomy should be considered.[37]

Considerations in Athletes

The operative approach chosen for an athlete with cervical radiculopathy may impact importantly on that athlete's ability to return to the premorbid level of activity and performance. In formulating an operative plan for the athletes that we have treated at the Kerlan-Jobe Orthopaedic Clinic, we have given strong consideration to the minimally invasive and biomechanically less destructive nature of microscopic posterolateral foraminotomy. Although no specific data related to athletes have been published, the evidence extrapolated from the scientific literature seems to support this approach. Certainly, an earlier return to sports is possible if the immobilization required to secure a rigid bony fusion is not necessary. The concern about returning to contact sports is also less of an issue after posterolateral foraminotomy versus anterior cervical fusion. Perhaps further study in this area will determine the scientific validity of this approach in athletes.

REFERENCES

1. Aldrich F: Posterolateral microdiscectomy for cervical monoradiculopathy caused by posterolateral soft cervical disc sequestration, *J Neurosurg* 72:370, 1990.
2. Boden SD et al: Abnormal magnetic resonance scans of the cervical spine in asymptomatic subjects: a prospective investigation, *J Bone Joint Surg* 72A:1178, 1990.
3. Brain WR, Wilkinson JL: *Cervical spondylosis and other disorders of the spine,* Philadelphia, 1967, WB Saunders.
4. Brown BM et al: Preoperative evaluation of cervical radiculopathy and myelopathy by surface-coil MR imaging, *AJR* 151:1205, 1988.
5. Davidson RI et al: The shoulder abduction test in the diagnosis of radicular pain in cervical extradural compressive monoradiculopathies, *Spine* 6:441, 1981.
6. Delamarter RB et al: Experimental lumbar spinal stenosis, *J Bone Joint Surg* 72A:110, 1990.
7. DePalma AF et al: Anterior interbody fusion for severe cervical disc degeneration, *Surg Gynecol Obstet* 134:755, 1972.
8. Dillin WH, Watkins RG: Cervical myelopathy and cervical radiculopathy, *Semin Spine Surg* 1:200, 1989.
9. Dillin W et al: Cervical radiculopathy, *Spine* 11:988, 1986.
10. Dyck P: Cervical foraminotomy: indications and technique. In Watkins RG, editor: *Surgical approaches to the spine,* New York, 1983, Springer-Verlag.
11. Epstein JA: The surgical management of cervical spinal stenosis, spondylosis, and myeloradiculopathy by means of a posterior approach, *Spine* 13:864, 1988.
12. Epstein JA et al: The importance of removing osteophytes as part of the surgical treatment of myeloradiculopathy in cervical spondylosis, *J Neurosurg* 30:219, 1969.
13. Farey ID et al: Pseudarthrosis of the cervical spine after anterior arthrodesis, *J Bone Joint Surg* 72A:1171, 1990.
14. Ferson M et al: Low natural killer cell activity and immunoglobulin levels associated with smoking in human subjects, *Int J Cancer* 23:603, 1979.
15. Friedenberg Z, Miller W: Degenerative disc disease of the cervical spine, *J Bone Joint Surg* 45A:1171, 1963.
16. Frykholm R: Cervical nerve root compression resulting from disc degeneration and root-sleeve fibrosis, *Acta Chir Scand (Suppl)* 160:5, 1951.
17. Garfin SR, Rydevik BL, Brown RA: Compressive neuropathy of spinal nerve roots: a mechanical or biological problem? *Spine* 16:162, 1991.
18. Gepstein R, Brown MD: Somatosensory-evoked potentials in lumbar nerve root decompression, *Clin Orthop* 245:69, 1989.
19. Greenbarg PE et al: Epidural anesthesia for lumbar spine surgery, *J Spinal Disord* 1:139, 1988.
20. Hedberg MC et al: Gradient echo (GRASS) MR imaging in cervical radiculopathy, *AJNR* 9:145, 1988.
21. Henderson C, Hennessy R: Posterolateral foraminotomy as an exclusive operative technique for cervical radiculopathy: a review of 846 consecutively operated cases, *Neurosurgery* 13:504, 1983.
22. Herkowitz HN, Kurz LT, Overholt DP: Surgical management of cervical soft disc herniation: a comparison between the anterior and posterior approach, *Spine* 15:1026, 1990.
23. Herron LD et al: Intraoperative use of dermatomal somatosensory-evoked potentials in lumbar stenosis surgery, *Spine* 12:379, 1987.
24. Holt E: Fallacy of cervical discography, *JAMA* 188:799, 1964.
25. Hult L: The Munkfors investigation, *Acta Orthop Scan Suppl* 16:1, 1959.
26. Hunter LY, Braunstein EM, Bailey RW: Radiographic changes following anterior cervical fusion, *Spine* 5:399, 1980.
27. Kelsey J et al: An epidemiologic study of acute prolapsed cervical intervertebral disc, *J Bone Joint Surg* 66A:907, 1984.
28. Kondo K et al: Protruded intervertebral cervical disc, *Minn Med* 64:751, 1981.
29. Larson EM et al: Comparison of myelography, CT myelography and magnetic resonance imaging in cervical spondylosis and disk herniation: pre- and postoperative findings, *Acta Radiol* 30:223, 1989.
30. Lees F, Turner J: Natural history and prognosis of cervical spondylosis, *Br Med J* 2:1607, 1963.
31. Lundborg G et al: Median nerve compression in the carpal tunnel: the functional response to experimentally induced controlled pressure, *J Hand Surg* 7:252, 1982.
32. Lunsford L et al: Anterior surgery for cervical disc disease, *J Neurosurg* 53:1, 1980.

33. McNab I: The mechanism of spondylogenic pain. In Hirsch C, Zotterman Y, editors: *Cervical pain,* New York, 1972, Pergamon Press.

34. Modic MT et al: Cervical radiculopathy: prospective evaluation with surface-coil MR imaging: CT with metrizamide and metrizamide myelography, *Radiology* 161:753, 1986.

35. Olmarker K, Rydevick B, Holm S: Intraneural edema formation in spinal nerve roots of the porcine cauda equina induced by experimental graded compressions. Paper presented at the thirty-fourth annual meeting of the Orthopaedic Research Society, Atlanta, Ga, Feb 1988.

36. Panjabi MM, White AA, Johnson RM: Cervical spine mechanics as a function of transection of components, *J Biomechan* 8:327, 1975.

37. Raynor RB, Pugh J, Shapiro I: Cervical facetectomy and its effect on spine strength, *J Neurosurg* 63:278, 1985.

38. Rees TD, Liverett DM, Guy CL: The effect of cigarette smoking on skin-flap survival in the face-lift patient, *Plast Reconstr Surg* 73:911, 1984.

39. Rodnitzky RL: *Pictorial manual of neurologic tests,* St Louis, 1984, Mosby.

40. Rothman R, Simeone S: *The spine,* Philadelphia, 1982, WB Saunders.

41. Simeone FA, Dillin WH: Treatment of cervical disc disease: selection of operative approach, *Contemp Neurosurg* 8:1, 1986.

42. Smyth MJ, Wright V: Sciatica and the intervertebral disc: an experimental study, *J Bone Joint Surg* 40A:1401, 1958.

43. Snyder GM, Bernhardt M: Anterior cervical fractional interspace decompression for treatment of cervical radiculopathy, *Clin Orthop* 246:92, 1989.

44. Spurling RG: *Lesions of the cervical intervertebral disc,* Springfield, Ill, 1956, Charles C Thomas.

45. Williams RW: Microcervical foraminotomy, *Spine* 8:708, 1983.

46. Wilson DW, Pezzuti RT, Place JN: Magnetic resonance imaging in the preoperative evaluation of cervical radiculopathy, *Neurosurgery* 28(2):175, 1991.

47. White AA, Southwick WO, Panjabi MM: Clinical instability in the lower cervical spine, *Spine* 1:15, 1976.

48. Yamamoto I et al: Clinical long-term results of anterior discectomy without interbody fusion for cervical disc disease, *Spine* 16:272, 1991.

49. Zdeblich TA, Bohlman HH: Cervical kyphosis and myelopathy: treatment by anterior corpectomy and strut-grafting, *J Bone Joint Surg* 71A:170, Feb 1989.

Chapter Eighteen

Microscopic Lumbar Discectomy

Robert G. Watkins

Microscopic lumbar discectomy provides an ideal way to remove a disc fragment. Some indications for this procedure are as follows:

1. Morbidity of sufficient severity and duration to warrant operative intervention
2. Presence of radicular leg pain, with more than 50% in the leg rather than the back and the leg pain in the distribution of a radicular nerve
3. Neurologic deficit, such as motor, sensory, or reflex loss, enabling the surgeon to determine which nerve is involved
4. Study results indicating an anatomic lesion that corresponds to the patient's symptoms, with the lesion in a location that corresponds to the symptoms, usually a herniated disc, extruded disc fragment, sequestral disc fragment, or segmental, localized lateral recess stenosis

In high-performance athletes, at the Kerlan-Jobe Orthopaedic Clinic we use microscopic operative techniques in order to:

1. Remove the disc fragment or stenosis from the canal
2. Visualize the nerve and blood vessels, providing better protection for both
3. Cause as little injury as possible to normal structures through better visualization, better lighting, and better exposure

We feel confident that, after removing a source of persistent radiculopathy such as an extruded fragment in conjunction with an excellent postoperative rehabilitation program, the potential is present to return athletes to their maximum performance.

OPERATIVE TECHNIQUE

With the patient's studies on the x-ray view box in the operating room, and after induction of general anesthesia, the patient is placed on the Andrews frame. The skin is prepared, and two to three needles are inserted in a paraspinous location (Fig. 18-1). A lateral x-ray film is obtained. By use of the needles and the position of the disc, the skin incision is placed directly over the disc space. Usually this is from just cephalad to the disc space, approximately 2 cm caudally. After the x-ray study is completed, the needles are removed and lines are drawn on the skin perpendicular to the spine with the marking pen to indicate the location of the pins. Full draping is carried out. The skin incision is made by using the lines to place the incision directly over the disc space.

Dissection is carried to the fascia. Then a Cobb elevator, approximately the width of the skin incision, is placed into the wound, and dissection is carried gently through the subcutaneous fat to the fascia to the spinous process. Then the lumbodorsal fascia is stretched over the edge of the spinous process with the Cobb elevator, and the fascial incision is made on the lateral edge of the bulbous tip of the spinous process (Fig. 18-2). The surgeon holds the fascia with the Cobb elevator with one hand and incises the fascia with the Bovie or knife. A generous fascial incision is made, and the Cobb elevator is placed into the wound onto the undersurface of the spinous process. With the curve of the blade facing medially and using gentle dissection to bone, the surgeon sweeps out laterally. A lateral-facing Cobb elevator may be inserted to pull laterally (Fig. 18-3). Palpation of the cephalad and caudad lamina allows the gentle sweeping of the muscles off the interlaminar area. With the muscle held back, the blade point of the Williams retractor is placed, exposing the interlaminar area. With the retractor in

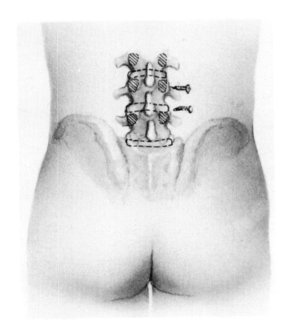

Fig. 18-1. Two needles are placed lateral to the spine at the approximate level of the disc space. The spinous process is not used as the marker because of its varying relationship to the disc space. (From Watkins RG, Collis JS Jr, editors: *Lumbar discectomy and laminectomy,* Rockville, Md, 1987, Aspen.)

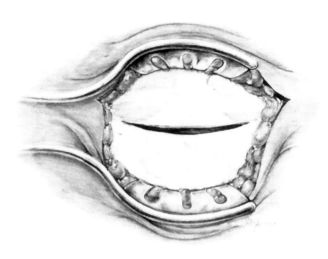

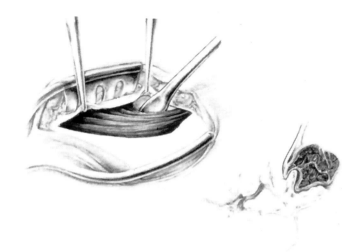

Fig. 18-2. Fascial incision of the skin on the lateral border of the bulbous tip of the spinous process. (From Watkins RG, Collis JS Jr, editors: *Lumbar discectomy and laminectomy*, Rockville, Md, 1987, Aspen.)

Fig. 18-3. Ellis clamps are used to open the leaves of the fascial incision. A Cobb elevator is inserted with the blade pointing mediodorsally under the bulbous tip to the spinous process. (From Watkins RG, Collis JS Jr, editors: *Lumbar discectomy and laminectomy*, Rockville, Md, 1987, Aspen.)

place, a Kocher clamp is placed in the interlaminar area (Fig. 18-4). There is no vigorous exposure of the area. Palpation alone allows one to determine the cephalad and caudad lamina and to place the Kocher in the interlaminar area. Then a final x-ray film is obtained, which indicates the appropriate interlaminar area. It should be remembered that the interlaminar area is caudal to the disc space. Therefore the Kocher should be caudal to the skin marks used to indicate the disc space and should be in the caudal portion of the incision and caudal to the disc space on the x-ray film. After return of the interlaminar marking x-ray film, we use a large pituitary rongeur to gently remove any soft tissue over the interlaminar area. The superficial ligamentum flavum is exposed.

The microscope is used from the time the second x-ray film is taken. With removal of the Kocher under direct visualization, the interlaminar area is seen. The superficial ligamentum flavum is incised laterally and dissected medially (Fig. 18-5, *A*); sometimes the edge of this superficial ligament can be trimmed. The deep ligamentum flavum is exposed (Fig. 18-5, *B*) and can be handled in one of two ways. One is to make a longitudinal incision in the lateral third of the ligamentum flavum. Then, protecting the nerve with the No. 4 Penfield dissector, the lateral third of the ligamentum flavum is resected with the Kerrison rongeur. We prefer to use a curette to detach the caudal attachments of the ligamentum flavum from the leading edge of the caudal lamina and the lateral wall of the facet (Fig. 18-6). The ligamentum flavum is gently dissected caudad to cephalad. The ligament, being elastic, shrinks up, helping this dissection. It is laterally detached and dissected cephalad. To ensure lateral exposure, a few millimeters of the medial aspect of the facet joint—first the inferior and then the superior facet—may need to be trimmed with a Kerrison

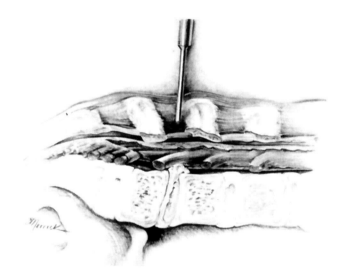

Fig. 18-4. Kocher clamp placed in the interlaminar area. (From Watkins RG, Collis JS Jr, editors: *Lumbar discectomy and laminectomy*, Rockville, Md, 1987, Aspen.)

rongeur (Fig. 18-7). Gentle palpation with the dental tool identifies the pedicle, which provides the surgeon with a distinct understanding of the intracanal structures. The pedicle is the key to intracanal anatomy (Fig. 18-8). With identification of the pedicle, it is known that the disc space is less than 1 cm cephalad. The traversing nerve root is immediately medial and the exiting foramen is caudal to the pedicle. The foramen below is caudal to the pedicle, and the foramen above is cephalad to the pedicle. The exiting nerve root of the segment above will be cephalad to the disc space and the pedicle. The traversing nerve root of a segment becomes the exiting root of the level below. For example, the fifth

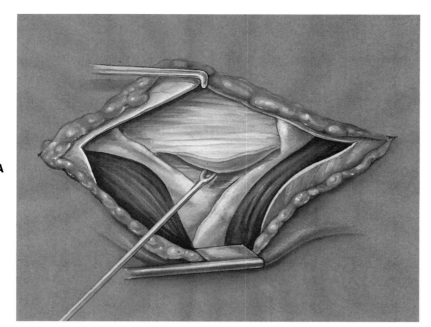

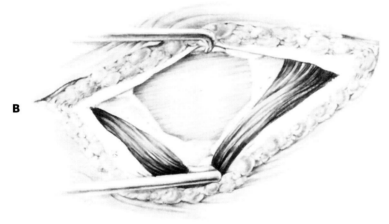

Fig. 18-5. Exposed interlaminar area of the right side. Removing the superficial layer of the ligamentum flavum by gently cutting the attachment of the superficial ligament to the facet joint capsule and dissecting it medially with the curette (A) exposes the yellow longitudinal fibers of the deep ligamentum flavum (B). (From Watkins RG, Collis JS Jr, editors: *Lumbar discectomy and laminectomy,* Rockville, Md, 1987, Aspen.)

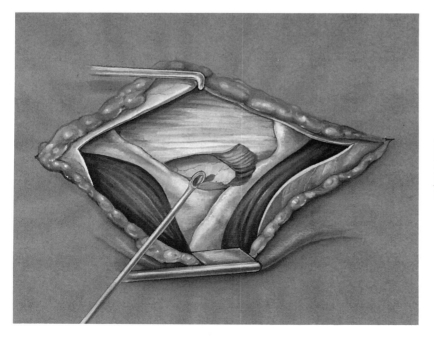

Fig. 18-6. A curette is used to detach the deep ligamentum flavum from the cephalad edge of the caudal lamina. (From Watkins RG, Collis JS Jr, editors: *Lumbar discectomy and laminectomy,* Rockville, Md, 1987, Aspen.)

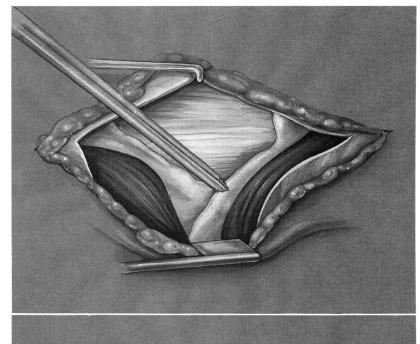

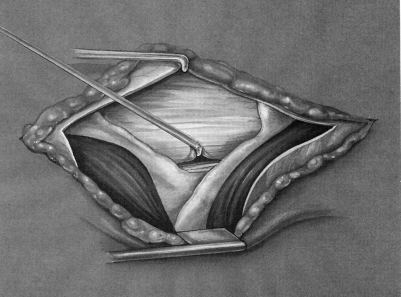

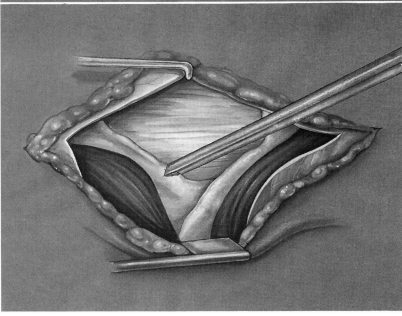

Fig. 18-7. A, The small Kerrison rongeur may be used to remove small areas of bone when segmental lateral recess stenosis exists. **B,** The caudal edge of the cephalad lamina can be removed before opening the ligamentum flavum and to allow entry into the epidural space for a cephalad-extruded disc fragment or an extruded fragment in the medial portion of the intervertebral foramen. Dissection into this cephalad lateral corner with the drill or Kerrison rongeur can allow exposure of the attachment of the ligamentum flavum, detachment of this attachment, and retraction of the ligamentum flavum to allow exposure of the disc. **C,** The Kerrison rongeur may be used caudally to open the entry zone of the caudal foramen at the critical angle — the junction of the caudal lamina and the superior facet. The nerve root exits under this critical angle. Removal of bone in this area is usually carried out after detachment of the ligamentum flavum from the caudal edge. (From Watkins RG, Collis JS Jr, editors: *Lumbar discectomy and laminectomy,* Rockville, Md, 1987, Aspen.)

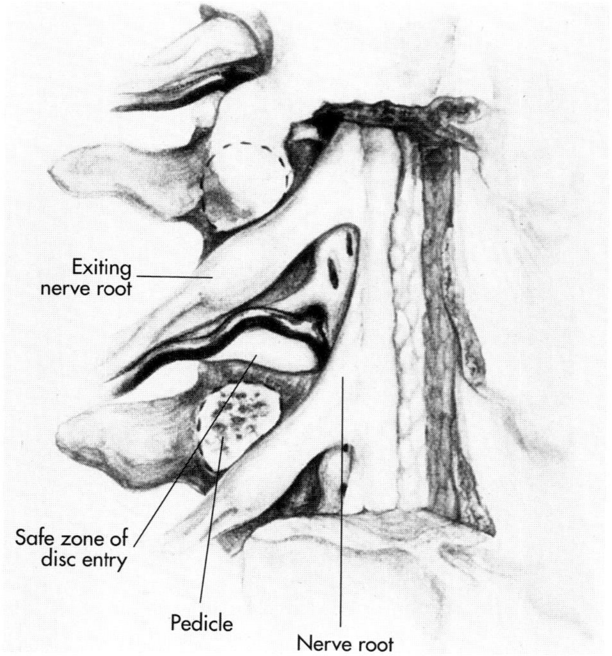

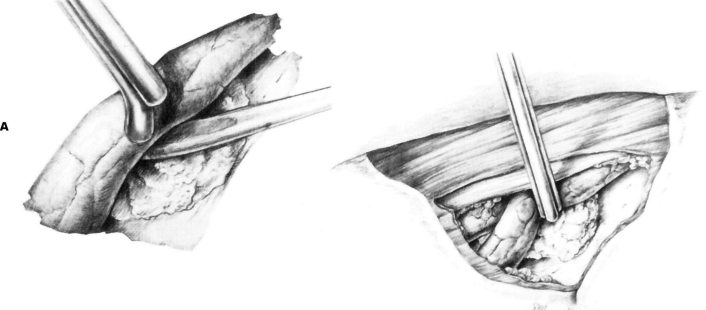

Fig. 18-8. Relationship of the pedicle to the disc and the nerve root (see text). (From Watkins RG, Collis JS Jr, editors: *Lumbar discectomy and laminectomy*, Rockville, Md, 1987, Aspen.)

nerve root is the traversing root of the L4-5 neuromotion segment (or level) and the exiting nerve root of the L5-S1 segment. The exiting nerve root of the L4-5 segment is the fourth nerve root.

The ligamentum flavum attaches to the leading edge of the caudal lamina and to no more than 50% of the surface of the cephalad lamina. It is not necessary to remove the ligamentum flavum in excising an extruded disc fragment. When there is lateral recess stenosis, a significant portion of the medial aspect of the facet may need to be removed, as well as more of the lateral ligamentum flavum.

With identification of the pedicle, a safe zone to enter the disc is immediately cephalad to the pedicle and lateral to the medial wall of the pedicle, because the traversing nerve root is not located at this site. This approach allows a lateral exposure of the disc. Then the surgeon tests the tension in the nerve root with the No. 4 Penfield dissector and the microsucker retractor and, if possible, gently elevates and retracts the nerve root (Fig. 18-9). We prefer that the surgeon do all the nerve root retraction, since this is a benign process and seldom causes bleeding. When the nerve root is very tight and cannot be retracted, five major alternatives are available:

1. Go lateral and remove more of the lateral recess out to the medial wall of the pedicle. Identify the medial wall of the pedicle, and remove bone cephalad and lateral to the medial wall of the pedicle. Remove the lateral ligamentum flavum and expose the disc in this area (Figs. 18-10 and 18-11). Punc-

A

B

Fig. 18-9. A, Whether from this lateral position or a much more medial position in a less critical situation, the No. 4 Penfield dissector is inserted with the right hand, and the Williams microsucker retractor is inserted with the left. **B,** The surgeon uses the microsucker retractor to gently retract and elevate the nerve root. (From Watkins RG, Collis JS Jr, editors: *Lumbar discectomy and laminectomy*, Rockville, Md, 1987, Aspen.)

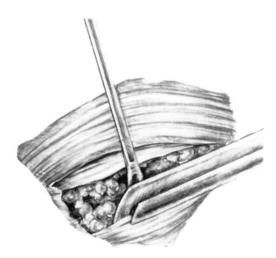

Fig. 18-10. When exposure is needed lateral to the nerve root, the No. 4 Penfield dissector is inserted under the lateral leaf of the ligamentum flavum. Between this lateral leaf of the ligamentum flavum and the dural sac, the dura is gently retracted away from the lateral leaf of the ligamentum flavum. This allows insertion of the small 40-degree-angle Kerrison rongeur to remove the lateral leaf of the ligamentum flavum. (From Watkins RG, Collis JS Jr, editors: *Lumbar discectomy and laminectomy,* Rockville, Md, 1987, Aspen.)

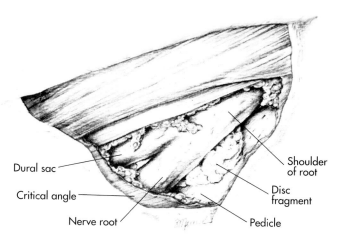

Fig. 18-11. Visualization of the nerve root, with a suggestion of nuclear fragments under the root, after removal of the lateral leaf of the ligamentum flavum. (From Watkins RG, Collis JS Jr, editors: *Lumbar discectomy and laminectomy,* Rockville, Md, 1987, Aspen.)

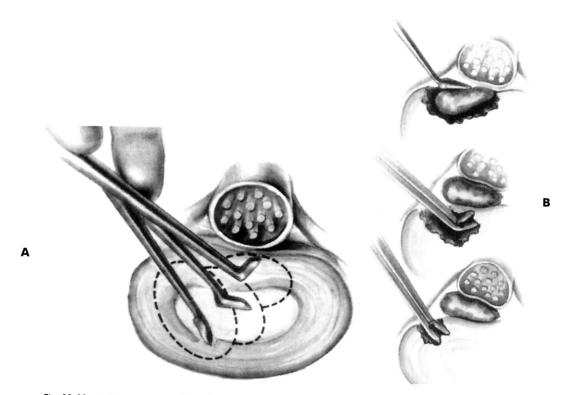

Fig. 18-12. **A,** The down-pushing Scoville curettes can be used to work disc material from under the nerve root down into the disc space, allowing safer removal of disc material lateral to the nerve root. **B,** By creating space in the disc space with disc removal, a fragment can be worked into the disc space to allow removal lateral to the nerve root. This is particularly important in large fragments medial to the nerve root wherein retraction of the nerve root against the fragment can produce significant nerve root damage. (From Watkins RG, Collis JS Jr, editors: *Lumbar discectomy and laminectomy,* Rockville, Md, 1987, Aspen.)

ture the disc, go underneath the annulus, push down with the Epstein or Scoville down-pushing curettes, and attempt to push disc material down to create a space in the disc space for removal of disc material (Figs. 18-12 and 18-13).

2. Check the axilla. Often a large, extruded, axillary fragment can be removed very early in the approach before any attempt is made to retract the nerve root. We do not significantly retract the nerve root until the fragment has been removed.

3. Remove bone at the critical angle, which is the junction of the caudal lamina and the superior facet, and perform an entry-zone foraminotomy of the traversing nerve root.

4. Perform a laminotomy of the cephalad lamina up to the insertion of the ligamentum flavum, and remove the most cephalad insertion of the ligamentum flavum. Approach the nerve root from the most cephalad aspect of the interlaminar area at the shoulder of the nerve root, and expose the back of the body above. Often the nerve root can be manipulated slightly more easily in this more cephalad position than in a more caudal position, which is closer to the pedicle around which the nerve root is exiting.

5. With a large extruded, more central lesion producing cauda equina compromise, several unusual steps may be necessary, such as first decompressing the opposite sides and then removing the fragment after a large laminotomy is performed on the lesion's more prominent side. Exposure of the extruded fragment is carried out with fine dissection and careful protection of the veins and epidural fat. It is not necessary to remove all epidural fat to identify the nerve root. Use the nerve hook to remove the fragment, then expose the disc space, identify the hole in the annulus of the disc, go into the disc space with the micropituitary, and remove any other loose pieces of disc material. We use the Schuler (a shortened Frazier) dissector and the dental tool to explore the spinal canal (cephalad and caudad), as well as the axilla and foramen, for any other loose pieces. The Schuler dissector can be used to push down on the annulus and allow further extrusion of intradiscal fragments. When the fragment is under the posterior longitudinal ligament, we use the No. 4 micro-Penfield dissector to puncture the posterior longitudinal ligament. Expand the hole with the regular No. 4 Penfield dissector, and identify disc contents before making a small cruciate incision with a No. 15 blade to facilitate exposure of disc material. We do not perform a large annulectomy or incision of the annulus, or a radical debridement or curetting of the disc space. We do only what is necessary to remove loose fragments of intervertebral disc and to accomplish the ultimate objective, which is freeing the nerve root. Retractability and lack of tension in the nerve root are the keys to the success of the operation and mark the end of the surgery.

When the nerve root is free, easily retractable, and

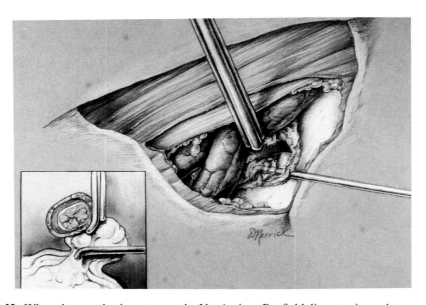

Fig. 18-13. When the annulus is not open, the No. 4 micro-Penfield dissector is used to puncture the annulus. A large No. 4 Penfield dissector is inserted, and the micropituitary dissector is inserted through the puncture wound in the annulus. Rarely, a knife cruciate incision is used. The nerve hook is used to identify extruded fragments and to retrieve sequestered fragments. (From Watkins RG, Collis JS Jr, editors: *Lumbar discectomy and laminectomy,* Rockville, Md, 1987, Aspen.)

without obstruction or nerve root tension and the canal is explored, then adequate decompression has been carried out, and it is time for irrigation and closure. This procedure can be performed on an outpatient basis (with special precautions) or with a 1- to 2-day hospital stay. Patients may walk the night of the operation or, at the latest, the next day. A Hemovac drain is used in every hospitalized patient and is removed the next day. Prophylactic antibiotics are administered for 24 hours.

Patients may shower at 10 days and swim at 3 weeks. The usual restrictions involve no driving for 3 to 4 weeks and no lifting anything heavier than a coffee cup for 3 to 4 weeks. We begin the postoperative rehabilitation program between 2 and 4 weeks and start over with the initial stages of the trunk stabilization program. We encourage the patients to walk as much as is comfortable and as often as possible from the time they wake up from the surgery. The water program is often expanded to a complete WetVest aerobic conditioning and water-resistance program. At the same time, the trunk stabilization program is expanded to an appropriate level of difficulty for the patient's anticipated level of activity.

TECHNIQUE FOR FORAMINAL HERNIATIONS

For foraminal herniations a small midline or paraspinous incision is made. Exposure of the intertransverse area is carried out using the McCulloch blade-point retractor and positioning the retractor on the pars interarticularis. The surgeon detaches the intertransverse ligament with the curette, identifies the most cephalad pedicle in the interlaminar area, and identifies the nerve root as the nerve root exits around this pedicle. The bipolar electric cautery is used to quickly coagulate the foraminal vessels. The nerve root is exposed and is often seen to be tented over the extruded fragment of disc. We usually explore cephalad to the nerve root first, using gentle pressure with the No. 4 Penfield dissector and microsucker retractors, but often the fragment is removed from caudal to the nerve root. If additional exposure is needed, the pedicle below is identified. The disc space is directly cephalad to the pedicle below, and exposure to the caudal pedicle allows adequate exposure of the intervertebral disc itself. Most foraminal spurs occur on the caudal edge of the body above, which is the cephalad margin of the disc space, often directly under

the exiting nerve root. Any attempt to remove foraminal spurs from the floor of the canal should first be preceded by entering, excising a portion of the disc, using a curette to create a space in the disc space and end-plate and under the spur, and then pushing the spur into the disc space. Often the lateral border of the superior facet is slightly trimmed back with the Kerrison rongeur. Occasionally the outer border of the pars is slightly trimmed, but this is usually not necessary. The postoperative restrictions are the same as those indicated in the first procedure discussed.

Use of the microscope definitely provides better lighting and visibility. The technique of using the scope—getting used to moving the scope around for proper view of the interlaminar area—allows a surgeon to accomplish several goals.

With excellent lighting and visibility, virtually any operation medial to the medial wall of the pedicle can be performed effectively through the scope. By moving the scope around, positioning it, and looking into the interlaminar area from several different angles, there should be no lack of visibility of the interlaminar area and its contents but, rather, enhanced visibility. Techniques of exploration of the interlaminar area are enhanced with the microscope. Understanding the anatomy, palpating the back of the body above and the back of the body below, exploring the axilla, and palpating the exiting foramen, are all techniques necessary with any disc excision. Adequate care must be taken with draping of the scope and prevention of contamination of the scope. Mastery of these techniques, which allow a small incision and smaller exposed area, should reduce the risk of infection. Use of the autofocus scope and zoom lens enhances visibility. We often use the drill under the scope. The drill can be used to perform the medial facetectomy or limited laminotomy with great effectiveness. The small incision, far from being simply a cosmetic advantage, is a result of not needing any larger incision to accomplish an effective removal of a herniated disc and thereby protecting normal tissue that is unnecessarily damaged with an expansive exposure.

Chapter Nineteen

◆

Posterior Lumbar Spine Surgery

Robert G. Watkins

The initial important aspect of the approach to the posterior lumbar spine is to attain proper "depth perception thinking"—that is, by identifying posterior structures, be able to know the location of anterior structures in relation to these posterior anatomic landmarks (Fig. 19-1).

Three-dimensional thinking is important in identifying levels of surgery. At the Kerlan-Jobe Orthopaedic Clinic we recommend that at least one intraoperative x-ray film be taken to establish the level of the operation in each lumbar spine approach.

The spinous process may be large and bulbous, extending well below the disc or interlaminar space. Although this can be used as a general guideline for a large skin incision, it is not the best landmark for locating a disc or even a fusion level. For a limited exposure, such as with a microscopic lumbar discectomy and facetec-

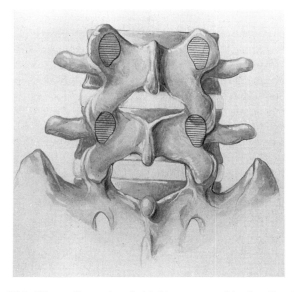

Fig. 19-1. Three-dimensional thinking starts with visualization and palpation of the spinous process and extends to the anterior column of the spine, the intervertebral disc, the vertebral bodies, and neurologic structures. The usual posterior approach to the lumbar spine begins with the spinous process. Dorsally, the critical angle marks the location of the exiting nerve root. The critical angle is the junction of the cephalad edge of the caudal lamina with the base of the superior facet. The nerve root exits immediately under this point. (From Watkins RG: *Surgical approaches to the spine,* New York, 1983, Springer-Verlag.)

tomy, two 18-gauge or 20-gauge spinal needles are placed approximately three fingerbreadths lateral to the spine after appropriate sterile preparation. These are inserted directly vertically, and a transtable lateral x-ray film is obtained. With use of the needles relative to the disc space, the surgical approach is planned to be positioned exactly over the disc space itself—not the interlaminar area nor the spinous process. This allows the best visualization of the disc space for a limited-exposure disc excision.

For a broader, more extensive exposure, the x-ray film is obtained after subperiosteal dissection and clearance of one side of the spine. The laminar and interlaminar areas are exposed out to the facet joint, self-retaining retractors are placed, and an instrument such as a Kocher clamp is placed in the interlaminar area. After exposure of the lamina, the facet joint is visualized. Location of the facet joint allows one to distinguish the inferior facet from the superior facet. The base of the superior facet leads to the transverse process. Visualization of the superior facet and the transverse process in the interlaminar area can lead to very specific locations of the pedicle. To identify the spinal level, we prefer using the interlaminar area as the key anatomic landmark. The interlaminar area is just caudal to the disc space and the neuromotion segment involved. Using the spinous process and the lamina as landmarks can result in deception.

In summary, for a limited exposure, we use lateral paraspinous needles for the skin incision, followed by a Kocher clamp placed in the interlaminar area of the disc to be exposed. Opening the interlaminar area allows access to the disc space, which is just cephalad.

Three-dimensional thinking also is important in determining the location of the intervertebral disc in relation to the interlaminar area. Even though the L5-S1 disc is at the level of the interlaminar area, as one progresses cephalad, the disc space, proportionately, is in a more cephalad position in relation to the interlaminar area. Therefore exposure of the L3-4 disc requires more removal of the caudal edge of the L3 lamina than would exposure at L5-S1. The disc will be in a more cephalad position compared with the interlaminar area the higher one progresses in the lumbar spine. When the transverse process is to be exposed, an 18-gauge needle is inserted dorsally over the proposed pedicle or at the base of the transverse process, which, on the lateral view, would be identifying a pedicle. The marker establishes the levels to be fused, and because a fusion should be from pedicle to pedicle, this identification provides the best marker. Using the spinous process may result in confusion inasmuch as the transverse process is very far cephalad to the spinous process of the level to be fused.

Discussion of specific anatomic structures is best undertaken while the approach is presented, and the approach begins with positioning. The ideal position should avoid any abdominal pressure, either from the side or directly volar. We prefer the Andrews frame for most decompressions. Both the hips and the knees are at 90 degrees. Touching the frame are the chest, knees, and chin. There are two well-padded, lateral thigh pads. The abdomen hangs entirely free. In operations involving internal fixation of the lower lumbar spine, however, positioning the patient with the proper amount of lumbar lordosis is a critical factor. Thus, if the patient's hips are at 90 degrees, the amount of lumbar lordosis may be insufficient. In cases in which this is critical, we use the four-poster frame, allowing the hips to be extended, which may produce a greater amount of lordosis.

APPROACH FOR A LAMINECTOMY AND FUSION

The actual approach for a laminectomy and fusion begins with a straight midline incision through the dermis only; 20 ml of 1:500,000 epinephrine is injected through the dermal incision into the subcutaneous tissue and the subfascial muscle layer. The "deep" knife extends the incision through to the fascial layer. Self-retaining Gelpi retractors are placed gently. A great deal of care is taken not to crush the subcutaneous fat tissue, and every attempt is made to avoid creating an unnecessary dead space in this very important layer.

With the fascia exposed in the midline and the preoperative decision having been made as to whether to take a midline approach or a paraspinous fascial approach, the exposure is extended subfascially by one of the following two means.

When the spinous process is to be removed, the electrocautery is used to cut directly down onto the bone of the spinous process, and the fascia is opened in this midline area. With the Bovie cautery the surgeon attempts to remove as much of the fascial insertion as possible from the bone to allow a better postoperative repair when the spinous process is removed. The surgeon uses two Cobb elevators to sweep the tissue off the tip of the spinous process, exposing the bone alone, and then dissects over the bulbous tip of the spinous process onto the lamina and removes all soft tissue while sweeping out laterally on the lamina with the two Cobb elevators. The assistant follows with the Bovie cautery and the cell-saver sucker. The lateral dissection ends at the medial portion of the facet joint capsule, and self-retaining retractors are then placed.

A second approach to the spine involves operations in which the spinous process is to be preserved. In these instances the Cobb elevator is used to gently sweep out

lateral to the bulbous tip of the spinous process, and a paraspinous fascial incision is made just off the bulbous tip of the spinous process. This leaves a medial leaf of lumbodorsal fascia to sew back to. It allows the Cobb elevators to be introduced under this fascial leaf and to dissect laterally on the lamina to the medial portion of the facet joint capsule. Exposure of the interlaminar area is carried out with the Cobb elevators, and a self-retaining Williams retractor or similar retractor is placed. The point of the retractor extends medially, usually just caudal to the spinous process, and the blade exposes the interlaminar area. In cases of lateral recess stenosis, in which an interlaminar operation is to be performed with preservation of not only the spinous process but most of the laminae, exposure of the interlaminar area is all that is needed. The caudal portion of the lamina above is identified; the caudal edge of the cephalad lamina laterally becomes the medial portion of the inferior facet. The cephalad edge of the caudal lamina laterally becomes the medial edge of the superior facet. Then the lateral border of the interlaminar area is the facet joint.

The facet joint is another important landmark exposed during the initial stages of the posterior approach. After the facet joint is identified, one should keep in mind that the superior articular process is underneath, anterolateral, or volar-lateral to the inferior articular process, which is the first bone encountered in the more dorsal position. The facet joint may be markedly distorted in cases of spinal stenosis. A huge, hypertrophic facet joint with a hypertrophic capsule and a synovial cyst that protrudes into the interlaminar area is not an uncommon occurrence. As the lamina is cleared, the same motion is used to sweep the inferior surface of the lamina with Cobb elevators. With identification of the inferior facet and the facet joint capsule, the next step is to identify the medial articular surface of the superior facet and the pars interarticularis. To identify the articular surface of the superior facet, the medial portion of the inferior facet must undergo osteotomy with a chisel, or a burr can be used to reveal the glistening dorsal surface of superior facet. Care is taken to protect most of the facet capsule. After the dorsal surface of the pars interarticularis is swept with a small Cobb elevator, the Bovie cautery is used to clear off the pars interarticularis itself. There are always significant bleeders just lateral to the pars interarticularis. These can be avoided, as well as excessive bleeding, by not extending the dissection lateral to the pars interarticularis in this area.

With a total laminectomy or significant foraminotomy or facet arthropathy, we allow time to expose the pars interarticularis, which provides a reasonable idea of the most lateral extent of the dissection. With the pars interarticularis exposed and the interlaminar area defined, self-retaining Wiltse retractors are used to hold back the muscle mass. Identification of the facet joints reveals the location of the transverse process. With spinal fusion the initial stages of the exposure consist of extending the Cobb elevators over the facet joint, initially preserving the capsule, and onto the transverse process. The transverse process extends caudally and laterally from the facet joint. The surgeon dissects over the facet joint capsule, feeling gently with the Cobb elevator, and then sweeps down laterally with the two Cobb elevators—one cephalad and one caudad to the transverse process—and exposes the transverse process. The electrocautery, on a low setting, is used to dissect the soft tissue from the dorsal surface of the transverse process. Again, the Wiltse self-retaining retractor provides the best exposure of these areas lateral to the facet joint.

With the spine exposed, after x-ray localization, the removal of the facet joint capsule may be carried out in cases of spinal fusion with exposure of the articular surfaces to allow removal of the lateral portions of the articular cartilage and impaction of bone into a portion of the facet joint.

The borders of the interlaminar area are cephalad lamina, caudal lamina, the spinous process medially, and the facet joint laterally. The floor is the ligamentum flavum, which consists of two layers, the superficial layer and the deep layer (Fig. 19-2). The deep layer has the typical vertical striations of ligament and is typically thought of as the yellow ligament. The insertion of the ligamentum flavum is approximately 50% cephalad on the undersurface of the cephalad lamina to the edge of the caudal lamina. It blends with the facet joint capsule laterally and then extends out over the nerve root to form a portion of the roof of the intervertebral foramen. A portion of the roof of the lateral recess forms the undersurface of the superior facet, the roof of the lateral recess, and the roof of the entry zone of the foramen. The ligamentum forms a major portion of the soft tissue lateral recess. There is a cleft in the middle of the ligamentum flavum, creating two leaves, one from the right side and the other from the left. In passing sublaminar wires, the surgeon often takes advantage of this interval beneath the two leaves of ligamentum flavum.

The ligamentum flavum can be detached from its insertion by dissection with a sharp curette. It can be completely detached by dissection cephalad with a curette under the cephalad lamina—removing the most cephalad attachment of the ligament—and laterally on the medial and volar surface of the superior facet. This is quite far underneath the cephalad lamina and requires use of the curette completely out of view, relying on tactile sensation for staying on the undersurface of the lamina. Although the caudal portion of the ligamentum flavum attached to the cephalad edge of the caudal

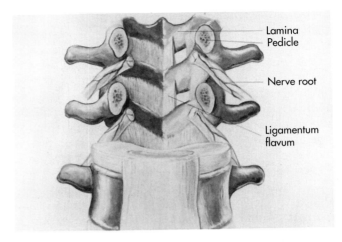

Fig. 19-2. The ligamentum flavum inserts approximately midway under the cephalad lamina and on the cephalad edge of the caudal lamina. This underview of the posterior elements from the intervertebral canal demonstrates the ligamentum flavum and its insertion on the lamina. (From Watkins RG: *Surgical approaches to the spine,* New York, 1983, Springer-Verlag.)

ligament is easier to detach, it must be remembered that the nerve root exits exactly under this attachment. The critical angle is the junction of the caudad lamina and superior facet. The nerve root exits directly under the critical angle. Therefore, it is important to stay directly on the bone of the caudal lamina and base of the superior facet in detaching the ligament without injuring the nerve root. In some cases of stenosis, the entire ligamentum flavum can be removed by detaching it at its periphery and excising it. With use of a 40-degree angled Kerrison rongeur, the lateral portion of the ligamentum flavum is removed between the nerve root and the lateral leaf of the ligamentum flavum.

The more limited approach used for the microscopic discectomy involves detaching the ligament caudally and laterally and then retracting it medially and cephalad, allowing a good exposure of the root and disc.

After opening the ligamentum and entering the epidural space, the surgeon first identifies the pedicle. The key to understanding intracanal anatomy and pathology is the pedicle (Fig. 19-3,*A*). To understand the intracanal anatomy and pathologic conditions as they are related to clinical symptoms, it is important to understand the concept of individual neuromotion segments. A neuromotion segment is defined as the vertebra, disc, ligament, facet joints, nerves, and vessels of one spinal level. Each segment has only one pedicle. The pedicle itself is immediately anterior to the base of the superior articular facet. The transverse process, the superior

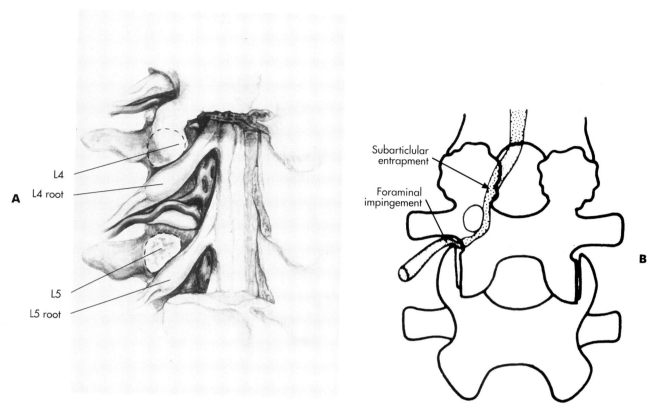

Fig. 19-3. A, The pedicle is the key to understanding intercanal anatomy and pathology (see text). **B,** A lateral recess stenosis of the traversing fifth root at L4-5 produces symptoms similar to those of a foraminal stenosis on the fifth root at L5-S1. (**A** from Watkins RG, Collis JS Jr, editors: *Lumbar discectomy and laminectomy,* Rockville, Md, 1987, Aspen.)

facet, and the pedicle form a triplane structure, with the pedicle projecting anteriorly in the transverse plane, the transverse process projecting laterally in the coronal plane, and the superior articular facet projecting cephalad in the parasagittal plane. Knowing the location of the pedicle provides the following information:

1. The disc space is less than 1 cm cephalad to the pedicle, often appearing immediately cephalad.
2. Just medial to the pedicle is the traversing nerve root. The key to identifying the traversing nerve root of that neuromotion segment is identification of the pedicle. The traversing nerve root of a segment (i.e., the fifth root at L4-5) becomes the exiting nerve root of the level below (the fifth root at L5-S1) (Fig. 19-3, *B*). The exiting nerve root traverses around the pedicle to exit caudally in the intervertebral foramen. A significant number of vessels surround the base of the pedicle.
3. Immediately dorsal and cephalad to the pedicle is the superior facet. The superior facet of L5 is

immediately dorsal and cephalad to the pedicle of L5. The superior facet is the roof of the intervertebral foramen for the exiting nerve root above and a portion of the roof of the lateral recess for the traversing nerve root. The superior facet is covered on its undersurface by the facet joint capsule and ligamentum flavum.

4. The intervertebral foramen is just caudal to the pedicle.

Exiting nerve root and *traversing nerve root* are important terms. For example, the traversing nerve root at L4-5 is the fifth nerve. The exiting nerve root at L5-S1 is the fifth nerve. If the patient has a foraminal stenosis at L5-S1 and has S1 symptoms, it is not caused by an interpedicular foraminal stenosis at L5-S1. That would affect the L5 root, not the S1 root. A foraminal stenosis at L4-5 should have no direct effect on the L5 nerve root because the exiting nerve root through the intervertebral foramen at L4-5 is the fourth nerve. Therefore one must describe not only the anatomic abnormalities of the spinal column, such as the location of an area of stenosis,

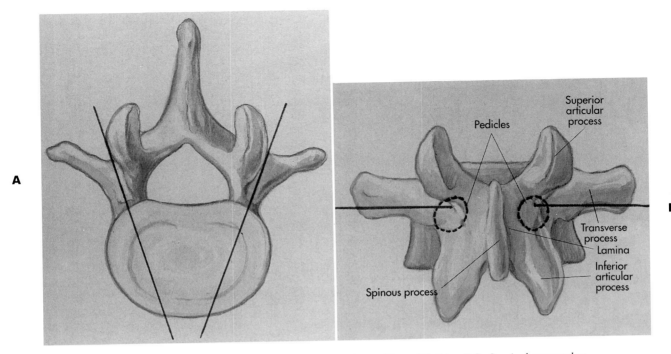

Fig. 19-4. Angle of the pedicle in the transverse plane. (From Watkins RG: *Surgical approaches to the spine,* NewYork, 1983, Springer-Verlag.)

but also relate that information to the neurologic column and the symptoms produced by these anatomic structures. The relationship of the nerve root to the pedicle and the intervertebral foramen is an important concept in identifying the location of anatomic lesions and their relationship to clinical symptoms. For example, the nerve exiting around the pedicle is numbered the same as that pedicle in relation to the spine.

The tube of the pedicle can be identified by localization of structures on the dorsal elements (Fig. 19-4). The projection of the tube of the pedicle is found by identifying a point formed by a line bisecting the center of the transverse process in the transverse plane and a perpendicular line just medial to the lateral wall of the superior articular facet in the parasagittal plane. From this point the direction of the pedicle may vary from 15 to 25 degrees from the midline angled medially to laterally. The angle of the pedicle decreases as one progresses cephalad in the lumbar spine, and the tube of the pedicle may become elliptic in the upper lumbar spine. Palpation in the canal for the pedicle with, for example, a dental tool may produce significant bleeding in this area and should be gentle and just enough to identify the cephalad and caudad border of the pedicle. Often, with significant hypertrophy of the superior facet, the medial border of the superior facet is mistaken for the pedicle, and only with more volar palpation is the full

lateral extent of the pedicle appreciated. With identification of the pedicle and then the nerve root, the lateral recess is better appreciated.

The boundaries of the lateral recess are as follows:
1. *Cephalad* — The cephalad tip of the superior facet
2. *Caudad* — The caudal border of the pedicle
3. *Roof* — The superior facet and ligamentum flavum
4. *Floor* — The disc and vertebral body medial to the medial wall of the pedicle

The lateral recess exists medial to the medial wall of the pedicle, and lateral recess stenosis involves impingement of the traversing nerve root medial to the medial wall of the pedicle (Figs. 19-5 and 19-6). The intervertebral foramen is divided into the entry zone, which starts at the critical angle — the junction of the caudal lamina and superior facet. The lateral recess is the foramen medial to the medial edge of the pedicle. The interpedicular portion of the intervertebral foramen, which is just lateral to the medial wall of the pedicle, is situated between the two pedicles. The pedicles form the cephalad and caudad border of the intervertebral foramen. The lateral portion of the intervertebral foramen is the portion starting just lateral to the lateral caudal wall of the pedicle.

It must be remembered that the pedicle is in the cephalad half of the intervertebral body. The initial stages of exposure should expose the pars interarticu-

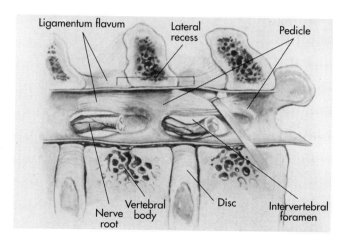

Fig. 19-5. Understanding the intervertebral foramen and the tissues present in the foramen is of critical importance. The far lateral portion of the intervertebral foramen is lateral to the lateral wall of the pedicle. The foramen begins at the medial border of the pedicle and extends laterally from that point. (From Watkins RG: *Surgical approaches to the spine,* New York, 1983, Springer-Verlag.)

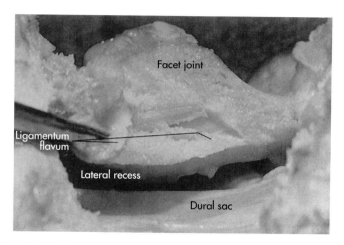

Fig. 19-6. The lateral recess is medial to the wall of the pedicle. The obstruction occurs from the superior facet and ligamentum flavum pressing the nerve root down on the disc or floor of the spinal canal medial to the pedicle. (From Watkins RG: *Surgical approaches to the spine,* New York, 1983, Springer-Verlag.)

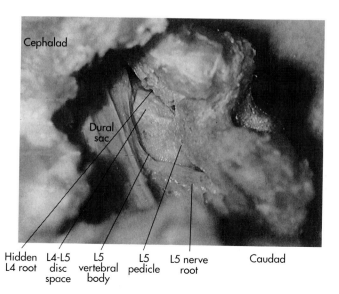

Fig. 19-7. A specimen cleaned of veins shows the relationship of the disc to the pedicle as visualized from a partial hemilaminectomy. The nerve root exits around the pedicle, and the disc space is immediately cephalad to the pedicle. (From Watkins RG: *Surgical approaches to the spine,* New York, 1983, Springer-Verlag.)

laris. This defines the lateral limits of the bony posterior column and allows the surgeon to leave adequate bone to prevent fracture when cutting the pars interarticularis with the laminectomy. The pars interarticularis is best thought of as the base of the superior facet.

The annulus of the disc covers the volar spur or herniation, and the floor of the intervertebral foramen frequently is the annulus of the disc. The roof of the intervertebral foramen is covered by the ligamentum flavum and the facet joint capsule. Interoperatively, soft tissue will be present in the roof of the intervertebral foramen—the ligamentum flavum of the facet joint capsule.

Identification of the pedicle leads immediately to identification of the traversing nerve root. In cases of spinal stenosis and disc herniation, the traversing nerve root may be tight against the medial wall of the pedicle. The nerve root should not be retracted against major resistance. Gentle palpation with the No. 4 Penfield dissector and the microsucker retractor allows one to test the tension in the nerve root medial to the medial wall of the pedicle. It is safer to attempt to gently retract and test for nerve root tension more cephalad than the pedicle at the disc space level, closer to the shoulder of the nerve root.

If the nerve root is tight, several measures can be used to avoid injuring the nerve root by retracting it. The key is knowledge of the anatomy. Knowing the exact location of the pedicle in the canal is the most significant first step in avoiding injury to the nerve (Figs. 19-7 and 19-8).

The surgeon exposes the disc cephalad to the pedicle and slightly lateral to the medial wall of the pedicle. This involves a partial medial facetectomy. Removal of the medial portion of the superior facet allows easy palpation and even visualization of the medial wall of the pedicle. Extending the exposure more cephalad results in running into the exiting nerve root of the segment above. There is usually a safe area immediately cephalad and lateral to the medial wall of the pedicle well caudad

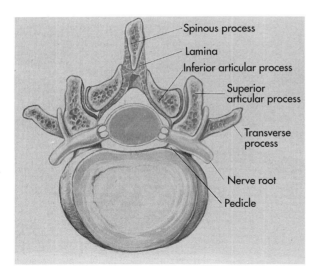

Fig. 19-8. Transverse plane section of the lumbar neuromotion segment emphasizing the orientation of the transverse process, superior articular process, and pedicle as a three-pronged structure. The facet joint is seen as the roof of the lateral recess. The nerve exits below the pedicle at each level. The nerve branches into a dorsal primary ramus that innervates from one to three facet joints at adjoining spinal levels. The ventral primary ramus is responsible for limb function and sensation. (From Watkins RG: *Surgical approaches to the spine,* New York, 1983, Springer-Verlag.)

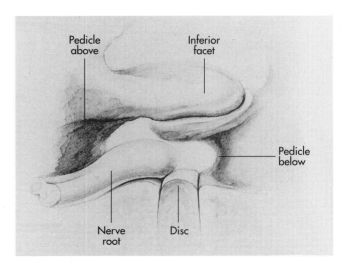

Fig. 19-9. Distortions in rotation and hypertrophy of the facet joint can produce a narrowing of the intervertebral foramen from two major sources: (1) hypertrophy of the tip of the superior facet pressing down and cephalad on the nerve root and (2) the marginal osteophyte on the back of the body above, producing obstruction volar to the nerve root. The nerve root has been retracted cephalad to show the disc.

to the nerve root exiting above and lateral to the traversing nerve root. Therefore the first step is to obtain a more lateral exposure until the medial wall of the pedicle can be easily visualized or palpated and then expose the floor and disc of the canal just cephalad and lateral to the pedicle. The traversing nerve root should not be in this area inasmuch as the root is medial to the medial wall of the pedicle. The disc space is entered lateral to the nerve root in the safe area. The surgeon tries to pull out disc material and decompress the nerve root from that area and then gently work under the nerve root, removing disc material from medial to lateral. Another step is to explore the axilla of the traversing nerve root with a No. 4 Penfield dissector. This may require removal of more of the cephalad edge of the caudad lamina, but exploration of the axilla may allow removal of a fragment that will prevent any medial retraction of the nerve root. Bleeding may be encountered in this area as well.

Another approach is to extend the exposure cephalad, removing more of the caudal lamina of the cephalad vertebra—possibly up to the most cephalad insertion of the ligamentum flavum. This should provide adequate clearance of the cephalad portion of the root. The foraminotomy may also need to be extended caudally on the nerve root, around the pedicle, with removal of bone from the critical angle. The critical angle is the junction

of the caudal lamina and the superior facet, under which the nerve root exits. The surgeon opens up this area, follows the nerve root around that pedicle as it exits, and performs an entry-zone foraminotomy. The roof of the canal is removed over the nerve as it exits around the pedicle. A foraminotomy of the foramen below may allow better retraction of the nerve root.

After opening the lateral recess, the surgeon identifies the root and the pedicle and follows the root around the pedicle past its medial wall to enter the intervertebral foramen (Fig. 19-9).

The boundaries of the intervertebral foramen are as follows:

1. The cephalad boundary is the caudal surface of the most cephalad pedicle.
2. The caudal boundary is the cephalad portion of the most caudal pedicle.
3. The roof of the intervertebral foramen is the superior facet and pars interarticularis.
4. The floor of the intervertebral foramen is the caudal portion of the vertebral body above and the intervertebral disc.

With rotational deformities of the neuromotion segment, the superior facet may be subluxated anteriorly downward, pressing against the pedicle above and the posterior caudal portion of the vertebral body above (Fig. 19-10). It must be remembered that not only the bone of the facet joint but also the ligamentum flavum and the facet joint capsule may contribute to a soft tissue stenosis in that area. A vertical subluxation of the tip of

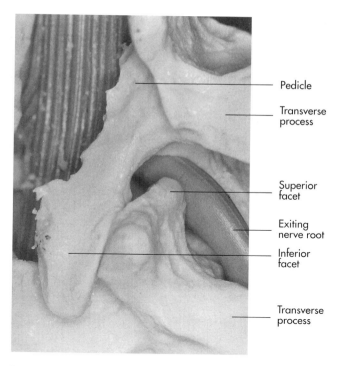

Fig. 19-10. Laminotomy demonstrating the transverse process inferior facet and superior facet of a subluxated facet joint projecting into the exiting nerve root as it courses in the intervertebral foramen. (From Watkins RG: *Surgical approaches to the spine,* New York, 1983, Springer-Verlag.)

the superior facet certainly can impede the nerve root against the pedicle above. When performing a foraminotomy, one usually removes the undersurface of the superior facet to provide an adequate opening of the foramen. Removal of the most cephalad tip of the superior facet can be performed with a chisel from lateral to the joint outside the spinal canal. The facet joint is exposed and the superior facet identified—just lateral to the pars interarticularis and caudal to the transverse process above (i.e., the most cephalad extent of the facet joint). With the chisel the surgeon cuts in a caudal and medial direction, removing the cephalad one third of the superior facet and leaving the capsule in the floor of the portion removed to protect the nerve root from the chisel. At times, a significant bony spur arising from the caudal portion of the more cephalad vertebral body (under the nerve root in the floor of the intervertebral foramen) must be removed. This is best accomplished by opening the intervertebral disc below and using a curette under the spur, creating a space in the end-plate. The spur can be pushed down into the space created in the inferior surface on the caudal portion of the body above (Figs. 19-11 to 19-14; see also Fig. 19-8).

Extraforaminal ligaments may bind the exiting nerve root to the floor of the intervertebral foramen and

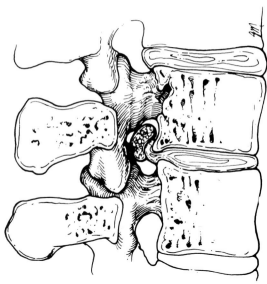

Fig. 19-11. Foraminal disc herniation and bone spur on the back of the body above. The left foramen viewed from inside the spinal canal shows the volar pressure on the nerve root itself.

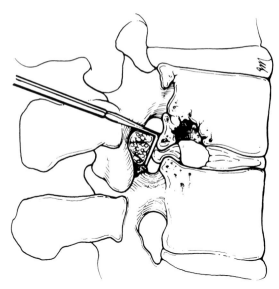

Fig. 19-12. The first step in relieving pressure is to burrow under the marginal osteophyte, creating room and space for impaction of the osteophyte. The surgeon must enter the intervertebral disc to create room between the intervertebral disc and the curette and burrow through the end-plate under the spur to create room for the spur.

provide a significant obstruction of the intervertebral foramen and the nerve root. Changes in anatomy as a result of degenerative disease may allow these structures to become a significant part of the potential obstruction to the lateral portion of the intervertebral foramen.

The vascular leash extends from the central portion of

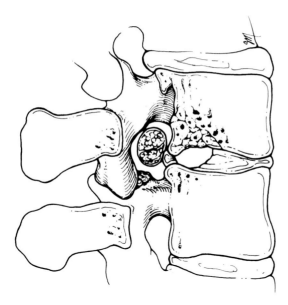

Fig. 19-13. Removal of a herniated fragment and impaction of the spur down into that space may relieve the volar pressure under the nerve root.

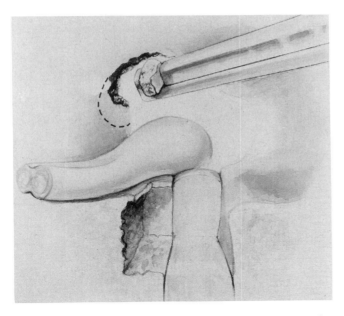

Fig. 19-14. Space created by the evacuation of the spur under the nerve root, as well as demonstrable relief of the obstruction over the nerve root. (From Watkins RG, Collis JS Jr, editors: *Lumbar discectomy and laminectomy,* Rockville, Md, 1987, Aspen.)

the canal out the intervertebral foramen, usually caudal to the exiting nerve root, and over the intervertebral disc, caudal to the nerve root. Significant veins extend vertically under the lateral portion of the dura. Obviously, identification of the vascular leash in extensive exposures of the floor of the spinal canal is important. Often these vessels are thick and not easily appreciated

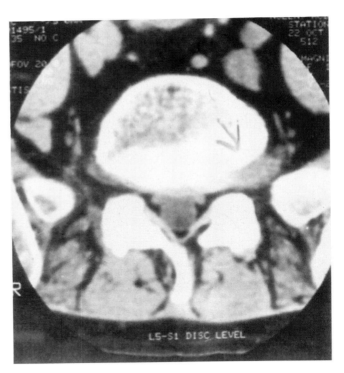

Fig. 19-15. Intertransverse approach showing a large extruded disc far laterally under the L5 spinal nerve as it exits the foramen. This disc was removed through a paraspinal approach. The nerve was exposed and retracted, and the fragment removed. The lateral approach is preferable to a medial laminectomy for removing this lateral fragment.

as vascular structures. They may mimic the nerve root and/or a conjoined or accessory nerve root. The key is that the structures coursing transversly just cephalad to the pedicle, over the disc space, are usually vascular, whereas the nerve root exits in the cephalad portion of the intervertebral foramen, just caudal to the pedicle above. The vessels exit around the cephalad edge of the pedicle and the caudal portion of the intervertebral foramen.

An extensive exposure of the disc, such as that needed for a posterior lumbar interbody fusion, requires that one ligate and transect the vascular leash. Because significant medial retraction of the dura is necessary, cephalad retraction of the exiting nerve root and a full exposure of the disc necessitate that the vascular leash be excised through this area. In standard disc excisions the vascular leash can be dissected bluntly, caudal to cephalad, and retracted cephalad to the disc to allow adequate opening of the disc and removal of the significant portion of intradiscal material.

PARASPINOUS APPROACH

The paraspinous approach to the spine may be used to excise a lateral disc herniation (Fig. 19-15), to perform a foraminotomy from the outside in, to expose the transverse process and pedicles for pedicle screw inser-

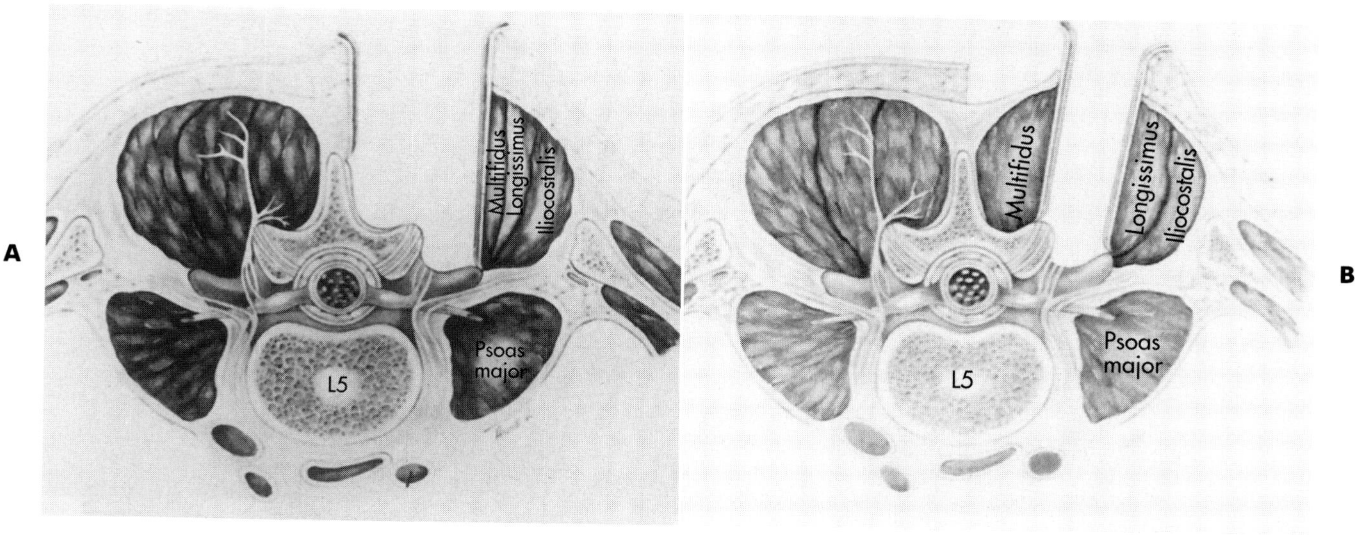

Fig. 19-16. A, Standard medial approach to the posterior lumbar spine with retraction of the paraspinous musculature laterally from the midline. This exposes the interlaminar area very well; from this position the transverse process can be exposed, and a facet fusion and posterolateral fusion can be carried out. **B,** The paraspinous approach uses a midline skin incision, a lateral fascial incision, and direct approach between the multifidus and longissimus muscles down to the transverse processes, the ala, and the facet joints. (From Watkins RG, Collis JS Jr, editors: *Lumbar discectomy and laminectomy,* Rockville, Md, 1987, Aspen.)

tion, or to expose the transverse process and outer portion of the facet for a posterolateral fusion, or any combination of these.

We prefer a midline skin incision with adequate length to allow lateral retraction of the skin, exposing the lumbodorsal fascia and the bulk of the paraspinous muscle mass. Then a paraspinous fascial incision is made at that point (Fig. 19-16). For lateral exposure of a disc herniation or for an outside-in foraminotomy, the fascial incision is in the midline and the muscle mass is retracted laterally. For pedicle screw insertion in which a laminotomy is used, the fascial incision is two fingerbreadths off the midline. For a more extensive posterolateral exposure (several levels for fusion), we use a curvilinear incision, three fingerbreadths from the midline in its center portion down to one fingerbreadth at the caudad and cephalad extent of the exposure. The paraspinous incision is a muscle-splitting incision. After the fascia is incised with a Bovie cautery, fingers are used to vertically separate the muscle fibers down to the lateral portion of the facet and the transverse process.

A tendency is to proceed too medially and end up on the lamina. Going directly down in a lateral position puts one onto the transverse process. After muscle spreading with the finger is completed, the self-retaining Wiltse retractors are inserted. Then the Cobb elevators are used to expose the transverse processes, with the assistant from the opposite side of the table using a Bovie cautery on a low setting and a sucker to aid in the exposure of these lateral structures. Exposure of the disc

from the lateral approach is carried out by identifying the transverse processes above and below the intertransverse area to be explored—for an L4-5 disc, the L4 and L5 transverse processes. Dissection on the cephalad transverse process proceeds medially to the base of the transverse process. The caudal lamina is exposed, and the superior facet is identified. The pars interarticularis will be more dorsal in the wound, but this should be exposed. The borders of the intertransverse area are as follows:

1. *Cephalad*—The cephalad transverse process
2. *Caudad*—The caudad transverse process
3. *Laterally*—The intertransverse ligament
4. *Medially*—The superior facet and the pars interarticularis
5. *Volarly*—Anteriorly the most lateral portion of the intervertebral disc and vertebral body and the nerve, vessel, and retroperitoneal space structures (Fig. 19-17, *A*)

The next step is to detach the intertransverse ligament from the cephalad transverse process, proceeding immediately along the pars interarticularis and then out on the cephalad portion of the caudal transverse process (Fig. 19-17, *B*). This can be dissected free with a curette, gently clamped, and retracted medially to laterally. Use of the Bovie and magnification at that point is important. We specifically use the bipolar Bovie on the vessels exiting with the nerve root from the spinal canal out into the intervertebral foramen and intertransverse area. The nerve root is identified by following the caudal surface of

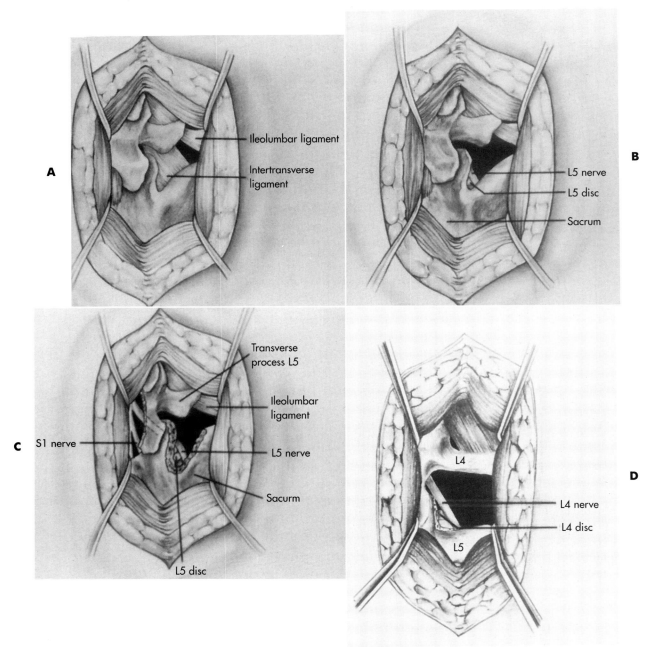

Fig. 19-17. **A,** Alar transverse area viewed from the paraspinous approach; the intertransverse and iliolumbar ligaments can be seen. **B,** Removal of the intertransverse ligament. As can be seen, additional bone removal at the alar transverse area is usually necessary in order to fully expose the nerve. **C,** This view shows more bone removal, as well as the nerve, demonstrating the point of identification cephalad at the pedicle of L5 and tracing it caudally. The L5-S1 disc is seen herniating into the nerve root, and removal of the ala is necessary for removal of that fragment. **D,** Similar intertransverse approach at L4-5. Again, identifying the pedicle at L4 allows one to identify the fourth nerve and then protect it while safely removing a foraminal herniation in that area. (From Watkins RG, Collis JS Jr, editors: *Lumbar discectomy and laminectomy,* Rockville, Md, 1987, Aspen.)

the cephalad transverse process medially to the lateral caudal wall of the pedicle. This leads to the nerve root exiting just caudal to the caudal wall of the pedicle (Fig. 19-17, C). Therefore the transverse process above and then the pedicle above are used to find the exiting nerve root. Identification of the nerve root in an avascular field after bipolarization of the vessels is the key to protecting the nerve root while exposing the intertransverse area. Identification of the nerve root at this point often reveals the intrusion onto the nerve root by the facet or other obstructing structures (Fig. 19-17, D). A disc fragment is sometimes seen directly volar to the exiting nerve root, and the tension and retractability of the nerve root are gently tested. To allow exposure of this exiting portion of the nerve root, it may be necessary to use the chisel and Kerrison rongeur to resect a lateral portion of the superior facet. This excision does not cause major damage to the facet joint. Of course, if this joint is going to be included in a fusion, much more of the superior facet can be resected quicker. After exposure of the nerve root, the pathologic condition may require additional exposure of the pedicle below. By approaching medially on the caudal transverse process to the caudal pedicle, one can certainly identify the intervertebral disc, which is always immediately cephalad to the caudal pedicle. Often the nerve root will be coursing over the intervertebral disc in this area, but additional exposure above and below the nerve root may aid in the foraminotomy and/or excision of disc material. A large lateral, volar spur may be removed by entering the disc space, creating a hole in the end-plate under the nerve, and impacting the spur into the hole.

Chapter Twenty

◆

Anterior Lumbar Spine Fusion

Robert G. Watkins
Salvador A. Brau

EVALUATION OF STUDIES

Numerous problems exist in evaluating fusion studies in general, including anterior lumbar fusion studies. Numerous methods have been used for spinal fusion, but the anterior lumbar fusion appears to be, theoretically, an ideal way to stop motion in any neuromotion segment. Because of potential complications with the approach and technical difficulties, the popularity of the operation has never matched that of similar operations, such as anterior cervical fusion.

In the past, studies of the results of anterior lumbar fusions have varied from very high fusion rates to low fusion rates and from very high clinical success rates to low clinical success rates. Several problems exist in evaluating these papers, as well as those detailing other fusion methods. In prospective studies, comparing results in fusion patients with those in nonfusion patients is quite difficult. Most studies making this comparison use patients having decompression for radicular symptoms, where the outcome depends primarily on the adequacy of the decompression, not the fusion. A better comparison would probably be between results in fusion patients and results in patients who are not treated or are treated nonoperatively.

Several measures can be used to properly review results of a specific operation without double-blind prospective comparisons:
- A. Identification of the sample
  1. Properly assess the preoperative morbidity and psychosocial factors.
  2. Establish a diagnosis.
- B. Standardization of method
  1. Establish a safe, reproducible operative technique and postoperative plan.
- C. Unbiased, consistent, comprehensive postoperative assessment evaluation
  1. Properly assess postoperative morbidity.
  2. Determine the structural result (e.g., of fusion).
  3. Fully discuss complications.
  4. Play the role of unbiased observer.
  5. Use comparable controls.

A good composite of reports of this kind shows the results to be expected and allows one to choose some factors responsible for success, as follows:
1. Experience
2. Good grafting technique
3. Safe approaches

In our review of one surgeon's work, severely disabled patients (those with at least 32 months of preoperative disability) were treated with anterior lumbar fusion[1] based primarily on discographic results. Postlaminectomy patients showed improvement equal to that of primary surgical patients, possibly indicating that anterior lumbar fusion is a reasonable choice for postlaminectomy patients because most other operative methods would have a lower success rate compared with primary surgery. Also, worker's compensation cases with the severest morbidity had an excellent recovery rate, indicating that anterior lumbar fusion has a role as a salvage operation for patients with difficult problems. With the strict fusion criteria used, the full bony union rate was low (60%), but 90% of the patients showed excellent clinical improvement.

OVERVIEW OF ANTERIOR APPROACHES AND TECHNIQUES

After deciding that an anterior approach is needed, the exact type must be determined. The position of the patient and the skin incision are the first considerations. The flank approach with the patient in the lateral decubitus position is commonly used for pathologic conditions of the thoracolumbar junction. The best exposure for the L1-2 area is the twelfth-rib approach. The approach with the greatest area of exposure is the tenth-rib thoracoabdominal approach. Any time poor visualization is anticipated in an approach to the upper lumbar spine, the lateral position should be used, the kidney rest raised, the table cracked in the middle, the twelfth rib removed, and the twelfth-rib bed opened extrapleurally and retroperitoneally.

For L1-2, the lateral position, twelfth-rib excision is used. The incision begins over the twelfth rib, extends to the twelfth-rib tip, and then curves down along the rectus sheath as far distally as needed. For the L2-3 disc space, the patient is placed in the supine position, and the incision is begun in the midlateral line over the twelfth rib and extended as a curvilinear incision to just above the umbilicus. For L3-4 and below, the incision begins equidistant between the twelfth rib and the iliac crest. The curvilinear, or oblique, incision ends at the umbilicus for L3-4, at the junction of the upper and middle third of the distance between the umbilicus and the pubis for L4-5, and at the junction of the middle and lower third of the distance between the umbilicus and the pubis for L5-S1.

The lateral position in obese patients allows the pannus to fall away from the spine, even over the edge of the table, leaving a minimum of tissue between the skin and the spine. If the skin incision begins in the midlateral line, the flank approach allows easy recognition of the peritoneum for the retroperitoneal approach. Gravity assists with retraction of the peritoneal sac with a flank approach.

The supine approach has the patient positioned on his or her back over the kidney rest. The medialmost extent of the skin incision is to the midline at the same point as that used for the flank approach. It is usually extended 8 to 14 cm toward the midlateral line above the iliac crest.

Cosmetically, the transverse, low, short incision is best, but the curvilinear, or oblique, incision, especially in the upper lumbar spine, allows more versatility and exposure.

The chief advantage of the supine position rather than the lateral position is the ability to extend the table, opening the disc space and giving a greater distraction and visibility of the disc space. Extending the table with the patient in the lateral decubitus position also opens the disc space and allows grafts to be held under tension. Also, the space may open unevenly, more on the left than on the right. Disc space distraction and graft fixation is better in the supine position. For reduction of a major deformity, the flank approach may offer advantages. In scoliosis, the convexity is positioned up, and excellent exposure of the apex is obtained. In reduction of a spondylolisthesis, the position is determined by the method of reduction to be used. We usually use the supine approach, but others use the flank approach.

Visualization of the posterior disc space and the spinal canal is important in certain operations in the thoracolumbar junction area. In the flank approach, the patient is rotated up to 45 degrees out of the true lateral decubitus position to allow better direct visualization of the spine. In the upper lumbar spine in the supine position, the spinal exposure is more directly anteroposterior (AP), but this approach is limited by the ability to retract the rib cage cephalad in the upper lumbar spine or the peritoneal sac far enough to the right to get a true AP view. Cutting the rectus sheath and rectus muscle and extending the skin incision across the midline can enhance exposure in the midline, but this is rarely needed. Knowing how to use the retractors is critical to direct AP visualization with either approach. Exposure of the dural sac from the anterior approach can be accomplished in two ways. The first is by approaching the canal laterally, exposing a pedicle and the lateral annulus, and separating the annulus from the dura laterally. This is commonly done in the thoracic spine by following the rib to the rib head to the disc space to the canal. The second method is to go directly down the middle, exposing the back of the vertebral body end-plate, and dissecting the annulus off the dura as the disc is excised from anterior to posterior—much like an anterior cervical fusion with canal exploration. The flank approach may be more suitable for the former, and the supine approach may be more suitable for the latter. We prefer the supine approach with maximum table extension and direct annular excision in cases where the canal is to be exposed in the lumbar spine and the lateral approach in cases where the canal is to be exposed in the thoracic or thoracolumbar spine.

The retroperitoneal approach has fewer complications and is easier than the transperitoneal approach. The transperitoneal exposure is used for more difficult cases with extreme lumbar lordosis because the disc space is angled caudally, making full visualization of the space difficult. A midline transperitoneal approach allows exposure as distally as possible and gives the best direct AP view. Extreme retroperitoneal scarring may necessitate a transperitoneal approach. Although the retroperitoneal approach is preferred because it is fast and effective, it retracts the ureters with the sac, and it allows easy exposure to the vessels, the transperitoneal approach allows good visualization in difficult cases.

The standard anterior retroperitoneal flank approach to L4-5 of the lumbar spine is as follows.

The patient is positioned supine on the table with the top of the iliac crest positioned at the flexion point and the kidney rest on the table. The heels and the lower extremities are carefully padded, and TED hose are applied before the patient enters the operating room.

The surgeon stands on the patient's left; the assistant stands on the patient's right. The level of the incision varies according to the level of the spine approached. Incisions for L5-S1 start at the midline at the junction of the lower third and middle third of the distance between the umbilicus and the pubis. Incisions for L4-5 in the midline are at the junction of the upper and middle third of that distance. Incisions for L3-4 are just below the umbilicus, and those for L2-3 are just above. The length of the incision varies from 8 to 14 cm. The incision is extended laterally on a line equidistant between the lowest rib and the superior iliac crest. The skin incision is made to the midline. With self-retaining retractors, the skin is spread and the subcutaneous tissue is opened. The electrocautery is used to cut down to the outer fascial layers of the abdominal wall.

The subcutaneous tissues are incised to the fascia extending beyond the ends of the skin incision, especially laterally to expose the external oblique aponeurosis.

The rectus sheath is incised obliquely from medial to lateral and at the lateral edge is incised vertically for 1 to 2 cm to allow for adequate mobilization of the rectus muscle. This incision is then carried laterally to incise the external oblique fascia, which fuses with the rectus sheath near its lateral border and should stop as the aponeurosis becomes muscular. The rectus muscle is

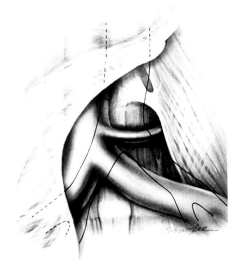

Fig. 20-1. The iliolumbar vein is a branch off the vena cava or left iliac vein that courses right to left, joining the left ascending venous system. Tearing of this vein is the most common source of significant bleeding. (From Watkins RG, Collis JS Jr, editors: *Lumbar discectomy and laminectomy,* Rockville, Md, 1987, Aspen.)

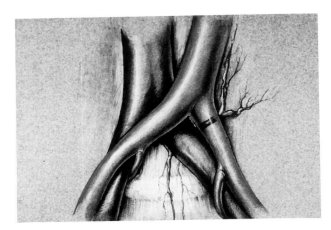

Fig. 20-2. Location of the left iliolumbar vein and the left iliac vein on the left side of the spine. (From Watkins RG, Collis JS Jr, editors: *Lumbar discectomy and laminectomy,* Rockville, Md, 1987, Aspen.)

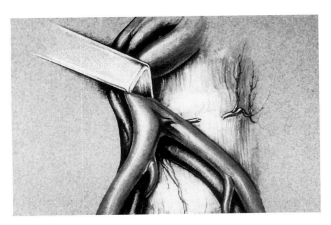

Fig. 20-3. Retraction from left to right of the vena cava and aorta may produce an avulsion of the iliolumbar vein, resulting in tremendous bleeding. The iliolumbar vein should always be ligated for an approach to L4-5. (From Watkins RG, Collis JS Jr, editors: *Lumbar discectomy and laminectomy,* Rockville, Md, 1987, Aspen.)

then mobilized without being transected and with care taken not to injure inferior epigastric vessels. The muscle is then retracted toward the midline, and the posterior rectus sheath is carefully incised. This layer is at times very tenuous, and care must be exercised to prevent lacerating the peritoneum. This incision should be as close to the lateral edge of the rectus sheath as possible without cutting into the internal oblique muscle. With careful blunt dissection, the peritoneum is then separated from the posterior rectus sheath toward the midline first and then laterally under the internal oblique muscle. At this point the dissection is turned posteriorly, and the peritoneum is mobilized medially until the psoas muscle is identified. The dissection is then continued along that plane toward the midline until the left iliac artery is identified (Fig. 20-1). The ureter is usually identified at this point and is carried upward with the peritoneum as the peritoneum is swept off the retroperitoneal structures.

For exposure to L4-5, the prevertebral structure is approached medially from the psoas. The dissection is taken deep and lateral to the iliac artery to expose the iliac vein (Fig. 20-2). Further deep dissection is carried out to expose the iliolumbar vein(s), which can then be doubly ligated and transected (Fig. 20-3). This allows for medial mobilization of both iliac vessels, exposing the left side of the disc. The dissection is then carried anterior to the disc toward the right side to properly expose the area. Again, a needle is inserted into the disc, and an x-ray film is taken to verify the level. Simultaneous exposure of L4-5 and L5-S1 can usually be obtained with this approach, since once the iliolumbar

veins are tied and transected, the vessels can often be mobilized far enough to the right to allow it.

When L5-S1 cannot be exposed from the left of the left iliac artery, the dissection is continued anterior and medial to the left iliac artery. The L5-S1 disc is palpated in the bifurcation. Sharp and blunt dissection exposes the disc between the iliac vessels. The left iliac vein is identified below and medial to the artery and swept away from the anterior surface of the spine using very careful dissection to expose the left side of the disc. Care is taken here to preserve any sympathetic fibers that may be encountered just anterior to the disc. The dissection is then carried to the right side of the disc to fully expose it. A needle is then inserted into the disc, and an x-ray film is taken to verify the level.

Exposure for L3-4 is similar to that for L4-5, except that on occasion the iliolumbar veins may not have to be taken to provide adequate exposure.

In addition to knowing the disc level, one must discern the location of the bifurcation of the aorta. With a very high bifurcation of the aorta, it could be necessary to approach the L4-5 disc within the bifurcation, but in the vast majority of instances the bifurcation is at L5 or lower and the approaches to L4-5 and L3-4 are to the left of the aorta and vena cava.

Dissection on the anterior surface of the spine consists of gentle stretching and pulling of structures, usually blunt dissection rather than sharp, cutting dissection. Because direct pressure over small bleeding vessels usually produces hemostasis, a minimum of electrocautery should be used. Often the branches between the preaortic and paraspinous sympathetic chains must be divided, but they should be preserved if possible. With identification of the disc space, the vessels and retroperitoneal tissue are swept from left to right and held to the right side of the spine. Our standard retraction is to use a malleable retractor of appropriate width and have the tip turned up in the opposite direction. This turned-up tip is fitted to the side of the spine opposite the approach (usually the right side with a left approach) and allows adequate retraction and full, clear visibility of the spine. If the abdominal contents obscure direct work on the disc space, it may be necessary to enlarge the skin incision. By placing this malleable retractor and several others around the spine, it is possible to isolate the disc space and allow adequate visibility for the work to be done. These retractors can be relaxed when work is not being directly carried out in the disc space. They also provide protection from instruments that can slip out of the disc space and potentially injure the retracted vessel.

An alternate method of retraction fixes retractors to the spine. Freebody-Steinmann pin retractors have rubber sleeves and are mounted on a Steinmann pin holder. Four of these pin retractors can be placed into the vertebral bodies adjacent to the disc space—two left and two right. The pin should be stabilized on the tip of the finger and laid directly on the vertebral body under direct visualization so that there is no chance of the wall of the vena cava or left iliac vein being punctured at the time of insertion of the Steinmann pin tip. With the surgeon holding the pin, the assistant hammers it into the vertebral body. The angle of the pin should not be directed toward the disc space or else the pin will project into the disc space and obscure the work on the disc space. At the same time, it should be far enough away from the disc space to allow adequate retraction of the soft tissue. There are excellent combination pin-blade retractors available that have the advantage of stationary, broad blade, protective retraction.

The order of placement is usually superior right, then

inferior right, then superior left, then inferior left, if needed. Some of the left pins are not always needed for the exposure, and the right pins carry the great burden of retracting the major vessels. Often it is advisable to pad the pins and use malleable retractors between the Steinmann pins to add additional protection to the vascular structures.

ANTERIOR RETROPERITONEAL TRANSVERSE APPROACH TO L5-S1

The approach is very similar to that of the L4-5 disc except that the skin incision begins at the junction of the middle and distal third of the distance between the symphysis and the umbilicus and extends laterally for approximately 8 to 12 cm toward the iliac crest. The next steps are as follows:
1. Separate the abdominal musculature.
2. Identify and reflect the peritoneum.
3. Identify the psoas muscle.

After the point of identification of the psoas muscle, it is usually best to proceed directly medially to identify the spine. As the peritoneal sac is bluntly dissected off the retroperitoneal structures, the spine and blood vessels are identified. The ureter comes with the peritoneal sac and will be found on the back of the retracted sac. First, a higher disc is palpated to the left of the vessels in the area of L4-5 to find the spine and become oriented. The surgeon should feel gently the pulsations of the aorta and left iliac artery. It is very important at this time to determine the approximate level of bifurcation of the aorta. Most of the time this is over the L4-5 disc or the L5 vertebral body. Next the aorta and left iliac artery are identified. The surgeon then proceeds to the bifurcation of the aorta and evaluates this visually and with palpation. The surgeon feels the disc bifurcation, even if it is through the left iliac vein. After palpating the left common iliac artery, the surgeon continues on to the L5-S1 disc and identifies the disc again by its raised white appearance and softer feel. The plane is developed just to the right of the left common iliac artery by blunt dissection. Blunt and occasionally sharp dissection are used to develop the plane down to the intervertebral disc surface.

It is very important to be aware of the structures that lie within the bifurcation of the aorta.

The *superior hypogastric plexus* is a continuation of the preaortic, sympathetic chain extending down from the thoracic area, anterior to the aorta and spine in the retroperitoneal space. The inferior hypogastric plexus is approximately at L3, and the superior hypogastric plexus extends from L4 down over the promontory of the sacrum. The size and consistency of the superior hypogastric plexus vary considerably. There may be a plexiform of multiple strands of nerve tissue or a single large nerve trunk. When one nerve trunk is very prominent, it is referred to as the presacral nerve. This plexus extends over the sacral promontory into the pelvis. The superior hypogastric plexus contains sympathetic nerve fibers that course to the urogenital mechanism in the perineal area.

Ejaculation is a combined sympathetic and parasympathetic function, whereas erection is predominantly a parasympathetic function under the control of the seminal muscle and vasculature. Disruption of the sympathetic plexus may result in retrograde ejaculation. These sympathetic fibers have some effect on the motility of the vas deferens, which is important in the transportation of spermatozoa from the epididymis to the seminal vesicle, but the main effect of interruption of the superior hypogastric plexus is a lack of closure of the bladder neck with ejaculation. This allows the semen to be ejected into the bladder rather than out the penis. Technically, if the retrograde ejaculation persists, sterility is the consequence, but the incidence of any ejaculation problem is rare. The prognosis for recovery from retrograde ejaculation, when it does occur, is excellent.

Impotence, or failure of erection, is not produced by damage to the superior hypogastric plexus. The parasympathetic fibers responsible for erection are supplied by the L1 to L4 nerve roots and arrive at that area through the pelvic splanchnic nerves. Somatic function from the S1 to S4 levels is carried through the pudendal nerve.

Methods to avoid damage to the superior hypogastric plexus are as follows:

1. Always use blunt dissection: open the prevertebral tissue in the bifurcation of the aorta. Dissect longitudinally first, just to the left of the left iliac artery, and then dissect bluntly from left to right across the L5-S1 disc, longitudinally spreading and retracting, dissecting left to right until the prevertebral tissue is removed intact from the front of the disc space.
2. Use no electrocautery in the aortic bifurcation or on the L5-S1 disc. Electrocautery produces symptoms much more frequently in this sympathetic tissue.
3. Do not make transverse scalpel cuts on the front of the L5-S1 disc until the annular tissue is clearly identified.

The second structure is the *left iliac vein*. The left iliac vein courses in the bifurcation of the aorta, from right to left, cephalad to caudad. It can be easily damaged and must be carefully identified. It is often compressed by the left iliac artery and may be very prominent in the wound. Anomalous formation of this vein can produce a huge three-vessel structure that demands careful handling for approach to the L5-S1 disc. Usually the left iliac vein must be retracted cephalad and is usually tightly draped around the retractor. Care must be taken to protect the left iliac vein as much as possible.

The third structure is the *middle sacral artery and vein*. These small structures rarely cause significant bleeding.

They can be bluntly dissected with the superior gastric plexus swept to the side and retracted without risk of major bleeding. If this is a prominent structure, it should be clipped with vascular clamps and ligated, not cauterized. The last of the soft tissue is dissected off the spine with the fingertips or a blunt dissector. The malleable retractor is placed to the right of the L5-S1 disc space. Occasionally a blade-point or Steinmann pin retractor is used on the left side of the lumbar spine to retract the left iliac vein cephalad. To use the Steinmann pin or pin-blade retractor, the surgeon puts the tip of the pin between the fingers and holds it against the vertebral body. The pins are inserted first into L5 on the left to safely retract the left iliac vein. The tip of the pin is inserted carefully so that it does not injure the vein. After the L5 pin is placed, an additional lap or malleable retractor is placed caudally when necessary. If the left iliac vein and artery are dissected caudally and to the right, the malleable retractors can be positioned caudally to isolate the vein and artery from the disc space.

In summary, the major steps are as follows:
1. Identify the peritoneum.
2. Identify the psoas muscle.
3. Identify the disc space.

Special precautions in exposure should be taken for discs that have a large, reactive anterior lipping. The vena cava is often adherent to the anterior surface of the disc because of prior or current inflammation. It is easy to tear the vena cava unless special precautions are taken in anticipation of adhesions between the vena cava and the surface of the inflammatory disc. Large osteophytic spurs and anterior lipping are associated with technical difficulties in the exposure. In cases with calcification in the aortic bifurcation, great care must be taken to avoid clotting of arterial structures during retraction. The left iliac artery is of particular concern, since this is often tightly retracted during the procedure. Under these circumstances, it is important to use a malleable retractor, frequently releasing the compression on the aorta. Always, especially when the pin stay retractors are necessary, the surgeon must be certain to evaluate the pulse in the artery at the time the retractors are removed.

After isolating the anterior surface of the disc space, the surgeon makes sure all the retroperitoneal soft tissue is off the annulus. With the disc space cleared off, the limits of the disc space can be defined with a needle. A spinal needle is used to feel the end-plates for a better idea of the exact margins. Then the surgeon proceeds 5 mm on each side of the bony margins and cuts a rectangle approximately 3 cm wide and 5 mm cephalad and caudad to the edge of the vertebral body. The disc space is opened by extending the table maximally, adjusting the table to allow adequate visualization of the depths of the disc space. Extending the table tightens the vessels around the retractors (Fig. 20-4). If the retractors are to be removed, the table is flattened to replace them.

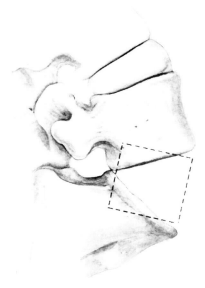

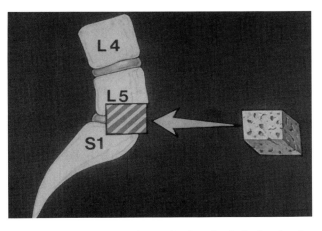

Fig. 20-5. The technique of anterior interbody fusion involves putting a rectangular bone graft into an often-rectangular disc space. (From Watkins RG, Collis JS Jr, editors: *Lumbar discectomy and laminectomy,* Rockville, Md, 1987, Aspen.)

Fig. 20-4. With hyperextension of the lumbar spine to produce distraction for graft placement, there is often a "fish mouth" effect—especially at the L5-S1 disc space. The surgical technique is to rectangularize the open triangular disc space to allow the rectangular graft to be inserted. (From Watkins RG, Collis JS Jr, editors: *Lumbar discectomy and laminectomy,* Rockville, Md, 1987, Aspen.)

The major portion of the inner annulus and the bulk of the nucleus are removed with the Hodgson rongeur.

Either a rectangular slot is cut in the annulus or a flap is made of anterior annulus, to be sutured down after the fusion (Fig. 20-5). If fibula grafts are used, the composite fibula graft is round. Rounding the cut into the lateral annulus is appropriate with fibula grafts. With rectangular grafts or a round femoral ring, the lateral portions of the annulus are preserved with a slot 3 to 4 cm wide. This width of graft bed allows adequate graft contact but retains sufficient strength in the annulus to allow distraction resistance and better graft fixation. Disc and cartilaginous end-plate are removed with the uterine curette, and the large Hodgson rongeur or luxel is used to remove cartilage and disc from the disc space. The angled curette is used to remove some of the tissue; a thrombin-soaked Gelfoam pad is then packed into the disc space, and a 4 × 8 pad is packed behind it to provide some tension to allow the Gelfoam to impregnate the bleeding articular surface of the bone. A drill is used to rectangularize the disc space by drilling down the sides and the posterior surface. A posterior protective shelf is left. The depth of the cut should produce bleeding bone but still preserve the subchondral strength of the bone. Using a chisel can produce a very smooth, level graft bed surface of bleeding, strong subchondral bone.

Two major carpentry factors remain: the depth of the slotted disc space and the uniformity of the graft bed surface. The rectangular slot graft measurer is put to the maximum depth. An x-ray film may be obtained to pro-

vide a good idea of how deep one is. A chisel is used to remove the remaining posterior portion of the end-plate, leaving a small bridge of bone. Usually the posterior third of the vertebral body bleeds more. Curettes, angled and straight, are used for the very back of the disc space. The surgeon can reach into the depths and pull forward rather than driving an instrument toward the spinal canal. A small, angled curette can be slipped over the back edge of the vertebral body to identify the canal. In some cases removal of the back of the annulus, decompression of the canal, and visualization of neurologic structures may be indicated. This is a demanding procedure requiring great skill and experience. Magnification is imperative. In most cases, removal of subannular material to within 1 cm of the dura, distraction, and immobilization of the disc space produces the desired results without resecting the posterior annulus.

The drill can be used safely for leveling the graft bed surface, especially posteriorly in the depths of the space, but visualization can be difficult. The ring and uterine curettes are less likely than an angled curette to gouge out a hole in the bed surface. We use the chisel for fine adjustments.

The dowel method of cutting the disc space is probably the fastest. Dowel cutters that allow a large bone graft to be impacted into the disc space are cut into the vertebral body to bleeding bone and allow clearing of the disc space with curettes and the Hodgson rongeur.

The most difficult, intrinsic problem with the articular surface is its natural concave shape. The problem is worse when Schmorl's nodes are present, necessitating more precise carpentry. The outer rim must be cut down. If long iliac crest plugs or round femoral rings are used, there may be minimal contact in the center. With fibula grafts one starts by putting grafts as lateral as possible and then using taller center grafts. One must be sure to get all of the articular cartilage off the center without gouging it deeper.

Preparation of the end-plate having been completed, the disc space is measured very precisely, with the posterolateral corners usually being the shallowest areas. The slot graft measurer is used for both the height and the rectangular shape of the space.

The choice of graft material depends on its healing ability, strength, ease of insertion, and potential for donor site pain. The following are three of the graft substances that can be used:

1. *Partially decalcified femoral ring packed with cancellous autograft* — This is our choice. It is fast, easy to insert, strong, and appears to unite well. The ring is cut to the desired height, and the edges are beveled.
2. *All fibula* — Each of the fibula plugs should be fashioned to fit next to each other with the nooks and crannies of the fibula and positioned in a perfect vertical fashion. We recommend against using bank bone fibula until the risk of nonunion is further assessed.
3. *Combined fibula and iliac crest* — We have used the fibula grafts and have inserted a central iliac crest tricortical plug down the middle of the slot to wedge the fibular pieces out laterally against the annulus. Our attempts to use allogenous iliac crest in combination with autogenous fibula have not been successful. The bank bone crest apparently requires compression and stimulation for resorption and healing. The fibula is so resistant to compression that it removes the normal stimulus for the iliac crest graft. When used with fibula, the iliac bank bone crest has dissolved, leaving only minimal fibula contact.

After the fusion is completed, the flap of anterior annulus, if preserved, is closed. The peritoneum is allowed to return to its anatomic position, and then all the fascial levels are approximated with running absorbable sutures, with special care taken to close the vertical slits in the anterior rectus sheath. Skin closure is then performed.

FIBULA GRAFT

In taking the fibular graft, great care must be used to avoid creating donor site problems. The fibular length is measured very exactly, from the top of the fibular head to the tip of the lateral malleolus. One uses the middle third, cheating slightly to the proximal third of the fibula under tourniquet. A long, straight skin incision is made with the knife down to the subcutaneous area, and the electrocautery then opens the incision to the lateral fascia. An incision is made just anterior to the lateral intramuscular septum and into the posterior aspect of the lateral compartment. Dissection is carried down to the fibula by direct palpation. At this point, one or two Army retractors are put into the wound but are carefully

positioned on the fibula itself, pulling directly vertically, not retracting hard into the soft tissue. Excessive longitudinal retraction against the cephalad margin of the wound is avoided, since this may produce a peroneal nerve palsy without actually cutting the nerve. The bipolar cautery is used to cauterize any blood vessels coursing across the surface of the fibula. The intramuscular septum is followed directly to the fibula.

The periosteum is incised, and the Lagenbach elevator is used to carefully clear the periosteum off the lateral surface of the fibula. The curved-tip rib elevator can be passed over the anterior and posterior surfaces of the fibula, clearing additional periosteum. Of course, the edge of the fibula is often very sharp, and dissection is slow.

At this point 1-inch-wide brain bands, preferably laminated ones around the fibula, are passed. By keeping the tension off the compartments while retracting them, the surgeon can curve the brain band to wrap around the bone, producing protection for the soft tissues from the saw but at the same time not retracting against the muscle, nerves, and vessels.

A measurement is taken of the exact amount of fibula needed; usually this is a 6- to 8-cm portion. An attempt is made to take all the graft that is needed in one piece, since returns to the wound for additional bone are traumatic. The surgeon cuts directly with the end-cutting saw through the bone to the brain band and removes the segment of fibula when partially decalcified femoral rings are used.

The cancellous autograft used to pack the center of the femoral rings is obtained while the level-marking x-ray film is being processed. Depending on the extent and location of the abdominal skin incision, we may use a small, separate incision or the abdominal incision, either going outside the external oblique fascia or between the external oblique fascia and the internal oblique fascia. The Cloward chisel is used to cut a rectangle into the top of the anterior iliac crest. The rectangular window is removed, and a gouge is made between the tables of the iliac crest. The walls of the slot are preserved, and the insides of the crest are removed through the window in its dorsal surface. Finally, the fascia is irrigated and closed.

Postoperatively, we attempt ambulation on the first postoperative day. For fusions above L5, we use a custom LSO as soon as the pain from the incision lessens enough to allow it. For levels to S1, we usually use an LSO with a leg extension. For a single-level L5-S1, we may use only a lumbosacral corset.

MUSCLE-SPARING APPROACH TO L3-4, L4-5, AND L5-S1

The skin incision is placed obliquely from the midline to the anterior axillary line just lateral to the rectus, with the location in the cephalocaudad plane depending on

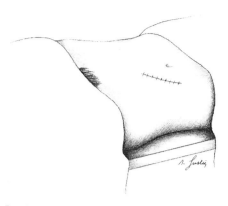

Fig. 20-6. Placement of the skin incision.

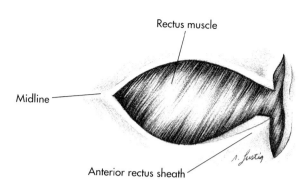

Fig. 20-7. The rectus sheath is incised to allow for adequate mobilization of the rectus muscle.

the level (Fig. 20-6). For L3-4 this is from just below the umbilicus to a point midway between the iliac crest and the twelfth rib. For L4-5 the location is from just above midway between the symphysis pubis and the umbilicus to a point just above the iliac crest. For L5-S1 it is from just below midway between the symphysis pubis and the umbilicus to a point level with the iliac crest.

The subcutaneous tissues are incised to the facies extending beyond the ends of the skin incision, especially laterally to expose the external oblique aponeurosis.

The approach we use today uses approximately a 4- to 5-inch obliquely placed incision. The rectus sheath is incised, the rectus muscle is protected, and the rectus sheath is repaired carefully at closure. The approach is between muscle valleys, avoiding any direct transection of the abdominal musculature. Careful retroperitoneal dissection exposes the intervertebral disc with malleable retractors. Not only does the approach have to be fast and safe, but there should also be no residual pain due to transection of structures during the approach.

The rectus sheath is incised obliquely from medial to lateral and at the lateral edge is incised vertically for 1 to 2 cm to allow for adequate mobilization of the rectus muscle (Fig. 20-7). This incision is then carried laterally to incise the external oblique fascia, which fuses with the rectus sheath near its lateral border, and should stop as the aponeurosis becomes muscular. The rectus muscle is then mobilized without being transected and with care taken not to injure the inferior epigastric vessels. The muscle is then retracted toward the midline, and the posterior rectus sheath is carefully incised (Fig. 20-8). The integrity of this layer is at times very tenous, and care must be exercised to prevent lacerating the peritoneum. The incision should be as close to the lateral edge of the rectus sheath as possible without cutting into the internal oblique muscle. With careful blunt dissection the peritoneum is separated from the posterior rectus sheath toward the midline first and then laterally toward and then under the internal oblique muscle (Fig. 20-9). At this point the dissection is turned posteriorly, and the

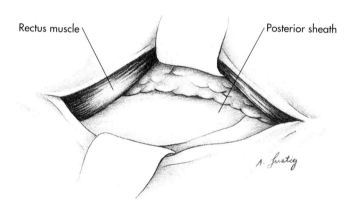

Fig. 20-8. The rectus muscle is mobilized and retracted toward the midline, and the posterior rectus sheath is incised.

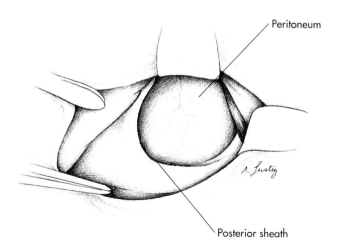

Fig. 20-9. The peritoneum is exposed.

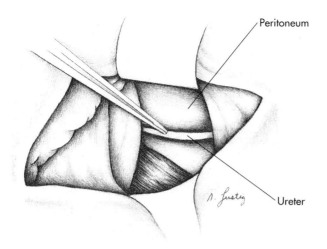

Fig. 20-10. The ureter is carried upward with the peritoneum.

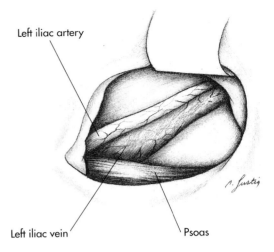

Fig. 20-11. The iliac vein gets swept away from the anterior surface of the spine with dissection to expose the left side of the disc.

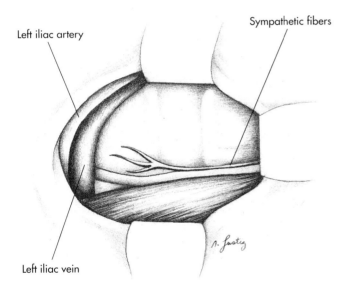

Fig. 20-12. Dissection is carried to the right side of the disc to fully expose it.

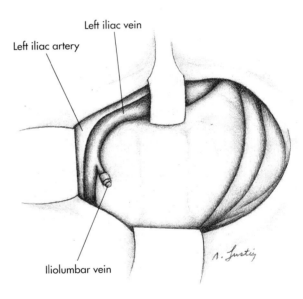

Fig. 20-13. Further deep dissection is carried out to expose the iliolumbar vein(s).

peritoneum is mobilized medially until the psoas muscle is identified. The dissection then continues along that plane toward the midline until the left iliac artery is identified. The ureter is usually identified at this point and is carried upward with the peritoneum (Fig. 20-10).

For exposure of L5-S1, the dissection is continued anterior to the left iliac artery. At this point the L5-S1 disc is palpated, and dissection is carried toward it with sharp and blunt dissection between the iliac vessels. The iliac vein is identified below and medial to the artery and swept away from the anterior surface of the spine with

very careful dissection to expose the left side of the disc (Fig. 20-11). Care is taken here to preserve any sympathetic fibers that may be encountered just anterior to the disc. Dissection is then carried to the right side of the disc to fully expose it (Fig. 20-12). A needle is inserted into the disc, and an x-ray film is taken to verify the level.

For exposure of L4-5, the dissection is taken deep and lateral to the iliac artery to expose the iliac vein. Further deep dissection is carried out to expose the iliolumbar vein(s), which can then be doubly ligated and transected

(Fig. 20-13). This allows for medial mobilization of both iliac vessels, exposing the left side of the disc. The dissection is then carried anterior to the disc toward the right side to properly expose the area. Again, a needle is inserted into the disc, and an x-ray film is taken to verify the level. Simultaneous exposure of L4-5 and L5-S1 can usually be obtained with this approach, since once the iliolumbar veins are transected, the vessels can be mobilized far enough to the right to allow for it.

Exposure of L3-4 is similar to that for L4-5, except that on occasion the iliolumbar veins may not have to be transected for adequate exposure.

After the fusion is completed, the peritoneum is allowed to return to its anatomic position, and then all the fascial levels are approximated with running absorbable sutures, with special care taken to close the vertical slits in the anterior rectus sheath.

Skin closure is then performed.

REFERENCE

1. Watkins RG: Results of anterior interbody fusion. In White AA, Rothman RH, Ray CD, editors: *Lumbar spine surgery: techniques and complications,* St Louis, 1987, Mosby.

SUGGESTED READINGS

Schneiderman G et al: Magnetic resonance imaging in the diagnosis of disc degeneration: correlation with discography, *Spine* 12:276, 1987.

Selby DK et al: Anterior lumbar fusion. In Cauthen J, editor: *Lumbar spine surgery: indications, techniques, failures, and alternatives,* ed 2, Philadelphia, 1988, Williams & Wilkins.

Watkins RG: Anterior lumbar interbody fusion complications. In Garfin S, editor: *Complications of spine surgery,* Philadelphia, 1988, Williams & Wilkins.

Chapter Twenty-One

◆

Spinal Endoscopy

Christopher R. Edwards
Robert G. Watkins
Jocylane M. Dinsay

The latest development in the treatment of spinal disorders has been the development of the spinalscope in a procedure referred to as spinal endoscopy. Technologic advances in the area of fiberoptics have resulted in a steerable fiberoptic visualization filament that can be used to inspect neuroforaminal anatomy and pathologic conditions in the extradural space. If proved successful and safe over an adequate trial period, its potential advantages could be enormous. Orthopaedic surgeons would finally have a tool that could be used to safely diagnose spinal problems and potentially remove an extruded fragment percutaneously.

The newest imaging system is the direct visual working cannula, which is a working channel scope wherein a flexible fiberoptic imaging bundle is actually housed within one of the side walls of the cannula. This allows direct visualization of the pathologic area and enables the examiner to address it through the cannula with instruments such as pituitary forceps or rongeurs under direct fiberoptic visualization. Certainly, this does not supplant the rigid wide-lens systems that are currently used for intradiscal endoscopy, since the rigid systems provide an image with a higher resolution, as well as a greater depth and field of view than the fiberoptics. Both have advantages and disadvantages, as listed in Table 21-1. However, the working cannula with visual capabilities adds a new dimension that has allowed us to address pathologic conditions not only within the disc itself but also within and through the intravertebral foramen.

The concepts and techniques in spinal endoscopy are still in a state of evolution. The purpose of this chapter is to describe our experience, which has focused on insertion techniques and clear identification of the

anatomy, as well as pathologic areas, in cadaveric specimens. Our goal is to make the spinalscope more user friendly, thereby decreasing the learning curve for general use in spinal procedures.

TECHNIQUES AND APPROACHES

As already mentioned, the recent development of small fiberoptic imaging bundles has allowed the surgeon to visualize and remove fragments from the epidural space. However, this concept is still in its fundamental stages, and new surgical approaches, portals, and techniques are continuing to be developed. With the basic goals of developing and evaluating insertion techniques, identifying anatomy and pathologic areas, and continuing to evaluate and develop percutaneous surgical procedures, our institution procured 15 cadaveric specimens that included thoracic, lumbar, and sacral spine segments with associated dorsal skin and musculature. The initial phase of our investigation was to test the optical and visual capabilities of the spinalscope and familiarize ourselves with its use. The four basic approaches we used with the spinalscope were as follows:

1. Open procedure (laminotomy and laminectomy)
2. Sacral coccygeal
3. Posterolateral (transdiscal)
4. Foraminal

Open Procedure

Our initial investigation began with the simplest approach, the open procedure. We used models before attempting each cadaveric dissection. We used standard dissection techniques to gain access down to the posterior elements of the lumbar spine. We then performed laminotomy over the L4-5 interspace using standard tools to gain access to the epidural space. With this approach, an introducer set is not necessary.

Initially we began by using the Murphy ball-style probe with the imaging bundle housed within. This gave us the ability to palpate the underlying pedicles between the adjacent spinal segments, thus providing a reference for examination. Under fiberoptic visualization, we were able to clearly see the pedicles and the exiting nerve roots, as well as the thecal sac and associated disc space. We inserted the ball-style probe and imaging bundle as a probe into the spinal canal. We first palpated the pedicles and then visualized them, receiving a clear

Table 21-1. Comparison of the Different Capabilities of Fiberoptics Versus a Rigid Wide-Lens Scope

Rod Lens Scope		Fiberoptics	
Field of view	90 degrees	Field of view	70 degrees
Depth of field	0-25 mm	Depth of field	2-8 mm
Resolution	20 + pix	Resolution	10-15 pix
Size	> 2.7 mm	Size	1-3 mm
Flexible	No	Flexible	Yes

image. We could also see the associated nerve root exiting just caudal to the structure. Careful probing into the intervertebral foramen allowed us to follow the nerve root almost completely out to the exit zone (Fig. 21-1). This gave us a clear advantage in determining whether a nerve root actually was decompressed when we were performing a foraminotomy. To document the position of the probe, we took a radiograph that clearly showed the probe with the imaging bundle exiting past the pedicle. We then maneuvered the probe back up to the cephalad aspect of the pedicle at the level of the disc space. We documented its location with the use of imaging and could also see it under direct visualization. Our attention then turned to the disc, which we could clearly see with the fiberoptic imaging bundle and easily identify by the white fibrous bands of the overlying annulus. Immediately adjacent was the nerve root, as well as the thecal sac. We repeated this procedure until we were quite comfortable with identifying neurologic structures, discs, and pedicles.

The next stage in this procedure is the use of the flexible sterile imaging bundle. We passed the imaging bundle and catheter under direct visualization on the ventral surface of the spinal canal to the three levels above the laminotomy site. We flexed the tip both medially and laterally and slowly withdrew it over each level in an effort to try to identify neurologic and bony structures. Our initial scope was one of the older models that did not give us as clear a picture, but the structures were discernible. We were able to identify the pedicle and thecal sac, as well as associated nerve roots and the area that appeared to be the disc (Fig. 21-2). To document that we were indeed seeing the structures, we placed an instrument through the disc at a level verified radiographically. We then attempted visualization, and on repeated passes of the flexible fiberoptic scope, we could clearly see the instrument as it pushed through the disc space. We checked the position of the endoscope

with the use of radiographic imaging, which allowed us to repeatedly identify the segmental levels, beginning with L1 down to our laminotomy site of L4-5. To ensure that we were indeed looking at what we thought we were seeing, we marked each structure on different occasions by various means for visual confirmation. After using an open technique with this instrument, we became comfortable enough with identifying neurologic structures, discs, and bony landmarks within the spinal canal to move on to a closed technique.

Sacral Coccygeal Approach

First we used the sacral coccygeal approach, which is similar to the approach that is used for caudal blocks and that can be found in many reference books, especially those used in anesthesiology. The approach is described briefly here.

To introduce the scope through this caudal percutaneous insertion point, an introducer set is available, which consists of a Touhy needle, short and long flexible guide wires, and a series of dilators. The sequence of introduction into the epidural space is similar to the placement of a central angiocatheter. First the Touhy needle is introduced into the caudal insertion point as would be done during a spinal block. Following this, a flexible guide wire is passed through the needle onto the ventral surface of the epidural space. Dilators are then passed over the wire to free the surrounding tissue. Fluoroscopic control is needed to ensure that the guide wires are taking a ventral course relative to the thecal sac. Once the guide wire has been directed up into the lumbar canal, insertion of the scope can begin. The 2.6-mm catheter is passed over the guide wire (Fig. 21-3),

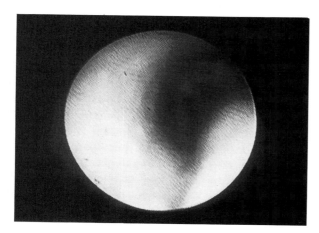

Fig. 21-1. Pedicle neuroforamen and exiting nerve root.

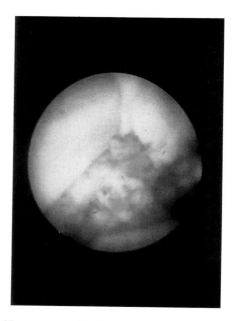

Fig. 21-2. Nerve root and underlying fragment at the disc level.

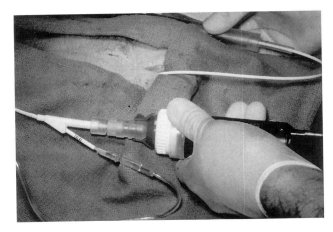

Fig. 21-3. Insertion of the flexible spinalscope through the sacral coccygeal hiatus.

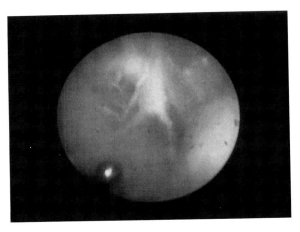

Fig. 21-4. Pedicle as pointed out by the probe and the underlying associated nerve root.

again under direct fluoroscopic control. Next the guide wire is removed, the imaging bundle is passed through the cannula sheath, and visualization of the spinal canal is begun. To get a clear image and to improve the field of view, it is important that the irrigation system that passes fluid through the scope is functioning.

We took similar steps to those used in the open technique to identify the nerve roots, thecal sac, pedicles, and neural foramina. We flexed the catheter tip to approximately 40 degrees, allowing visualization of both the exiting nerve root and the thecal sac. We could easily confirm the direction and level of the catheter tip with the use of fluoroscopic imaging. Again, to confirm and clearly document the structures that we were identifying, we opened the spinal canals of multiple specimens, clearly identifying and marking bony landmarks, as well as neural structures and discs. We then passed the scope during multiple, repeated procedures to again document that we could clearly visualize and with confidence identify structures within the neural canal (Fig. 21-4).

Of note during this approach is the fact that on different specimens, especially those with degenerative lumbar spine disease and degenerative scoliosis, the guide wire would on occasion hang up at the L5-S1 level on the posterior osteophytes, making passage much more difficult. Another drawback to this procedure is the fact that 15% of the population may not have a sacral coccygeal opening to allow insertion of the spinalscope using this approach. Therefore our indications for using the sacral coccygeal approach have been quite limited, and at this point we have abandoned this approach for routine studies. Other approaches allow for much clearer visualization with fewer complications.

Posterolateral (Transdiscal) Approach

The next approach we used was the transdiscal, or posterolateral, approach, which is used in combination

with rigid discoscopy during percutaneous discectomy procedures. There are multiple percutaneous techniques to gain entrance into the anterior disc space. However, the technique that we selected for our study was posterolateral as originally described by Craig[1] and later modified by Kambin and Schaffer[3] and Schreiber et al.[11] As with the previous approaches, this procedure was initially performed on several models and then in cadaveric specimens.

In this approach the patient is placed in a prone position and is lightly sedated. A site approximately 8 to 12 cm lateral to the midline is selected, and a long 18-gauge needle is inserted percutaneously through the skin into the annulus at an angle of approximately 45 to 60 degrees (Fig. 21-5). The correct positioning of the needle is crucial and should be done under fluoroscopic control. To get a true view without rotation, the anteroposterior (AP) image must demonstrate that the spinous processes are in the middle of the vertebral body. On the lateral view the image must demonstrate that the end-plates of the disc space are parallel and located in the middle of the screen. The needle is then advanced until the tip lies on the posterior vertebral body line and is parallel and midway between the end-plates (Fig. 21-6). This is the key starting point and position of reference on the lateral view to ensure that the needle is in the safe entry zone of the posterior aspect of the annulus. On the AP image the needle is advanced between the lateral border of the vertebral bodies and a line connecting the medial border of the corresponding pedicles (Fig. 21-7). Care must be taken not to advance the needle further than this point, because it may place the surgeon unnecessarily close to the thecal sac. If this technique is followed precisely, it allows for the correct placement of the needle in the posterior central aspect of the disc. Key factors to be aware of are as follows:

1. Always flex the patient's hips during positioning,

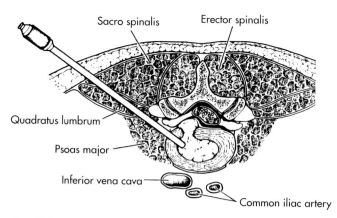

Fig. 21-5. Percutaneous insertion of the guide wire. (From Kambin P, Brager MD: *Clin Orthop* 223:145, 1987.)

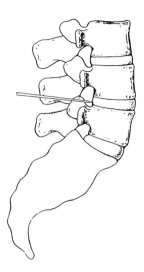

Fig. 21-6. Insertion of the needle on the lateral image until the tip lies on the posterior vertebral body line (PVBL).

which allows the nerve root to move forward, thereby increasing the safe zone during entry.

2. Do the initial placement and advancement of the needle on lateral imaging, which allows compensation for lordosis.

3. Check the needle placement on two views, especially if the position has been changed, which will confirm the correct placement and eliminate any unwanted surprises (Fig. 21-8).

Once radiographic confirmation is achieved, a blunt-tipped tissue dilator is passed over the wire to move away any nearby associated soft tissues. This is followed by a large cannula, which is passed directly over the tissue dilator and docked onto the posterolateral aspect of the vertebral disc. The annulus cutting jig is then inserted within the cannula and is turned clockwise, thereby gaining entrance through the annulus into the disc space. Once this is complete, the suction dissector is inserted and discectomy is begun. A mirror image of these maneuvers is performed on the opposite side, which allows for triangulation of the instruments within the disc space. One should be able to feel the tips of both instruments abutting each other within the disc space and confirm their position on an image (Fig. 21-9). Key points include the following: once the cannula is inserted on the opposite side, the rigid discoscope is inserted on the ipsilateral side with the dissector now being inserted on the opposite side under discoscopic visualization. This allows continuation of the discectomy under direct discoscopic visualization (Fig. 21-10). More important, if at any point during this procedure the patient experiences any radicular pain, the procedure should be aborted and the sequential steps performed again.

Once the disc space has been completely evacuated, a 70-degree discoscope can be turned up to look at the overlying annulus and/or disc protrusion. Ratcheted curved forceps, which have a bendable arch of approximately 80 degrees, are inserted under direct visualiza-

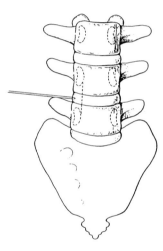

Fig. 21-7. Insertion of the needle on the AP image with tip advancement to the mid–pedicular line.

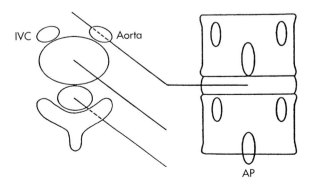

Fig. 21-8. Good placement on the AP image. However, actual placement may be in an unwanted location.

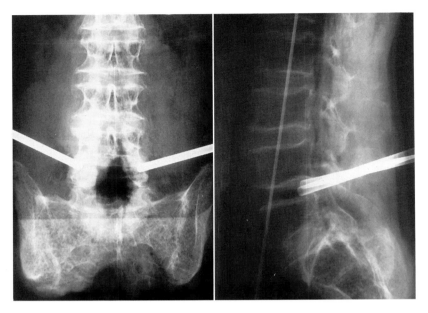

Fig. 21-9. AP and lateral x-ray film with appropriate triangulation of working cannulas within the disc space.

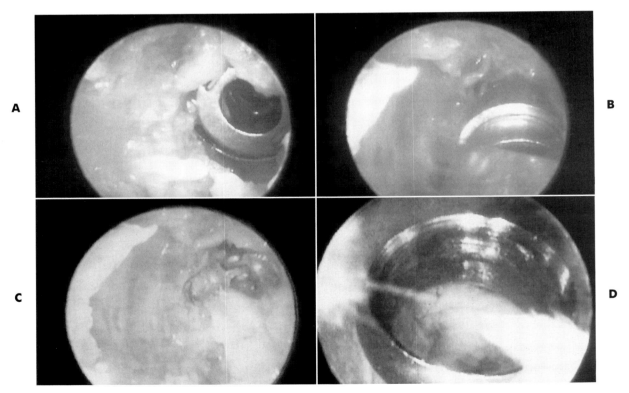

Fig. 21-10. A, Cannula within the disc space. **B,** Reciprocating suction dissector. **C,** Pituitary forceps extracting disc material. **D,** Ring currette removing remaining disc and end-plate.

tion and can be used to grasp either the annulus above or the pathologic area (Fig. 21-11). From this point, the rigid discoscope is replaced by the fiberoptic imaging bundle that is housed within a working cannula, allowing a clear picture of the area directly in front of the cannula. First the cannula is inserted into the disc space to confirm that the disc has been adequately decompressed. If any remaining disc material needs to be removed, grasping forceps or pituitary rongeurs are passed through the cannula into the disc space under fiberoptic visualization, allowing one to extract the remaining material through the cannula. After adequate decompression, the cannula is slowly withdrawn, with the imaging bundle and the tip of the cannula pointed toward the ventral surface of the overlying disc and the exiting nerve roots. This, too, can be clearly identified with the use of the fiberoptic imaging cannula. If a herniated disc fragment remains within the spinal canal, it can be sequentially removed with the grasping forceps or pituitary rongeurs under direct cannula visualization

with care being taken not to injure the associated thecal sac and nerve roots.

This new imaging instrument has been very beneficial in our cadaveric studies, allowing us to not only document residual fragments within the canal but also address them safely without further neurologic injury. It is our expectation that the fiberoptic imaging cannula will be one of the workhorse instruments in the continued development of spinal endoscopy.

Foraminal Approach

The last approach that we evaluated during this cadaveric study was transforaminal. The insertion technique is essentially identical to the preceding one with some minor modifications. On withdrawal of the fiberoptic imaging cannula from the disc space, it is directed toward the foramen, and the foramen with the exiting nerve root is clearly identified (Fig. 21-12). The scope can then be advanced slightly within the exiting zone of the foramen. At this point two options remain: (1) a straight probe can be inserted that can mildly probe the area in and around the nerve root to see if there are any obstructions remaining, or (2) a fiberoptic imaging bundle can be passed down the cannula, through the foramen, and onto the ventral surface of the spinal canal. This second option allows visualization of the thecal sac, as well as of the exiting nerve root and foramen located on the opposite side of the canal. Because the fiberoptic imaging bundle is flexible and steerable, it can also be used to inspect the disc levels that are located above this insertion site. The working channel scope is now used to remove both foraminal and posterolateral herniations via the transforaminal approach.

◆ ◆ ◆

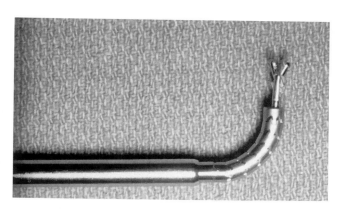

Fig. 21-11. Ratcheted curved forceps.

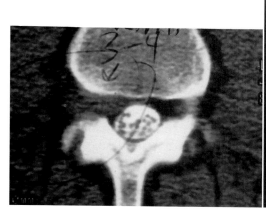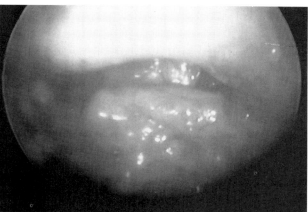

Fig. 21-12. A, Lateral disc herniation that can be approached and corrected using this technique. **B,** Posterolateral aspect of the disc with the exiting nerve root.

One can clearly see the potential use of this instrument as was demonstrated in this study. At our institution we have become quite comfortable with its use. We do suggest that before using these approaches in the actual operating theater, the surgeon should become familiar with the equipment and the approaches through cadaveric study.

CLINICAL APPLICATIONS AND CURRENT USES

Currently the spinalscope and the rigid working channel scope is accepted as a versatile surgical tool that can be used in the diagnosis and treatment of intraspinal problems. There is a potential reduction in surgical trauma with this minimally invasive procedure, and it is certainly worthy of our attention in the treatment of back disorders. The techniques described are innovative and are continually being refined at various institutions. However, the current indications for the use of the spinalscope are as follows:
1. Documentation of pathologic conditions
2. Documentation of decompression of structures
3. Direct nerve root inspection
4. Inspection of internal fixation
5. Delivery of therapeutic agents

These indications are a result of the work performed by Stoll et al.,[13] who participated in FDA Study 150-K in 1989. In a multicenter evaluation, patients underwent spinalscopic examination as an adjunct to open surgical procedures. As a result, the investigators clearly proved that they were able to document existing problems, verify their correction, and, most important, show that there were no complications with the use of this new surgical instrument. The work has continued to evolve in these various institutions, and some of the clinical applications and results have been, to say the least, impressive. The current uses of the spinalscope and endoscopy in clinical practice have evolved to the following:
1. Closed decompression of nerve roots
2. Use with lasers—closed technique
3. Epidural biopsy
4. Percutaneous interbody fusion
5. Decompression of thoracic disc herniations
6. Removal of foraminal and posterolateral extruded disc fragments

In 1986 Schreiber et al.[11] attempted trans–discoscopic percutaneous discectomy in a total of 40 patients with 49 disc herniations. At that time they were able to use modified arthroscopy equipment only, and their indications were limited to patients with lumbago who had positive myelographic findings. Even with these nonspecific conditions and limited indications, however, they were able to show good or very good results in the majority of their patients and believed that this would improve to even better results with better instrumentation, more specific indications, and more experience. Mathews[6] used spinalscopic assisted percutaneous in-

terbody fusions in 21 patients and noted that 20 of these patients were able to return to their jobs within 6 months, with only 1 patient showing no improvement whatsoever over an average follow-up time of 5 months. There were three complications, which included one infection and two seromas, which were resolved quite easily. Overall, they considered this an excellent technique that gave them an added option for the treatment of segmental instability.

Interest has been rising in the use of spinalscopic principles and techniques in the treatment of thoracic spine problems (Fig. 21-13). In our study we evaluated the use of the spinalscope and working channel scope in the treatment of thoracic disc herniations and other thoracic spine problems using the basic technical concepts described by Landreneau et al.[4] and Regan et al.[10] Of course, modifications were made in order to apply these concepts to thoracic spine surgery.

The patient is placed in a lateral decubitus position, and the table is maximally flexed in order to drop the hip and upper torso away from the operative field. This promotes increased widening of the intercostal spaces, allowing for ease of instrument insertion while at the same time reducing the amount of levering of instruments against the underlying ribs. Access to the pleural cavity is usually established in the fifth or sixth intercostal space at the mid to posterior axillary line. A 10-mm rigid 30-degree-angle spinalscope is then placed through this initial trochar portal, and exploration of the thoracic cavity is begun. The immediate view of the thoracic cavity is the same as that seen during thoracotomy, with the anterior mediastinal structures seen on one side and the posterior structures seen on the other side of the screen (Fig. 21-14). As the scope is turned more posteriorly, the sympathetic chain and stellate ganglion can be seen as they cross over the heads of the ribs just lateral to the vertebral bodies. These ganglions appear as slight bulges at each of the intercostal levels. Of note during this procedure when we performed it was the development of some fogging of the lens when the scope was initially placed. To avoid this, an antifogging solution was used that readily rectified the problem and allowed for a clear video image.

After initial exploration of the pleural cavity is complete, a second and/or third trochar is placed, usually at the same level. Placement of these trochars is guided by the location of the problem, with each port being placed as far away as possible from the camera and from each other so as to prevent abutment of instruments in the thoracic cavity. A very useful concept that we adopted illustrated quite nicely the principles of triangulation; this was to imagine a baseball diamond in which the scope port was home base, the pathologic lesion was second base, and the working ports were first base and third base (Fig. 21-15). However, portals can be placed in any position that will allow for ease of

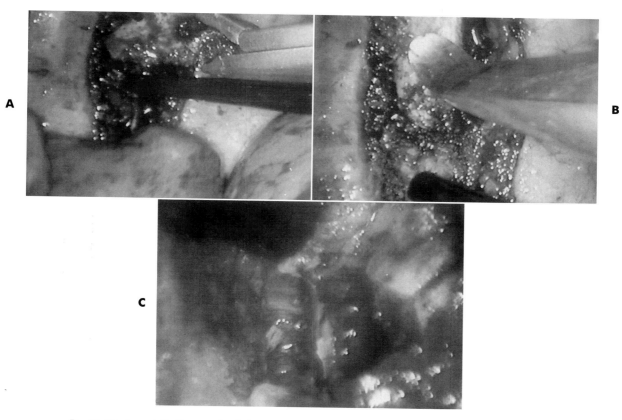

Fig. 21-13. A and **B,** Removal of the rib head with pituitary forceps. **C,** The disc has been removed back to the dura.

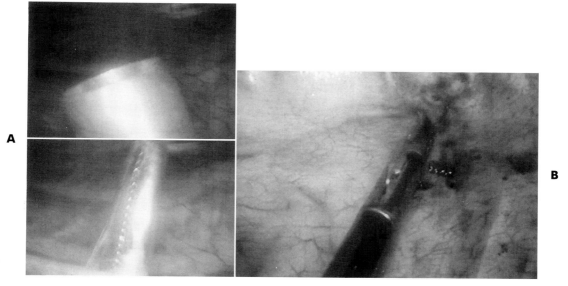

Fig. 21-14. A, Insertion of the trochar into the thoracic cavity. **B,** The ribs, lung, and segmental vessels as seen through the spinalscope at the beginning of the procedure.

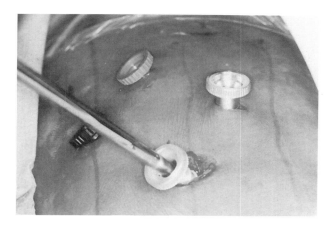

Fig. 21-15. Baseball diamond configuration with the scope at home plate, the disc path at second base, and the working ports at first base and third base.

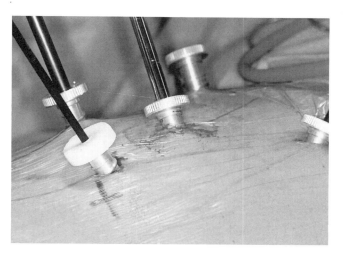

Fig. 21-16. Portal positions.

instrument manipulation in the pleural cavity (Fig. 21-16). Once general exploration has been complete, the disc can usually be identified as the white prominent structure that is relatively avascular. The correct level can be determined by counting the ribs inside the chest or by inserting a needle into the disc space and getting radiographic confirmation. The anatomy of the spine at this point is obscured by the reflection of the parietal pleura as it covers the structures over the spinal column. The pleura is then dissected off with the use of electrocautery or endoscopic scissors (Fig. 21-17). Intercostal veins and arteries cross the midportion of each vertebral body and may be ligated with the use of an endoscopic clip, thereby preventing any significant bleeding.

Thoracic discectomy is begun by first identifying and removing the head and proximal 2 cm of the rib at the appropriate disc level (Fig. 21-18). This is done by using an osteotome to divide the rib laterally and then dissecting it free from the surrounding muscle. The rib is then disarticulated at the transverse process of the vertebral body, allowing access to the corresponding pedicle. The superior portion of this pedicle is then carefully removed with the use of rongeurs or a high-speed burr through the working portal. The herniated nucleus pulposus is then clearly identified and removed from the epidural space by using careful curettage and rongeurs (Fig. 21-19). On completion of the discectomy, a fusion can be accomplished by using bone chips that are then placed in the evacuated disc space. With this procedure multilevel anterior releases can also be accomplished in a similar fashion. This may not require removal of the rib head.

In performing this study, we determined that by using these techniques, a spine surgeon could safely address pathologic conditions of the thoracic spine using spinalscopic principles and techniques. This fact has been

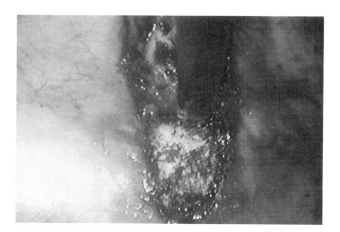

Fig. 21-17. Rib being dissected free with cautery and modified instruments.

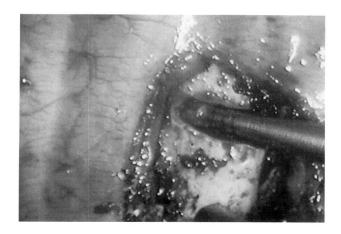

Fig. 21-18. Osteotomy of the rib with a high-speed burr, 2 cm proximal to the head.

borne out by the reports of success by other institutions that have also begun their use in clinical practice.[5,10]

The current indications for use of the spinalscope in the thoracic spine are as follows:
1. Biopsy, debridement
2. Drainage of abscess
3. Corpectomy
4. Thoracic disc excision
5. Interbody fusion
6. Anterior spinal release

The current contraindications to using these techniques are as follows:
1. Previous thoracotomy
2. History of pleurodesis
3. History of empyema
4. Severe chronic obstructive pulmonary disease (COPD)

Recent reports have shown that high success rates with this procedure can and should be expected when the above criteria are followed. This has been demonstrated in one of the more recent articles by Mack et al.[5] They performed this procedure, which was referred to as "video-assisted thoracoscopy" in 10 patients for various thoracic spine problems (Table 21-2). They reported success in all cases, with no mortality, and only one case of postoperative pneumonia. Work at their institution has continued, with reports of all procedures successfully being completed using this technique. Again, in a series of 12 patients there was no mortality, and morbidity consisted of only a persistent fever, pleural effusion, and atelectasis in one patient who was found to be a heavy smoker undergoing correction of 105-degree scoliosis. Crawford[2] has also expressed good early results in pediatric cases.

One of the most important findings is the fact that no patients have been found to have any evidence of postthoracotomy pain syndrome. Certainly, this is a major advantage when compared with open thoracotomy

procedures. Research and development are ongoing, and we expect the results to be comparable to the experience of the sports medicine physicians who developed knee arthroscopy versus arthrotomy. Further experience and instrument modification will be needed, but at this point application of spinalscopic techniques in the thoracic spine has proved to be a great success.

Finally, the last spinalscopic techniques that we evaluated were those used in concert with anterior and retroperitoneal laparoscopy. The use of the laparoscope in general and gynecologic surgery is well known and has proved to be quite safe and effective.[12] Modifications of these techniques have now been applied to spinal surgery.[9] The first approach that we evaluated in our study was the transperitoneal approach to the L5-S1 disc space.

To begin, the laparoscope is inserted via a Hassan trochar using a periumbilical incision. Carbon dioxide can then be used to insufflate the peritoneum to 16 cm of water pressure. The laparoscope is inserted through the umbilicus because this is the thinnest area of the anterior abdominal wall. The patient is then placed in the Trendelenburg position, which allows the abdominal contents to fall away in a cephalad direction, thus revealing the posterior abdominal cavity and the sacral promontory. Two 5-mm trochars are placed midway between the umbilicus and the symphysis pubis 6 to 8 mm from the midline equidistantly. These are inserted under direct or endoscopic visualization with care taken not to injure any underlying structures that may not have been moved away. Various retractors can be inserted to move and hold the bowel contents away from the anterior ventral aspect of the L5-S1 disc space. Laparoscopic identification of the bifurcation of the great vessels should be made, followed by identification of the ureters, middle sacral vein and artery, and the sympathetic plexus.

The middle sacral vein and artery are ligated in an

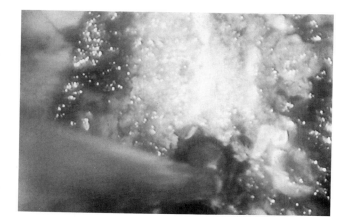

Fig. 21-19. Disc space being evacuated by sharp curettes.

Table 21-2. Use of the Spinalscope in the Thoracic Spine

Procedure	No. of Patients
Anterior release (discectomy) with fusion for correction of kyphosis/scoliosis plus thoracoplasty (1 case)	3
Discectomy for herniated nucleus pulposus	3
Biopsy/debridement collapsed vertebral body/discectomy	1
Drainage of disc space abscess	1
Biopsy of collapsed vertebral body	1
Fusion of disc space	1
TOTAL	10

From Mack MJ et al: *Ann Thorac Surg* 56:736, 1993.

effort to control bleeding. Once all of these structures have been identified and the surgeon is oriented in the cavity, the spinal part of this operation is begun. A suprapubic portal is made, and a 5-mm cannula is placed in this position. Graspers are then used to grab the posterior peritoneal lining, and a longitudinal incision is made with cutting shears down to the level of the disc space. The annulus is clearly identified, and a Steinmann pin is placed in the disc space, allowing for radiographic confirmation of the correct level. The annulus is then incised with either an endoscopic scapula or an ultrasonic knife. The disc space can then be excavated with long pituitary rongeurs and uterine and/or ring curettes in the usual manner. Following this, the disc space is inspected by first using a 30-degree endoscope, checking each end-plate carefully. Any remaining disc material can be removed at this time. A 0-degree scope is then placed in the suprapubic site, and the posterior disc space is inspected. All disc material that can be identified can safely be removed, and inspection of the end-plate should reveal bleeding bone. Appropriate interbody spacers are then selected to determine the correct height, depth, and width of the excavated disc space. X-ray films are again obtained to ensure that the surgeon is parallel with the end-plate at the S1 location. An allograft bone block or a fusion cage filled with cancellous bone is then inserted and tamped securely into the disc space. The operating room table should be maximally cracked so as to open the disc space when the interbody fusion material is being inserted. Once this material is tamped into place, the table is then cranked back into a neutral position, thus locking the device into place. The fusion device is then checked to make sure that it is quite secure, and final x-ray films are taken to confirm appropriate placement. Following this, the peritenon should be sutured closed, achieving a watertight closure in an effort to prevent any postoperative hernias.

Although we believe that this technique is effective and safe when performed according to these guidelines, we still encourage each surgeon to participate in either cadaveric study or live animal laboratory studies before using it in the actual operating theater. A laparoscopic approach to L5-S1 is an acceptable alternative to treatment of a pathologic condition found in this disc space area. However, we believe that pathologic findings in the remaining lumbar disc spaces should be approached using either a posterolateral or retroperitoneal technique.

With a retroperitoneal approach, the patient is placed in a left lateral decubitus position. At this point the tip of the twelfth rib can easily be identified, and a small incision is made in this area. The internal and external oblique muscles are then identified and subsequently spread apart in the direction of their fibers. The transversalis fascia is then identified and opened. Blunt

finger dissection is used to dissect in the retroperitoneal space with care taken to feel the posterior course of the twelfth rib and the transverse process of the corresponding spine. It is at this point that we use a balloon that is secured to the end of a catheter. The balloon is insufflated with approximately 300 to 400 ml of saline, creating a large space in the retroperitoneal area. The balloon is subsequently drained and removed, and a 12-mm trochar is inserted in its place. The laparoscope is then inserted, and the procedure is begun.

The first step is to select appropriate additional portals. These portals are usually 5 mm and are inserted under direct endoscopic visualization with care taken not to injure any of the underlying retroperitoneal contents. A fan retractor is then placed in the retroperitoneal space, mobilizing the peritoneal contents in an anterior direction. Blunt dissection through the third portal is then used to gently tease any remaining fibers off of the lumbar spine. This allows a straight shot when one is inserting a spinal needle and other instruments into the disc space. The spinal needle is inserted under endoscopic control through one of the percutaneous portals. Radiographic confirmation is then obtained to confirm that this is indeed the correct level. Similar techniques to those described for the laparoscopic approach are then used. The annulus is taken down with a surgical cutting knife or an ultrasonic knife, and the disc space is evacuated using various instruments, including pituitary rongeurs, ring curettes, and uterine curettes.

What we found very helpful is that the working cannula can be inserted right down to the level of the disc space, permitting the instruments to be passed through directly onto the disc space, thereby minimizing any possible injury to the segmental vessels or abdominal contents. Of note is the fact that these segmental vessels can be ligated with standard surgical techniques and dissected away from the surgical field if necessary. Once the disc space is evacuated, a 30-degree-angle scope is used to visualize the disc space and to confirm that all disc material has been removed. Following this, the portal is placed directly into the opening of the excavated disc space, and cancellous bone graft can be inserted, or as was done with the laparoscopic techniques, a bone block or fusion cage can be tamped into place. Although we were quite comfortable and satisfied with this technique and its applications, we advocate having the assistance of a general or vascular surgeon when using the laparoscope.

REFERENCES

1. Craig FS: Vertebral body biopsy, *J Bone Joint Surg* 38A:93, 1956.
2. Crawford A: Personal communication, 1994.
3. Kambin P, Schaffer JL: Percutaneous lumbar discectomy: review of 100 patients and current practice, *Clin Orthop* 238:24, 1989.
4. Landreneau RJ et al: Video-assisted thoracic surgery: basic technical concepts and intercostal approach strategies, *Ann Thorac Surg* 54:800, 1992.

5. Mack MJ et al: Application of thorascopy for diseases of the spine, *Ann Thorac Surg* 56:736, 1993.

6. Mathews H: Personal communication, Oct 1993.

7. Ooi Y, Satoh Y, Morisaki N: Myeloscopy, *Int Orthop* 1:107, 1977.

8. Ooi Y, Satoh Y, Morisaki N: Myeloscopy: the possibility of observing the lumbar intrathecal space by use of an endoscope, *Endoscopy* 5:901, 1973.

9. Regan JJ, Aronof RJ: *Thorascopy and laparoscopy of the spine,* Workshop, Dallas, 1994.

10. Regan JJ et al: Technical report of video-assisted thorascopy in thoracic spinal surgery, Manuscript submitted for publication, 1994.

11. Schreiber A et al: Does percutaneous nucleotomy with discoscopy replace conventional discectomy? *Clin Orthop* 238:35, 1989.

12. Semmo K: Die pelviskopische appendecktomie, *Dtsch Med Wochenschr* 113:3, 1988.

13. Stoll J et al: *Midwest spinal center,* Milwaukee, 1989, FDA-IDE Study.

Chapter Twenty-Two

Intradiscal Therapy

Gurvinder S. Uppal

The number of patients seeking care for back and radiating leg pain is increasing each year. The impact of lumbar disc disease on the socioeconomic state of society is tremendous—both in pain and suffering and in days lost from work. Studies from all over the world show the ever-increasing societal impact of low back disorders.[8] This has led to interest in minimizing the effect and magnitude of low back disorders by improving both nonoperative and operative treatments. The potential morbidity of open spine surgery has created interest in percutaneous procedures that would decrease the morbidity yet allow adequate treatment of the disc abnormality. These percutaneous intradiscal procedures include chemonucleolysis, intradiscal arthroscopic microdiscectomy, automated percutaneous lumbar discectomy, and laser discectomy.

CHEMONUCLEOLYSIS

Percutaneous removal of intervertebral discs has been performed with a variety of enzymatic and mechanical techniques for the past two decades.[16] These have in common the removal of all or part of the nucleus pulposus to induce more rapid healing and restabilization of the degenerating lumbar disc. It has been assumed that patients would experience decreased pain and disability as a result.

At one time chemonucleolysis was widely used. This procedure consisted of the injection of chymopapain into the symptomatic degenerating intervertebral disc. Chymopapain is a proteolytic enzyme that disrupts the protein mucopolysaccharide component of the nucleus pulposus, causing rapid reduction in its viscosity and molecular weight.[5,6,18-21,23,25] After its injection into the disc, nuclear tissue dissolves at the rate of 1 g of wet tissue/hr/mg of chymopapain at pH 7.4. The glycosaminoglycan degradation products of the nucleus are found in significant concentrations in blood and urine. Because chymopapain has little effect on collagen, the annulus fibrosus remains intact after the dissolution of the nucleus. The empty disc space is replaced by fibrous tissue, resulting in restabilization of the disc and relief of symptoms.

Severe problems have arisen with the use of chymopapain on a clinical basis. Most patients experience moderately severe discomfort when 1 ml or more is injected into the disc space. Up to 85% have back pain and muscle spasm for several days or weeks after the procedure. A serious problem with chemonucleolysis is

anaphylaxis caused by presensitization to chymopapain. Cauda equina syndrome,[11] subarachnoid hemorrhage,[3] acute encephalopathy,[2] and paraplegia[15,17] have occurred as complications of chemonucleolysis. The serious complication rate appears to be less than that of open surgery.[4,6,22] Overall, significant complications with chemonucleolysis occur in 2% to 4% of patients who have the procedure. Successful pain relief occurs in 70% to 80% of patients in the various reported series, and some authors suggest that chemonucleolysis is the last step in conservative treatment before an open surgical procedure is considered. Alexander et al.,[1] for example, noted that 18% of patients who had chemonucleolysis continued to have symptoms sufficiently severe to require surgery. After laminectomy and disc excision, the rate of satisfactory outcome was 90% for their entire group of chemonucleolysis patients as compared with an 80% success rate in patients treated with surgery alone.[24] Other studies have shown surgery to be slightly more effective.[15]

ARTHROSCOPIC INTRADISCAL MICRODISCECTOMY

Mechanical techniques require the insertion of instruments with much larger diameters than the needles used in enzymatic chemonucleolysis or automated percutaneous lumbar discectomy. Arthroscopic intradiscal microdiscectomy was introduced by Hijakata[10] and by Kambin and Saliffer.[13] The outside diameter of the cannulas used in their procedures was 6 to 8 mm, and some surgeons now recommend a biportal technique. Arthroscopic intradiscal microdiscectomy, therefore, is more invasive and a procedure of greater magnitude than chemonucleolysis. Its advantages lie in the surgeon's ability to enter the disc under direct vision, remove more tissue, and directly visualize a protruding disc fragment from inside the disc and remove it. Certain automated techniques are being developed that increase scope and directional capabilities.

AUTOMATED PERCUTANEOUS LUMBAR DISCECTOMY

Automated percutaneous lumbar discectomy (APLD) involves the insertion of a motorized probe (nucleotome) into the disc space (Fig. 22-1). With fluoroscopic control and the patient under local anesthesia, the device is passed through a 2.8-mm cannula. A continuous saline lavage under strong suction removes particles of disc material caught in the reciprocatory cutter. The blunt configuration of the tip of the nucleotome with a

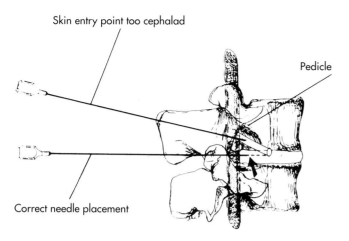

Skin entry point too cephalad

Pedicle

Correct needle placement

Fig. 22-1. Correct needle placement for automated percutaneous lumbar discectomy (APLD).

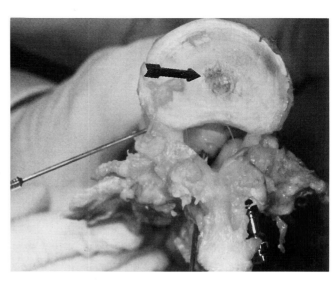

Fig. 22-2. Cadaveric lumbar spine segment after laser discectomy; 1200 J of energy was used with a Ho:YAG laser. The arrow points to the area of ablation.

side-cutting port is said to prevent damage to the annulus and provide for safe removal of nuclear contents only. Onik et al.[18] described the results of this procedure in 327 patients. They noted a 75% success rate in appropriately selected patients and found that complications occurred in only 1% of patients. These included psoas hematoma, discitis, vasovagal reaction, and postoperative spasm. Kahanovitz et al. showed the APLD to be less effective.[12,14]

The procedure has been criticized on several grounds. Relatively little disc material may be removed by APLD, and in experimental animals the disc appears unchanged several months after the procedure has been performed.[7,9] Increasing the amount of disc removed may improve results.

◆ ◆ ◆

Assuming that some patients with protruding or prolapsed discs do not spontaneously improve within a suitable time after the onset of symptoms, it would seem appropriate to have a procedure available that might control symptoms. Chemonucleolysis, arthroscopic intradiscal microdiscectomy, automated percutaneous lumbar discectomy, and, more recently, laser nucleotomy[26] all offer the advantage of percutaneous surgery, with minimal morbidity, local anesthesia, and outpatient care to minimize the expense of the procedure.

Enzymatic chemonucleolysis has the reported disadvantage of exposing the patients to the risk of anaphylaxis and neurologic damage. Arthroscopic intradiscal microdiscectomy requires the use of large-bore devices and repetitive reentry into the disc space with hand instruments, thus increasing the risk of infection. APLD may be less efficacious in removing degenerative disc material, although the reciprocating cutter can be inserted through a much smaller cannula than with the arthroscopic interdiscal microdiscectomy technique.

LASER DISCECTOMY

Laser discectomy can be performed through a small-bore needle, and the defect in the center of the disc is usually safely, accurately, and predictably configured. Furthermore the creation of the defect does not require the injection of material into the disc, as is the case with chemonucleolysis. The intraoperative discomfort of the enzymatic technique is avoided because there is no addition of volume to the disc. The laser procedure carries no risk of anaphylaxis, and the instrumentation is smaller than that used in any of the mechanical percutaneous discectomy operations.

LASER (light amplification by stimulated emission of radiation) has been successfully used to ablate the intervertebral disc. The laser is a photothermal device that transfers light energy to heat and causes an ablation of tissue (Fig. 22-2). Different types of laser differ in their wavelength and thus the light characteristic. Tissue absorption of these different wavelengths of light determines to what degree tissue ablation occurs. The neodymium: yttrium aluminum garnet (Nd:YAG), potassium titanyl phosphate (KTP), and holmium (Ho:YAG) lasers have been used to ablate the intervertebral discs. Animal studies and clinical trials show that the Ho:YAG laser is the preferred laser for this task. The depth of thermal penetration of this 2.1 μm–wavelength laser's energy is 2 mm.

Indications for laser discectomies include contained herniated discs in patients with radiculopathy unresponsive to conservative nonoperative programs (Figs. 22-3

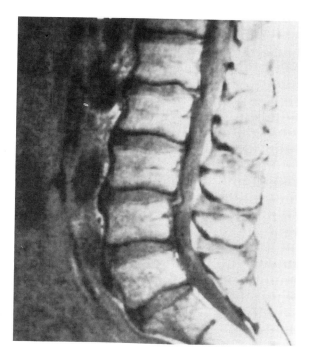

Fig. 22-3. Sagittal-view MRI of the lumbar spine showing a contained herniated disc at L3-4.

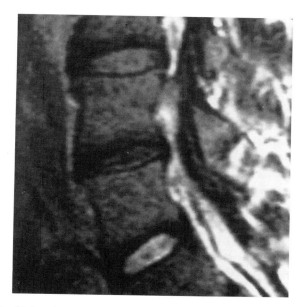

Fig. 22-5. T2-weighted image showing a dehydrated disc at L4-5. The discs at L3-4 and L5-S1 are relatively normal.

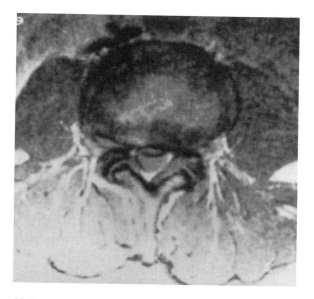

Fig. 22-4. Axial-view MRI showing a central contained herniated disc.

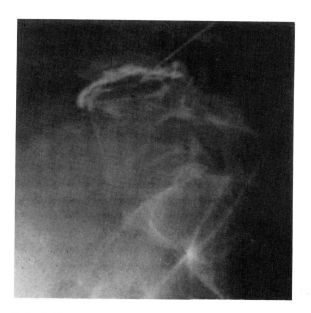

Fig. 22-6. A discogram at L4-5 in the same patient reproduces the usual back pain. The disc morphology is also abnormal.

and 22-4). Approximately 77% of patients who have this procedure have good to excellent results. A subset of patients on whom we have performed this procedure includes those with internal disc disruption. These patients have more back pain than leg pain. Nonoperative programs consisting of physical therapy, nonsteroidal antiinflammatory drugs (NSAIDs), and epidural cortisone injections are unsuccessful. The plain radio-

graphs of these patients usually show normal findings; yet their magnetic resonance imaging (MRI) scans show a black, dehydrated disc on the T2-weighted image (Fig. 22-5). A discogram performed at that level completely reproduces their pain (Fig. 22-6). Approximately 60% of these patients who have laser discectomies have good to excellent results.

Ho:YAG laser discectomy is performed with the

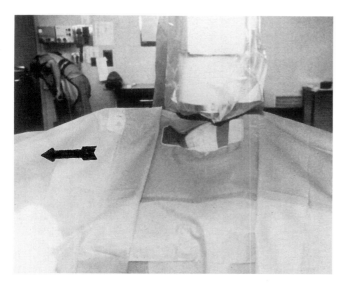

Fig. 22-7. Properly positioned and draped patient. The arrow points cephalad.

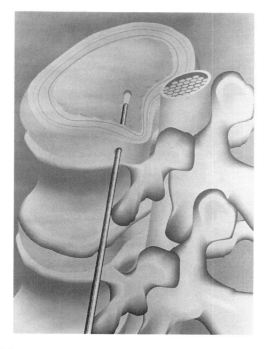

Fig. 22-8. The straight-fire tip refers to the laser beam exiting straight from the end of the laser fiber. (Courtesy Trimedyne, Inc.)

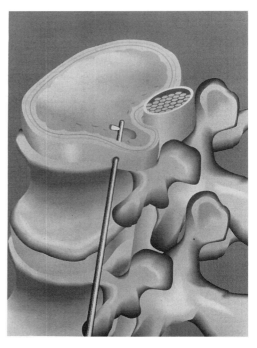

Fig. 22-9. The side-fire tip refers to the laser beam exiting from the side of the laser probe. (Courtesy Trimedyne, Inc.)

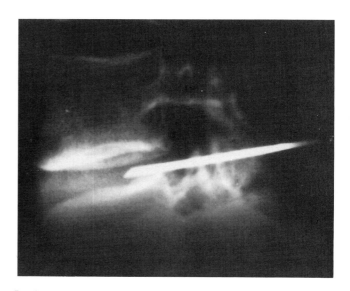

Fig. 22-10. Laser introduction needle in the center of the L4-5 disc on the lateral view.

patient in either the prone or the lateral decubitus position. We prefer the latter so as to avoid injury to the colon (Fig. 22-7). The skin is prepared with a povidone-iodine solution and sterile draping. A sterilely draped C-arm is used for fluoroscopic control throughout the procedure. Intravenous antibiotics are given for prophylaxis. Intravenous sedation is used in conjunction with

local lidocaine at the needle entry site. Lidocaine is injected into the skin 10 cm laterally to the disc space, and a 160-gauge needle is inserted at approximately 45 degrees to the coronal plane down to the annulus. If the patient experiences leg pain, the needle is withdrawn slightly and redirected. Once the annulus is engaged, the needle is passed through the annulus and into the

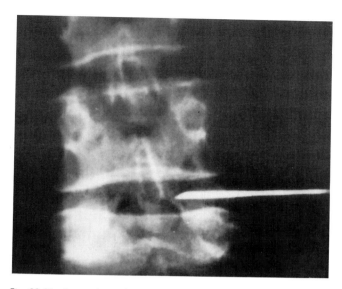

Fig. 22-11. Laser introduction needle in the center of the L4-5 disc on the AP view.

nucleus. The stylet in the needle is then withdrawn, and a laser fiber with either a side-fire or straight-fire tip is passed through the needle into the nucleus (Figs. 22-8 and 22-9). The side-fire probe offers a more circumferential ablation of the disc with rotation of the fiber. This allows a greater ablation of the disc with fewer thermal changes to the adjacent disc. The tip of the fiber is radiopaque so that its position can be easily identified fluoroscopically.

Once the positioning is confirmed on both anteroposterior (AP) and lateral radiographs (Figs. 22-10 and 22-11), the laser is activated with the use of 1.5 W/pulse at 10 Hz. It is imperative that the introducing needle be in the center of the disc before laser ablation. No more than 5 J of laser energy should be imparted to the nucleus at one time. Approximately 2 seconds are allowed to elapse between each period of laser activation to prevent excessive heat buildup of the surrounding tissues. The products of vaporization escape through the needle that contains the laser fiber. Throughout the procedure the position of the needle and the laser fiber is continually checked to avoid misplacement of the laser energy. A total of 1200 J of laser energy is imparted to the nucleus in each patient. After completion of the ablation, the fiber and needle are withdrawn and an adhesive bandage is used to cover the needle site.

The patients are started on a trunk stabilization physical therapy program 5 to 7 days after surgery.

Percutaneous discectomy can be performed with chymopapain, APLD, or arthroscopic intradiscal microdiscectomy, or with one of several available lasers. Experimentally, lasers have been shown to cause a

reduction of intradiscal pressure by altering the osmotic pump mechanism of the intervertebral disc, as well as changing the healing response of the herniated disc. These qualities may be responsible for the clinical efficacy of the procedure noted.

REFERENCES

1. Alexander AH et al: Chymopapain chemonucleolysis versus surgical discectomy in a military population, *Clin Orthop* 244:158, 1989.
2. Anderson BA: Acute encephalopathy and third-nerve palsy after chymopapain injection, *Can Med Assoc J* 139:412, 1988.
3. Benoist M et al: Chemonucleolysis for disc rupture, *Spine* 12:421, 1987.
4. Bouillet R: Treatment of sciatica: a comparative survey of complications of surgical treatment and nucleolysis with chymopapain, *Clin Orthop* 251:144, 1990.
5. Branework P et al: Tissue response to chymopapain in different concentrations, *Clin Orthop* 67:52, 1969.
6. DATTA: Diagnostic and therapeutic technology assessment: laminectomy and microlaminectomy for treatment of lumbar disc herniation, *JAMA* 264:1469, 1990.
7. Fater EA: The neurosurgical management of lumbar spine disease, *N Dev Med* 3:5, 1988.
8. Frymoyer JW: Back pain and sciatica, *N Engl J Med* 35:291, 1988.
9. Gunzburg R et al: An experimental study comparing percutaneous discectomy with presentations. Paper presented at the annual meeting of the International Society for the Study of the Lumbar Spine, Boston, June 16, 1990.
10. Hijikata S: Percutaneous nucleotomy: a new concept technique and 12 years experience, *Clin Orthop* 238:9, 1989.
11. Javid MJ: Cauda equina syndrome following chemonucleolysis, *J Neurosurg* 68:317, 1988 (letter).
12. Kahanovitz N et al: A multicenter analysis of percutaneous discectomy, *Spine* 15:713, 1990.
13. Kambin P, Saliffer PL: Percutaneous lumbar discectomy: reviewing 100 patients and current practice, *Clin Orthop* 238:24, 1989.
14. Lavyne MH: Complications of percutaneous laser nucleolysis, *J Neurosurg* 76(6):1992.
15. Muralikuttan KP et al: A prospective randomized trial of chemonucleolysis and conventional disc surgery in single level lumbar disc herniation, *Spine* 17:381, 1992.
16. NacNab I, McCulloch JA, Weiner DS: Chemonucleolysis, *Can J Surg* 14:280, 1971.
17. Nordby EJ, Wright PH, Schofield SR: Safety of chemonucleolysis: adverse effects reported in the United States 1982-1991, *Clin Orthop* 293:122, 1993.
18. Onik G et al: Automated percutaneous discectomy: a prospective multi-institutional study, *Neurosurgery* 26:228, 1990.
19. Parkinson D: Late results of treatment of intervertebral disc disease with chymopapain, *J Neurosurg* 59:990, 1983.
20. Smith L: Chemonucleolysis, *J Bone Joint Surg* 54A:1795, 1972.
21. Smith L et al: Enzyme dissolution of the nucleus pulposus, *Nature* 198:1311, 1963.
22. Spengler DM et al: Elective discectomy for herniation of a lumbar disc: additional experience with an objective method, *J Bone Joint Surg* 72A:230, 1990.
23. Watts C, Knighton R, Roulbec G: Chymopapain treatment of intervertebral disc disease, *J Neurosurg* 42:374, 1975.
24. Weber H: Lumbar disc herniation: a controlled prospective study with 10 years of observation, *Spine* 8:131, 1983.
25. Wiltse LL: Chemonucleolysis in the treatment of lumbar disc disease, *Orthop Clin North Am* 14:605, 1987.
26. Yonezawa T et al: The system and procedures of percutaneous intradiscal laser nucleotomy, *Spine* 15:1175, 1990.

Section Five

◆

Prevention, Treatment, and Rehabilitation

Chapter Twenty-Three

♦

Exercise Therapy Program After Prolonged Disability

Raymond W. Steffanus

The objective of the exercise therapy program is to return the patient who has had prolonged disability to a normal way of life as soon as possible. This is best achieved by establishing two necessary goals. The patient must rigidly follow the therapeutic exercises discussed in this chapter, as well as strive to develop and maintain a positive mental attitude throughout the rehabilitation period.

IMPORTANCE OF A POSITIVE ATTITUDE

Because of the negative events associated with a back injury, a confident state of mind is a vital supplement to the healing process. The injured person, unable to move without pain, is adversely affected in all aspects of lifestyle. These patients cannot sleep, sit, stand, or walk with any comfort. If they are unable to work, the additional financial pressure inevitably raises the level of stress in their lives. When surgery is planned, the patient is usually very anxious, fearful, or depressed—the common emotions that accompany this condition.

After the ordeal of surgery, these patients wake up and find themselves in bed not knowing whether they can move without pain or what their limitations are. They are apprehensive about what the future holds. At this point a good mental attitude is very important, especially when the time comes for the therapeutic exercise program. Patients know that the exercise program takes effort and that in the beginning it is somewhat painful because the muscles, especially in the legs and the back, are very stiff. The stiffness is due to prolonged lying and sitting in awkward positions. In addition, the psychologic stress brought on by the pain makes the muscles more tense.

The surgery and the muscle stiffness are perceived by the patient as very painful. This condition makes the person more tense and fearful of moving. This fearful resistance to movement causes the patient to lie in bed or sit in a chair to avoid as much of the pain as possible. Such inactivity is detrimental because the muscles of the body remain stiff, and it protracts the healing process by increasing tension and pain. This condition could turn into a psychologic problem. The motivation to move becomes diminished in the patient who is depressed, which is why a good mental attitude is so important. The ability to relax and become active is vital if the healing process is to take place quickly.

PHASES OF THE EXERCISE PROGRAM

When it is time for exercise therapy, it should be initiated in three phases. In the first phase confidence building is required to reduce patients' fearfulness, which will help reduce their pain and motivate them to move. The second phase consists of increasing the range of motion in their muscles and joints. In the third phase the goal is to strengthen the muscles in the back and legs, as well as in the rest of the body, and to increase the endurance of the muscles and the cardiovascular system.

The body, a dynamic entity, is designed to move. When the body does not get exercised daily, it becomes stiff, which places pressure on the spine, joints, ligaments, and muscles, and results in pain. To help patients overcome the fear of pain and inactivity, the recommended exercises are mild and prolonged. The best exercise at first is to walk, but it must be done correctly, which requires discipline.

Phase 1: Walking

Walking correctly will accomplish the following goals: (1) to get the patient mobile slowly with as little pain as possible, (2) to increase maximum blood flow throughout the body and speed up the healing process, (3) to give the muscles in the body an increased range of motion, (4) to increase the strength of the muscles in the body, and (5) to balance the increased motion and strength evenly on both sides of the body. To accomplish these five goals the patient must walk on a flat surface, such as a sidewalk, and avoid angled driveways. Walking across the uneven angle of a driveway will overload one side of the body and place unequal stress on the spine and pelvic girdle. Soft surfaces such as sand must also be avoided because the muscles in the back and legs will have to work too hard to stabilize the body.

In the beginning of exercise therapy it is best for the patient not to walk on a treadmill because the speed of the treadmill belt is too constant. No one walks at a constant speed; when we walk from site A to B, we walk at an uneven speed. For example, if we walk 2 mph, during one walk period, we walk quickly and we walk slowly. On a treadmill, however, the belt would move at a constant of 2 mph, which could fatigue the muscles in the back and legs and result in muscle spasms. If a person were to trip, shock waves throughout the body would

260

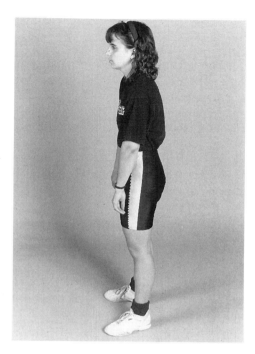

Fig. 23-1. Incorrect standing. The shoulders are forward and the feet are turned out, which places tremendous stress on the lower back.

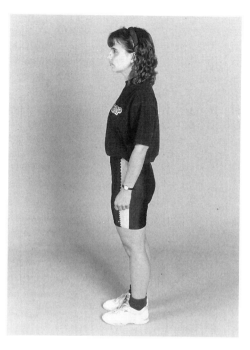

Fig. 23-2. Correct standing. The shoulders are back, and the toes and knees are lined up. There is no stress on any part of the properly balanced body.

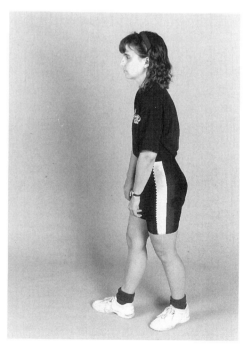

Fig. 23-3. Incorrect walking technique. The shoulders are slumped forward and the feet are pointed out, which creates stress on the lower back.

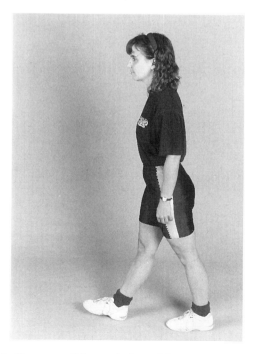

Fig. 23-4. Correct walking technique. The shoulders are back, the toes and knees are lined up, and the back is straight. The person comes down on the heel and walks over the ball of the foot.

increase the muscle tension. Treadmills are helpful only after patients gain confidence, are stronger and more relaxed, and have less pain.

Before starting to walk, patients should look at themselves in a mirror and see if they are standing straight with their shoulders even, making sure that one is not lower than the other. A look at their body profile will ensure that they are not leaning forward. Patients who lean forward could be overloading their posterior muscles, ligaments, and joints. The body must be straight and in an upright position, with the shoulders back, the weight equally distributed on both sides of the body, and the feet straight, with the toes lined up with the knees (Figs. 23-1 and 23-2).

As stated, during the beginning stage of walking, patients should walk with their knees and feet lined up, extending the leg at the knee, coming down on the heel, and walking over the foot and pushing off on the toes. The body should be erect and not bent forward (Figs. 23-3 and 23-4). It is important that there is no muscle imbalance on one side of the body, which places more pulling force on one side than on the other and produces pain. The whole idea of walking straight is to take the stress off the spine and pelvic girdle and to equalize the muscle load while the legs are in the flexion and extension phases of walking. This will help to stretch out the muscles in the buttocks and the legs. In addition, when these muscles are fully stretched out, pressure will be removed from the pelvic girdle and spine. With this removal of stress, there will be a reduction in pain and the patient will start to relax.

It should be emphasized that it is extremely important that the walking be gentle. The whole idea is to relax the body so that the pain will be quickly decreased. Pain creates psychologic tension in the body and makes the muscles stiff, and this tension, with the fear that the pain will return, is what brings the pain back quickly. This can become a vicious cycle of fear, tension, and pain and must be prevented. After the pain has been reduced, the exercise program can become more aggressive.

At the beginning of exercise therapy there might be an increase in pain. Icing the painful areas for 20 to 30 minutes after the exercise session will counteract the pain by decreasing the inflammation in the nerves and muscles. Sitting in a hot tub or Jacuzzi will further relax the muscles and increase their range of motion.

It is important to remember that patients are going to have good days and bad days (i.e., less pain on some days and more on others). On good days when the pain is less severe or even nonexistent, patients should not become overconfident and overexert themselves during physical activity, and on bad days when the pain is at its maximum, they must keep faith and persevere with the program.

Phase 2: Gentle Stretching

After 2 or 3 weeks of gentle, balanced walking during which the person is feeling better, phase 2 can begin. Some gentle stretching exercises can slowly increase the range of motion in the back and leg muscle groups.

The hamstrings constitute the first muscle group to be stretched because these muscles tend to be the tightest and will usually produce pain in the back while the person is standing or walking. To stretch the hamstrings, the patient sits in a chair and places one foot on another chair, trying to keep the leg extended at the knee with the toe and knee in line. Through contraction of the quadriceps muscle to further extend the knee, the hamstring muscle will be stretched (Fig. 23-5). The process is repeated with the other leg. This stretch is to be performed five times with each leg.

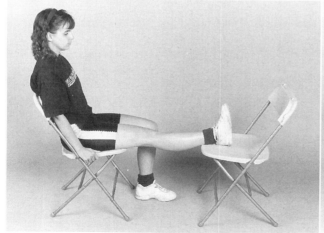 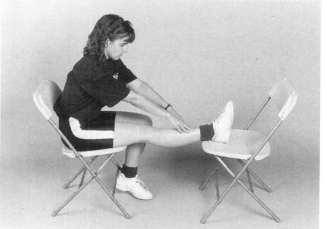

Fig. 23-5. Hamstring stretch. **A,** The foot is placed on the chair, and the quadriceps muscles are contracted. **B,** If the hamstring stretch in **A** is done easily, additional stretch to the hamstring can be achieved by bending forward at the hip and reaching for the toes.

The next muscle group to be stretched consists of the muscles in the lower back and buttocks. The person lies on the back on a hard surface, such as the floor or a hard bed, and gently pulls one leg by the knee to the chest, being careful not to stretch to the point of pain. One leg is stretched at a time. To stretch out the buttocks muscles, the person takes one leg by the knee with the opposite hand and pulls it across the body toward the shoulder on an oblique angle. For example, placing the left hand on the right knee and pulling it gently toward the left shoulder will cause a stretch in the right buttock. This is repeated five times on each side, with the person taking care not to stretch to the point of pain. The physician should be consulted before the person does any flexing or bending-stretching exercise in a standing position. In some back surgeries, such as spinal fusions, the spine should be stable, with no bending, until it heals. All stretching exercises should be performed slowly and never to the point of pain. Stretching to the point of pain causes the muscles to tighten back up, the pain to increase, and the healing process to be slowed.

Phase 3: Strengthening Exercises

It should take an average of 6 to 20 weeks, depending on the degree of tightness present in all the major muscle groups, to reduce pain and to achieve full range in all planes of movement. When this is accomplished, phase 3 can begin by introducing some gentle strengthening exercises to strengthen all the major muscle groups in the legs, the abdomen, and the back.

Jerking must be avoided during the strengthening exercises because it may tighten the muscles and cause a spasm. In addition, all strengthening exercises should include sufficient resistance throughout 15 repetitions, with resistance being the strongest on the last 3 repetitions. This will add strength and endurance to the muscle groups being exercised. Again, if pain occurs during a strengthening exercise that is being done correctly, either the weight should be reduced or the exercise terminated altogether. It might be too early in the exercise program for that particular exercise. It can be put back into the exercise routine later. Sometimes going slowly is the fastest way to achieve the goal.

Combining the Three Phases

Once all three phases are in the exercise routine, my preference is to stretch all the muscles that relate to the back and legs and then strengthen all the muscle groups involved at that time. After the strengthening exercises, my patients walk for 20 to 40 minutes. The exercise session is concluded with the stretching exercises used in the beginning. The back or painful area is iced for 20 to 30 minutes, and then heat is applied; the person either sits in a hot tub or Jacuzzi or takes a warm shower, depending on the individual situation.

The reason for this sequence of exercises is to stretch out and relax the muscles first. This prepares the muscles, tendons, and ligaments for the strengthening exercises to follow. The strengthening exercises tighten up the muscles and produce a waste product in the muscles caused by the breakdown of energy. The waste product is toxic to the system and can cause pain, which could result in tight muscles or spasm. Walking for 20 to 40 minutes increases the blood flow throughout the body, removes the waste product, and increases the range of motion in the muscles. The exercise session ends with a stretching phase so that the muscles will be relaxed at the end of the session.

A good beginning program for a patient who is working alone is to walk 5 days a week for about 20 to 30 minutes per session for about 2 to 4 weeks. Then if the pain has been reduced, stretching exercises may be introduced for 4 weeks. When all the muscle groups have full range and there is no pain, the patient can increase the walking by distance or speed. At this point phase 3 begins, with the addition of leg-strengthening exercises and the use of light weights. The leg press or extension, leg curls, side leg raise, and calf press all make the legs stronger and provide good support to the back. Upper body–strengthening exercises, with the use of light hand weights, can then be included. To strengthen the upper body and lower back muscles, the military press, side arm raises, and front arm raises are added.

Adding Stomach-Strengthening Exercises

When the program has been successfully achieved, and the physician has given permission, stomach-strengthening exercise, such as lower back stabilization exercises, may be added.

A good therapeutic exercise program must be carried out in close association with the attending physician to achieve the maximum benefit to the patient. The physician should be aware of what the goals are for each stage of the program and know the specific details of the exercise therapy in process.

SUGGESTED READINGS

Cinque C: Back pain prescription: out of bed and into the gym, *Physician Sportsmed* 17(9):185, 1989.

Halpern BC, Smith AD: Catching the cause of low back pain, *Physician Sportsmed* 19(6):71, 1991.

Halvorson GA: Therapeutic heat and cold for athletic injuries, *Physician Sportsmed* 18(5):87, 1990.

Johnson RJ: Low back pain in sport, *Physician Sportsmed* 21(4):53, 1993.

Schatz MP: Walk your back to health, *Physician Sportsmed* 19(5):127, 1991.

Chapter Twenty-Four

♦

Rehabilitation of Athletes With Spinal Pain

Arthur H. White

The term *stabilization* has become widely accepted by practitioners of spinal therapy throughout the United States. To some, stabilization has come to mean *a series of exercises* rather than a way of life. However, stabilization training is not an exercise program. It is an athletic endeavor in itself. As with any other athletic endeavor, certain patterns of movement are practiced until they become finely tuned natural motions that require no conscious thought. They become basic reflex mechanisms. One of the goals of this book is to demonstrate the changes in basic body mechanics that athletes should make to ensure safety of the spine and therefore years of successful athletic life in their particular sport.

Stabilization effected in one sport does not automatically carry over to other sports any more than do the skills of a talented football passer who wants to play as a baseball pitcher. Learning stabilization exercises in the gym or clinical setting is a far cry from perfecting stabilization on the pitcher's mound. Various chapters of this book provide very specific techniques for the rehabilitation and training of injured athletes. Some generalizations that should be underscored are presented here, along with certain principles that seem to hold true for high-level athletes in any sport who are trying to continue playing their sport with a back injury.

PRINCIPLE OF ALTERING BODY MECHANICS

Most people believe that there is only one way to use the body to accomplish a given task. Athletes may develop patterns of movement that have proved successful for their sport but that are not necessarily safe for their backs. Marathon runners who have not participated in other athletic activities are good examples of this mistaken strategy. These runners may start running and find that they do it well, even though they do not have experience with the protective body mechanics they might have developed as participants in football or wrestling. Solely as runners, they have not developed the protective mechanism for the lumbar spine that such sports as boxing and the martial arts provide. Without this protective mechanism, the excessive forces that are applied to the lumbar spine as these runners cover thousands of miles take their toll. The result is injured runners with no knowledge or experience of stabilization.

It is difficult to take world-class athletes away from their normal training routines and ask them to perform such mundane activities as sit-ups and balancing on a ball. It is even more difficult to convince and train ath-

letes to walk, run, jump, throw, and hit in a different fashion from the one that has been responsible for their past success. Top-speed running provides the best example. When any of us run at our top speed, we cannot imagine altering the body mechanics of our knee movement to protect the knees from trauma. We cannot, for example, consciously run knock-kneed and still maintain our top speed. When swinging a bat at a ball, it is generally all we can do to hit the ball, much less worry about whether our wrists are cocked and our elbows or shoulders are rotated. It is extremely hard to alter such biomechanics and not interfere with performance. On the other hand, while we are learning a sport and perfecting our technique, a trainer can help us make minor changes that will improve our game. It is only after these early suggestions have been ingrained by years of play that they become difficult to change.

The first step, then, in rehabilitating athletes with spinal injuries is to have them alter their playing technique to protect their backs. In most cases the alterations that are going to be made will also improve the athlete's performance. Athletes must be convinced that they will not only relieve their back pain but will also improve their performance by participating in a few weeks of sport-specific spinal training.

IMPORTANCE OF TRUNK STABILIZATION

Athletes who are hard to convince or unwilling to listen can profit from an explanation of the efficiency of movement and increased power produced by trunk stabilization. This explanation can be made for any sport so that the athlete better understands the concepts of stabilization. In martial arts, for example, most people understand the concept that one individual is transferring energy through the body to affect another individual. This transfer occurs through a blow or throw that displaces or injures another person. The energy force created by the martial artist usually begins with the feet and legs against the ground. The energy is then carried through the trunk to the upper extremities that deliver the blow. If the martial artist has a weak trunk that bends or twists during these activities, energy will be dissipated and the desired effect will be lessened.

Even after athletes have been evaluated and trained, it is surprising to see how few of them use trunk stabilization to their advantage. Only boxers and martial artists routinely improve their effectiveness through trunk stabilization.

DEFINITION OF TRUNK STABILIZATION

In its simplest form, trunk stabilization may be defined as tightening the abdominal muscles or creating an increased interabdominal corset by using the diaphragm to increase interabdominal pressure. Such a maneuver is typically protective for a boxer who is being hit hard in the abdomen. This abdominal setting, however, is only part of the program. The most important part of the program is having the athlete hold the spine in a neutral, balanced position while performing active athletic endeavors. In swinging a golf club or baseball bat, it is quite natural to swing through the waist using maximal rotatory spinal capabilities. In football and basketball it is typical to use the full range of flexion and extension of the lumbar spine for various forms of blocking, jumping, and throwing. These forceful extremes of the range of motion of the spine eventually take their toll. They are also inefficient mechanisms for producing the desired result. Athletes can learn to set their abdominal muscles, place their spine in a neutral and balanced position, and use substitute body mechanics to accomplish any given task. Substitute body mechanics entail bending from the hips rather than from the lumbar spine and blocking the spinal motion that results from excessive lumbar lordosis and rotation. Athletes learn these new body mechanics very quickly and can control and prevent most spinal problems.

EFFECT OF STABILIZATION ON PERFORMANCE

The power and endurance required to maintain neutral spine stabilization for an extended period of time come from development of the gluteal muscles, the paraspinals, and the abdominal musculature. Many athletes who have learned the principles of stabilization soon find that they are able to play that way during the early parts of their sporting event, but eventually they reach the limit of their endurance and stop. Although the muscles that are required to perform their particular sport well may be very strong, few athletes have concentrated on strengthening the muscles that are required for spinal stabilization, and few have built up the coordination and endurance to maintain the biomechanics of a neutral spine for long periods of time. Once they make the connection as to what biomechanics are needed for spine-safe play, they can then monitor their own progress as they strengthen the appropriate muscles and practice stabilizing during their athletic endeavors.

OTHER BASIC PRINCIPLES

Other basic principles in the stabilization training of athletes are as follows:

1. Build stabilization into all activities of daily living. Stabilization should become a way of life, not just a mechanism athletes turn on and off when they think they need it.
2. Adjust to the athlete's time frame and capabilities.

If you are not accustomed to the temperament and endurance of athletes, you may try to slow them down to the pace that most of your patients are accustomed to maintaining. There is nothing worse for athletes than such statements as *stop running, live with it, just do what you can*. This type of statement frustrates athletes who are anxious to get back to their sport. If they do not see some fairly rapid improvement, they are quite likely to seek alternative care out of frustration.

3. Make use of the off season. Many professional athletes will *let themselves go* during the off season. They have been working and training so hard that they feel they deserve a break. They do not have the time to devote to their back problems during the playing season. To make great strides in spinal control and strength, several months of intensive spinal training for 2 or 3 hours a day are needed.
4. Use trainers who understand the athlete's sport, as well as the spinal body mechanics necessary for its performance. Good physical therapists or athletic trainers who understand spinal training and body mechanics may fall short when training athletes in the performance of sports that they have not played themselves. The high-level intricacies of the sport are what need fine tuning. Therefore trainers who have been actively involved, such as Olympic swimmers, skiers, ex-football players, dancers, and martial artists, should be selected, if possible, for sport-specific stabilization training.
5. Remember that spinal problems are different from other injuries. Many professional athletes have had five or six operations on their knees, and most return to their sport after surgery on their ankles, elbows, or shoulders. However, only about 50% of patients return to high-level professional athletics after spinal surgery. Rehabilitation and stabilization can increase that percentage significantly.

TAILORING THE REHABILITATION PROGRAM

Rehabilitation must be tailored to the particular athlete's situation. Even highly trained spinal therapists or trainers need to understand the psychology of the patient involved, the intricacies of the athletic endeavor being pursued, and the underlying pathologic condition that is being addressed.

We need to know not only the sport-specific techniques presented in this text, but also the unique circumstances that are brought to us by athletes with spinal injuries. We need to know the specific patho-anatomy and pain generators of the injuries. We need to know the physical and mental strengths and weaknesses of these patients. We need to understand the social, economic, and legal aspects of the injury affecting these patients and their individual sport.

Chapter Twenty-Five

Aerobic Conditioning

Gurvinder S. Uppal
William H. Dillin

Aerobic conditioning refers to exercise that occurs at a level at which the body can supply adequate oxygen to allow energy production via the Krebs cycle and yet is not strenuous enough to signal anaerobic recruitment of glycosides to meet the added energy requirement. Generally the exercises have a lower associated injury rate than do the more strenuous anaerobic exercises. Sustained physical activity results in lactate accumulation, and fatigue ensues with the development of breathlessness whenever oxygen utilization exceeds supply. This is termed *lactate* or *anaerobic threshold*. Patients increase the lactate threshold with aerobic conditioning so as to maintain maximal physical activity close to their maximal oxygen uptake (Vo_{2max}).

General conditioning is not a novel concept; we are all aware of the axiom that exercise promotes health. However, the scientific basis of the benefits of aerobic conditioning varies as to its causal relationship. Some benefits have no proven basis and are promoted by our exercise-conscious society. This chapter demonstrates the impact of aerobic conditioning not only on patients' cardiovascular system and general metabolic state, but also on their mental state and pain perception. We hope this altered pain perception can be added to the conservative care of chronic back pain.

GENERAL GUIDELINES

Guidelines for a specific aerobic exercise program should be individualized to meet a person's age, fitness level, and aerobic capacity (Vo_{2max}). Modes of aerobic conditioning, discussed later in this chapter, are individualized to each patient. Before a program is initiated for inactive patients older than 35 years of age, a complete medical evaluation is recommended to screen for previously undetected heart disease. Inactive patients need to improve oxygen delivery before they undertake aggressive aerobic conditioning. Therefore a gradual increase in conditioning is recommended.

Variables that can be easily controlled by physical therapy prescription in aerobic conditioning include frequency, intensity, and duration. The recommended frequency of exercise programs varies from 3 to 5 days per week.[11,15] Less-frequent programs are associated with less adaptation to training programs and gradual lack of acceptance. More frequent regimens are associated with increased incidence of certain overuse syndromes and also lead to a gradual lack of acceptance of

the conditioning. A simple method of assessing an acceptable intensity level for conditioning, measured as the percentage of maximal aerobic capacity, is to maintain the heart rate at 130 beats/min for 10 minutes.[14] The Karvonen formula is used to set the appropriate training heart rate:

$$TRH = RHR + IF\ (MHR - RHR)$$

where

TRH = Targeted heart rate
RHR = Resting heart rate
IF = Intensity factor
MHR = Maximal heart rate

Estimation of the maximal heart rate is achieved by use of the following formula:

$$MHR = 220 - Age$$

The intensity factor can be altered by varying the rate or duration of the exercise program. The optimal intensity factor recommended by the American College of Sports Medicine (ACSM) ranges from 70% to 85% (0.7 to 0.85). Therefore an average 20-year-old man should perform aerobic exercise to maintain 70% to 80% of his maximal heart rate:

$$MHR = 220 - 20 = 200$$
$$70\% - 80\% \times 200 = 140 - 160$$

Duration of aerobic conditioning depends on the intensity of the exercise. In general, less-intense exercise should be performed for a longer period of time to achieve the same optimal intensity factor. Optimal duration of exercise tends to range from 15 to 60 minutes per session.[1] Attempts to decrease the duration by increasing the intensity are associated with decreased compliance and increased injury rate.[2]

CARDIOVASCULAR EFFECTS

General aerobic conditioning has been investigated for many years. In the fifth century BC Hippocrates said: "All parts of the body which have a function, if used in moderation and exercised in labors in which each is accustomed, become thereby healthy, well-developed and age more slowly, but if unused and left idle they become liable to disease, defective in growth, and age quickly." In the 1950s, published studies demonstrated that British bus conductors with a more active job (better aerobically conditioned) had fewer manifestations of coronary artery disease than the more sedentary bus drivers. Many authors have suggested that persons with increased physical activity at work and during leisure time experienced less incidence of fatal and nonfatal cardiac problems. To date there have been no randomized studies to document whether healthy, symptom-free, sedentary persons who enter an aerobic conditioning program benefit by showing a decreased incidence of heart disease in the future.

The potential benefits of aerobic conditioning include alteration in cardiac output, decreased incidence of ventricular dysrhythmias, altered coagulation, and decreased hypertension.

Animal studies have demonstrated that conditioned rats had hearts that showed increased resistance to ventricular fibrillation in a state of normoxia and hypoxia.[8] Epidemiologic studies show a direct correlation between physical activity and decreased risk of sudden cardiac death for lethal dysrhythmias in human beings.[4] This may be due partially to decreased obesity in aerobically conditioned patients. Early studies have shown that exercise conditioning decreases the platelet aggregation and increases fibrinolytic activity and thus may result in a decreased incidence of thrombus formation at a site of preexisting atherosclerotic plaque in the coronary artery.

Epidemiologic studies show that a well-balanced aerobic conditioning program is beneficial in preventing hypertension.[7] Patients with preexisting hypertension have shown an average decrease in their systolic blood pressure by 10.8 mm Hg and in their diastolic blood pressure by 8.2 mm Hg. Although the exact mechanism for the decrease in the blood pressure is not yet clear, data suggest that it may result from reduction in cardiac output and peripheral vascular resistance. It has been shown that the amount of blood pressure reduction does not correlate with the intensity of activity.[7]

METABOLIC EFFECTS

Aerobic conditioning was once limited to cardiac conditioning. However, changes occur in the body's metabolism to handle the added requirement of the aerobic metabolism of skeletal muscle.

Maximal oxygen uptake (Vo_{2max}) is the product of cardiac output and extraction (arteriovenous oxygen difference):

$$Vo_{2max} = CO \times AVo_2$$

where

CO = Cardiac output
AVo_2 = Arteriovenous oxygen difference

Vo_{2max} represents the use of oxygen by different tissue at the body's maximal rate of metabolism. Measurement of Vo_2 usually is performed in pulmonary laboratories by measuring the fraction of inspired and expired oxygen and multiplying their difference by the ventilation rate. With aerobic conditioning the ability of the body to utilize oxygen (as represented by Vo_{2max}) improves, and Vo_{2max} increases by 10% to 20% in just 3 to 6 months of training.[11]

Maximal aerobic power (MAP) is a term that was developed to reflect (1) the ability of the lungs to bring oxygen into the body, (2) extraction of oxygen by tissues, and (3) a person's use of aerobic power (via Krebs' cycle). Aerobic conditioning has been reported to increase MAP from 5% to 100%.

Needle biopsy specimens of the quadriceps muscle before and after aerobic conditioning show that the rate of muscle glycogen depletion in trained persons is lower than in untrained persons at the same relative work level.[14] This occurs because the conditioned person has a higher rate of oxygen consumption than does a nonconditioned person at a given level of work.

Aerobic training also increases oxidation of both fat and carbohydrates in the muscles. However, aerobic conditioning allows the body to derive a greater percentage of energy from the oxidation of fatty acids and less from carbohydrates. This is represented by a lower respiratory quotient in conditioned persons.[1]

The myoglobin content reflects the body's respiratory capacity and therefore its increase with aerobic training. After 12 weeks of training, there is an 80% increase in myoglobin content. The importance of this change is that myoglobin improves the muscle's oxygen diffusion capacity. The capillary density in muscles also increases in aerobically conditioned muscle. Utilization of oxygen in conditioned muscle is also improved, as represented by increased concentration of mitochondria and citric acid cycle enzymes within each cell.

In summary, aerobic conditioning changes the metabolism in such a manner as to reduce peripheral resistance and to allow greater blood flow to muscles. At the cellular level, oxygen diffusions and utilization are optimized.

PSYCHOLOGIC EFFECTS

It is well documented in the literature that electroencephalographic (EEG) changes occur with exercise.[4,5,10] A comparison of personality types (type A versus type B) on the basis of EEG changes after exercise reveals that type A persons show greater production of alpha activity in their EEGs. Although there has been no direct demonstration of the presence of alpha activity associated with mood alteration, it is known that conditioned runners (who achieved 80% of their maximal exercise heart rate during exercise) show EEG alpha activity in association with lower levels of anxiety.[10] Therefore exercise does affect the central nervous system in such a manner as to produce changes in the EEG.

Endogenous opiates are a class of neuropeptides

produced in many tissues, including brain tissue. The endorphins are a subclassification of these opiates that produce a potent psychologic and physiologic effect.[6] Beta-endorphins (β-En) are a subclassification of the endorphins whose effects can be reversed with naloxone. The binding sites for these opioid-like substances are found throughout the spinal gray matter, with the highest concentration in the dorsal horn, thus accounting for their involvement in pain perception. There is a significant rise in β-En in response to exercise in both human beings and in animals. The reported euphoria and mood alteration experienced by many in the postexercise period prompted numerous researchers to link these changes to β-En.[3,5,7] Self-reported mood elevation after aerobic exercising was shown by Mihevic[12] and then Morgan.[13] Janal, Colt, and Clark[9] reported that indirect evidence exists to support the mood alteration phenomenon in the postexercise period, which can be reversed after naloxone administration.

The serum levels and range of β-En in normal persons are from 30 to 1024 pg/ml; however, the value at rest ranges from 15 to 40 pg/ml. Circulating β-En levels during acute graded exercise show a nonlinear increase with exercise intensity (Fig. 25-1). Reports vary on the degree of β-En elevation in response to exercise—from twofold to fivefold.[4,7,8] Although it would be tempting to assume that greater exercise intensity leads to greater β-En elevation, no relationship between exercise intensity and level of β-En elevation has been proved. Generally, there is no consistent elevation in β-En with low-intensity exercise of 60% Vo_{2max}. There exists an exercise-intensity threshold so that a significant elevation in β-En occurs only after this threshold is reached. To date, however, no such threshold has been discovered, and it is still unclear if this threshold can be universally applied to all patients.

An alteration in psychologic states after exercise occurs that correlates with the concomitant rise in β-En. This assumes that there is a correlation with peripherally circulating β-En and central nervous system adjustment. To date no studies have verified this adjustment. Injec-

tion of β-En systemically has not universally altered mood states. Janal and colleagues[9] reported that aerobic exercise that causes 85% Vo_{2max} leads to feelings of joy and euphoria that are reversed with naloxone, although other studies report no evidence of mood alteration with the administration of naloxone after exercise. These studies suggest that not all postexercise mood alterations can be attributed to β-En. However, most studies that test mood alteration are so subjective that their results are not consistent.

Pain experience has been correlated with low levels of β-En in the cerebrospinal fluid (CSF). Patients with rheumatoid arthritis showed an elevation in systemic β-En levels and reported decreased pain after aerobic training periods. This finding was not verified by clinical or radiographic changes in the level of the disease.[6] Women who underwent aerobic training during pregnancy had lower levels of pain during labor, with a concomitant elevation in serum β-En levels. It has also been demonstrated that there are decreased levels of β-En in the CSF of persons with postoperative chronic pain. This suggests the possibility that aerobic conditioning may decrease pain that is associated with increasing levels of β-En. A direct correlation between systemic and CSF β-En levels would help us to understand the effects of aerobic conditioning and β-En on pain management. However, such a study would be very difficult to undertake in a controlled fashion.

Catecholamine (epinephrine and norepinephrine) levels are also elevated after exercise. Elevated catecholamine levels are associated initially with feelings of anxiety, followed by an increased capacity to cope with stress.[5]

Exercise is helpful in decreasing depression, especially among persons in institutions, as well as providing an excellent adjuvant to psychotherapy. It is well known that chronic pain is associated with a significant component of depression. Pain control through aerobic exercise and/or antidepressant medication may help with pain management. Intellectual functioning (memory and imagination) has also been shown to be augmented with exercise programs.

LOW BACK PAIN

Our current interest lies in using aerobic conditioning programs in treating patients with low back pain. Potential benefits of aerobic exercise for patients with low back pain include strengthening bone, tendons, ligaments, and muscles, as well as enhanced oxidation capacity of skeletal muscle, cartilage, and intervertebral discs. The CSF of patients with postoperative chronic low back pain shows decreased β-En levels. This decreased β-En level can be elevated, at least in theory, by aerobic exercising and could account for some decreased perception of pain.

An analysis of the relationship among fitness, low

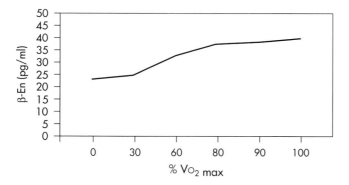

Fig. 25-1. Serum beta-endorphin level increases with increasing Vo_{2max}.

back pain, and depression reported that (1) stronger persons with low back pain are less limited by their pain and (2) higher aerobic work capacity was generally observed in more active patients.

MODES OF AEROBIC CONDITIONING

The exercise prescription in aerobic conditioning is adequate only if the patient is motivated to comply with the regimen. We make every effort to educate the patient to the exact mode of exercise in terms of duration, frequency, intensity, and potential benefits of the regimen. Great care is taken to set realistic goals for the patient.

Several methods of aerobic exercise are available to our patients. An age-appropriate maximal target heart rate of 80% for 10 to 15 minutes optimizes cardiopulmonary benefits and β-En elevation. In certain patients this involves simple brisk walking or running. In patients afflicted with various arthritides, we have had considerable success with water running (Fig. 25-2). This involves wearing a life vest and running in place in the deeper end of a pool.

Treadmills (Fig. 25-3) vary in their options, but the underlying goal is maintenance of 80% maximal heart rate for 10 to 15 minutes. Appropriate conditioning can

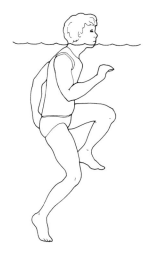

Fig. 25-2. Stationary running in the deep part of a swimming pool. A life vest is worn.

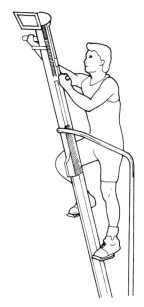

Fig. 25-4. The stair climber has a higher incidence of overuse injuries.

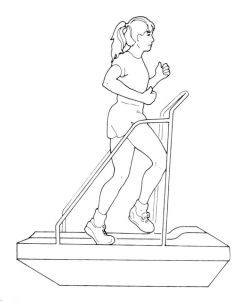

Fig. 25-3. Treadmills range from simple to highly sophisticated models that allow an uphill run and calculation of calories used.

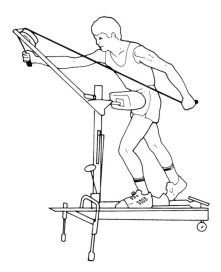

Fig. 25-5. Ski machines allow upper and lower extremity exercise while providing an aerobic workout.

be accomplished with a stair climber (Fig. 25-4). Although asynchronous recruitment of large muscle groups tends to be inefficient, continuous climbing at 75 degrees on the machine will promote higher oxygen consumption at submaximal work and elevated blood lactate levels at just 5 minutes of exercise (anaerobic exercise). However, this mode of conditioning is associated with a higher injury rate than the more aerobic modes such as the treadmills. A ski machine (Fig. 25-5) allows aerobic conditioning without the repetitive loading of the knee or ankle joint. The manufacturers of these machines claim there is greater Vo_{2max} elevation with a far lower incidence of overuse syndrome. The maximal oxygen consumption is equivalent to the traditional bicycle ergometer and treadmill.

This mode of exercise must be tailored to (1) the patient's acceptance, (2) availability to the patient, and (3) associated physical limitations. The various kinds of commercially available equipment have the same basic criterion: to maintain a target heart rate for a set time.

REFERENCES

1. Braun LT: Exercise physiology and cardiovascular fitness, *Nurs Clin North Am* 26:135, 1991.
2. Brill PA, Burkhalter HE, Kohl HW: The impact of previous athleticism on exercise habits, physical fitness, and coronary heart disease risk factors in middle-aged men, *Res Q Exerc Sport* 60:209, 1989.
3. Burckhardt CS, Clarke SR, Padrick KP: Use of the modified Blake treadmill protocol for determining the aerobic capacity of women with fibromyalgia, *Arthritis Care Res* 2(4):165, 1989.
4. Czajkowski SM, Hindelang RD: Aerobic fitness, psychological characteristics, and cardiovascular reactivity to stress, *Health Psychol* 9:676, 1990.
5. DeGeus EJ, VanDoornen LJ, DeVisser DC: Existing and training induced differences in aerobic fitness: their relationship to physiological response patterns during different types of stress, *Psychophysiology* 27:457, 1990.
6. Hicks JE: Exercise in patients with inflammatory arthritis and connective tissue disease, *Rheum Dis Clin North Am* 16:845, 1990.
7. Hofstetter CR, Hovell MF: Illness, injury, and correlates of aerobic exercise and walking: a community study, *Res Q Exerc Sport* 62:1, 1991.
8. Jackson AS, Blair SN, Mahar MT: Prediction of functional aerobic capacity without exercise testing, *Med Sci Sports Exerc* 22:863, 1990.
9. Janal M, Colt W, Clark WC: Pain sensitivity, mood and plasma endocrine levels in man following long distance running: effects of naloxone, *Pain* 19:13, 1984.
10. Lennox SS, Bedell JR, Stone AA: The effect of exercise on normal mood, *J Psychosom Res* 34:629, 1990.
11. McCutcheon MC, Sticha SA, Giese MD: A further analysis of the 12-minute run prediction of maximal aerobic power, *Res Q Exerc Sport* 61:280, 1990.
12. Mihevic P: Anxiety, depression and exercise, *Quest* 33:140, 1981.
13. Morgan W: Affective beneficience of various physical activity, *Med Sci Sports Exerc* 17:94, 1985.
14. Sallis JF, Patterson TL, Morris JA: Familial aggregation of aerobic power: the influence of age, physical activity, and body mass index, *Res Q Exerc Sport* 60:318, 1989.
15. Steptoe A, Moses J, Mathews A: Aerobic fitness, physical activity, and psychophysiological reactions to mental tasks, *Psychophysiology* 27:264, 1990.

Chapter Twenty-Six

◆

Water Workout Program

Robert G. Watkins
William Buhler

A healthy back has a natural curve. From a side view the curve of the spinal column looks like the letter *S*. To maintain this healthy S shape requires that one stand with the chest forward, the shoulders back, and the head over the spine. Too often, however, the pursuit of human endeavors does not do much for our posture. Working behind a desk can be worse for the back than many sports. Everyday activities such as driving and watching television can be harmful as well. When the head is pitched forward, the round-shouldered position changes the curve of the spine. It flattens the lower back and flexes the thoracic and cervical spine. This posture turns the spine from an S to a C shape, placing more stress on the muscles, joints, and intervertebral discs.

Most back problems would be alleviated if correct posture were maintained. In particular, keeping the head over the shoulders instead of letting it just out in front of the body greatly reduces the strain on the back muscles and bones. The farther forward the head is placed, the greater the length of the lever arm between the spine and the head, with increased stress on the cervical vertebrae. The weight of the head cannot be changed, but this lever arm can be eliminated by bringing the head and neck back over the body.

Once the head is over the neck, it is easier to keep the chest forward and the shoulders back. This puts the curve back in the lumbar spine and puts the entire back into its healthy S shape again. This means the muscles and bones are not subjected to undue stress.

Maintaining good posture requires strong back and abdominal muscles. The back muscles, because they are always used to hold the body upright, are usually much stronger than the abdominal muscles. A weak abdomen can wreak havoc on the posture. One can think of the trunk muscles as a girdle. For the entire girdle to provide support, it must be tight all around. If the front part of the girdle is weak, the body will sag in that direction. This is exactly what happens if the abdominal muscles are weak. The abdomen sags forward, exaggerating the curve of the lumbar spine, which, in turn, leads to back pain.

Water exercise is excellent for the back. In the water the force of gravity is about one tenth of that on land, and the stress on the body is reduced. At the same time the back and abdominal muscles are constantly working to stabilize the trunk in the water. This makes the girdle that surrounds the spine much stronger. These exercises are specifically designed to strengthen the muscles of the back and abdomen, thus helping to maintain a healthy posture, which in turn will reduce back pain.

The use of water for relaxation and rehabilitation is not a new concept. The Romans had their baths, the ancient Greeks had the sea, and modern civilization has backyard and neighborhood swimming pools. Today water is primarily thought of as a place to swim, frolic with the kids, or float on an air mattress and soak up the sun. Yet water exercise—designed to tone the muscles and get the heart and lungs in shape—is being discovered as a fresh approach to fitness.

Water rehabilitation in a swimming pool is a fairly new idea. For about 20 years, physicians and physical therapists have been telling injured athletes to work out in the pool until their injuries have healed, but the "workout" has never really been defined. For some, working out means swimming laps, but many athletes find lap swimming boring and difficult. It is not an alternative for athletes who cannot swim or for those who are afraid of water. Telling an athlete to "use the pool" without assigning a specific workout usually means the pool exercise will be abandoned after two or three sessions. This chapter gives athletes a plan—goals and exercises—to help them stay with the recovery program until they are better and ready to return to their sport.

Athletes who have worked hard getting into shape and who really love their sport find it discouraging to be suddenly rendered inactive because of an injury. They will want to stay in shape and return to their dry-land exercise program as quickly as possible. Water exercise will allow them to accommodate both of these goals.

Research has shown that persons lose fitness twice as fast as they gain it. For example, if a young woman has been exercising for 2 months and sprains an ankle, in 4 weeks she is going to be right back where she started if she does no physical activity during her recovery time. When an ankle is badly sprained—the most common sports injury—it may take 4 weeks for the swelling to go down and for the athlete to be able to work out on land without pain. The pool provides an alternative. The woman in our example can work out in the water without hurting her ankle. She will be able to maintain her level of fitness, keep her muscles strong and in tone, and actually speed her recovery from the sprain.

The exercises in this chapter are based on our experience in working with athletes and in rehabilitating our own sports injuries. We have talked to many athletes who have used the pool to recover from injury, and they have shared their ideas with us. We have discovered in our interviews and professional contacts with these athletes that a water recovery program works. We also discovered that in many cases the plan for these programs was hit-and-miss. It has usually been left up to the motivation and imagination of the injured person to come up with a workout. To take the guesswork out of water rehabilitation, we wanted to create a plan that would establish an intelligent, safe, and effective workout program for the injured athlete during the weeks of recovery.

Water is virtually a risk-free exercise environment for joints, muscles, and bones. This is one of the reasons swimming has become the most popular sport in the country, with 72.6 million participants. During immersion in water the body is about one tenth as heavy as it is on dry land. A person who weighs 160 pounds out of the water weighs only 16 pounds underwater. Water is as close to zero gravity as one can get without traveling into outer space. Space shuttle astronauts learn how to operate equipment in space by training submerged in a 30-foot-deep swimming pool.

The exercises in this chapter do not take place totally underwater, but even when a person is only neck- or chest-deep in water, that person's weight is a fraction of what it is on land. Buoyancy allows one to exercise in water sooner than on land. With the water supporting the muscles, joints, and bones around the injury, there is none of the impact stress that occurs during exercise.

Exercising the injured part—strengthening and rehabilitating the area around the injury—can be done much more safely in the water, and this is what has made water rehabilitation so popular with physicians and physical therapists. A decade ago, physicians told the injured athlete to rest for a few weeks until the injury healed. Now we know that rest and inactivity may be the worst thing for an injury. The muscles atrophy and weaken, and the athlete loses physical condition and often becomes depressed and anxious. For most injuries, however, normal exercise is not possible. Water exercise is the perfect alternative. A sensible water exercise program will actually strengthen the injured part and speed the healing process by increasing the circulation to the injured area. It will allow the athlete to maintain a high level of physical conditioning and a positive attitude during the recovery.

Water is a risk-free weight-training facility. As one moves the body through the water, it resists movement, causing the muscles to work harder. Thus the natural resistance of water facilitates muscle toning and strengthening. The level of resistance is increased the faster one moves against the water. This is why we suggest that the athlete move in a controlled, slow manner when first learning the exercises. As the person becomes stronger, the speed of the moves is increased, thereby increasing the resistance the water exerts on the muscles.

Many athletes are nonswimmers. Some positively abhor exercising in the water. One of us (W.B.) has coached several Los Angeles Dodgers reluctant to get their feet wet and has found the following advice to these athletes helpful:

1. Go to a pool that has a lifeguard. (The athlete will feel more secure knowing there is a trained person on hand to provide help.)
2. Do not work out alone. Find someone who can swim with you. Make sure this person knows you are a nonswimmer or are nervous in the water and that assistance may be needed.
3. Exercise in the shallow end. (All of these exercises, with the exception of water running and cycling, are done in the shallow end of the pool. Even the deep-end activities can be replaced with water walking or running in chest-deep water, provided that contact with the bottom does not aggravate the injury.)
4. Wear a flotation device—even in the shallow end. (Flotation will give the athlete more confidence and control. A waterskiing belt, vest, or specially designed WetVest* is excellent. The flotation device should allow freedom of movement in the arms and legs.)
5. Rather than doing the exercises the first day, begin by walking back and forth in the shallow end. (The training partner should be by the athlete's side in the water. Once the athlete feels comfortable in the water, the exercises are begun.)

A pool of any size can be used, from the Olympic to the backyard variety, as long as it has a shallow and a deep end. In a small pool the slope of the bottom should be checked. It should be level where the athlete is standing in chest-deep water. It can be difficult to maintain a solid footing on a slanted bottom. The temperature for a pool workout should be 78° to 90° F.

The most challenging aspect of the water recovery program is knowing how to plan the workout. There may be a question as to whether to add an exercise to the program. The important rule here is "if it hurts, don't do it." You cannot work through pain and make yourself better. This kind of attitude can only aggravate the injury. The athlete who, in a non–weight-bearing position, is free of the symptoms of the injury should be able to handle the exercise program. The person who has had surgery can usually begin the program 3 weeks after the operation.

The exercises are shown in ascending order of difficulty. The first one is less challenging to the injured part than the second, and so on. The first week of the program should begin with the water cycling or water jogging

---

* Bioenergetics, 2841 Anode Lane, Dallas, TX 74220.

warm-up, followed by three exercises. One or two exercises are added per week until the person is doing a full program of all the exercises. The athlete should never do an exercise if it causes pain. One word that should be kept in mind throughout the program is *cadence*. The speed with which the limbs move through the water determines the amount of resistance. If the movement is quick, the muscles work harder. If the movement is slow, the muscles can relax a little. Altering this cadence will greatly change the difficulty of the workout.

The program should begin with slow movements. As the weeks progress, the movements can gradually increase in speed, or cadence, and thereby increase the strength building in the injured area. If the injured player moves too quickly too soon, there is the risk of putting additional stress on the injury. We recommend the first few repetitions of the exercise be done very slowly, to learn the level of tolerance, as well as the position the body should be in for the exercise.

We recommend a maximum of four sets of 10 repetitions for each exercise. To increase the difficulty of the exercise, one increases the speed with which it is performed. Concentration on form and technique is important no matter how quickly the movements are performed. It is important to exercise both sides of the body, not just the injured side. This will allow the athlete to maintain muscle balance and prevent reinjury.

WATER WARM-UP

Before beginning the water exercise program, one of the warm-ups in this section should be completed.

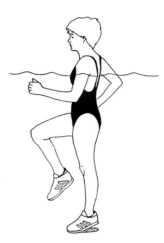

Water jogging. Stand in chest-deep water. Run slowly from one side of the pool to the other. Continue for 5 minutes. NOTE: It may be more comfortable to wear a pair of athletic shoes in the water during this warm-up.

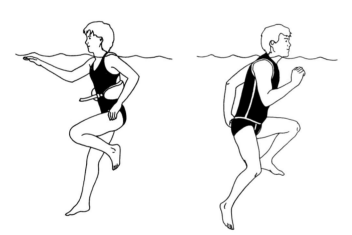

Water cycling. While wearing a flotation device, such as a waterskiing belt, vest, or WetVest, go into the deep end of the pool and gently move your legs in a cycling motion. It is easier to keep your head above water if you keep your hands in the cupped position. Move your arms back and forth, as if you were running slowly. You may find yourself bending at the waist, so concentrate on keeping the body upright in the water. Continue for 5 minutes. NOTE: Aerobic conditioning can be maintained during the recovery period by doing a program of water running. Rather than running mileage or interval training on land, the activity can be duplicated in the pool.

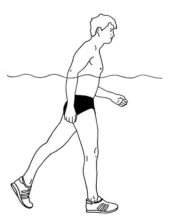

Water walking. Stand in chest-deep water. Slowly walk from one side of the pool to the other. NOTE: You may want to wear shoes while walking in the water. It will increase the support and reduce the impact with the pool bottom.

WATER EXERCISES

Arm fanning. Stand in shoulder-deep water with the legs apart to shoulder width and the knees slightly bent. With the hands open and palms forward, place your arms straight out at the sides, parallel to the surface of the water. Bring your arms together, keeping them straight and parallel to the surface. Return to the starting position, pulling your arms away from the midline of the body. This completes one repetition.

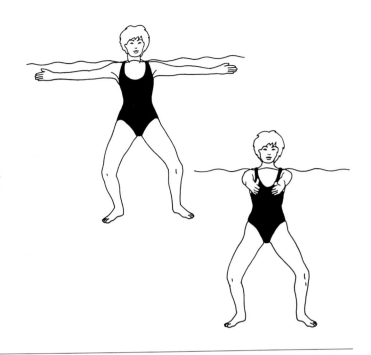

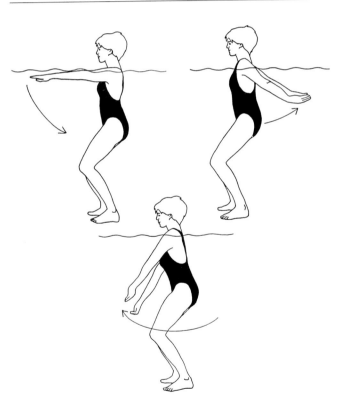

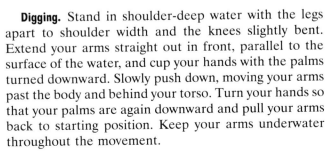

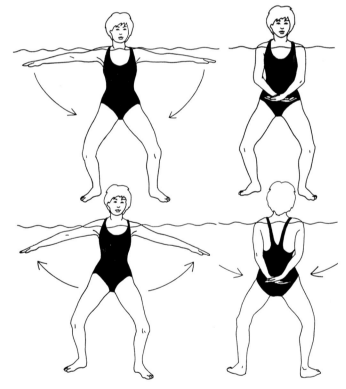

Digging. Stand in shoulder-deep water with the legs apart to shoulder width and the knees slightly bent. Extend your arms straight out in front, parallel to the surface of the water, and cup your hands with the palms turned downward. Slowly push down, moving your arms past the body and behind your torso. Turn your hands so that your palms are again downward and pull your arms back to starting position. Keep your arms underwater throughout the movement.

Arm crossing. Stand in shoulder-deep water with the legs apart to shoulder width and the knees slightly bent. Begin with the arms parallel to the surface of the water and straight out to the sides. With the hands cupped and palms downward, swing your arms down in front of the body and then return to the parallel position. Swing your arms down behind the body and then return to the parallel position. This completes one repetition. The arms remain underwater throughout the movement.

Knee lifts. Hang by your arms from the side of the pool. Your feet should not touch the bottom. Keeping your buttocks against the pool wall, extend your legs straight below you. Bend your knees to your chest. Return to the starting position. One lift is equal to one repetition.

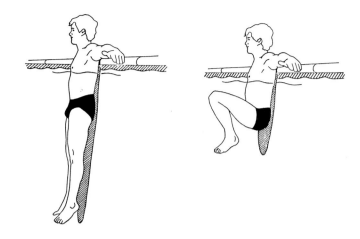

On-the-wall leg raises. Hang by your arms from the side of the pool. Your feet should not touch the bottom. Keeping your buttocks against the pool wall, extend your legs straight below you. Slowly raise both legs to the surface until they are parallel to the bottom. Keep the legs straight and together. Return to the starting position. One lift is equal to one repetition.

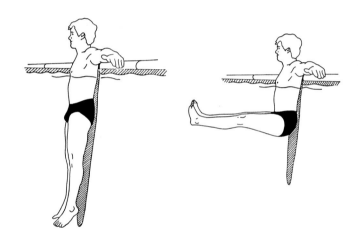

Wall sit-ups. Rest your calves on the pool deck and float on your back in the pool. Cross your arms on your chest. Gently curl upward so that your shoulders just break the surface of the water. Hold for a count of 10 and return to the starting position. NOTE: Do not hold your breath. Gently breathe in and out as you count to 10.

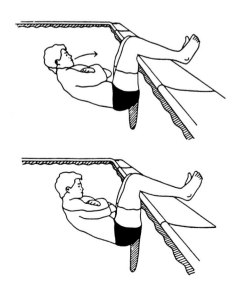

SWIMMING

Swimming is one of the best exercises for the back. The muscles of the abdomen and back work to keep the body on top of the water. The stress of gravity on the back is eliminated because the body weight is suspended in water. For some patients we have recommended only swimming for their back injury. A few minutes of swimming, in addition to the water exercises presented in this chapter, will greatly relieve pain and will speed the recovery. Patients who do not know how to swim should not attempt to learn these strokes while they are injured.

Strokes that permit the patient to float on the back are advised at the beginning because they are easy on the spinal column. The freestyle stroke tends to extend the lower back, which can aggravate an injury. One should wear a waterskiing belt, as well as a snorkle and mask, when doing the freestyle. It should be remembered that the breaststroke places considerable stress on the lumbar spine.

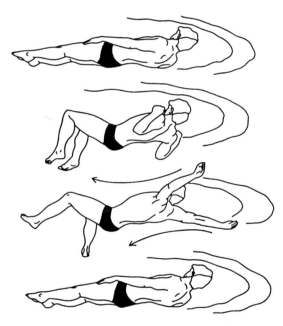

Elementary backstroke. The arm motion of the elementary backstroke works all the major muscles of the back as the abdominal muscles work to keep the body parallel to the surface. It is the perfect stroke to begin with if laps are to be included in the workout after the water exercises have been completed.

Continue for up to 10 minutes, but not to the point of muscular fatigue or pain.

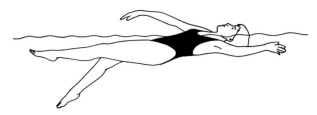

Backstroke. The backstroke works the back and abdominal muscles. If you find that the elementary backstroke is too slow or awkward, try the backstroke for a while. Do the lap swimming after the water exercise program. Continue for up to 10 minutes, but not to the point of muscular fatigue or pain.

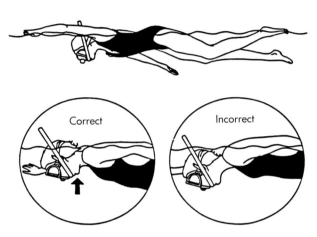

Freestyle. Swimming facedown tends to accentuate the curve of the lower back, which is why we recommend the backstroke. Swimming the freestyle—or the front crawl—is perfectly safe if a few simple guidelines are followed:

1. Wear a snorkle and mask when swimming. You will be able to keep your spinal column straight, rather than constantly rotating to breathe.
2. Wear a waterskiing belt or WetVest to help support your lower back and increase buoyancy. This is especially helpful to patients who are not strong swimmers.
3. If you do not have a waterskiing belt or WetVest, keep your abdomen tucked when swimming and do not let your back sag toward the bottom of the pool.
4. Keep your head in line with your spine. Do not let your neck and head sag toward the bottom of the pool. Swim for up to 10 minutes after the water exercises are completed. If your back, especially the lumbar spine, hurts, stop swimming.

TOTAL-BODY AEROBIC WORKOUT

Once the athlete is healthy and participating in the sport, the pool exercises can be continued. The pool running program will not replace running on land, but it will reduce stress on the body, cut down the risk of injury, and provide the benefits of running for aerobic conditioning.

Aerobic exercise makes the heart, lungs, and circulation system work more efficiently. To attain the fitness and health benefits of aerobic exercise, the athlete must work out within what experts refer to as the "training heart rate range." When the heart is beating at a certain rate—and this rate varies from person to person—it is working at an aerobic level that will improve fitness. Research from the American College of Sports Medicine shows that if exercise is performed within the training heart rate range three to five times a week for a minimum of 15 minutes, the participant will experience the mental and physical benefits of aerobic exercise.

Determining the heart rate range for aerobic training takes a few minutes of simple calculations:

1. Find your resting pulse rate. Take your pulse for 1 minute in the morning before getting out of bed. The morning pulse is the minimum heart rate, or resting pulse. Now that you have your resting heart rate, you can complete the rest of the calculation.
2. Subtract your age from 220. This figure is your maximum heart rate.
3. Subtract the minimum (resting) heart rate from the maximum heart rate. This figure is your heart rate reserve. Calculate 60% and 90% of the heart rate reserve by multiplying it by 0.6 and 0.9. Add the 60% figure to the minimum (resting) heart rate. This number is the *low end* of the training heart rate. Add the 90% figure to the minimum heart rate. This figure is the *top end* of the training heart rate. (See box above, right.)

The pulse should be taken midway through the aerobic pool workout and immediately after finishing the workout. The heart rate should be within the training range. If the pulse has been regularly monitored during aerobic exercise on land, the heart rate will be slightly lower in the pool even though the exerciser believes that the same effort is being exerted. Recent research has shown that the heart rate will be 8 to 10 beats/min lower in the pool than it would be for the same level of exertion on land. This occurs because of the physiologic effects of

---

Training Heart Rate

Low End

220
Minus the patient's age
Equals the maximum heart rate
Minus the resting heart rate
Equals the maximum heart rate reserve
Times 0.6
Equals 60% of the maximum heart rate reserve
Plus the resting pulse
Equals the low end of the training heart rate

High End

220
Minus the patient's age
Equals the maximum heart rate
Minus the resting heart rate
Equals the maximum heart rate reserve
Times 0.9
Equals 90% of the maximum heart rate reserve
Plus the resting pulse
Equals the high end of the training heart rate

---

buoyancy and water pressure on the circulation system and the heart. As long as it is within the heart training rate range, the patient will receive the benefits of aerobic exercise.

We have included two types of workouts in this program. The first is a *contact* workout, which means that the feet touch the bottom of the pool. Unlike the running workout, which involves only the running motion, the contact workout has a variety of exercises. It is designed to strengthen and tone the major muscle groups of the body and improve aerobic fitness.

The second is the *noncontact* workout; the exerciser wears a buoyancy device while doing the exercises in the deep end of the pool. It is relatively easy to maintain the head out of the water with the use of a proper buoyancy vest.

Pool running allows patients to maintain aerobic conditioning despite their injuries. Because they are not in contact with the bottom of the pool, there is no impact stress on the muscles and joints. As long as pool running does not cause pain at the injury site, it can be used as a method of maintaining aerobic fitness during recovery.

Contact Workout

The contact workout has been designed to include all of the major muscle groups.

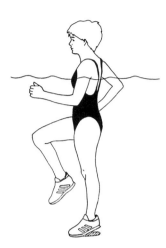

Warm-up. Stand in chest-deep water. Run slowly from one side of the pool to the other. Continue for 4 to 5 minutes.

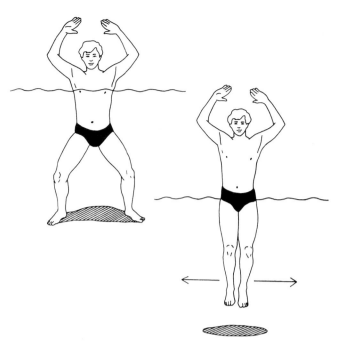

Standing jumping jacks. Stand in chest-deep water with the legs apart to shoulder width and the knees slightly bent. Raise your arms over your head and keep them out of the water throughout the exercise. Jump up and bring your legs together. Immediately spread them apart again, landing with the legs apart to shoulder width and the knees slightly bent. Your feet should not be touching the bottom of the pool when your legs are together. Continue for 1 minute.

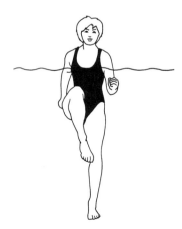

Sprinting in place. Stand chest-deep in water. Run vigorously in place, bringing one knee up to the point at which the thigh is parallel to the pool bottom. Keep the arms bent at a 90-degree angle and bring the elbow back as you raise the opposite knee. Continue for 2 minutes.

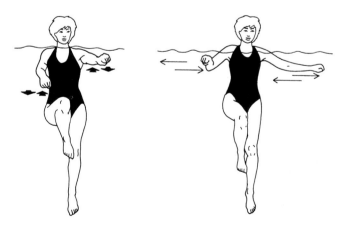

Run and punch. Stand in shoulder-deep water. Sprint in place, punching your arms to the front, underwater, to a count of 8. As you raise your right knee, punch forward with your left arm. Alternate left and right for a count of 8. Then continue sprinting and punch your arms to the side in the same manner to a count of 8. Alternate punching front and side for 2 minutes.

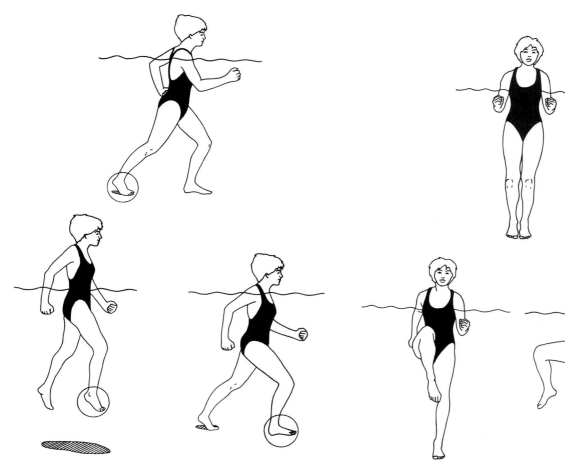

Lunges and leaps. Stand in chest-deep water with the left knee bent and the body weight over the left foot. Extend the right leg back, with the toes touching the pool bottom. Jump up and bring the right leg forward and the left leg back, landing with the weight on the right foot, the knee bent, the left leg extended behind, and the left toes touching the bottom of the pool. Keep the arms bent at 90 degrees and move them in the opposite direction of the corresponding leg: left leg back, right elbow back, and so on. Continue for 1 minute.

Front and side knee lifts. Stand with the legs together in chest-deep water. Raise the left knee four times, keeping the other leg straight. Rotate the left leg to the side and raise the knee four times. Return to the starting position and repeat with the right side. This completes one repetition. Continue for 2 minutes.

Bounding. Stand in chest-deep water with your back to the pool wall. Bound from one side of the pool to the other, driving the right knee forward while pushing off with the left leg and foot. Then drive the left knee forward while pushing off with the right leg and foot. Keep the arms bent at a 90-degree angle and move them vigorously back and forth, bringing the right arm forward when the left knee drives forward and then bringing the left arm forward with the right knee. Continue for 2 minutes.

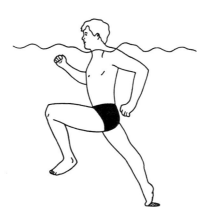

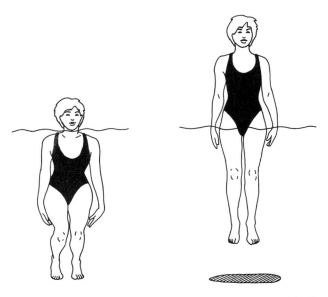

Double-leg jumps. Stand in chest-deep water with the legs together and the knees slightly bent. Keep the arms at the sides. Jump up as high as possible. Bend the knees when landing and immediately do another jump. Continue for 1 minute.

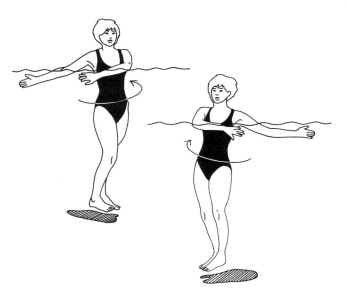

Rotations. Stand in chest-deep water with your body erect. Bend your arms 90 degrees and face both palms in the same direction, with one thumb up and one thumb down. Lock your trunk in a neutral position. Jump up and turn your legs and body to the right. At the same time, sweep your arms in the opposite direction, pushing against the water with the hands. After you land, jump up and rotate your body to the left while sweeping your arms to the right. Continue for 2 minutes.

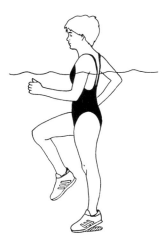

Cool-down. Jog slowly from one side of the pool to the other for 5 minutes.

Noncontact Workout

It is relatively easy to maintain the head out of the water with the use of a proper buoyancy vest, such as the WetVest. The general routine of these exercises involves water running followed by abduction scissors, jumping jacks, hand clapping, bent-knee trunk twists, vertical trunk twists, and sit-ups.

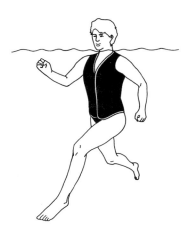

Water running. Water running, a non-weight-bearing activity, takes place in the deep end of the pool (8 to 10 feet of water). Wearing a flotation device to keep the head above the water line, the exerciser runs, just as on dry land. If long-distance running is the usual program or if maintenance or improvement of cardiovascular fitness is the goal, running for 15 minutes or more after the warm-up is appropriate. If the running program involves short, fast distances—a type of running called interval training—this can be done in the pool with the assistance of a tether attached to the side of the pool. Water running places no stress on the lower extremities or the spine and is an excellent conditioning method that avoids the jarring effect of running.

A pair of old tennis shoes can be worn, and a buoyancy vest or life jacket can be of great help. A kitchen timer is used right beside the pool. The stride is that of a full sprint. Keep the back straight. Bring the knees up in a high-step sprint. Begin with 15-second intervals of full-out sprinting in the water. You can usually maintain a static position in the water, with your face out of the water.

Week 1

1. Jog slowly for 15 minutes.
2. Run hard for 30 seconds and sprint for 15 seconds.

Week 2

1. Jog slowly for 15 minutes (warm-up).
2. Run hard for 2 minutes and sprint the last 15 seconds.
3. Run hard for 1½ minutes and sprint the last 15 seconds.
4. Run hard for 1 minute and sprint the last 15 seconds.
5. Run hard for 30 seconds and sprint the last 15 seconds.
6. Run hard for 30 seconds and sprint the last 15 seconds.
7. Run hard for 1 minute and sprint the last 15 seconds.
8. Run hard for 1½ minutes and sprint the last 15 seconds.
9. Run hard for 2 minutes and sprint the last 15 seconds.
10. Jog slowly for 5 minutes (cool-down).

Weeks 3 to 16

Repeat week 2 routine.

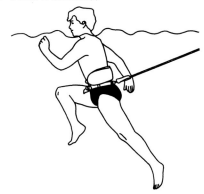

Water sprinting. Water sprinting can be done in the deep end of the pool. Sprint training is not aerobic. It involves running at full tilt for a short time, resting for a few seconds, and then sprinting again. This type of conditioning is necessary for sports that involve short, explosive bursts of speed, such as volleyball, football, and baseball. The sprint/rest/sprint technique is called interval training. The best way to sprint in the pool is to run against a tether secured around the waist, with the tether positioned in the middle of the back. The other end is held by the trainer or tied to the pool ladder, which allows the sprinter to run against resistance.

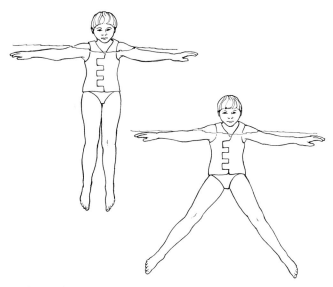

Abductor scissors. Wearing a buoyancy device, in the deep end of the pool extend your arms to the sides to provide control in the water and some buoyancy. Place your legs together, straight up and down. Keeping the knees stiff, spread your legs apart to shoulder width and then pull them together to the starting position. This is one repetition. Continue for 2 minutes.

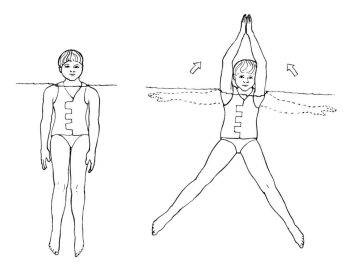

Jumping jacks. Wearing a buoyancy device, in the deep end of the pool float on your back with your arms spread down at the sides of your body and your legs straight and together. Bring your hands over your head, keeping them parallel to your trunk in the water, and clap them together while spreading your legs. Return to the starting position, bringing your legs together again and your arms down to the sides. This is one repetition. Continue for 2 minutes. You will need a large area of the pool for this exercise.

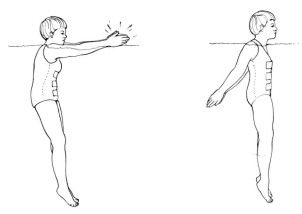

Hand clapping. Wearing a buoyancy device, in the deep end of the pool spread your arms out to the sides to allow control in the water and some buoyancy. Keep your legs straight up and down. Swing your arms forward, keeping the elbows straight and the arms parallel to the water, and clap in front of your body. Swing your arms back from this position and clap behind your body. Return your arms to the side-extended position. This is one repetition. Continue for 2 minutes.

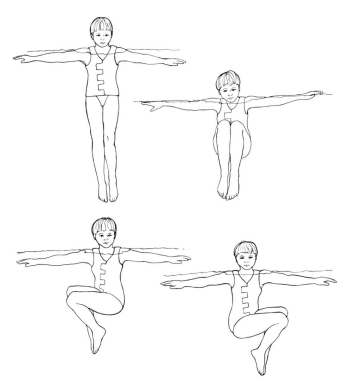

Bent knee trunk twists. Wearing a buoyancy device, in the deep end of the pool spread your arms out to the sides to allow control in the water and some buoyancy. Keep your legs straight up and down. Keeping your arms extended to the sides, bring your knees up to your chest, swinging them first to the right, then across to the left, and finally returning back to the center and back to the extended position. This is one repetition.

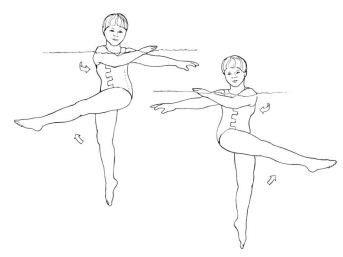

Vertical trunk twists. Wearing a buoyancy device, in the deep end of the pool spread your arms out to the sides to allow control in the water and some buoyancy, with your legs straight up and down. Keeping your arms extended to the sides and your legs straight, swing your left foot across your body and up toward your right shoulder while swinging your right arm across the front of your body toward your left shoulder, keeping the elbow straight. Return to the starting position, and repeat with your right foot and left arm. This is one repetition. NOTE: These twisting types of exercises should be done with firm muscle control of the trunk.

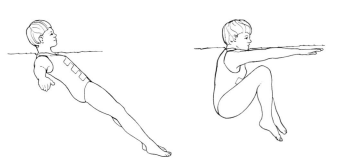

Deep-water sit-ups. Wearing a buoyancy device, in the deep end of the pool spread your arms out to the sides to allow control in the water and some buoyancy, with your legs straight up and down. Incline your body to a 45-degree angle. Bring your arms together in front of your body, keeping the elbows straight and the arms parallel to the water while bringing your knees to your chest at the same time. Return to the starting position. This is one repetition.

SUGGESTED READING

Watkins RG, Buhler B, Loverock, P: *Water workout recovery program,* Chicago, 1988, Contemporary Books.

Chapter Twenty-Seven

♦

Spinal Exercise Program
Robert G. Watkins

TRUNK STABILIZATION PROGRAM

Our trunk stabilization program has been divided into five levels of eight categories. The graduated nature of this exercise program allows a patient to go from a neutral, pain-free position for the spine (a very safe, controlled position) to very advanced strengthening exercises conducted in a somewhat precarious position, requiring balance and coordination. The therapist's objective is to teach the patient how to do the exercises and to take the patient through the program in a safe and graduated manner. Questions such as "When can I return to certain activities?" is determined by when the patient can do a certain level in the program. Often, the patient will advance more quickly in one category than in another. Patients may be doing level 3 in "dead-bug" exercises, yet only level 2 in prone exercises. The therapist will advance the patient more quickly through exercises that the patient is better able to perform and has less pain doing. For example, in category A the sit-ups are done with the feet on the floor, the back in the neutral, pain-free position, and the arms clasped across the chest, followed by an elevation of the head and back, a slight hold, and a return to the neutral position. The difficulty of the exercise is then progressively increased; weights are added to the chest, and then finally the exercise is done with the arms extended forward. There is a minimal amount of back motion in this exercise. There is no need to fully sit up; extending the legs merely increases hip flexor strength, just as hooking the feet increases hip extensor strength.

From the initial stage of identifying the neutral position and maintaining it, the patient proceeds through a series of unsupported arm and leg motion exercises that are made progressively difficult through increasing weights on the arms and legs, increasing the time unsupported, and finally keeping both legs off the ground.

Partial sit-ups are begun with the hands on the chest. Eventually they are done with weights on the chest and unsupported weights over the head and behind. These exercises increase in frequency, duration, and intensity.

The bridging exercises are done by lifting the pelvis off the floor, but maintaining the neutral, pain-free position. The lifting is done with the legs. The back is not arched into a hyperextended position. Holding this bridged position helps isolate trunk musculature in a different manner than in the dead-bug exercises.

Pain with this maneuver is often a result of too much hyperextension in the lumbar spine and not properly using the gluteal muscles to stabilize the pelvis and back. This exercise progresses to a one-leg bridge on the ball, and weights may be added to the trunk and extended legs.

In patients with extreme pain with hyperextension, the prone exercises are begun with a cushion under the stomach to allow a little less hyperextension when the exercises are begun. Again, the idea is to hold the back in a neutral position, not hyperextend from the position. Alternate arm and leg extensions require good trunk control to prevent hyperextension.

"Quadruped" exercises begin with the patient on all fours, knees and hands. This is an unusual position for learning trunk stabilization and how to hold the neutral position. It is a very common area for relaxation of the trunk muscles. The patient must learn to hold the back in this position, with the trunk musculature tight, slowly lifting one arm, then one leg, then alternate arms and legs, then increasing weights, with the final stages being with the body blade across the back, not letting that tip or bend in either direction while still maintaining good, tight trunk control.

The wall slide exercises can begin with a gentle flexion of the knees and with no real lower extremity or back strain. These are easy exercises, initially, that can be begun in the immediate postoperative period. Quadriceps strength is directly proportional to the ability to work in a bent-forward position while lifting. The quadriceps exercises are a reflection of the ability of patients to use their legs for bending and lifting, rather than their back. Patients with weak quadriceps muscles lock their knees and bend at the waist, which is exactly the opposite of what we want for a patient with back pain. The wall slide progresses through a full 90 degrees, with longer periods of holding. The addition of weights and extended arms increase the difficulty of the maneuver.

The ball exercises are begun by balancing on the ball to get a feel for movement. Some people certainly have much more agility and ability to control their trunk on the ball than others. The leg press is the easiest way of improving balance on the ball. The leg press begins with just a simple balancing exercise, rolling on the ball and maintaining control of the ball throughout the motions. Eventually being able to do sit-ups on the ball and make

Table 27-1. Watkins-Randall Scale: Functional Activities

Functional Activities	Cannot Do	Perfect With Cueing	Perfect Without Cueing	Point Scale
Sit-stand	0	1	2	Stab* 1: 6-12 points
Sit-lie	0	1	2	Stab 2: 13-18 points
Roll	0	1	2	Stab 3: 18-22 points
Reach overhead	0	1	2	Stab 4: 22-25 points
Bend/stoop	0	1	2	Stab 5: 25-27 points
Throw	0	1	2	Function 1: 1-4 points
Hit	0	1	2	Function 2: 5-7 points
Lift	0	1	2	Function 3: 6-10 points
Run	0	1	2	Function 4: 10-14 points
				Function 5: 14-18 points

*Stab, Stabilization.

resistive use of pulleys and sticks evolves into many of the sport-specific exercises, such as using the baton with resistance from the therapist to pull through in one direction and then pull through in the other direction.

The key to good aerobic exercise is diversification. That is, running and jogging or doing one specific exercise exclusively may produce a tendonitis or strain because of constant activity in one particular posture or body position. Diversification includes walking on land or in water. We begin having patients walk in the pool as early as 3 weeks postoperatively because of the body being unweighted and the water providing gentle resistance to forward-and-back motion. We progress to using the exercycle because the bent-forward position usually provides stability. We then move the patient to swimming or using a ski machine, but only if the patient has the ability to do one or the other and has the balance and coordination to do it properly. Flailing in the water is hardly good exercise for the back, whereas swimming properly can be a tremendous exercise for a spinal patient. With stair climbers the key is to have the appropriate-height step. We use a stair climber with a very narrow step. The aerobic conditioning is there without the pelvic tilting that results with too high of a

step. The same is true with the exercycle. The seat should be low enough that the feet are not reaching down for the peddles, producing rocking of the pelvis on the seat. Although running is important, it is a stiffening exercise, prone to development of contractures and weaknesses in isolated areas that are not used. A bad running posture can produce an abnormal posture. Good running technique is critical. Skipping rope is an excellent technique for trunk strength. Maintaining the slightly bent-forward flexion, locking the back in a neutral position, and maintaining trunk control while performing this aerobic exercise can produce very tight trunk control while providing aerobic conditioning. The shorter the rope, the better.

The functional activity levels have been expanded from the original scales to include sports activity that allows a greater rating for return to full sports activity. The stabilization scores, likewise, have been increased. The original three-stage scale used by Arthur White, M.D., and Jeff Saal, M.D., has been better adapted, we feel, to more intense training and stabilization exercises, allowing higher levels of accomplishment for advanced exercisers and advanced-stage athletes (Tables 27-1 and 27-2).

Table 27-2. Watkins-Randall Scale: Specific Exercises

Dead-Bug (A)	Partial Sit-Ups (B)	Bridging (C)	Prone (D)	Quadruped (E)	Wall Slide (F)	Ball (G)	Aerobic (H)
Supported, arms over, 2 min, marching	Forward—hands on chest, 1 × 10	Slow reps,* double-leg, 2 × 10	Gluteal squeeze, alternating arm/leg lifts, 1 × 10 reps	Upper or lower extremity, hold, 1 × 10	Less than 90 degrees, reps, 10 ×	Balance on ball, leg press	Walk, land and water
Unsupported, arms over head/one leg extended, × 3 min	3 × 10, forward—hands on chest	Slow reps, double-leg, weight on hips, 2 × 20	Alternating arm/leg lifts, 2 × 10, hold	Arm and leg, 2 × 10, hold	90 degrees, hold 20 sec, 10 ×	Leg press with arms over head, sit-ups forward, no hold	10 min, cycle, water run
Unsupported, arms 7 min over alternate leg, extended with weights	3 × 10 forward, 3 × 10 right, 3 × 10 left	Single-leg, 3 × 20, hold, double-leg with weights, double-leg on ball	Ball flies, swims, superman, 2 × 10	Arm and leg, 3 × 20, hold 5 sec, with weights	90 degrees, hold 30 sec, 10 ×, lunges/no weights	Ball sit-ups, ×20, forward, right, left	20-30 min, swim and ski machine
Unsupported, upper extremity and/or lower extremity, 10 min, alternate leg extended	3 × 20 forward, 3 × 20 right, 3 × 20 left, weights on chest	On ball, single-leg, 4 × 20, hold, double-leg with weights, feet on ball, double-bridge	Ball, 10 × 20, hold, superman with weights, prayer, push-ups, walk-outs	Arm and leg, 2 × 20, hold 10 sec with weights, body blade	90 degrees, hold 15 sec, with weights, × 10, lunges with weights	Ball, sit-ups, forward, right, left, with weights, 3 × 20, wand, manual resistance, pulleys	45 min, stair climber, skip rope
Unsupported, bilateral lower extremity extended, 15 min total, increased weights, bilateral upper extremity with bilateral lower extremity extension	3 × 30 forward, 3 × 30 right, 3 × 30 left, unsupported, weights over head and behind	On ball, single-leg, 5 × 20, with weights, hold, double-leg with feet on ball and bilateral knees flexed	Ball, all exercises with weights, 4 × 20, body blade	Arm and leg, 3 × 20, hold 15 sec with weights, body blade	90 degrees, hold arms extended, × 10, lunges with weights, hold 1 min	Ball over head and lateral, pull-through sports, stick, pulleys, body blade	60 min, run

*Repetitions.

STABILIZATION EXERCISES

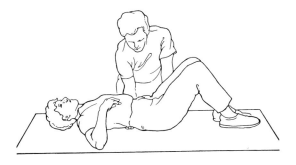

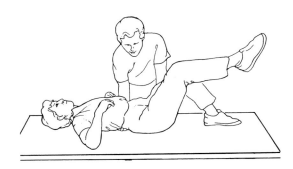

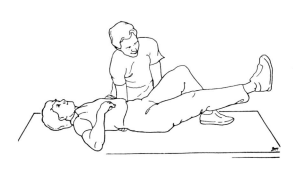

We begin our identification of the neutral spine position with the dead-bug exercises. Dead-bug exercises are done supine with the knees flexed and the feet on the floor. With the assistance of the trainer or therapist, the player pushes the lumbar spine toward the mat by tightening the abdominal muscles until a moderate amount of force is exerted on the examiner's hand. This is not exaggerated, back-flattening, extreme force but a mild to moderate amount of painless force on the examiner's hand. The player is then taught to maintain this same amount of force through abdominal and trunk muscle contraction while doing the following:

1. Raising one foot
2. Raising the other foot
3. Raising one arm
4. Raising the other arm
5. Raising one leg
6. Raising the other leg
7. Doing a leg flexion and extension with one foot
8. Doing a leg flexion and extension with the other foot

These same exercises can be performed with weights on the arms or legs.

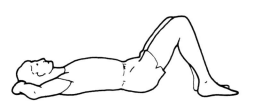

Hold the spine in the pain-free neutral position. Maintain it for a count of 10 and relax. Abduct the arms in an extended position alongside the head and do the abdominal bracing maneuver by tightening into the pain-free neutral position. Isometrically hold the trunk muscles for a count of 10 and relax.

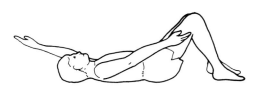

Hold the spine in the pain-free neutral position, feet firmly on the ground, and alternately flex and fully extend the arms while maintaining the neutral, pain-free trunk position. Slowly alternate the arms to a count of 10, and return to the neutral, relaxed position.

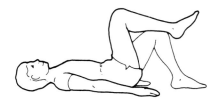

Tighten the trunk musculature in the neutral, pain-free position and bring one leg off the ground to the 90/90 position (hips at 90 degrees, knee at 90 degrees) while maintaining the neutral, pain-free position. The arms may be positioned at the sides, with palms to the floor for balancing. Hold for a count of 10 and then reposition the foot to the floor. Alternate legs.

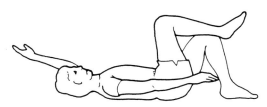

Combine the preceding two maneuvers with alternate arm extensions and hip flexion: left arm, right leg; then right arm, left leg—all while maintaining tight trunk control in the neutral, pain-free position. Return the feet and hands to the floor after each maneuver.

Shoulder Flexion

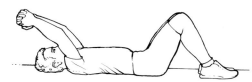

Basic shoulder flexion. Assume the supine position with the back locked in neutral, the hands clasped, the arms extended over the chest, the knees bent, and the feet on the ground. Extend the arms over the head. Hold and return.

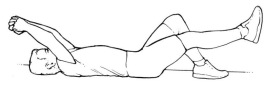

Shoulder flexion with alternate lower extremity extension— supported. This exercise can also be done with the arms at the sides, with alternate lower-extremity extension— supported.

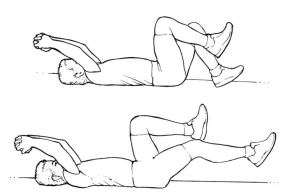

Shoulder flexion with alternate lower extremity extension— unsupported. Do this slowly, concentrating on keeping the back pressed to the ground.

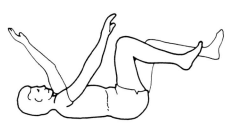

Alternate shoulder flexion with alternate leg extension— unsupported. With the feet off the ground, alternately extend each leg as you extend the opposite shoulder. Do this slowly, concentrating on keeping the back pressed to the ground. For increased difficulty, add weights.

PARTIAL SIT-UPS

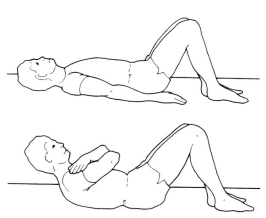

Place the feet firmly on the floor with the arms beside the body and the palms to the floor. Begin abdominal bracing. Place the arms across the chest and raise the shoulders and back off the floor while maintaining the neutral pain-free position of the spine. As long as the unsupported head does not strain the neck, hold the shoulders off the ground for a count of 5, and then return. The amount of time the shoulders are held off the ground may vary from 2 to 10 seconds. The speed with which the maneuver is done may vary from a resting count of 1 to 2 seconds. Repeat this in three sets of 30 times each. Weight may be added to the chest. This exercise is the key to increasing abdominal tone and strength. It may be done with the arms behind the head, alternating shoulders.

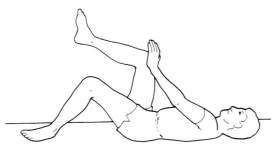

Maintain the neutral spine position. Tighten trunk muscles and do alternate knee pushes: the left hand against the right knee, alternating with the right hand against the left knee. Hold the push for 10 seconds, and return to the neutral position. Then alternate sides.

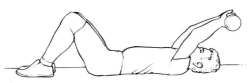

Maintain the neutral spine position, and, holding a weight, extend the arms up over the body. Slowly extend the arms over the head. Hold for a count of 10. Then slowly return to the starting position.

BRIDGING

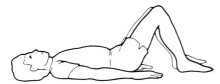

Starting in the supine neutral position, raise the hips 1 inch off the floor and maintain the neutral, pain-free position for a count of 10. Then return the hips to the floor.

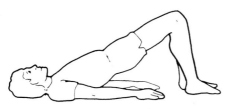

Raise the hips further off the floor to the maximum height allowed while maintaining the neutral position and hold for a count of 10. Then return the hips to the floor. This is not meant to be a back-arching exercise, so maintain trunk control in the neutral, pain-free position throughout the exercise.

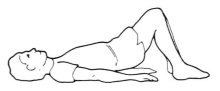

Raise the hips off the floor approximately 3 inches and hold for a count of 10. Then return the hips to the floor.

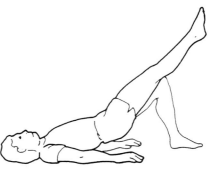

Raise the hips off the floor approximately 3 inches and hold. Extend one leg while maintaining the back in the neutral pain-free position. Hold for a count of 10. Place the foot back on the floor and relax the hips back to the starting position. Repeat with the other leg. Light weights can be added to the leg in this position, and the legs may also be crossed over in a flexion/abduction/external rotation of the leg while the neutral, pain-free position is maintained.

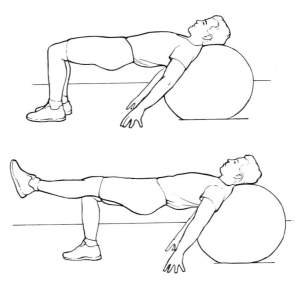

Supine green ball bridging. Position the ball at the upper back position, with the chin tucked, the head up, the knees at 90 degrees, and the feet on the ground. Bridge by bringing the pelvis up, locked in the neutral position. Maintain, then relax. Add alternate extension of one lower extremity in the bridged position. Hold for a count of 10 and relax.

PRONE EXERCISES
Prone: Floor

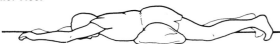

Neutral position. Because the prone position may be painful in certain back conditions, it is suggested that the prone exercises begin with a pillow under the trunk to prevent too much lumbar extension.

Rigidly tighten the trunk musculature into the neutral, pain-free position while maintaining the arms and legs in an extended position. Hold for a count of 10 and relax.

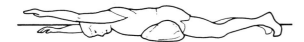

Prone with single-arm lifts. Maintain the original abdominal bridging position in the neutral pain-free position while extending one arm off the ground. Hold for a count of 10 and relax. Repeat with the other arm.

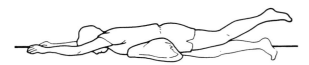

Prone with single-leg lifts. Maintain the original abdominal bridging position in the neutral pain-free position while extending one leg off the ground. Hold for a count of 10 and relax. Repeat with the other leg.

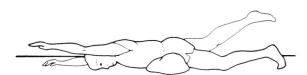

Prone with alternate arm and leg lifts. Maintain the original abdominal bridging position in the neutral pain-free position while lifting the opposite arm and leg off the ground. Hold for a count of 10 and relax. Repeat with the other arm and leg.

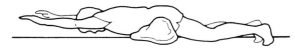

Prone with double-arm lifts. Maintain the original abdominal bridging position in the neutral pain-free position while extending both arms off the ground. Hold for a count of 10 and relax.

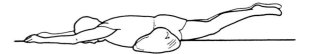

Prone with double-leg lifts. Maintain the original abdominal bridging position in the neutral pain-free position while extending both legs off the ground. Hold for a count of 10 and relax.

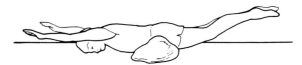

Prone with double-arm and double-leg lifts. Maintain the original abdominal bridging position in the neutral pain-free position while lifting both arms and both legs off the ground. Hold for a count of 10 and relax.

Prone: Ball

In the prone position, roll out with the abdomen resting on the ball, with the feet apart and the toes on the floor in the push-up position. Flex the arms at the shoulder and down to the floor. Roll forward slowly, extending the trunk out into midair while maintaining tight trunk control. Hold for 10 seconds; then roll back to the starting position.

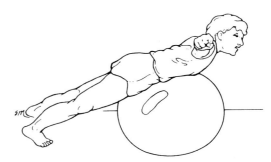

A variation of the exercise is to extend the arms parallel to the shoulders. Roll out slowly, hold for 10 seconds, and roll back. Weights can be held in the hands to increase the difficulty of the exercise.

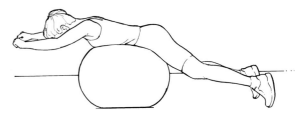

Superman. Start prone in the kneeling position with the ball approximately at chest level. Lock the spine in the neutral position, with the elbows at 90 degrees. Roll out on the ball and extend the elbows and knees at the same time. Hold; then roll back. Keep the neutral position tight and the trunk under tight control throughout this maneuver.

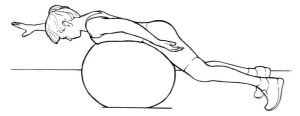

Swimming. In the prone position, place the ball approximately under the abdomen. Lock the spine in the neutral, pain-free position, with the feet and legs extended and the toes on the ground. Alternate arm extension at the shoulder with full arm reach—first the right arm and then the left arm.

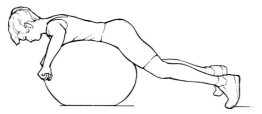

Green ball shoulder abduction. Position the ball prone on the stomach, with the legs apart and the toes on the ground. With the elbows at 90 degrees, extend the elbows back, hold, and return to the original position.

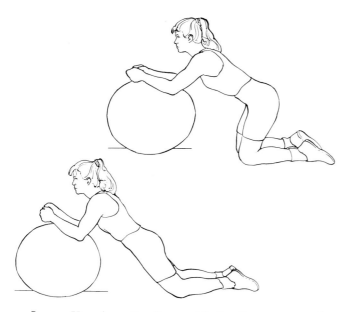

Prayer. Kneel on the floor with the forearms on the ball. Keep the spine in the neutral position, with tight muscle control. Rock forward, maintain the spinal position, and rock back. Do not allow lumbar motion to occur with this exercise.

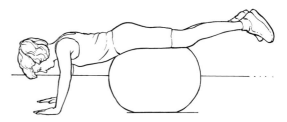

Push-up prone on the ball. In the prone position, place the ball approximately under the abdomen. Lock the spine in the neutral, pain-free position, with the arms extended to the floor, the palms down, the feet and legs extended, and the toes off the ground. Slowly lower the upper portion of the body to the floor, maintaining neutral-position trunk control. Then return to the starting position.

QUADRUPED EXERCISES

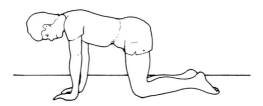

In the all-fours position, with the knees and hands on the floor, tighten the trunk musculature and hold the spine in the neutral, pain-free position for a count of 10. Then relax.

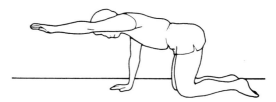

In the all-fours position, with the knees and hands on the floor, tighten the trunk musculature and hold the spine in the neutral, pain-free position. Extend one arm, hold for a count of 10, and relax. Repeat with the other arm.

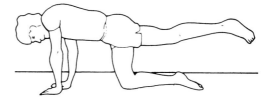

In the all-fours position, with the knees and hands on the floor, tighten the trunk musculature and hold the spine in the neutral, pain-free position. Extend one leg, hold for a count of 10, and relax. Repeat with the other leg.

In the all-fours position, with the knees and hands on the floor, tighten the trunk musculature and hold the spine in the neutral, pain-free position. Extend one arm and one leg, hold for a count of 10, and relax. Repeat with the opposite arm and leg.

The difficulty of the quadriped exercises can be increased with the use of light weights on the extremities or the balancing of the bar across the back.

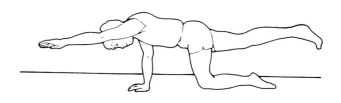

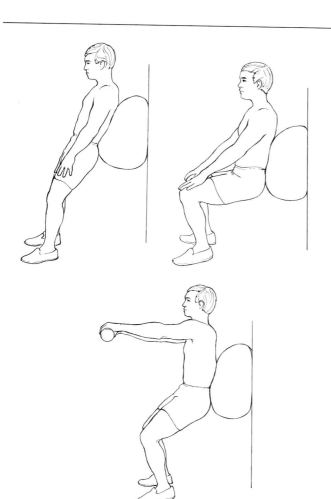

WALL SLIDES

Position a green exercise ball behind the back against the wall, with the legs slightly apart and the arms at the sides. Roll your body down the ball into a sitting position and maintain this sitting position for a count of 10. Return to the beginning semistanding position. Begin with only a slight knee flexion and a partial squat. Eventually you can proceed to a full 90/90 position—90 degrees of hip and knee flexion.

Throughout the exercise, maintain the trunk in the neutral, pain-free position with tight abdominal bridging. This exercise combines trunk strengthening with a functional quadriceps-strengthening maneuver.

After you can maintain a full 90/90 position for three sets of 30 times each, holding the position for 10 seconds, you can do the maneuver while standing on the toes, with the option of holding a weight.

LUNGES

Maintaining the neutral, pain-free position, stride forward with one foot, bending the knee, and partially kneel with the opposite knee. Hold for 3 seconds and return to the starting position. Repeat with the other leg. This can be done with the addition of weights on the arms or with a stick across the shoulders. This exercise is not appropriate for anyone with knee problems.

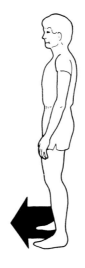

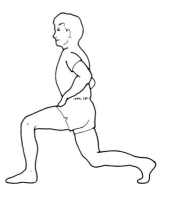

SUPINE GREEN BALL EXERCISES
Stabilization Exercises

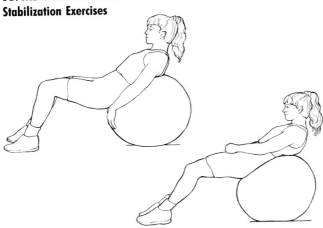

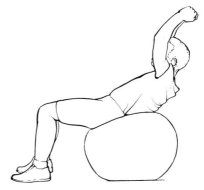

Supine quadriceps press. Sit against the ball with the ball placed in the small of the back. Keep your chest and stomach tight. Keeping your feet in the same position, roll back on the ball by straightening your legs. Keep your chin tucked in so as not to strain your neck. Keep your back in neutral and your chest up off the ball. Return to the starting position by bending your knees and rolling back down on the ball.

Supine green ball shoulder flexion. Alternating shoulders, flex the shoulders with the arms over the head: first do a right-arm hold, then a left-arm hold. Do this with or without weights.

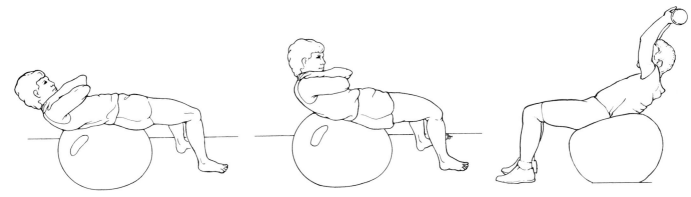

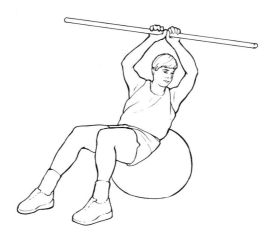

Supine ball sit-ups. Maintain a supine position with the lower back on the ball, the arms folded across the chest, the knees bent, and the feet flat on the floor. Tighten the trunk into the neutral, pain-free position. Keep the pelvis stabilized and level, using your abdominal and buttock muscles. Lift your shoulder blades and upper back off the ball, keeping your lower back in a neutral position. Walk backward on the ball so that more of the trunk is off the ball, projecting out into the air. Hold for a count of 4 to 8 while keeping the trunk rigid. Weights may be held to the chest to increase resistance. Repeat the maneuver of rolling the chest off the ball. With the arms positioned behind the head, rotate the left shoulder, pointing the elbow toward the right knee. Alternate with the right elbow pointing toward the left knee, again maintaining tight, rigid trunk control.

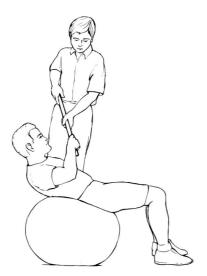

Resistance. The trainer or therapist uses a baton or a towel and pulls against the person on the ball, providing resistance for a count of 8 to 10. This resistance can be provided alternately across the chest, to the side, or over the head with a baton, weighted stick, or pulleys.

AEROBIC CONDITIONING

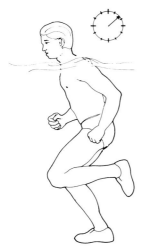

Water running. Water running is a non–weight-bearing activity that places no stress on the lower extremities or the spine. It is an excellent conditioning method that avoids the jarring of running. It is done in 8 to 10 feet of water. The stride is that of a full sprint. A pair of old tennis shoes can be worn. A kitchen timer is used right beside the pool. Usually a static position in the water can be maintained with the face out of the water. A buoyancy vest or life jacket can be of great help. Begin with full-out sprinting in the water for 15-second intervals. Keep the back straight. Bring the knees up in a high-step sprint.

Week 1
1. Jog slowly for 15 minutes.
2. Run hard for 30 seconds and sprint for 15 seconds.

Week 2
1. Jog slowly for 15 minutes (warm-up).
2. Run hard for 2 minutes and sprint the last 15 seconds.
3. Run hard for 1½ minutes and sprint the last 15 seconds.
4. Run hard for 1 minute and sprint the last 15 seconds.
5. Run hard for 30 seconds and sprint the last 15 seconds.
6. Run hard for 30 seconds and sprint the last 15 seconds.
7. Run hard for 1 minute and sprint the last 15 seconds.
8. Run hard for 1½ minutes and sprint the last 15 seconds.
9. Run hard for 2 minutes and sprint the last 15 seconds.
10. Jog slowly for 5 minutes (cool-down).

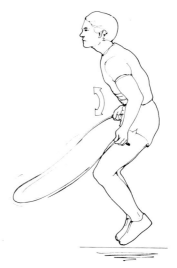

Skipping rope. The sequence of rope skipping is based on the three exercise levels of experience (noted below). Skipping rope begins with a two-step jump, counting the number of jumps. It progresses to an alternate step-jump and eventually to a shorter rope. The shorter the rope, the tighter the abdominal contraction is during the time of jumping. With experience, one should be able to progress to skipping rope for specific intervals of time.

Start by counting the jumps. Begin with 15-second intervals and progressively increase by 15-second intervals.

Level 1: 25 jumps—5 times
Level 2: 50 jumps—5 times
Level 3: 15 minutes of jumping

WEIGHT TRAINING

In the transition from the trunk stabilization exercises to use of a weight-type machine, it is essential to maintain the neutral, pain-free position while using the different types of weight machines, such as those exercising the pectoralis or latissimus muscles or a bench press machine. The person using the machine tightens the trunk in the neutral, pain-free position and performs the exercise following the program appropriate to the type of machine being used, relaxing the position between sets. As with free weights, control is a vital part of any weight machine program. For example, the forward lunge can be done with or without weights, but, obviously, maintenance of a proper neutral position is of paramount importance while the exercise is performed.

UPPER EXTREMITY POSTURAL EXERCISES

The slip-shouldered, round-forward posture is probably the most typical cause, or extenuating factor, in delay of recovery from neck and arm pain. This position produces a lever-arm effect to the head, using the weight of the head—it closes in the intervertebral foramen because of extension in the cervical spine and closes the thoracic outlet.

The basis for our cervical treatment at the Kerlan-Jobe Orthopaedic Clinic is the same as that for our lumbar spine treatment—the trunk stabilization program. We begin with the same lumbar-neutral position assumed in the dead-bug exercises. To produce a "chest-out" posture the patient must be doing trunk isometric exercises, because an adult's posture cannot be changed without active exercising to increase tone (the chest-out posture is done with the trunk).

The chest-out posture removes the lever-arm effect in the weight of the head and opens the thoracic outlet and an intervertebral foramen. All exercises to strengthen the upper extremity should be designed to produce the isometric strength necessary to maintain this position. Neck therapy should never begin by stretching or moving a painful neck; instead, careful head control, positioning, modalities, and posture realignment are used.

We frequently use a basic group of preventive exercises designed for neck and shoulder problems. The key to these exercises is emphasizing the chest-out posture, which enhances head and neck alignment. The chest-out posture accomplishes three objectives:

1. It increases the thoracic outlet. This is the area through which the artery, veins, and nerves pass from the trunk out the arm.
2. It puts the weight of the head over the neck, which eliminates the lever-arm effect the head has on the spine when the head's center of gravity is shifted off-center, decreasing the neck strain required to resist that weight.
3. It opens the intervertebral foramen and provides more clearance for the nerve as it exits the spine.

A general exercise program might include the shoulder and rotator cuff exercises, as well as dorsal glides, midline neck isometrics, shoulder shrugs, arm rolls, and a weight program. An important point to remember is that the patient just thrusts the chest out, without attempting to hold the shoulders back and/or forcefully tuck the chin, using instead the muscles of the chest, abdomen, and buttocks. The important factor is the chest-out posture.

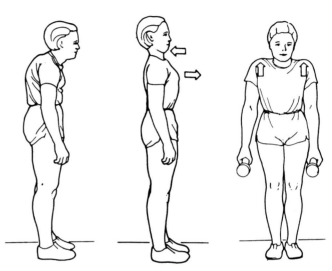

Shoulder shrugs and shoulder rolls. Shrug the shoulder and relax; shrug the shoulders and relax. Roll the shoulders and relax; roll the shoulders and relax. Weights may be added to increase the difficulty.

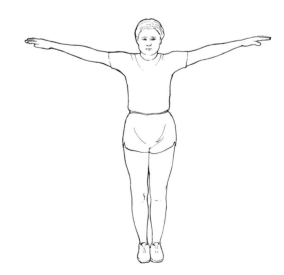

Arm roll. With proper alignment of the spine, stand facing the mirror with the arms extended out to the sides. Do a small arm roll, first with the fingers pointed out, then with the thumbs pointed down, and finally, with the thumbs pointed up.

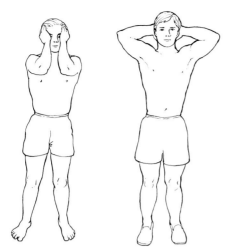

Elbow touch. The arms and elbows are at 90 degrees, with the hands pointing up. Bring the elbows together in front and then extend them as far back posteriorly as possible. Touch the hands behind the back and hold for a 10-second count.

Arm abduction (not shown). Standing in the same legs-apart, spine-neutral position, touch the palms over the head. Repeat this 10 times. Then alternate with the arms at 10 o'clock and 4 o'clock. Rotate first clockwise, then counterclockwise. Then alternate arms, first clockwise, then counterclockwise. Hold at the extremes for a 10-second count.

Alternate arm-over (not shown). Touch the palms over the head. Repeat this maneuver 10 times. Then, with the arms clasped, rotate to the right, then to the left.

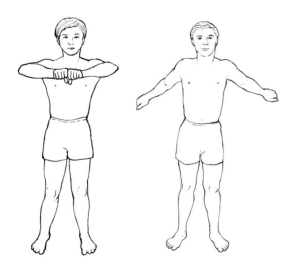

Chest-pull. Stand in the same legs-apart, spine-neutral position, facing the mirror. The shoulders and the elbows are at 90 degrees, with the body parallel with the ground and the hands touching. Spread the arms apart to full maximum length, and bring the hands back together.

EXTREMITY-STRENGTHENING EXERCISES
Isoband Exercises

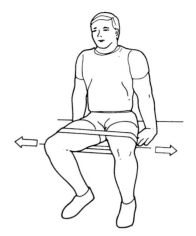

Hip abduction. Lie down supine with the knees bent and the feet unhooked, or sit up. Wrap the isoband around the thighs. Abduct the thighs as far apart as possible and hold for a count of 8 seconds.

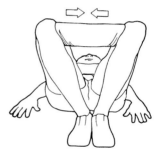

Hip adduction. Lie down supine with the knees bent and the feet unhooked. Place a soft, noncompressible roll, approximately 9 inches in length, between the knees and squeeze in adductor tension for a count of 8. NOTE: Abduction/adduction exercises should be performed with the abduction exercises done first in a series of 20, followed by adduction exercises in a series of 10. This sequence is then repeated.

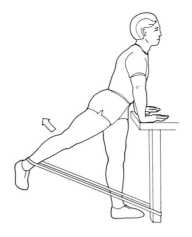

Hip extension. Grip the table and lean slightly over the table. Hook the isoband from the leg of the table around the ankle and extend the hip, holding for a count of 4 to 8. Vary the position of the stance leg for comfort, thus providing different ranges of motion and resistance. It is not advisable to hyperextend the back and leg to obtain strength. This position may cause discomfort. Stand upright, pull back, and hold for 4 to 8 seconds.

Alternate methods
1. Hook the isoband around the stance leg with the knee slightly flexed.
2. Use a sling attachment to the wall pulleys to lift increasing amounts of weights.

EXTREMITY-STRETCHING EXERCISES

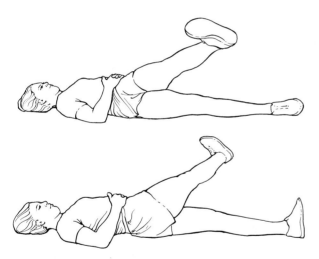

Alternate supine arm and leg twist. With the arms out at the sides, rotate the head opposite from the angle in which one leg crosses over another, gently producing a rotatory stretch of the body. Keep the spine and hips parallel and flat on the ground.

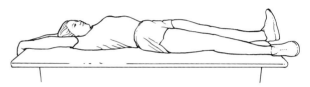

Alternate supine arm and leg stretch. Lie supine with the back protected in a neutral position. Fully extend the outstretched arm and leg of the alternate sides, with the wrist and ankle dorsiflexed to their maximum. Stretch, hold 10 seconds, and then relax. Then alternate with the opposite side in a series of 10 alternate stretches.

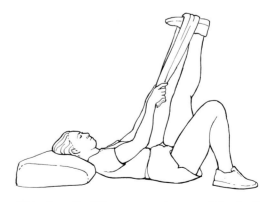

Hamstring strength. Wrap a towel around the bottom of the foot and extend the leg with the towel while immobilizing the pelvis on the ground. Maintain good trunk control and slowly stretch out the hamstring, using tight muscle control. An alternate method, which provides less control, is to lie in a doorway, placing the leg up on the back of the doorway.

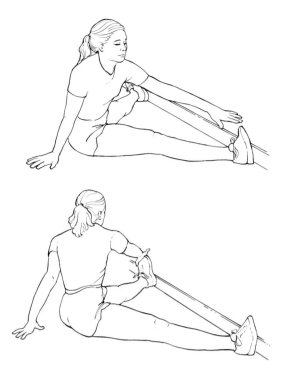

Sitting. Sit with the back against the wall or the feet against the wall. Fully extend the leg and dorsiflex the foot. Reach out and touch opposite toes with hands: left hand to right toe, then right hand to left toe. This may irritate sciatic conditions.

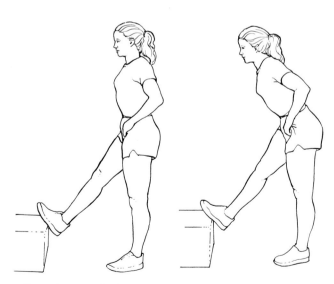

Hamstring stretch. Standing with the back locked into a neutral position, bend forward at the hip and place the foot on a block or stool, 6 to 10 inches high. Extend forward at the hip, with the knees unlocked, until the hamstring tightens. Hold and then reestablish the upright posture.

Indian squat, supine (not shown). Lie in the supine position. Immobilize the spine in the neutral position, and bring the legs up, with the feet touching and knees flexed. This produces considerable stretch on the adductors and quadricep areas. Slowly work into this position from the Indian-squat, sitting maneuver.

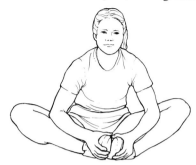

Indian squat, sitting. Sit in an Indian-squat position and bend slightly forward. Bring the legs back, with the soles of the feet touching each other and the legs stretched and the knees bent. Hold this position 10 seconds and then relax. Bending forward slightly requires more stretch. Do not rotate the toes up.

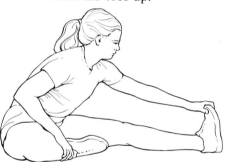

Sitting position, leg-extended stretch. Reach out and touch alternate toes.

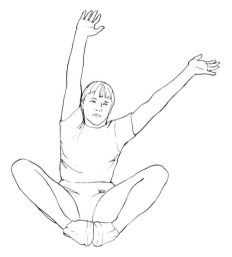

Indian squat, reach. In the Indian-squat position, bend first to the left and then to the right. Hold approximately 10 seconds and return to neutral.

Indian squat, arm-over (not shown). In the Indian-squat sitting position, flex your arm, first fully to the left then to the right. This can also be done with the legs extended, flexing the arms. The spine must be maintained in the correct position. Do not roll the lumbar spine out.

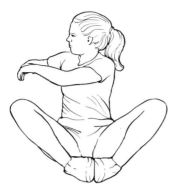

Sitting twist. This spine-mobility exercise allows a slow turn and hold. Maintain the spine in the correct position and do not roll the lumbar spine out.

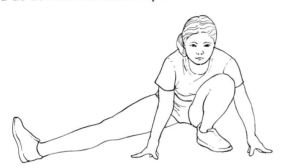

Karate squat. This exercise stretches the gastrocnemius and hamstring muscles. Stand in a neutral position with the legs apart. Squat first onto the right heel, with the buttock touching the heel and the heel on the ground. Then squat to the left, with the buttock touching the heel and the heel on the ground. Because the heel tends to rise up, it may take time to slowly develop the ability to sit in this manner. Hold down for approximately 10 seconds and then return. This exercise is very hard on the knees.

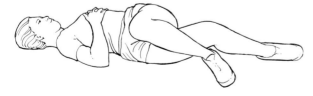

Leg roll. Lie supine on the floor. Hook the left leg behind the right knee, providing a gentle rotatory twist to the lumbar spine. Use muscle control, and stretch slowly out for a count of 6 to 8. Alternate with the right leg, placing it behind the left knee and carrying out rotation in the opposite direction. This may be done with the arms fully abducted or extended at the sides.

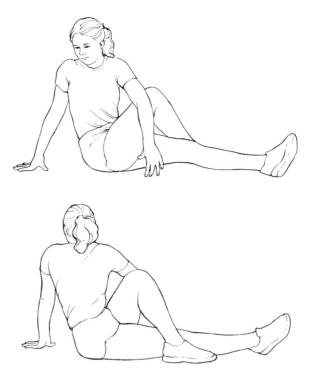

Sitting hip stretch. Sit with the knees and heels on the floor and cross the right leg over the left leg. Bend the right knee and place the right foot on the floor outside the left knee, with the left elbow outside the right knee. Pull slowly for 10 seconds.

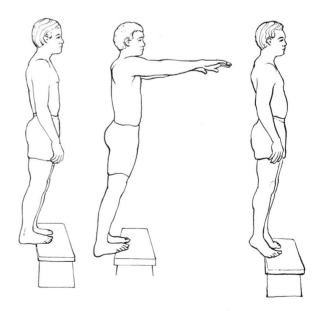

Gastrocnemius, foot over the step. Using any step-up device, slowly let the gastrocnemius stretch out by allowing the heel to be stretched over the end of the step. Hold 10 seconds and then return. The recommendation is to do one foot at a time for more stability; the foot not being stretched rests fully on the step.

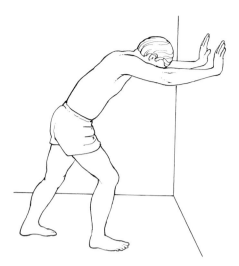

Gastrocnemius, leaning forward. With the feet in the neutral position and the hands on the wall, lean forward, stretching out the back gastrocnemius. Press heels to the floor and keep the spine neutral. Push up against the standing wall, stretching out both gastrocnemius muscles at the same time.

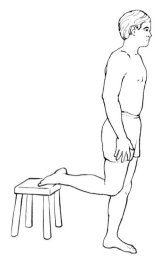

Alternate femoral stretch, standing. Place a chair or a bench behind you at approximately knee height. Place one foot on the bench and stretch forward.

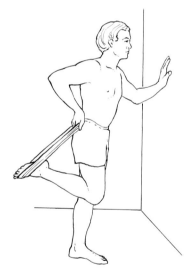

Femoral stretch, standing. Reach behind and grab one foot (a towel can be used). Stretch the front of the leg by pulling up on the foot.

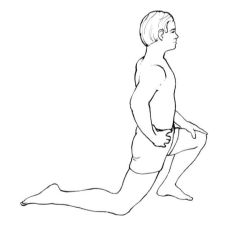

Femoral stretch, kneeling. Kneel down on one knee and rock forward on the knee, with the spine in a neutral position. Stretch out the quadriceps of the knee touching the ground.

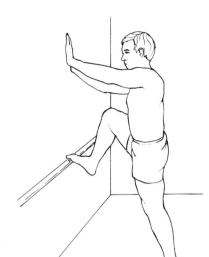

Runner's stretch on the wall rail. Pick a wall rail of appropriate height. Place one foot on the wall rail and bend forward into the foot. This stretch for the calf of the foot on the ground also stretches the hip extenders of the foot on the rail.

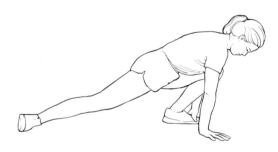

Runner's stretch squatting. In a squatting position, extend one leg out with the palms on the floor for support. Gently stretch the extended leg for a count of 10 and release. Repeat with the other leg.

ASSISTED ROTATIONAL EXERCISES

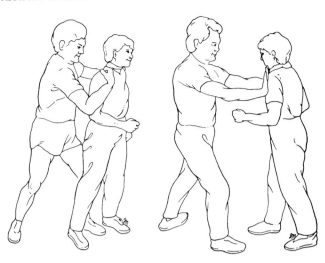

Retraining an athlete to rotate while maintaining tense abdominal control with the spine in a safe, neutral position requires learning to rotate properly. Start by removing the ball, bat, or athletic equipment. Perform the resistive rotational exercises while varying the position from supine to prone, sitting to standing. Use prone, alternate, resistive arm and leg extension; kneeling and sitting resistive rotation; and progressing to simulated athletic activity. Two examples of these assisted rotational exercises are as follows:

1. With the therapist standing behind the player, the player assumes a neutral spine position, resisting rotation by the therapist.
2. With the therapist standing in front of the player, the therapist resists the player's rotation through full range of motion.

Do these resistive exercises with a broom handle or baton. This is an example of moving the spine through a full range of motion while resisting force. This trains trunk muscle control with trunk motion. It should be noted that trunk motion against resistance can cause injury, so be careful and stay under control.

TRUNK-STRETCHING PROGRAM

It is easy to repeat the sequence of the following exercises; do the modified push-up, then the alternate arm/leg exercise, the cat/cow exercise, the Moslem prayer exercise, and then start over with the modified push-up.

There should be no bouncing at the full extended range of motion of these exercises. The exercises should be held for a set number of seconds, usually 4 to 8.

Stretching exercises should be done without holding the breath or straining. It is important to relax and breathe during the 4 to 8 seconds of the full stretch.

Lumbar Prone Exercises

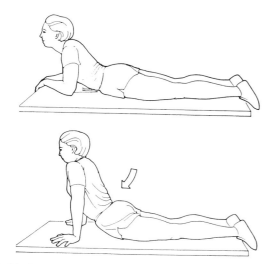

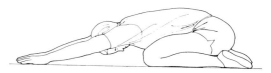

Moslem prayer. Proceed from the cat/cow exercise to the Moslem prayer exercise, which is a forward-kneeling position with the buttocks on the back of the legs, the arms extended forward, and the head down. As range of motion increases, stretch and reach out as far as possible. This is done in a series of 10.

Modified push-up. Lie prone on the table or the floor, using the arms to produce a modified push-up, with the pelvis remaining on the table. Hold in the arm-extended position for a count of 8, then relax. This is done in a series of 10. Players with back problems may need to start by lying on their stomachs only, then progress to their elbows and finally to a full "sagging push-up."

Lumbar Flexion Exercises

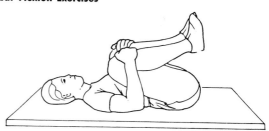

Bilateral knee-to-shoulder stretches. Lie supine on the table, and pull the right knee to the right shoulder. Bring the knee lateral to the shoulder—not in—over the abdomen, where the thigh produces abdominal compression. Hold behind the knee to avoid compressing the knee cap. Hold for a count of 8. Extend or flex the other leg, depending on the comfort level. Then alternate to the left side and repeat with the left knee to the left shoulder. This is done for a series of 10.

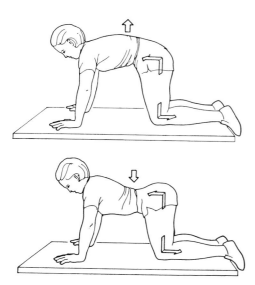

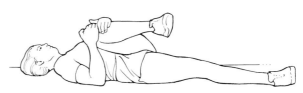

Cat/cow. From the prone position of the modified push-up, proceed to the hands and knees position. Arch the back for the *cat* portion of the exercise and then sag for the *cow* position. Each of these positions is held for a count of 4. Start gently and exaggerate the exercise as mobility increases.

Lumbar flexion rotation. Pull the left knee to the right shoulder. Hold and release. Hold behind the knee to avoid compressing the knee cap. Repeat with the right knee to the left shoulder. Hold and release.

Chapter Twenty-Eight

♦

Spinal Manipulation

Scott Haldeman
Tammy Rubenstein de Koekkoek

As recently as 10 years ago, manipulation of the spine was usually available only to athletes in private hotel rooms and corridors while they were participating in major sporting events. Many athletes would obtain manipulation between events in the offices of local chiropractors, osteopathic physicians, or the few physical therapists and medical physicians who specialized in this treatment modality. This often took place without the knowledge or approval of their sports physicians or coaches. Although a few celebrities such as Babe Ruth made no secret of their use of chiropractic services, most athletes had very little understanding of what was meant by spinal manipulation, thus limiting its availability.

The situation has changed drastically over the past decade.[13] At the 1992 Olympic games, chiropractors and physical therapists who practice manipulation were appointed to the national teams of the United States, the Unified teams, and the teams of many other competing countries. Entire sports teams such as the Detroit Pistons have chiropractors in attendance.[53] Celebrities are now openly acknowledging spinal manipulation in the public news media. For example, Joe Montana, the football Superbowl winning quarterback in 1990, was seen on national television receiving a manipulation during the pregame show. *Time* magazine reported the use of manipulation in athletes in its article on the topic. Other athletes who have publicly acknowledged the benefit of manipulation include Jeff Reardon of the Montreal Expos, who acclaimed its success in treating his neck and arm pain, and Ladies' Professional Golf Association (LPGA) champion, Barbara Bunkowski, who stated that she was able to go back on tour after 2 months under chiropractic care rather than after the 6 months originally projected by her treating physician. In 1989 the national powerlifting champion and record setter, Dave Pasanella, deliberately sought inclusion of manipulation in his program so that he could improve his performance.[22] Similarly, Alexi Grewal, a cyclist of national and international renown, has suggested that spinal manipulation allows him to maintain a rigorous training schedule, as well as alleviating the pains that result from strenuous training. Spinal manipulation is now publicly associated with a wide variety of sports, including cycling, football, powerlifting, track and field, swimming, bowling, and many others.[40,69] Fig. 28-1 illustrates the types of facilities for manipulation that can be found at certain sports events.

From these examples, it can be seen that not all athletes perceive the benefits of manipulation in the same way. Athletes consider its value to be primarily the following: (1) that manipulation relieves back and neck pain that may occur during training or competition, (2) that manipulation can reduce the period of disability and pain resulting from injury and thereby prevent deconditioning and loss of competition, and (3) that manipulation somehow can enhance or improve performance and thereby provide an edge during competition. These claims have resulted in increasing demand for manipulation by athletes both during and between sporting events.

The problem faced by sports physicians is to sort out the myths that surround manipulation and to determine exactly when it is reasonable to recommend this treatment in addition to, or instead of, other treatments. This requires an understanding of the current scientific literature and the theoretic basis for manipulation. It must be assumed that any physician involved in the treatment of athletes has a working knowledge of manipulation, if for no other reason than to be able to discuss it and advise athletes. It is essential that sports physicians be able to separate reasonable expectations

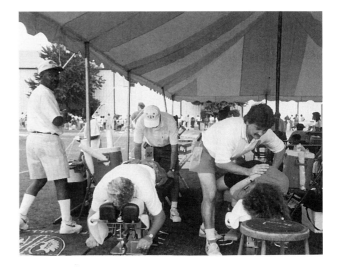

Fig. 28-1. Example of facilities for manipulation now available at major sports events. Note two types of manipulation being offered: a prone manipulation on a special table and a side-posture adjustment. (Courtesy Richard Kowalske, D.C., Georgia State Games, 1992.)

for manipulation from anecdotal claims and mythic connotations.

This chapter presents a brief overview of manipulation, addresses the three basic claims for manipulation, and reviews the clinical trials and experimental research on which the various theories have been based.

MANIPULATION TECHNIQUES

Massage and manipulation fall into the larger field referred to as manual medicine, manual therapy, or manipulative therapy. All techniques in which the hands are used to touch, feel, massage, or manipulate tissue therapeutically to directly benefit a patient can be included under these headings. There are multiple methods, variations, and techniques of massage and manipulation. Clinicians who use manual therapy to treat athletes begin to modify methods they have been taught very early in their career and adapt their approach to the particular patient and tissue they are treating. Techniques are also adapted to suit a clinician's level of strength, dexterity, training, and confidence.

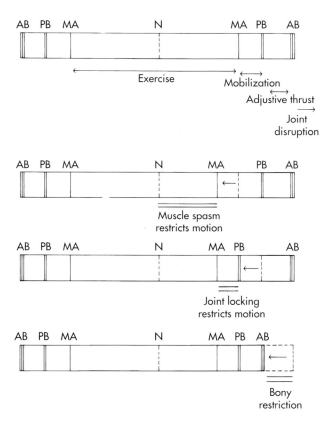

Fig. 28-2. Conceptual model illustrating the range of motion of a joint, including its so-called barriers. Note the manner in which muscle spasm, joint locking, and bony restriction is thought to limit motion. The positions within the range of motion at which exercise, mobilization, and the adjustive thrust is applied are noted. *N*, Neutral position; *MA*, limit of muscle activity; *PB*, physiologic barrier; *AB*, anatomic barrier.

There are, however, a number of principles that allow for a classification of the multiple massage and manipulation techniques.

The most common classification of manual techniques is based on a differentiation between massage, passive movement, mobilization, and the manipulative or adjusting techniques. These techniques are applied at different positions within a specific range of motion of a joint as shown in Fig. 28-2.

Massage

Massage can be considered the touching or application of forces to soft tissues, usually muscles, tendons, or ligaments, without causing movement or change in position of a joint. These techniques are the most passive and are often used for relaxation and toning of muscles. They are performed with the joint in the neutral position.

Stroking or effleurage. This is the light movement of the hands over the skin in a slow, rhythmic fashion. The hands mold to the contour of the area being massaged and are in constant contact with the skin. The hands may gently stroke the skin or influence deeper tissues, depending on the amount of pressure exerted. Light stroking tends to be nonpainful and soothing. Deeper pressure techniques can be slightly uncomfortable and are taught always to be in the direction of venous or lymph flow with the stated goal of reducing edema.[20]

Connective tissue massage. This technique uses deeper stroking motions and is presumed to free subcutaneous connective tissue adhesions. The technique, developed in Germany, involves deep stroking in specifically defined patterns, resulting in a sensation of warmth and hyperemia of the skin.[19]

Kneading and pétrissage. This technique requires the clinician to grasp, lift, squeeze, or push the tissues being massaged. The skin moves with the hands over the underlying tissues. This differs from stroking, in which the hands move over the skin. Commonly this technique is applied to muscles that can be gripped, alternately compressed, and then released before the masseur moves on to another area.

Friction and deep massage. The theoretic goal of this technique is the loosening of scars or adhesions between deeper structures such as ligaments, tendons, and muscles; therefore it is one of the most common techniques used in athletes. This procedure is presumed to aid in the absorption of local effusion within the tissues. The direction of movement of the fingers over the tissues being massaged is described by Wood[70] as circular, whereas Cyriax[16] insists that the movement should be transverse across the fibers of the structure being massaged. The massage is continued until a muscle is mobilized from its surrounding tissues or any palpated effusion or thickening in a ligamentous structure is dispersed. It may require several sessions to achieve this result, and the massage should be followed by exercise to maintain mobility.

Tapotement (percussion or clapping). This technique consists of a series of gentle taps or blows applied to the patient.[34] It has been described as hacking (using the ulnar border of the hand), clapping or cupping (using the palm either flat or concave), tapping (using the tips of the fingers), or beating (using the fists). These percussive movements have been used primarily in postural drainage of the lungs to obtain muscle contraction and relaxation or to increase circulation. They are generally not recommended for the treatment of pathologic tissues[70] and are commonly used on athletes to tone and relax muscles.

Shaking and vibration. This massage method requires the clinician to take hold of a portion of the patient's body and apply either a coarse shaking or a fine vibration motion. It is not widely used except in postural drainage of the lungs.

Passive Movement

The passive motion of a joint falls into the category of manual therapy although these procedures are often performed by trainers, nurses, or family members. These movements are briefly mentioned here to demonstrate the wide spectrum of manual therapeutic techniques. The techniques are relatively simple to teach and perform. They require an understanding of the different directions of movement a joint may traverse. The clinician takes hold of the peripheral arm of the joint and systematically moves the joint through each of its normal motions from the neutral point to the point of resistance or pain. No attempt is made to force the joint, but the entire length of the range of motion must be traversed, and each direction of potential motion must be included. The procedure is repeated and performed several times a day. The goal is to prevent stiffening or shortening of the ligamentous structures, as well as to maintain motion and lubrication in the joint and surrounding tissues.

The natural progression from passive range of motion is to active range of motion or exercise. Exercise is performed within the same boundaries of joint motion as is passive range of motion, although not all directions of motion that can be achieved passively can be reproduced by exercise. Exercise has the additional advantage of including muscle activity and developing strength and coordination.

Mobilization and Stretching

Mobilization includes those manual procedures that attempt to increase the range of motion beyond the resistance barrier that limits passive range of motion or exercise (see Fig. 28-2). Certain mobilization methods include stretching of muscles and ligaments, whereas others include movement of joints in nonphysiologic directions of motion. Mobilization differs from manipu-

lation or adjustments by the absence of a forceful thrust or jerking motion.

Graded oscillation or mobilization. This technique was popularized by Maitland,[45] who proposed four levels or grades of mobilization. Grade I is a fine oscillation with very little force or depth. Grade II is a mobilization with greater depth but within the first half of the range of motion. Grade III is a deeper mobilization at the limits of the motion, whereas grade IV is a deep fine oscillation at the limits of potential motion. The clinician tends to start at grade I and increase to grade IV as greater motion becomes possible.

Progressive stretch mobilization. This technique requires the application of successive short-amplitude stretching movements to the joint. The depth of the stretching into the resisted range of motion is increased as permitted by the joint. Again, four grades or depths are described,[50] but in this situation the grades refer to each quarter of the potential motion of the joint. This technique is used primarily to overcome soft tissue restriction to joint motion.

Sustained progressive stretch. This is a sustained stretching motion with progressively increasing pressure. This sustained-force technique is recommended to stretch shortened periarticular soft tissues and is performed slowly and carefully to avoid tearing of tissues.

Spray and stretch. This technique has been taught widely by Janet Travell[65] and John Mennell[49] for the treatment of painful muscular trigger points. The muscle being treated is placed on a light stretch, and a fluoromethane spray is applied to the muscle in a specific pattern. This results in a cooling of the skin as the fluoromethane evaporates. The muscle can then be stretched further, allowing increased range of motion and theoretically the elimination of the trigger point.

Muscle energy. This method requires the use of muscle activity and subsequent relaxation to set the stage for increasing range of motion. In peripheral joint mobilization it has been called the "hold-relaxation" technique. The clinician places the muscle in light stretch. The patient then contracts the muscle against resistance applied by the clinician. The contraction is held for a brief period, and the patient then relaxes. The clinician can then increase the stretch on the muscle and joint. Certain osteopathic physicians[27,41] have modified these techniques with sophisticated positioning of the patient to allow for specific directional mobilization or manipulation of vertebrae.

Manipulation or Adjustive Thrusts

The distinction between mobilization and manipulation or adjustment is based on the application of a high-velocity, low-amplitude thrust to the joint. Many chiropractors believe that there is a difference between nonspecific manipulation and the classical adjustment that has specific direction, force, and presumed physiologic effects. Other clinicians include mobilization techniques and muscle-energy techniques under the heading of manipulation. There is, however, a fairly clear difference between the previously described non-thrust techniques and the thrusting techniques described under this heading. Thrusting techniques force the joint beyond the physiologic range of motion, through the paraphysiologic space, and to the anatomic limits of motion (see Fig. 28-2). The thrust is commonly followed by a "click" or "pop" that is audible and thought to be related to release of gases within the joint space.

Nonspecific long-lever manipulations. These techniques are becoming less popular because of the potential for exerting large forces that theoretically could damage bones, ligaments, or discs. Force is applied through use of a long bone as a lever. Commonly a shoulder or leg is used to exert force into the spine.[12,16] In the past these techniques were commonly used with the patient under anesthesia, which allowed the exertion of strenuous forces to a joint. In large patients treated by small clinicians, the use of long levers with directed force may be the only way in which a joint can be manipulated.

Specific spinal adjustment. The application of high-velocity, small-amplitude thrusting techniques to short levers of the spine, such as a spinous or transverse process, has been the mainstay of traditional chiropractic practice (Figs. 28-3 and 28-4). The goal has been variously described as correcting misalignments or subluxations, increasing intersegmental motion, and bringing about a variety of neural and muscular reflex changes. Numerous techniques have been described in textbooks.[28,30,31,43,62] To allow for control of the depth and direction of the force to be applied, each vertebra can be adjusted in a number of different directions, and the patient can be placed in very specific positions before the administration of an adjustment. It has yet to be

established, however, that such precise application of force does in fact bring about specific vertebral movements as claimed. A number of chiropractic techniques require specialized tables for patient positioning.

Toggle-recoil. Certain chiropractic techniques[64] require the patient to be placed on a table that is constructed so that one vertebral segment is locked or blocked while a rapidly controlled force is applied to the adjacent vertebra. The portion of the table supporting the vertebra being adjusted then drops approximately 1 cm, allowing for a concussion or recoil effect. Properly performed, high-velocity forces can be applied very specifically to a vertebra without the clinician exerting much force or effort.

Joint play. John Mennell[49] has been instrumental in teaching techniques of moving joints in directions not commonly moved during exercise. Most joints have some degree of play at rest because of ligamentous elasticity. When joints cease to have this play because of tightening of the ligaments and especially if the joint is locked in a slightly abnormal position, Mennell recommends that the joint be manipulated in specific directions to increase the play. A number of manipulation techniques for increasing joint play in both vertebral and peripheral joints have been described.

Traction and distraction. Manual traction and the combination of mechanical traction or distraction with manipulation techniques are commonly accompanied by pulling or thrusting methods while the patient is in traction.[14] These techniques are widely used by chiropractors under the label "adjustments." Manual traction without thrusting is also used as a standard physiotherapeutic technique and could be included under mobilization methods. Other practitioners use elaborate pieces of equipment to exert traction to the spine.

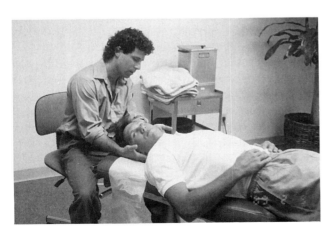

Fig. 28-3. Cervical adjustment or mobilization. (Courtesy Rich Speizer, D.C., and Yarro Dachniwsky, professional soccer goalie, Atlanta Attack.)

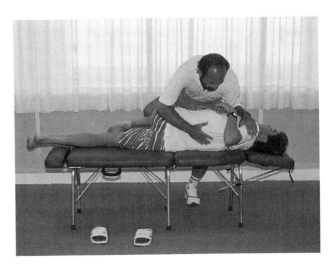

Fig. 28-4. Lumbar adjustment. (Courtesy Leroy Perry, D.C., and Andre Cherkasov, 1992 Bronze Medalist, Olympic men's single tennis, Unified team.)

RELIEF OF BACK AND NECK PAIN

By far the greatest amount of clinical research available on manipulation has to do with the relief of spinal pain. The primary reason why spinal manipulation has gained acceptance as a treatment modality is the number of published clinical trials on the topic. It has been stated that as of 1992 there are more controlled trials on the effectiveness of manipulation in the treatment of low back pain than on any other treatment method. This does not mean that the exact role of manipulation is understood or that it is possible to predict the outcome of manipulation. As in any body of scientific research, the results of clinical trials on manipulation are sometimes contradictory or equivocal. There are, however, many critical reviews of the topic that address the strengths and weaknesses of this research.[6,52]

A recent consensus study carried out by the Rand Corporation[58] has resulted in a document that is of particular importance in outlining the potential indications for manipulation. This document includes an extensive literature review, which together with a recent meta-analysis published in the *Annals of Internal Medicine,*[59] provides a beginning analysis of indications for manipulation. These findings were derived from a consensus process established by the Rand Corporation to assess other medical treatment protocols. Most of the studies and reviews have divided pain into acute and chronic stages, with and without sciatica.

Acute Pain

A number of clinical trials have shown a beneficial short-term effect of manipulation in patients with acute low back pain compared with a placebo and a number of passive treatment methods. The earlier trials by Coyer and Curwen,[15] Rasmussen,[55] and Evans et al.[21] suffered from serious research design problems, although they did attempt to establish controls. The more recent studies, however, are much more sophisticated, although not without criticism. The studies by Glover, Morris, and Khosla[25,26] used a placebo in a single blind trial. The studies by Buerger[7,8] and by Buerger and Tobis[26] were the first attempt to create a double-blind research protocol. These studies all showed a short-term positive effect of manipulation. Like the studies by Sims-Williams et al.,[60,61] most of these clinical trials demonstrated that the greatest effect was obtained either immediately after the manipulation or was evident within the first 2 to 4 weeks. Within this period the natural improvement of most patients caught up with the beneficial effect of manipulation. Until recently, long-term benefits were not noted. This is, however, not unexpected as by far most persons with back pain spontaneously improve without any treatment. Nonetheless, the short-term benefit of manipulation in relieving pain is of particular interest to athletes who do not want to delay training while they spontaneously get better.

There are now sufficient published prospective controlled clinical trials for meta-analyses. The most recent meta-analysis is by Shekelle et al.,[59] who reviewed 29 controlled trials of manipulation for low back pain. After completion of the meta-analysis on the seven comparable trials, the researchers reached the conclusion that manipulation caused a 34% improvement in recovery.

Considerably fewer prospective trials have been published on the effectiveness of manipulation in treating neck pain and headaches. Nonetheless, the seven randomized clinical trials on this topic have tended to support the claims that manipulation is beneficial in these conditions.[5] These studies have had great variability in design, patient population, and outcome and are therefore difficult to analyze. Certain outcome parameters, such as headache severity and immediate pain levels, have been reported as improved after manipulation, whereas others, such as long-term pain relief and electromyographically verified frontalis muscle activity, did not.[4,35,36] These trials often intermixed patients with acute and chronic pain.

Chronic Pain

There are considerably fewer studies on the effectiveness of manipulation in chronic back pain. The past few years have, however, seen the publication of a few prospective controlled or comparative trials addressing this issue. Evans et al.[21] studied patients with a median pain period of 4 years. They performed manipulation three times in 3 weeks with a crossover trial design and noted that the manipulation group showed significantly less use of narcotics and had greater pain relief than the controlled groups. The trial by Waagen et al.,[67] was also a simple short-term trial on patients with chronic or recurrent low back pain. These investigators demonstrated that patients undergoing manipulation had better pain relief compared with patients who were treated with standard bed rest, unsupervised exercises, and analgesic medication.

Long-term benefits of manipulation are now being suggested from a few trials. In a 6-month assessment, Arkuszewski[1] reported significant benefit from manipulation compared with a control group. The problem with this study was that the assessment was not blinded, and the outcome parameters were not well defined. Two-year studies have been carried out in two centers that suggest, but by no means prove, a long-term effect of manipulation. The study by Meade et al.[48] compared chiropractic treatment in an office setting with physical therapy in a hospital setting. The actual treatment regimen in each center was not controlled, but the chiropractic group inevitably underwent high-velocity manipulation. The researchers noted that certain beneficial effects of manipulation could be demonstrated up to 2 years after the treatment was discontinued. Similar results were noted in the long-term follow-up trial by Waagen et al.[68] These investigators found that patients who had undergone chiropractic treatment described, on a 2-year follow-up, a higher level of confidence in the treatment and expressed greater satisfaction that the treatment had been of value. The problem in this study is that, like most clinical trials in the United States, only 50% of patients were available for follow-up, thus clouding the significance of the results.

REDUCTION IN THE PERIOD OF DISABILITY

Probably no issue is more important to the athlete than the time of recovery and period of restricted training after an injury. Unfortunately, there is no information in the literature that addresses this problem directly. The only studies that may have some relevance are those relating to periods of disability-related absence from the workplace by nonathletes who have been injured. The comparative trials by Arkuszewski,[1] Sims-Williams et al.,[60,61] and Lewith and Turner[42] all demonstrated an earlier return to work for those persons who underwent manipulation than for control subjects. These trials, however, suffer from design flaws and have been the subject of considerable criticism. Nonetheless, they do show a consistent bias toward reducing the period of disability, which is shared by many patients and athletes.

IMPROVED PERFORMANCE

The area of improved performance generates perhaps the greatest possible controversy and speculation for which there is as yet no answer. As in many athletic endeavors, the very mythology surrounding manipulation may be sufficient to cause the psychologic boost necessary to achieve better performance. Charms, religion, astrology, and similar belief systems have been used by athletes in the past and have been claimed to enhance performance. Manipulation has the additional benefit of having documented high-satisfaction rates among patients. Furthermore, practitioner confidence, which is often the hallmark of practitioners who offer manipulation, can translate into successful management of back pain.

This factor was first noted by Kane, Olsen, and Leymaster[39] in 1974 when they demonstrated significantly greater satisfaction in the care received from chiropractors as compared with medical care. Recent studies by Pope et al.[54] also demonstrated a high confidence level in patients receiving manipulation as compared with other passive modalities. These researchers compared the effect of manipulation, massage, corsets, and transcutaneous electrical stimulation on a number of physical and psychologic parameters associated with back pain. Although there were no significant

differences in the effect of these treatments on the physical parameters, patients showed much more satisfaction and compliance with manipulation and massage, with increasing satisfaction as the treatment progressed. This could potentially translate, in the athlete, into a perception of being cared for adequately, with an accompanying feeling of emotional well-being or relaxation, that might translate into improved performance.

THEORIES OF MANIPULATION

It should be stated at the outset that the exact mechanism by which manipulation reduces back pain is not fully understood. This is partly because the factors that produce back pain in a large section of the population are also not understood. Nonetheless, there is a developing body of knowledge that is beginning to shed some light on the matter. In an attempt to build a useful model to explain the effects of manipulation, the discussion here is limited to the possible theories currently being used to describe the reported benefits to the athlete.

Relief of Pain

Inasmuch as the most obvious and reproducible effect of manipulation is the acute relief of pain, this has been the subject of the initial research efforts in manipulation theory. Terrett and Vernon[63] reported a change in the pain tolerance in patients undergoing treatment. They found that patients undergoing manipulation showed a 140% increase in the level of paraspinal cutaneous pain tolerance compared with control subjects. This led to the theory that there might be a release of endorphins after manipulation. Initial studies reported such changes.[66] Other authors, however, have not been able to confirm this.[11,56]

As the search in spinal research for the pain-producing factors has progressed over the past years, there has been extensive speculation as to how such factors or pathology may be affected by manipulation. The intense scrutiny of the intervertebral disc as a source of back pain has led numerous authors to propose theories on how disc lesions may be affected by manipulation. Matthews and Yates,[46] using epidurography as an evaluative tool, reported that disc herniation could be reduced by manipulation. Chrisman, Mittnacht, and Snook,[10] however, were unable to show changes in myelographic defects after manipulation of the anesthetized patient. Maigne, Rime, and Delignet[44] have reported that disc herniations diminish in size after other nonsurgical treatments, which may reflect simply the passage of time and the resolution of symptoms with any treatment rather than a specific effect of manipulation.

Others have contended that pain relief after manipulation is a result of changes in muscle function: Grice,[29] Diebert and England,[18] and Shambaugh[57] reported

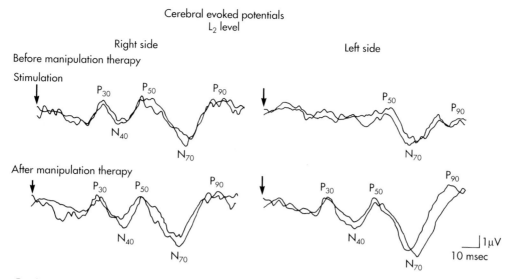

Fig. 28-5. Changes in cortical evoked responses elicited on magnetic stimulation of paraspinal muscles in a patient with unilateral back pain and muscle spasm. Note the change in the response on the left side after manipulation. (Courtesy Y. Zhu, A. Starr, and S. Haldeman, University of California, Irvine.)

reduced paraspinal muscle activity after manipulation, suggesting that the relief of muscle spasm may occur. However, the relationship between muscle spasm and back pain and even the proposition that muscle spasm is a cause of back pain have been seriously questioned. Recent research by Zhu et al.[71] may shed some light on the matter. These researchers compared back pain on the symptomatic side with that on the asymptomatic side and with that of pain-free control subjects. They found that demonstrable changes occurred in the cortical evoked responses of the magnetically induced paraspinal muscle contractions. In a small number of patients undergoing manipulation there was a normalization of these responses (Fig. 28-5). These responses seem to be elicited from the muscle spindles, and it may be that in certain persons with low back pain, there is a disturbance of muscle spindle function that returns to normal either after manipulation or with the resolution of pain. Similar studies have not been carried out on a comparative group of patients undergoing other forms. Thus it is not yet clear whether manipulation does in fact have a direct effect on muscle. This research, however, raises that possibility above the level of mere speculation.

The other popular theories concerning manipulation include effects on the posterior facets, sacroiliac joints, interosseous hypertension, and ligamentous injuries, and all revolve around the presumption that manipulation increases range of motion.[3] The support for this premise is discussed in the next section.

Reduced Disability

The primary theories to explain reduced disability have to do with relief of pain and the psychosocial effects of manipulation. The assumption is that in most persons, and especially in athletes, the period of disability rarely exceeds the period of pain. It is, however, important not to discard the psychologic effects of any treatment method in the management of patients with low back pain. Patients who have confidence that they will get better and have a close working relationship with their physician are likely to improve faster than patients who feel neglected. This assumption is supported by the observation of Pope et al.[54] that confidence levels after manipulation are considerably higher in patients undergoing manipulation or massage than in those wearing corsets or undergoing treatment with transcutaneous muscle stimulation. These researchers also found that confidence scores increased with repeated manipulation and massage treatments but not with the other treatment approaches.

Improved Function

The primary function that is presumed to improve after manipulation is range of movement. The data supporting this, however, are not yet that impressive. Intersegmental movement of facets is assumed to be the explanation for the click or pop that is commonly associated with manipulation, a phenomenon based primarily on research on peripheral joints, which has shown that a release of gases in the joint space accompanies the noise. This occurs when a joint is moved beyond its physiologic range.[9]

Rasmussen,[55] in measuring the C7 to S1 distance on standing and forward flexion, described improvement in range of motion after manipulation. However, more accurate measurements of gross movement by Pope et al.[54] failed to show significant changes in basic range-of-motion parameters after manipulation of the lumbar spine when results were compared with those of patients who did not receive manipulation. Jirout,[37,38] on the other hand, reported increased cervical range of motion after manipulation as measured on motion x-ray films. In a number of studies, increased range in straight leg raising has also been reported after manipulation. Fisk[24] demonstrated a statistically verified improvement in straight leg raising in patients with low back pain as compared with the effects of manipulation in control subjects. Hoehler, Tobis, and Buerger[33] also demonstrated improved straight leg raising after manipulation but only when pelvic motion was used as an end point. Bergquist-Ullman and Larsson[2] and Matthews et al.[47] similarly reported improved straight leg raising after manipulation.

Another interesting observation is that by Herzog, Conway, and Willcox,[32] who recorded changes in gait patterns after manipulation using a force platform. These researchers noted that asymmetric gait patterns were measurable in patients diagnosed as having sacroiliac syndrome and that these patterns became symmetric after manipulation. The possible relationship of these gait patterns to coordination is, however, not known.

A MODEL FOR THE BENEFICIAL EFFECTS OF MANIPULATION IN ATHLETES

Fig. 28-6 is an attempt to combine the multiple theories regarding manipulation into a single model that may help to explain some of the claims being made for the use of this modality in athletes. It must be realized that the support for some of the steps in this model remains quite weak. At the same time, this model does allow a combination of factors to be taken into account and avoids the pitfall of assuming that a single theoretic approach to the problem holds all the answers.

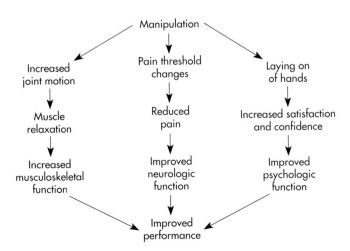

Fig. 28-6. Model used to explain the effects of manipulation in athletes.

This model assumes three distinct categories of effects of manipulation: biomechanical, neuromuscular, and psychophysiologic. The biomechanical effects are primarily changes in joint function and range of motion, with possible effects on gait. The neuromuscular effects are those associated with relief of pain, either by a change in pain threshold or secondary to the mechanical changes. The psychophysiologic effects are possibly related to the effects on endorphins—assuming there is such an effect—as well as the effects of patient confidence and belief in the beneficial effects of manipulation. These effects are probably interactive and combine to explain why athletes seek out chiropractic and manipulative treatments with increasing enthusiasm.

COMPLICATIONS OF MANIPULATION

To fully understand any treatment protocol, it is necessary to review indications, as well as contraindications and potential complications. In the case of manipulation in athletes, the complication rate is extremely small. The rarity of complications and inability to document them even in clinical studies on large numbers of patients make it difficult to obtain an accurate assessment of the frequency of serious complications in the general population.[50] It has been stated that manipulation is one of the safest active treatment approaches to patients with back pain.

A number of the reported complications would not be evident in most athletes. Very few athletes, for example, would be expected to have severe osteoporosis, active inflammatory rheumatoid disease, or significant bleeding disorders. In most athletes the likelihood of encountering a destructive bone or joint lesion such as osteomyelitis or malignancy is extremely small. All these conditions are obvious contraindications for high-velocity thrust manipulation.

Other potential contraindications must, however, be kept in mind before the clinician attempts manipulation in an athlete.

Acute Bony Fracture

Acute bony fracture is probably the most likely contraindication to be encountered in dangerous sports. The application of a force into an area of fracture, especially certain spinal fractures, can cause serious and irreversible harm. Whenever a situation is encountered in which a fracture could have occurred, x-ray films or other studies should be considered before manipulation.

Acute Ligamentous Disruption

Again, it is inadvisable to exert a force into a joint that has lost its ligamentous integrity. One hopes that most practitioners of manipulation would be able to assess this possibility as part of the premanipulation clinical examination. When the situation is not clear, however, appropriate stabilization and imaging studies to confirm the integrity of the joint should be considered before a course of manipulation is begun.

Acute or Progressive Neurologic Deficit

Neurologic deficit is a clear contraindication to manipulation, at least until the cause of the deficit is known. It has not yet been demonstrated that manipulation can cause cauda equina syndrome or myelopathy, but a few unrecognized cases of these problems have been reported to progress while patients were undergoing manipulation.

Vertebral Artery Occlusion

Rapid jerking movements of the neck, especially rotation and extension, can result in occlusion of the vertebral artery. Although this usually is not accompanied by symptoms, in rare instances the vertebral artery may go into spasm or a dissecting aneurysm can occur with concomitant brainstem or cerebellar ischemia. Permanent residual effects have been reported after manipulation of the cervical spine, although the currently acknowledged incidence is reported at one in a million manipulations of the neck. In the athlete it is probably prudent to avoid manipulation of the cervical spine after a neck or head injury accompanied by symptoms of brainstem or cerebellar dysfunction.

REFERENCES

1. Arkuszewski Z: The efficacy of manual treatment in low back pain, *Man Med* 2:68, 1986.
2. Bergquist-Ullman M, Larsson U: Acute low back pain in industry: a controlled prospective study with special reference to therapy and vocational factors, *Acta Orthop Scand Suppl* 170:11, 1977.
3. Bogduk N, Jell G: The theoretical pathology of acute locked back: a basis for manipulation, *Man Med* 1:78, 1985.
4. Brodin H: Cervical pain and mobilization, *Man Med* 20:90, 1982.
5. Bronfort G: Effectiveness of spinal manipulation and adjustment. In Haldeman S, editor: *Principles and practice of chiropractic*, Norwalk, Conn, 1992, Appleton & Lange.
6. Brunarski DJ: Clinical trials of spinal manipulation: a critical appraisal and review of the literature, *J Manipulative Physiol Ther* 7:243, 1984.
7. Buerger AA: A clinical trial of rotational manipulation, Paper presented at the second world congress on pain, International Association for the Study of Pain, Montreal, 1978.
8. Buerger AA: A clinical trial of spinal manipulation, *Fed Proc* 38:1250, 1979.
9. Cassidy JD, Kirkaldy-Willis WH, McGregor M: Spinal manipulation for the treatment of chronic low back and leg pain: an observational study. In Buerger AA, Greenman PE, editors: *Empirical approaches to the validation of spinal manipulation*, Springfield, Ill, 1985, Charles C Thomas.
10. Chrisman OD, Mittnacht A, Snook GA: A study of the results following rotatory manipulation in the lumbar intervertebral disc syndrome, *J Bone Joint Surg* 46A:517, 1964.
11. Christian GF et al: Immunoreactive ACTH, beta-endorphin and cortisol levels in plasma following spinal manipulative therapy, *Spine* 13:1411, 1988.
12. Coplans CW: The conservative treatment of low back pain. In Helfet AJ, Gruebel Lee DM, editors: *Disorders of the lumbar spine*, Philadelphia, 1978, JB Lippincott.
13. Corwin J: The current status of chiropractic in the world of sports medicine, *ACA J Chiropract* 25(2):32, 1988.
14. Cox JM: *Low back pain*, ed 3, Fort Wayne, Ind, 1980, Author.
15. Coyer AB, Curwen IHM: Low back pain treated by manipulation: a controlled series, *Br Med J* 19:705, 1955.
16. Cyriax J: Diagnosis of soft tissue lesions, vol 1, ed 6, *Textbook of orthopedic medicine*, London, 1971, Bailliére Tindall.
17. Reference deleted in proofs.
18. Diebert P, England R: Electromyographic studies. I. Consideration in the evaluation of osteopathic therapy, *J Am Osteopath Assoc* 72:162, 1972.
19. Ebner M: *Connective tissue massage: therapy and therapeutic application*, Baltimore, 1960, Williams & Wilkins.
20. Elkins EC et al: Effect of various procedures on the flow of lymph, *Arch Phys Med* 34:31, 1953.
21. Evans DP et al: Lumbar spinal manipulation on trial. I. Clinical assessment, *Rheum Rehabil* 17:46, 1978.
22. Ezzell M: Dave Pasanella: on top of the world, *Today's Chiropract* 19(3):37, 1990.
23. Farrell JP, Twomey LT: Acute low back pain: comparison of two conservative treatment approaches, *Med J Aust* 1:160, 1982.
24. Fisk JW: A controlled trial of manipulation in a selected group of patients with low back pain favouring one side, *NZ Med J* 645:288, 1979.
25. Glover JR, Morris JG, Khosla T: Back pain: a randomized clinical trial of rotational manipulation of the trunk, *Br J Ind Med* 31:59, 1974.
26. Glover JR, Morris JG, Khosla T: A randomized clinical trial of rotational manipulation of the trunk. In Buerger AA, Tobis JS, editors: *Approaches to the validation of manipulation therapy*, Springfield, Ill, 1977, Charles C Thomas.
27. Goodridge JP: Muscle energy technique: definition, explanation, methods of procedure, *J Am Osteopath Assoc* 81:249, 1981.
28. Greco MA: *Chiropractic technique illustrated*, New York, 1953, Jarl Publishing.
29. Grice AA: Muscle tonus changes following manipulation, *J Can Chiroprac Assoc* 19(4):29, 1974.
30. Haldeman S: *Modern developments in the principles and practice of chiropractic*, New York, 1980, Appleton-Century-Crofts.
31. Haldeman S: *Principles and practice of chiropractic*, Norwalk, Conn, 1992, Appleton & Lange.
32. Herzog W, Conway PJW, Willcox BJ: Effects of different treatment modalities on gait symmetry and clinical measures for sacroiliac joint patients, *J Manipulative Physiol Ther* 14:104, 1991.
33. Hoehler FK, Tobis JS, Buerger AA: Spinal manipulation for low back pain, *JAMA* 245:1835, 1981.
34. Hofkosh JM: Classical massage. In Basmajian TV, editor: *Manipulation, traction and massage*, ed 3, Baltimore, 1985, Williams & Wilkins.
35. Howe DH, Newcombe RG, Wade MT: Manipulation of the cervical spine—a pilot study, *J R Coll Gen Pract* 33:574, 1983.
36. Hoyt WH et al: Osteopathic manipulation in the treatment of muscle contraction headache, *J Am Osteopath Assoc* 78:332, 1979.
37. Jirout J: Changes in the sagittal component of the reaction of the cervical spine to lateroflexion after manipulation of blockade, *Cesk Neurol Neurochir* 35:175-180, 1972.
38. Jirout J: The effect of mobilization of the segmental blockade on the sagittal component of the reaction on lateral flexion of the cervical spine, *Neuroradiology* 3:210, 1972.
39. Kane R, Olsen D, Leymaster C: Manipulating the patient: a comparison of the effectiveness of physician and chiropractor care, *Lancet* 1:1333, 1974.
40. Kaplan E: The professional's professional, *ICA Int Rev Chiropract* p 22, Nov/Dec 1991.
41. Kimberly PE: *Outline of osteopathic manipulative procedures*, Kirksville, Mo, 1979, Kirksville College of Osteopathic Medicine.

42. Lewith GT, Turner GMT: Retrospective analysis of the management of acute low back pain, *Practitioner* 226:1614, 1982.
43. Logan HB: *Textbook of Logan basic methods,* St Louis, 1950, LBM.
44. Maigne JY, Rime B, Delignet B: Computed tomographic follow-up study of 48 cases of nonoperatively treated lumbar intervertebral disc herniation, *Spine* 17:1071, 1992.
45. Maitland GD: *Vertebral manipulation,* ed 3, London, 1973, Butterworth.
46. Matthews JA, Yates DAH: Reduction of lumbar disc prolapse by manipulation, *Br Med J* 20:696, 1969.
47. Matthews JA et al: Back pain and sciatica: controlled trials of manipulation, traction, sclerosal and epidural injections, *Br J Rheumatol* 26:416, 1987.
48. Meade TW et al: Low back pain of mechanical origin: randomized comparison of chiropractic and hospital outpatient treatment, *Br Med J* 300:1431, 1990.
49. Mennell JM: *Back pain — diagnosis and treatment using manipulative therapy,* Boston, 1960, Little, Brown.
50. Nyberg R: The role of physical therapists in spinal manipulation. In Basmajian JV, editor: *Manipulation, traction and massage,* ed 3, Baltimore, 1985, Williams & Wilkins.
51. Nyiendo J, Haldeman S: A prospective study of 2,000 patients attending a chiropractic college teaching unit, *Med Care* 25:516, 1987.
52. Oltenbacher K, DiFabio RP: Efficiency of spinal manipulation/mobilization therapy: a meta-analysis, *Spine* 10:833, 1985.
53. Panter J: The rigorous role of Dan McNeal, *Today's Chiropract* 19(4):60, 1990.
54. Pope MH et al: A prospective randomized three week trial of spinal manipulation, transcutaneous muscle stimulation, massage and corset in the treatment of subacute low back pain, Unpublished manuscript.
55. Rasmussen GG: Manipulation in low back pain: a randomized clinical trial, *Man Med:* 1:8, 1979.
56. Sanders GE et al: Chiropractic adjustive manipulation on subjects with acute low back pain: visual analog pain scores and plasma beta-endorphin levels, *J Manipulative Physiol Ther* 13:391, 1990.
57. Shambaugh P: Changes in electrical activity in muscles resulting from chiropractic adjustment: a pilot study, *J Manipulative Physiol Ther* 10:300, 1987.
58. Shekelle PG et al: (1991)*The appropriateness of spinal manipulation for low back pain,* Santa Monica, Calif, 1991, Rand Corp.
59. Shekelle PG et al: Spinal manipulation for low back pain, *Ann Intern Med* 117:590, 1992.
60. Sims-Williams H et al: Controlled trial of mobilization and manipulation for patients with low back pain in general practice, *Br Med J* 2:1338, 1978.
61. Sims-Williams H et al: Controlled trial of mobilization and manipulation for patients with low back pain: hospital patients, *Br Med J* 2:1318, 1979.
62. States AZ: *Spinal and pelvic technics: atlas of chiropractic technic,* ed 2, Lombard, Ill, 1968, National College of Chiropractic.
63. Terrett ACJ, Vernon H: Manipulation and pain tolerance: a controlled study of the effects of spinal manipulation on paraspinal cutaneous pain tolerance levels, *Am J Phys Med* 63:217, 1984.
64. Thompson JC: *Thompson technique,* Davenport, Iowa, 1973, Author.
65. Travell J: Myofascial trigger points: clinical view, *Adv Pain Res Ther* 1:919, 1976.
66. Vernon HT, Dhami MSI, Annett R: Paper presented at the symposium of low back pain, Canadian Foundation for Spinal Research, Vancouver, BC, March 15-16, 1985 (abstract).
67. Waagen GN et al: Short term trial of chiropractice adjustments for the relief of chronic low back pain, *Man Med* 2:63, 1986.
68. Waagen GN et al: A prospective comparative trial of general practice medical care, chiropractic manipulative therapy and sham manipulation in the management of patients with chronic or repetitive low back pain. Paper presented at the International Society for the Study of the Lumbar Spine, Boston, 1990.
69. Weine H: FICS fills international sports void, *Am J Chiropract,* p 27, June 1989.
70. Wood EC: *Beard's massage principles and techniques,* Philadelphia, 1974, WB Saunders.
71. Zhu Y et al: Paraspinal muscle evoked cerebral potentials in patients with unilateral low back pain. Manuscript submitted for publication, 1992.

Section Six

◆

Specific Sports

Chapter Twenty-Nine

♦

Neck Injuries in Football

Robert G. Watkins

Football is a violent sport that requires superior skill, great strength and agility, excellent eye-hand coordination, and outstanding conditioning. It is a unique sport involving (1) high-velocity collisions among players unequal in size, skills, and preparation; (2) use of the helmet and head for spearing, face tackling, and blocking; and (3) unexpected deforming loads on the head and shoulder alignment. There are a large number of participants in the United States, and the sport is spreading to other parts of the world, achieving reasonable popularity in Europe. Whether at the grade school, high school, college, or professional level, football makes tremendous demands on its participants, requiring a rare combination of strength, size, speed, violence, and understanding of the details and techniques of the game. A great deal of protective equipment is worn, including helmets, face masks, shoulder pads, hip pads, and rib pads, to absorb the tremendous shocks and blows delivered in the sport. The size of the players and the use of artificial surfaces have increased the velocity of the collisions occurring in the sport, and body contact is responsible for a significant number of injuries. In football, violent head and shoulder contact is incorporated into the techniques of the game, producing significant lower extremity injuries, as well as some of the most violent injuries possible in sports, including fractures of the pelvis, dislocated hips, fracture dislocations of the cervical lumbar spine, open fractures in any extremity, and fracture dislocations in any joint.

SCOPE OF THE PROBLEM

There is no universally accepted definition of what constitutes an injury or how to measure the severity of an injury in football accidents.[44] In some research, offensive players were identified as having an increased incidence of neck injury,[21,42] whereas one study specified defensive and tackling players.[34] Compared with other sports, football and rugby show the highest rate of neck injury.[15,30] In a critical review of the available literature on the risk of injury to high school football players, Halpern et al.[26] identified the proportion of head and neck injuries to be 7.4% of all injuries in approximately 5109 injured football players. In a clinical study Hill et al.[30] reported that football-related injuries represented 8% of all pediatric injuries.

Probably the best review of the mechanical forces operative in cervical spine injuries among football

players and other athletes is offered by Alexander.[2] The study by Albright et al.[1] probably is the most thorough in documenting neck injuries in football players. These researchers found that 50% of high school football players had significant neck pain before injury occurred. Results of the study revealed a 4% incidence of lost time as a result of neck injury, with neurologic involvement in 45% of these players. The estimate of non–lost-time injuries was approximately twice that of the lost-time injury rate.[45] Although serious injuries are rare, recurrences are common.

Injuries to the intervertebral disc affect downlinemen with a higher incidence and are usually associated with weight-lifting training rather than with playing the game.[18,46] The incidence of spondylolisthesis is high in all positions of football, with no established difference in positions despite some suggestion that interior linemen are at greater risk. The thoracic and thoracolumbar spine in football players, as well as in other athletes, suffers a higher degree of compressive and rotatory stresses. Because of cartilaginous vertebral body structures, a great deal of repetitive injury may occur, especially in the young, growing athlete.[27] There are demonstrated incidents of Schmorl's nodes and related compressive injuries and anterior cartilaginous growth plate injuries. Abnormalities of this kind were noted in 36% to 55% of all athletes, with football, wrestling, gymnastics, soccer, and tennis represented.[23,41]

In the last 20 years the volume of sports medicine literature related to football injuries has increased in response to the popularity of football in the United States. As many as 1.5 million players participate in American football. It is estimated that 1 million football-related injuries are sustained annually. Most occur during practice contact and in the training period rather than during the game. Spinal injuries account for 40% of football trauma. An overall review of common football injuries by Saal[40] outlines injuries to the extremities and the spine, as well as the training techniques and equipment used to prevent injury.[1,36-48,50]

The occasional catastrophic outcome of severe neck injuries and the medical-legal issues involving coaches, physicians, and players have heightened public awareness of neck injuries in football. From 1931 to the peak of injuries in 1968, most football fatalities were due to head injuries. In 1976 the rules changed, making it illegal to block or tackle with the head, and improved football helmet standards went into effect in the mid-1970s. The incidence of serious head injuries has decreased.[13] However, brain injuries have occurred and will continue to occur.[9] The National Football Head and Neck Injury Registry[45] clearly demonstrates that most cervical fracture dislocations are due to axial loading. As a result, there is a great push toward changing the rules again to eliminate the deliberate use of the head as an offensive weapon. Rules against spearing, which involves using the helmet as an initial point of contact, have been implemented at the high school and college level, with a resultant decrease in the number of cervical quadriplegic incidents from 34 in 1976 to 5 in 1984.

Cerebral stroke has occurred in relation to vertebral artery trauma in the cervical spine.[27] Bilateral traumatic rotatory dislocation of the axis on the atlas[34] and paresthesias in the trigeminal nerve from upper cervical spine injuries have been reported.[19]

Reports in the literature have noted anatomic characteristics of the cervical spine that can be identified radiographically and have been associated with an increased severity of neurologic injury in cervical spine trauma.[10,50] No studies to date have identified a reliable screening tool that can be used as a predictor of future neurologic injury in athletes.

The physician who cares for football players must understand the syndromes involved, the gravity and breadth of the problems, and how to prevent, as well as how to treat, neck injuries. Areas to be emphasized are the immediate care of these problems, the transport of the injured player, and thorough work-up of the case so that an intelligent assessment of future risk can be made.

RESEARCH FINDINGS
Kerlan-Jobe Orthopaedic Clinic Study

At the Kerlan-Jobe Orthopaedic Clinic we evaluated and treated[67] football players over a 3-year period for neck injuries sustained during football games and in organized, supervised play. The players ranged in age from a 12-year-old junior high school player to an experienced 42-year-old professional. The average age was 19.6 years, with most players involved in high school–level play.

We adapted the guidelines for data acquisition established by the National Football Head and Neck Injury Registry to our routine evaluation.[45] All the information was collected during a detailed history and physical examination in an office setting. The players were seen in the office after the precipitating traumatic event and carefully questioned regarding treatment given at the time of injury and the intervening symptomatic course. The initial presenting complaint was recorded for all patients. The mechanism of injury, including the position of the head and the direction of applied load, was recorded when the player was able to

recall the details of the incident. Additional factors included the duration of the initial symptoms, any loss of upper extremity or neck function as it related to football, any history of recurrent episodes, and the presence of any neurologic deficits.

In all players, standard lateral radiographs were obtained. The radiographs were reviewed for evidence of clinical instability as defined by White et al.,[48] who describe clinical stability as the ability of the spine to limit its patterns of displacement under physiologic loads so as not to damage or irritate the spinal cord or the nerve roots. Their radiographic criteria for instability include (1) horizontal displacement exceeding 3.5 mm between motion segments or (2) angulation of the vertebra in question that is more than 11 degrees greater than the angulation of either normal adjacent vertebra, which indicates clinical cervical spine instability. Radiographic abnormalities were documented, including subluxation, instability, foraminal narrowing, degenerative changes, and congenital anomalies. The diameters of the spinal canal and the vertebral body were measured radiographically by means of a computerized digitization technique that has been described and validated by Odor et al.[35] This method was used for all cervical vertebral levels evaluated.

The computerized measurement allowed us to accurately determine and reproduce the mid–sagittal diameter of the canal, as well as to calculate the ratio of the sagittal canal diameter to the vertebral body diameter, using the technique published by Torg and Pavlov.[44] Using plain lateral radiographs, we also calculated the sagittal canal–to–vertebral body ratio, which compares the sagittal diameter of the spinal canal measured from the midpoint of the posterior vertebral body to the nearest point on the spinolaminar line of the same level with the anteroposterior (AP) diameter of the corresponding vertebral body at its midpoint. The measurements were made in all 67 players with neck injuries from the second to the seventh cervical vertebra. A total of 372 cervical spine levels were evaluated and computer digitized. Individual players who had undergone cervical spine surgery or had any injury that altered the structural contour of the bony landmarks were excluded from this analysis.

Results. All 67 players had neck pain, often accompanied by paraspinal cervical muscle spasm. Thirty-four players had only neck pain or spasm without any associated neurologic symptoms or objective neurologic deficits. However, 29 players had subjective neurologic complaints or objective neurologic findings, with 20 of these players describing varying degrees of radiating upper extremity pain or paresthesias in one or both arms. Five players had numbness in one or both upper extremities, and 11 players had motor involvement in addition to the sensory complaints, with 2 players having an episode of neurapraxia of the spinal cord with transient quadriparesis. One player with a cervical (C5-6) fracture dislocation secondary to an axial loading injury with complete quadriplegia was eliminated from the study. All 11 of the players with a motor loss described the characteristic sharp, lancinating upper extremity pain characteristic of stingers, or burners, in association with weakness in upper extremity function (see Chapter 30).

The mechanism of injury of the incident causing the presenting complaint of neck pain or neurologic injury was known in 42 of the 67 players. The remaining 21 patients could not reliably recall the direction of forces applied to the head or the position of the head at the time of the injury. Twenty-two patients described an axial loading mechanism of injury, with the predominant force applied to the top of their helmet while the neck was relatively straight. Fourteen players described a force applied to the head that caused a hyperextension movement about the cervical spine. These 14 players all believed that a component of axial loading and possibly rotation, in addition to the hyperextension, contributed to their symptoms. Three players described a flexion force applied to the head, and three players described a lateral rotation and bending direction of the applied load, with neck symptoms felt at the extremes of motion. There was no identifiable correlation between the mechanism of injury—whether axial loading, extension, flexion, rotation, or a combination—and the description of the subsequent symptoms or the presence of a motor deficit.

Nine players were found to have demonstrable muscle group weakness that persisted until the time of the office visit. Two players had weakness of the deltoid. One player had biceps weakness. No players had only triceps weakness, and one player had weakness of the intrinsic muscles of the hand. In addition, five patients had a combination of the aforementioned muscle group weaknesses, with a pattern of radiculopathy that involved more than a single cervical nerve root level. Two players had four-extremity involvement with temporary weakness of the arms and legs lasting less than 5 minutes in both cases. Neither player with transient neurapraxia of the spinal cord had residual motor loss at the time of the office visit.

Six players did not accurately describe whether they had a history of recurrent neck injury. Of those players who were able to describe their history of recurrent episodes of neck injury, 25 did not recall any prior episodes of neck injury, neck pain, or neurologic symptoms related to the upper extremities. Thirty-two players described one or more prior episodes of neck injury; 11 thought they had at least five such episodes before the current injury. These prior incidents ranged from minor neck pain without neurologic manifestations to more severe neck pain and spasms with sensory complaints consistent with burners and stingers. Four

players had five prior episodes, two players had four prior episodes, five players had two prior episodes, and 10 players could recall only a single prior episode.

The radiographs obtained at the initial office visit usually included AP, lateral, flexion, extension, oblique, and open-mouth odontoid views. Thirty-five players had completely normal findings on cervical spine radiographs. Twenty-three had varying degrees of intervertebral disc space narrowing, foraminal narrowing, or degenerative spurs. Two players were found to have congenital fusions of one or more motion segments. Two players had radiographic evidence of healed fractures, and three players had mild to moderate subluxation or instability of adjacent motion segments.

Evaluation. The findings of this study suggest that axial loading and hyperextension are the most frequent mechanisms of injury of the neck in football. We found that hyperextension with an element of rotation toward the painful arm is a common mechanism of injury in the production of stingers (see Chapter 30).

Other Studies

The prevention of catastrophic neurologic injury remains a stimulus to the publication of sports medicine reports related to cervical spine injuries in athletes. Injuries related to football play have been studied from a cost-benefit, as well as a humanitarian, viewpoint.[1,45] These studies demonstrate that major preventive efforts to decrease the incidence of serious injuries in athletes are justified, and the benefit to the individual, as well as to society, outweighs the potential cost of these preventive efforts. The mechanisms by which the team physician, trainer, or coach may implement this goal are many. They include the identification of risk factors for neurologic or neck injury (e.g., the individual player's radiographic spinal anatomy, aerobic conditioning, muscular strength and body size, playing conditions, mechanics of injury, and prior injury history).[1]

The identification of a reliable radiographic or anatomic marker that is helpful in predicting a person's chance of sustaining neurologic impairment also has been studied[6,10,50] (see later section on measurement of cervical stenosis).

MANAGEMENT
Initial Care

The decision-making process begins the moment the player injures his neck. If the patient is conscious and up and running toward the bench, he should be taken to the bench, seated, questioned about his symptoms, and evaluated immediately on the bench. If the player is lying down on the field, standard practice calls for the trainer to go to the player, start the evaluation, and summon the physician.

The chief diagnostic obligation of a clinician is to diagnose a potentially unstable cervical spine that could lead to a major neurologic deficit after injury. The player down on the field with neck and arm pain should be examined closely to determine first if there is cervical spine injury. The physician determines the potential for an unstable spine and assesses the patient's condition. This leads to a therapeutic plan, beginning with assurances of vital function and protective transportation (see Chapter 9).

An unconscious player is treated as having an unstable cervical spine injury until it is proved otherwise. If his symptoms totally resolve, the player is usually walked to the sidelines and then reexamined on the bench or taken for an immediate x-ray film. If he is not totally symptom free, it is important to ensure a proper airway. If the airway is a problem, if there is choking or evidence of a swallowed tongue, or if the mouth is not clear, the mouth must be cleared and the patient turned onto his back as for an unstable spinal cord injury.

The diagnostic evaluation begins with a determination as to whether the patient has had motor-sensory loss. Does he have spinal pain? Was he unconscious? Is there neck or arm pain? Is there spine and leg pain?

The initial history and physical examination are critically important. Many times decisions concerning continued play to be made months later depend on the facts obtained during this crucial initial period. The patient must be carefully questioned as to what sensations he felt, including whether he had weakness, numbness, tingling, or inability to move his legs or toes, squeeze his hands, or move his arms. The length of time of involvement of the symptoms must also be carefully documented. Neck stiffness can be a sign of an occult fracture.

Follow-Up Evaluation

At the bench or in the locker room, decisions must be based on the history and key physical findings. For example, players are not returned to play with any symptoms of motor weakness in the arm. Physical examination includes a complete neurologic examination, head compression test, Spurling's and Adson's maneuvers, resistive head pressure, and cervical range of motion. If there is any doubt, it is far safer to leave the helmet in place, pending satisfactory findings on lateral radiographs. If suspicion of serious cervical spine injury remains, the helmet can be removed in the hospital, where definitive treatment modalities are available. If it is safe to remove the helmet on site, the procedure is the same as that used when an unstable spine is suspected: The face mask is cut off, and the examiner reaches inside the helmet-shoulder interval from the anterior, holding the occiput to the trapezius with his hands. Two assistants pull out the sides of the helmet and remove it in a cephalad direction; then the examiner's hands are moved into the standard position.

Key findings. Neurologic deficit, leg involvement, radiating arm pain, loss of function, paresthesias, and weakness are key findings. Radiating arm pain and neurologic deficit can indicate a serious problem, such as spinal instability, that can lead to permanent neurologic deficit, either cord or radicular in nature. A painful neck is important, but loss of cervical range of motion, with or without a lot of pain, could be the only residual sign of an unstable cervical spine lesion. Pain perception may be altered by the emotion of the game, and a stiff neck with or without pain should be reason enough to remove the athlete from play. These symptoms may indicate an occult fracture. Other signs of fracture can be neck pain with head compression and pain on resisting hand pressure to the head.

A "numb all over" feeling may indicate a loss of consciousness, a transitory quadriplegia, or nothing. Usually, if it lasts 1 to 5 seconds and there are no residual symptoms, the player leaves the field. Any lingering symptoms or persistent lower extremity weakness or numbness should be examined closely and the player transported as for a spinal injury. Players are not sent back into the game with residual numbness, tingling, dysesthesias, weakness, or pain radiating into the arm. Lower extremity numbness and tingling or abnormal gait should eliminate the player from competition until diagnostic evaluation can be obtained. If there is lower extremity involvement (even transitory) that can definitely be identified as characteristic of myelopathy, the player should not be allowed to return to the game that day. If there is transitory neurapraxia in the arm, the player can return. Loss of cervical range of motion and neurologic deficit are the chief criteria for removing a player from the game; no return should be permitted as long as these symptoms persist.

X-ray evaluation. If locker room x-ray facilities are available, AP, lateral, two oblique (when possible), and flexion/extension films should be obtained, beginning with a transtable lateral view to evaluate for fracture or signs of instability. In a patient with residual neck stiffness, the flexion-extension films may be worthless because they could fail to disclose a subtle ligamentous instability and/or partial subluxation resulting from a facet fracture. The flexion/extension film should be considered valid only if a good full range of flexion-extension motion is seen on the films. It is important to see the entire cervical spine, including C7. This can be difficult in football players. The Boger straps are passive stretch straps that are unequaled in terms of their ability to demonstrate a full x-ray view of the cervical spine in patients with shoulder pads and large shoulders. We have not found a circumstance in which the Boger straps did not show the C7 segment under these emergency conditions.

If the Boger straps are not available, an assistant standing at the foot of the x-ray table can place the

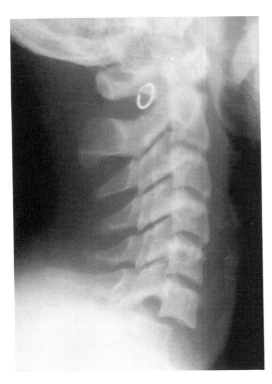

Fig. 29-1. A bilateral facet dislocation that could be missed if a full visualization of C7 is not obtained with the proper lateral x-ray film.

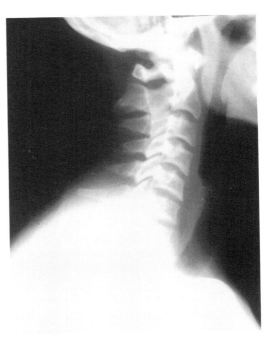

Fig. 29-2. X-ray film of a 20-year-old university-level running back who had a severe episode of transient quadriparesis with significant residual neurologic deficit lasting several months. His congenital cervical canal stenosis could easily be measured on a standardized-distance x-ray film or confirmed with a more detailed study, such as MRI or a CT scan.

patient's feet onto his chest and grasp the patient's hands. By pulling distally on the hands against the resistive force of his own chest to the patient's lower extremities, the assistant can effectively uncover the C7 segment otherwise hidden from radiographic view (Fig. 29-1). With adequate findings on flexion/extension and plain x-ray films, as well as normal cervical range of motion and some mild residual neck pain, the patient can return to the game.

Ligamentous instability on the flexion/extension lateral films are measured by drawing lines parallel to the inferior end-plates of each vertebral body. The angle between any two adjacent lines should not be greater than 11 degrees greater than the angle measured between the pair above *or* below. Horizontal translation greater than 3.5 mm may be another indication of ligamentous instability. Dynamic instability may also be noted if only the flexion films shows translation. This may be due to facet fracture, pillar fracture, or major ligamentous injury.

One difficult aspect of the radiographic evaluation is to determine if this is an acute injury, an old injury, or an asymptomatic finding. One complicating factor is the presence of a hypermobile segment over stiff, arthritic segments. Many athletes who do neck-strengthening exercises on a regular, consistent basis, especially starting at a young age, have relative osteoarthritic changes

at certain lower cervical levels. The stiffness at these levels produces a relative increase in mobility at levels just above these stiffened segments (Fig. 29-2).

The ideal would be to help identify an area of ligamentous instability resulting from a recent injury. Because this seldom happens, it must be determined whether the hypermobile segment is the result of recent injury. This determination can be effectively accomplished by use of the averaging technique for the amount of kyphotic displacement; that is, if there is no motion in the lower segments, it should be even harder to produce a dynamic instability measuring greater than 11 degrees' difference on film. A fixed deformity rarely meets criteria for instability.

Additional tests. Magnetic resonance imaging (MRI) or a computed tomography (CT) scan should be ordered if the patient has a quadriparetic or quadriparesthetic episode or if radicular dysfunction persists. Of course, myelopathy requires work-up by a spinal consultant as soon as possible.

The clinician who orders the study should be prepared to ascertain the significance of the results, which requires the ability to relate them as specifically as possible to the clinical findings. It should be remembered that in the general population at least 30% of CT scans will show abnormalities and cervical CT scans of football players inevitably show abnormalities.

The clinician uses the same criteria in ordering diagnostic tests for football players as for any patient. Any time there is reason for concern about the patient's status, the tests should be ordered. On the other hand, x-ray examination is unnecessary if the results would not change the diagnosis, the treatment, or the prognosis.

Any diagnostic study may reveal asymptomatic lesions that have nothing to do with the current problem but that in themselves necessitate serious decision making concerning their effect on the patient. The clinician should be prepared to treat lesions found on diagnostic studies and to make recommendations about potentially symptomatic lesions that do not match the clinical syndrome. X-ray changes can affect the future of a football player. Recommendations about future disability and compensation must be made about each anatomic lesion and symptom. Often the prognosis is particularly important to athletes. To make appropriate roster adjustments, teams need to know as exactly as possible how long the patient will be disabled. The player, agent, and team also need to know what to expect in the future (i.e., what effect an injury will have on the level of play). Again, the safest course is to order diagnostic studies in terms of the best medical diagnostic and treatment plan for the patient involved.

Diagnosis

The diagnosis on which the treatment is based is very important. A common problem involves referring to a symptom complex as a strain, such as cervical or lumbar strain, and subsequently having results of a diagnostic study such as a CT scan show a disc herniation. This can be a difficult situation for the clinician and the patient. This sequence can be avoided by making an open, flexible clinical diagnosis or by pinpointing the exact anatomic problem before any diagnosis is made. It is best to be as specific and detailed as possible as soon as necessary.

Decisions About Continued Play

When the neck is injured because of violent athletic contact, the team physician or health care provider for the team is often called on to make a clear-cut decision regarding the player's ability to safely return to active participation. Thus the team physician can be exposed to tremendous pressure from those persons who may attempt to compromise his authority. The obvious economic realities of professional sports and the subtle social pressure, as well as family and peer pressure on high school and college players, can be enormously influential factors. The athlete's ego and drive to play must also be considered in the evaluation of the player's symptoms and findings on examination. Overall, however, the team physician must remain completely objective and focus only on the medical facts to avoid any diminution in the quality of medical care provided to the player.

The decision to return a football player to full contact football depends on the diagnosis, prognosis, and certain circumstances peculiar to football. Crucial to the continued play recommendation is an understanding of the game. The full velocity of a large, speeding body is delivered through the rigid plastic battering ram of a helmet. Totally unexpected collisions can occur and can be resisted with tremendous force. The collision response requires superb conditioning, and many athletes are maximally conditioned to participate in collisions. The higher the skill level, usually the greater is the ability to deliver and receive the blow. High school football, with both skinny 14-year-old boys and mature 19-year-old men, differs significantly from professional football. Discrepancies in skill level and age may make a certain decision easy, such as removing an immature high school boy from contact.

Decision-making physicians should understand not only the potential for injury but also the ability of highly conditioned athletes to avoid injury. For example, football players have larger necks for a very good reason: to be able to avoid neck injuries. Relating the risk of cervical injury in football players to that in the general population is not a comparison of similar samples. The closer the physician is to the game and the players, the better he will understand all the factors. Neck pain is common, and once injured, the athlete is more likely to be injured again, although serious injuries are uncommon.

Often a spinal consultant is asked to rule on the potential risk to the patient (or the team) of incapacitating injury or future symptoms that would impair play. The opinion of consultants should be divided into risk categories, and the risks involved in continued play should be fully explained to the athlete and the team. Risks may be expressed in terms of permanent injury (e.g., death, cord injury, permanent root injury with resulting chronic pain and neurologic deficit) or as the possibility of recurrence of symptoms that would hinder future play. The risk categories are as follows:

1. *Minimal risk*—There is a very small increased chance of risk as compared with play before the injury.
2. *Moderate risk*—There is a reasonable chance that the patient will have a recurrence of symptoms and is at some risk for some permanent injury.
3. *Extreme risk*—The patient runs a high risk of recurrence of symptoms and permanent damage.

It is critical that all factors related to the player's symptoms, history of injury, radiographic findings, results of any special studies needed, and expectations be included in the ultimate recommendation regarding the likelihood of injury if the player returns to football. Examples of each category are offered here as guidelines for appropriate decision making.

Minimal-risk category. Undisplaced fractures that heal without any residual deformity are at a low risk for

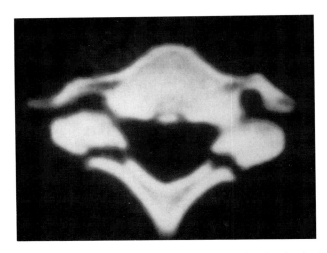

Fig. 29-3. CT scan of a 26-year-old professional defensive back with severe neck pain after an acute tackling episode, revealing a three-level laminar fracture, an unusual clay shoveler type of injury. It healed fully, and the patient returned to football with no significant risk for future contact.

reinjury and the player can be returned to play. Clay shoveler fractures are avulsion fractures of the tip of the spinous process of C7 caused by strong muscular contractions of the trapezius and shoulder muscles (Fig. 29-3). They present with point tenderness, otherwise negative study findings, and dual rigidity. Lateral mass fractures always heal but may have a slight subluxation of one vertebra on another. The degree of risk depends on the degree of subluxation. Ligamentous damage rarely occurs with this injury. Laminar fractures that heal without deformity carry only a minor risk. Disc herniations that have been asymptomatic over many months or years are not significant except in relation to how they have narrowed the central canal. Foraminal stenosis is important when symptoms are present, but because of the high incidence of asymptomatic foraminal stenosis, we would not consider a nerve root to be endangered just because radiographic foraminal stenosis is present.

Thus minimal-risk injuries can be categorized as follows:
1. Asymptomatic bone spurs
2. Certain healed facet fractures
3. Stingers, or burners
4. Healed disc herniation
5. Healed laminar fracture
6. Fractured tip of the spinous process
7. Asymptomatic foraminal stenosis

Moderate-risk category. Fractures of the cervical facet or pillar fractures through the lateral mass may present as a facet dislocation because of the anterior subluxation of one vertebral body on another, which occurs frequently. For these fractures the ultimate recommendation as to return to play depends most significantly on any residual

deformity that persists after healing has occurred, as well as any residual instability or cervical stiffness that is manifested after appropriate treatment has been completed.

Herniated cervical discs are reasonably common in adult football players. Most of the herniated cervical discs that we identify in athletes have a lingering or persistent radiculopathy or occur in those players with a first-time severe burner at the professional or college level. Because the incidence of asymptomatic disc bulges and herniations in the general population is significantly high, in a football player the finding of a herniated cervical disc that was completely asymptomatic for related signs and symptoms of cervical myelopathy or radiculopathy would not place that player at an increased risk of injury. However, players who have evidence of radiculopathy are in a moderate-risk category. It is often difficult to determine whether a disc herniation is acute, chronic, hard (as in a cervical osteophyte), soft, a free fragment, or simply a contained disc bulge. It is important that (1) any radiographic diagnostic imaging abnormalities in these players be closely correlated with the physical findings and (2) the physical findings match the herniation for an accurate prognosis to be made, inasmuch as peripheral nerve lesions can mimic a cervical radiculopathy. The treatment for herniated, extruded cervical discs is an anterior cervical discectomy and fusion. After such treatment, we often place the player in a mild-risk category, secondary to the biomechanical alterations that must necessarily occur above and below the fused cervical motion segment. If given the appropriate clinical indications, we might recommend a microscopic cervical foraminotomy for the treatment of monoradiculopathy secondary to foraminal stenosis in an athlete involved in contact sports. For the athlete with significant intermittent radiculopathy, a positive result on Spurling's hyperextension test, and foraminal stenosis, a posterolateral foraminotomy is a reasonable approach. The technique of this operation is adopted from Robert Warren Williams[51] and includes a minimal resection of the posterior wall of the foramen only until nerve root pulsations are clearly present. Return to football is contraindicated after a significant facet resection. Kyphotic deformity after treatment or as a preexisting condition associated with a disc herniation increases the risk to the player.

Examples of moderate-risk injuries are as follows:
1. Facet fractures
2. Lateral mass fractures
3. Nondisplaced healed odontoid fractures
4. Nondisplaced healed ring of C1 fractures
5. Acute lateral disc herniations
6. Cervical radiculopathy because of a foraminal spur

Extreme-risk category. Fractures of the first cervical vertebra (Jefferson fractures) generally represent an axial loading injury, often resulting from a player's head-on collision with the opponent or the ground. The Jefferson fracture is disruption of the ring of the first cervical vertebra and may be identified on the open-mouth AP view as eccentric or excessive overhang of the lateral mass of the first cervical vertebra on the second cervical vertebra. A CT scan can provide precise identification of the configuration of a C1 fracture. At the level of the atlas, there is considerable room for the spinal cord secondary to the large central spinal canal at that level. Thus neurologic injury resulting from a Jefferson fracture is unusual. The mechanism of injury involves axial loading that forces the occipital condyles into the lateral masses of the atlas, resulting in failure of the ring of the atlas, often at the thinner region just medial to the trough that lies at the level of the vertebral artery.

Certainly, return to play after a recent Jefferson fracture is contraindicated. It is only after bony healing has occurred and appropriate tests for ligamentous stability can be obtained that a recommendation about return to play can be made. If the bone completely heals, if a full, normal range of motion is present, and if no residual instability is noted on flexion/extension views, then return to play is possible. Certainly if there is any residual instability, residual neck stiffness, or discomfort, then return to play places that player in an extreme-risk category. Occasionally, C1 ring fractures heal with a fibrous union as evidenced on a CT scan. In this event a player with no residual neck stiffness or pain could be placed in a moderate-risk category for return to play (Fig. 29-4). A rotation subluxation occurring in an adolescent can produce a residual deformity that would make any additional axial loading injury potentially dangerous.

Transverse ligament ruptures, which result from high-velocity axial loading injuries, are quite rare and occur in only 3% of all cervical spine injuries.[17] The odontoid is held snugly against the back of the atlas by the strong fibers of the transverse ligament. These fibers arise from the lateral masses of the atlas, just behind the origin of the accessory ligament. Rupture of the transverse ligament is identified by abnormal motion between the atlas and the odontoid on the flexion/extension views or by an atlantodens interval of greater than 5 mm on the neutral lateral film. Partial tears of the transverse ligament may be identified by an atlantodens interval of from 2 to 5 mm. We have treated an athlete with a partial tear of the transverse ligament who played as a starting professional defensive tackle and who suffered a high-velocity injury resulting in residual stiffness and pain in his neck. This player was believed to be in an extreme-risk category for further play. We have also treated a 17-year-old high school football player with a significant neck injury that resulted in upper cervical spine stiffness and pain. A V-shaped atlantodens interval was present,

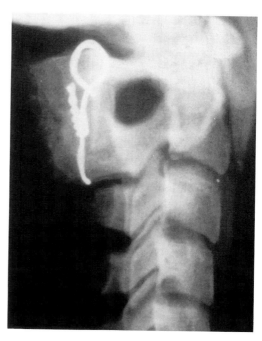

Fig. 29-4. X-ray film of a patient who wanted to return to football after a C1-2 fusion. The decision was that a contact sport would place him at considerable risk for cervical spine injury.

and the player's diagnosis was a partial transverse ligament tear, even though this entity has been considered an incidental finding. Our recommendation to this young man and his parents was that he would be at an increased risk of neurologic injury from continued participation in football.

The open-mouth view, used to identify odontoid fractures, can be classified according to the system of Anderson and D'Alonzo[3] into one of the following three types. Type I includes the tip of the odontoid and is believed to be a stable fracture configuration, whereas type II is a fracture through the base of the odontoid and is the least stable and most likely to lead to nonunion. Type III is an odontoid fracture that involves a variable component of the vertebral body of C2 and is likely to lead to early union. Odontoid fractures that heal completely, without deformity and with free, unrestricted, pain-free neck motion, are considered to place the player at mild risk for secondary injury from continued play. However, any residual deformity or the suggestion of a fibrous union between the odontoid and the body of C2 is considered a potentially unstable situation; significant biomechanical stress on that fracture is to be expected, which would place the player in an extreme-risk category.

Fracture of the pedicle of C2 is called a "hangman's fracture" because of its association with the sudden, hyperextension provided by the hangman's noose. Hangman's fractures have been classified according to the system of Effendi et al.[21] and modified by the system proposed by Levine and Edwards.[32] Type I injuries, which are considered stable, are fractures through the pars interarticularis with less than 1 to 2 mm of displacement at that fracture site. Type II injuries often have some degree of displacement and occur through the isthmus. In these fractures there may also have been some rebound flexion, with associated disruption of the posterior ligamentous structures or the C2-3 disc, resulting in residual angulation and subluxation.

Type IIA fractures, introduced by Levine and Edwards,[32] include fractures that have less displacement but more angulation than the type II injury of Effendi et al.[21] These fractures may have been associated with primary flexion force and are particularly prone to increased angulation and displacement when traction is applied. Type III fractures are generally secondary to flexion injury and may be associated with facet capsule disruption between C2 and C3. This allows for fracture through the pars interarticularis. If the hangman's fracture heals completely, with no fibrous union, and satisfactory reestablishment of the posterior arch of C2 occurs, the player's risk for subsequent injury is considered minimal. However, any suggestion of fibrous union or significant residual deformity after bony union would increase the chance of injury and thus place the player at extreme risk. Often the soft tissue injury involves the posterior and middle columns, and occasionally the anterior column as well, and the risk is extreme.

Congenital abnormalities of the cervical spine sometimes place the player at an increased risk for neurologic damage, depending on the precise morphology of the abnormality. Os odontoideum, which has been documented in the literature as most likely secondary to a traumatic lesion, can be a significantly unstable condition that places the player at extreme risk for injury. Not infrequently, os odontoideum presents in the younger player as an asymptomatic and incidental finding and, as such, can be a particularly difficult problem to explain in the otherwise young, healthy, high-caliber athlete. Multiple levels of failure of segmentation, as found in the Klippel-Feil syndrome (Fig. 29-5), place the adjoining spinal motion units at an increased biomechanical disadvantage secondary to the compensatory increased motion that occurs adjacent to the fused levels. Generally, we would list the risk factor of this constellation of segmentation defects as moderate to extreme, depending somewhat on the findings on flexion/extension films, as well as on the distribution of the fused segments. Sprengel's deformity in association with Klippel-Feil syndrome is not unusual and is considered an extreme-risk category.

The hidden flexion injury of McSweeney can be identified as a subtle subluxation on the flexion view that is actually a total ligamentous disruption. This diagnosis is made on the lateral or flexion film.[47] The x-ray findings

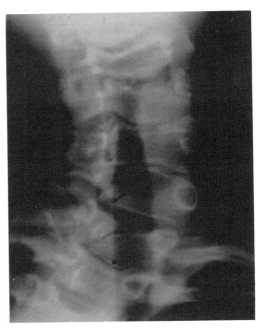

Fig. 29-5. X-ray film showing a patient with Klippel-Feil syndrome who requested clearance for high school–level football. Extensive congenital anomalies of this type place the patient in a high-risk category.

may include a gaping of the spinous processes, a localized end-plate deformity, or a subtle avulsion fracture of the anterior edge of the vertebral body. The symptoms may be quite subtle, and the radiographic findings may take several weeks to become apparent because of the residual stiffness and spasm present immediately after the accident. Failure to diagnose this residual ligamentous instability and allowing these players to return to play would place them at extreme risk. Herkowitz and Rothman[28] have documented this particular ligamentous and radiographic finding after cervical spine trauma. Delay in the diagnosis and treatment of this injury can also lead to a fixed kyphotic deformity, placing the patient permanently in an extreme-risk category.

Fractures of the vertebral bodies C3 to C7 can be associated with compression and flexion forces, as well as torsional forces, that may leave the player with a significant cervical spine instability. Vertebral burst fractures, which can include significant spinal cord injury, are occasionally associated with facet dislocations that place the player at significant risk for serious neurologic injury. Certainly, there is not always a good correlation between the degree of spinal cord injury and the amount of bony injury or dislocation on the plain films. The prognosis for return to play after vertebral burst fractures, which sometimes include subluxation or dislocation in the cervical spine, depends on the neurologic injury and the residual deformity present after complete healing. If, of course, there is no residual neck pain or stiffness, no residual neurologic deficit, no residual associated cervical instability, and no residual deformity or canal narrowing, then players who are recovered from cervical spine compression or burst fractures may be allowed to return to play, although they are still in the mild-risk category.

Facet dislocations, bilateral and unilateral, can occur with head compression and flexion-rotation injury. The facet dislocation that reduces completely and heals with no residual deformity or instability would place the player in a moderate-risk category because of the damage to ligamentous support for that segment. Healed facet dislocations with any residual deformity or instability would certainly place the player at an extreme risk of further injury.

Disc herniations involve a number of different categories. Certain disc herniations, especially central disc herniations producing transitory quadriparesis or cervical myelopathy, certainly carry extreme risk. If they produce a significant amount of spinal stenosis, even with healing, the risk is certainly greater than in lateral disc herniation with fewer radicular symptoms.

In summary, among the most common injuries that place the player in the extreme-risk category are the following:

1. Os odentoideum
2. Ruptured transverse ligament C1-2
3. Occipitocervical dislocation
4. Odontoid fracture
5. Total ligamentous disruption of a neuromotor segment of the lower cervical spine
6. Unstable fracture dislocation
7. Unstable Jefferson fracture
8. Cervical cord anomaly
9. Acute large central disc herniation

Recommendations. In conclusion, the decision-making process that each team physician uses in approaching the football player with a cervical spine injury must be based on the medical facts and current medical knowledge. Attention to detail, with structured preplanning and a practiced, on-the-field routine, is critical to ensuring that the injured player suffers no additional damage after the accident. Counseling the player and other concerned persons must be consistent and should include only the medical facts. It is important to remember that the team physician's role is to convey the medical information and to instruct and train the players, coaches, and trainers in techniques that will be useful to prevent player injury or further injury once a player is down on the field. There are no strict guidelines that are considered the standard of care. An understanding of the relative risk of a spinal disorder or injury to an individual player, both at the time of injury and in allowing a return to play, must come from advanced training in sports-related spinal injuries or

from clinical experience in the care of athletes on a regular basis.

CERVICAL STENOSIS

Cervical spinal stenosis and its associated transient neurapraxia of the cervical spinal cord is a source of great controversy with regard to recommendations for continued play. Grant and Sears[25] first described the clinical entity of cervical spinal cord neurapraxia with transient quadriplegia. Torg and Pavlov[44] describe the clinical picture as an acute transient neurologic episode of cervical cord origin with sensory changes that may be associated with motor paresis involving either both arms, both legs, or all four extremities after forced hyperextension, hyperflexion, or axial loading of the cervical spine. The sensory changes include burning pain, numbness, tingling, loss of sensation, and motor changes that consist of weakness or complete paralysis.

Congenital cervical spinal stenosis is associated with a decreased AP diameter of the cervical spinal canal as measured from the posterior vertebral body to the anterior spinal laminar line on the lateral radiograph. Acquired spinal stenosis is more likely to occur in the professional football player with multiple levels of degenerative disc disease and osteophyte formation, disc bulging, disc herniation, and hypertrophy of both the ligamenta flava and the facet joints. This combination of degenerative and hypertrophic changes in the professional football player is not unusual.

The absolute minimum sagittal diameter of the cervical spinal canal that can accommodate the spinal cord without cord compression is somewhere between 11 and 13 mm, depending on the relative diameter of the spinal cord. The classic work of Penning[38] documented that if the sagittal diameter is less than 11 mm in extension, there is a strong suspicion of spinal cord compression. It was Penning who illustrated the "pincers mechanism," in which the spinal cord is pinched between posterior vertebral osteophytes off the lip of the vertebral end-plate and the posterior lamina. Certainly, this mechanism of injury is commonly responsible for causing the central cord syndrome in persons with preexisting degenerative disc disease and osteophyte formation who suffer a hyperextension injury of the head and neck. However, there is ample clinical experience in dealing with professional football players with sagittal cervical spine canal diameters of less than 11 mm and yet have no signs or symptoms of spinal cord compression. Therefore, as with all radiographic findings, precise clinical correlation of the radiographic findings with the patient's history and physical examination, as well as a basic understanding of the mechanical considerations of the patient's sport, must be considered before the clinician makes a judgment as to the individual player's risk category.

Torg[44] has concluded that on the basis of his data,

which involved the evaluation of 32 patients in whom an acute transient neurologic episode resulted from forced hyperextension, hyperflexion, or axial loading of the cervical spine, those persons with developmental spinal stenosis are not predisposed to more severe injuries with associated permanent neurologic sequelae. However, he believed that athletes with developmental spinal stenosis and demonstrable cervical spinal instability or with acute or chronic intervertebral disc disease should not be allowed further participation in contact sports.[42] We believe that many factors must be considered before making such a determination.

Types

The three basic types of cervical stenosis are congenital, developmental, and acquired.

Congenital stenosis is typified by the short pedicles and funneling shape to the basic bony structure of the spinal canal, observable on the lateral x-ray film.

Developmental stenosis develops over years and may be the result of thickening of the bone as a result of increased stress. For example, upper body–weight lifters, strengtheners, and persons who perform upper body– and neck-strengthening exercises produce a larger cervical spine bone, just as they produce larger muscles in the neck and upper extremity; as a result the spinal canal may narrow as the bone increases in size. However, Herzog et al.[29] showed that football players have the same size spinal canals as everyone else, although they do have larger retrieval bodies. The concept of bone size increasing as a result of muscle stimulation and strengthening is an unproven concept. It may be that developmental cervical stenosis does not exist—that it is only an illusion that football players have an increased incidence of narrowing of the spinal canal at the vertebral body level.

Acquired cervical stenosis is due to cervical spondylosis with development of bone spurs, disc bulges, and bulges of ligamenta flava, as well as disc space narrowing and osteophytes on the facet joints. Of course, a patient may have more than one type of cervical stenosis. Athletes who perform neck-strengthening exercises will acquire premature degenerative changes in the cervical spine and in the resulting acquired cervical spine stenosis.

Measurement

Various techniques are available for measuring the size of the spinal canal to assess the presence and degree of cervical stenosis. Torg and Pavlov[44] described a sagittal diameter ratio of the central canal to the vertebral body that can be measured on lateral x-ray films to correct for x-ray magnification. These researchers determined that a ratio of 0.8 or less is indicative of cervical stenosis, but the determination was based on symptoms of transient cord neurapraxia in persons with a ratio of 0.8 or less and a lack of symptoms in those with ratios higher than that.

In a group of patients with myelopathy and radiculopathy who did not play football, Odor et al.[35] compared results of the ratio formula with diameters obtained from CT scans of the central canal in patients with myelopathy and found that the 0.8 ratio provides an extremely sensitive but less specific measurement. Every patient with a 0.8 ratio or less had 10 mm or less of central canal diameter, but there were patients with 10 mm or less who had a ratio higher than 0.8. With 17 ± 5 mm considered by most to be the normal sagittal diameter,[49] 10 mm is considered to be abnormally small. The contrast CT scan used in this study is the definitive technique for measuring central canal diameter. It allows one to measure not only the central canal diameter but also a functional central canal diameter. The functional central canal diameter in the sagittal plane can be defined as the amount of canal available for the dural sac and spinal cord. The trefoil-shaped canal, or the canal with the small, peaked empty space, exactly in the midline, does not allow full expansion of the dural sac and cord throughout its central diameter. Thus inclusion of a small, peaked area of space that could account for 2 mm of measurement, yet will not accommodate the dural sac, provides a measurement that is of little consequence to cord function. This is certainly true in the lumbar spine in which lateral recess stenosis very commonly produces a major compression on the entire sac, leaving an empty dorsal portion of the spinal canal.

Herzog et al.[29] found the Torg ratio to be of no value when they measured vertebral bodies and canals in football players and found that the vertebrae are larger in football players as compared with the normal population. Their study of the CT scans of a large number of players revealed that 78% of those with an abnormal Torg ratio had a normal-sized spinal canal. The football players had larger vertebral bodies, therefore rendering the ratio useless in identifying players with cervical stenosis. These authors also found that a carefully distance-corrected plain x-ray film determines the bony canal diameter as accurately as a CT scan. The conclusion is that the canal diameter can be determined from a plain lateral cervical spine x-ray film. The use of myelography, CT, or MRI is needed before the clinician can advise an athlete whether it is safe to play. Thus the Torg ratio is of no value in screening or decision making.

The contribution made by Torg cannot be underestimated. He spent 20 years in acquiring records concerning injuries to football players, which provided great insight into the overall problem of cervical paralysis in football players. Although many cases show distinct differences and have characteristics of a number of different injuries, it was Torg's impression and understanding that no instances of permanent quadriplegia in football players could be traced to disc herniations or

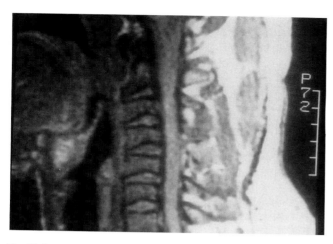

Fig. 29-6. This running back suffered one episode of transient quadriparesis and has a significant amount of cervical stenosis. He ultimately went back to play an additional 2 years with no episodes.

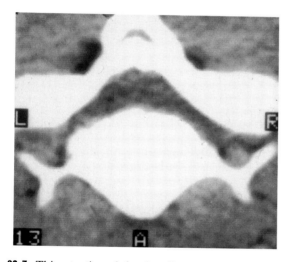

Fig. 29-7. This starting defensive lineman in the National Football League had one several-minute episode of transitory quadriparesis and quadriparesthesia. He had obviously been playing for some time with a 6- to 8-mm spinal canal, which demonstrates the ability to function with severe spinal stenosis.

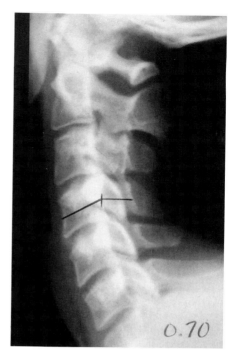

Fig. 29-8. The Torg ratio is a vertebral body-to-canal size ratio obtained from a standard x-ray film. Because football players have larger vertebral bodies, the ratio, if positive—less than 8 mm—wrongly predicts spinal stenosis in 80% of cases. The Torg ratio is of no value in screening x-ray films or in decisions about continued play.

spinal stenosis only.[45] Certainly, some cases of fracture dislocations may have had characteristics of stenosis or a disc herniation, but there is no record of any football player having been totally paralyzed as a result of these two entities alone. The 0.8 ratio should not be used as a screening tool because the finding has no correlation to permanent neurologic deficit. With an episode of transient quadriparesis, there is a 90% chance that the ratio will be 0.8 or less. However, the incidence of transient quadriparesis (Figs. 29-6 and 29-7; see also Fig. 29-2) has been estimated to be 7 in 10,000 ball players; thus the presence or absence of a 0.8 ratio cannot be statistically correlated with any increased chance of

transient neurapraxia or permanent deficit. The Torg ratio is of little value for screening and should not be used for decisions concerning continued play (Fig. 29-8).

Matsurra et al.[33] at Rancho Los Amigos Hospital found a strong correlation between the shape (meaning flatness of the cord) of the spinal canal and the predisposition to spinal cord injury resulting from trauma. Using the ratio of sagittal to transverse diameter, they found a strong positive correlation between this ratio and spinal cord injury when compared with control subjects. Although the transverse diameter was inversely proportional and the sagittal diameter was directly proportional to the spinal cord injury, the area of the spinal canal was not. The exact mean ratio varied at different levels but was best correlated at the three most important levels, C4, C5, and C6. The control mean was approximately 0.6, and the spinal cord injury mean was 0.5. These researchers found the Torg ratio to be less powerful a discriminator than the sagittal diameter. Ogino et al.[36] used the sagittal-to-transverse "compression" ratio (Fig. 29-9) as an indicator of cord damage in patients with myelopathy. This study, performed on cadaveric specimens, shows a relationship between compression ratio and the degree of cord damage in persons with cervical stenosis and myelopathy (Fig. 29-10).

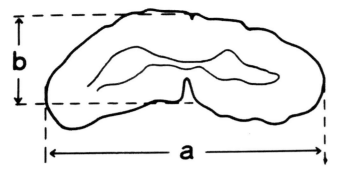

Fig. 29-9. The compression ratio described by Ogino et al. (AP compression ratio = b/a × 100) is a measure of the flatness of the cord. This has been correlated strongly with pathologic changes at autopsy and with neurologic deficit in fracture dislocation. This measurement may be more important than a true central canal diameter.

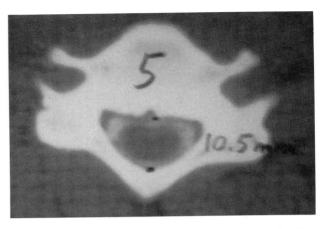

Fig. 29-10. This rookie offensive lineman at the professional level sustained clonus in both legs and had florid cervical myelopathy and upgoing toes. His myelopathy became more obvious in the three-point lineman stance with neck extension, producing sustained clonus in his leg. His central canal diameters were not severely abnormal; 10.5 to 12 mm is a very large, round cord. The area of the cord in this patient demonstrates significant relative constriction of the spinal cord. There is no scientifically consistent measurement for area of cord versus area of canal.

The area of the canal as related to the area of the body has been found to be important in evaluating radiculopathy and myelopathy. One can measure surface area of the dural sac versus the canal to determine the surface area of canal available for the sac. The lateral portions of the canal and the area of the nerve root sleeves that will not accommodate much dural expansion should not be included in the area available for dural expansion.

There are cases with larger or smaller spinal cord–to–sac ratios. Measuring exact cord shapes depends on exact radiologic technique. The presence of a large volume of dye circumferentially around the cord is a good sign, and the obliteration of dye ventrally can be an important sign of ventral compression. A flat cord is a poor sign.

The amount of motion in the cervical spine is probably proportional to the degree of risk from stenosis. Dynamic MRI has been used to demonstrate the narrowing of the cervical canal that occurs with extension.[14] It is well known that the cervical spinal canal can narrow up to 2 mm in full extension as compared with neutral or flexion. Neurologic tissue in the spine becomes slack and loose in extension and taut in flexion, whereas the spinal canal narrows in extension and opens in flexion.[8] Numerous clinical syndromes depend on the effect of these dynamic factors on spinal cord and nerve root function in addition to exact central canal measurements and ratios. The biomechanics of the spinal column and neurologic tissue motion must be considered in decisions concerning continued play for athletes with cervical stenosis.

Bohlman[6] has pointed out the importance not only of canal diameter but also of blood flow to the cord and cervical motion as three important factors in the determination of symptoms of cervical myeloradiculopathy. Exact quantification of vascularity to the cervical cord is difficult to assess clinically, but vascular abnor-

malities and insufficient areas of flow can certainly predispose an individual patient to neurologic injury.

Batzdorf and Batzdorf[4] showed that patients with a hyperlordotic cervical spine had more neck pain and a poorer response to laminectomy for cervical myelopathy than did patients with a lordotic cervical spine.

There are several facts known about cervical stenosis in persons who do not play football. Eismont et al.[22] found that the greater degree of cervical stenosis with a specific cervical spine injury, the greater the neurologic deficit. Matsurra et al. found, as already noted, that it was not just the central canal diameter but the shape of the canal that is important. The greater the compression ratio, the greater the chance of neurologic deficit with a spinal injury. Edwards and LaRocca[20] demonstrated that a person with cervical canal stenosis is more likely to require surgery with a cervical disc herniation and less likely to recover without surgery. Radicular pain is more common in smaller canals.[50]

In the study by Epstein et al.[24] 20 patients of the 200 admitted to an acute spinal cord injury unit had neither fracture nor dislocation but had complete neurologic deficit. Among these cases were various diagnoses, such as cervical spondylosis and congenital stenosis, but results of the study indicated that permanent neurologic deficit can occur with spinal stenosis. Depending on the sample studied, the incidence of permanent quadriplegia in spinal column injury has varied from 4% to 70% of pediatric neck injuries. Some researchers have hypothesized that causative factors in quadriplegia without fracture dislocation might be a combination of injury to

<table>
<tr><td>

Conclusions Regarding Cord Injury

1. The presence of a narrow canal significantly influences the morbidity and prognosis of an injury.
2. Patients with the lowest AP diameters have the most severe myelopathy after trauma.

</td></tr>
</table>

microvascular blood supply, longitudinal traction on the cord, acute disc prolapse, or compromise of the arterial system of the spine.[3,5,28,44,47] A common pathologic condition in these cases is a central cord infarct.[7] The incidence of permanent cord injury in football is rare (see box above).

Effect of Transient Quadriparesis

Numerous factors affect decision making in cases of traumatic quadriparesis and spinal canal stenosis. Among them are severity of the episode, extent of neurologic deficit, severity of the symptoms, age, player position, and neck size. The numerous methods of assessing cervical canal size bear consideration. Regardless of the canal diameter, there is certainly greater danger to someone who suffers a greater neurologic injury with the episode. A person with symptoms of myelopathy over a 6-month period is obviously at greater risk for return of those symptoms than someone who had the episodes for 5 seconds. Each case varies in terms of the severity of the symptoms, the type and extent of the neurologic deficit, and the longevity of the symptoms. Thus there can be no set standard for measuring all cases. The hemiparetic symptoms are different from unilateral arm dysesthesia. The important factors are history and physical examination during which the clinician must document very carefully exactly what happened. To identify and quantify the deficit, the neurologic examination must be meticulously performed.

The severity of the episode is important, and we have found the following rating system to be helpful in this assessment.

Extent of neurologic deficit

1 — Unilateral arm — numbness or dysesthesia, loss of strength
2 — Bilateral upper extremity loss of motor and sensory function
3 — Ipsilateral arm and leg and trunk loss of motor and sensory function
4 — Transitory quadriparesis
5 — Transitory quadriplegia

Time

1 — Less than 5 minutes
2 — Less than 1 hour
3 — Less than 24 hours

4 — Less than 1 week
5 — Greater than 1 week

Any existing neurologic deficit caused by a cord neurapraxia should result in the athlete's exclusion from play. As a general guideline, less than 4 is a mild episode, 4 to 7 is a moderate episode, and 8 to 10 is a severe episode. When combined with canal size, the severity of the episode can lead to some guidelines for recurrence.

Narrowing of the central canal diameter

1 — Greater than 12 mm
2 — Between 10 and 12 mm
3 — 10 mm
4 — 10 to 8 mm
5 — Less than 8 mm

Return-to-Play Decision

Armed with the history of the player's injury, results of his initial physical examination, radiographic studies, additional test findings, and knowledge of the major risk factors (extent, time, and narrowing), the team physician can formulate a reasonable recommendation. Each case is unique, but in general, up to six additive risk points for all three factors would be considered minimum risk for return to play: 6 to 10 moderate, 10 to 15 severe. For example, a brief episode with a 4-mm canal may absolutely preclude future play. The rating scale is only a guideline. Clinically we use the rating scale, but we also evaluate extenuating factors such as level of play and the risk versus benefit to the patient, which is often an unquantifiable factor.

With cervical stenosis and a prior episode of transient quadriparesis, an informed consent concerning continued play should include an accurate assessment of as many known facts as possible. The incidence of permanent paralysis in professional football is rare, and when it occurs, it is most related to blocking and tackling techniques. An episode of transient quadriplegia does not necessarily precede an incident of permanent neurologic loss. Cantu[12] was the first author to clearly identify and report cases of permanent paraplegia resulting after episodes of transient quadriparesis. Thereafter it was noted that cases of significant cord injury do occur with a prior episode of transient quadriparesis. Torg[43] followed up on Cantu's report and identified four cases. Each of these four cases, Torg believed, had some evidence of structural injury: two had an old compression fracture, a third showed ligamentous laxity, and the fourth sustained injury of the C5 limbus vertebra. Torg identified several factors in these patients — both normal findings and those predominantly centered around the evidence of structural injuries in the spinal column through abnormal findings on flexion/extension films and loss of normal cervical lordosis. A stiff, painful neck, structural injury, and a straight cervical spine without proper motion in lordosis are key factors. Returning athletes to play with a painful, stiff neck without normal range of motion after a significant episode of transitory quadriparesis can lead to further injury. However, a diagnosis of stenosis does not mean the player will smash someone with his head, have a fracture dislocation, and become a permanent quadriplegic. Indeed, the condition may have no specific relation to a future incident.

An example of an adequate consent would be to inform those concerned that the athlete with stenosis is not automatically predisposed to sustaining the fracture dislocation that typically paralyzes football players. The football player should be given the same information provided to the general patient population.

Reinjury is *always* a risk when the player returns to the football field. Although every position on the field carries some risk of head trauma, the most dangerous are the impact positions of defensive back and linebacker. Blocking and tackling techniques can rarely be changed at the professional level. If the player is a head hitter, he usually stays a head hitter. Albright et al.[1] showed that at the high school level, the reinjury rate after all neck injuries—one third of which had extremity or neurologic symptoms—was 17.2%. The twice-injured players at all levels of play had an 87% chance of future injury. After a time-lost injury, the recurrent injury rate was 42% in the current season; 62% in the following season; and 67% in future seasons. Therefore there is a significant recurrent injury rate, regardless of the type of injury received, and it is higher with the time-lost neck injury.

What can be done to prevent this recurrence? Conditioning can prevent injury. Preconditioned response to predicted head stresses can allow an increased protective muscle reflex response to ward off even relatively unexpected blows.[32] Neck strengthening can help protect the player from neck injury.[16] Probably the greatest testimonial to conditioning is the ability of professional football players to deliver or receive high impact blows with the frequency they do without sustaining injury.

Diagnostic Test Results

At our clinic we assess the potential risk of returning an athlete to play by using various diagnostic tests, such as the rating scale plus the compression ratio, functional central canal diameter, Torg ratio, area of the cord, myelographic defect, foraminal and disc changes, and disc herniations. Soft tissue disc herniations are at considerably greater risk for further extrusion and myelopathy than is a chronic hard disc herniation. The difficulty is telling them apart. The use of spinal cord somatosensory evoked potential, electromyography, and neurologic checks play a less well defined role in decision making. We are not inclined to restrict play when the EMG shows abnormal findings but results of the clinical examination are normal.

Responsibility is always a consideration, and it is important to emphasize that the physician who performs the player's physical examination and clears him to play has certain obligations. Through proper informed consent, the patient and his family are also responsible. In any worker's compensation situation the team's owner, as employer, is liable for the employees' health, as well as for managing an effective team. Again the concept of risk versus benefit to the patient applies. The benefit of continued play to the patient will be well known to the patient, family, agent, team members, and others. The real risk to the patient can be difficult to determine. Unlike provable facts, predictions are basically educated guesses. Nevertheless the physician must communicate the risks to the patient as specifically as possible.

PREVENTION

Use of the head for contact with another player triggers mechanisms that elicit cervical injury.[6,8,11,14,31] Most of the injuries are self-limiting, however, and most players can return to the sport. The following factors are important in preventing injury: shoulder pad modifications, chest-out posturing, and thoracic outlet obstruction exercises. (See Chapters 23, 24, and 27 for a discussion of the latter two.)

Protective Gear

Protective gear is limited to good shoulder pads with a high neck roll that is built up on the lateral portion of the neck. The posterior rolls are not as helpful as the side rolls because the shoulder pads are more likely to be posterior at contact and the neck is more likely to be straight. The spine straightens with slight flexion to deliver the axial loading blow with the top of the head. Although the mechanism of pure extension has been implicated as a source of serious injury,[51] others believe that it is not a significant source of major cervical injury in football. The lateral pads can help with lateral flexion and rotation toward the painful arm, so common with stingers, or burners, the majority of which involve root injury, specifically at the C6 level.

Training and Rehabilitation

Neck strengthening is important. Use of the head in football generally and the chance or planned use of the head in blocking and tackling necessitate that the football player have good neck strength, agility, and technique—factors that prevent neck injuries during head contact. An apt comparison is the boxer with a reputation for defensive fighting by virtue of his talent for avoiding the opponent's punches; the football player's proper use of the head can mean the difference between a serious injury or no injury. Proper preparation for the game requires much training. Maintaining good head position for eye focus and agility, for seeing the opponent, and for seeing the ball—these all are vital parts of the game.

Having the eyes in the right place at the right time starts with agility at the center axis of the entire body. All training techniques should concentrate on this core axis of agility and muscle function. That is why football training techniques are designed to teach the player to continually block, roll, catch, tackle, fake, make contact and come up in an agile, head-forward position, and be ready to visualize the opponent or the next step in the play. Any neck-strengthening technique must concentrate on agility and total body function.

Neck and radicular pain causes muscle weakness and dysfunction in the muscles that support the head. The same emphasis on quadriceps strengthening for knee injuries should be applied to neck muscles in neck injuries, but it must be done carefully. Resistive neck exercises are begun very slowly so that the compressive load on the cervical spine does not produce pain. Neck isometrics should be done with the head in the midline only, and resisting forces should be applied perpendicularly to the head from every direction. When the player is completely pain free on midline strengthening, the head can be taken out of the midline very slowly. However, extremes of head flexion—anteriorly, posteriorly, or laterally against resistance—are seldom indicated for adequate neck strengthening. Our emphasis has been on midline isometric strengthening and stretching through a full range of motion.

Stretching exercises are of some importance in giving the cervical spine a protective flexibility and range of motion. Cervical stiffness is produced by nerve, ligament, or disc injury. If not corrected, the reactive stiffness can produce chronic contractures and a loss of range of motion. These contractures should be relieved and a protective range of motion restored with a program of cervical stretching and range-of-motion exercises, working in painless areas initially, and then slowly into the painful areas. Extension is usually the most painful but cannot be neglected. Neck motion exercises have to be used with caution, since they can strain an injured joint. Remember that the chest-out posture should be used during the exercises.

The key factor at this phase of rehabilitation is the return of neck strength and suppleness, with accompanying return of shoulder and upper extremity function. We believe that the reinjury rate is substantially decreased by following this guideline.

CASE ILLUSTRATIONS

Figs. 29-11 to 29-26 illustrate cases involving neck injuries in football players.

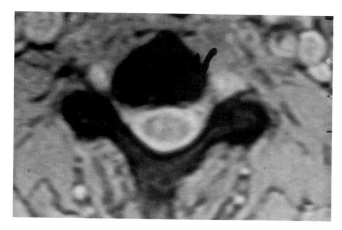

Fig. 29-11. This college offensive lineman suffered recurrent burners until he was moved to the opposite side of the line, where his head sustained knocks in the opposite direction, preventing extension/rotation toward the side with foraminal stenosis. Thus chronic burners were relieved with a change in position.

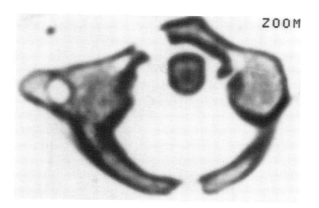

Fig. 29-12. This head compression resulted from a head-first tackle. There is a 7-mm total overhang of the ring of C1 on C2. This represents a Jefferson fracture with a partial tear of the transverse ligament, shown on the CT scan.

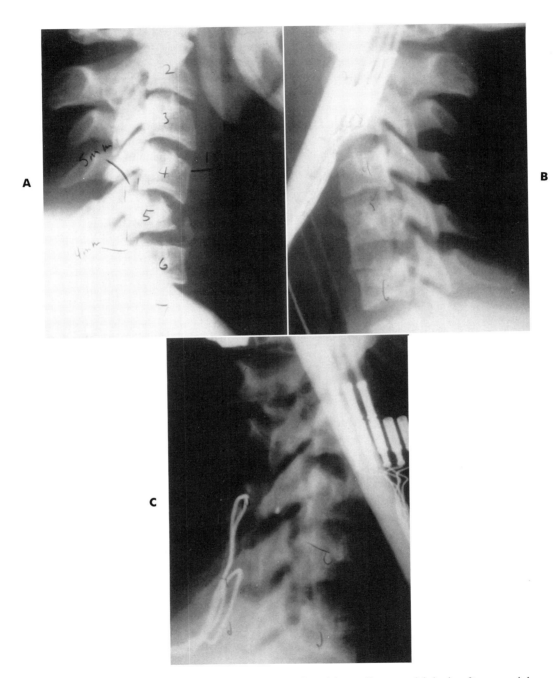

Fig. 29-13. This junior college defensive back suffered immediate quadriplegia after an axial loading injury. His neurologic deficit did not improve after an anterior vertebrectomy and posterior fusion. **A,** Flexion/rotation injury. **B,** Patient in traction. **C,** Internal fixation and fusion with external fixation.

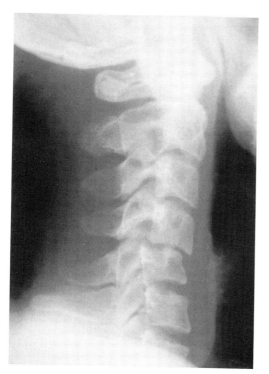

Fig. 29-14. The hidden flexion injury of McSweeney occurs secondary to an axial loading and/or flexion lesion. It produces the characteristic segmental kyphotic deformity. There is splaying in the spinous processes, which is a kyphotic deformity through one disc segment. Angulation that is 11 degrees greater at this segment than at the adjacent segments indicates a rupture of the interspinous ligament, the ligamentum flavum, and the posterior longitudinal ligament. It is important to identify the lesion because progressive kyphotic deformity can occur unless the condition is properly treated. This is an acutely unstable lesion. Because of its ligamentous nature, it is best treated first with careful evaluation for disc material in the spinal canal and then by open reduction and internal fixation.

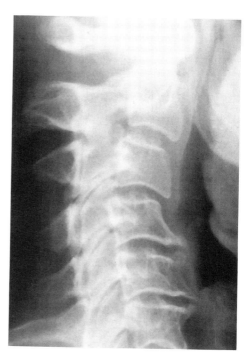

Fig. 29-15. Flexion/extension films showing a ligamentous instability often indicate only the segment that has the most motion rather than revealing an acute ligamentous injury. This film of a 52-year-old former wrestler and football player demonstrates a hypermobile segment above the level of an osteoarthritic stiff segment. Resultant pain may very well be at the hypermobile segment or the stiff osteoarthritic segments. If this person were involved in a traumatic episode, it would be very difficult to distinguish this chronic condition from an acute ligamentous injury. Active professional football players have more subtle amounts of arthritis and stiffness in certain spinal segments, often with hypermobile and stiff segments that must be evaluated for acute injuries.

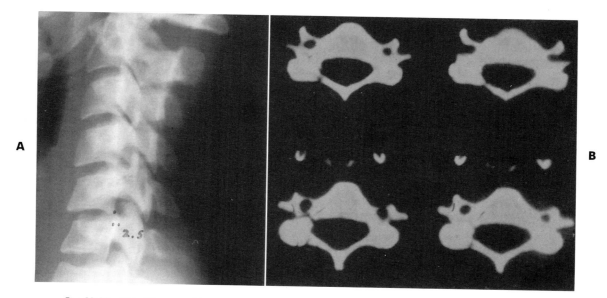

Fig. 29-16. This 25-year-old professional defensive back suffered a lateral mass fracture from an axial loading injury sustained in a professional football game. **A,** The slight offset on the lateral view of the x-ray film is a sign of potential facet fracture. **B,** The CT transverse section outlines the injury.

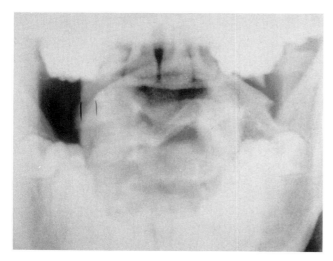

Fig. 29-17. This high school football player sustained mild torticollis resulting from an axial loading head injury. X-ray films revealed a rotatory subluxation, and the advice was not to return to contact sports until physicians were able to correct the problem.

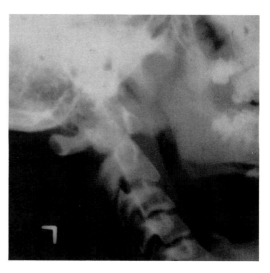

Fig. 29-18. This professional football defensive lineman had a resulting stiffness and pain in his neck secondary to an axial loading injury. X-ray films revealed a partial tear of the transverse ligament of C1-2.

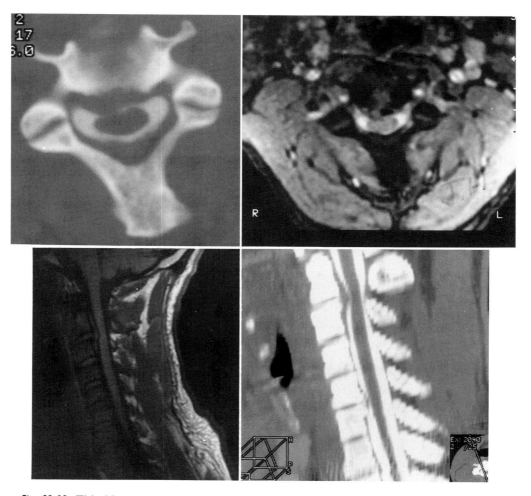

Fig. 29-19. This 25-year-old professional linebacker with a central herniation, stenosis, and transient quadriparesis from a central herniation at C2-3 underwent a successful anterior cervical fusion and returned to contact and professional sports in 6 months.

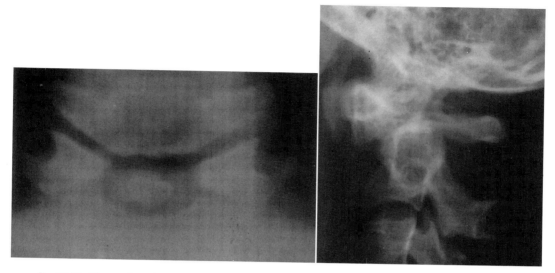

Fig. 29-20. Even after the athlete undergoes fusion at the C1-2 level, return to a sport, such as football, that involves axial loading carries a potentially significant risk.

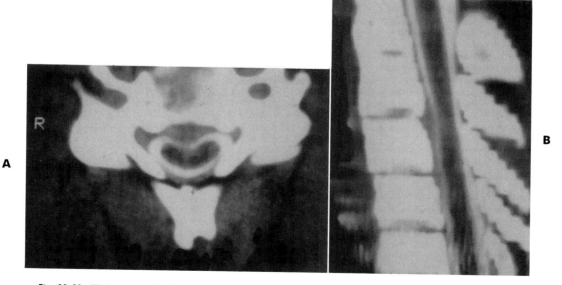

Fig. 29-21. This university-level defensive back suffered a transient quadriplegic episode from an axial loading injury. X-ray films demonstrated a soft tissue herniation at C3-4 with considerable distortion of the spinal cord. This player retired from football. **A,** CT scan. **B,** Parasagittal view on the contrast CT scan.

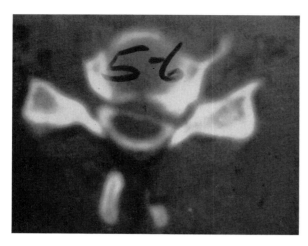

Fig. 29-22. This 32-year-old professional football player had intense C6 radiculopathy that was unresponsive to nonoperative treatment. He underwent an anterior cervical fusion, and because of persistent radiculopathy, was advised to retire.

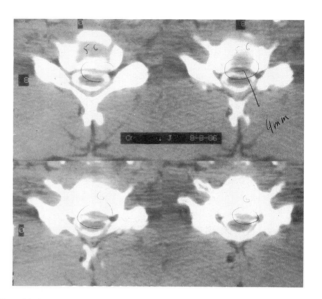

Fig. 29-24. This 29-year-old professional linebacker had a peripheral axillary nerve lesion confirmed by EMG and nerve conduction study. The contrast CT scan revealed an asymptomatic soft tissue disc herniation. It was not a major decision-making factor in his case.

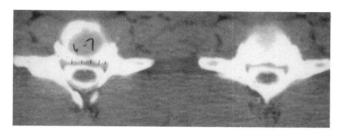

Fig. 29-23. This 30-year-old professional defensive back with strong symptoms of C7 radiculopathy retired from professional football because of the injury. Had this patient had neck pain only, it would not have been a career-ending injury.

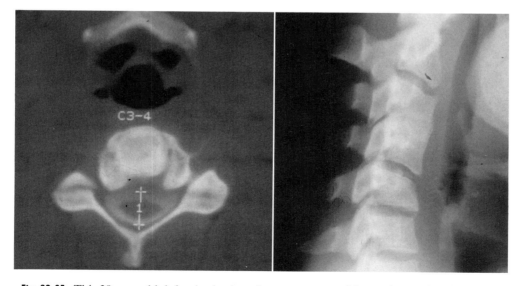

Fig. 29-25. This 30-year-old defensive back underwent a successful anterior cervical fusion for an extruded C3-4 disc fragment. His overall central canal diameters were 11 mm, which, after a successful fusion in that area, allowed him to return to play professional football. The kyphotic deformity below the fusion indicates some potential problem at that level, and the widening in the spinous process at C4-5 signals that a major head compression injury could cause abnormal loading in that area.

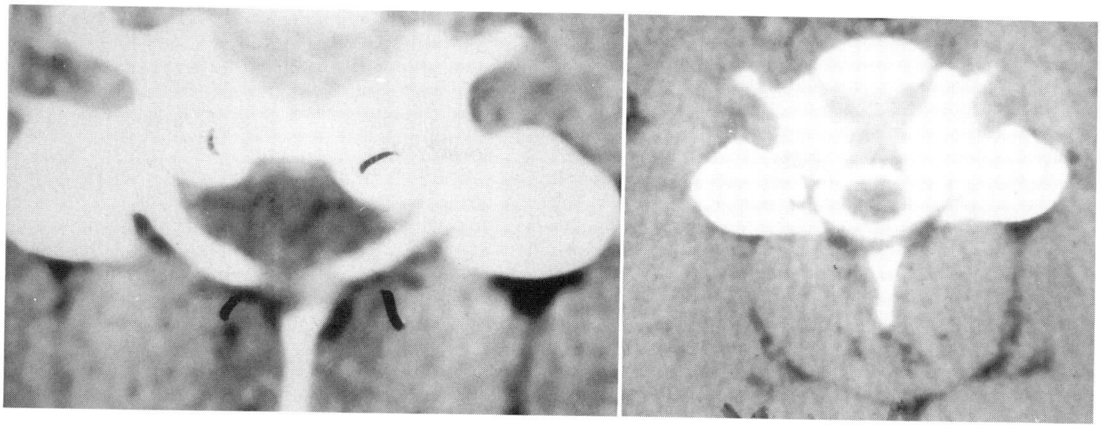

Fig. 29-26. This professional wide receiver had one short transitory episode of quadriparesis. **A,** The noncontrast CT scan shows a significant amount of canal stenosis. **B,** The contrast CT scan shows a round, plump cord, which portends minimal risk for continued play.

REFERENCES

1. Albright JP et al: Non-fatal cervical spine injuries in interscholastic football, *JAMA* 236:1243, 1976.
2. Alexander MJ: Biomechanical aspects of lumbar spine injuries in athletes: a review, *Can J Appl Sports Sci* 10(1):1, 1985.
3. Anderson LD, D'Alonzo RT: Fractures of the odontoid process of the axis, *J Bone Joint Surg* 56A:1669, 1974.
4. Batzdorf U, Batzdorf A: Analysis of cervical spine curvature in patients with cervical spondylosis, *Neurosurgery* 22:827, 1988.
5. Bergfeld JA, Hershman EB, Wilbourn AJ: Brachial plexus in sports, a five year followup, *Orthop Trans* 12:743, 1988.
6. Bohlman H: Cervical spondylosis with moderate to severe myelopathy, *Spine* 2:151, 1977.
7. Bracken MB et al: A randomized controlled trial of methylprednisolone or naloxone in the treatment of acute spinal cord injury, *N Engl J Med* 322:1405, 1990.
8. Brieg A, Turnbull I, Hassler O: Effects of mechanical stresses on the spinal cord in cervical spondylosis, *J Neurosurg* 25:45, 1966.
9. Bruce DA, Schut L, Sutton LN: Brain and cervical spine injuries occurring during organized sports activity in children and adolescents, *Prim Care* 1:495, 1982.
10. Burke DC: Traumatic spinal paralysis in children, *Paraplegia* 11:268, 1974.
11. Cantu RC: Head and spine injuries in the young athlete, *Clin Sports Med* 7:459, 1988.
12. Cantu RC: Cervical spinal stenosis: challenging an established detection method, *Physician Sportsmed* 25:1082, 1993.
13. Cantu RC, Mueller FO: Catastrophic injuries and fatalities in high school and college sports, fall 1982–spring 1988, *Med Sci Sports Exerc* 22:737, 1990.
14. Cervical Spine Research Society meeting, Key Biscayne, Fla, 1988.
15. Clancy W, Brand R, Bergfeld J: Upper trunk brachial plexus injuries in contact sports, *Am J Sports Med* 5:209, 1977.
16. Clark KS: The survey of sports related spinal cord injuries in schools and colleges: 1973-1975, *J Safety Res* 9:140, 1977.
17. Davis D et al: The pathologic findings in fatal craniospinal injuries, *J Neurosurg* 34:603, 1971.
18. Day AL, Friedman WA, Indelicato PA: Observations on the treatment of lumbar disk disease in college football players, *Am J Sports Med* 15:72, 1987.
19. Dyer PV: An upper cervical spine injury producing paresthesia in the distribution of the mandibular division of the trigeminal nerve, *Br J Surg* 29:374, 1991.

20. Edwards W, La Rocca H: The developmental segmental sagittal diameter of the cervical spinal canal in patients with cervical spondylosis, *Spine* 8(8):20, 1983.
21. Effendi B et al: Fractures of the rim of the axis, *J Bone Joint Surg* 63B:319, 1981.
22. Eismont FJ et al: Cervical sagittal spinal canal size in spine injuries, *Spine.*
23. Elattrache N, Fidali PD, Few H: American football: thoracolumbar spine fracture in American football player, *Am J Sports Med* 21:157, 1993 (case report).
24. Epstein J et al: Cervical myelopathy caused by developmental stenosis of the spinal canal, *J Neurosurg* 51:362, 1972.
25. Grant J, Sears W: Spinal injury and computerized tomography; a review of fracture pathology and a new approach to canal decompression, *Aust NZ J Surg* 56:299, 1986.
26. Halpern B et al: High school football injuries: identifying the risk factors, *Am J Sports Med* 16(suppl 1):S113, 1988.
27. Hellstrom M et al: Radiological abnormalities of the thoracolumbar spine in athletes, *Acta Radiol* 31:127, 1990.
28. Herkowitz H, Rothman R: Subacute instability of the cervical spine, *Spine* 9:348, 1984.
29. Herzog RJ et al: Normal cervical spine morphometry and cervical spinal stenosis in asymptomatic professional football players: plain film radiography, multiplanar computer tomography, and magnetic resonance imaging, *Spine* 16(suppl 6):S178, 1991.
30. Hill SA et al: Pediatric neck injuries: a clinical study, *J Neurosurg* 60:700, 1984.
31. Jackson DW, Lohr FP: Cervical spine injuries, *Clin Sports Med* 5:373, 1986.
32. Levine AM, Edwards CC: The management of traumatic spondylolisthesis of the axis, *J Bone Joint Surg* 67A:217, 1985.
33. Matsurra P et al: Comparison of computerized tomography parameters of the cervical spine in normal control subjects and spinal cord injured patients, *J Bone Joint Surg* 71A:183, 1989.
34. Mazur JW, Stauffer ES: Unrecognized spinal instability associated with seemingly simple cervical compression fractures, *Spine* 8:687, 1983.
35. Odor JM et al: Incidence of cervical spinal stenosis in professional and rookie football players, *Am J Sports Med* 18:507, 1990.
36. Ogino K et al: Canal diameter, anteroposterior compression ratio and spondylitic myelopathy of the cervical spine, *Spine* 8:1, 1983.
37. Pang D, Wilberger JE Jr: Spinal cord injury without radiographic abnormalities in children, *J Neurosurg* 57:114, 1982.

38. Penning L: Some aspects of plain radiography of the cervical spine in chronic myelopathy, *Neurology* 12:513, 1962.
39. Robertson PA, Swan AJ: Traumatic bilateral rotatory facet dislocation of the atlas on the axis, *Spine* 17:1252, 1992.
40. Saal JA: Common American football injuries, *Sports Med* 12(2):132, 1991.
41. Sward L et al: Back pain and radiological changes of the thoracolumbar spine of athletes, *Spine* 15:124, 1990.
42. Thomas JC: Plain roentgenograms of the spine in the injured athlete, *Clin Sports Med* 5:353, 1990.
43. Torg J: Spear tackler spine, *Am J Sports Med* 21:640, 1993.
44. Torg JS, Pavlov H: Cervical spinal stenosis with cord neurapraxia and transient quadriplegia, *Clin Sports Med* 6:115, 1987.
45. Torg JS et al: The National Football Head and Neck Injury Registry: 14 year report on cervical quadriplegia, 1971-1984, *JAMA* 254:3439, 1985.
46. Virgin HW: Football injuries to the skeletal system, *Compr Ther* 11(1):19, 1985.
47. Watkins RG: Neck injuries in football players, *Clin Sports Med* 5:215, 1986.
48. White AA III et al: Biomechanical analysis of clinical stability in the cervical spine, *Clin Orthop* 109:89, 1975.
49. Wilkenson H, Lemay M, Ferris E: Roentgenographic correlations in cervical spondylosis, *Am J Roentgenol* 105:370, 1969.
50. Williams JPR, McKibben B: Cervical spine injury in the rugby union football, *Br Med J* 2:1747, 1978.
51. Williams RW: Microcervical foraminotomy: a surgical alternative for intractable radicular pain, *Spine* 8:708, 1983.

Chapter Thirty

◆

Stinger Injuries in Football

Andrew B. Dossett
Robert G. Watkins

In violent participant sports, such as football, hockey, wrestling, and rugby, there exists an indistinct clinical entity know colloquially as the "stinger" or "burner." It is the prototype of neck injury sustained in these settings and appears to cover a spectrum of clinical entities. Typically the player complains of transient loss of function accompanied by searing, lancinating pain starting at the trapezius/shoulder area and coursing down the arm. There is temporary paralysis, but symptoms usually last only 10 to 15 minutes, although trace neurologic deficit may persist for months. As the symptoms of arm weakness and burning resolve, a C6 distribution of numbness (thumb, index, and ring finger) persists. Motor deficits may be found in shoulder abduction, as well as in wrist and finger extension.

Players may complain of recurrent stingers and burners throughout the season and in the off-season. Generally, when symptoms recur, the same dermatomal pattern is present, the same motor deficit occurs, and the same biomechanical mechanisms of injury are responsible. However, it is not unusual for a multiroot pattern to be found. Repeated episodes over a season may cause significant weakness of the deltoid and biceps.[5] A residual neurologic deficit may persist for days or months after more severe episodes.

MECHANISMS OF INJURY

Several different mechanisms have been described for this syndrome, including axial load, hyperextension and rotation (Spurling's maneuver), and lateral neck flexion combined with shoulder depression. Each mechanism produces distinct characteristics, as follows:

Axial load injury—Bilateral arm pain and temporary quadriparesis[9,10]; pathophysiology secondary to cervical stenosis

Lateral neck flexion and shoulder depression injury—Longer-lasting pain (sometimes more than 15 minutes) and dense paresthesias ("dead arm" sensation); pathophysiology related to brachial plexus traction injury[2-4,6,11,13]

Hyperextension/rotation injury—Discrete radicular pain in a dermatomal distribution[11] that is transient, sometimes with an apparent resulting motor weakness

In professional football players, the mechanism most often producing injury is an off-center axial load that is applied to the head, forcing it uncontrollably into both extension and lateral flexion. The movement of the head to the ipsilateral side causes the stinger. The extension of the spine produces a slackening of the cord and spinal nerves, whereas the lateral flexion increases nerve tension. With extension and bending of the cervical spine toward the involved shoulder and arm, the neural foramina are abruptly narrowed, allowing the bony walls of the neural foramina or the intervertebral disc or osteophytes to pinch the nerve root as it exits the spinal canal. This mechanism of injury is equivalent to performing Spurling's maneuver,[11] a diagnostic sign elicited in patients with cervical radiculopathy. It consists of extension of the head, as well as lateral bending and rotation of the head and neck toward the painful side. If pain is reproduced in the patient's shoulder and arm, the sign is positive and indicates cervical foraminal stenosis due to either soft disc herniation or osteophyte encroachment of the neural foramina. The ipsilateral rotation and axial loading mechanism of injury seen with stingers implies that the pathomechanics involve a multilevel root contusion from narrowing of the canal and foramina. A contrast computed tomography (CT) scan or magnetic resonance imaging (MRI) may demonstrate this narrowing. However, in some cases even complete diagnostic evaluation with MRI, CT/myelography, and electromyographic (EMG)/nerve conduction studies fails to reveal the source of the condition.

Stingers can also be produced by an abrupt stretching of the exiting cervical nerve roots or the adjacent brachial plexus. The head is forced away or to the opposite side of the depressed shoulder and symptomatic arm. The brachial plexus tautness is increased with this mechanism. While this is associated with transient signs and symptoms, the potential for long-term neurologic deficit is present.

CLASSIFICATION

Two distinct and useful classification systems of stingers, or burners, have been described by Seddon[8] and by Clancy, Brand, and Bergfeld.[2] In Seddon's classification system, neurapraxia is the mildest lesion that has identifiable histologic findings and corresponds to demyelinization of the axon sheath without intrinsic axonal disruption. Recovery of neural functioning generally occurs within 3 weeks. Axonotmesis includes disruption of the axon and the myelon sheath with preservation of the fibrous epineurium. The epineurium serves as a conduit for the regenerating axon in axonotmesis. In most healthy adults the rate of recovery in axonotmesis can be expected to be approximately 1 mm per day, with an initial 7-day delay from the time of injury. This expected rate of recovery is measured from the site of injury to the motor end-plate to which the nerve supplies motor impulses. Neurotmesis corresponds to complete nerve transection. In neurotmesis, there is generally no possibility of distal nerve regeneration without surgical repair and reapproximation of the nerve sheath.

Clancy and colleagues used Seddon's classification system for differentiation of the stinger syndrome from brachial plexus injury. Grade I injuries have an initial recovery of motor and sensory function generally within several minutes of injury and a complete recovery within 2 weeks. These injuries correspond to Seddon's definition of neurapraxic lesions. Grade II injuries can result in motor loss to the deltoid, biceps, interspinales, and supraspinatus muscles. Weakness can last from weeks to months and corresponds to axonotmesis. Grade III lesions are quite rare and are more typically seen in trauma patients who have suffered a penetrating injury to the neck or shoulder region from a motor vehicle accident, knife fight, gunshot wound, or shrapnel injury from an explosion. Also falling within this category of injuries is scapulothoracic dissociation injury, which is associated with high-energy trauma and results in avulsion and separation of the shoulder girdle from the thorax. Scapulothoracic dissociation is also associated with significant trauma to the traversing major blood vessels, neurologic structures, and muscular structures.

ROLE OF ELECTROMYOGRAPHIC STUDIES

EMG studies will show abnormalities in type II and type III lesions. Generally, type I or grade I lesions (neurapraxia) will not show EMG or nerve conduction velocity abnormalities. The long-term EMG findings in a group of 20 athletes with stingers were studied by Bergfeld, Hershman, and Wilbourn.[1] These researchers selected a group of players with clinical findings who had severe neurologic involvement after athletic injuries that caused stingers. In this study, the EMG findings were generally localized to the upper trunk of the brachial plexus, as well as to cervical nerve root and peripheral nerve root levels. The study demonstrated that the EMG abnormalities lagged behind the motor strength recovery of the individual as the injury resolved; it also demonstrated that using EMG studies as a criterion for return to play after a stinger is an inaccurate and ineffective prognostic measure.

PREVENTION

The primary means of preventing stingers is by wearing properly fitting shoulder pads. Shoulder pads should accomplish four basic functions: (1) absorb shock, (2) protect the shoulders, (3) fit the chest, and (4)

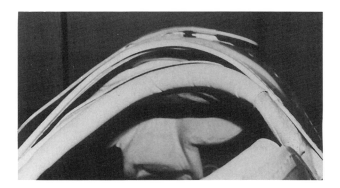

Fig. 30-1. Typical shoulder pad of a professional football player.

align and afix the midcervical spine to the trunk. The typical shoulder pad, seen in Fig. 30-1 and worn by a professional defensive lineman, is a soft arc that consists of a very thinly padded material with questionable shock-absorbing properties. It fits the chest in a semi-arc type of configuration. The fixation of the shoulder pads to the chest is less than ideal and allows sliding of the shoulder pads on the shoulder during contact. To fit the chest properly, the pad should be more of an A-frame with very rigid, long anterior and posterior panels. The shoulder pads should conform to the subxiphoid portion of the chest and fit snugly around the chest. A proper shoulder pad should encompass many of the characteristics of a proper cervicothoracic orthosis.

Because afixing the head to the chest area is impossible in a football player, modifications to the ideal have to be made. Immobilization of the cervical spine in any type of cervical brace requires rigid fixation of the brace to the chest. All studies evaluating fixation methods that include only the neck, such as a hard or soft cervical collar, demonstrate poor fixation and limitation of cervical spine motion. It is only when the base is extended and held firmly against the chest, as in a proper cervicothoracic orthosis, that restriction of cervical spine motion occurs. Some support, however, can be provided between the chest and base of neck by the use of properly fitting neck pads, which effectively elevate the shoulder pad at the base of the neck, thereby "supporting" the lower cervical segments.

The majority of neck rolls are inadequate in that they are attached at the top of the shoulder pads and rotate away approximately 6 inches from the neck at the moment of contact (Fig. 30-2). This rolling back of the shoulder pads adds to a lack of protection for the cervical spine, especially in resisting compression. This mechanism of injury is commonly seen in serious neck injuries and plays a major role in the stinger syndrome. As the shoulder pad rolls back, the head coils into the hole in the shoulder pad. There is no protection against head compression in injuries or in the extension, compression,

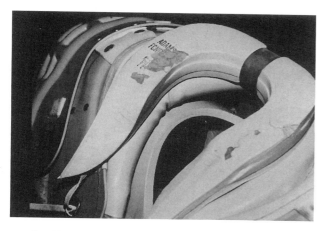

Fig. 30-2. Modified shoulder pads with a neck roll.

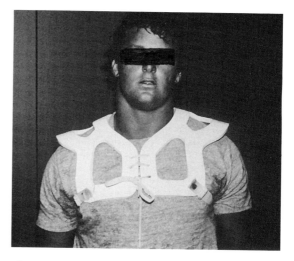

Fig. 30-3. Lifters provide additional neck support.

and rotation mechanism of a stinger. It is very difficult to get a collar roll on the back of the shoulder pads that can block extension during contact. One professional player used a stiff cervical collar that was tied tightly around his neck posteriorly and attached to shoulder pads by strings tied to the laces on the front of the pads. This was an attempt to prevent the failure to block the extension seen with collar rolls.

Thick, comfortable, stiff pads at the base of the neck are the key. It is this support laterally at the base of the neck that offers fixation to the cervical spine. Some posterior support could be helpful but is very difficult to obtain. Higher, thicker, lateral pads that are tighter at the base of the neck can improve fixation of the cervical spine, especially when the pad fits the chest and shoulders well.

A common method of adapting pads is to add lifters (Fig. 30-3), which provide a pad at the base of the neck that supplements the typical shoulder pad. Often the combination of lifters, the preexisting pads, and the neck roll all add to the improved fit of the pad laterally at the base of the neck. Because most of the rotation of the cervical spine occurs at C1-2, it is believed that this support should not limit the player's visibility and should provide some added support in the mid and lower portions of the cervical spine. Fig. 30-4 shows a shoulder pad that provides good pads for the base of the neck. Also, the tighter fit to the chest can be seen in the shape of the shoulder portion of this pad.

Regarding the shock-absorbing capability of the shoulder pad, proper fit to the chest is important in distributing the shock to the shoulders evenly over the pads and into the thorax. Better resistive padding and better plastics in the outer shoulder pads will absorb shock and allow the use of the shoulder in proper blocking and tackling techniques. Better shoulder protection should allow one to deemphasize the use of the head as a blocking and tackling instrument.

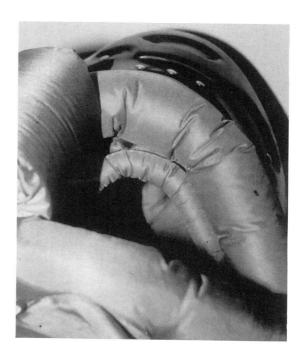

Fig. 30-4. Well-constructed shoulder pad with a neck roll.

TREATMENT

Figs. 30-5 to 30-8 illustrate foraminal stenosis as a source of stinger injury in collegiate football players and the various forms of treatment.

In addition to prevention, treatment is critical. Once the symptoms occur, proper trunk stabilization, chest-out posturing, and neck-strengthening (thoracic outlet obstruction) exercises should be emphasized. These increase intraforaminal dimensions of the cervical spine, allowing for dynamic decompression of the nerve root and, ultimately, decreased inflammation due to decreased mechanical pressure.

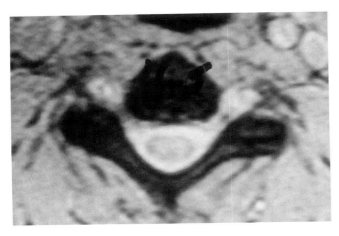

Fig. 30-5. This 20-year-old, 6-foot 2-inch, 290-pound left offensive guard with recurrent stingers radiating into his right upper arm was noted to have decreased sensation along the C5 dermatome with some deltoid and some biceps weakness. The player underwent intensive rehabilitation with trunk stabilization, a neck-strengthening program, and chest-out posturing, along with equipment modification. Despite this, the player had recurrent symptoms when blocking. An MRI scan of the cervical spine showed right C4-5 foraminal stenosis. Treatment options included retirement, therapy, and/or surgery. A fourth alternative—the player switching from playing left offensive guard to playing right offensive guard—was employed. This simple but effective change stopped the stingers, since the opposing players were now creating a predominantly Spurling's maneuver to the left. The player participated for 2 more years without problems.

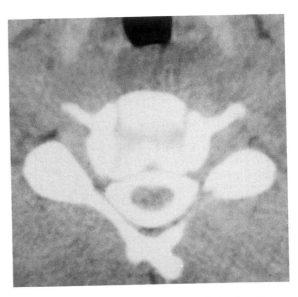

Fig. 30-6. This 19-year-old college fullback had a history of recurrent neck and arm pain in high school that became worse in college. A hyperextension/rotation injury occurred to his right side during blocking and caused a stinger. The player was treated with rest and rehabilitation. The following season the player had the same injury mechanism while blocking on a sweep to the right. The player experienced the same sensation, but it was more prolonged. On physical examination there was pain with Spurling's maneuver to the right, a decreased right biceps reflex, and a 3/8-inch wasting of the right bicep. EMG showed a right C5 denervation while CT myelography of the cervical spine showed right C4-5 foraminal stenosis. The player underwent microscopic cervical foraminotomy with complete resolution of his symptoms. He returned to football without problems and started all 12 games his senior season without recurrence of symptoms.

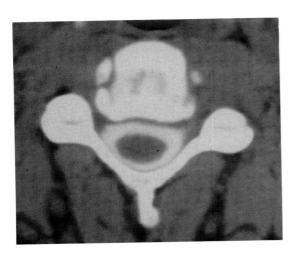

Fig. 30-7. This 6-foot 5-inch, 280-pound college offensive tackle who developed stingers radiating into his left upper extremity during spring practice sat out the remainder of spring practice and underwent a trunk stabilization and neck-strengthening program. The player returned to activity in the fall but had a recurrent injury. Physical examination showed a positive Spurling's maneuver on the left and weak left shoulder internal rotation (subscapularis—upper subscapular nerve). The pain drawing showed a C5 distribution while the CT scan showed a left C4-5 foraminal stenosis. This player chose medical retirement from intercollegiate sports.

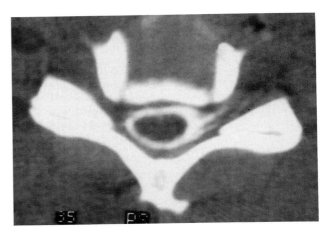

Fig. 30-8. This 20-year-old, 6-foot 6-inch, 255-pound college tight-end developed recurrent stingers and underwent a diagnostic work-up. On examination there was a positive Spurling's maneuver on the right, a decreased right brachial radialis reflex, and decreased sensation of the right C6 distribution. EMG demonstrated denervation and renervation of the right C6 root. CT myelography of the cervical spine showed right C5-6 foraminal stenosis. The player underwent microscopic cervical foraminotomy at that level in January and played the entire following season without recurrent symptoms.

Other means of treatment include anterior cervical fusion. This procedure will increase the foraminal dimension and eliminate the problem,[7] but fusing the cervical spine in a healthy young football player who expects to return to the sport introduces the problems of a stiff motion segment and adjacent-level breakdown, as well as the inherent risk of axial load injury and possible catastrophic trauma to adjacent motion segments. Thus an alternative surgical treatment was proposed by Williams,[12] namely the microscopic cervical foraminotomy for the treatment of unilateral cervical radiculopathy secondary to foraminal stenosis. We have used this procedure successfully in returning collegiate football players to competition.

The procedure described here is based on that developed by Williams.[12] Note that a thorough knowledge of the anatomy on the part of the surgeon and the presence of a discrete lesion that is amenable to surgical correction are required for this procedure to be successful.

Operative Procedure

Surgical microscope and instrumentation. A Zeiss Opmi I microscope with straight binoculars and a 300-mm lens is used when retraction is accomplished with a self-retaining retractor having a 1 × 5 cm blade. In addition to a scalpel, electrocoagulator, and periosteal elevator, the instruments required are a 90-degree blunt microhook, a 45-degree 1.5-mm rongeur, and a 45-degree and 90-degree 1-mm rongeur and microcurette.

Patient preparation, anesthesia, and positioning. In addition to a complete medical evaluation, patients receive povidone-iodine (Betadine) showers, shampoos, and positive-pressure pulmonary treatments preoperatively. The operation is performed with the patient in the sitting position under general endotracheal anesthesia with mechanical ventilation, arterial and venous pressure monitoring, and cardiac Doppler for detection of air emboli (Fig. 30-9). The legs are wrapped, and systolic pressures are maintained above 120 mm Hg.

Operating time. Operating time can be estimated as 1 hour from entrance to exit in a single foraminotomy. For each additional root decompressed, the procedure is extended by 1/2 hour.

Surgical approach. Since a minimal surgical approach is used, accurate placement of the posterior skin mark, using radiographic control, is stressed. The deep location of the sixth root can be estimated by finger palpation of the spinous process of C5, and the location of the seventh root can be estimated by palpation of C6, etc. After reaching the intralaminar space, the anatomic level is exposed again and confirmed by a lateral radiograph.

Procedure

Dissection to the lamina. A 1-inch posterior midline skin incision is adequate for foraminotomy at two levels. The fascia is separated from the spinous process by electrocautery, and gentle periosteal retraction displaces the muscle laterally. Self-retaining retractors are inserted for exposure. Hemostasis is accomplished by electroco-

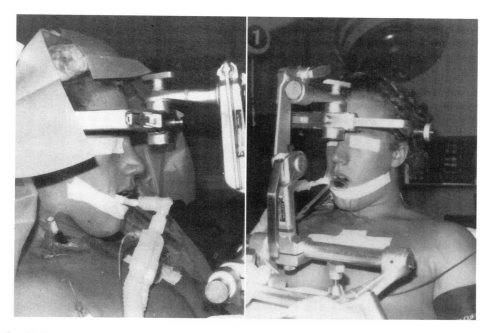

Fig. 30-9. The operation is performed with the patient in the sitting position under general endotracheal anesthesia with mechanical ventilation, arterial and venous pressure monitoring, and cardiac Doppler monitoring for detection of air emboli. The legs are wrapped, and systolic pressures are maintained above 120 mm Hg.

agulation, with care being taken to avoid contact with the ligamentum flavum.

Foraminotomy. The ligamentum flavum is separated from its most lateral attachment to the upper lamina with the use of a microcurette. An appropriate microrongeur is inserted under the lateral laminar shelf, and bone is removed in an upward direction until the foramen entrance can be identified by microhook palpation. Most important, the rongeur is not turned laterally into the facet or its synovium.

Once a foramen entrance has been located, additional judgment can be made as to possible stenosis, density of root sleeve adhesions to the posterior and inferior foraminal walls, and the angle by which the neural tube exits the spine. During foraminal decompression, perineural soft tissues are protected, manipulation of the nerve root is strictly avoided, and the cervical disc is rarely visible. Coagulating instruments should not be used for hemostasis once neural structures are exposed.

When the foramen entrance seems significantly stenosed, as determined by magnification and microhook palpation, it is safe to proceed with only a microcurette. Extremely gentle maneuvers are used to initiate an exact anatomic plane between the perineural soft tissue and bone. Resculpturing of posterior and inferior foraminal walls proceeds along the plane from inside out, avoiding mechanical pressures on the root. Motor responses should not occur when the plane of dissection is accurate. Once tight stenotic lesions have been relieved by microcurette technique, microrongeurs are used to widely hollow the foraminal walls from entrance to outlet. Osteophytes in the root axilla are removed by similar technique. At the termination of the procedure, the nerve root should be clearly visible, pulsatile, and widely decompressed on its posterior and inferior surface. Cerebral spinal fluid has not been encountered with this technique, and entrance into the facet and synovium are minimal. Blood loss rarely exceeds 100 ml. No attempt is made to visualize intervertebral discs or treat bony lesions anterior to the root. Wound closure is in layers, and care is taken to do a multilayer closure.

POSTOPERATIVE CARE

The same rehabilitation program that is used preoperatively is recommended postoperatively. It is expected that the patient will continue the trunk stabilization and neck-strengthening program after surgery.

Postoperatively the patient is placed in a soft collar for 2 weeks for comfort of the soft tissues and can resume therapy at 3 weeks.

It is believed that by using the microscope and being able to make visualization of the pulsating nerve our end point for decompression, we are able to resect a minimal amount of bone, thus preserving cervical stability. Zdeblick[14] has shown that resecting less than 50% of the facet causes no clinical instability. During the aforementioned procedure, significantly less than 20% is resected. With this in mind, we believe that the player may have a safe return to the contact sport without increased risk of cervical spine damage.

REFERENCES

1. Bergfeld JA, Hershman EB, Wilbourn AJ: Brachial plexus in sports, a five year follow-up, *Orthop Trans* 12:743, 1988.
2. Clancy WG, Brand RL, Bergfeld JA: Upper trunk brachial plexus injuries in contact sports, *Am J Sports Med* 5:209, 1977.
3. DiBenedetto M: Electrodiagnostic localization of traumatic upper trunk brachial plexopathy, *Arch Phys Med Rehabil* 65:15, 1984.
4. Hershman EB: Acute brachial neuropathy in athletes, *Am J Sports Med* 17:655, 1989.
5. Jackson DW, Lohr FP: Cervical spine injuries, *Clin Sports Med* 5:373, 1986.
6. Poindexter DP: Football shoulder and neck injury: a study of the "stinger," *Arch Phys Med Rehabil* 65:601, 1984.
7. Robinson RA: Anterolateral cervical disc removal and interbody fusion for cervical disc syndrome, *Bull Johns Hopkins Hosp* 96:223, 1955.
8. Seddon H: *Surgical disorders of the peripheral nerves,* Edinburgh, 1972, Churchill Livingstone.
9. Torg JS: Neurapraxia of the cervical spinal cord with transient quadriplegia, *J Bone Joint Surg* 68A:1354, 1986.
10. Torg JS: Spear tackler's spine, *Am J Sports Med* 21:640, 1993.
11. Watkins RG: Neck injuries in football players, *Clin Sports Med* 5:215, 1986.
12. Williams RW: Microcervical foraminotomy, *Spine* 8:708, 1983.
13. Vereschagin K: Burners, *Physician Sportsmed* 19(9):96, 1991.
14. Zdeblick TA: Cervical stability after foraminotomy, *J Bone Joint Surg* 74A:22, 1992.

Chapter Thirty-One

◆

Lumbar Spine Injuries in Football

Robert G. Watkins

ROLE OF BACK STRENGTH

Football players require tremendous strength in the upper body and the legs. Some football players, of course, rely on great agility, jumping ability, throwing ability, and eye-hand contact, but strength is the backbone of football. Every year, every professional team needs heavier, stronger, and faster athletes. When training camp begins, players, especially the offensive line, experience a period of mechanical back pain as blocking drills begin. It is difficult in the off-season to adequately prepare an athlete for the extreme and rapid extension of the back against weight that is necessary for offensive-line blocking. It is similar to the weight-lifting position that requires raising weight over the head except that in football the force must be generated with forward leg motion and off-balance resistance to the weight while the athlete is trying to carry out specific maneuvers, such as blocking a player in a specific direction. Extension jamming of the spine produces facet joint pain, spondylolysis, and spondylolisthesis. Thus specific training in back-strengthening exercises is required to prevent lumbar spine injuries.

Weight training and weight lifting are important tools in developing the strength and power necessary to play football. However, safety precautions must be a primary consideration; it has been estimated that more injuries may actually occur in training than in competition. The player must be protected by thorough instruction in proper weight-lifting techniques. Thus football coaches and training staff personnel play important roles in designing training programs that will prevent lumbar spine injuries.

TYPES OF INJURIES

In addition to extension and lifting-type forces, football involves sudden off-balance rotation, which is caused by tremendous loads in an unprotected position. This rotation may produce transverse process fractures, torsional disc injuries, and tears in the lumbodorsal fascia. Another hazard is the athlete's vulnerability to receiving unexpected, severe blows to the lumbar spine, which can produce contusion or fracture. A helmet in the ribs produces rib fractures, whereas a helmet in the flank can produce renal contusion, retroperitoneal hemorrhage, injury to the transverse process, spinous process fractures, and transverse shear injuries to a neuromotion segment. Many acrobatic receivers and runners suffer

spondylitic defects for the same reasons that make gymnasts and ballet dancers vulnerable.

As already noted, one of the distinguishing characteristics of football players, as compared with many other athletes, is their tremendous upper body muscular development and body weight. Certainly, the strength acquired and developed in football players is an advantage in protecting the spine. The muscle mass and muscle strength provide added stability to the cervical, thoracic, and lumbar spine.

Unfortunately, the catch-22 is that when a player develops an injury to one of the discs in the lower lumbar spine (e.g., an injury to the L4-5 joint), the resultant pain produces a loss of coordinated muscle activity and progressive weakness. The inflammation causes a reflex muscle spasm and stiffness around the joint. At this point the upper body weight and muscle mass become detrimental to proper healing of the injured L4-5 joint. A chain is only as strong as its weakest link. If there are 250 pounds of body weight above an injured L4-5 joint, the resulting lever-arm effect of this body weight with any motion or activity produces continued injury through an injured joint without proper muscular protection. Although the principle on which treatment is based may be sound, a good result can be difficult to achieve.

PREVENTION

The solution to the above dilemma is based on the same hard work and determination that produced the muscle mass in the beginning: to adhere to a properly developed trunk-stabilization and rehabilitation program. Intensive practice or training is one of the hallmarks of football. For the number of minutes spent actually playing the game, there are many hours of hard, grueling work in training. Thus the trainer and therapist, using proper trunk rehabilitation techniques, can take advantage of the well-developed work ethic of the successful football player. This focus more than compensates for any deleterious effects of body weight.

APPROACH TO INJURIES

The history and physical examination of a football player with an injury consist of the elements discussed in Chapters 5 and 7. Is it a back pain problem? Is it a leg pain problem? What makes the pain worse? The basic principles of the history are followed by a standard physical examination. Is there neurologic deficit? Are there neurologic symptoms? Are underlying disease processes contributing to the pain? Each question is answered in terms of the four objectives of the history and physical examination:

1. Quantify the immobility.
2. Eliminate psychosocial factors.
3. Eliminate tumor, as well as infections and neurologic catastrophies.
4. Identify the clinical syndrome.

Diagnosis and Treatment

A complete diagnosis should be made as early as possible, and a strategy is planned on the basis of findings. Spinal injuries in football are similar to those that occur in every life-style and every sport. Discogenic injuries and injuries to the lumbar joints are common in football players. Stress fractures, spondylolisthesis, and disc herniations make up the bulk of football injuries; stress fractures and acute injuries should be ruled out. Magnetic resonance imaging, myelography, and contrast computed tomography scanning are used as for any patient.

Trunk Stabilization Training

At the Kerlan-Jobe Orthopaedic Clinic our nonoperative treatment of football players is based on the trunk stabilization program. Trunk stabilization fits perfectly into the heavy weight lifting that is required of many football players. The modification of weight lifting in a player with a back injury is a program that is designed in terms of the maximum mechanical advantage for the lumbar spine. Eliminated are exercises designed to put the lumbar spine at the greatest mechanical disadvantage; emphasized are weight-lifting techniques that best protect the lumbar spine.

The need for tremendous strength has been emphasized in football, and certainly that is the public perception. However, coaches, trainers, and players fully understand the key role of balance and coordination. Levers and balance are vital in dealing with a 300-pound adversary. The success of the 190-pounders on the field depends on coordination, and the possession of balance and coordination separates the most successful 300 pounders from the least successful 300 pounders.

The principles of stabilization are vitally important in football. Sport-specific stabilization exercises vary according to the player's position. The transition from a rehabilitation program following injury to practicing the sport still involves the basic adaptation of power and balance for the lumbar spine: the weight is centered, and the midportion of the body is balanced. The power of the legs and fine control of the arms are used for leverage. Each of the basic maneuvers that the athlete uses—whether this player is a linebacker, defensive lineman, offensive lineman, or quarterback—is analyzed according to what the player is going to do in the game. The transition of these maneuvers is made from the floor in

the rehabilitation area, to the green exercise ball, and then to the slide and balance boards, with emphasis on neutral-position trunk control against resistance.

Surgery

Many indications for surgery are the same as in other high-performance athletes. Spinal fusion takes a long time to heal, and the ultimate result may not place the athlete at the greatest mechanical advantage for what the sport requires. On an empiric basis, fusion appears to be a more supportable concept in a professional football player than in a top-flight professional golfer; however, the indications for surgery are much the same. For patients with a significant problem that will cause long delays in return to function or considerable time missed from the sport—thus leading to deterioration in skill level—or for those with significant radicular or neurogenic pain that prevents proper rehabilitation, surgery rather than rehabilitation is considered. The operative technique is much the same as for any number of other athletes at the professional level. The surgeon does as little harm as possible in removing or changing the source of the offending pain with as little destruction to normal tissue as possible. The surgeon should remember at all times the importance of a dynamic postoperative rehabilitation program, which is intended to produce spinal stability through muscle control. For example, a large, extruded fragment should be removed with as little damage and as little contact with normal tissue as possible. The rehabilitation program can be relied on to restore strength, stability, and proper mechanical functioning to the injured joint.

CASE ILLUSTRATIONS

Figs. 31-1 to 31-10 illustrate cases involving lumbar spine injuries in football players.

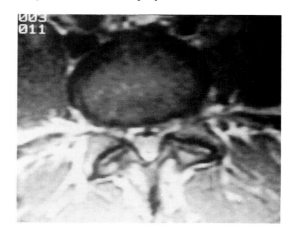

Fig. 31-1. This 29-year-old professional football receiver reported left-sided L5 radicular pain. The transverse section CT scan revealed a small extruded fragment trapping the nerve root under the lateral recess. The player was unresponsive to nonoperative care and underwent a microscopic lumbar discectomy and small medial facetectomy, which resulted in complete relief of symptoms and return to play the next season.

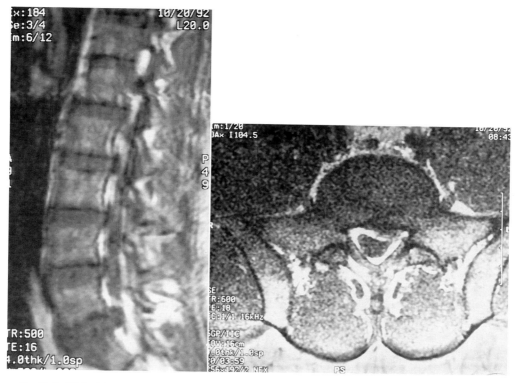

Fig. 31-2. This 6-foot 5-inch, 270-pound professional defensive tackle suffered an acute onset of left S1 radiculopathy. The player attempted a course of nonoperative care that did not produce a sufficient resolution of his symptoms. When he returned to running or any vigorous activity, his radiculopathy recurred. He underwent microscopic lumbar discectomy at L5-S1 and returned to play 5 months later with no further symptoms.

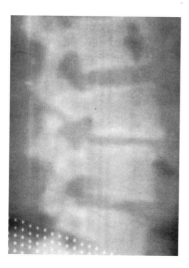

Fig. 31-3. This 38-year-old former professional football player reported severe back and radiating leg pain. X-ray films revealed a severely degenerated L3-4 disc with spondylitic spondylolisthesis. Fusion was considered, and multilevel discography reproduced all of the patient's symptoms at L4-5. Therefore a two-level fusion was the only recommended surgery for this problem. The patient decided against surgery.

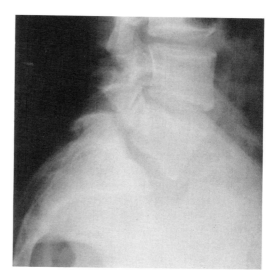

Fig. 31-4. Spondylolisthesis. This is a typical lumbar finding for a number of athletes, including football players, and is not considered a significant factor in their return to play. In most instances the use of strengthening techniques can overcome the symptoms of spondylolisthesis. We have not had, to date, a professional football player whose career was shortened solely because of a spondylolisthesis that was treated nonoperatively.

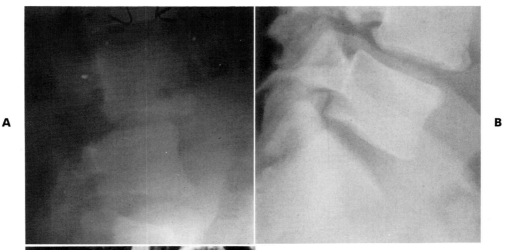

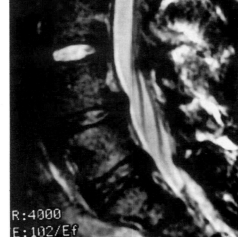

Fig. 31-5. This 24-year-old professional wide receiver reported back and radiating leg pain. Lateral flexion/extension films (**A** and **B**) revealed a hypermobile dynamic spondylitic spondylolisthesis at L4-5. The patient was found to have two-level degenerative disc disease and a pseudodisc at the olisthetic L4-5 level (**C**). He was treated nonoperatively with trunk stabilization exercises and returned to play within the same season.

Fig. 31-6. This starting professional linebacker reported weakness in his leg, radiating dysesthesia, and mild pain. He felt that he had lost his mobility and strength as a linebacker. He was unable to respond quickly to the plays. He had a weakness in his leg that fatigued as the game went on. The physical examination revealed positive findings on straight leg raising, neck flexion, and the Cram test, but the actual pain was not as severe as the loss of function and the inability to respond and move laterally as quickly as possible. A microscopic lumbar discectomy was carried out. The patient returned the next season, fully functioning as a starting linebacker in the National Football League, with no symptoms and full agility and response.

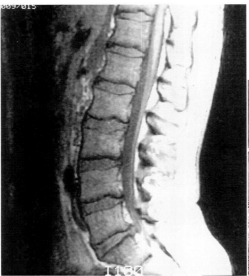

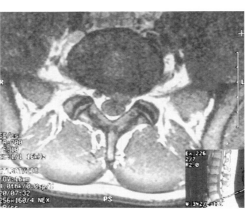

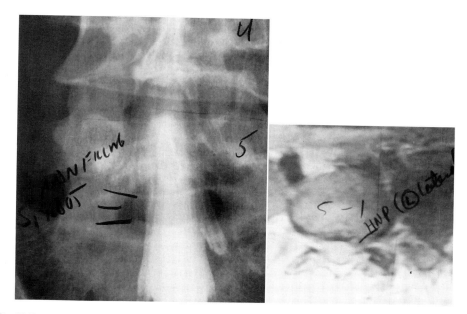

Fig. 31-7. This 29-year-old professional lineman reported severe radiating right leg pain for the last 6 weeks of the football season. There was considerable weakness, numbness, and inability to push off on his leg, and he was having a great deal of difficulty. The diagnosis was disc herniation. He underwent a microscopic lumbar discectomy, returned the next season at the start of the fall season, played for several years, and has continued to perform at an all-professional level.

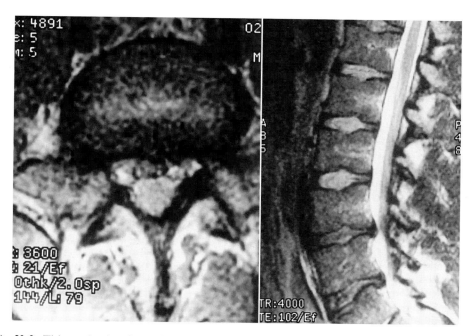

Fig. 31-8. This professional running back had consistent right buttock and radiating leg pain, with positive signs of sciatica and nerve root tension on physical examination. He underwent a microscopic lumbar discectomy.

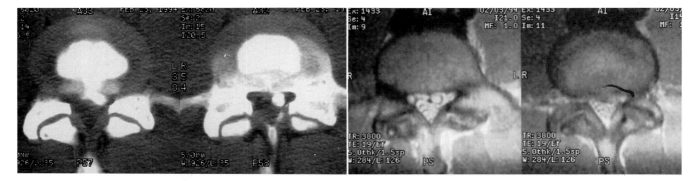

Fig. 31-9. This running back had consistent pain in his leg and was unable to sit for a considerable period of time. He had a nagging, gnawing pain in the leg that was unresponsive to nonoperative treatment. Although he could run with the lesion, he experienced weakness and intermittent but considerable problems with it. The patient underwent a microscopic lumbar discectomy.

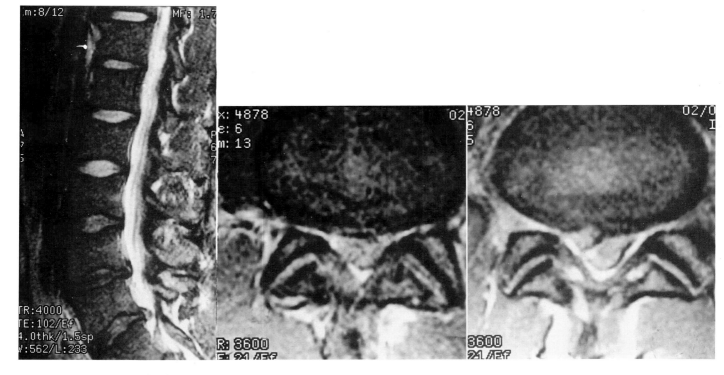

Fig. 31-10. This defensive end had severe pain throughout the season. He was forced to miss several games during the season because of radiating leg pain. Near the end of the season, appreciable radiculopathy was present, but he played the last three games of the season despite significant pain and weakness, and he decided to play at the play-off level. He subsequently underwent a microscopic lumbar discectomy, which revealed an extruded fragment at L5-S1 with lateral recess stenosis at L4-5. His physical examination demonstrated both L5 and S1 radiculopathy.

Chapter Thirty-Two

◆

Trunk and Lower Extremity Strengthening for Football

Robert Ward

It is absolutely essential at the very beginning of training to establish a philosophy of training based on science to integrate the desired trunk and leg training benefits with their functional use on the football field. This concept differs from one based only on strengthening the trunk and legs through increasing individual tissue strength. It suggests that an effective program involves a meaningful relationship between performance, increased strength, and a decrease in football injuries. Admittedly, this goal cannot be achieved easily. Forces on the field can affect the athlete in such a way that no training program could provide adequate preparation. This recognition launched me on a 15-year search for strategies to counter these forces, which led right back to the football field and the skills required of the player — where the solution had been all along.

The technology of video and computer graphics is being used to determine the actual force levels generated by players in game situations. Logically, such information will help the team physician, coach, and football player develop intelligent prevention and rehabilitation programs to effectively meet these on-field demands.

Acceleration is the two-edged sword that produces great feats on the field and that generates the great forces that cause injuries to players. This evidence supports a long-held belief that acceleration, or the more common term *quickness,* is the most critical factor in football, not only for high levels of performance but for protection. Essentially it is the ability to repeatedly start, stop, and change direction at will. Football is a contact sport and by its very nature increases the effects of this acceleration on a player during the contact phase. Actions of this kind place a great amount of force on the body. Therefore the football player must strengthen the whole body to a threshold level. The trunk and legs account for approximately 80% of the total body weight and therefore need to be trained to effectively absorb, transmit, or direct the energy in a harmless direction.[8] In fact, the most important protective element in playing football is not the strengthening of tissues but the way their collective strength is used. I have observed many elite football players over the years who overtrained the structural components (e.g., bench press plus 500, power clean plus 400) at the expense of nervous system control.

Efficient use of the athlete's body movements would dramatically reduce the negative impact of improper handling of energy on the field, thereby reducing injuries and increasing performance.

Many coaches waste valuable time and effort by spending too much time, especially during the preseason, on isolated factors (e.g., speed, strength, agility drills) and not enough on their integration into the game itself. Certainly, basic elements comprise the minimum skills required for a specific performance level. However, an increase in any one element does not guarantee a commensurate improvement in the skill.[5] One must remember that performance is a complete process that defies fragmentation.[12] Therefore the method presented here provides a possible solution to maximizing the effectiveness of trunk and leg strengthening for football.

NATURE OF MOTION IN FOOTBALL

The integrity of any structure is primarily determined by the soundness of its supportive structures. The supportive structures in this case must be defined in a broad, all-encompassing context — from the smallest unit to the sum of all the units: the total system. Our bodies certainly follow this principle. Therefore it is imperative that a training program be designed around this fundamental principle. In my opinion one of the most productive methods for training program development is based on the ancient concept of centering.

Centering (the first dimension of seven dimensions discussed later) is a term used to describe a physical and mental dynamic that is in a constant state of flow. This concept has been expressed by many dissimilar groups in various disciplines or sports. It can be likened to the calm in the eye of the hurricane or the internal attention of the master performer in any skill. Uncommon performances require the summoning up of all the desirable and necessary internal and external resources we possess in order to optimize our chances of reaching that elusive point of mental or physical balance that determines the quality of our performance. The essence of our training must weave a supportive fabric through this point, or maximum benefits will not be accrued.

The centering point of focus for our purposes here is the center of gravity of the body. It is the literal crossroad of energy transport from lower to upper in the case of

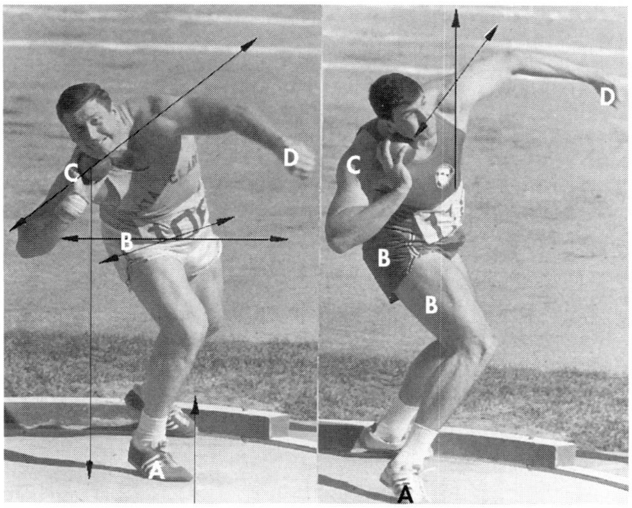

Fig. 32-1. Note the "X" formed by the shoulders and hips of these two shot-putters. This position maximizes the forces required for throwing the shot put. It is evident that shot-putters must have a powerful trunk and legs.

ground-originating forces, or vice versa in the case of hand-originating forces. Fig. 32-1 shows this dynamic interplay of forces acting on the upper and lower extremities of the body—from the ground through the center of gravity and anatomic planes of two shot-putters. Consequently, an efficient training program focuses on exercises that function along the same patterns of flow, biomechanically and physiologically.

The focus of any training program is to increase the capacity of the energy transfer system of the body. First, however, it is important to understand the nature of the motions involved in the game, emphasizing the obvious fact that the actual playing time is only about 12 minutes in a 60-minute game. Furthermore, the skills required in football are needed in a very short time span and at high speed (Table 32-1).

A review of the literature reveals that human engineers have looked at events in relation to a time base, which I have extended to the game of football (Table 32-2).

Table 32-1. Analysis of a Football Game*

Factors	Time/Distance
Game duration (gross)	3 hr +
Game time	60 min
Plays per game	50 to 70 plays
Play time = snap of the ball to end of play	
Actual playing time (8%-12%)	5-7 min
Passing time % of total (52%)	2.6-3.6 min
Passing time/play	2.3-5 sec
Running time % of total (48%)	2.4-3.4 min
Running time/play	2-5 sec
Special teams	
Kickoffs (4/game)	45 yd
Punts (6/game)	40 yd

Data from OFAS On-Field-Analysis, Orlando, Fla.; Dallas, Tex.
*Statistics give a broad estimate of the composition of a football game.

Table 32-2. Time Duration by Functional Categories Applied to Football

Category	Event Time
Impact	100 msec
Reaction/force	100-300 msec
Quick play	30 msec-2 sec
Play time (average)	2-10 sec
Prolonged play	10-60 sec

Table 32-3. Static Strength Relative to Speed of Motion

Speed of Motion	Radians/Sec	Degrees/Sec	Static (%)
Slow	0.26	15	50
Medium slow	2.60	150	40
Medium	9.00	516	33
Fast	13.00	745	30
Very fast	17.00	974	20

Table 32-4. Analysis of a One-Arm Striking Inertial Exercise

Platform Weight (lb)	Travel Distance (in)	Repetitions/Sec	Average Power/Rep*	Approximate Duration to Fatigue	Maximum Reps/Session	High-Range Degree/Sec	Stopping Time (msec)	Starting Time (msec)	Maximum Velocity (fps)
28.5	42	1.43	106.34	2 min	85.96	1078.76	46	108	6.45
13.5	34	2.91	410.78	10 sec	29.07	2127.77	22	32	10.10
11.0	32	3.03	424.88	10 sec	30.30	2543.69	18	28	9.48
8.5	29	3.62	425.05	10 sec	25.36	3012.04	18	28	10.81
6.0	24	4.07	345.00	20 sec	81.30	1977.74	18	26	10.64
3.5	21	5.15	336.15	20 sec	103.09	1617.87	18	24	12.79

Data from Davidson S, Engineering Marketing Associates, Newman, Ga (data collected from exercise with the Impulse Inertial Exercise System).
*Rep, repetition; fps, power in foot pounds per second.

A comparison of Tables 32-1 and 32-2 indicates that the game requires the football player to have the ability to repetitively deliver high levels of energy in short bursts with recovery periods of approximately 60 seconds, a skill required in most sports[11] (Table 32-3).

The ability to exert maximum strength diminishes as the speed of motion increases.[15] Furthermore, through proper exercise it is possible to educate the body's energy transport system by using total body actions that tax the nervous system and the muscle, tendon, and ligament complex. The exercises best suited for the development and delivery of high levels of this kind of athletic power transmit energy from the ground to the hands or point of contact. These exercises involve both sides of the body, such as punching, hitting, or twisting actions. Careful observations reveal a symphony of explosive rhythms in the torquing of the legs, hips, and shoulders. Coaches will see this as an extension of the concept of crossing the X. The shoulders and hips form an X in the process of good throwing or hitting action—hence the name. Each exercise is performed at extremely high speeds. Studies that I did with Steve Davidson[4] while I was with the Dallas Cowboys showed that equivalent field forces were being duplicated on the inertial impulse machine. Table 32-4 analyzes a one-arm striking inertial exercise similar to what would be used on the football field.

Our data support the following findings:

1. More power is generated at a platform load of 8.5 to 13.5 pounds.
2. Endurance decreases as the power output increases.
3. Football players can be taught to hit with greater force. A training program using lighter platform weights was implemented to see if it is possible to train power hitting. Preliminary results are showing that inertial exercise is an effective strategy to teach football players to hit at higher forces within a short period of training time.

These findings concerning the value of inertial exercise in improving the coordinated action of the trunk and legs justify its being given a high-level priority for inclusion in the training facility. Explosive power delivery exercises for the legs and trunk, such as single- and double-hand striking patterns, need to be added to the traditional programs that work at a basic tissue-strength level only. Table 32-5 shows that athletic joint motions have extremely high instantaneous angular speeds.

The additional physiologic benefits derived from inertial impulse training are as follows:

1. Toning of tendons and ligaments
2. Increased muscle-anaerobic endurance
3. Transfer of energy across joints

These new dimensions of exercise require that additional terminology be incorporated into the exercise prescription process. Even the traditional terms take on different magnitudes. For instance, doing one repetition in an exercise of 400 pounds is certainly different from one that requires 5 to 20 pounds. Speed is the missing ingredient that keeps the force levels lower in the example of 400 pounds and many fast repetitions. Explosive quickness, which is driven by the ability to accelerate, is the single most important quality required in sports. The ability to generate explosive power requires that a high degree of body acceleration be available for use. This quality is best seen on the field when the player is able to start, stop, and change directions effortlessly. I have discussed acceleration in conversations with Jim Counsilman, noted swim coach from Indiana University, who has termed his work in this area *programmable acceleration*. Counsilman believes that this training technique, which is still in development, can be of great value to modern training programs. Programmable acceleration requires that exercises be described with additional terms or with a different understanding of the presently used terms. The following additional terms can help define the rationale for use of an exercise:

1. *Maximum workout loads*—Loads range from 5 to 20 pounds
2. *Maximum time*—Time ranges from 10 to 30 seconds
3. *Repetitions per second*—Attempting to do as many as possible
4. *Dominant equivalence*—Improving the nondominant side
5. *Time to maximum repetitions*—Improving time to maximum
6. *Repetitions in the first second*—Developing quickness

SEVEN DIMENSIONS OF TRAINING

The program presented in this section is based on the following seven dimensions of training: (1) centering, (2) specificity, (3) efficiency, (4) planes and tensions, (5) balance focus, (6) exercise selection, and (7) program development.

Dimension 1: Centering

See discussion on p. 349.

Table 32-5. Educating the Energy Transfer System of the Trunk and Legs (Total Body Action With Inertial Impulse Training)

Level (degrees/sec)	Loads	Time
1. 200-600	Platform (one-tenth slug—3¼ lb) + 15 lb	Extended
2. 600-1000	Platform + 5-10 lb	30-60 sec
3. 1000-2000	Platform + 5-10 lb	10-30 sec
4. 2000-4000	Platform + 1¼ lb	7-10 sec

Dimension 2: Specificity

There is a tendency to view specificity as a modern concept. However, if a thorough historical study were conducted, it would reveal that human beings have used it from the beginning of time. For example, if drum skills are the desired outcome, it takes only common sense to practice on the drums, not the violin. An understanding of the principles of music certainly helps, but there is no substitute for hands-on practice time with the instrument to develop the neuromuscular processes involved. That the literature reveals many advocates of this principle is a given. The question, however, is how to apply it in the training program. Again, the answer is simple: practice the skill, and the necessary training benefits will develop accordingly.

Dimension 3: Efficiency

The law of efficiency is a natural effect of applying the first two dimensions. It guarantees the athlete the most efficient use of training time. The training effects produced will have the greatest direct impact on the skill or sport. Because precise stresses are being placed on all the body's systems, the effects will be efficiently developed. Consequently the tissues required for the task are being strengthened in the exact patterns of usefulness.

Dimension 4: Planes and Tension

Most athletic skills are multidimensional. Thus it would seem that training should be guided by the principle of planes and tension. Consequently the exercises that move through the three anatomic planes with optimum tension are given a higher priority. Most exercise programs do not stress the horizontal plane that runs parallel to the ground, and few exercises include a twisting motion around the vertical axis (see Fig. 32-1). Alternating dumbbell exercises designed to produce these motions provides excellent training. An outstanding summary of multi-plane motion, along with other related concepts concerning the biomechanics of the trunk and legs, can be found in Logan and McKinney's book titled *Kinesiology.*[9]

Dimension 5: Balance Focus

The best source of the balance dimension is Plagenhoef's work.[11,12] Exercises that isolate and develop only one body part produce specific adaptations to the forces imposed on the body, a phenomenon that can be seen by comparing the throwing arm of the quarterback with his opposing arm, revealing the differences in muscle and bony structure. Therefore Plagenhoef recommends that proper muscular balance be maintained to combat any cumulative pathologic condition that could develop over time. My opinion is that a natural body wisdom produces the anatomic changes best suited for the skill. However, a fine line exists between this ideal and a condition that would create an imbalance or undesirable adaptation in the body.[2]

Table 32-6. Comparison of Maximum Knee Extension Strength by Joint

Exercise	Maximum (%)	Minimum (%)
Lower Extremities		
Raise on toes (foot extension)	116	53
Knee extension (lower leg)	100	87
Knee flexion (leg curl)	99	33
Hip extension	134	47
Hip flexion	68	29
Hip abduction (outward)	100	27
Hip adduction (inward)	100	47
Trunk flexion (back extension)	59	52
Trunk extension (start of sit-up)	78	78
Upper Extremities		
Upper arm extension (pullover)	57	17
Upper arm flexion	38	18
Upper arm abduction	62	21
Upper arm adduction	80	3
Upper arm horizontal adduction (pectorals)	39	16
Elbow extension (triceps)	21	14
Elbow flexion (biceps)	24	12
Shoulder girdle elevation (shoulder shrug)	80	49

Data from Plagenhoff S: *Patterns of human motion,* Englewood Cliffs, NJ, 1971, Prentice-Hall.

A total body balance test should be given on biomechanically sound machines. These machines should follow the person's anatomic strength curves as closely as possible; otherwise a true measure of the athlete's strength will not be reflected.[3] In addition, the test position, or joint angle, will determine the amount of maximum joint strength displayed. Table 32-6 shows the strength ranges for 17 different commonly executed exercises relative to maximum knee extension. The test data can be evaluated to determine the relative strengths of all the major muscle groups of the body. The subsequent assessment of these tests provides a sound basis for a comprehensive exercise prescription. Sophisticated computerized machines are available to meet these requirements. However, equipment of this kind is not available to many athletes, and a set of dumbbells would be the best alternative for determining upper extremity measurements. Certainly, a barbell can be used under the direction of a trained teacher or coach to collect the necessary information for the upper and lower extremities. Plagenhoef[12] has compared the relative strength of the muscle joint actions with knee extension in the test exercises recommended for total body balance, which are discussed in the next section. However, they apply only if the testing machines used follow the aforementioned biomechanical criteria and the athlete is tested at the same joint angles.

Dimension 6: Exercise Selection

The selection of exercises is based on the specific objectives of each level of the *seven-step model*,[4] which is discussed under dimension 7. Therefore an exercise that is effective at one level may be less so at another level unless it can be modified to meet the criteria for that level. Remember, each of the seven dimensions must be considered along with the seven-step model as a basis for selecting exercises. This model was developed to integrate all the dimensions of training into a processing structure that assists in organizing and administering the training program.

Adrian and Cooper[1] suggest four elements that can serve as criteria for selecting exercises to include in the training program. These elements are categorized according to biomechanical design:

1. Exercises that improve strength and power of muscles, ligaments, and bones
2. Exercises that improve anaerobic and aerobic capacity
3. Exercises that increase range of motion
4. Exercises that improve neuromuscular functioning, agility, balance, and coordination

Dimension 7: Program Development

The seventh dimension integrates the individual parts, or dimensions, of program development. The seven-step model, used to develop and organize a training program, evolved after many years of training and coaching athletes. The program suggested for trunk and lower extremity training is based on this model. For various reasons, too many programs have failed to coordinate all the essential training resources into a comprehensive program. Thus this model may expedite a solution to this problem in programming. In addition, further studies may reveal that much of our so-called scientific training regimens are unnecessarily fragmented and/or redundant and therefore have little value except for adding variety to our programs. Examples of applications of the seven-step model (Table 32-7) illustrate how it can be used in both the preseason and the playing season (Table 32-8), thereby providing a better understanding of how the model can be used in developing a sound trunk and leg training program for football.

Step 1: Basic training. The purpose of basic training[6] is to develop all the player's personal resources required for football to the *threshold level*. The threshold level is that amount of a resource that is required to perform at a particular grade level. Increased skill does not guarantee better performance. Basic training conditioning provides a solid base to build each successive step. Many of us have forgotten that *repetition is the mother of learning*. The first step of basic training establishes this principle. According to martial artist Dan Inosanto,[7] "skills must be repeated a minimum of 3000 times to begin a neuromuscular grooving." The types of programs included develop body control, pure strength/muscle endurance, and sustained effort (muscular and cardiovascular exercises involving all of the body's energy systems in an integrated manner).

Step 2: Functional strength/power training. Functional strength/power training[6,14] employs explosive movements against medium to heavy resistance. Maximum power is developed by working in an intensity range of 55% to 85% maximum. The Olympic lifts and their variations that use either the Olympic bar or dumbbells are the essence of this step. A key principle is to train the total body chain (hands to feet) all at once. Therefore the snatch, jerk, and the clean and jerk are excellent because they require the football player to manage the forces across all the body's segments from the hands to

Table 32-7. Seven-Step Model*

Step	Basic Elements†	Time of Year‡		
		Preseason	Season	Postseason
7	Overspeed	0-1-0	2	0-3
6	Sport speed	0-1-0	1-2	0-3
5	Sport load	0-1-0	2	0-3
4	Plyometrics	0-1-0	2	0-3
3	Ballistics	0-1-0	2	0-3
2	Power	0-1-0	2-0	0-3
1	Basic training	0-1-0	2-0	0-3

*The best assessment is one that can be determined during the game; those qualities not adequately developed on the field should be assessed off the field at the times indicated.
†Activities used to develop each of the resources at each of the steps.
‡*0*, assessment; *1*, develop; *2*, maintain; *3*, restore/active rest.

Table 32-8. Seven-Step Model Applied to Preseason and Season*

		Day of the Week‡						
Step	Basic Elements†	M	T	W	T	F	S	S
Preseason								
7	Overspeed	7	7	7	0	0	0	0
	Training volume	3	2	3	0	0	0	0
6	Sport speed	6	6	6	6	6	0	0
	Training volume	3	2	3	3	2	0	0
5	Sport load	0	0	1	1	1	0	0
	Training volume	0	0	2	3	2	0	0
4	Plyometrics	6	6	6	0	0	0	0
	Training volume	1	2	1	0	0	0	0
3	Ballistics	6	6	6	6	0	0	0
	Training volume	1	3	1	3	0	0	0
2	Power	6	0	6	0	0	0	0
	Training volume	2	0	3	0	0	0	0
1	Basic training	6	6	6	6	6	0	0
	Training volume	1	1	1	3	3	0	0
Season								
7	Overspeed	0	0	7	0	0	0	0
	Training volume	0	0	1	0	0	0	0
6	Sport speed	5	0	6	6	5	4	0
	Training volume	2	0	3	2	1	0	G
5	Sport load	0	0	5	6	5	0	0
	Training volume	0	0	3	1	0	0	0
4	Plyometrics	0	0	6	6	0	0	0
	Training volume	0	0	1	1	0	0	0
3	Ballistics	0	0	6	6	0	0	0
	Training volume	0	0	1	1	0	0	0
2	Power	4	0	5	0	0	0	0
	Training volume	1	0	1	0	0	0	0
1	Basic training	5	0	5	4	0	0	0
	Training volume	2	0	2	1	0	0	0

*The best assessment is one that can be determined during the game *without disturbing the athlete;* those qualities not adequately developed on the field should be assessed off the field at the times indicated.

†Activities used to develop each of the resources at each of the steps.

‡*7,* 100% repetition maximum (RM); *6,* 100%-90% RM; *5,* 90%-80% RM; *4,* 80%-70% RM; *3,* 70%-60% RM; *2,* 60%-50% RM; *1,* 50%-40% RM; *0,* nothing. Volume: *3,* high; *2,* medium; *1,* low; *0,* none; *G,* game.

the feet at the ground. Remember, all that is required is that threshold amount—no more, no less.

Step 3: Ballistics training. High-speed sending and receiving movements are included in ballistics training.[4,6] Medicine balls weighing between 4 and 23 pounds serve as excellent devices for throwing or catching. Proper throwing action requires that the thrower use the legs and the trunk. A comprehensive program incorporates single- and double-arm actions. Although state-of-the-art materials has allowed the manufacturing of functional and durable balls, many other implements can also be used, such as shots, weights, and discuses. Every motion of the body should be included in this section of training.

Step 4: Plyometrics training. Step 4 includes a variety of explosive exercises, such as hopping, jumping, bounding, hitting, and kicking.[4,6,13]

Step 5: Sport-loaded training. Sport-loaded training[6,10] includes activities of precise loading at high speed. The intensity ranges are from 90% to just under 100% of maximum speed. Research conducted with Ralph Mann[10] has verified the biomechanical applicability of using blocking sleds, weight-pulling sleds, and other more sophisticated devices, such as the power trainer (a specially designed loading system), for increasing initial driving power required in football.[6,10] Biomechanical evaluation of players using the power trainer showed that it forces the player to maintain an effort that closely matches the first four steps of a start, which is exactly what is wanted. Selected loads should impede the player's speed by no more than 5% to 10% for the particular skill in question.

Step 6: Sport speed/quickness/speed endurance. The sixth step includes actual participation in the sport and/or skills involved in the sport.[6] Participation in related games that involve repetitive, quick, explosive starting and stopping, as well as catching, throwing, hitting, or kicking, can be included in this step. For example, basketball, handball, court soccer, martial arts, and badminton provide outstanding cross-training opportunities.

Step 7: Overspeed training. Overspeed training includes any activity that is performed at levels beyond the normal competitive speed.[6] A systematic program should be developed that trains the nervous system with activities that exceed the maximum performance speeds anywhere from 5% to 10%. Various training techniques and devices can be used. A danger in overspeed training is to assume that going faster is the only answer. Force platform studies I conducted with Dave Wilson[16] confirmed the hypothesis that football players being pulled at high speeds will break at each step. In other words, they are attempting to slow down at each step. This movement has an effect opposite from that desired in training. The emphasis should be on turnover (moving the legs faster and getting the foot closer to the center of gravity).

My opinion is that when the proper thresholds have been attained in training to maximize football skills, most training time should focus on steps 5 through 7. Surely, maintenance programs must be instituted to hold any desirable personal resource at a level perceived to be essential for the sport or skill. Remember, the perception of what is to be accomplished can be based on either psychologic or physiologic factors.

SEVEN-STEP MODEL FOR TRUNK AND LOWER EXTREMITY TRAINING

Specific exercises are suggested for each of the seven steps to provide a guide to the types of exercises recommended. Although there are many ways to structure intensity, sets, and repetitions, some common principles are presented for each step (Table 32-9).

Table 32-9 Rating Intensities of the 1 Repetition Maximum (1RM) for Exercise Prescription

1RM (%)	Rating	Quality Developed*
90	Very heavy	Strength
80-90	Heavy	Strength/strength endurance
70-80	Medium	Power/strength endurance
60-70	Medium light	Power/muscle endurance
50-60	Light	Power/muscle endurance
40-50	Easy	Threshold of training effect

Data from Ward B, Ward P: *Encyclopedia of weight training,* Laguna Hills, Calif, 1991, PPT Publications, 1991.
*The speed of movement will determine the amount of power developed at any one intensity level.

Step 1: Basic Training

Purpose	Exercise	Planes*	Sets/Reps†
Legs/back	Deadlift (Fig. 32-2)	2	Recommended strength, 78%-100% Sets: 3-6 Reps: 1-5
	Squat back (Fig. 32-3)	2	Muscle endurance, 40%-78% Sets: 3-6 Reps: 6-12 +
	Squat front (Fig. 32-4)	2	
	Step-ups (a)	2	
	(b)	2	
	Leg sled	2	
	Leg press	2	
	Extension	2	
	Flexion	2	
	Toe raises	2	

*Activities noted as plane 3 involve a greater rotational element in the action.
†Repetitions.

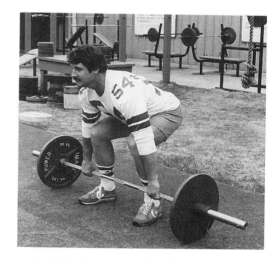

Fig. 32-2. Starting position for the deadlift.

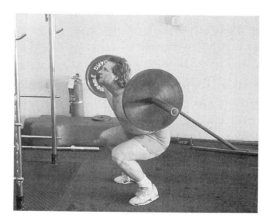

Fig. 32-3. Back squat. The bar is kept over the base; the legs are bent; the back is tight; the head is up.

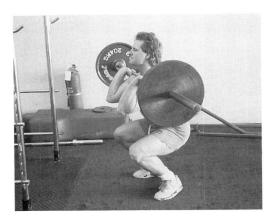

Fig. 32-4. Front squat. The bar is held on the front part of the shoulders; the elbows are up; the bar is kept over the base; the legs are bent; the back is tight; the head and eyes are up.

Purpose	Exercise	Planes*	Sets/Reps†
Trunk/ abdomen	Bent press 1 dumb-bell (Db) (Fig. 32-5)	3	Same as for legs/back
	Sit-ups (Fig. 32-6)	2-3	
	(All variations straight, rotating with and without loading)		
	Swingball exercises 3 (medicine ball or Db)		
	Horizontal bar		
	Leg raises	2	
	Leg raises (alternate)	3	
	Leg circles	3	
	Leg swings	3	

Step 2: Functional Strength

Purpose	Exercise	Planes*	Sets/Reps†
Legs/back	Pulls (Fig. 32-7)	2	Recommended power, 55%-85 + %
	Dumbbell (Db) swings (Fig. 32-8)	2	Sets: 3-6
	Cleans (Fig. 32-9)	2	Reps: 1-52
	Snatches (Fig. 32-10)	2	
	Jerks (Fig. 32-11)	2	
	Clean and jerk	2	
	Snatch 1 Db	3	
	Jerk 1 Db	3	
	Clean and jerk 1 Db	3	

Step 3: Ballistic Training

Purpose	Exercise	Planes*	Time
Total body	Hammer and related exercises	3	About 30 min for any exercise selected
	Weight throws	3	
	Shot	3	
	Discus	3	
	Medicine ball	2-3	
	Throws and catches	2-3	

*Activities noted as plane 3 involve a greater rotational element in the action.
†Repetitions.

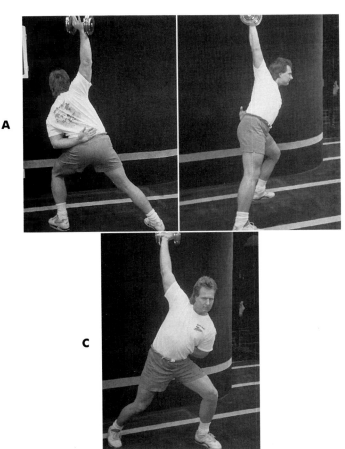

Fig. 32-5. Bent press. The dumbbell is held over the base of support; the left leg bends; the trunk is being rotated, placing rotary stress on the trunk and hips (accomplished bent-pressers have been observed with a 90-degree trunk-leg angle); the free arm can be held as shown or in front of the body. **A,** Rear view. **B,** Side view. **C,** Front view.

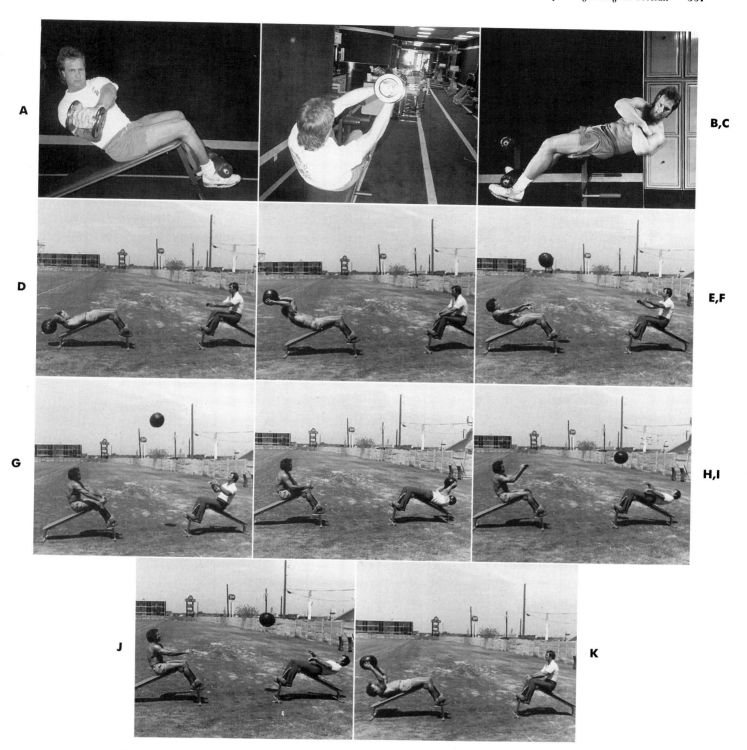

Fig. 32-6. **A** and **B,** Russian twist with dumbbell being done on an abdominal bench (**A,** side view; **B,** rear view). The dumbbell is held at 90 degrees arms-to-trunk; the trunk is held at a 90-degree angle to the thighs; the dumbbell is rotated as far as possible side-to-side; the feet can be held by any means. **C,** Russian twist (side view) being done on an abdominal bench. The arms are held across the chest, with the trunk being held over the end of the bench at about a 20-degree angle during the exercise; the trunk is rotated side-to-side as far as possible. **D** to **K,** Medicine ball abdominal board sit-ups. The athlete on the left throws the ball to the receiver on the right in the act of sitting up; the ball is thrown randomly to the receiver's center, left and right. The receiver keeps the energy of the ball going and returns it to the thrower as shown.

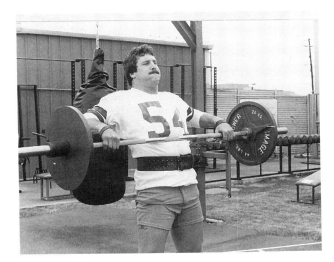

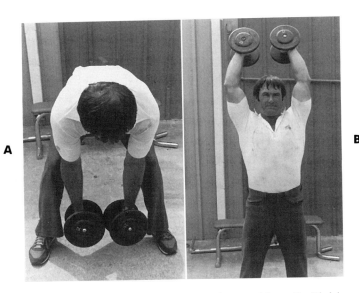

Fig. 32-7. Pull exercise. The pull can be done with or without straps. The pull can be started from the ground as shown in Fig. 32-2 or from the knees or thighs. Using the legs and back, the bar is pulled as high as possible. The elbows are kept up as shown. The athlete returns to the starting position and repeats the exercise.

Fig. 32-8. Dumbbell swing. **A,** Starting position. **B,** Finish position, standing erect. On the return, the legs are bent while the back is kept tight. The athlete returns to the starting position following the same arc of the upswing.

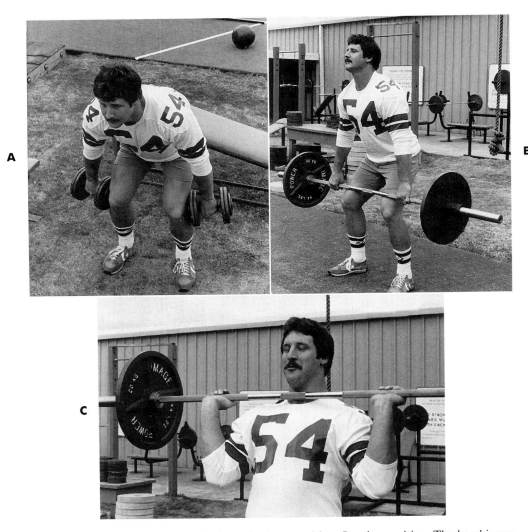

Fig. 32-9. A, Cleans with dumbbells from the hang position. Starting position. The head is up; the back is straight; the body is straightened using an explosive jumping action; the elbows are kept high. **B** and **C,** Cleans with a barbell from the hang position. **B,** Starting position. The head is up, the back is straight; the body is straightened using an explosive jumping action; the elbows are kept high. **C,** Rack position. The weight is on the shoulders; the elbows are through farther than shown to ensure resting on the shoulders; the head is up; the back is straight.

Step 4: Plyometric Training

Purpose	Exercise	Planes*	Time/Sets/Reps†
Total body	Inertial impulse (Fig. 32-12)	2-3	1-3 sets, levels 4-1 (see Table 32-5) Maximum rest recovery; maintain maximum speed possible with proper technique
Explosion	Machine		30 min (duration of session); much of this work can be part of warm-up
	Standing triple	2-3	
	Standing long jump	2	
	Hopping one leg	2	
	Bounding	2	

*Activities noted as plane 3 involve a greater rotational element in the action.
†Repetitions.

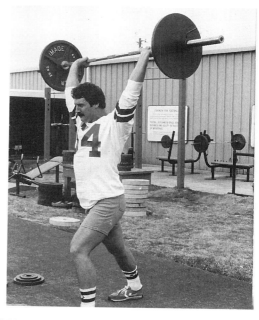

Fig. 32-11. Jerk finish using the split—shoulder-width hand grip. The weight is over the base; the chest is up; the athlete returns to the rack position and repeats the exercise.

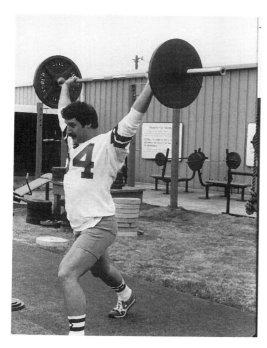

Fig. 32-10. Snatch finish using the split—wide hand grip. The weight is over the base; the chest is up; the athlete returns to the standing position and repeats the exercise.

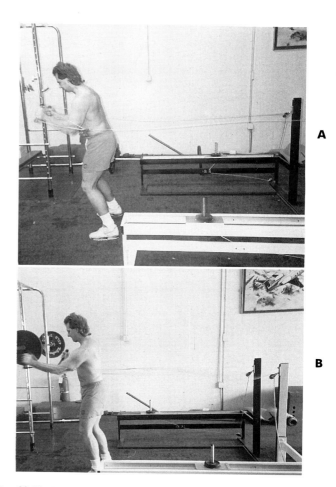

Fig. 32-12. Inertial impulse. **A,** Two-hand punching action exercise. **B,** One-hand punching action exercise.

Step 5: Sport-Loaded Exercises

Purpose	Exercise	Planes*	Time
Total body power output	Hills	2	30-60 min (duration of session)
	Stadiums	2	
	Surgical tubing	2	
	Sled/weighted	2	
	Power trainer (Fig. 32-13)	2	
	Heavier implements (shot, discus, javelin, baseball, football, soccer ball)	3	

*Activities noted as plane 3 involve a greater rotational element in the action.

Step 6: Sport Speed

Sport speed is the single most important dimension of the training program. The successful execution of the actual skill in competition *validates* the training program's expected benefits. Performance blends all of the player's personal resources, which are unrecognizable in their pure form. All skills should be practiced in similar or identical circumstances as those that would be encountered in the actual competition. It is acceptable to incorporate other activities, such as basketball, handball, court soccer, badminton, and martial arts, in practice sessions. High levels of decision making and quickness should be emphasized during play, with the implementation of as many skills per unit of time as possible.

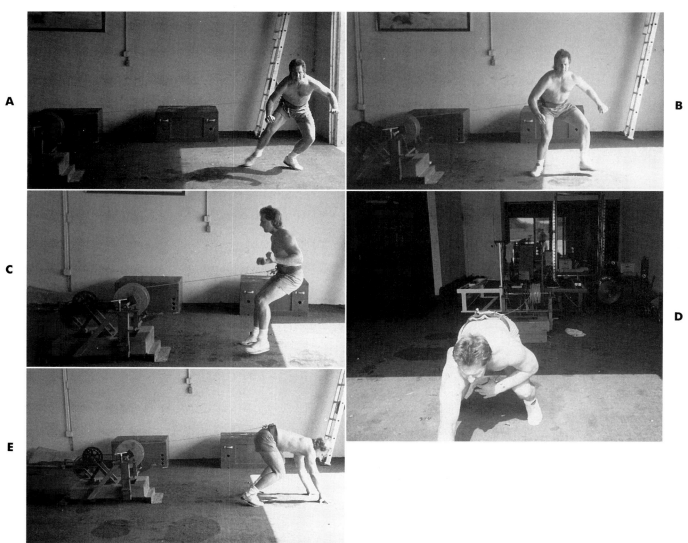

Fig. 32-13. Power trainer. **A,** Start of the lateral sliding exercise for the legs and hips. Both left and right actions are done. **B,** Lateral sliding exercise for the legs and hips. Both left and right actions are done. **C,** Back pedal exercise for the legs and hips. **D** and **E,** Forward running exercise for the whole body (**D,** front view; **E,** side view). This is an excellent exercise for developing starting power for all sports.

Step 7: Overspeed

The focus of overspeed training is on the nervous system. To accomplish this goal, it is necessary to work at lightened or assisted levels. The degree of change from the normal competitive condition is not well established to date. It is recommended that a 5% to 10% variance from normal not be exceeded. Further studies are required to determine the precise levels that produce the greatest training effect. In my opinion, however, there is a very narrow range of overspeed or sport-loaded training that is translatable or of benefit to the actual skill. This range could easily fall within plus or minus 5% of the actual performance speeds, which makes it possible to increase the rate at which the action of any skill can be completed. Good mechanics are extremely important in training and should never be disregarded during any level of work; however, they become absolutely essential in overspeed training.

SPEEDWEEK

Speedweek is a concept I developed during my years with the Dallas Cowboys. This experience demonstrated that a high-performance program of football training requires development of many human strengths. The difficulty is in allocating the proper amount of time to each of these strengths in a systematic way. Speedweek, therefore, became one possible solution to programming the players' activities during the week. Its logic is simple: work on speed and quickness when the players are fresh and rested and on endurance when they are fatigued. The more zealous players would invariably take the approach that if a little is good, more is better. Consequently, the intensity level of their total program would shift the targets from building quickness, speed, power, and strength levels to building muscle endurance or aerobic levels, which is the exact opposite effect from that desired. Certainly, the net training effects would swing to the endurance side of the training continuum. Speedweek is a three-phase concept that was developed to help players work intelligently toward the development of quickness in their on-field actions (see box above, right).

Three Phases of Speedweek Cycle

Phase 1: High-Intensity Training (Monday Through Wednesday)

Purpose: Forces the nervous system to function faster through nonfatiguing efforts and long recovery time*

Exercises

1. Overspeed
2. Sport speed
3. Body control
4. Hitting
5. Power—cleans/jerk/snatch
6. Leg work/squats done last

Phase 2: Stamina Training (Thursday and Friday)

Purpose: Forces the nervous system to sustain high-power output levels

Exercises

1. Power
2. Speed endurance
3. Muscle balancing program/muscle endurance

Phase 3: Recovery (Saturday and Sunday)

Purpose: Restoration of the body's energy stores
Saturday: Active recovery day with light intensity workloads
Sunday: Rest day that allows the body's fuel supplies to be restored

---

*No specific leg work until Wednesday's high-intensity work is completed, an interval termed *breakpoint.*

REFERENCES

1. Adrian MJ, Cooper JM: *Biomechanics of human movement,* Indianapolis, 1989, Benchmark Press.
2. Albert M: *Eccentric muscle training in sports and orthopaedics,* Edinburgh, 1991, Churchill Livingstone.
3. Chaffin D, Anderson G: *Occupational biomechanics,* New York, 1984, John Wiley & Sons.
4. Davidson, S: Unpublished data, Newman, Ga, 1991, Engineering Market Associates.
5. Dintiman G, Coleman G, Ward B: Speed improvement for baseball, *Sports Fitness,* p 25, May 1985.
6. Dintiman G, Ward R: Sport speed: the #1 speed improvement program for all athletes, *Sports Fitness* p 23, 1988.
7. Inosanto D: Unpublished data, Los Angeles, Inosanto Academy of Martial Arts.
8. Kondraske G, Ward R: *Talent assessment using a new resource economic strategy: concepts and demonstration with NFL quarterbacks* (Tech Rep 90-001R), Arlington, Tex, 1985, University of Texas at Arlington.
9. Logan GA, McKinney WC: *Kinesiology,* Dubuque, Ia, 1970, Wm C Brown.
10. Mann R: Unpublished data, Orlando, Fla, 1988, Compusport at Grand Cypress.
11. Plagenhoeff S: *Patterns of human motion,* Englewood Cliffs, NJ, 1971, Prentice-Hall.
12. Plagenhoff S: *Anatomy for rehabilitation,* Englewood Cliffs, NJ, 1987, Bennett Ergonomic Laboratories.
13. Radcliffe J, Farentino R: *Plyometrics: explosive power training,* Champaign, Ill, 1985, Human Kinetics.
14. Ward B, Ward P: *Encyclopedia of weight training,* Unpublished manuscript, 1991.
15. Ward B, Nase R: Sport speed, *Training Models in Sport,* p 6, April 1987.
16. Wilson D: Unpublished data, Newton, Mass, Advanced Medical Technologies.

Chapter Thirty-Three

Swimming

Andrew J. Cole
David R. Campbell
Dvera Berson
Richard A. Eagleston
Marilou Moschetti
Steven A. Stratton
Joseph P. Farrell

Swimming attracts athletes of all ages and all levels of conditioning. For this reason, a discussion of the diagnosis, treatment, and prevention of back and neck injuries in swimmers must cover a broad spectrum of spine care, varying from care of young swimmers, who have an amazing ability to train for hours without any injury, to care of Masters-level swimmers (referring to the U.S. Masters Swimming group), who may have to endure low back pain from lumbar facet joint arthrosis or intervertebral disc dysfunction and disease to reach their desired conditioning goals. Swimming is a particularly interesting sport for the physician, therapist, or trainer who treats patients with spinal dysfunction, spinal arthritis, or spinal injury. When incorporated into a program of trunk stabilization exercises with chest-out posturing and aerobic conditioning, certain swimming strokes are a very useful adjunct in the treatment of low back pain and neck pain. However, when a swimmer is involved in the high-mileage and long hours of training required in modern competitive swimming, chronic overuse of the shoulder, neck, back, and knees may lead to a troublesome cycle of pain, inflammation, tissue injury, and more pain.

This chapter deals with spinal problems in competitive swimmers, as well as in middle-aged and elderly persons with degenerative or inflammatory arthritides. Truly competitive swimmers strive for and expect a high level of functioning from their bodies and expect their treating physician, physical therapist, or trainer to be familiar with the treatment of spinal disorders. The more mature patient who has disabling deformity or pain from a crippling arthritic condition has more limited expectations and needs a safe and effective rehabilitation program that will increase strength while decreasing pain.

Portions of this chapter are modified from Cole AJ, Eagleston RE, Moschetti M: Swimming. In White AH, Schofferman JA, editors: *Spine care*, vol 1, *Diagnosis and conservative treatment*, St Louis, 1995, Mosby.

INCIDENCE OF SPINAL INJURIES IN COMPETITIVE SWIMMERS

As with other sports causing repetitive stress on specific anatomic structures, the incidence of injury in competitive swimmers increases proportionately with an increased duration of stress applied to the tissue or an increased number of cycles during which the tissue is subjected to stress. In swimmers the shoulder particularly is subjected to repetitive injury with subacromial and coracoclavicular ligament impingement of the rotator cuff. Impingement may originate because of glenohumeral subluxation resulting from weakness of the surrounding musculature or injury to the glenoid labrum. Intrinsic damage to the rotator cuff resulting in rotator cuff tendinitis is commonly reported in freestylers and butterfly swimmers.

In a study of shoulder injuries in competitive American swimmers, Richardson, Jobe and Collins[102] refer to shoulder pain as the most common orthopaedic problem. A study of Japanese elite competitive swimmers and synchronized swimmers found that 100% had some type of chronic musculoskeletal injury and 60% had an active chronic injury for which they were undergoing treatment. The distribution of injury according to anatomic site in the competitive swimmers was surprising. Low back pain accounted for 37% of the complaints, whereas shoulder problems accounted for only 31%.[91] The authors recognized the differences between their observations of Japanese swimmers and the published reports of American swimmers,[62,102,103] indicating that Americans have a greater incidence of shoulder problems. They concluded that the difference in the injury distribution may be because Japanese swimmers place more emphasis on their kick than their American counterparts. In the same study, low back injuries were also the most prevalent among the elite synchronized swimmers evaluated, with 45% complaining of some type of chronic back pain. The authors point out the high level of training their athletes followed, with each swimmer averaging 8 years of specialized training beginning at age 10.[91]

Richardson and Miller[103] have studied swimming and its relationship to the older athlete. They point out that degenerative arthritis of the spine is much more common in this population. The combination of degenerative disc disease with disc space narrowing, facet joint subluxation, and arthrosis alters the normal biomechanical functioning of the spinal motion unit. This can lead to worsening of back pain, radiculopathy, or neurogenic claudication if the older swimmer accentuates the normal lordotic sagittal contour of the lumbar spine with the freestyle or the butterfly stroke. This hyperextension of the lumbar spine narrows the neural foramina and spinal canal, causing foraminal stenosis with nerve root entrapment. It may also narrow the transverse and sagittal diameters of the spinal canal, leading to central or lateral recess spinal stenosis with the symptoms of neurogenic claudication.

Even though it is performed in a non-weight-bearing environment, Richardson and Miller[103] believe that competitive swimming is a "spine-intensive" activity because it requires extension and twisting of the neck and lower back. The groups of competitive swimmers most at risk for spinal pain include the more mature Masters-level swimmers with preexisting degenerative disc disease or spinal stenosis and the elite freestyle, butterfly, and breaststroke swimmers, who may swim 10,000 to 20,000 m per day in addition to cross-training with weights and running. Younger swimmers are more at risk for back and neck pain if they have underlying disc dysfunction or spondylolysis of the lumbar spine.

BIOMECHANICS OF SPINAL INJURY

Of the four competitive strokes, the freestyle and backstroke increase lumbar segmental axial rotation and thus torque forces the most and therefore place the annulus fibrosis in particular jeopardy.[7,39,40,50] This risk factor would seem to decrease in importance with the improved stroke technique seen in elite swimmers who seek to decrease head drag by having their hips follow directly behind their shoulders by rolling their bodies as a single unit. By training their bodies and thus their spines to roll as a single unit (nonsegmentally),[19-22,113] they minimize torque force across individual lumbar motion segments. However, the forces that elite swimmers develop during training and competition probably subject their lumbar spine motion segments to greater force per stroke, thus paradoxically increasing the chance of injury due to repetitive microtrauma.[7,12-15,25,80] The risk of lumbar zygapophyseal joint pain increases with strokes that include an accentuated lumbar extension, such as the butterfly and breaststroke.[113] In the performance of these two strokes, the elite athlete in particular is at risk because of an exaggerated undulation that increases sagittal motion (i.e., extension and flexion). This undulation compounds the risk of zygapophyseal injury due to repetitive microtrauma. Even

with the breaststroke, traditionally a controlled swimming style, recent advances in stroke technique have resulted in a significant increase in sagittal plane motion by emphasizing undulatory rather than linear, plane, and horizontal motion.[63] Although injury to the pars interarticularis may be seen more frequently in competitive divers,[104] many swimmers with a quiescent spondylolysis may develop symptoms because of the repetitive extensions that occur with the breaststroke, butterfly stroke, starts, and turns. Furthermore, the risk of developing a pars stress reaction, spondylolysis, or spondylolisthesis caused by stress placed on the posterior column of the spine by these strokes remains unclear.

Although injuries to the thoracic spine seem to occur less frequently and appear to be more easily rehabilitated, these structures are nonetheless at risk. Most common is thoracic zygapophyseal pain, especially with strokes that generate a great degree of increased segmental rotatory motion at particular thoracic motion segments, such as the freestyle and backstroke. The extension required in the butterfly and breaststroke may cause zygapophyseal joint dysfunction and pain. The pain and concomitant inflammation result from repetitive zygapophyseal joint compression, distraction, and shear forces.[19,21,24] During the pull phase, compressive forces are generated by the ipsilateral latissimus dorsi, scapular, retractors, and long thoracic spinal extensor muscle groups. Ipsilateral thoracic spinal muscle groups produce thoracic spinal extension to counter the thoracic spinal flexion created by the latissimus dorsi. The contralateral thoracic spinal muscle groups stabilize the thoracic spine, preventing untoward lateral flexion toward the pull-phase side. Passive distractive forces affect the ipsilateral zygapophyseal joint during the recovery phase because of activation of the ipsilateral scapular protractors, relaxation of the scapular retractors, inactivation of the latissimus dorsi, and relative relaxation of the thoracic spinal extensor muscle groups.[14,15,92,98,109]

Thoracic costovertebral joints may be injured as a result of a significantly increased vital capacity and enhanced chest wall and rib motion. These joints may be further compromised by arm elevation and the consequent increased tension on the rib system. In addition, faulty stroke mechanics resulting in increased rotation through the thoracic spine may also contribute to costovertebral joint pain.

The cervical spine is subjected to continuous repetitive microtrauma from the mechanics of breathing. Annular as well as zygapophyseal injuries are most commonly seen with the freestyle stroke because of the significant rotation required for side breathing.[14,15,24] Occasionally a side-breathing technique is used during the butterfly stroke, also placing the cervical segments at increased risk. Extension, which is seen with the breaststroke and butterfly stroke, increases the chance of cervical posterior element injury, resulting in cervical zygapophyseal pain. Cervical extension may also increase intradiscal pressure, compromising the intervertebral disc.[54] Although the backstroke requires little rotation for breathing, exceptional stabilization of the cervical segments in a relatively neutral position is needed to decrease drag forces. Therefore fewer intrinsic cervical segmental injuries occur with this stroke. However, muscular strain to the cervical dynamic stabilizing soft tissues, such as the paraspinal muscle groups, sternocleidomastoid muscles, and upper trapezius, is common. Note should be made of the risk of catastrophic cervical spine injury due to impact loading.[2,51,64,68] The greatest potential for this type of injury occurs with faulty start mechanics and, less commonly, with impact loading of the cervical spine during a missed turn—particularly during the backstroke, where the oncoming wall is not seen and overhead warning flags are not observed.[12,13,90]

GENERAL SPINAL ABNORMALITIES

Patients with Scheuermann's kyphosis were found to develop increased pain during swimming, particularly during the butterfly stroke, as seen in a study by Wilson and Lindseth.[123] Of the four competitive strokes, the butterfly includes the greatest end-range extension of the diseased, less-mobile thoracic motion segments. Increased pectoral and associated chest and abdominal muscle contractions during the pull phase of a stroke such as the butterfly may cause additional compressive forces that further damage anterior column structures.[5] However, because these muscles are also significantly active during the pull phase of the freestyle stroke and breaststroke,[11,89,92,97,98] repetitive end-range extension microtrauma may be the primary biomechanical source of pain in the butterfly stroke. Although kyphotic patients can be managed conservatively with daily bracing, additional time out of the brace was suggested to allow continued swimming. So long as the butterfly stroke was avoided, no deleterious change was noted.[123] In addition, because of the swimmer's horizontal position in the water and the buoyant effect of the water, the axial compressive forces on the spine[89] are significantly reduced. This positioning and buoyancy may therefore significantly mitigate any potential mechanical risk factors that may cause this condition to progress.

The prevalence of adolescent idiopathic scoliosis is approximately 2% to 3%.[119] In the athletic population, the average frequency of idiopathic scoliosis has been reported to be 2%,[73] and the incidence of functional scoliosis 33.5%.[71] The higher incidence of functional scoliosis in the athletic population may be due to larger unilateral torque forces developed in particular activities such as serving and throwing.[73] Becker[3,4] showed a 6.9% incidence of idiopathic scoliosis and a 16% incidence of functional scoliosis in the screening of 336 swimmers at

the Junior Olympic Swimming Championships, East, 1983. The 6.9% figure is roughly three times the reported incidence of structural idiopathic scoliosis, but the 16% figure is below the incidence reported by Krahl and Steinbruck.[71] However, 100% of the functional curves were toward the dominant-hand side, which, according to Yeater et al.,[128] consistently produces greater pull-phase peak forces than the nondominant side. Further studies summarized by Becker revealed histologic and morphologic changes in the paraspinal and gluteus muscles, secondary adaptation of supporting vertebral soft tissues, and adaptive changes in muscles to meet specific repetitive functional demands.[3] However, if curve progression is truly facilitated by the asymmetric functional demands swimming places on the spine, a therapeutic exercise program could theoretically be designed to counter them. Moreover, exercise alone is unable to inhibit the progression of a scoliotic curve,[3] and it remains to be shown whether it can accelerate curve progression. In addition, the most recent advances in swimming technique (especially in the freestyle stroke) emphasize symmetric motion (e.g., alternate-side breathing) and minimize repetitive unilateral torsion and lateral flexion. Proper coaching should help to further deemphasize the potential effect of a stronger dominant side on the spine. Swimming is not contraindicated for the adolescent with functional or idiopathic scoliosis if there is appropriate training by the patient's therapist and coach, both of whom should know swimming technique and mechanics. In fact, with proper technique, aquatic activity may help the scoliotic patient to maintain flexibility, strength, and endurance while minimizing axial compressive forces and shear forces on the spine.

PERIPHERAL JOINT DYSFUNCTION

Peripheral joint dysfunction can set off a cascading series of motion changes throughout the spinal axis. The cervicothoracic and thoracolumbar transition zones are the most commonly affected because they are the junction between the more mobile and less mobile sections of the spine.[22,96] Fig. 33-1 presents the "motion cascade," originally described by Cole and Herring.[19] For example, a shoulder injury such as rotator cuff tendinitis results in guarding and decreased shoulder range of motion.[19,23,24,26] The swimmer's arm cannot abduct and extend as it normally would[60] during recovery, resulting in decreased body roll, increased lumbar segmental motion, and an abnormally low head position from which to breathe.[20] Compensatory adaptive changes include crane breathing (increased cervical suboccipital extension [OA] and rotation [AA], cervical extension [C2 to C7], and cervical rotation [C2 to C7]) (Fig. 33-2), as well as even more extension and rotation from C3 to C5.[24] The C5 to T1 segments ultimately become hypomobile to compensate, and mid- and

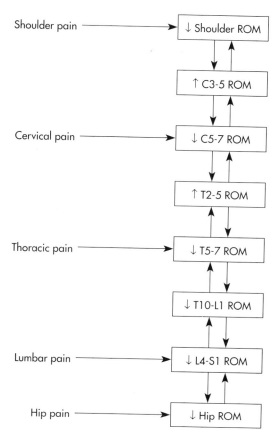

Fig. 33-1. Peripheral joint dysfunction can set off a "motion cascade" throughout the spinal axis; conversely, spinal dysfunction can create peripheral joint dysfunction. ↓, Decreased; ↑ increased; *C,* cervical; *T,* thoracic, *L,* lumbar; *S,* sacral; *ROM,* range of motion. (From Moschetti M: *Aquaphysics made simple,* Aptos, Calif, 1989, AquaTechnics Consulting Group.)

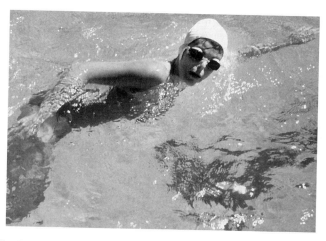

Fig. 33-2. Crane breathing during the freestyle: a biomechanical adaptation that improves access to air by increasing capital and cervical spine extension and rotation. It can occur for a variety of reasons, most commonly as a result of a poor body roll. (From Moschetti M: *Aquaphysics made simple,* Aptos, Calif, 1989, AquaTechnics Consulting Group.)

low-cervical pain results. Compensatory hypermobility from T2 to T5 and hypomobility from T5 to T7 and T10 to L1 begin. Primary cervical, thoracic, and lumbar injuries and pain influence the spinal axis in a similar fashion. Hip,[122] pelvis, and lumbar spine pain result in hypomobility at L4 to S1 and ultimately at the T10 to L1 transition zone. Adaptive changes then proceed up the axis and may even set the stage for a compensatory change in shoulder mechanics and ultimately cause a shoulder injury. Identification of the initial injury is important so that treatment can eliminate that problem, as well as the secondary compensatory sites of dysfunction.[19,24,65]

NECK INJURIES

The orientation of the cervical spine anatomy is such that hyperextension of the neck with a resultant accentuation of the normal cervical lordosis causes a narrowing of the diameter of the central spinal canal and a narrowing of the neural foramina. In the swimmer with preexisting cervical disc disease, the position of neck extension and head elevation, coupled with torsion of the neck for breathing, may aggravate cervical facet pain or nerve root entrapment. The resultant neck and arm pain may be quite problematic in the high-level performer.

A more common complaint among competitive swimmers involves pain from a chronic overuse syndrome, with burning pain in the back of the neck and at the cervicothoracic junction, often radiating caudally to the interscapular region. This may be more of a diagnostic challenge, especially if most of the pain is present at the levator scapula and rhomboid musculature region. The athlete with discogenic symptoms may have no objective neurologic findings but will complain of neck pain and possibly referred pain to the anterior chest, shoulders, posterior cervical region, and scapular regions. Posterior occipital headaches and occipital neuralgia from greater occipital nerve irritation may occur. It has been suggested that stimulation of the adjacent sensory receptors of the sinovertebral nerve in the annulus fibrosis and the anterior and posterior longitudinal ligaments is responsible for these referred pain patterns. The most caudal cervical spine motion units refer pain to the interscapular region of the upper back. However, local muscle, tendinous attachments, and bursae can also be irritated from chronic overuse in the swimmer, leading to a similar clinical picture.

Paris[96] has stressed the importance of considering the thoracic outlet as a potential site of pathologic entrapment of neurovascular structures in the swimmer. The overhead activities with extremes of abduction and external rotation of the shoulder can lead to entrapment of neurovascular structures from either the anterior and middle scalene muscles or a first cervical rib. This may occur in an individual with enlarged scalene musculature or a variation of normal anatomy. The thoracic outlet syndrome may have a varied and imprecise clinical presentation with parasthesias, pain, or weakness in many different combinations, leading to a difficulty in diagnosis if the syndrome is not considered.

BACK INJURIES

The differential diagnosis for a young competitive swimmer with back pain is significantly different from the differential diagnosis for a mature athlete with spinal or referred leg pain. An appropriate and complete history of any injury or of the factors leading up to the development of back pain is critical. Often no one single injury can be recalled by the athlete, only a long history of pain and discomfort that is made worse by a particular stroke or noticed when there is an acceleration in the level of training. In the young competitive swimmer, pars interarticularis stress fractures with spondylolysis or spondylolisthesis, facet joint capsule or posterior spinal ligamentous inflammation, Scheuermann's kyphosis, osteoid osteoma, inflammatory/infectious discitis, annulus fibrosis tears, annular disruption with herniation of the nucleus pulposus, and muscular sprains and strains may be similar in their clinical presentation. Pain with accentuation of the normal lumbar lordosis in spinal hyperextension is characteristic of spondylolysis and spondylolisthesis. Facet joint capsule irritation or tendinitis and ligament inflammation from chronic overuse may also cause pain with prolonged extension of the lumbosacral spine, as occurs with the freestyle stroke or breaststroke. The abrupt change from spinal flexion to extension with an aggressive butterfly stroke or breaststroke may exacerbate low back pain. Scheuermann's kyphosis, a spinal disorder characterized by an increase in the normal curve of the thoracic spine, has been associated with backaches that were particularly aggravated by swimming the butterfly stroke, according to a report by Wilson and Lindseth.[123] They coined the term "adolescent swimmer's back" to describe this syndrome.

Severe pain out of proportion to the objective clinical findings, with the pain relieved by aspirin-containing products, is characteristic of osteoid osteoma. Progressive, severe, and constant back pain, perhaps with a fever and elevated erythrocyte sedimentation rate, may be found with childhood discitis. Back pain, paraspinal muscle spasm, and leg pain with positive nerve tension signs can be found in the unusual child or adolescent with a herniated lumbar disc and sciatica or femoral neuritis. There seems to be a familial association in the occurrence of herniated lumbar intervertebral discs in youngsters.

The older swimmer/athlete with spinal or leg pain requires a careful history, physical examination (including rectal examination), and diagnostic studies to safely exclude serious disease. Nonmechanical or resting spinal pain can be caused by primary or metastatic tumors, vertebral osteomyelitis, inflammatory arthritides, referred pain from expanding or dissecting aortic aneurysms, visceral tumors, or other intraabdominal or intrapelvic pathology. Fever, night sweats, recent weight loss, and a history of coexisting disease must be sought from the mature athlete with spinal pain. These patients may also have complaints of referred arm or leg pain in a discogenic or radicular pattern.

Structural spinal disorders in the mature swimmer include degenerative disc disease; segmental spinal instability with spondylolisthesis or scoliosis, including vertebral subluxation in the sagittal, coronal, or axial planes; spinal stenosis, including central, lateral recess, or foraminal stenosis; and facet joint arthropathy. The mature athlete with a structural spinal disorder may complain of mechanical spinal or leg pain associated with standing, walking, or swimming the freestyle stroke, butterfly stroke, or breaststroke. These activities position the lumbar spine in extension with resultant narrowing of the neural foramina and the spinal canal.

Neurogenic claudication must always be differentiated from vascular claudication in the mature swimmer. The onset of cramping leg pain after exercising with the spine in extension, or even after just walking, can be due to spinal stenosis or peripheral vascular disease. Appropriate clinical questioning will generally indicate the cause of this type of leg pain. With neurogenic claudication caused by lumbar spine stenosis, the leg pain is caused by the narrowing of the spinal canal with bone and soft tissue encroaching into the canal. The increased mechanical pressure on the nerve roots traversing the constricted area leads to progressive venous stasis, arterial compromise, or direct mechanical deformation of the nerves, with resultant leg pain. Spinal flexion relieves these symptoms by increasing the area available for the nerve roots. Swimming the backstroke or a modified sidestroke, following the Berson program[6] for arthritic patients (described at the end of this chapter), or riding an exercise bicycle while leaning forward will enable the spinal canal to increase in diameter.

The pain of vascular claudication typically starts below the knee and has a reproducible onset after a certain distance or duration of exercise. The pain progresses proximally up the limb after starting in the foot or calf. It is described as being more of a cramping-type pain than the aching pain of neurogenic claudication. It is generally relieved within 1 to 5 minutes after stopping the exercise or after having stopped walking. It is not relieved by spinal flexion and is associated with diminished pedal pulses. Neurogenic claudication typically starts in the posterior buttock, thigh, or calf and progresses distally to the foot. It cannot be relieved by simply stopping the activity but requires a change in position from spinal extension to spinal flexion. It may take many minutes to resolve and may be associated with more complaints of prolonged numbness.

Pure back pain is not uncommon with structural disorders of the spine. Segmental spinal instability with abnormal and pathologic motion between adjacent spinal motion units may cause incapacitating spinal pain that is exacerbated by activities. Lumbar spine–bending films are instrumental in making the diagnosis of segmental spinal instability. Discography is a helpful diagnostic tool in patients with incapacitating spinal pain after lumbar surgery if surgical arthrodesis is being contemplated. In addition, contrast-enhanced computed tomography scans, contrast-enhanced (gadolinium) magnetic resonance imaging, and electromyograms/nerve conduction studies are essential components of the evaluation with failed lumbar spine surgery. Postlaminectomy patients present particularly difficult diagnostic problems because radicular and back pain can be produced by nerve root scarring and adhesions to the posterior wall of the vertebral body, by recurrent disc herniation, by persistent postoperative nerve root entrapment or compression, or by segmental spinal instability due to loss of the intrinsic supporting structures both within and adjacent to the intervertebral disc.

The mature swimmer with predominantly sciatic or femoral distribution leg pain requires the classic diagnostic differentiation between a herniated disc with sciatica and spinal stenosis with neurogenic claudication. The differential diagnosis is between a structural abnormality causing nerve root tension from a herniated intervertebral disc and nerve root compression from spinal stenosis. Activities that increase nerve root tension in patients with a herniated disc in the lower lumbar spine with sciatica include spinal flexion, hip flexion, knee extension, neck flexion, and foot dorsiflexion. A more cephalad herniated disc, causing femoral nerve root pain, produces nerve root tension and pain with hip extension and knee flexion. Sitting, coughing, sneezing, and straining increase intradiscal and intraspinal pressure, exacerbating the symptoms of a disc herniation. Positive findings of a straight leg raising test, together with positive findings of a crossed, straight leg raising test, is characteristic of nerve root tension from a herniated lumbar disc, especially with the patient sitting at the edge of the examining table.

DIAGNOSIS AND TREATMENT

The work-up and diagnosis of spinal pain in swimmers is no different from that for any other athlete. The astute clinician has a thorough understanding of anatomy and stroke-specific functional biomechanics that enables development of a thorough treatment plan, including a complete rehabilitation program. The rehabilitation program must address the primary injury, as well as any secondary sites of dysfunction.[24,55,66,99] In addition, the physician must be cognizant of the great physiologic and psychologic needs of elite competitive athletes. For example, highly competitive athletes require alternate training regimens during their rehabilitation programs to maintain peak flexibility, strength, and aerobic conditioning. Recreational swimmers may be more flexible in this regard. Therefore the aggressiveness of the work-up and rehabilitation program should be geared to the level of the athlete's need. The need to make changes in land-based training and specific stroke mechanics as part of the rehabilitation process requires close cooperation among the patient, therapist, and coach.*

Dynamic land-based stabilization training is a specific type of therapeutic exercise that can help patients gain control of segmental spine forces, eliminate repetitive injury to their motion segments (i.e., discs, zygapophyseal joints, and related structures), encourage healing of injured motion segments, and possibly alter the degenerative process. The underlying premise is that motion segments and their supporting soft tissues react to minimize applied stresses and thereby reduce the risk of injury.[106] The details of dynamic land-based stabilization training are described elsewhere in the text. The goals of aquatic stabilization exercise and swimming programs incorporate these elements but take into account the unique properties of the aqueous medium so that risk of spinal injury is minimized (see also Chapter 26). In particular, aquatic stabilization programs help develop an athlete's flexibility, strength, and body mechanics so that a smooth transition to aquatic stabilization swimming programs may occur. Aquatic stabilization swimming programs then help the injured swimmer to minimize segmental trunk motion and shear forces; reinforce lumbar control; encourage hip, knee, and ankle propulsion; develop head and neck stability; and establish arm control and strength.[14,15,19-22,27]

Rehabilitation Environment: Land Versus Water

Accurate diagnosis of patients' spinal injuries and observation of their initial response to land-based stabilization help determine further therapeutic exercise treatment options. A transition from dry to wet exercise conditions eliminates dry-land risks, establishes a supportive training environment, provides a new therapeutic activity, decreases the risk of peripheral joint injury, and allows a return to a prior activity. Moving from dry to wet environments should also be considered if patients have an intolerance for axial or gravitational loads or require increased support in the presence of a strength or proprioceptive deficit. Remaining in a water-supported environment is appropriate if the dry environment exacerbates symptoms or the patient has a preference for the water. Transition from a wet to a dry environment should occur if patients are doing well in the water and need to return to land to most efficiently meet functional training needs in order to attain their ultimate competitive

*References 16, 19, 21, 22, 24, 100, 106, 113.

Contraindications to Aquatic Rehabilitation

1. Fever
2. Cardiac failure
3. Urinary tract infections
4. Bowel and/or bladder incontinence
5. Open wounds
6. Infectious diseases
7. Contagious skin conditions
8. Excessive fear of water
9. Uncontrolled seizures
10. Colostomy bag or catheter used by patient
11. Cognitive/functional impairment that creates a hazard to the patient or others in pool
12. *Severely* weakened or deconditioned state that poses a safety hazard
13. *Extremely* poor endurance
14. *Severely* decreased range of motion that limits function and poses a safety hazard

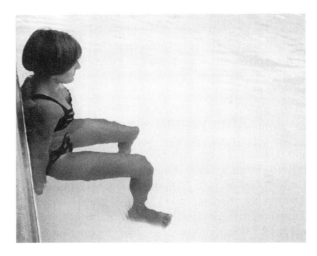

Fig. 33-3. The wall sit develops isometric strength primarily in the quadriceps and hamstring groups. Abdominal muscles are trained to hold an appropriate dynamic posture. (From Moschetti M: *Aquaphysics made simple,* Aptos, Calif, 1989, AquaTechnics Consulting Group.)

goals.[12-15] See box above for specific contraindications to aquatic rehabilitation.[16,21,100]

Aquatic Stabilization Techniques

The same principles of spinal stabilization that have been discussed for land programs are applicable to aquatic programs. Certain exercises that can be performed on land cannot be reproduced in water and vice versa. Aquatic programs can be designed for those unable to train on land or for those whose land training has plateaued. Aquatic stabilization was first described by Eagleston[37] in 1989.

The advantages that aquatic programs offer are directly related to the intrinsic properties of water, including buoyancy, resistance, viscosity, hydrostatic pressure, temperature, turbulence, and refraction. The details regarding these properties are described elsewhere.[13,15,18,20-22] Graded elimination of gravitational forces through buoyancy allows the patient to train with decreased yet variable axial loads and shear forces. In essence, water increases the safety margin of patient postural error by decreasing the compressive and shear forces on the spine. The velocity of motion can be better controlled by water resistance, viscosity, buoyancy, and the training devices used. Buoyancy increases the available range of training positions. The psychologic outlook of athletes can be enhanced because rehabilitation occurs in their competitive environment. Many believe that a certain degree of pain attenuation takes place in the water because of the "sensory overload" generated by hydrostatic pressure, temperature, and turbulence.*

* References 12, 13, 29, 30, 53, 67, 69, 72, 73, 80, 83-85, 89, 92, 94, 97, 98, 104-106, 111.

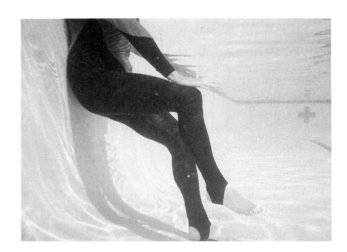

Fig. 33-4. Level 1 partial wall sit-ups train muscles activated in the wall sit and also challenge contralateral gluteals, ipsilateral hip flexors, and rotational abdominals and paraspinals. (From Moschetti M: *Aquaphysics made simple,* Aptos, Calif, 1989, AquaTechnics Consulting Group.)

A set of six core aquatic stabilization exercises with three levels of difficulty has been designed to provide graded training of stabilization skills.[12,13,15,20-22,28] Table 33-1 and Figs. 33-3 to 33-16 illustrate a typical aquatic exercise progression for a patient with lumbar discogenic pain. Programs must be customized to meet the needs of each patient's unique spinal problem, related musculoskeletal dysfunction, and comfort with the aquatic environment. Once mastered, a more advanced program is provided. Eventually, the swimming athlete works through a series of transitional aquatic stabilization

Table 33-1. Aquatic Stabilization Exercises: Progression for Lumbar Discogenic Pain

Exercise	Level 1	Level 2	Level 3
Wall sit	Isometric 90-degree hip 90-degree knee 1-min hold	Isometric 90-degree hip 90-degree knee 3-min hold	Isometric 90-degree hip 90-degree knee 5-min hold
Partial wall sit-up	Isometric Hip flexion Unilateral Alternating 90-degree hip 90-degree knee 5-sec hold 60-sec per side	Isotonic Hip flexion Bilateral Simultaneous 45-degree hip 90-degree knee Repetitions: 2 min	Isotonic Hip flexion Bilateral Simultaneous 45-degree hip Knee: full extension Repetitions: 3 min
Modified superman	Face wall Hip extension to 20 degrees Knee: 45-degree static Unilateral 60 sec per side	Face wall Hip extension to 20 degrees Knee: full extension Unilateral 2 min per side	Face wall Hip extension to 20 degrees Knee: full extension Unilateral 3 min per side 3-lb ankle cuffs
Water walk backward	Palms at side 3 min Slow speed*	Palms forward Abduct arms 45 degrees 5 min Moderate speed†	Palms forward Abduct arms 45 degrees Hand paddles 10 min Fast speed‡
Water walk forward	Palms at side 3 min Slow speed*	Palms forward Abduct arms 45 degrees 5 min Moderate speed†	Palms forward Abduct arms 45 degrees Hand paddles 10 min Fast speed‡
Quadruped	Therapist assistance Prone Mask/snorkle Alternating arms only, 1 min Alternating legs only, 1 min	Therapist assistance Prone Mask/snorkle Simultaneous or alternating arms/legs 3 min	No assistance Ski belt Prone Mask/snorkle Simultaneous or alternating arms/legs 5 min

*Slow = 50% of potential maximum velocity.
†Moderate = 70% of potential maximum velocity.
‡Fast = 85% of potential maximum velocity.

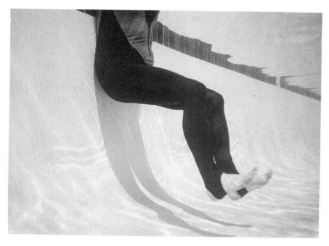

Fig. 33-5. Level 2 partial wall sit-ups train hip flexors and hip extensors bilaterally and isotonically. Higher-level isometric conditioning continues for abdominal and paraspinal muscle groups. (From Moschetti M: *Aquaphysics made simple,* Aptos, Calif, 1989, AquaTechnics Consulting Group.)

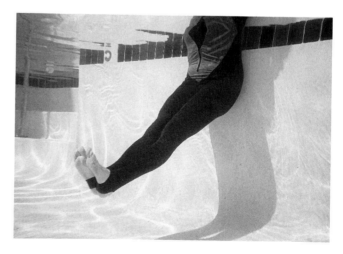

Fig. 33-6. Level 3 partial wall sit-ups provide an incrementally greater challenge to all groups described in Fig. 33-5. (From Moschetti M: *Aquaphysics made simple,* Aptos, Calif, 1989, AquaTechnics Consulting Group.)

exercises that help reestablish a spine-stabilized swimming style that minimizes the risk of further spinal injury and helps maximize swimming performance.[12-15]

Prone swimming. Once patients' stabilization skills have progressed to the point where a return to swimming is possible, a thorough analysis of stroke technique and its effect on spinal motion is critical. The following overview focuses on lumbar spine injury and indicates the role that the cervical spine plays in the mechanics of lumbar

aquatic motion. The detailed case presentation that follows focuses on the cervical spine.

Stroke mechanics analysis, like gait analysis, should be done in an ordered sequential manner so that all deficits and the relationships among them are carefully scrutinized. The analysis typically begins with the head and continues distally.

In prone swimming, the head should be midline. Breathing should occur by turning the head (i.e., rotating

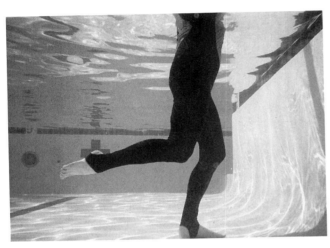

Fig. 33-7. Level 1 modified "superman" develops strength in the ipsilateral hip flexors and extensors and the contralateral gluteus medius, as well as isometric strength in the abdominal and paraspinal stabilizers. (From Moschetti M: *Aquaphysics made simple,* Aptos, Calif, 1989, AquaTechnics Consulting Group.)

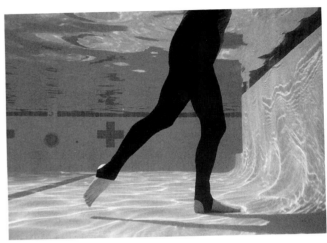

Fig. 33-8. Level 2 modified superman provides an incrementally greater challenge to all groups described in Fig. 33-7. (From Moschetti M: *Aquaphysics made simple,* Aptos, Calif, 1989, AquaTechnics Consulting Group.)

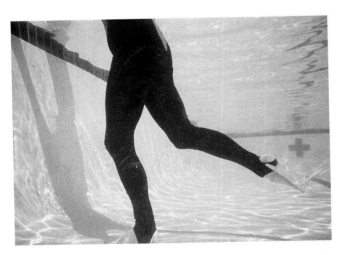

Fig. 33-9. Level 3 modified superman again incrementally enhances resistive exercise and training duration of activity for muscle groups previously described for this component of the progression. (From Moschetti M: *Aquaphysics made simple,* Aptos, Calif, 1989, AquaTechnics Consulting Group.)

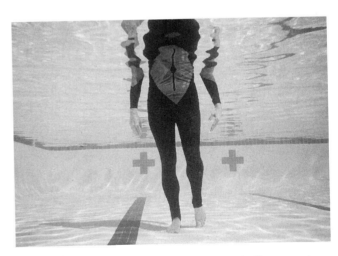

Fig. 33-10. Level 1 walking forward isometrically strengthens the abdominal muscle groups and those groups involved in maintaining proper posture. Isotonic strengthening occurs in those muscles dynamically involved in gait. Walking backward provides a similar strengthening pattern with greater emphasis on isometric paraspinal muscle conditioning. (From Moschetti M: *Aquaphysics made simple,* Aptos, Calif, 1989, AquaTechnics Consulting Group.)

the head along the axial plane). There should be no craning (i.e., suboccipital cervical extension [OA] and rotation [AA], or cervical extension and rotation [C2 to C7] (see Fig. 33-4). The body roll also contributes to proper breathing mechanics and is essential to minimize dysfunctional cervical positioning and subsequent pain. The cervical spine should be kept in the neutral position along the sagittal plane, since excessive extension causes the legs and torso to drop in the water, whereas excessive flexion can cause a struggle for air.[12-15,20-22,24]

Upper body arm position is evaluated by stroke phase (see box at right). The freestyle stroke is divided into

---

Swimming Stroke Phases (Freestyle)

Entry Phase
1. Hand entry
2. Hand submersion ("ride")

Pull Phase	Recovery Phase
1. Insweep	1. Exit
2. Outsweep	2. Arm swing
3. Finish	

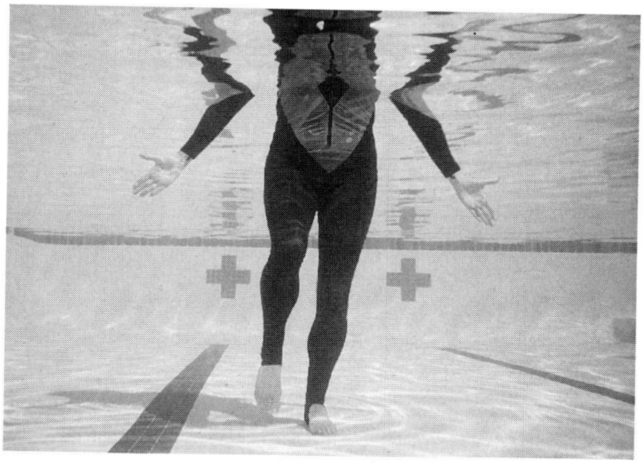

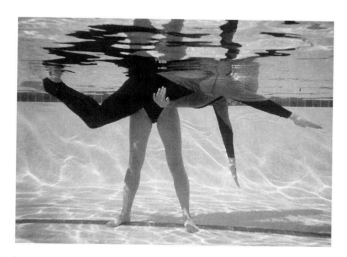

Fig. 33-11. Level 2 walking forward and backward provides incrementally greater challenge to all groups described in Fig. 33-10. (From Moschetti M: *Aquaphysics made simple,* Aptos, Calif, 1989, AquaTechnics Consulting Group.)

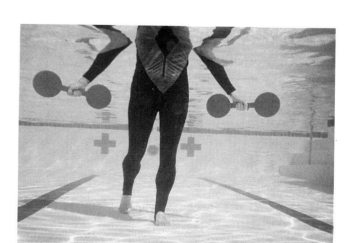

Fig. 33-12. Level 3 walking forward and backward incrementally enhances resistive exercise and training duration of activity for muscle groups previously described for this component of the progression. (From Moschetti M: *Aquaphysics made simple,* Aptos, Calif, 1989, AquaTechnics Consulting Group.)

Fig. 33-13. Level 1 quadruped activities (arms only) challenge lumbar spine stabilizer groups isometrically and upper extremity shoulder groups that produce flexion and extension isotonically. (From Moschetti M: *Aquaphysics made simple,* Aptos, Calif, 1989, AquaTechnics Consulting Group.)

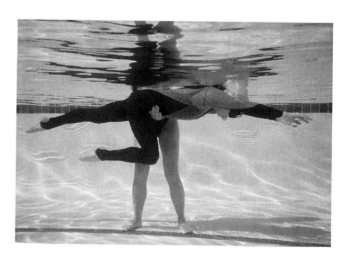

Fig. 33-14. Level 1 quadruped activities (legs only) challenge lumbar spine stabilizer groups isometrically and lower extremity hip flexors and extensors isotonically. (From Moschetti M: *Aquaphysics made simple,* Aptos, Calif, 1989, AquaTechnics Consulting Group.)

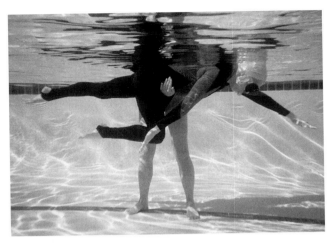

Fig. 33-15. Level 2 quadruped activities incrementally and isometrically challenge lumbar spine stabilizer groups and continue to isotonically train the upper and lower extremity groups previously described in Figs. 33-13 and 33-14. (From Moschetti M: *Aquaphysics made simple,* Aptos, Calif, 1989, AquaTechnics Consulting Group.)

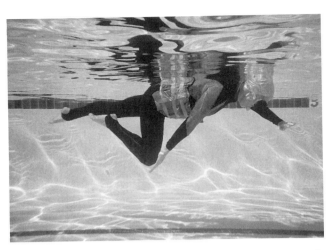

Fig. 33-16. Level 3 quadruped exercise again increases the training intensity progression by requiring greater independence during performance of the exercise. (From Moschetti M: *Aquaphysics made simple,* Aptos, Calif, 1989, AquaTechnics Consulting Group.)

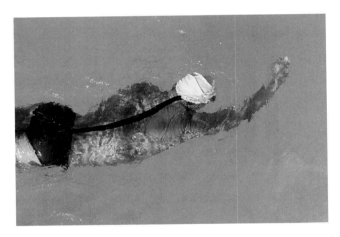

Fig. 33-17. The swimmer's arm abducts beyond 180 degrees during the entry phase of the freestyle. This stroke defect creates lateral lumbar flexion and lumbar segmental rotation. (From Moschetti M: *Aquaphysics made simple,* Aptos, Calif, 1989, AquaTechnics Consulting Group.)

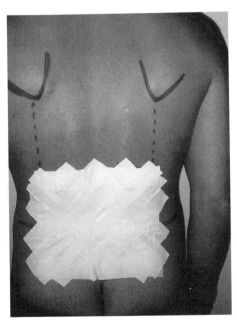

Fig. 33-18. Waterproof strapping tape can be applied to the lumbar spine to reinforce lumbar proprioceptive awareness and help minimize lumbar rotation and lateral flexion. (From Moschetti M: *Aquaphysics made simple,* Aptos, Calif, 1989, AquaTechnics Consulting Group.)

three phases. The entry phase includes both hand entry and hand submersion ("ride"). The pull phase incorporates insweep, outsweep, and finish components. The recovery phase includes the exit and arm swing.[113] There are several stroke defects that can cause poor lumbar mechanics. If the arm abducts beyond 180 degrees, lateral lumbar flexion and rotation are produced (Fig. 33-17). During the pull phase, decreased body rotation can cause lateral lumbar flexion and rotation, which stresses the lumbar motion segments, particularly the annular fibers surrounding the nucleus pulposus. Inadequate triceps strength during the finish phase results in

low arm recovery, which in turn generates secondary lateral flexion and rotation through the lumbar spine. During recovery, an inadequate body roll causes the neck to crane, which results in a struggle for air and accompanying lateral flexion and rotation through the lumbar spine.[12-14,19,22,24]

Table 33-2. Freestyle Stroke Defects

Primary Peripheral Joint Stroke Defect	Secondary Effect	Reaction of Spine
Head high	Lower body sinks	Increased cervical extension Increased lumbar extension
Head low	Upper body sinks	Increased lumbar flexion
Crane breathing	Lower body sinks Contralateral shoulder sinks	Increased cervical and suboccipital extension Increased cervical rotation Increased lumbar lateral flexion and rotation
Crossover hand entry	Lateral body movement	Increased lumbar lateral flexion and rotation
Wide hand entry	Contralateral shoulder roll	Increased cervical rotation Increased lumbar lateral flexion and rotation
Inefficient pull power	Upper body sinks Difficulty breathing	Increased cervical rotation Increased cervical extension Increased lumbar extension Increased lumbar lateral flexion and rotation
Increased hip flexion	Decreased kick propulsion Lower body sinks	Increased cervical extension Increased lumbar extension Increased lumbar lateral flexion and rotation
Crossover kick	Decreased kick propulsion Increased hip roll Lower body sinks	Increased cervical extension Increased lumbar extension Increased compensatory lumbar lateral flexion and rotation
Increased knee flexion	Decreased kick propulsion Lower body sinks	Increased cervical extension Increased lumbar extension
Increased ankle dorsiflexion	Decreased kick propulsion Increased hip roll Lower body sinks	Increased cervical extension Increased lumbar extension Increased compensatory lumbar lateral flexion and rotation

Trunk motion is closely monitored for any primary or secondary lumbar flexion, both sagittal and coronal, or for axial rotation. If abnormal motion is not corrected by simple changes in stroke mechanics, additional proprioceptive cues can be provided by taping the lumbar spine region. The tape pulls on the skin each time the lumbar spine moves in a segmental manner (i.e., when the patient generates excessive lumbar rotation or lateral lumbar flexion[27] [Fig. 33-18]). Table 33-2 delineates how these and other primary peripheral joint freestyle stroke defects and secondary effects can create abnormal spinal mechanics during swimming that may cause or exacerbate a painful spinal dysfunction.

Flip turns are discouraged. Instead, stabilized turns are employed in which the patient initially comes to a vertical position before turning. This vertical position allows the patient the opportunity to stabilize the spine in preparation for changing direction. Eventually, a horizontal spin is incorporated into the turn, and the vertical position is eliminated. Flip turns may then be resumed.[12-15,20-22,113]

Supine swimming. In the supine position, starting with a simple kicking program is best, with the arms at the sides, since adequate stabilization can be easily maintained. The use of fins is often suggested to improve propulsion. While the patient is supine, extension of the cervical

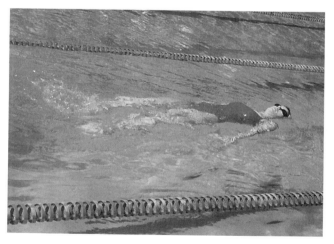

Fig. 33-19. Cervical spine extension induces lumbar extension while the patient is supine. (From Moschetti M: *Aquaphysics made simple,* Aptos, Calif, 1989, AquaTechnics Consulting Group.)

spine will induce lumbar extension (Fig. 33-19). On the other hand, cervical flexion will cause the patient to "sit" in the water with a lowered leg position and decreased propulsion (Fig. 33-20). Extreme cervical extension or flexion is to be avoided in favor of a more neutral stabilized cervical posture.[12-15,19-22,24,113]

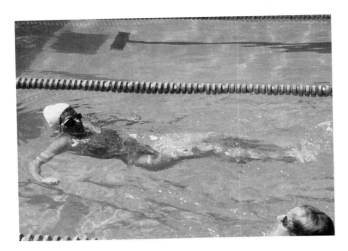

Fig. 33-20. Cervical spine flexion induces lumbar flexion, and the patient "sits" in the water. (From Moschetti M: *Aquaphysics made simple,* Aptos, Calif, 1989, AquaTechnics Consulting Group.)

Problems with stroke technique can usually be solved with simple changes in stroke mechanics or by the addition of adaptive equipment. For example, a struggle for air can be resolved by the addition of a mask and snorkel. Trunk position can be improved by using the taping technique already mentioned. Poor propulsion can be remedied with an appropriate choice of fins. Hand paddles can provide better kinesthetic awareness of hand and arm position.[12-15,20,21]

CASE PRESENTATION

History

The patient is a 20-year-old Division I college swimmer. His events are the 200- and 500-yard freestyle. He has a history of chronic right shoulder rotator cuff tendinitis. This injury recently had an acute flare-up. His regular physician prescribed 2 weeks of rest and oral nonsteroidal antiinflammatory drugs (NSAIDs). Shortly after he resumed regular training, right shoulder pain recurred, in conjunction with an acute onset of right-sided upper and lower cervical pain. There was also associated pain in the right upper trapezius and behind his right ear. His pain was exacerbated with right-side breathing, making breathing and concentration difficult. His racing times increased, soon prompting him to see a sports medicine physician.

Physical Examination

The sports medicine physician's physical examination was thorough and focused and was guided by his understanding of swimming biomechanics. His evaluation also took into account the way in which repetitive microtrauma can damage particular structures in the spine and shoulder complex. The patient had a typical swimmer's posture—an exaggeration of the forward head posture. The severity of the swimmer's rounded shoulder posture and the degree of lumbar lordosis were notable. Cervical active range of motion was restricted in right rotation, lateral flexion, extension, and extension/rotation, with reproduction of pain in all of these planes of motion, but particularly with extension/rotation. Other cervical active range of motion was normal. His cervical pain was decreased with manual traction (with the cervical spine in 20 degrees of flexion) and increased with compression.

Manual examination of the patient's cervical spine revealed tenderness to palpation and motion restrictions at the right occipitoatlantal, atlantoaxial, and C5-6 zygapophyseal joints with reproduction of pain on motion and associated overlying soft tissue changes. Decreased soft tissue flexibility was noted in the capital extensors, cervical extensors, scalenes, levator scapulae, upper trapezius, and humeral internal rotators—especially the subscapularis, latissimus dorsi, and pectoralis minor and major. Trigger points and tight bands were palpated in the upper trapezius, cervical extensors, scalenes, levator scapulae, latissimus dorsi, and pectoralis minor and major. There was a muscular strength imbalance between the cervical flexors and the stronger cervical extensors. There was also a muscular strength imbalance between the stronger capital extensors and the weaker cervical extensors.

Evaluation of the patient's right shoulder complex revealed normal right shoulder active range of motion with pain in the anterolateral acromial region at roughly 90 degrees of abduction, as well as pain at the end ranges of forward flexion and abduction. Anterior glenohumeral instability was present. Scapulothoracic mechanical dysfunction was noted, and the patient had an abnormal slide test. Significant muscular strength imbalances were identified, with particularly weak scapular depressors (e.g., the lower trapezius), weak scapular retractors (e.g., the rhomboid minor and major as well as middle trapezius), and weak humeral external rotators (e.g., the teres minor and infraspinatus).

With the exception of the strength imbalances noted, the patient's neurologic examination was completely normal in both his upper and lower extremities.

Radiographic evaluation was deferred, since the patient had a recent set of shoulder films from his last episode of shoulder pain. There was no significant indication for cervical films based on the physician's initial cervical evaluation.

Tissue Injury Cycle

The tissue injury cycle assisted the sports medicine physician in defining all aspects of this patient's total injury complex. The patient had an acute cervical zygapophyseal joint injury superimposed on a chronic postural dysfunction. The cervical zygapophyseal joint injury was also superimposed on an acute exacerbation of a chronic rotator cuff tendinitis that was due to extrinsic impingement secondary to glenohumeral instability.

His cervical and postural *tissue overload complex* consisted of eccentric overload of the capital and cervical flexors, scalene muscles, thoracic spinal extensors, humeral external rotators, and scapular depressors and retractors. Concentric overload of the capital and cervical extensors, humeral internal rotators, the capital and cervical extensors, upper trapezius, and levator scapulae also characterized his injury. Included in this complex were the posterior occipitoatlantal fascia and intermuscular fascia surrounding the named muscle groups.

The joint capsules of the right occipitoatlantal, atlantoaxial, and C5-6 zygapophyseal joints were also involved. The postural and cervical *tissue injury complex* included a synovitis and capsulitis of the right occipitoatlantal, atlantoaxial, and C5-6 zygapophyseal joints. Additional components of the tissue injury complex included myofascial changes in the upper trapezius, cervical extensors, scalenes, levator scapulae, latissimus dorsi, and pectoralis minor and major muscle groups. The *clinical sign and symptom complex* included myofascial pain, trigger points, and tight bands in those muscles subserving the postural abnormality. These myofascial changes especially affected the upper trapezius, cervical extensors, scalenes, levator scapulae, latissimus dorsi, and pectoralis minor and major muscle groups. Other components of this complex were pain, tenderness, and segmental motion restrictions localized to the right occipitoatlantal, atlantoaxial, and C5-6 zygapophyseal joints. The right occipitoatlantal, atlantoaxial, and C5-6 zygapophyseal joints referred pain to the right cervical spine posterior to the ear, the right upper cervical spine, and the right upper shoulder from C3 to T1 above the level of the scapular spine, respectively.

The *functional biomechanical deficits* included decreased cervical active range of motion with extension and the coupled, complex motions of right lateral bending, right rotation, and right extension/rotation. Tight humeral internal rotators and tight capital and cervical extensors were also part of the functional biomechanical deficit complex. The tight humeral internal rotators and forward position of the scapula due to the shortened pectoralis minor created a functional narrowing of the supraspinatus outlet, exacerbating the dynamic subacromial impingement. Strength imbalances also affected the swimmer's performance, with weak cervical flexors in comparison with cervical and usually stronger capital extensors, weak scapular depressors (e.g., lower trapezius) in comparison with scapular elevators, weak scapular retractors (e.g., rhomboid minor and major, as well as middle trapezius) in comparison with scapular protractors, and weak humeral external rotators (e.g., teres minor and infraspinatus) in comparison with very powerful humeral internal rotators, (e.g., subscapularis, pectoralis major, and latissimus dorsi).

The *subclinical adaptation complex* included an increased body roll to enhance access of the mouth to air, a decreased but maximum cervical suboccipital spinal extension and cervical rotation, and an increased mid- and lower cervical and upper thoracic extension to ensure that his head rode higher out of the water. All of these subclinical adaptations ensured the patient's adequate access to air. These changes in stroke biomechanics resulted in increased head drag and ultimately slowed the patient's swimming speed, thus increasing his performance times.

The patient's shoulder injury complex was also noted by the physician. The *tissue overload complex* consisted of tensile loading of the posterior shoulder capsule and muscles, as well as the scapular stabilizers. The *tissue injury complex* included rotator cuff tendon dynamic impingement, anterior glenoid labrum attrition, and anterior capsule stretch and inflammation. The *clinical sign and symptom complex* included dynamic subacromial impingement pain and anterosuperior glenohumeral instability. The *functional biomechanical deficits* were tight internal rotators, rounded shoulders, and strength deficits in the right shoulder scapular stabilizers. Decreased strength in the external rotators was found when the external and internal rotators were compared, indicating a strength differential that created a muscle strength imbalance. The *subclinical adapta-*

tion complex included a recovery phase using a shortened and lowered right arm, and a shortened and less powerful pull phase using decreased internal rotation of the shoulder. Entry, pull, and recovery phases made with right arm lateral drift from the midline and continued humeral external rotation of the right arm were also part of this complex.

The tissue injury cycle helped the physician to understand the relationship between the three components of the patient's examination. The patient's chronic postural dysfunction produced tight humeral internal rotators. The tight, shortened pectoralis minor, in particular, caused the patient's scapula to assume a forward, protracted position, which created a functional narrowing of his supraspinatus outlet. When he began regular swim training, he developed laxity in his anterior glenohumeral capsule. The glenohumeral laxity superimposed on the functional narrowing of his supraspinatus outlet yielded extrinsic impingement secondary to glenohumeral instability, the source of his recurring shoulder pain. His altered shoulder mechanics superimposed on his postural dysfunction resulted in his newest problem, the zygapophyseal injury complex, which caused his cervical pain.

This patient's freestyle stroke underwent many adaptations to avoid further pain due to impingement. The patient lowered his arm above water during the recovery phase and externally rotated his humerus, thus allowing his hand to enter the water palm down rather than thumb down. He also allowed his hand to enter the water farther away from the midline. By lowering his arm during the recovery phase, he increased his upper body roll in order to breathe. In an effort to moderate the amount of segmental roll through his spine to gain access to sufficient air for right-side breathing, he began right crane breathing. Because of his underlying postural dysfunction, the patient was already functioning at near end-range capital and cervical extension. The additional stress placed on his tight and weak capital and cervical extensors and rotators due to crane breathing allowed him to function at end-range active motion for a short period of time. Soon he began to strain the noncontractile tissue supporting those joints that allow crane breathing to occur—the zygapophyseal joint capsules of the right occipitoatlantal, atlantoaxial, and C5-6 zygapophyseal joints. The patient recruited his C5-6 joint to increase his cervical extension and rotation more than was already being provided by the occipitoatlantal extension and atlantoaxial rotation. The tissue overload of the occipitoatlantal, atlantooccipital, and C5-6 zygapophyseal joints created capsulitis and synovitis.

The result of the increased body roll had additional biomechanical consequences. The patient found it impossible to move the lumbar, thoracic, and cervical parts of his spine as a unit (i.e., using log-rolling or nonsegmental motion. This biomechanical adaptation resulted in an increase in segmental rotation through his lumbar spine. Because he externally rotated his humerus to minimize further loss of supraspinatus outlet space and to minimize his subacromial impingement, his hand entered the water palm down, resulting in an increased amount of segmental motion (i.e., twist) through his lumbar spine. Widening the entry phase position caused his trunk to rotate away from the entry phase side, thus increasing lateral flexion and segmental motion through the lumbar spine. The patient also adopted a crossover kick to offset the segmental rotation produced through his lumbar spine. Unfortunately, the crossover kick only served to further increase the amount of lateral flexion and segmental motion through his lumbar spine.

Rehabilitation Program

According to Kibler, Chandler, and Pace,[66] the rehabilitation of soft tissue injuries and their associated deficits can be divided into three parts: (1) an acute phase, (2) a recovery phase, and (3) a maintenance phase. Each phase is designed to sequentially address specific aspects of the tissue injury cycle. This describes the rehabilitation process for the patient in the preceding case presentation. However, the details of the rehabilitation process of rotator cuff tendinitis in a competitive swimmer are described earlier in the chapter and are not repeated here. It is most important to realize that the rotator cuff tendinitis program, as well as the posture and cervical spine program, must occur in a coordinated and simultaneous manner to address all components of the patient's injury and minimize the chance for a recurrence.[18,19]

Acute phase. During the acute phase of rehabilitation the tissue injury and clinical sign and symptom complexes are treated. A description of the acute phase of rehabilitation is presented in the box below. The goals of this phase are to reduce pain and inflammation, reestablish nonpainful range of motion, improve neuromuscular cervical spine postural control, and retard the development of any muscular atrophy of the cervical spine muscle groups, postural muscles, and muscle groups subserving the upper extremity and scapulothoracic articulation.

Pain and inflammation can be reduced by the judicious use of NSAIDs that are prescribed by the physiatrist. The antiprostaglandin effect of NSAIDs may control an injury's inflammatory response and provide pain relief. The duration of an NSAID's analgesic effect may be different from its antiinflammatory effect.[56] Some authors have expressed concern that NSAIDs may actually interfere with the later stages of tissue repair and remodeling, whereas prostaglandins still help mediate debris cleanup.[61] The dosage, timing, and potential side effects of NSAIDs should be evaluated. Patient responses to a particular NSAID cannot be predicted on the basis of its chemical class or pharmacokinetics.[32]

The physical therapist has a variety of techniques available to further control inflammation and pain. Acute injury is best treated by therapeutic cold, which decreases pain and muscle spasm and causes arteriolar and capillary blood flow to diminish, thus helping to control edema. The time required to cool an injured structure is directly dependent on the depth of intervening fat and may vary from 10 to 30 minutes.[38,76,77] Cryotherapy is easily applied to the cervical spine at home or in the clinic and may be used in conjunction with other treatment techniques. In addition to providing pain relief and controlling inflammation, physical modalities have other benefits. Ultrasound can stimulate tissue regeneration, promote soft tissue repair, increase blood flow to damaged tissue to provide needed nutrients to the healing tissue and aid in the removal of inflammatory by-products, increase soft tissue distensibility, and decrease muscle spasm and pain.[17,36,47,129]

Electrical stimulation is another extremely useful modality that is particularly helpful in modulating acute pain. It can also help decrease muscle spasm by inducing posttetanic relaxation, as well as increasing circulation, which helps remove inflammatory waste products.[35] Electrical stimulation techniques, including transcutaneous electrical nerve stimulation (TENS), high-voltage pulsed galvanic stimulation (HVPGS), interferential electrical stimulation, and minimal electrical noninvasive stimulation (MENS), have been reported to promote analgesia, muscle relaxation, resolution of edema, and wound healing, as well as to retard inflammation and muscle atrophy.[124]

The recent application of electroacuscope and low-energy lasers, which are newer and less traditional modalities for the management of pain associated with sports injuries, awaits well-controlled prospective studies to determine their mechanism of action and their efficacy.[35]

Joint protection techniques offer another way to help reduce pain by minimizing repetitive cervical motion into painful ranges of motion. This can be accomplished passively by providing a soft cervical collar that can be worn for as long as 10 to 12 days and then weaning the patient from the collar as rapidly as possible to help avoid psychologic dependence and help prevent further muscular weakness and decreased soft tissue flexibility.

Acute Phase of Rehabilitation

Complexes Involved

Tissue injury
Clinical signs and symptoms

Therapeutic Activities

Active rest
Conditioning of other areas
NSAIDs
Physical therapy modalities
Manual therapy approaches
Protected range of motion/stabilization
Isometric muscle strengthening

Criteria for Advancement

Increased cervical range of motion
Decreased cervical pain
Decreased muscle spasm
Decreased adaptive muscle and other soft tissue changes

Weaning should allow increasing periods of daytime removal, with continued use at night to prevent injury during sleep.[99,110] Once the patient has been weaned from daytime collar use, nighttime use may also be discontinued. Active joint protection techniques are part of the initial phase of a cervicothoracic stabilization program. Cervicothoracic stabilization training is a specific type of therapeutic exercise that can help the patient to (1) gain dynamic control of cervicothoracic spine forces; (2) eliminate repetitive injury to the motion segments (i.e., discs, zygapophyseal joints, and related structures); (3) encourage healing of an injured segment; and (4) possibly alter the degenerative process. The underlying premise is that the motion segment and its supporting soft tissues react to minimize applied stress and thereby reduce the risk of injury. During the initial phase of stabilization training, the patient is taught how to find a neutral position, or a position of optimal function—the least painful cervicothoracic spine position that minimizes segmental biomechanical stress. As the patient's condition improves, a series of flexibility and strengthening exercises are initiated to help correct postural dysfunction, inflexibilities, and muscle strength deficits and imbalances.[116]

Manual therapy techniques can also help decrease pain and improve mobility and function to the point that the patient may begin to exercise in a painless manner. The techniques may also be used to help determine the source and relative contribution of various aspects of a patient's pain and dysfunction. These techniques include massage of the soft tissues, manually sustained or rhythmically applied muscle stretching, traction applied to the longitudinal axis of the spine, passive joint mobilization, and, as the patient's pain begins to subside, specific or general high-velocity manipulation.[41,43,93] High-velocity manipulation can be particularly helpful to treat painful dysfunctions that are aggravated by repetitive oscillatory movements.[42] Manual therapy techniques would be targeted to the patient's occipitoatlantal, atlantoaxial, and C5-C6 zygapophyseal joints, as well as all supporting structures in the cervical and thoracic spine and associated joints, including the glenohumeral joint and scapulothoracic articulation. The neurologic effects of manual therapy that can help attenuate pain include restoration of axonal transport due to mechanically induced deformation of spinal nerves,[41,70] stimulation of large-fiber joint afferents conveyed by joint receptors that depend on the gate-control theory,[41,127] and stimulation of clinically effective levels of endorphins.[41,117] Increased intraosseous pressure can cause pain; this pressure may be influenced by both joint position and intraarticular pressure. End-range passive mobilization techniques may help decrease intraarticular pressure, thereby reducing pain.*

* References 1, 8, 41, 44, 48, 79.

There are other benefits of manual therapy. Repetitive passive joint oscillations carried out at the limit of the joint's available range can have a mechanical effect on joint mobility, thus improving a vertebral motion restriction.[41,81,88,95,126] Mechanically controlled passive or active movements of joints can improve the remodeling of local connective tissue, the rate of tendon repair, and gliding function within tendon sheaths during the repair process.[9,41,75,78,125] Passive joint motion has been shown to stretch joint capsules, lubricate tissues, and induce metabolic changes in soft tissue, cartilage, and bone.[41,46] Manipulation, if needed, would most likely involve the occipitoatlantal, atlantoaxial, and C5-6 zygapophyseal joints.

If the patient's pain is not significantly relieved during the acute phase of the rehabilitation program, trigger point injections may help lessen trigger zone and referred pain and help improve muscular flexibility.[101,112] Oral steroids also may be used. Or, contrast-enhanced fluoroscopically guided zygapophyseal joint injections using a combination of steroid and local anesthetic at the site of pain may help to significantly decrease the patient's pain. These injections may allow rehabilitation to progress more rapidly.[31,33,34,75,99]

The second goal of the patient's acute phase of rehabilitation is to reestablish nonpainful active and passive ranges of motion of the cervical spine, thoracic spine, and associated joints, including the glenohumeral joint and scapulothoracic articulation. Passive joint mobilization techniques are usually the most successful during the early portion of the acute phase of rehabilitation. Then, as the patient's condition improves, a gradual shift to an active program is made to ensure rapid recovery and patient independence. Passive mobilization of the occipitoatlantal, atlantoaxial, C2-3, and C5-6 vertebral motion segments mobilizes their respective zygapophyseal joints and stretches their zygapophyseal capsules and is initiated for reasons previously cited.[41] Soft tissue techniques, including lateral stretching, linear stretching, deep pressure, traction, and/or separation of muscle origin and insertion[49,52] can help decrease pain, muscle spasm, and soft tissue inflexibility, as well as improve circulation and remove inflammatory by-products.[10,52] Myofascial techniques can be used to help stretch the noncontractile portion of the soft tissue.[118] Inhibition techniques, such as positional release, can help to modify increased muscle tone, thus helping to restore balanced muscular flexibility and strength.[58,59,74]

Varying combinations of these techniques would be directed primarily at those muscles that have become tight and painful secondary to the acute underlying zygapophyseal joint pain. Treatment would also be directed to the muscles and other soft tissues chronically affected by poor posture to help restore them to normal length and flexibility. These muscles include those that are shortened, less flexible, and weak—the capital and cervical extensors, sternocleidomastoid, upper trapezius, and levator scapulae. These techniques could also be used to help restore normal flexibility, strength, and length to the muscles that have been eccentrically lengthened and are weak—the scalenes, cervical and capital flexors, middle and lower trapezius, and rhomboid minor and major. The muscles, fascia, and other soft tissue components responsible for creating a functionally narrowed supraspinatus outlet and a rounded shoulder posture should be treated: pectoralis minor and major, subscapularis, serratus anterior, latissimus dorsi, anterior deltoid, and thoracic musculature. While stretching these muscles, particular care should be taken to avoid inadvertently stretching the anterior glenohumeral joint capsule and ligaments so that the patient's anterior glenohumeral instability is not worsened. Finally, an active stretching program for those muscles that stabilize and support the lumbar spine is implemented at this stage of rehabilitation.[86,107]

The last two goals of the patient's acute phase of rehabilitation must also be addressed: improving neuromuscular control of the cervical spine and retarding weakness and increasing the strength of the cervical spine muscle groups and those that support the glenohumeral joint and scapulothoracic articulation. Improved neuromuscular control is developed for static positions first and then progresses to include control during dynamic and functional activities. This type of training is included in the cervicothoracic dynamic stabilization program.[116] Various proprioceptive neuromuscular facilitation techniques can be performed within the pain-free portion of the weakened or limited cervical and shoulder complex range of motion. As the patient improves, the extent of the movement pattern is increased both for range of motion and for the amount of resistance that is manually applied.[108,116,140]

Cervical spine strengthening should begin with isometric exercises in the neutral position determined during previous stabilization training. Single-plane isometric strengthening with resistive forces applied perpendicularly to the head to strengthen the cervical flexors, extensors, rotators, and lateral flexors is initiated with the patient supine; strengthening then progresses with the patient in the seated, then standing position. By varying the patient's positioning and direction relative to gravity, direct stabilization of the cervical spine results.[99,116] As the patient's pain permits, an increasing range of isometric strengthening occurs. When strengthening progresses to isotonic strengthening, care should be taken during the initiation of combined cervical movements, such as lateral bending and rotation, to avoid an increase in symptoms due to the increased zygapophyseal joint and muscular requirements needed to perform these movements. When symptoms permit, concentric isotonic strengthening of all the cervical spine

muscles should begin and should emphasize those muscle groups that have been stretched and weakened as a result of poor posture—the cervical and capital flexors and scalenes—thus providing improved muscular balance and flexibility.

Strengthening programs must also include the thoracic muscle groups, middle and lower trapezius, and rhomboid minor and major to provide strength to the thoracic spine and scapulothoracic articulation to help lessen postural thoracic kyphosis and scapular protraction and elevation. Balanced flexibility and strength will allow the patient to assume a more mechanically correct posture from which to develop further segmental mobility and dynamic functional strength. Finally, special emphasis should be placed on strengthening the humeral external rotators, including the teres minor, infraspinatus, and latissimus dorsi. This strengthening will improve strength balance with the disproportionately strong internal rotators of swimmers that also contribute to poor posture and functional narrowing of the supraspinatus outlet.[18,45,87]

A low-level program of aerobic conditioning may be instituted depending on the patient's level of pain and function. This low-level program can help the patient avoid significant cardiovascular deconditioning. Stationary bicycle, treadmill, or stair climber exercise provides excellent cardiovascular training without requiring upper extremity involvement. Water running using only the legs is particularly appropriate because it involves only the lower extremities.[120,121] These low-level programs will allow the patient to continue training in his competitive environment without potentially compromising his shoulder function.

The patient should be advanced to the recovery phase when his cervical pain has almost completely resolved, his passive and active cervical range of motion and neuromuscular control have significantly improved, and the muscles and other tissue maintaining his postural adaptive changes have improved.

Recovery phase. The recovery phase of rehabilitation addresses the tissue overload and functional biomechanical deficit complexes. A description of the recovery phase of rehabilitation is presented in the box on p. 379. The goals of this phase are to completely eliminate the patient's pain; improve and normalize his cervical, thoracic, glenohumeral, and scapulothoracic passive and active ranges of motion; improve and normalize his cervical, thoracic, glenohumeral, and scapulothoracic strength and neuromuscular control; continue to improve his posture; and initiate swim-training progressions. Complete resolution of the tissue injury and clinical symptom complexes is necessary in the early recovery phase. NSAIDs are probably unnecessary in this phase. Manual therapy, including manipulative and soft tissue techniques, may still be needed to help eliminate vertebral motion restrictions and improve the

<table>
<tr></tr>
</table>

Recovery Phase of Rehabilitation

Complexes Involved

Tissue overload
Functional biochemical deficit

Therapeutic Activities

Appropriate loading
Protected range of motion
Resistive exercise
  Local
  Balance
  Kinetic chain
Functional exercises

Criteria for Advancement

Full nonpainful range of motion
  Cervical
  Thoracic
  Lumbar
Scapulothoracic
  Glenohumeral
Improved spine posture
  Cervical
  Thoracic
Improved cervical, thoracic, scapulothoracic
  Neuromuscular control
  Strength
Improved strength and flexibility of the supporting
  Muscles
  Joints
Improved stroke mechanics

flexibility, length, and motion of the soft tissues so that cervical, thoracic, glenohumeral, and scapulothoracic active and passive ranges of motion are normalized. The improved active and passive ranges of motion permit further normalization of the patient's posture as muscular strength and balance are enhanced to help maintain the improved posture during daily activities, as well as athletic training and competition. Strength training using independent single-plane and complex multiple-plane coordinated motions are performed through varying combinations of concentric and eccentric isotonic, isokinetic, tube, pulley, and isolation exercises. A Theraband* or Sportcord† can be used to allow training at home. The specific type of strengthening depends on the joint and particular muscles targeted. Emphasis is first placed on improving the strength balance and neuromuscular control of the force couples that govern proper cervical, thoracic, glenohumeral, and scapulothoracic mechanics. For example, cervical and

* Hygenic Co., Akron, Ohio.
† Sportcord, Inc., Irvine, Calif.

capital flexor and extensor strength balance is improved; then those force couples that control the scapulothoracic articulation, including the scapular protractors and retractors, elevators and depressors, and upward rotators and downward rotators, are trained; and then the force couples that govern glenohumeral mechanics, including humeral internal and external rotators, abductors and adductors, and elevators and depressors, are trained. These training techniques are extended to the entire kinetic chain.[23,26,57] Appropriate strength should be developed throughout a particular range of motion to help minimize the potential of future injury.[26] Multiple-plane and combined motions that create cervicothoracic, scapulothoracic, and glenohumeral rhythms are emphasized to help improve general and sport-specific coordination and strength.[114] Muscular reeducation may be necessary to help the patient isolate individual muscles and coordinate the firing of muscles involved in complex rhythmic sequences.[108] Muscular reeducation should be done early in strength training to ensure that proper muscle-firing patterns and neuromuscular control are maintained during higher-level function. This reeducation can be facilitated with a variety of electronic biofeedback devices that use surface electrodes to monitor muscular activity. Strengthening techniques that simulate the freestyle stroke are initiated later in this phase of treatment.

Toward the end of this phase of rehabilitation, while continuing the aerobic cross-training begun during the acute phase of rehabilitation, the patient begins freestyle specific retraining progressions. First, while lying on a bench, he simulates the freestyle stroke with his coach, physical therapist, trainer, and physician present. Retraining of his stroke mechanics is initiated with special emphasis on head position during breathing to ensure that crane breathing is eliminated and cervical rotation and nonsegmental body roll are incorporated. This retraining will help prevent reinjury of his cervical zygapophyseal joints. The normal engram for proper arm mechanics is established to help avoid an exacerbation of his rotator cuff tendinitis. After his land-based swim stroke mechanics are normalized, the patient begins aquatic retraining. At first, a mask and snorkel are used to avoid a struggle for air so that arm and body mechanics can be trained. Then the mask and snorkel are removed, and hypoxic training is begun. Hypoxic training limits the number of breaths per length so that the mechanics of each breathing cycle can be analyzed and perfected. Finally, the patient is trained to breathe on alternate sides to minimize the repetitive microtrauma from single-side breathing. Because the patient uses all four competitive strokes—freestyle, backstroke, breaststroke, and butterfly—during training, review of these strokes' mechanics is also imperative to ensure that reinjury does not occur as a result of the biomechanical consequences of a different stroke's mechanics.

Criteria for advancement to the maintenance phase of rehabilitation include full, nonpainful active and passive cervical, thoracic, glenohumeral, and scapulothoracic ranges of motion; significantly improved posture; normal neuromuscular control; significantly improved strength and strength balance; and improved stroke mechanics.

Maintenance phase. Maintenance is the final phase of rehabilitation. A description of the maintenance phase of rehabilitation is presented in the box below. The goals of this phase are to increase and improve balance, power, and endurance of the cervical, thoracic, scapulothoracic, and glenohumeral muscle groups, as well as other muscles in the kinetic chain; normalize posture; normalize multiplane coupled neuromuscular control to eliminate subclinical adaptations; and enable the patient to return to unrestricted sport-specific aquatic activities.

Soft tissue flexibility and proper balance of flexibility and strength are emphasized to allow the patient to assume and maintain a biomechanically correct posture. Power and endurance training is initiated and focuses on maintaining normal multiplane coupled cervical motion and normal scapulothoracic and glenohumeral joint mechanics and control. Patterned motion training using tubing is particularly helpful because it permits enough freedom of movement to mimic swimming patterns. These activities can be performed in front of a wall mirror to further enhance proprioceptive feedback. The

Swim Bench,* a particular type of land-based swim-training equipment, can be used to develop strength, endurance, and specific stroke mechanics. Continued use of tubing and a Theraband or Sportcord is recommended for home use. Freestyle, backstroke, breaststroke, and butterfly stroke retraining continues with increased workout times and difficulty. Bilateral breathing is maintained for the freestyle. Starts and turns are reviewed to ensure that proper mechanics are used to avoid reinjury.

Criteria for this patient's return to unrestricted competition include no pain, normal physical examination findings that ensure that provocative testing (such as the cervical quadrant and overpressure tests[112]) does not produce the patient's symptoms, normalized posture, and normal stroke mechanics.

REHABILITATION OF CHRONIC SPINAL PAIN IN SWIMMERS WITH ARTHRITIS

A very separate issue from the competitive age-group, collegiate, or Master's level swimmer is the population of middle-aged and elderly individuals who are afflicted with chronic, disabling arthritis. The use of aquatic-oriented rehabilitative exercises for the severely afflicted arthritic patient was documented as far back as the days of the Roman Empire. Spa therapy has been practiced throughout history. In a review of the current principles of rehabilitation for patients with rheumatoid arthritis, Sutej and Hadler[115] point out that for Aesculapius, the spa was the focal point for medicine; for the Romans water therapy was incorporated into the fabric of society. However, modern medicine has developed a plethora of nonaquatic therapeutic modalities to treat the chronic arthritic, including oral and injectable medications, surgery, exercises, splinting and rest, thermal therapy, transcutaneous electrical nerve stimulation, acupuncture, mobilization techniques, manipulation, traction, massage, and appliances to assist in grasp and ambulation. Many of these therapeutic modalities have potential side effects, some of which are serious and life-threatening. Many of the treatments are prohibitively expensive for the Medicare patient living on a fixed income. Most important, the value of some of these modalities remains to be scientifically validated.

The swimming pool exercises presented in this section are for those afflicted with any of the numerous arthritides to incorporate into their therapeutic regimen. The biomechanical theory behind these exercises centers around the chronic joint inflammation and disuse that is characteristic of most of the arthritides. This leads to a progressive loss of the normal flexibility of the surrounding joint capsule, supporting ligaments, and intrinsic musculature. In the spine, disc degeneration

---

Maintenance Phase of Rehabilitation

Complexes Involved

Functional biochemical deficit
Subclinical adaptation

Therapeutic Activities

Strength and flexibility balance
Endurance
Functional aquatic progressions

Criteria for Return to Play

Normal cervical coupled multiplane active range of motion
Normal cervical muscular strength and muscle balance
Normal cervical, thoracic, glenohumeral, and scapulothoracic
  Muscular passive range of motion
  Active range of motion
Negative clinical examination, including negative provocative tests
  Quadrant testing
  Overpressure testing
Normal and balanced strength and neuromuscular control
  Shoulder complex
  Upper extremities
  Thoracic spine and associated structures

---

* Biokinetic Fitness Laboratories, Berkeley, Calif.

with disc space narrowing leads to progressive facet joint subluxation, facet arthrosis, and neural canal compromise. These aquatic exercises have been designed to gradually relax, stretch, and strengthen the muscle surrounding the involved joints and spinal motion units.

The Berson program[6] has proved particularly useful because it is designed for patients who have painful arthritis and does not exacerbate any of the preexisting symptoms attributable to the arthritis while progressing through the program. This series of exercises does not require the supervision of a physician, physical therapist, trainer, or coach and is therefore readily accessible to any individual with access to a swimming pool.

The rationale for using water as the medium in which to rehabilitate patients with neck pain, back pain, and other musculoskeletal arthritic disorders relies on the natural buoyancy of the human body in water. The natural buoyancy afforded by the water reduces body weight to only 10% of the normal weight on dry land. Walking in water subjects the axial skeleton to one-and-a-half times the normal body weight, and jogging can increase the mechanical load on the axial skeleton up to three times that on land. Water is a very forgiving medium for patients who have back or neck pain or who are disabled and unable to perform any out-of-water exercises. Water therapy is effective at strengthening and stretching diseased joints, ligamentous supporting structures, and muscles because it offers four times the resistance of air while maintaining the individual in an almost weight-free environment. (This characteristic of water also benefits overweight patients and pregnant women.) Marchbanks and Lambert[82] have developed an aquatic exercise program called Aquamotion that permits a balanced workout that further reduces the risk of injuries that may result from the overdevelopment of antagonist muscle groups. This concept is probably most valid for the more active and strong individual, rather than the severely afflicted arthritic patient.

In addition to the benefits of the buoyant effects of water, the water temperature and the heat-conductive properties of water allow the individual to stay comfortably cool while participating in even vigorous aerobic conditioning programs.

Berson Program[6] of Water Exercises

The Berson program is not intended to increase aerobic capacity or cardiovascular fitness but does so as a beneficial side effect for the majority of arthritic patients who are not aerobically fit when they start the program. The program is primarily and specifically designed for the treatment of muscular deconditioning and loss of mobility secondary to one of the arthritides.

Beginners' exercises. These simple flexibility exercises involve standing comfortably in the pool in chest- or shoulder-deep water, near the edge for those less adept at swimming, and not exercising beyond fatigue or

comfort. The exercises should be performed five times a week initially, until the patient is pain free; thereafter a maintenance program of three times a week may suffice. The duration of each exercise is dependent on the level of general conditioning and fatigability present when the program is initiated. If systemic diseases are present that may place the patient at risk from an exercise program, then early consultation with an appropriate physician is recommended. Advancement through this series of exercises will vary widely, from weeks to months, depending on the severity of the disease and the general debility of the patient.

The beginner's exercises include 25 individual and separate active motions of the upper and lower extremity joints (see Fig. 33-21 for an example). All small and large joints are moved through a full range of motion underwater using the increased resistance of the water to generate force against the movement, providing for stretching, strengthening, and then relaxation of the muscles surrounding each joint.

Intermediate exercises. Intermediate and advanced exercises are especially beneficial to people who have arthritis in more than one area. The intermediate and advanced exercises can be started when the patient is comfortable and not fatigued or experiencing pain when performing the exercises. Intermediate exercises that involve floating and swimming should be performed initially in shallow water for safety. If the patient is afraid of the water and/or not naturally buoyant enough to float effortlessly, then he or she should wear a flotation aid, such as a water-ski belt. There are five intermediate exercises that incorporate combined active range of

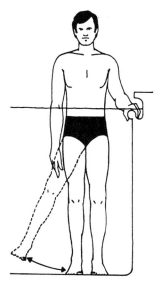

Fig. 33-21. The purpose of this beginners' exercise in the Berson program for hip joints is to further relax, stretch, and strengthen muscles surrounding hip joints by raising and lowering each leg sideways. (From Berson D, Roy S: *Pain-free arthritis,* Boca Raton, Fla, 1982, S & J Books.)

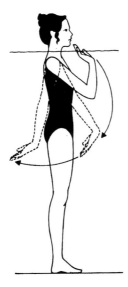

Fig. 33-22. This intermediate exercise in the Berson program involves exercising three joints. Its purpose is to further relax, stretch, and strengthen muscles surrounding the wrist, elbow, and shoulder joints. It is performed as follows: Raise your arm and bend back your wrist as if you were a waiter carrying a tray. Then, push down with both your arm and your hand below the wrist. Move them both as far back and down as they will comfortably go. On the return upward motion, raise both your arm and your hand below the wrist so that you resume the position of a waiter carrying a tray. (From Berson D, Roy S: *Pain-free arthritis,* Boca Raton, Fla, 1982, S & J Books.)

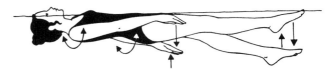

Fig. 33-23. This advanced exercise in the Berson program is performed as follows: In the floating position, with your hands by your sides and your legs close together, raise and lower your arms and legs. Your right arm and right leg should move downward as your left arm and left leg move upward. Then, your right arm and right leg should move upward as your left arm and left leg move downward. This up-and-down movement of the arms and legs causes the hips and shoulders to roll from side to side. (From Berson D, Roy S: *Pain-free arthritis,* Boca Raton, Fla, 1992, S & J Books.)

motion of the upper and lower extremities (see Fig. 33-22 for an example).

Advanced exercises. All of the advanced exercises are performed without the support of the bottom of the pool. When the patient reaches this stage in the program, then these exercises replace most of the beginners' and the intermediate exercises. There are four advanced exercises that should be alternated with one another to form a comprehensive back and neck exercise program (see Fig. 33-23 for an example). The general recommendation is that the length of time that the advanced exercises are done should be gradually increased until the patient is pain free.

General considerations. Unlike other water exercise programs, it is not suggested that optimal results can be achieved by doing a fixed amount of repetitions, such as 10, 20, or 30. Instead, patients should start with a very small amount of exercise that will gradually get the patient used to exercise but not cause strain. Over a period of weeks and months, the amount of exercise is gradually and progressively increased until the patient is relaxing, stretching, and strengthening muscles enough to become pain free.

It is not possible to predict how much exercise will be necessary to make different individuals pain free. For someone with relatively mild symptoms, gradually build-

ing up to doing 50 repetitions might be enough to achieve freedom from pain. But for people who are more seriously afflicted, 50 repetitions might be only enough to achieve minor improvement. Such individuals should not be satisfied with minor improvement or conclude that they cannot be helped very much. What they should do is gradually build up to doing much more exercise. Similarly, individuals who achieve major improvement from doing a relatively large number of exercise repetitions (100 or 200, for instance) should not necessarily conclude that they have improved all they can. What they should do is keep on increasing their exercise.

As with the amount of repetitions, the optimal amount of exercise time varies widely with different individuals. If an individual has relatively mild symptoms confined to one joint, 10 or 15 minutes a day of exercise might be enough. For more serious symptoms involving multiple joints, 1 to 2 hours might be required. In extreme cases even more time might be required.

What also varies widely is the length of time it takes different individuals to become pain free. Generally speaking, the milder the symptoms are to start with, the faster a full recovery is achieved. The more severe the symptoms, the longer it takes. For very mild cases, 3 to 4 weeks of gradually increased exercise may be all that is necessary. Much more severe cases might take 6 months to 1 year.

A minimum requirement for a rehabilitation exercise is that it should put a joint and/or muscle group through its full range of motion. The mechanics of Olympic-style swimming strokes are such that they do not put all or even most of the neck and back muscles through their full range of motion. Thus the advice that patients should "try swimming" is not specific enough to provide consistent results for most people. A combination of advanced exercises on the Berson Program[6] does put the back and neck muscles through their full range of motion and has been found to be particularly helpful for arthritis and chronic disc problems; it may also be very beneficial as a preventive measure. One should consider the theoretic probability that such a program may be of great value in preventing some or even most of the back problems that are commonly encountered by people who do large amounts of exercise, including professional athletes in many different sports.

ACKNOWLEDGMENT

Thanks go to Anne Geddes (Scientific Publications Office, Baylor Research Institute, Dallas, Tex.) for reading and editing a major portion of this manuscript.

REFERENCES

1. Arnoldi C et al: The effect of joint position in juxtaarticular bone marrow pressure, *Acta Orthop Scand* 51:893, 1980.
2. Bailes JE et al: Diving injuries of the cervical spine, *Surg Neurol* 34:155, 1990.
3. Becker TJ: Scoliosis in swimmers, *Clin Sports Med* 5:149, 1986.
4. Becker TJ: Personal communication, 1991.
5. Benson D, Wolf A, Shoji H: Can the Milwaukee brace patient participate in competitive athletics? *Am J Sports Med* 5:7, 1977.
6. Berson D, Roy S: *Pain-free arthritis,* Boca Raton, Fla, 1982, S & J Books. Also available from S & J Books: *Berson program for pain-free arthritis* (videotape).
7. Bogduk N, Twomey LT: *Clinical anatomy of the lumbar spine,* ed 2, New York, 1991, Churchill Livingstone.
8. Bustrode C: Why are osteoarthritic joints painful? *J R Nav Med Serv* 62:5, 1976.
9. Cantu R, Grodin A: *Myofascial manipulation: theory and clinical application,* Rockville, Md, 1992, Aspen.
10. Cantu R, Grodin A: Soft tissue mobilization. In Basmajian JV, Nyberg R, editors: *Rational manual therapies,* Baltimore, 1993, Williams & Wilkins.
11. Clarys JP, Piette G: A review of EMG in swimming: explanation of facts and/or feedback information. In Hollander AP, Huijing PA, deGroot G, editors: *Biomechanics and medicine in swimming,* Champaign, Ill, 1983, Human Kinetics Books.
12. Cole AJ: Aquatic stabilization strategies. Paper presented at the American Academy of Physical Medicine and Rehabilitation annual meeting, San Francisco, Nov 16, 1992.
13. Cole AJ: The intrinsic properties of water. Paper presented at the American Academy of Physical Medicine and Rehabilitation annual meeting, San Francisco, Nov 16, 1992.
14. Cole AJ: Spinal pain in the elite competitive swimmer. Paper presented at the Steadman Hawkins Foundation, Vail, Colo, Dec 4-5, 1992.
15. Cole AJ: Spine injuries in the competitive swimming athlete. Paper presented at the American College of Sports Medicine annual meeting, Seattle, Wash, June 4-5, 1993.
16. Cole AJ: When to call for help, *J Phys Educ Recreation Dance,* 64(1):55, 1993.
17. Cole AJ, Eagleston RE: The benefits of deep heat: ultrasound and electromagnetic diathermy, *Physician Sportsmed* (in press).
18. Cole AJ, Eagleston RE, Moschetti M: Swimming. In White AH, Schofferman JA, editors: *Spine care,* vol 1, *Diagnosis and conservative treatment,* St Louis, 1995, Mosby.
19. Cole AJ, Herring SA: The role of the physiatrist in the management of lumbar spine pain. In Tollison DC, editor: *The handbook of pain management,* ed 2, Baltimore, 1994, Williams & Wilkins.
20. Cole AJ, Moschetti M, Eagleston R: Getting backs in the swim, *Rehabil Manage,* 8:62, Aug/Sept 1992.
21. Cole AJ, Moschetti ML, Eagleston RE: An aquatic sports medicine approach for lumbar spine rehabilitation. In Tollison DC, editor: *The handbook of pain management,* ed 2, Baltimore, 1994, Williams & Wilkins.
22. Cole AJ, Moschetti ML, Eagleston RE: Aquatic rehabilitation applications for spine pain, *J Back Musculoskel Rehabil* (in press).
23. Cole AJ, Reid M: Clinical assessment of the shoulder, *J Back Musculoskel Rehabil* 2(2):7, 1992.
24. Cole AJ, Stratton SA, Farrell JP: Cervical spine athletic injuries: a pain in the neck, *Phys Med Rehabil Clin North Am* 2:1, Feb 1994.
25. Cole AJ, Weinstein S: *Lumbar spine pain: a clinical approach,* Boston, Andover Medical Publishers (in press).
26. Cole AJ et al: Electromyographic study of the subscapularis, *Arch Phys Med Rehabil* 71:790, 1990.
27. Cole AJ et al: Lumbar torque: a new proprioceptive approach. Poster presented at the annual meeting of the North American Spine Society, Keystone, Colo, Aug 1-3, 1991.
28. Cole AJ et al: The Portola Valley Scale: a classification system for aquatic exercise, Manuscript submitted for publication.
29. Costill D, Cahill P, Eddy D: Metabolic responses to submaximal exercise in three water temperatures, *J Appl Physiol* 22:628, 1967.
30. Councilman J: *The science of swimming,* Englewood Cliffs, NJ: 1968, Prentice Hall.
31. Cousins MJ, Bromage PR: Epidural neural blockade. In Cousins MJ, Bridenbaugh PO, editors: *Neural blockage in clinical anesthesia and management of pain,* New York, 1988, JB Lippincott.
32. Dahl S: Nonsteroidal anti-inflammatory agents: clinical pharmacology/adverse effects/usage guidelines. In Williams RF, Dahl SL, editors: *Therapeutic controversies in the rheumatic diseases,* Orlando, Fla, 1987, Grune & Stratton.
33. Derby R: Cervical injection procedures. Paper presented at The Cervical and Lumbar Spine: State of the Art '91, San Francisco, March 24, 1991, San Francisco Spine Institute.
34. Dreyfus P: The cervical spine: nonsurgical care. Paper presented at Tom Landry Sports Medicine and Research Center, Dallas, Tex, April 8, 1993.
35. Dreyfus P, Stratton S: The use of the low energy laser, electroacuscope, and neuroprobe in sports medicine: a current review, *Physician Sportsmed* 21(8):47, 1993.
36. Dyson M: Therapeutic applications of ultrasound. In Nyberg WL, Ziskin MC, editors: *Biological effects of ultrasound: clinics in diagnostic ultrasound,* New York, 1985, Churchill Livingstone.
37. Eagleston R: Aquatic stabilization programs. Paper presented at the Conference on Aggressive Nonsurgical Rehabilitation of Lumbar Spine and Sports Injuries, San Francisco, March 23, 1989, San Francisco Spine Institute.
38. Eldred E, Lindsky D, Buchwald J: The effect of cooling on mammalian muscle spindles, *Exp Neurol* 2:144, 1960.
39. Farfan HF: Effects of torsion on the intervertebral joints, *Can J Surg* 12:336, 1969.
40. Farfan HF et al: The effects of torsion on the lumbar intervertebral joints: the role of torsion in the production of disc degeneration, *J Bone Joint Surg* 52A:468, 1970.
41. Farrell JP: Cervical passive mobilization techniques: the Australian approach, *Phys Med Rehabil State Art Rev* 4(2):309, 1990.
42. Farrell JP: Personal communication, April 1993.
43. Farrell JP, Soto JY, Tichenor CJ: The role of manual therapy in spinal rehabilitation. In White AH, Schofferman JA, editors: *Spine care,* vol 1, *Diagnosis and conservative treatment,* St Louis, 1995, Mosby.
44. Ferrel W, Nade S, Newbold P: Interrelation of neural discharge, intraarticular pressure, and joint angle in the knee of the dog, *J Physiol* 373:353, 1986.
45. Fowler PJ, Webster MS: Rotation strength about the shoulder: establishment of internal to external strength ratios. Paper presented at the American Orthopaedic Society for Sports Medicine annual meeting, Nashville, Tenn, July 1985.
46. Frank C et al: Physiology and therapeutic value of passive joint motion, *Clin Orthop* 185:113, 1984.
47. Gann N: Ultrasound: current concepts, *Clin Manage* 11:64, 1991.

48. Giovanelli-Blacker B, Elvey R, Thompson E: The clinical significance of measured lumbar zygoapophyseal intra-capsular pressure variation. In *Proceedings of manipulative Therapists Association of Australia,* Brisbane, Australia, 1985.

49. Glossary of osteopathic terminology, *J Am Osteopath Assoc* 80:552, 1981.

50. Goldstein JD et al: Spine injuries in gymnasts and swimmers: an epidemiologic investigation, *Am J Sports Med* 19:463, 1991.

51. Good R, Nickel V: Cervical spine injuries resulting from water sports, *Spine* 5:502, 1980.

52. Greenman P: Principles of soft tissue and articulatory (mobilization without impulse) technique. In *Principles of manual medicine,* Baltimore, 1989, Williams & Wilkins.

53. Hansson T, Keller T, Manohar M: A study of the compressive properties of lumbar vertebral trabeculae: effects of tissue characteristics, *Spine* 12:56, 1987.

54. Hattori S, Oda H, Kawai S: Cervical intradiscal pressure in movements and traction of the cervical spine, *J Orthop* 119:568, 1981.

55. Herring SA: Rehabilitation of muscle injuries, *Med Sci Sports Exerc* 22:453, 1990.

56. Huskisson E: Non-narcotic analgesics. In Wall PD, Melzach R, editors: *Textbook of pain,* New York, 1984, Churchill Livingstone.

57. Inman V, Sanders J, Abbott L: Observations of the function of the shoulder joint, *J Bone Joint Surg* 26A:1, 1944.

58. Jones L: Spontaneous release by positioning, *DO* 4:109, 1964.

59. Jones L: *Strain and counterstrain,* Newark, Ohio, 1981, American Academy of Osteopathy.

60. Kadaba MP, Cole AJ: Intramuscular wire electromyography of the subscapularis, *J Orthop Res* 10:394, 1992.

61. Kellett J: Acute soft tissue injuries—a review of the literature, *Med Sci Sports Exerc* 18:489, 1986.

62. Kennedy JC, Hawkins R, Krissoff WB: Orthopedic manifestations of swimming, *Am J Sports Med* 6:309, 1978.

63. Kenney S: Personal communication, Palo Alto, Calif, 1991, Head Swim Coach, Stanford University Men's Swim Team.

64. Kewalramani L, Taylor R: Injuries to the cervical spine from diving accidents, *J Trauma* 15:130, 1975.

65. Kibler WB: Clinical aspects of muscle injury, *Med Sci Sports Exerc* 22:450, 1990.

66. Kibler WB, Chandler TJ, Pace BK: Principles of rehabilitation after chronic tendon injuries, *Clin Sports Med* 11:661, 1992.

67. Kirby R et al: Oxygen consumption during exercise in a heated pool, *Arch Phys Med Rehabil* 65:21, 1984.

68. Kiwerski J: Cervical spine injuries caused by diving into water, *Paraplegia* 18:101, 1980.

69. Kolb M: Principles of underwater exercise, *Phys Ther Rev* 37:361, 1957.

70. Korr I: Neurochemical and neurotrophic consequences of nerve deformation. In Glasgow EF et al, editors: *Aspects of manipulative therapy,* Melbourne, Australia, 1985, Churchill Livingstone.

71. Krahl H, Steinbruck K: *Sportsachaden und Sportverletzungen and der Wirbelsaule Arztebl Deutsch,* 12:19, 1978.

72. Kreighbaum E, Barthels K: *Biomechanics: a qualitative approach for studying human movement,* ed 2, Minneapolis, 1985, Burgess.

73. Kuprian W: *Physical therapy for sports,* Philadelphia, 1982, WB Saunders.

74. Kusunose R: Strain and counterstrain. In Basmajian JV, Nyberg R, editors: *Rational manual therapies,* Baltimore, 1993, Williams & Wilkins.

75. Kvist M, Jarvenen M: Clinical, histochemical and biochemical features in repair of muscle and tendon injuries, *Int J Sports Med* 3:12, 1982.

76. Lehmann J: Therapeutic heat and cold, *Clin Orthop* 99:207, 1974.

77. Lehmann J, deLateur BJ: Diathermy and superficial heat and cold therapy. In Kottke EJ et al, editors: *Krusen's handbook of physical medicine and rehabilitation,* Philadelphia, 1982, WB Saunders.

78. Lester JP, Windsor RE, Dreyer SJ: *Medical management of the cervical spine,* New York, Churchill Livingstone (in press).

79. Levick J: An investigation into the validity of subatmospheric pressure recordings from synovial fluid and their dependence on joint angle, *J Physiol* 289:55, 1979.

80. Maglischo E: *Swimming even faster,* Sunnyvale, Calif, 1982, Mayfield.

81. Maitland G: *Vertebral manipulation,* ed 2, London, 1986, Butterworth.

82. Marchbanks P, Lambert C: *Aquamotion,* Santa Barbara, Calif, 1988, Santa Barbara Cottage Hospital.

83. Martin R: Swimming: forces on aquatic animals and humans. In Vaughan CL, editor: *Biomechanics of sport,* Boca Raton, Fla, 1989, CRC Press.

84. Martin W et al: Cardiovascular adaptations to intensive swim training in sedentary middle-aged men and women, *Circulation* 75:323, 1987.

85. McArdle W, Katch F, Katch V: Energy expenditure during walking, jogging, running, and swimming. In McArdle W, Katch F, Katch V, editors: *Exercise physiology: energy, nutrition, and human performance,* Philadelphia, 1986, Lea & Febiger.

86. McClure M: Flexibility training. In Basmajian JV, Nyberg R, editors: *Rational manual therapies,* Baltimore, 1993, Williams & Wilkins.

87. McMaster WC, Long SC, Caiozzo V: Isokinetic torque imbalances in the rotator cuff of the elite water polo player, *Am J Sports Med* 19:72, 1991.

88. Mennel J: *Back pain,* Boston, 1960, Little, Brown.

89. Miller F: Fluids. In *College physics,* ed 4, New York, 1977, Harcourt Brace Jovanovich.

90. Moschetti ML, Cole AJ: Risk management and facility issues in aquatic rehabilitation, *J Back Musculoskel Rehabil* (in press).

91. Mutoh Y, Miwako T, Mitsumasa M: Chronic injuries of elite competitive swimmers, divers, water polo players, and synchronized swimmers. In Ungerecht VB, Wilke K, editors: *Swimming science,* Champaign, Ill, 1988, Human Kinetics Books.

92. Nuber G et al: Fine wire electromyography analysis of muscles of the shoulder during swimming, *Am J Sports Med* 14:7, 1986.

93. Nyberg R, Basmajian JV: Rationale for the use of spinal manipulation. In Basmajian JV, Nyberg R, editors: *Rational manual therapies,* Baltimore, 1993, Williams & Wilkins.

94. Panjabi M et al: Spinal ability and intersegmental muscle forces: a biomechanical model, *Spine* 14:194, 1989.

95. Paris S: Mobilization of the spine, *Phys Ther* 59:988, 1979.

96. Paris SV: The spine and swimming. In Hochshuler SH, editor: *Spinal injuries in sports,* Philadelphia, 1990, Hanley & Belfus.

97. Piette G, Clarys JP: Telemetric EMG of the front crawl movement. In Terauds J, Bedingfield W, editors: *Swimming,* vol 3, Baltimore, 1979, University Park Press.

98. Pink M et al: The normal shoulder during freestyle swimming: an electromyographic and cinematographic analysis of twelve muscles, *Am J Sports Med* 19:569, 1991.

99. Press JM, Herring SA, Kibler WB: Rehabilitation of musculoskeletal disorders. In *The textbook of military medicine,* Borden Institute, Office of the Surgeon General (in press).

100. Reister VC, Cole AJ: Start active, stay active in the water, *J Phys Educ Recreation Dance* 64(1):52, 1993.

101. Reynolds M: Myofascial trigger point syndromes in the practice of rheumatology, *Arch Phys Med Rehabil* 6:111, 1981.

102. Richardson A, Jobe F, Collins H: The shoulder in competitive swimming, *Am J Sports Med* 8:159, 1980.

103. Richardson AB, Miller JW: Swimming and the older athlete: sports medicine in the older athlete, *Clin Sports Med* 10:301, 1991.

104. Rossi F: Spondylolysis, spondylolisthesis and sports, *J Sports Med Phys Fitness* 18:317, 1978.

105. Saal JA, Saal JS: Later stage management of lumbar spine problems, *Phys Med Rehabil Clin North Am* 2:205, 1991.

106. Saal JS: Rehabilitation of the injured athlete. In DeLisa J, editor: *Rehabilitation medicine: principles and practice,* ed 2, Philadelphia, 1993, JB Lippincott.

107. Saal JS: Flexibility training. In Saal JA, editor: *Physical medicine and rehabilitation: rehabilitation of sports injuries,* Philadelphia, 1987, Hanley & Belfus.

108. Saliba VL, Johnson GS, Wardlaw CF: Proprioceptive neuromuscular facilitation. In Basmajian JV, Nyberg R, editors: *Rational manual therapies,* Baltimore, 1993, Williams & Wilkins.

109. Scovazzo M et al: The painful shoulder during freestyle swimming: an electromyographic cinematographic analysis of twelve muscles, *Am J Sports Med* 19:577, 1991.

110. Shelokov A: Evaluation, diagnosis and initial treatment of general disc disease. In *Spine State Art Rev* 5(2):67, 1991.

111. Shirazi-Adl A, Ahmed A, Shrivastava S: Mechanical response of a lumbar motion segment in axial torque alone and combined with compression, *Spine* 11:914, 1989.

112. Simons D: Myofascial trigger points: a need for understanding, *Arch Phys Med Rehabil* 62:97, 1981.

113. Sinnett E, Cole AJ: The biomechanics of the freestyle, backstroke, breaststroke, and butterfly swim strokes, *J Back Musculoskel Rehabil* (in press).

114. Stratton SA, Bryan JM: Dysfunction, evaluation, and treatment of the cervical spine and thoracic inlet. In *Orthopaedic physical therapy,* ed 2, New York, 1993, Churchill Livingstone.

115. Sutej PG, Hadler NM: Current principles of rehabilitation for patients with rheumatoid arthritis, *Clin Orthop* 265:116, 1991.

116. Sweeney T et al: Cervicothoracic muscular stabilization techniques. In *Phys Med Rehabil State Art Rev* 4(2):335, 1990.

117. Ward R: Headache: an osteopathic perspective, *J Am Osteopathic Assoc* 81:458, 1982.

118. Ward R: Myofascial release concepts. In Basmajian JV, Nyberg R, editors: *Rational manual therapies,* Baltimore, 1993, Williams & Wilkins.

119. Weinstein SL: Adolescent idiopathic scoliosis: prevalence and natural history. In *Instructional Course Lectures,* vol 38, Park Ridge, Ill, 1989, American Academy of Orthopaedic Surgeons.

120. Wilder RP, Brennan DK: Physiological responses to deep water running in athletes, *Sports Med* 16:374, 1993.

121. Wilder R, Brennan D, Schotte DA: Standard measure for exercise prescription for aqua running, *Am J Sports Med* 21:45, 1993.

122. Wilder RP et al: Overuse injuries of the hip and pelvis in sport, *J Back Musculoskel Rehabil* (in press).

123. Wilson F, Lindseth R: The adolescent swimmer's back, *Am J Sports Med* 10:174, 1982.

124. Windsor RE, Lester JP, Herring SA: Electrical stimulation in clinical practice, Physician *Sportsmed* 21:85, 1993.

125. Woo S and others: The effects of exercise on the biomechanical and biochemical properties of swine digital flexor tendon, *J Biomech Eng* 103:51, 1981.

126. Wright V, Dawson N: Biomechanics of joint function. In Holt PLJ, editor: *Current topics in connective tissue disease,* Edinburgh, 1975, Churchill Livingstone.

127. Wyke B, Polacek P: Articular neurology: the present position, *J Bone Joint Surg* 57B:401, 1975.

128. Yeater R et al: Tethered swimming forces in the crawl, breast, and back strokes and their relationship to competitive performance, *J Biomech* 14:527, 1981.

129. Ziskin MC, McDiarmid T, Michlovitz SL: Therapeutic ultrasound. In Michlovitz SL, editor: *Thermal agents in rehabilitation,* Philadelphia, 1990, FA Davis.

Chapter Thirty-Four

Waterskiing

Glenn R. Rechtine
Michael W. Reed

Over the last decade the popularity of waterskiing has grown by the tens of millions in the United States and throughout the world. Enjoyed by young and old alike, waterskiing has many psychologic and physical benefits. However, because of the forces involved, there is also the risk of injury, which can vary in severity from minor strains and sprains to fractures, dislocations, and even death. This chapter focuses on the different types of waterskiing, the types of forces involved in each subset, and the subsequent types of spinal problems encountered in each subset.

TYPES OF WATERSKIING

Waterskiing is enjoyed by people of all ages—from those as young as 1 year of age to those in their nineties. Most are involved in recreational skiing, but many participate in competitive skiing. Recreational skiers commonly ski on either two skis, one ski, or, for the adventuresome, no skis. Competitive skiing comprises several categories. One is tournament skiing, which consists of slalom skiing, jumping, and tricks. Another subset is "barefooting" (i.e., skiing without the benefit of waterskis). This was first performed in 1947 and has become increasingly popular. Since 1963 it has been organized into a tournament event consisting of starts, wake slalom, tricks, and jumping. Another type of competitive skiing is speed skiing, in which skiers are pulled for long distances with ropes behind hydroplanes at speeds of up to 80 mph.

SPINAL INJURIES

As skis became smaller and boats faster, waterskiing became increasingly popular. With this increasing popularity, however, different types of injuries have become more prevalent.

The most serious injuries are the result of falls in shallow water; collisions with inanimate objects such as a boat, dock, or ski jump; or high-velocity falls. By following boating and waterskiing regulations, as well as using common sense, most skiers can prevent these injuries. The types of spinal injuries that occur in both the adult and juvenile skier—cervical, thoracic, and lumbar spine—often depend on the type of skiing activity taking place. These injuries range from strains and sprains to more severe osseoligamentous injuries, depending on the amount of force involved and the mechanism of injury. The most common spinal injury occurring in waterskiing is to the cervical spine. This injury results from either a fall in shallow water or a fall with enough velocity to produce an osseoligamentous injury.

Thoracic Injuries

Thoracic spine injuries are unusual except for the dystrophic changes that can occur from long exposure to competitive jumping.[14]

Lumbar Injuries

Injuries in the lumbar area, which occur frequently, most commonly consist of strains and sprains as a result of the forces across the low back. The beginning skier usually starts off with two skis. The anatomic starting position for the beginner has the skier floating in the water, with arms fully extended, holding the tow rope. The upper body should be slightly reclined with the lumbar spine flexed approximately 40 degrees, the hips flexed at 100 degrees, the knees flexed to 90 degrees, and the ankles dorsiflexed to approximately 20 degrees. As the boat accelerates, the skier begins to come out of the water, the lumbar spine continues to flex, and the trapezius, latissimus dorsi, erector spinae, gluteus maximus, and hamstring muscles undergo eccentric contraction until the skis have begun to plane on the water. At this point the beginner has the tendency to remain with the knees in an extended position and the lumbar spine in a flexed position to maintain balance. This places undue strain on the hamstrings, gluteus maximus, and erector spinae. This anatomically unsound position on top of the skis results in a high number of skiers with muscle soreness, as well as a large number of strains that occur in beginners. Proper execution by a beginning skier accelerating out of the water requires the concentric contraction of the gluteus maximus, hamstrings, erector spinae, and latissimus dorsi. Once the skier is planing on the water, the muscular forces across the back can be minimized by maintaining an anatomically correct position over the skis, with the upper body erect, the arms extended, and the hips, knees, and ankles slightly flexed. Injuries can also be minimized through proper conditioning, instruction, and warm-up exercises.

Cervical Injuries

Waterskiing injuries to the cervical spine are most commonly the result of a forward fall at high speed. This head-first position can occur in any type of skiing but is more common in falls during slalom and barefoot skiing. Depending on the magnitude of the force encountered, injuries vary from soft tissue injuries to fractures or dislocations. The mechanisms of injuries common to the cervical spine are compressive extension injuries, vertical compression, and compressive flexion injuries.[1] These injuries are named according to the initial dominant force vector leading to failure and also to the presumed attitude of the cervical spine at the time of failure.

Soft tissue injuries. The most common soft tissue injury to the cervical spine is acceleration hyperextension, or whiplash of the neck. In this injury the motion of the head and neck is stopped when the back of the head strikes the upper spine, which has continued to move forward. Falls directly on the face can produce sudden extension of the neck and cause injuries ranging from mild muscular strain to dislocation. Most severe injuries are noted with hyperextension because the potential range of motion is greater.[6] When the neck is caused to flex anteriorly or laterally, the head strikes the shoulder or chest.[12] The soft tissues of the neck are protected by this limitation of motion. Symptoms and signs of soft tissue injury are variable. Often the skier experiences severe pain immediately after the injury, but this may be delayed up to 24 hours. The most common finding after the injury is muscular tenderness both anteriorly and posteriorly. Injury to the strap muscles of the neck can cause difficulty in lifting and rotating the head.[11,17] Pain may radiate down the neck into the shoulders and down the arms or to the inner scapular area, chest, and occipital region. These patterns of referred pain are nonneurogenic and may be produced by chronic irritation of the musculoligamentous, joint, and intervertebral disc structures.[12] Pain radiating down the arm does not necessarily indicate nerve root compression. Frank disc herniation is unusual from soft tissue injury alone. One frequent complaint is numbness along the ulnar border of the hand, with concomitant objective sensory changes. This often is due to scalenus spasm rather than a true ulnar neuropathy.[13,15]

Treatment of soft tissue cervical injuries should be adjusted to the severity of the injury and directed toward early mobilization. Immobilization of the neck in a contoured soft cervical collar may be useful in the early postinjury period to rest the traumatized tissues. Increasing the time spent out of the collar, along with gentle active range of motion, should be encouraged. Local heat may help relieve early symptoms of stiffness and soreness, and antiinflammatory medications can be helpful.[7,9] Injuries to the C1-2 complex are related to one another by several facets of anatomy, the mechanism of injury, and the methods of treatment. Injuries most commonly caused by force applied to the spine through the base of the skull, common in motor vehicle accidents, are less apt to occur in waterskiing.

Compressive flexion injuries. Most waterskiing injuries in the cervical spine occur in the lower cervical spine and are the result of indirect forces originating on the head or trunk that cause compressive forces to act on the neck. The first group of injuries to be considered in the lower cervical spine are those of the compressive flexion category. These result from a force vector directed inferiorly and anteriorly to the lower cervical spine. This particular category has five recognizable stages.[17] The first two stages of injury in this compressive flexion category result in loss of some of the anterior height of the vertebral body, but there is no posterior element damage. As this compressive force increases with the spine in flexion at the time of injury, there is an increasing shear in the posterior elements. This links the more severe anterior compression injury with increasing posterior shear and ligamentous failure. Injuries in which there is posterior ligamentous disruption often show late instability if they are treated primarily with halo traction or by anterior stabilization alone.[4,5] Patients whose injuries cause neurologic damage and who show signs of anterior compression will need staged anterior decompression and fusion along with posterior stabilization.

Vertical compression fractures. Another group of cervical spine injuries in skiers is vertical compression fractures, or "burst fractures." These are caused primarily by an axial load. In this injury the neck is in a neutral position when the force is first applied. The neck goes into flexion, the posterior elements are placed under tension, and posterior ligamentous injury occurs. If the neck remains in neutral or becomes slightly extended, the posterior elements are placed under compressive loads and may fracture. In vertical compression injuries, restoration of alignment is the primary goal. Surgical stabilization is rarely indicated unless instability is demonstrated at a later date.[10]

Compression extension injuries. A third mechanism of injury seen in cervical spine injuries in waterskiing is that of compression extension. In this injury the major injury vector is directed toward the trunk, stressing the posterior elements in compression. These injuries can range from unilateral vertebral arch fractures to bilateral laminar fractures. More severe injuries consist of anterior ligamentous disruption, with displacement of one vertebral body on another.[17] The compression extension mechanism is the most common cervical injury seen in waterskiing and is commonly associated with high-speed slalom falls or forward falls in barefoot skiing.

Upper Thoracic Injuries

Severe injuries to the thoracolumbar spine in waterskiing are less common. Considerable violence is necessary to produce a fracture or dislocation of the upper thoracic spine, which is more rigid than other parts of the spine and is stabilized by the contiguous rib cage.

Bending and extension are markedly resisted because the anatomy of the facets and lamina restricts rotational motion.[2,3] The thoracolumbar junction is the region at greatest risk of sustaining a fracture. The thoracolumbar junction is the first mobile area distal to the stabilizing influence of the ribs, and it acts as the fulcrum of the motion for the thorax. It is situated between the distal end of the relatively long lever arm of the thoracic complex and the highly mobile lumbar spine. It sits in an area of transition from the kyphotic thoracic spine to the lordotic lumbar spine. The thoracolumbar junction is also the point at which the facets are in the process of changing their orientation from the coronal plane to the sagittal plane.[15,16]

Incidence

Waterskiing fractures outside of the cervical spine region are very unusual. However, the axial compressive forces that occur during competitive jumping can cause some injury to the thoracic and thoracolumbar spine. In competitive waterskiing the transient deceleration forces on the body are far greater than the forces encountered in other sports.

In an unpublished study of Canadian waterski jumpers, J.G. Reid, of the Biomechanics Laboratory of Queens University, found that men who jumped 40 m at a take-off velocity of 26.5 m/sec experienced forces of 3944 N (5.0 g/94 m/sec) on landing in water. Boys younger than 14 years old using a 5-foot-high ramp rather than the adult 6-foot ramp experienced less stress on take-off — 2945 N (3.9 g/95 m/sec), but on landing the impact forces were greater in both groups, with 4174 N (5.6 g/95 m/sec) in boys and 4956 N (6.7 g/95 m/sec) in adults. In competition this degree of force will be exerted on a rigid spine several times daily.

A radiographic survey of 117 competitive waterski jumpers was conducted to determine whether the sport can cause spinal column damage and, if so, whether the damage is more likely to occur in those who participate during the period of spinal growth and development (15 years or younger). This review revealed a high prevalence of two types of abnormalities: Scheuermann's osteochondrosis was present in 26% of the skiers, and vertebral body wedging occurred in 34%. The prevalence of adolescent spondylodystrophy increased with the number of years of participation in the sport before the age of 15 years. Of the participants in this age group who had skied for 5 years or more, 57% showed adolescent spondylodystrophy. Of those in the same age group who had skied for 9 years or more, 100% were affected. Wedged vertebrae increased as participation time increased, regardless of the age at which exposure began.

A biometric and skeletal study involving 83 international waterskiers revealed that many skiers had episodes of low back pain, and 41% showed radiographic evidence of degenerative spinal changes. Although the spondylodystrophy changes are not as devastating as a thoracic or thoracolumbar fracture, it has been shown that persons with this stress spondylodystrophy have more back pain later in life.

TURNING

In either recreational or competitive slalom skiing, the turn can be broken down into three phases: the deceleration phase, the reach phase, and the acceleration phase.

Deceleration Phase

In skiing, deceleration occurs when the skier begins to slow the ski down to start a turn. Normally it occurs as soon as the skier has crossed the second wake behind the boat. However, at slower boat speeds, the skier may have to wait 7 to 10 feet after the second wake. In other words, deceleration and the changing of the edge of the ski help facilitate the deceleration, and this process varies according to boat speeds and rope lengths. The faster the skier travels, the sooner the deceleration phase must begin.

The anatomic position of the shoulders should be erect, facing square to the shore, with the knees and ankles bent as far down as possible, the ski handle in close to the body, and the arms flexed. This motion requires a sustained isometric contraction of the quadriceps, gluteus maximus, latissimus dorsi, biceps, and forearm flexors. This body position is maintained by continuous contraction of the rectus abdominis, trapezius, erector spinae, hip flexors, gluteus maximus, and the gastrocsoleus complex. From this body position the edge change is smooth and quick. The speed that is accumulated from the pull through both wakes will keep the momentum going to begin the deceleration phase. At this point the ski begins its roll over onto its inside edge. This motion puts weight on the front of the ski, placing more surface area of the ski into the water, which begins deceleration for the turn. The knees are pushed forward while the body is maintained in an erect position. This motion requires the eccentric contraction of the quadriceps while the hip flexors and extensors control the motion of the shifting of the ski to the inside edge. At the same time the edge is changed, the outside hand comes off the handle to begin the reach phase of the turn.

Reach Phase

The reach phase begins as the skier starts to extend the inside arm toward the direction of the pull of the boat. The arm is extended to its full position. This involves a concentric contraction of the latissimus dorsi, pectoralis major, and biceps of the leading arm. During this portion of the turn, the upper body remains erect, which requires the isometric contraction of the erector spinae, gluteus maximus, neck extensors, rectus abdominis, quadriceps, hamstrings, and gastrocsoleus complex. As the skier reaches, the ski continues to roll onto its inside edge, slowing the ski and setting up the final phase of the turn, the acceleration phase.

Acceleration Phase

The final phase, or acceleration phase, is begun by bringing the handle in quickly to the outside hip to ensure proper body alignment for the pull. Pulling the handle straight in toward the outside hip uses a concentric contraction of the latissimus dorsi, biceps, and forearm flexors. The outside elbow is elevated to shoulder height to keep the body up and balanced. At the same time, this outside arm reaches for the handle, meeting it halfway. This motion of the outside arm helps to turn the shoulders toward the wake in the direction of the pull and will begin the acceleration phase. Positioning of the arms and pulling the handle to the hip require the concentric contracture of the latissimus dorsi, trapezius, deltoids, biceps, and forearm flexors. Simultaneously the gluteus maximus and erector spinae undergo concentric contraction to maintain the correct anatomic position as the force of the pull increases. During this acceleration phase the erect position is maintained through the isometric contracture of the leg muscles, hamstrings, quadriceps, and gastrocsoleus complex.[8]

PREVENTION OF INJURY

A large number of spinal injuries that occur in skiing are due to poor judgment and carelessness and therefore are preventable. Other spinal injuries are more difficult to prevent and occur as part of the natural risk involved in the many facets of this sport. They commonly occur in falls in barefoot waterskiing, slalom skiing, and competitive jumping because of the high speeds required. Falls in these events are rarely predictable and often are uncontrollable. Certain precautions can be taken to minimize the risk of injury from falling. In a forward fall in barefoot skiing, the best thing to do is to tuck the head and roll over a shoulder. Some of the worst falls are caused by holding onto the handle a moment too long after catching a toe. This prevents the skier from tucking and allows a hard face-first slam into the water, placing a compressive extension force on the spine. Thus once a skier begins a forward fall, the rope should be released as soon as possible.

Again, most injuries are preventable or can at least be minimized by adhering to some of the following rules. Skiers should wear a snug-fitting life jacket; a loose vest can be dangerous. Water-tight shorts should be worn to prevent injection of water into unwanted places. Equipment should be checked regularly so there are no protruding or sharp objects to snag or cut the skin. The skier should warm up properly, be in good physical condition, and obtain proper instruction before practicing a new skill. The boat driver and skier should have a

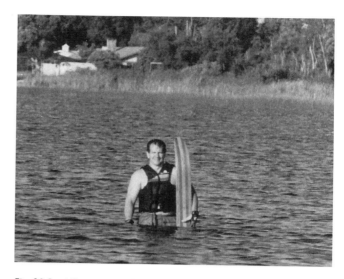

Fig. 34-1. All concerned should be familiar with the underwater terrain inasmuch as sandbars or other underwater obstructions may exist far from shore.

set of signals understood by both for proper communication. The driver should be competent, understand the signals, and be aware of the surrounding terrain. The ski line should not be placed around the hand, arms, or neck. The terrain should be checked for shallow water, with a minimum safety depth of 5 feet for any skiing (Fig. 34-1). The boat driver should maintain the skier well away from shore, and the skier should stay away from unfamiliar water. Both the driver and the skier should watch for floating debris. Not all injuries are avoidable; however, the risk of a serious spinal injury is significantly reduced by the use of common sense.

REFERENCES

1. Allen BL, Fergusion RL: Cervical spine trauma in children. In Bradford D, Hensinger R, editors: *The pediatric spine,* New York, 1985, Thieme.
2. Bohlman HH: Current concepts review: treatment of fractures and dislocations of the thoracic and lumbar spine, *J Bone Joint Surg* 67A:165, 1985.
3. Bohlman HH, Freehafer A, Dejak J: The results of treatment of acute injuries of the upper thoracic spine with paralysis, *J Bone Joint Surg* 67A:360, 1985.
4. Capen DA, Zigler J, Garland DE: Surgical stabilization in cervical spine trauma, *Contemp Orthop* 14:25, 1987.
5. Capen DA et al: Surgical stabilization of the cervical spine: a comparative analysis of anterior and posterior fusions, *Paraplegia* 25:111, 1987.
6. Deng YC, Goldsmith W: Response of a human head/neck/upper torso replica to dynamic landing. II. Analytic/numerical model, *J Biomech* 20:487, 1987.
7. Dunn EJ, Balzar S: Soft tissue injuries of the lower cervical spine. In Griffen PP, editor: *Instructional course lectures,* Chicago, 1987, American Academy of Orthopedic Surgeons.
8. Eberhardt T: An anatomical description of the slalom turn in water skiing and how to condition for this sport, *Natl Strength Cond Assoc J* 10,(6):80, 1988.
9. Gassman J, Seligson D: The anterior cervical plate, *Spine* 8:700, 1983.

10. Grady MS et al: Use of the Philadelphia collar as an alternative to the halo vest in patients with C2-C3 fractures, *Neurosurgery* 18:151, 1985.
11. Harns JH, Edeiken-Monroe P, Kopaniky DR: A practical classification of acute cervical spine injuries, *Orthop Clin North Am* 17:15, 1986.
12. Hohl M: Soft tissue injuries of the neck, *Clin Orthop* 109:42, 1975.
13. Hohl M: Soft tissue injuries of the neck in automobile accidents: factors influencing prognosis, *J Bone Joint Surg* 56A:1675, 1984.
14. King AG: Spinal column trauma. In *AAOS instructional course lectures,* vol 35, St Louis, 1986, Mosby.
15. McNab I: Acceleration and extension injuries of the cervical spine. In Rothman RH, Simeone FA, editors: *The spine,* ed 2, Philadelphia, 1982, WB Saunders.
16. White AA, Panjabi MM: *Clinical biomechanics of the spine,* Philadelphia, 1978, JB Lippincott.
17. White AA III et al: Biomechanical analysis of clinical stability in the cervical spine, *Clin Orthop* 109:85, 1975.

Chapter Thirty-Five

Diving

Nathan H. Lebwohl

Diving accidents are the fourth most common cause of spinal cord injury after motor vehicle accidents, gunshot wounds, and falls. In Miami, Florida, diving injuries account for 6% of admissions to our spinal cord rehabilitation center. Across the country, approximately 9% of admissions for spinal injuries are due to diving accidents. More cases of quadriplegia have been caused by diving accidents than by injuries from all other sports combined. Paradoxically, organized competitive diving is rarely associated with catastrophic spinal injury.

INJURIES IN COMPETITIVE DIVING

Competitive diving is an organized sport with strict rules regarding safety, training, and supervision. Despite the potential for injury, there has been no report of a fatality or catastrophic injury during supervised training or competition in 80 years of competitive diving in the United States.[8] Internationally, two fatalities in accomplished divers occurred when the divers struck their heads on the platform during difficult maneuvers.

There are three components to each dive during which a diver can be hurt.[4] The first, and most dangerous, component is during takeoff from the board or platform. The diver must achieve adequate horizontal and vertical velocity so as to clear the end of the board without hitting his or her head. The second component is during entry to the water. Diving has been described as a water entry collision skill. Vertical entry is the goal. Horizontal entry can result in pain and injury, although rarely does a serious injury occur as a result of collision with the water surface. The third component is the possibility that the diver may hit the pool bottom or some other object after entering the water.

TAKEOFF

Years ago, diving boards were made of wood and were angled upward[26] to help the diver gain height. As a result, if the diver remained in contact with the board too long, the recoil of the board would result in a backward-directed force. It was fairly common for the diver to hit the tip of the board with his or her head (Fig. 35-1). Today's aluminum boards are mounted level so that this problem occurs less frequently, but if the diver remains in contact with the board too long to achieve greater height, horizontal velocity may not be adequate and the board may not be cleared. An important design feature is to make the tip of the board as lightweight as possible. In theory, the perfect board would be weightless, so that a collision with the diver's head would not result in an injury.

Certain types of dives, especially inward and reverse dives, pose a higher risk of striking the board or diving platform. In an inward dive, the diver stands at the tip of the board facing backward and after takeoff rotates inward with the head moving toward the board. The risk of colliding with the board is obvious if adequate horizontal velocity is not achieved at takeoff. In a reverse dive, the diver stands at the tip of the board facing forward and after takeoff rotates backward with the head moving toward the board. Again, the risk of collision with the board is obvious. The angular momentum for the somersault in both the inward dive and the reverse dive must come from the horizontally oriented takeoff force of the diver's feet pushing off the board (Fig. 35-2). If the takeoff force is vertically oriented, the diver's head will strike the board. In a reverse dive, if the angular momentum is initiated by the diver pulling the head and shoulders backward during takeoff instead of pushing off forward with the feet, adequate horizontal velocity will not be achieved and the head will strike the board.[10]

Both of the divers who were killed as a result of striking their heads on diving platforms were attempting reverse, multiple somersault dives. The rare occurrence of severe injury is a testimony to the careful training of competitive divers. This represents not only the intensive

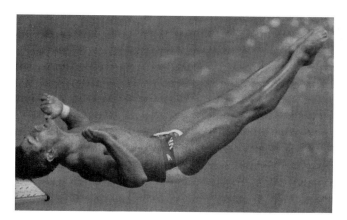

Fig. 35-1. U.S. Olympic champion Greg Louganis struck his head on the diving board during the Summer Olympics in Seoul. Fortunately, no serious injury occurred. Two fatalities have been reported in international competition because of similar injuries. (© 1988 Brian Smith.)

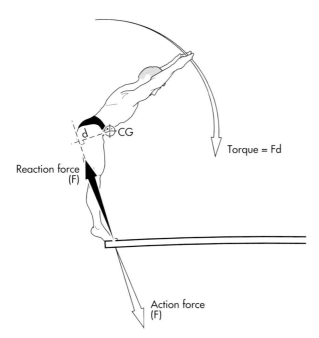

Fig. 35-2. In an inward dive the takeoff force must be adequately oriented in the horizontal plane or the diver will strike the board. The torque for the inward somersault is achieved by the force of takeoff from the board, multiplied by the distance from the center of gravity. Rotation should not be achieved by pulling the upper body toward the board. (© 1995 Tim Krasnasky. Redrawn from Manual JG, editor: *U.S. diving safety,* 1990, U.S. Diving.)

practice of these athletes but also the importance of the coaches who progress the divers carefully to dives requiring greater skill and emphasize performer readiness to avoid injury.

WATER ENTRY

Vertical, or near-vertical, water entry is the goal of every dive. Horizontal entry, or landing flat, results in rapid deceleration and can result in severe injury, including detached retinas, rib fractures, internal bleeding, and ruptured viscera. Although divers practice and perfect vertical entry with every dive, horizontal entry does occur, especially during training. An air-bubbling system, known as an air sparger, has been devised to minimize injury during water entry. The air sparger, located at the pool bottom, injects air at high velocity to create a 50/50 mixture of air bubbles and water.[7] Because air is much more compressible than water, the bubbles form a cushion into which the diver enters. The impact force can be reduced by as much as 80%. This means that landing flat from 10 m would result in about the same impact as landing flat from 2 m on solid water.

COLLISION WITH THE POOL BOTTOM OR IN-WATER OBSTACLES

Collision of the diver's head with the pool bottom is the primary cause of spinal cord injury in recreational swimming pool diving accidents. However, this has never been the cause of injury in competitive diving. Competitive diving always takes place at the deep end of an appropriately constructed pool. Competitive divers steer underwater to avoid striking the pool bottom. Although buoyancy and drag will slow a diver's descent, underwater steering is required to avoid hitting the bottom in all but the deepest pools. Albrand and Walter[1] filmed divers underwater to determine their speed at various depths. They found that a diver jumping from a 1-m springboard entered the water at more than 25 feet/sec. At a depth of 10 feet, the diver was still moving at more than 10 feet/sec. Gabrielson[9] showed that an untrained diver using a running start could achieve a horizontal distance of 20 feet from the end of a 1-m board before entering the water, demonstrating the ability of the diver to overshoot the deep end of a pool. Stone,[29] in a study funded by the National Swimming Pool Foundation, concluded that within practical limits of pool design "it is not possible to rely solely on the slowing effect of water to ensure that the diver will not hit the bottom of the pool at dangerous velocities (Fig. 35-3). The diver must steer underwater to avoid collision with the bottom.

What is the minimum safe depth in which to dive? There is no universally agreed-on answer. Albrand and Walter[1] estimated a maximum reaction time of 0.5 seconds to begin underwater steering. Using their underwater deceleration curves, the maximum depth reached from a 1-m platform dive at 0.5 seconds was 9 feet. Based on this and other reports, a depth of 12 feet underneath the tip of a 1-m board has been commonly accepted for new pool construction. However, what about existing pools? The New York State Department of Health recently reviewed their experience with 212 high school pools and found no evidence of significant injury. Their decision was to continue using pools with 9 feet of depth under a 1-m board.

NONCATASTROPHIC SPINAL INJURIES
Lumbar Spine

In a radiographic study of over 1400 athletes, Rossi[23] determined that diving was the sport most commonly associated with spondylolysis. In 30 divers he reported an 83% incidence of abnormalities of the pars interarticularis. In 63% there was a definite spondylolysis, and of those, 16% had spondylolisthesis. This compared with an overall 16.7% occurrence of spondylolysis for all athletes studied. After interviewing the athletes, Rossi suggested that hyperextension during water entry was the maneuver most likely to have caused the injury. The description of sudden onset of violent pain suggests that acute fracture of the pars may occur, rather than the fatigue fracture most commonly associated with spondylolysis.[19] Hyperextension during water entry is a technical error. It can be due to overrotation during forward dives, with the lower extremities continuing to rotate after the trunk

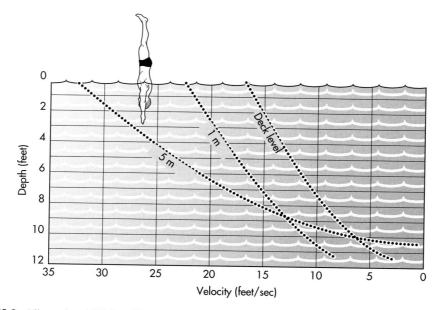

Fig. 35-3. Albrand and Walter filmed divers underwater to determine the slowing effect of the water on their descent. When jumping from the side of the pool, the divers were still moving at 7 feet/sec when they reached a depth of 10 feet, indicating that divers cannot rely on the water alone to prevent them from hitting the bottom of the pool. ((© 1995 Tim Krasnasky. Redrawn from Albrand OW, Walter J: *Surg Neurol* 4:461, 1975.)

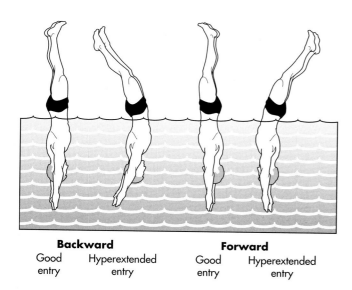

Fig. 35-4. In a backward dive the diver must hyperextend to achieve a vertical entry. This predisposes to pars interarticularis injury. Similarly, lumbar hyperextension can occur in a forward dive if the lower extremities "fall over" as a result of overrotation. (© 1995 Tim Krasnasky.)

has entered the water. More commonly, it is the result of a backward dive in which rotation is inadequate. The diver hyperextends the spine in order to achieve a vertical entry (Fig. 35-4). Our experience at the University of Miami suggests that the incidence of spondylolysis

is not as high as that reported by Rossi. This is most likely due to differences in training and technique.

Hyperextension of the spine during takeoff from the diving board, and the repetitive flexion (piking) and extension (arching) that are common during diving have been implicated as important causative factors in low back pain, which is frequent in divers.[25] Treatment is centered around rest, stretching, strengthening, and technique modification to avoid reinjury.[2]

Cervical Spine

Neck injuries can occur as a result of forces applied to the head during water entry with poor alignment. Injuries are more common in platform divers because of the greater energy on water contact. These strains and sprains are relatively uncommon because of the protective effect of the arms during entry. Rubin[24] has reported that, on occasion, severe rotational force can be applied to the neck, resulting in a brachial plexus traction injury.

The biomechanical forces acting on the cervical spine during diving may be more significant than those implied by the mild injuries commonly seen among competitive divers. In a study of patients with cervical disc herniation, designed to identify risk factors, recreational diving was found to be the single most important risk factor.[16] A person who reported diving from a board more than 10 times in the 2 years before the onset of symptoms was found to be 2.3 times more likely than a nondiver to suffer from cervical disc disease. When the frequency of diving was more than 25 times in 2 years, the risk increased to 6.4 times that of the nondiver. This risk was greater than that found in persons who reported heavy lifting more than 25 times daily (4.9 times the risk of the nonlifter).

In a classic study of high divers in Acapulco, Mexico, Schneider, Papo, and Alvarez[28] demonstrated the importance of diving technique in preventing cervical spine injury. These divers performed approximately 1000 dives annually from a height of 130 feet into water with a depth of 15 feet. One of the divers was known to have sustained a thoracic compression fracture when a gust of wind caused him to twist and hit the water sideways. There was no clinical history of neck injury in any of the divers. Schneider obtained radiographs of six divers and found that in three of them there was evidence of multiple cervical compression fractures with spontaneous anterior fusion. One additional diver had a mild compression fracture of C5, and the remaining two divers had no evidence of cervical spine abnormality. The three divers with severe radiographic changes all entered the water with their hands outstretched. As a result, their heads struck the water directly, sustaining the full impact. The other three divers entered the water with their hands locked together, above their heads. Thus their hands protected their heads from the full force of initial impact with the water.

CATASTROPHIC SPINAL INJURY IN RECREATIONAL DIVING

Unlike competitive diving, in which injuries are uncommon and rarely catastrophic, cervical spine injuries that occur during recreational diving are devastating (Fig. 35-5). More than 90% of the injuries result in quadriplegia. More than half are complete injuries. According to the Centers for Disease Control, 1000 new cases of spinal cord injury annually are the result of recreational diving.[20] Burst fractures and compression fractures are the most common injuries because of compression and flexion as the top of the head strikes the bottom of the pool, river, lake, or ocean. Facet dislocations are uncommon. Occasionally a thoracic fracture is reported.[30] C5 and C6 are the levels most commonly fractured.

The majority of reported injuries are the result of diving into shallow water or misjudging the depth of the water. Diving into natural bodies of water has been identified as being especially dangerous because of the presence of underwater obstacles and changing depths due to tides, shifting sand, and variations in rainfall.[27] For example, a threefold increase in diving accidents was reported in Wisconsin after a record-setting drought in 1988[22] lowered the water levels in lakes and streams. In coastal areas a running surface dive into the surf is a common mechanism of injury.[11]

Alcohol consumption has been identified as an important risk factor in diving injury.[15] In a series from the Regional Spinal Cord Injury Center at Northwestern

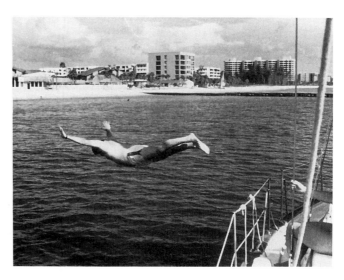

Fig. 35-5. This photograph of a recreational diver demonstrates several factors that predispose to catastrophic injury. He is diving into water of unknown depth that may contain hidden underwater obstacles such as rocks, coral, or wreckage. He is not protecting his head with his arms. Fortunately, this person escaped any injury.

University, alcohol played a role in 44.1% of the diving injuries.[3] Similarly, 38% of patients treated at Allegheny General Hospital had blood alcohol levels greater than 100 mg/dl.[18] Griffiths[14] described the case of a 27-year-old man who was fishing and drinking ouzo "at the rate of half a tumbler every 10 minutes." His boat went aground on a sandbar, and he failed to appreciate that this meant shallow water as he dove in to push the boat off. Burke[5] described the case of a young man who jumped off a sign warning against diving because of shallow water. Even small amounts of alcohol have been shown to contribute to diving accidents without the gross impairment of judgment described in these anecdotes. In a study designed to evaluate the effect of alcohol on the ability to safely perform a shallow-water entry dive, significant impairment was found at blood alcohol levels of 40 mg/dl. Divers were not aware of their degraded performance or of their increased risk of injury from diving after drinking.[21]

Evaluations of spinal cord injury resulting from accidents in swimming pools by Ennis et al.[6] and Green et al.[13] reveal additional risk factors. In 54 of 72 accidents, some form of contributory negligence by the victim was thought to have occurred. The most common problem was diving into shallow water, defined as a depth of 5 feet or less. Eighteen of those injured dove into the shallow end of an in-ground pool. The majority of the pools had no visible markings to indicate pool depth or which was the shallow end. Twenty persons were injured by diving into an above-ground pool. Above-ground pools never have adequate depth to allow

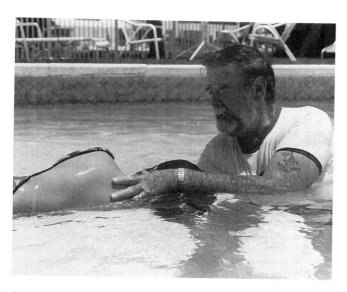

Fig. 35-6. If a victim is floating facedown in the water, the rescuer must stabilize the head to the torso before turning. In this figure note that the rescuer is grabbing the chest between his hands and stabilizing the head between his forearms while turning the victim.

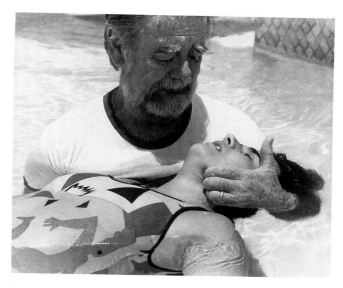

Fig. 35-7. A jaw thrust is appropriate to establish an airway. The neck should not be hyperextended. Note that the rescuer is cradling the victim's head and supporting the thoracic spine, maintaining cervical alignment. Artificial respiration can be started with the victim in the water.

safe diving. Six patients sustained injuries by entering shallow water headfirst from a pool slide.

RESCUE OF THE INJURED DIVER

Green et al.[13] also noted that 55 of the 72 patients were extricated from the pool by persons with no training in rescue techniques. They and other authors have raised the possibility that incomplete injuries may have been converted to complete injuries by improper handling. "It has been the unhappy experience of the authors that victims of diving accidents have reported initial motor function after impact but after being pulled over pool edges, rolled over or manipulated improperly, have lost this capability."[17]

It is imperative that the head and neck be aligned with the spine during the rescue. If the diver is facedown in the water, it is important to turn the person quickly to prevent drowning. A variety of techniques have been described to accomplish this while maintaining spinal alignment. One technique is to bring the victim's arms forward and splint the head between the arms. This allows a single rescuer to maintain alignment of the head, neck, and trunk while turning the victim. Another technique is to support the chin and occiput between the rescuer's two hands, stabilizing the forearms along the sternum and back of the victim. A final technique is to stabilize the head between the rescuer's forearms while holding the trunk between the hands. The victim is now turned, with pressure applied to maintain stability and alignment (Fig. 35-6).

After the victim is turned, an airway may need to be

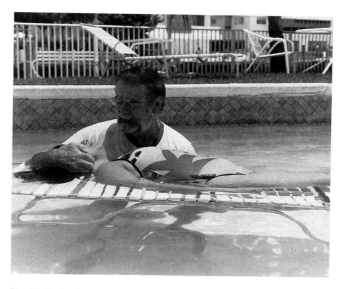

Fig. 35-8. A single rescuer cannot safely lift a victim from the water while maintaining spinal alignment without assistance. If a backboard is available, it is best to position it under the victim while the victim is still in the water. If a backboard is not available, effective substitutes such as lawn furniture can be used.

established. This should be accomplished by the jaw thrust maneuver, rather than by hyperextending the neck (Fig. 35-7). Artificial respiration can be started with the victim in the water. The rescuer should not attempt to move the victim out of the water without assistance, since this cannot be done while maintaining spinal alignment

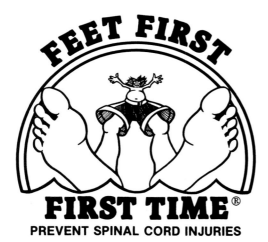

Fig. 35-9. Local community prevention programs have been effective in reducing the number of spinal cord injuries from careless diving. This logo on T-shirts and billboards helped raise awareness among young people in a highly successful program in northern Florida. It encouraged jumping feet first to determine water depth on the first plunge into the water. (Courtesy Feet First, First Time, Inc., Think First of Northwest Florida, 1985.)

and stability. It is best to use a spine board to lift the victim out of the water. If a spine board is not available, effective substitutes such as lawn furniture may be used (Fig. 35-8).

PREVENTION OF INJURY

Almost all spinal cord injuries caused by diving are preventable. Most are caused by failure to appreciate the depth of the water. During the Fourth of July weekend in 1980, seven patients were admitted to a single hospital in northwest Florida for quadriplegia sustained in diving accidents. This epidemic prompted Dr. Joseph John to initiate a public education program called "Feet First, First Time," directed at teenagers and young adults. Within 2 years the number of spinal cord injuries caused by diving in northwest Florida was cut in half.[12] Because of its success, the program was adopted by the American Association for Neurological Surgeons, as well as the Congress of Neurological Surgeons. Now known as "Think First," it provides a basic curriculum, available nationwide, emphasizing prevention of head and spinal cord injuries (Fig. 35-9).

ACKNOWLEDGMENT

I gratefully acknowledge the invaluable contributions to this chapter by Sherri Patchen, R.N., and James O'Heir.

REFERENCES

1. Albrand OW, Walter J: Underwater deceleration curves in relation to injuries from diving, *Surg Neurol* 4:461, 1975.
2. Alexander MJ: Biomechanical aspects of lumbar spine injuries in athletes: a review, *Can J Appl Sports Sci* 10:1, 1985.
3. Bailes JE et al: Diving injuries of the cervical spine, *Surg Neurol* 34:155, 1990.
4. Billingsley H: A philosophy of safety awareness in diving. In Gabriel JL, editor: *U.S. diving safety manual,* 1990, US Diving.
5. Burke DC: Spinal cord injuries from water sports, *Med J Aust* 2:1190, 1972.
6. Ennis JE et al: *Medical analysis of swimming pool injuries,* A study conducted for the US Consumer Product Safety Commission, summary report, Dec 1977.
7. Flewwelling H: Sparging system. In Gabriel JL, editor: *U.S. diving safety manual,* 1990, US Diving.
8. Gabriel JL: *Diving safety, a position paper,* 1988, US Diving.
9. Gabrielson MA: *Diving injuries: a critical insight and recommendations,* 1984, Council for National Cooperation in Aquatics.
10. Golden D, Miller DI: Biomechanics of safe diving. In Gabriel JL, editor: 1990, US Diving.
11. Good RP, Nickel VI: Cervical spine injuries resulting from water sports, *Spine* 5:502, 1980.
12. Green BA, Eismont FJ, O'Heir JT: Spinal cord injury—a systems approach: prevention, emergency medical services, and emergency room management, *Crit Care Clin* 3:471, 1987.
13. Green BA et al: Analysis of swimming pool accidents resulting in spinal cord injury, *Paraplegia* 18:94, 1980.
14. Griffiths ER: Spinal injuries from swimming and diving treated in the spinal department of Royal Perth Rehabilitation Hospital, *Paraplegia* 18:109, 1980.
15. Herman JM, Sonntag VKH: Diving accidents: mechanism of injury and treatment of the patient, *Crit Care Nurs Clin North Am* 3:331, 1991.
16. Kelsey JL et al: An epidemiologic study of acute prolapsed cervical intervertebral disc, *J Bone Joint Surg* 66A:907, 1984.
17. Kewalramani LS, Taylor RG: Injuries to the cervical spine from diving accidents, *J Trauma* 15:130, 1975.
18. Kluger Y et al: Diving injuries: a preventable catastrophe, *J Trauma* 36:349, 1994.
19. Letts M et al: Fracture of the pars interarticularis in adolescent athletes: a clinical-biomechanical analysis, *J Pediatr Orthop* 6:40, 1986.
20. Maiman DJ et al: Diving associated spinal cord injuries during drought conditions—Wisconsin 1988, *MMWR* 37:453, 1988.
21. Perrine MW, Mundt JC, Weiner RI: When alcohol and water don't mix: diving under the influence, *J Stud Alcohol* 55:517, 1994.
22. Raymond CA: Summer's drought reinforces diving's dangers, *JAMA* 260:1199, 1988.
23. Rossi F: Spondylolysis, spondylolisthesis and sports, *J Sports Med Phys Fitness* 18:317, 1978.
24. Rubin BD: Orthopaedic aspects of competitive diving. In *Proceedings of the U.S. Diving Sports Science Seminar,* 1985, US Diving.
25. Rubin BD: Orthopedic care. In Gabriel JL, editor: *U.S. diving safety manual,* 1990, US Diving.
26. Rude R: Diving equipment. In Gabriel JL, editor: *U.S. diving safety manual,* 1990, US Diving.
27. Scher AT: Diving injuries to the cervical spinal cord, *South Afr Med J* 59:603, 1981.
28. Schneider RC, Papo M, Alvarez CS: The effects of chronic recurrent spinal trauma in high diving. *J Bone Joint Surg* 44A:648, 1962.
29. Stone RS: *Diving safety in swimming pools,* 1981, Arthur D Little.
30. Wieclawek H, Kiwerski J: Thoracic spine injury after a plunge into water, *Chir Narzadow Ruchu Ortop Polska* 49(2):111, 1984.

Chapter Thirty-Six

◆

Water Polo

Terry A. Schroeder
Robert G. Watkins

Water polo was invented in England in the early 1870s to provide swimmers and divers with a new and exciting method of training and competition. In the late 1890s the game of water polo was introduced in the United States. It was a physically demanding game, called by many a cross between American football and underwater wrestling. It was not uncommon in the early days of water polo for players to have to be pulled from the water and resuscitated.

In the year 1900 the game was introduced into the Olympic games program on an exhibition basis. By the 1904 Olympic games in St. Louis, water polo had become the first team sport officially on the Olympic program. Since that time, water polo has become a very popular sport in the United States, especially on the West Coast in California. There are clubs in 46 of the 50 states and more than 10,000 registered participants. The U.S. Olympic team has won silver medals at the past two Olympic games, in Los Angeles in 1984 and in Seoul, Korea, in 1988. During the past 10 years the U.S. team has been consistently ranked among the top three teams in the world.

BASICS OF THE GAME

Today's game of water polo is most often described as a cross between basketball and soccer played in a pool. It is played in an all-deep pool that measures 30 × 20 m, although high school athletes may play in a pool that has a shallow end. There is a goal at each end of the pool, which is 1 m high and 3 m wide. Each team consists of seven players, six in the field and one in the goal, plus six additional team members, and substitutions may be made after a goal or at the quarter break. The players are not allowed to touch the bottom and, with the exception of the goalie, can touch the ball only with one hand at a time.

Much of the strategy in water polo is taken from basketball, with terminology such as zone defense, press defense, front court offense, counterattacks, and fast breaks in common. The ball is a yellow rubber ball slightly larger than a volleyball. The game is played in four 7-minute quarters with 2-minute intermissions between each quarter. These quarters are time measured; thus every time the referee blows a foul, the clock stops. Each quarter usually lasts a total of 15 minutes. The team that scores the most goals in the four-quarter game wins the contest.

There are four main positions in water polo: the 2-meter man, the drivers, the defenders, and the goalies. The 2-meter man is much like a center in basketball; he sits on a low post approximately 2 m from the goal. He draws fouls, makes assists, and is an occasional scorer. The 2-meter man is the quarterback of the offensive team and is one of the larger players on the team. The drivers are much like guards in basketball, usually smaller and quicker players than the 2-meter man. They usually lead the counterattack and are good scorers. The defenders tend to be large players with very good leg support. Their primary job is to defend against the opposing team's best players, either the 2-meter man or the drivers. As in any team sport, these players may not always get the credit, but good defenders win championships. The goalies are the final line in defense, and they are much like a soccer goalie—the quarterback of the defense. A good goalie can be an asset in offensive play and often makes the first outlet pass on the counterattack.

Almost all players in the United States have a strong swimming background. Each one of the 1984 and 1988 Olympic team members competed first in age-grouped swimming. It is not uncommon during the course of the game for a field player to swim up to 2 miles.

BIOMECHANICAL ANALYSIS

The sport of water polo requires a balance of strength, swimming speed, quickness, and great endurance. It is a team sport that also requires good game sense and good hand-eye coordination. The players must have the upper body strength to wrestle and hold a position on an opponent. During the course of the game they must also be able to swim end to end many times with speed and endurance. In addition to this wrestling and swimming, they must be able to simultaneously and effectively pass and shoot the ball.

The following basic skills of the game are analyzed in terms of body biomechanics to illustrate the stress placed on the human body during the sport of water polo:

1. Swimming with the ball (dribbling)
2. Swimming and changing directions, or changing from the horizontal (swimming position) to the vertical (shooting position)
3. The eggbeater kick and the ready position in water polo
4. The goalie lunge

5. Shooting the ball

It is important to note that because the human body contains a high percentage of water and has a specific gravity of very near 1.0, buoyant forces and gravitational forces very nearly cancel each other out for athletes in the water. Therefore no action is required to support the body against gravity, and the athlete can move through the water as though weightless. Consequently, a gravitational, or pounding, effect on the joints and soft tissue of a competitive aquatic athlete is diminished. The injury percentage of these athletes is relatively low, although certain areas of the body are placed under a great deal of stress.

Swimming

The water polo athlete uses the crawl stroke approximately 90% of the time. Because of the phenomenon of weightlessness, the strokes and kicks are designed to give the athlete horizontal rather than vertical propulsion. The upper extremity stroke action provides much of the power for the propulsion. In the crawl stroke, the arms are alternating in a pattern of entry, stretch, catch, pull, and recovery. As one hand enters the water and stretches to maximum extension in front of the body, the other hand is exiting the water and beginning the recovery phase of the stroke.

The major muscle groups involved in the propulsive phase of the crawl stroke are the flexors and internal rotators of the shoulder, specifically the pectoralis major, latissimus dorsi, teres major, and subscapularis. The triceps are also involved in extension of the arm at the elbow. Other muscles that actively participate in the crawl stroke are the deltoids, biceps, rotator cuff muscles, trapezius, rhomboids, and serratus anterior. This stroke is a highly repetitive motion. An average high school swimmer or water polo player may do 20,000 or more shoulder revolutions per week, which can be compared with an elite baseball or tennis player, who may do 1000 shoulder revolutions per week. The shoulder joint complex is by far the most vulnerable structure in the sport of swimming and water polo. The swimmers and water polo players tend to develop very strong, overpowering pectoralis major muscles. This results in a forward and downward pull on the shoulder and a kyphotic posture, placing the shoulder in a vulnerable position for impingement syndrome, which is very common among swimmers.

The muscles of the trunk participate in stabilizing the body during the crawl stroke. There is some degree of rotation around the thoracolumbar spine. Correct stroke biomechanics and strong trunk muscles will limit this rotation. Too much rotation causes wasted energy, unwanted body roll, and an inefficient stroke.

In the water polo stroke (Fig. 36-1), the head is held high in the water with the eyes out of the water so that the player can always see where the ball is and where the free man is. This puts an additional load on the cervical extensors and the extensors of the thoracic spine.

The crawl stroke involves a flutter type of kick, which helps to propel the body through the water. When the flutter kick is properly performed, the knee and ankle are dynamically stabilized. This implies a cooperative contraction of all muscles associated with the joint without maximal fixation of the joint involved. Most of the power and action of the flutter kick come from the hip flexors and hip extensors. Specifically, the rectus femoris, iliopsoas, tensor fasciae latae, and sartorius flex the hip, whereas the gluteus maximus, adductor magnus, semimembranosus, semitendinosus, and biceps femoris extend the hip. These muscles are alternately used to help propel the body through the water. The lumbar spine is in a slightly extended position, stabilizing the pelvis and rotating slightly back and forth with the alternating hip flexion and extension. Stabilization at

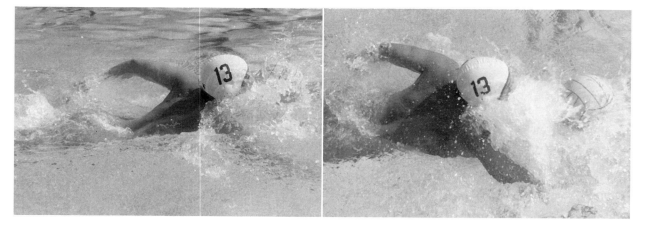

Fig. 36-1. Swimming with the ball (dribbling): side view and top view. The body is just below the waterline, and the head is held up above the water, with the swimmer looking straight ahead. The stroke used is a crawl stroke with a flutter kick.

the lumbar spine is important to minimize this rocking action and thus decrease drag. Overall, the muscles of the trunk and spine serve an important role in the crawl stroke. The cervical spine is extended, and the abdominal, erector spinae, and oblique muscles all participate actively in stabilizing and coordinating movement in the upper and lower extremity.

Change of Direction

The water polo athlete needs to be able to change directions quickly in the water (Fig. 36-2). This requires great strength from the trunk muscles, including the abdominal muscles, lumbar spine musculature, and the oblique muscles. The athlete needs to be able to change swimming directions and also be able to change quickly from a horizontal (swimming) position to a vertical (shooting) position in the water. The hip flexors and extensors, abdominal muscles, including the rectus abdominis, internal and external obliques, and the muscles of the lower back, provide the muscular action for these motions. Trunk rotation, flexion, extension, and lateral bending are all involved in changing directions

and going from a swimming position to a shooting position in the water.

Eggbeater Kick

When water polo athletes go into the vertical (shooting or passing) position, they rely heavily on a kick called the *eggbeater kick* to propel them up out of the water to catch, shoot, and pass the ball (Fig. 36-3). An experienced water polo player is able to propel the body upward using the eggbeater kick so that the entire torso, from the waist up, is above the water line. The players with the best legs, or eggbeater kick, are usually the better players in the sport. Players depend on their legs for stability and a base of support because there is no ground to stand on.

The eggbeater kick is much like the frog kick used in the breast stroke except that the eggbeater kick is executed one leg at a time. The hip flexors and extensors are used alternately, as well as the flexors and extensors of the knee. The ankle is alternately dorsiflexed and plantar flexed. The adductors of the leg are also heavily involved in this kick. The greatest propulsion stage of the

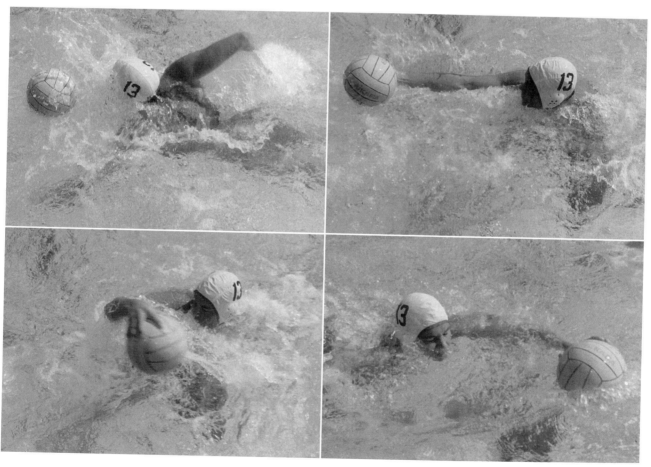

Fig. 36-2. Change of direction sequence: swimming with the ball and suddenly changing directions to swim in the other direction.

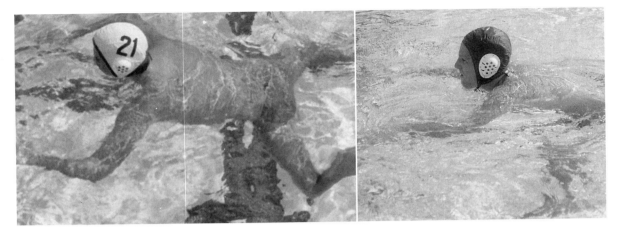

Fig. 36-3. The ready position (eggbeater kick): top view and side view.

kick involves the adductors, hip extensors, knee extensors, and the dorsiflexors of the feet. Specific muscles involved are the gracilis, adductor magnus, adductor brevis, adductor longus, pectineus, iliopsoas, and semimembranosus in adduction. The gluteus maximus, adductor magnus, semimembranosus, semitendinosus, and biceps femoris are used in hip extension. The quadriceps femoris, especially the rectus femoris, and the tensor fasciae latae provide powerful knee extension, whereas dorsiflexion is accomplished with the tibialis anterior, extensor digitorum longus, extensor hallucis longus, and peroneus tertius.

The position in water polo known as the ready position is similar to that assumed by volleyball or basketball players when they are on their toes with their knees slightly bent and their trunk slightly flexed forward. In this position, the athlete is ready to react and move toward the ball. The water polo athlete, in the ready position, is doing the eggbeater kick in a position that most resembles sitting in a chair. The legs are flexed up on the trunk, and the trunk is slightly flexed forward, placing more strain on the components of the lumbar spine. In this position the body is coiled, and the water polo athlete is ready to spring up in the water for a ball or to lunge, either forward or to the side, to begin swimming. The stabilizing power comes from the support of the eggbeater kick, as well as from the trunk flexors and abdominal muscles. From this position the body may explode into lateral flexion, rotation, flexion, or extension. The muscles of the trunk are involved in all of these motions.

Goalie Lunge

The goalies spend most of the game in the water polo ready position (Fig. 36-4). The eggbeater kick and sculling with the arms stabilize the body and keep it in this coiled position, ready to explode to either side or go into extreme lateral bending. The muscles used in these

movements are the rectus abdominis, the internal and external obliques, iliopsoas, erector spinae, and quadratus lumborum. The pectoralis major, latissimus dorsi, and trapezius also act to pull the shoulder toward the side of the contraction.

The goalie may also explode straight up in the water and hyperextend the spine. The muscles involved in this motion are the erector spinae, which effects a power contraction, or the gluteus maximus, latissimus dorsi, and trapezius, which act to pull the shoulders backward. Either action requires excellent leg support. The athlete's power to extend or bend laterally while coming up out of the water is generated by the eggbeater kick.

Shooting Motion

The final motion to be discussed is the water polo shot. There has been much research into the throwing action, particularly with baseball pitchers. Although some similarities between the baseball overhand throw and the water polo throw exist, there are also many differences. Perhaps the biggest difference is that the water polo athlete is not stabilized on the ground. The stabilizing point, or beginning of the kinetic chain, begins with the eggbeater kick propelling the upper torso out of the water. In water polo undoubtedly more stress and pressure are placed on the shoulder, and perhaps more of the velocity in throwing a water polo ball is generated by the arm. The ball is also much larger and heavier than a baseball, so that the biomechanics of the overhand throw are also altered. It should be pointed out, again, that the best water polo players can propel themselves out of the water from the waist up; thus in a throwing motion the upper torso meets no water resistance. The overhand throw is a highly complex motion that involves a coordinated movement of the shoulder girdle and torso.

The phases of the overhand throw in water polo can be compared with a baseball throw. The cocking phase

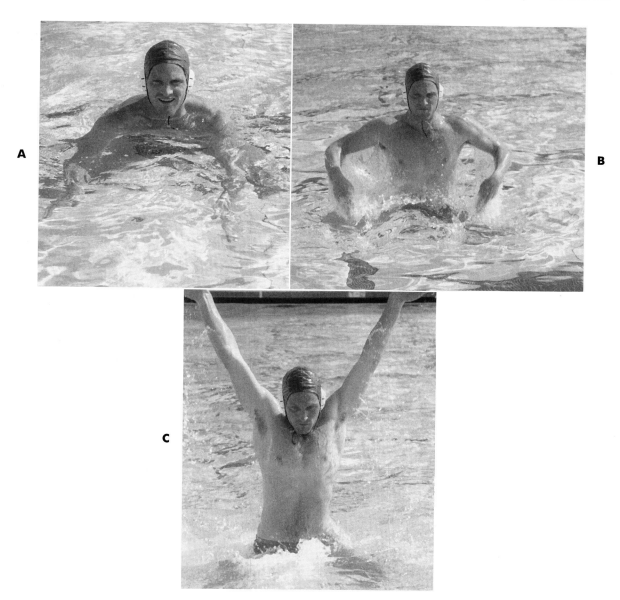

Fig. 36-4. Goalie lunge. **A,** Ready position. **B,** Midphase. **C,** Final phase in full extension.

(Fig. 36-5, *A*) involves bringing the ball up from the water at the moment in which the shoulder is in maximal external rotation. In this phase the water polo athlete is propelling the body out of the water with a strong eggbeater kick. The trunk is also being coiled for the throw. The hips are rotated to the same side as the throwing arm. There is also slight lateral bending to the same side and extension of the lumbar spine. The shoulder is brought into a position of abduction, horizontal extension, and maximal external rotation. The elbow is flexed to approximately 90 degrees, and the ribs are in a neutral position. The shoulder capsule is wound tight, like a coiled spring ready to release. The important aspect of the cocking phase is to place the

body in a position so that all segments may contribute to the propulsion of the ball.

Electromyographic studies have shown that in this stage of the overhand throw, the deltoids are very active in raising the shoulder above the head. The supraspinatus, infraspinatus, and teres minor muscles are also very much involved in bringing the shoulder into maximal external rotation. At the end of this phase the subscapularis fires to decelerate shoulder external rotation. The pectoralis major, latissimus dorsi, and serratus anterior muscles also are involved in decelerating external rotation with eccentric contractions.

The next phase of the overhand throw is the acceleration phase (Fig. 36-5, *B*). This phase begins with

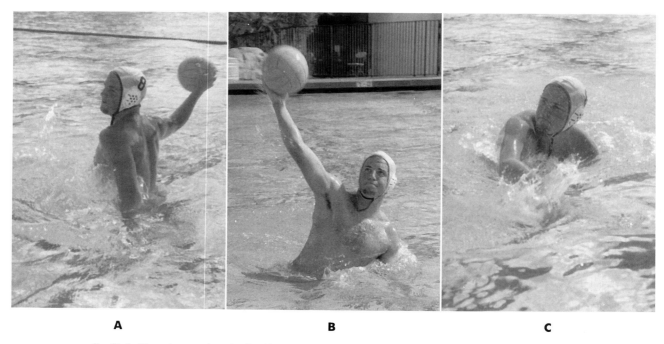

Fig. 36-5. Shooting motion. **A,** Cocking phase. **B,** Acceleration phase. **C,** Follow-through phase.

the arm in maximal external rotation and ends with the ball released. In the water polo athlete this phase also begins with the maximal leg kick, which is a combination of an eggbeater type of kick and a scissors kick. A right-handed thrower will end up with the left leg almost directly under the body. During the maximal leg thrust the energy is transferred to the trunk. In the acceleration phase the hips rotate ipsilateral to the throwing arm. There is trunk flexion and lateral bending away from the throwing side. Energy and movement are generated in the trunk by the abdominal, oblique, and erector spinae muscles. This energy is then transferred into the upper extremity and results in a more powerful throw. It has been estimated that in the baseball pitcher approximately 50% of the ball velocity comes from the step and the body rotation. Because in water polo there is no ground to stabilize the body and initiate the throwing motion, the kinetic chain in the water polo throw is potentially weaker and body rotation would most likely contribute a lesser percentage to ball velocity.

The active muscles of this phase are the abdominals, hip flexors, and obliques, the opposite internal oblique being one of the real keys to throwing strength. Right-handed throwers obtain much power from the left internal oblique. The shoulder motion involves muscular activity from the pectoralis major, latissimus dorsi, subscapularis, and many other muscles participating in a stabilizing role. The elbow is going from a flexed position to an extension, and the triceps are significantly involved. The wrist also flexes near ball release.

The final phase of the overhand throw is the follow-through phase (Fig. 36-5, *C*). This begins with ball release and continues until the motion of throwing has ceased. The purpose of this phase is to comfortably decelerate the throwing limb. The follow-through phase in water polo differs greatly from the baseball overhand throw in that the water provides a cushion to help decelerate the throwing limb as the hand and arm hit the water. The pectoralis major and latissimus dorsi still participate as forceful internal rotators and assist the subscapularis in carrying the arm across the chest. The external rotators of the shoulder fire again to decelerate internal rotation. The triceps are active as the arm continues to extend, and there is a decelerated trunk rotation and stabilization to regain balance in the water. Because the water poloist does not properly learn to follow through, and the muscles used to effect deceleration are not involved to the same extent as in a baseball throw, the water polo athlete is perhaps more prone to injury while participating in a dry land throwing activity.

The water polo athlete must develop trunk strength. The trunk helps to stabilize the body in the swimming position; that is, in a properly executed swimming stroke, it prevents excessive roll of the body. The extensors of the lower back are also important in stabilizing the kicking motion. The extensors of the thoracic spine and the cervical spine are critical in holding the head in an extended position as the water poloist swims with the head high in the water. As the water polo athlete changes directions in the water or goes from the horizontal (swimming) position to the vertical (shooting) position, the lower trunk becomes a pivot point around which the body rotates. The abdominal musculature and the muscles of the trunk must be extremely strong to perform these motions.

The goalie must be particularly strong in the trunk inasmuch as this player spends most of the game in the ready position with the body coiled, ready to explode into a position of hyperextension or extreme lateral bending to either side. The water polo shooter relies heavily on trunk strength and stability to transfer power from the legs to the upper extremity in the kinetic chain of the throwing motion. Because there is no ground to stabilize the thrower, the kinetic chain of the throwing motion depends on the trunk to generate power. In the overhand throw, less of the ball's velocity can be initiated by body rotation, and more stress and pressure are therefore placed on the shoulder joint. In water polo the shoulder is by far the most vulnerable joint and is prone to the overuse type injuries of swimming, in which a highly repetitive motion is required. The water polo athlete is also prone to shoulder problems as a result of the explosive nature of throwing a ball.

SHOULDER INJURIES

The most common injury to the water poloist involves the shoulder joint. The shoulder is placed under stress because of the large number of shoulder revolutions in swimming. This can result in an overuse type of injury to the shoulder. In addition, the joint is stressed during the overhand throw and can also be injured while the athlete wrestles for position with an opponent. The most common injury to the shoulder is the impingement syndrome. This occurs when a combination of swelling and repetitive motion impinges on the long head of the biceps or the supraspinatus tendon under the coracoacromial arch. Swimmers and throwers often develop imbalances in the pectoralis major muscle. The muscles become overdeveloped and cause a forward and downward pull on the shoulder joint. This can lead to a slightly kyphotic posture that places additional tension on the rotator cuff tendons, especially the supraspinatus, and may cause additional impingement.

Improper stroke mechanics may also be involved in the shoulder problems. A common mistake the swimmer makes is dropping the elbow below the hand on the underwater pull, which causes the head of the humerus to be jammed into the coracoacromial arch, further impinging on the soft tissues. Treatment includes rest to the injured joint, cryotherapy during the acute phase and after exercise, the teaching of proper stroke mechanics, and specific exercises to balance the body in the weight room. These exercises include a seated row to work the rhomboids and a seated front pull-down to work the trapezius, especially the middle trapezius and the latissimus dorsi muscles. Surgical tubing exercises

can also be very helpful in the treatment of shoulder injuries.

SPINAL INJURIES
Cervical Spine

Cervical spine injuries occur quite commonly in water polo: hyperextension injuries from swimming with the head up constantly and cervical sprain or strain injuries, especially to the 2-meter man when he is wrestling for position. The head, which is the only part of the body above the water, often gets grabbed, pulled, and hit. In the acute phase, treatment consists of rest and ice, as well as specific chiropractic manipulations to restore normal alignment and joint motion. Electrical stimulation, trigger point therapy, and massage therapy to reduce muscle spasm and pain can also be helpful. In addition, proper cervical spine flexibility exercises and strengthening exercises should be used.

Thoracic Spine

During the game tremendous rotational forces affect the thoracic spine in swimming, wrestling to hold position, and throwing. The thoracic spine is the stabilizing area in many of the activities of this sport. A common injury to this area is rotational sprain or strain with possible vertebral or rib subluxation. These injuries respond well to conservative therapy, specific chiropractic manipulation, and appropriate physical therapy.

Lumbar Spine

A common injury to the goalie in water polo is a hyperextension injury to the lumbar spine. Field players who are extending (jumping) high in the water to reach a ball are also prone to this type of injury. The extensors of the back must be strong, but the real key is maintaining a good balance between the abdominal musculature, the obliques, and the lumbar extensors. These muscles form a band around the waist and keep the trunk protected, stabilized, and strong. Conservative care is effective in treating lumbar spine injuries.

The water polo athlete may experience groin and knee injuries because of the forceful eggbeater kick used in the sport. Trunk strength is a critical factor. Many of the injuries to the upper and lower extremities may result from imbalances or weaknesses of the trunk musculature.

Rehabilitation can often be quickly achieved through use of hydrotherapy. Range of motion and water-resistance exercises can be helpful, especially to an athlete who is comfortable in the water. The injured athlete can usually begin range-of-motion exercises in the water shortly after an injury. To maintain aerobic fitness and retain their feel for the water, these athletes can always work the noninjured body segment. For example, an athlete with a shoulder injury can still get in the water and do sets of both the eggbeater and the flutter kicks until the shoulder is well enough to begin rehabilitation.

PREVENTION OF INJURY

As in any sport, prevention is the key to reducing the number and severity of injuries. Each sport should have specific exercises to increase strength, flexibility, and aerobic capacity. Strength training is an important part of a water polo athlete's regimen and should include the following concepts.

The athlete must work for balance in muscular strength. As has been discussed, most swimmers over-develop the pectoralis major muscle, which creates an imbalance in the upper extremity and the thoracic spine. Weight training, therefore, should be used to balance this problem. The water polo athlete should concentrate on building the muscles to counteract this imbalance. The middle trapezius, rhomboid major, rhomboid minor, latissimus dorsi, and upper thoracic extensor muscles should all be worked consistently in the weight room. Because the shoulders are overworked in the pool (swimming and throwing), they must be protected during all aspects of the athlete's weight training. Most exercises should be performed with a narrow grip (at shoulder width). This is especially important in exercises such as the bench press, pectoral flies, and lap pull-downs. It is also imperative that the shoulders be properly warmed up before any weight training is begun.

Weights should be used to build power. Strength is important, particularly upper body strength, but the swimmer does not want to develop too much bulk. A proper balance of strength, speed, and endurance must be found. Too much strength often results in decreased endurance. This concept should be considered in the design of a weight-training program.

Off-season workouts should be used to build strength, whereas weight training during the season should focus on power, speed, and maintaining strength with more repetition and less weight. A weight-training program should include trunk-strengthening exercises: front half sit-ups or crunches, side sit-ups to work the oblique muscles, and back extension exercises. The program should be designed so that the body parts are alternated, with the first set consisting of an upper body exercise and the second set consisting of a lower body exercise, and so on. This sequence maximizes the rest period for a particular body part in between sets.

The following sample weight-training program can be used in or out of the season by changing the number of sets, the number of repetitions, and the amount of weight. For most of the exercises, the athlete can do three sets of 10 repetitions with a fairly heavy weight three times a week. During the season the athlete should do two or three sets of 15 to 20 repetitions with a much lighter weight and at a faster speed. Remember, this program is designed to obtain a proper balance of strength, speed, and endurance.

1. Pullover machine (A Nautilus or a Universal type of machine can be used; an excellent exercise for swimmers and water polo players)
2. Leg press
3. Lap pull-down (Done in front of the body with a narrow grip to protect the shoulders)
4. Leg extension
5. Bench press (Can be performed on a Nautilus machine or with free weights, with use of a narrow grip to protect the shoulders)
6. Leg flexion
7. Pectoral flies (Free weights or dumbbells should be used, and a narrow grip should be maintained to protect the shoulders)
8. Sit-ups, 250 (five sets of 50), alternating sets: one set of 50 in front, one set of 50 each side, and then one set of 100 in front
9. Seated row: (Good posture is maintained, with special focus on the rhomboids)
10. Back-extension machine
11. Tricep extension
12. Sit-ups, 250, alternating front and sides
13. Wrist curls
14. Deltoid lifts, abductors of the shoulders
15. Adductors of the legs
16. Sit-ups, 250
17. Back-extension machine

Weight training for water polo tends to concentrate more on the upper body. Surgical tubing exercises, which help strengthen and improve the motion of throwing, can be done specifically for internal and external rotation, as well as for the supraspinatus muscle. Some surgical tubing exercises are based on a throwing motion, as well as a swimming crawl stroke motion. The most important factor in the use of weights and surgical tubing is to strive for good balance in the shoulder joint complex.

Leg work, or leg-strength training, must be stressed in the water because it is a key factor in developing a good water polo player. Many drills are available to improve leg strength, or power, in the eggbeater kick. In the pool, a teammate can sit behind another player's back and push down on the second player's shoulders while this player does the eggbeater kick. This can be done in intervals of 10 seconds on and 10 seconds off, or in intervals of 20 seconds on (pushing down) and 10 seconds off, for a total of 5 minutes. Diving bricks, weight belts, and water jugs may be used to increase resistance and build eggbeater leg strength. Walking laps with bricks, weight belts, or bottles will greatly improve leg strength. In another outstanding drill to build leg strength, the water polo athlete sits in the water in the ready position and does jumping exercises, side to side or straight up, using the eggbeater kick to further increase eggbeater power. These drills are also good to help build and coordinate trunk strength. Proper warm-up is critical before any leg-conditioning program is initiated.

Bicycling and stair climbing can also be used to build leg power, especially in the off season. It is critical in stair climbing work to protect the knees and joints of the body by walking down the stairs and running only up the stairs.

Flexibility

Flexibility is critical for preventing injuries. Most swimmers and water polo players have a problem with flexibility because it is difficult to stretch on a cold morning on the pool deck. Water polo players should be taught to stretch properly. Proper stretching can be done in the water after the athlete has swum a couple of laps to warm up the muscles. Care should be taken to properly stretch the shoulder, especially in internal and external rotation. Proprioceptive neuromuscular facilitation (PNF) is also useful in improving flexibility in a tight athlete. This method of stretching can be easily taught to all of the team members. During the stretching, the coach must carefully monitor the athletes because improper stretching will result in even more injuries. Another good time to stretch and work on flexibility is after weight training, when the muscles are very warm. This tends to help keep the athlete's muscles loose rather than tightening up as much. Stretching after weight training also helps the athlete retain a better feel for the water.

Endurance

Because endurance is such a key factor in water polo, aerobic exercise is essential. The most beneficial aerobic exercise is the most sport specific. To get in shape for water polo, the person has to play the game. Practice games and scrimmages are the most specific form of aerobic conditioning for water polo.

Lap swimming for conditioning, which is also important, varies in amount depending on the period of the water polo season. For example, in the early part of the season the coach may elect to do more sets of longer yardage. As the season goes on, the sets and yardage generally taper down. Early-season workouts may consist of 4 to 6000 yards or meters per day, whereas midseason and late-season workouts probably range from 2 to 3000 yards or meters per day. Most swimming sets consist of 200 yards or less. The athletes may do five times 200s on a 230 base, then 10 times 100s on the 130 base, then a kick set consisting of eggbeater and flutter kick 500 to 1000 yards, followed by 10 times 50s on the 45-second base, and finally some sprint work. It is important that the coach work kicking sets into the swimming conditioning. As mentioned before, the water polo athlete with strong legs usually is the better player in the game. Swim sets should also consist of some head-up swims because this is how a water polo player swims during the game.

Off-season aerobic conditioning is important. Running stairs and bicycling are both very good for building power and endurance in the legs. The athlete should always walk down the stairs to avoid the pounding on the joints that would occur in running down the stairs. Stair-climbing machines can be beneficial. Because water polo is a team sport, it is a good idea to play basketball in the off-season. This participation helps maintain aerobic fitness and at the same time develop better team skills.

Water-resistance exercises can be helpful in building specific muscle strength and in rehabilitating an injured athlete. Many products are available on the market that an athlete can wear on the arms or legs to increase resistance in the water. Shoulder stability and rotator cuff exercises should be stressed as part of any water-resistance exercise program for the water polo player. In addition, power walking in chest-deep water can be valuable in strengthening trunk musculature.

Chapter Thirty-Seven

Surfing

Gary L. Douglas
Michele Toomay Douglas

Hawaii affords an excellent opportunity to study spinal and spinal cord injuries generated by the surf that surrounds this eight-island chain. Hawaii has over 750 miles of shoreline and several hundred beaches.[13] In addition to year-round surfing, Hawaii has the longest rideable waves on the planet, and Hawaiian surfers have been riding waves for hundreds of years.[18] Hawaii has seen the evolution of board surfing, body surfing, body board surfing, skim boarding, wind surfing, and riding waves with canoes, kayaks and jet skis.[17,18,20] Tourists come to Hawaii unaware of the energy stored in waves formed by storms thousands of miles away. Many of the beaches have very dangerous shore breaks that possess a beautiful wave face that lands on the sand beach; these include Sandy Beach and Waimea Bay on the island of Oahu, and Kaanapali on the northwest coast of Maui.[21] Seventy-five percent of the spinal and spinal cord injuries occurring in surfers in Hawaii occur in body surfers on just four beaches.

TYPES OF SURFING

All forms of surfing attempt to take advantage of the stored energy of the wave to propel the surfer over the surface of the water. The surfer has to gather speed to catch up to the speed of the wave at the right moment when the surfer's surface friction can be exceeded by the force of gravity that propels the surfer down the face of a wave. Buoyancy reduces friction and makes it easier to catch the wave, ride down its face, and avoid being thrown over the falls in front of the wave.[3]

Board Surfing

Board surfing was first recorded in the Hawaiian islands by Lt. King when, arriving with Captain Cook in 1778, he described men flying across the surface of the water on a board:

The boldness and address with which we saw them perform these difficult and dangerous maneuvers was altogether astonishing and is scarce to be credited.[18]

It is obvious from this description that the Hawaiians had been surfing for a considerable time. Hawaiian surfboards ranged from a 34-inch-long child's board to an 18-foot-long, 180-pound board made of wiliwili or koa wood.[8] As the sport evolved, refinements were made, including reducing the length of the board, in an attempt to decrease the weight of the board and increase its

buoyancy. In 1929 the hollow surfboard was patented, reducing the weight of the board to approximately 60 pounds. In the 1940s combination surfboards were manufactured of balsa for lightness and redwood for strength and durability. By the 1970s the use of a fiberglass and balsa wood combination brought the weight of the surfboard down to 30 pounds and paved the way for the modern foam and fiberglass boards weighing less than 10 pounds.[25]

With the lighter board the addition of a leash or "dingstring" has enabled the surfer to stay with the board, thus decreasing the hazard to others and the recovery time of a loose board, but increasing the possibility of personal injury from the board. Skags or keels for the back of the surfboard provide more control and maneuverability but also contribute to an increased number of laceration injuries. Keels have been used since the early 1800s, the number increasing from a single skag in the midline to three, increasing the directional control. Board surfing is done at the first break of the wave, in deep water, to enable the participant to get a long ride. The maximum speed of a board surfer is 20 to 25 mph on the surface of the wave, but the wave also has a forward velocity of its own.[3]

Body Surfing

Body surfing is the most strenuous of the surfing activities, since there is no added buoyancy of a board and it requires treading water while waiting to catch a wave. The body surfer sprints to catch the wave, using the body as a board and the arms and hands as steering devices. A major advancement in body surfing was the development of the swim fin, which gives the surfer increased speed and quickness, decreasing the effort required to catch a wave and improving the surfer's ability to get off the wave. Body surfers have much less maneuverability on the wave. Inexperienced body surfers or surfers without fins frequently stay where they can touch bottom in order to get a push off to catch the wave and to be able to rest between waves. Inexperienced body surfers close to the shore may miscalculate when to enter a wave and pay the price of going "over the falls."[20]

Body Board Surfing

The body board is a further refinement of the surfboard; it is a much smaller, shorter board made of a combination of closed-cell soft foam. The body board adds lift and buoyancy to the rider, who lies down or kneels, making it easier to hydroplane on the surface but sacrificing the stability of a longer, stiffer board. The small size of the board substantially increases speed, enabling one to catch larger waves, and maneuverability on the wave face and offers the opportunity for stunts such as spins and flips. Early Hawaiians used short body boards,[8] but these did not become popular until the introduction of laminated light foam "boogie" boards by Morey in 1971. The board material is quite soft and less prone to producing injuries. The latest trend is toward firmer, stiffer boards that provide increased speed and control. Body board surfing is done in slightly deeper water and in the shore break.

Other offshoots of the surfboard are the skim board, the jet ski, and the windsurfer. The skim board is a small, circular piece of thin plywood that is thrown onto the receding wash of the waves; the person then jumps on it and hydroplanes across the beach. Windsurfing adds a sail to a larger surfboard for the purpose of wind-propelled surfing. This results in increased speed and maneuverability. The sail may also act as a parachute to buffer the descent of the surfer after jumping a wave. Windsurfers may attain speeds of up to 45 mph, nearly twice the speed of a board surfer. The jet ski is essentially a snowmobile for the water and travels at high speed.

WAVES: THE GREAT DECEPTION

An understanding of the mechanism of injuries acquired during surfing requires an appreciation of waves and beaches. Waves are graceful, glittering, transparent creations of nature that invite one to come and play in their bubbling billows. The reality however, is that waves have the stored energy of the wind that creates them. The energy stored in waves is enormous and deceptive.[3,9,36]

Waves are generated by the wind that blows across the surface of the ocean or lake. The wind creates a ripple. Ripples accumulate energy until they coalesce into a chop. As the wind blows the top off of a wave, the falling water transfers its energy to a larger and longer wave, which becomes a swell. The size of the wave depends on the velocity of the wind, the length of time the force of the wind is applied, and the depth of the water. As the distance between the crests of the swells or the wavelength increases, the speed of the waves increases. The energy stored in a wave is proportional to the square of its height. A wave of the same wavelength, whether it is 10 or 20 feet high, travels at the same speed, but the energy stored in the latter is four times the energy stored in the former.

Because waves are formed randomly, they may travel in the same direction but at different speeds and heights, creating the opportunity for formation of a very large, or rogue, wave, which is 2.2 times the average wave height; it occurs in 1:20,000 waves in the open ocean.[3]

The stored energy of the wave is released when the wave breaks. When an ocean-generated wave encounters the shallow water of the shore, the wave is slowed, causing the wavelength to decrease, the height to increase, and the wave to peak. When the depth of the water reaches 1.3 times the wavelength, the wave becomes unstable and begins to break. The maximum release of energy is at the foam line, where the falling wave has reached maximum velocity, almost 3.5 times the energy of a swell.[3] A 3-foot swell, traveling at about 32 mph, has 85 foot pounds of moment, whereas at the foam line the moment is 320 foot pounds.[3]

Beaches

Not all of the beaches in Hawaii are suitable for surfing. Those with a fringing reef to absorb the ocean's energy have no waves at the shore, but the large waves breaking offshore in deep water provide board surfers with a long ride and the opportunity to exit safely. These waves usually break over coral reefs. Body board surfers and body surfers have difficulty accelerating enough to catch these larger waves and generally prefer smaller waves (the second or third break) closer to shore. The steeper the incline of the bottom, the quicker the wave rises up and breaks, and the less distance between the breaking wave and the shore. This shore break is the most dangerous because practically all of the energy of the wave is spent on the beach.[3] Beaches with long, sloping bottoms cause the wave to break several times, resulting in a dissipation of the energy and a safer beach.

SPINAL INJURIES

Although spinal injuries caused by surfing are well known in hospitals near beaches, the injuries are not well documented in the medical literature. Blankenship[4] summarized the results of two studies conducted in 1964 and 1965 in the San Diego County area of California on board surfing injuries. Most of the injuries were the result of blunt trauma caused by the board, including one death by drowning after a concussion. A single thoracic compression fracture was reported. Blankenship noted that the injury pattern changed with increasing age. The younger, presumably inexperienced surfers, sustained injuries to the face and trunk, whereas the older, experienced surfers were more likely to injure the extremities or the back of the head. Similar findings were reported by studies in Australia,[25,26] where only two thoracic vertebral fractures were reported in 218 injuries in 1 year.[25]

Similar results were reported in a survey of hospitalizations for surfing injuries at a single hospital in Honolulu, Hawaii, over a 56-month period (1969 to 1975).[1] The mean age of the injured surfers was 20, with an age range of 8 to 38 years. Of 36 hospitalizations for surfing injuries (24 involving board surfers and 11 involving body surfers) 12 were for craniospinal injuries

(34%). Five of these were the result of being struck by a surfboard, and seven were the result of impacting the sand beach. Of the seven, six occurred during body surfing; there were five cervical spine injuries, one high thoracic injury, and one lumbosacral spine fracture. One individual had quadriplegia as a result.

In a more recent, 10-month, prospective, three-hospital study of all ocean-related injuries in Hawaii, 82 of 276 injured persons were board (27%), boogie (7%), or body (7%) surfers.[23] In the study interval, the board surfers accounted for 100% of the concussions, 75% of the internal injuries, and 61% of the lacerations. Sprains and fractures were also reported, but there were no injuries to the spine. Among the body surfers three suffered spinal column injuries.

In all of these studies the injured were predominately male, and there was a seasonal increase in the frequency of injury that coincided with summer, or the peak beach season. All researchers noted that the incidence of board surfing injuries decreased with the advent of lighter boards.[4,25,26] Board surfers sustain frequent soft tissue injuries, primarily caused by the board, and rarely have injury to the spinal column.[33] In contrast, body surfers sustain more serious and morbid injuries to the spine caused by impacting the sand.[26] Contrary to common thought, two thirds of the ocean-related injuries in Hawaii are sustained by the residents, not by tourists.[21,23]

Oahu Study

Types of injuries. An 11-year (1980 to 1990) retrospective study of spinal column injuries in surfers treated at Oahu area hospitals was initiated specifically for this chapter. Preliminary results have identified 83 persons with spinal column injuries; 73% of these were body surfers, 14% were persons entering or leaving the surf, and the remainder were board surfers, skim board surfers, and jet skiers. Overwhelmingly, the injured individuals were male, primarily because most surfers are male. The youngest individual with a spinal column injury was 9 years old, and the oldest was 66 years old; the mean age was 29 years. Spinal column injuries occurred equally in residents and tourists. There was an average of six surfing injuries per year in each of the six Oahu hospitals surveyed. Of the spinal column injuries recorded in this study, 53.7% occurred at body-surfing beaches on Oahu that are notorious for their shore breaks. Information on the prevailing surf conditions is difficult to obtain, but in the 12 cases where the information was available, the surf ranged from flat to 4 feet.

Distribution of injuries within the spinal column. Within this series the location of injuries paralleled the typical distribution of all spinal trauma.[30] Fig. 37-1 documents the distribution of injuries within the spinal column and the type of neurologic lesion sustained. More than 80% of the injuries were fractures and/or dislocations of the cervical spine. Fractures of the body, arch, or processes;

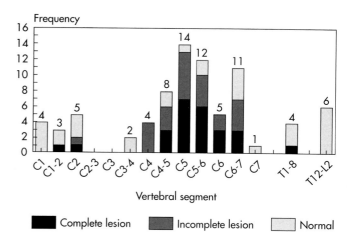

Fig. 37-1. Frequency distribution of spinal column injuries by vertebral level and neurologic function.

fracture-dislocations; disc herniation; facet dislocation; and neurologic impairment without fracture also occurred.

The patients with C1 vertebra fractures (n = 4) all had normal neurologic function, and all were treated with external immobilization. All were body surfers. Three had fracture dislocations of C1-2; two of these had normal neurologic function, and one person with ankylosing spondylitis had a complete lesion. All were treated with external immobilization although not necessarily appropriately (i.e., skeletal traction in bed versus use of a halo vest). There were a total of four odontoid fractures among the upper cervical lesions. One was a complete lesion, and all occurred in body surfers.

Two patients with incomplete lesions of the C3-4 segments subsequently improved after fusion and traction, respectively. A 44-year-old man suffered a herniated disc without bony injury and recovered after a discectomy. All of the C4 injuries (n = 4) were incomplete lesions; three of these patients had improved neurologic function. The fourth, with an anterior cord syndrome, or anterior vertebral artery syndrome, had a posterior spinal fusion and was unimproved. Patients with C4-5 injuries (n = 8) included three with complete lesions, three with incomplete lesions, and two with normal neurologic function. One of these was a 52-year-old man who recovered from a central cord lesion that was the result of an extension injury to a degenerative spine without fracture. In another case a skim boarder had complete spinal cord injury after unreduced bilateral facet dislocation.

The C5, C6, and C7 vertebrae (n = 42) were the most commonly injured segments. In this series patients with lesions at these levels were fairly evenly divided between those with complete and those with incomplete neurologic compromise, with nine (21%) having normal function.

In the cervical spine all levels may be affected. In most cases axial loading and flexion injury are the primary mechanisms, resulting from forced contact with the sand. Neurologic deficits are common, including nerve root and anterior cord impingements, central cord lesions, and complete paralysis. Surprisingly, some individuals are actually able to walk out of the water, go home, and present themselves to the emergency department on a subsequent day. The C4 to C7 cervical spine injuries are the most disabling of all of the injuries. There were no cervical spine injuries in children younger than 14 years of age in this study.

Less commonly seen are bony injuries of the thoracic spine. The T3 to T7 segments were affected in four persons in this series. The youngest person injured, a 9-year-old, sustained a thoracic fracture without neurologic injury. Only one person sustained complete motor loss, in an unstable spine requiring Harrington stabilization. The other fractures were untreated or braced.

There were seven thoracolumbar junction injuries, including two burst fractures of T12, four L1 compression fractures, and one extension injury to the L2 vertebra. There were six hyperflexion injuries and one extension injury. One burst fracture produced a conus lesion requiring reduction and Harrington distraction rod stabilization. The only two jet ski injuries encountered in this study were a Chance fracture of the L1 vertebra and a compression fracture of the lumbar spine.

Only two persons had concomitant injuries at different levels. One had a fracture of the C2 vertebra with a fracture-dislocation at C6-7. The other sustained a C4 teardrop fracture and a compression fracture of the L1 vertebra.

Of all of the patients with spinal column injuries, 39 had normal neurologic function, 29 had complete lesions, and 16 had incomplete injuries. Of the incomplete injuries five were central cord lesions, four were anterior cord lesions, three were Brown-Sequard syndromes, and four were nerve root impingements. All of these improved except for the anterior cord syndromes, which remained the same.

Mechanism of injury. The mechanism of spinal column injury in surfing is difficult to verify for many reasons. Often the victim is amnesic in regard to the injury and only remembers being airborne for a short interval or being tumbled as if in a washing machine until hitting the bottom. The injury is often unwitnessed or undocumented. The literature review emphasizes that board surfers are typically hit by their own board or by another surfer and/or board, sustaining lacerations, blunt trauma, fractures of the skull, and concussion with associated drowning.[1,4,25,26]

The number of injuries seems to be inversely proportional to the height of the waves; the larger the surf, the fewer the injuries. This may be because novice surfers, as well as waders and swimmers, are frightened and do not enter the water. In addition, larger waves tend to break further offshore in deeper water.

There are essentially three mechanisms of injury to the spinal column in body and body board surfing: vertical loading in extension, a neutral position, and flexion. Impacting on the face results in hyperextension of the neck and fracture of the odontoid, fracture of the pedicles of C2, lateral mass fracture, or a central cord contusion due to osteophyte impingement.[10] One rare hyperextension fracture of L1 was documented in a military man who did a "face plant" into the sand as his feet hit him in the back of the head.[16] If the impact is directly on the top of the head, then fracture of C1, or Jefferson fracture, results.[33] Hyperflexion injuries are caused by impacting on the back of the head and/or neck and result in fractures and dislocations of C4 through C7.* Hyperflexion of the neck is the most common mechanism of injury, occurring in 62% (55/84) of the injuries in this series. Cervical spinal injury is rare in children,[14] and none were recorded in this study.

Injuries to the upper thoracic spine also result from flexion.[24] When the cervical spine is supple, the load is transmitted to the upper thoracic spine (T4 to T8), as in the only person younger than 14 years old with a spinal column injury in this study. It is possible that impact on the back of the neck would fracture the upper thoracic spine, but this is not documented in the literature. Fractures in the thoracolumbar junction are axial loading compression injuries except for the hyperextension fracture noted above and a single Chance fracture, which is a flexion-distraction fracture.[32]

Biomechanical studies of spinal column injury mechanisms document that a double-facet dislocation can be produced in a 70-kg person by a fall on the head from a height of 9 inches.[30] A burst fracture of C5 will occur with a fall of 4 feet. As noted previously, there is more than enough force in a breaking wave to cause these injuries. Falling and hitting sand, which has a dampening effect, allows the force to be transmitted to the spinal column rather than being absorbed by the skull. Landing on a hard surface such as rock or coral produces concussions and fractures as the skull absorbs the force. This may explain why board surfers do not sustain spinal fractures and body surfers do.

The only board surfer who sustained a spinal fracture in this series was struck on the back of the head by his own large board (60 pounds) with enough force to break the board in two (Fig. 37-2). He saw the wave coming and "turtled" the board (i.e., turned the board upside down and held on underneath it so that the wave would break on the board); however, he was separated from the board and remembered nothing more.

Body board surfers are injured when they are unable to penetrate the wave to get through the surf. The

---

* References 5, 22, 31, 33, 34, 41.

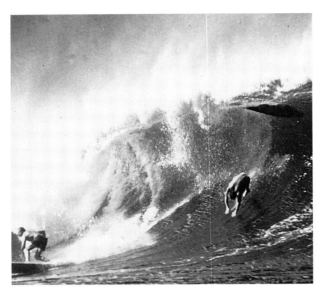

Fig. 37-2. Falling from a surfboard does not produce many spinal column injuries because of the depth of the water. Board surfers are vulnerable to injuries caused by hitting or being hit by the board. (Courtesy Jeff Divine.)

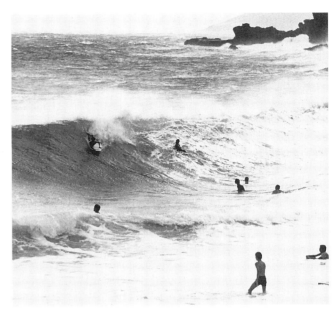

Fig. 37-3. Body board surfing is usually done closer to shore, where the waves travel more slowly. (Courtesy Jim Howe.)

leading surface of a wave is traveling upward, and with the added buoyancy of the foam board, extra force is needed to "sink" beneath the wave. The body board surfers in this study were essentially caught up on the leading edge of the wave and were tossed backward onto their heads. Body board surfing injuries occurred in three novice middle-aged men.

Body surfers are injured by going "over the falls" (n = 36) (Figs. 37-3, 37-4, and 37-5). The surfer is caught by the crest of the wave and thrown over to the bottom. It may be the result of catching the wave too late, failing to "duck out" in time, diving under the wave and coming up only to be caught by the wave, or not penetrating the wave. Diving under the waves and hitting the bottom also was a frequent mechanism of injury in this study (n = 14). The wave action on the shore often creates a hidden sandbar just at the breaking area, which the surfer may hit as he or she tries to dive beneath a breaker, or the surfer may misjudge the depth of the water available beneath the wave. Playing in the shore break and going out or coming in through the surf was another significant cause of injury in this study (n = 21). Frequently people exit the water facing the beach and are hit unexpectedly by a large wave and thrown to the bottom. Jet skiing injuries (n = 2) are sustained when an oncoming wave is jumped and the jet ski lands flatly on the other side, with the rider landing heavily on his or her buttocks on the machine. Injuries to the thoracolumbar junction are the most common.

In conclusion, the mechanism of injury in board and body surfers recorded in earlier studies is supported by the nature and level of the injuries documented in this

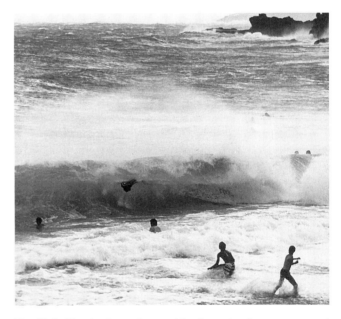

Fig. 37-4. The body surfer upside down in the wave crest is "going over the falls" and will be thrown onto the bottom. (Courtesy Jim Howe.)

study. No windsurfing, kayak, canoe or surf ski spinal column injuries were recorded in this study.

TREATMENT
At the Time of Injury

Frequently victims are fished from the water by a friend or bystander who recognizes they are injured. The

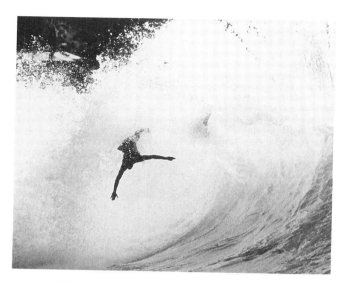

Fig. 37-5. The surfer is tossed over the falls and driven into the bottom. (Courtesy Jeff Divine.)

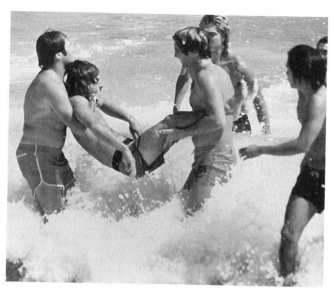

Fig. 37-6. Extrication of the unconscious or paralyzed victim from the surf zone is dangerous for both the victim and the rescuer. Every effort is made to minimize additional spinal cord injury. (Courtesy Division of Water Safety, City and County of Honolulu.)

coroner of Oahu reported no cases of drowning with associated spinal injury at autopsy during the period 1989 to 1993, supporting the prevalence of quick rescue times. However, extrication of the unconscious or paralyzed victim from the surf impact zone is dangerous for both the victim and the rescuer (Fig. 37-6). Every attempt is made to stabilize the spine from lateral bending, rotation, and flexion/extension to minimize additional spinal cord injury. Following rescue from the water, the victim is packed in sand until the ambulance and emergency medical technicians can place the victim on a spine board and transport him or her to the hospital.

Physical assessment of the injured individual to establish the extent of the injury and the neurologic status and associated problems is primary. Skeletal traction to stabilize the spine using Gardner-Wells tongs is the next step, followed by investigative studies to further delineate the extent and nature of the injury, including radiographs, a myelogram, a computed tomography (CT) scan, and/or a CT myelogram when necessary. Magnetic resonance imaging (MRI) is valuable to illuminate spinal cord injury when there is no radiographic evidence of bony injury, as is myelography.

Definitive Treatment

A high loading dose of steroids (30 g/kg) administered within 8 hours of injury followed in 45 minutes by an infusion of 5.4 mg/kg/hr for 23 hours[7] is standard.

C1 fractures and C2 pedicle and odontoid base fractures are best treated using a halo vest to maintain alignment and reduce the possibility of injury to the thecal elements. C1-2 instability due to ligamentous injury or fractures of the waist of the odontoid are best managed by posterior spinal stabilization and fusion.[5,6]

Unstable, axial-loading, flexion cervical spine fractures of the C3 vertebra and below are best treated by posterior stabilization and anterior decompression and fusion during a single surgical procedure.[27-29,39] When there is an incomplete neurologic lesion or evidence of extruded disc material anterior to the cord, the procedure sequence is reversed. When one is performing anterior decompression and fusion followed by posterior spinal stabilization, it is crucial to remember that anterior fusion without posterior stability is fraught with problems in achieving a stable end result.[33,34] When the posterior spine is compressed too tightly, the interval between the disrupted segments of the spine will increase anteriorly, and the strut graft or intervertebral dowel may be destabilized and extrude. Decompression anteriorly before posterior stabilization is likely to reduce the injury to an incomplete spinal cord lesion and is worth the risk.

In pure dislocation or in tiny teardrop fractures, if the lesion is complete with preservation of the nerve root exiting at the level of instability, then posterior stabilization and fusion alone will provide excellent stability. Comminuted vertebral body fractures with posterior instability and complete neurologic deficit are best approached posteriorly first, followed by corpectomy, canal decompression, and insertion of a strut graft.[6] Anterior decompression to preserve an additional nerve root is mandatory even if the injury has been previously neglected.

Facet dislocations, whether single or double, should be treated in traction, followed by posterior fusion using interspinous wiring or wiring of the facet joints to maintain reduction and stability. Closed reduction with the patient under general anesthesia, intravenous sedation, and muscle relaxants or paralytic agents to facilitate reduction are not recommended, in contrast to a report by Osti, Fraser, and Griffiths.[28] One C3-4 double facet dislocation with complete neurologic loss in the Oahu study was treated without reduction, resulting in autofusion in kyphosis.

Unstable fractures of the thoracic spine should be treated by posterior stabilization using a double-rod technique and fusing the entire rodded segment.[11-13,24] Unstable thoracolumbar and lumbar spine fractures should be stabilized by rodding long and fusing short.[2,19,40] Cottrel-Duboset contoured rods may be a better option for thoracolumbar junction fractures to preserve lordosis, although none of the patients in the Oahu study were treated in this manner.[15]

REHABILITATION

Rehabilitating body surfers to return to the sport was seldom accomplished with the patients in the Oahu study. Paraplegics were unable to participate, and novices often abandon the sport after injury. Surfing after fusion of a segment of the spine is not recommended. One body surfer who sustained a burst fracture of the C5 vertebra with radiculopathy at the age of 17 was so impressed by and grateful to the lifeguards who saved his life that he became one.

A complete discussion of the rehabilitation of the paralyzed patient is beyond the scope of this chapter. In our institution patients with neurologic deficits are admitted to the neurosurgical service and those without neurologic deficits are admitted to the orthopedic service. Having two surgeons of different services evaluate the patient aids the family in knowing that all that can and should be done is being done. This serves to allay the anger and fear experienced by the family of the traumatized individual.

Once patients are stabilized, they are transferred to a rehabilitation facility (after approximately 2 weeks). Consultation is initiated as soon as possible (1 day following surgery) so that the rehabilitation physician may evaluate and begin to plan the care of the patient. Psychologists, physical therapists, occupational therapists, and speech pathologists (for diaphragmatic paralysis) greatly enhance patients' affect and education about their injury. Range of motion, appropriate splinting, mobility aids, communication aids, and special eyewear all work toward decreasing the severity of the injury to the extremities and the psyche.

PREVENTION OF INJURY

Warning signs and informational brochures[37,38] are in use in Hawaii, but the perception is that the warnings are not heeded, perhaps because of the mindset of the

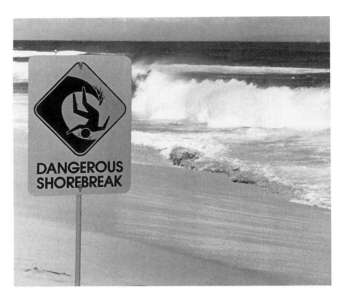

Fig. 37-7. Warning signs have been given high priority as a means of public education of the danger of particular beaches. The success of signs is difficult to assess. (Courtesy Division of Water Safety, City and County of Honolulu.)

vacationer (Fig. 37-7). Helmets, board noseguards, and redesign of the surfboard to blunt the nose have also been suggested,[35] but have failed to gain acceptance because of the psychologic perceptions of the sport of surfing. Recommendations have also been made to improve the warning systems, target specific beaches, and aim educational efforts at the age groups that are most prone to getting injured.[23] Efforts should be made to research and develop safer extrication methods and devices. On Hawaiian beaches that have lifeguards the beach may be closed during dangerous surfing conditions, but the guards have no authority to keep people from going into the water. Perhaps legislation to make violating beach warning signs a crime would help in deterrence. Videos on water safety should be shown on every arriving aircraft, and safety brochures should be in all hotel rooms in Hawaii. Residents and vacationers alike need to be warned about the specific beaches where most of the injuries occur, in addition to being warned about the possible severity of injury.

A survey of the incidence of spinal column injuries in all surfers documents the prevalence of severe spinal cord injury in body surfers. Although the incidence is not high relative to the number of participants and the number of beachgoers,[1] the suddenness and severity of the injury warrant specific concern.

ACKNOWLEDGMENTS

We would like to thank the following Honolulu hospitals for their assistance in this ongoing project: The Queen's Medical Center, Tripler Army Hospital, Rehabilitation Hospital of the Pacific, Kuikini Medical Center, Shriners Hospital for Crippled Children, and Kapiolani Medical Center for Women and

Children. Ralph Goto of the Division of Water Safety, City and County of Honolulu, and Janet West also provided invaluable assistance.

REFERENCES

1. Allen RH et al: Surfing injuries at Waikiki, *JAMA* 237:668, 1977.
2. Anden U, Lake A, Nordwall A: The role of the anterior longitudinal ligament in Harrington rod fixation of unstable thoracolumbar spinal fractures, *Spine* 5:23, 1980.
3. Bascom W: *Waves and beaches,* New York, 1980, Anchor Books.
4. Blankenship JR: Board surfing. In The *encyclopedia of sports science and medicine,* New York, 1971, Macmillan.
5. Bohlman HH: Acute fractures and dislocations of the cervical spine, *J Bone Joint Surg* 61A:1119, 1979.
6. Bohlman HH, Eismont FJ: Surgical techniques of anterior decompression and fusion for spinal cord injuries, *Clin Orthop* 154:57, 1981.
7. Bracken MB et al: A randomized controlled trial of methylpred-nisone or naloxone in the treatment of acute spinal-cord injury, *N Engl J Med* 322:1405, 1990.
8. Buck PH: *Arts and crafts of Hawaii,* Honolulu, 1964, BP Bishop Museum Press.
9. Cornish V: *Waves of the sea and other water waves,* Chicago, 1910, Open Court.
10. Daffner RH, Deeb ZL, Rothfus WE: "Fingerprints" of vertebral trauma—a unifying concept based on mechanisms, *Skeletal Radiol* 15:518, 1986.
11. Denis F: The three column spine and its significance in the classification of acute thoracolumbar spinal injuries, *Spine* 8:817, 1983.
12. Denis F: Spinal instability as defined by the three-column spine concept in acute spinal trauma, *Clin Orthop* 189:65, 1984.
13. Denis F et al: Acute thoracolumbar burst fractures in the absence of neurologic deficit, *Clin Orthop* 189:143, 1984.
14. Evans DL, Bethem D: Cervical spine injuries in children, *J Pediatr Orthop* 9:563, 1989.
15. Farcy JC, Weidenbaum M, Glassman SD: Sagittal index in management of thoracolumbar burst fractures, *Spine* 15:958, 1990.
16. Ferrandez L et al: Atypical multivertebral fracture due to hyperextension in an adolescent girl, *Spine* 14:645, 1989.
17. Filosa GF: *The surfer's almanac,* New York, 1977, EP Dutton.
18. Finney BR, Houston JD: *Surfing: the sport of Hawaiian kings,* Rutland, Vt, 1966, Charles E Tuttle.
19. Flesh JR et al: Harrington instrumentation and spine fusion for unstable fractures and fracture-dislocations of the thoracic and lumbar spine, *J Bone Joint Surg* 59A:143, 1977.
20. Gardner R: *The art of body surfing,* New York, 1972, Chilton.
21. Goebert DA et al: Traumatic spinal cord injury in Hawaii, *Hawaii Med J* 50:44, 1991.
22. Goldberg AL et al: Hyperextension injuries of the cervical spine, *Skeletal Radiol* 18:283, 1989.
23. Hartung GH et al: Epidemiology of ocean sports–related injuries in Hawaii: 'Akahele O Ke Kai,' *Hawaii Med J* 49(2):52, 1990.
24. Holdsworth F: Fractures, dislocations and fracture-dislocations of the spine, *J Bone Joint Surg* 52A:1534, 1970.
25. Kennedy M, Vanderfield G: Medical aspects of surfcraft usage, *Med J Aust* 2:707, 1976.
26. Lowdon BJ, Pateman NA, Pittman AJ: Surfboard-riding injuries, *Med J Aust* 2:613, 1983.
27. McAfee PC, Bohlman HH: One-stage anterior cervical decom-pression and posterior stabilization with circumferential arthrod-esis, *J Bone Joint Surg* 71A:78, 1989.
28. Osti OL, Fraser RD, Griffiths ER: Reduction and stabilisation of cervical dislocations, *J Bone Joint Surg* 71B:275, 1989.
29. Robinson RA et al: The cervical spine, *J Bone Joint Surg* 41A:1, 1959 (editorial).
30. Sances A et al: The biomechanics of spinal injuries, *Crit Rev Biomed Eng* 11:1, 1984.
31. Schneider RC, Kahn EA: Chronic neurological sequelae of acute trauma to the spine and spinal cord. I. The significance of the acute-flexion or "tear-drop" fracture-dislocation of the cervical spine, *J Bone Joint Surg* 38A:985, 1956.
32. Smith WS, Kaufer H: Patterns and mechanisms of lumbar injuries associated with lap seat belts, *J Bone Joint Surg* 51A:239, 1969.
33. Stauffer ES, Kaufer H, Kling TF: Fractures and dislocations of the spine. In Rockwood CA, Green DP, editors: *Fractures in adults,* ed 2, Philadelphia, 1984, JB Lippincott.
34. Stauffer ES, Kelly EG: Fracture-dislocation of the cervical spine, *J Bone Joint Surg* 59A:45, 1977.
35. Taniguchi R, Blattau J, Hammon W: Surfing. In Schneider RC et al, editors. *Sports injuries: mechanisms, prevention and treatment,* Baltimore, 1985, Williams & Wilkins.
36. Tricker RAR: *Bores, breakers, waves and wakes,* London, 1964, Mills & Boon.
37. United States Lifesaving Association—Hawaii Region: Beach map Oahu, water safety brochure 1986.
38. University of Hawaii Sea Grant College: Bodysurfing safety brochure, UNIHI-SeaGrant-AB-76-01, 1979.
39. Verbiest H: Anterolateral operations for fractures and disloca-tions in the middle and lower parts of the cervical spine, *J Bone Joint Surg* 51A(8):1489, 1969.
40. Wenger DR, Carollo JJ: The mechanics of thoracolumbar fractures stabilized by segmental fixation, *Clin Orthop* 189:89, 1984.
41. Yoganandan N et al: Injury biomechanics of the human cervical column, *Spine* 15(10):1031, 1990.

Chapter Thirty-Eight

Cricket

Christopher R. Weatherley
Philip Hobson Hardcastle
Daryl Hugh Foster
Bruce C. Elliott

Cricket is played in many countries. The game is reported in the *Guinness Book of Records* to have had its beginnings in approximately 1150 in Surrey, U.K. Since then, cricket has progressed to be the national game in many countries of the British Commonwealth. The traditional game is played over a 3- to 5-day period; however, recently, 1-day cricket has proved very popular. Each team is composed of 11 players, each with a specialist role—batsman, bowler (fast or slow), all rounder, or wicketkeeper. The game as it is now played involves two teams competing to achieve the highest score (runs). Similarities to baseball exist in that there is a fielding and batting side, with the facing batsman (batter) having the possibility of scoring runs after hitting balls delivered by the bowler (pitcher). An important difference in these two games is that the cricket ball is usually bounced off the ground in its delivery to the batsman, whereas in baseball it remains airborne. This contact with the ground introduces new possibilities for the bowler to confront and dismiss the batsman. Thus in addition to a curved or straight trajectory through the air at a selected pace (slow, medium, or fast), the contact with the ground (soft or hard, even or uneven) at a variable distance from the batsman and either at him (although this is not considered "cricket") or to either side creates such a range of possibilities (either intentional, fortuitous, or unfortunate) that two additional persons (umpires) are on the field to ensure fair play.

Bowlers become known for their ability to effect certain deliveries, and, of these, the fast bowler is certainly the most spectacular. "One can find many examples of outstanding individual performances, not only of skill and artistry but also of incredible determination and courage, for success in this great game frequently demands more than just natural ability. The intangible qualities of temperament and judgement are essential, but there is no line in the score book to record them." Although Sir Donald Bradman[2] referred to cricketers generally in this quote, the fast bowler more than any other player exemplifies the qualities expressed.

The most potent attacking force that a team possesses is its battery of fast bowlers. Fast bowling requires not only natural talent but also countless hours of training and technique practice, since the ball must be delivered at speeds of 80 to 100 miles an hour for long periods. The slower a bowler delivers the ball, the more he has to make it move either in the air or off the wicket to be successful. Each first-class bowler delivers between 500 and 1000 balls a week during a season lasting 5 to 6 months, and some may play in another country during the off-season.

The aim of fast bowling is to deliver a ball to the batsman accurately and, as indicated above, at great speed. The technique involves a run up to gain momentum, followed by release of the ball from the outstretched arm. In this release, the contralateral foot is planted and the body pivots around the extended leg, involving the lumbar spine sequentially in extension, rotation, and flexion (Fig. 38-1).

INCIDENCE OF INJURIES

The participation of children and adolescents in organized cricket has resulted in an increased number of injuries.[17] The young fast bowler has been described as the cricketer most susceptible to either traumatic or overuse injuries[19] due not only to the repetitive nature of the bowler's role in the game but also to faults in their basic action. Injuries to young fast bowlers, which may be a result of a combination of poor technique and overuse, are exacerbated by immature musculoskeletal development and inadequate muscle strength for the rigors of fast bowling.

It is common belief in Australia that many young fast bowlers are injured before they have a chance to reach their potential, and many senior bowlers continue to be plagued by injuries.[6,8,10] Payne et al.[19] reported that 50% of a sample of fast bowlers from one Australian A-Grade club followed over a 5-year period experienced a stress fracture. A subsequent study by Hardcastle et al.[14] confirmed this incidence of stress fracture or isthmic defect.

MECHANISM OF INJURY

Fast bowling is an impact activity wherein large forces are transmitted to the joints of the lower body while the trunk is extending, laterally flexing, and rotating in an

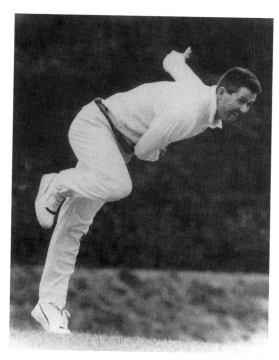

Fig. 38-1. Right-arm fast bowler after release of the ball (follow-through). (Courtesy *Sunday Independent*).

endeavor to achieve maximum delivery speed. As a result, the fast bowling action places stress on the lower back, which may result in injury. Furthermore, fast bowlers are usually required to perform for an extended period, which may precipitate an overuse problem. Therefore stress of the bowling action in combination with overuse may significantly increase the risk for a fast bowler to sustain a back injury. Sports that require repetitive lateral flexion, extension, or thoracic and lumbar rotation of the spine characteristically cause overuse back problems in young athletes. These injuries generally fall into one of three categories: a stress fracture of the pars interarticularis (spondylolysis), hyperlordotic low back pain, or disc herniation.[17] A fast bowler suffering from any one of these three problems experiences pain and restricted spinal movement, which may affect his bowling and daily activities. Consequently, it is of prime importance for all aspiring fast bowlers to reduce the possibility of this debilitating lower back injury.

Most injuries sustained by fast bowlers are due to poor technique, overuse, or poor physical preparation. Probably the most important factor, however, is technique, since no matter how physically fit a player is, if his technique involves hyperextension or excessive rotation, he is at significant risk of developing an overuse stress fracture or other pathologic conditions.

Elliott and Foster[4] completed a biomechanical evaluation of Australian side-on and front-on fast bowlers,

since it had been suggested that the front-on technique may be more susceptible to injury (see Figs. 38-9 and 38-11 for illustrations of the side-on and front-on actions, respectively). Results showed that bowlers using these techniques delivered the ball at a similar velocity (36 m/sec^{-1}) and were required to absorb similar maximum vertical ground reaction forces of approximately five times their body weight at front foot impact. Key differences in body segment orientation were identified at different phases of the bowling action.

A further study by Elliott, Foster, and Gray[8] showed that A-Grade level fast bowlers produced peak vertical and horizontal ground reaction forces of 4.1 and −1.6 body weights, respectively, at front-foot impact. The kinematic data presented showed that many current Australian fast bowlers, both senior and junior, use a "mixed" delivery action, which may be one of a number of reasons for the sudden rise in back injuries in fast bowlers.

PATHOLOGIC CONSIDERATIONS IN FAST BOWLING

Cricket is a noncontact sport, and the vast majority of injuries to fast bowlers are due to overuse, poor technique, poor physical fitness, or a combination of these factors. Soft tissue injuries or strains causing myofascial pain are quite common. Disc protrusions and facet dysfunction syndromes do occur, but the most common problem that will prevent a bowler from continuing his career is the stress fracture to the pars interarticularis, particularly in the lumbar area. This may be due to an underlying congenital predisposition, such as a spina bifida occulta, or arise as a direct result of repetitive hyperextension and rotation of the spine during the delivery action.

A prospective MRI study of 22 Western Australian young fast bowlers between 18 and 20 years of age demonstrated that 14 had degenerative disc disease, 7 had stress fractures, and 4 were diagnosed as having spondylolisthesis.[14] The pattern of degeneration was quite interesting (Fig. 38-2). The degenerative change was either in the upper lumbar spine at T12-L1, L1-2, or L2-3 or in the lower lumbar spine at L4-5 and L5-S1. Degeneration was usually at two or more levels but was present in only about 50% of bowlers with stress fractures and 75% of bowlers with a spondylolisthesis. This would suggest that the stress fracture is not related to degeneration and that the causes of the high incidence of degeneration and spondylolysis are different.

Stress Fractures

Stress fractures become apparent between the ages of 12 and 20 when a bowler increases his work load. They can occur anywhere in the lumbar spine, but in the study of young fast bowlers by Hardcastle et al.,[14] they generally were apparent at the L4 or L5 level. Unilateral fractures occur on the opposite side to the bowling arm

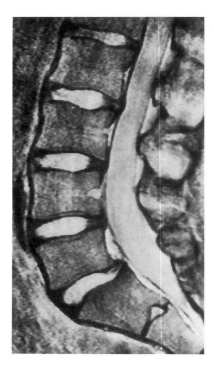

Fig. 38-2. MRI scan of a young 21-year-old international fast bowler demonstrating spondylolisthesis at L5-S1 due to a stress fracture. Note also the loss of signal from the L1-2 intervertebral disc and associated disc space narrowing.

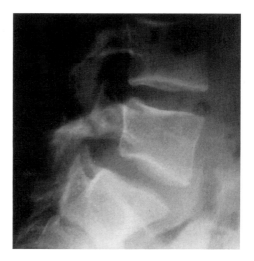

Fig. 38-3. Plain radiograph clearly showing a stress fracture at L5 with a relatively high intervertebral disc, indicating that this intervertebral segment permits a reasonable amount of sagittal plane movement, which is best assessed on flexion/extension views.

in about 80% of cases, which would suggest that hyperextension does not cause these unilateral fractures, since hyperextension occurs on the same side as the bowling arm. Therefore it is probably the repetitive rotation that causes these unilateral fractures. Spondylolisthesis may then result from hyperextension in the young bowler. Anatomic studies have suggested that sheer stresses are greater in the pars when the lumbar spine is extended. Young fast bowlers face an additional problem in that the pars is thin and the neural arch has not reached its maximum strength and the intervertebral disc is less resistant to sheer.[4] The pars interarticularis thickens and becomes stronger with age, and those fast bowlers who survive can continue bowling over long periods of time. There is no reported case of a stress fracture occurring in a bowler over the age of 25.

Symptoms in the early phase are minor. The bowler usually complains of some discomfort on the side he normally rotates away from (i.e., the left lower lumbar area in a right-arm fast bowler) after bowling. This discomfort gradually increases, and eventually the bowler is unable to bowl, although he is relatively pain free unless he bowls at near top pace. Early diagnosis and assessment of the stress fracture is important, since there are different causes and different patterns of fracture. Many overuse or repetitive strain stress fractures will heal over a few months, particularly at L4 and above. The player must cease bowling in this period, but

he can still undergo a strengthening program. Dennis Lillee, Australia's main pace bowler from 1969 to 1983, suffered a stress fracture at L2. He was treated by immobilization in a plaster jacket and then a long period of physical rehabilitation to strengthen his spine and change his bowling action. He returned to first-class cricket for another 10 years, and radiographs in 1989 were normal apart from pars interarticularis sclerosis.

The following factors need to be assessed before management decisions can be made concerning the stress fracture.

Clinical aspects. First, the anatomic location of the pain must be assessed, and the possibility of any nerve root compression must be considered. Second, the bowler's muscle strength must be measured to detect any major imbalance between flexors and extensors of the lower limb or between flexors and lateral deviators of the trunk. A number of bowlers have very good action, but when they tire toward the end of a spell of bowling, the support from their musculature is reduced such that they may abnormally hyperextend and rotate their spine during the delivery action in an endeavor to maintain their pace. The influence of muscle fatigue at the end of a long spell or near the completion of a day's play must therefore be taken into consideration when assessing a player's action.

Anatomic considerations. There are considerable anatomic variations in the lumbar spine, particularly at the lumbosacral junction. Plain x-ray films will demonstrate any associated congenital anomalies, such as spina bifida occulta, although radiographs of 45 first-class fast bowlers did not show any players with spina bifida occulta or other congenital anomalies, and it is presumed

Fig. 38-4. A, Here L5 lies below a line drawn across the cranial aspect of the iliac crest. In this situation L5 is probably a stable segment. **B,** In this view an intercrestal line crosses through the body of L5; if L5 has a wide disc space and small transverse processes, then the presence of a pars fracture creates a much more potentially unstable situation than in **A.**

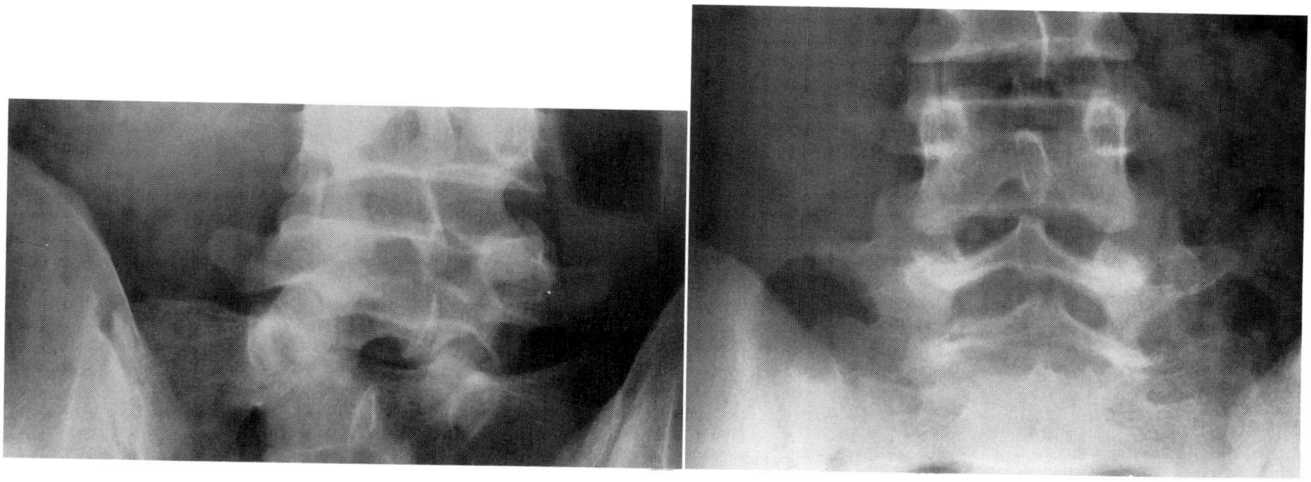

that players with spina bifida occulta do not become fast bowlers because of the stresses involved at a young age. The higher or wider an intervertebral disc space, the greater the potential for movement at that particular joint (Fig. 38-3). The bowler with the greater movement has the potential to elicit greater stress at that joint.

The relationship between the iliac crest and L5 is also important. Fig. 38-4 shows variations in the relationship between L5 and the iliac crest. If L5 lies entirely below a line drawn across the most cranial portion of both iliac crests, then the lumbosacral joint is much more likely to be stable than it would be if this line went through the vertebral body. There are a number of variations, but this aspect is particularly important in assessing the stability of the fracture if it involves L5. Another radiologic factor that is important in assessing stability is the size of the transverse processes; a very large transverse process is more likely to be associated with a stable mobile segment. The lumbosacral angle is also important, since the more lordotic this angle is, the more likely one is to develop pars stress.

Radiologic factors. Assessment with plain x-ray films may not demonstrate the site of the fracture in the spine or the number of fractures. Technetium-99m bone imaging is the best diagnostic method available for the diagnosis of stress fractures. However, reverse-gantry computed tomography (CT) scans give a much better radiologic assessment of the fracture itself, and these may also detect abnormal stress concentrations. The amount of displacement is important, since in the true stress fracture, particularly in the early phases, there is no forward displacement of the vertebra as opposed to the situation with a long-standing fracture, wherein 2 to 3 mm of forward displacement often occurs. In growing

adolescents pars elongation may occur as a result of healing stress fractures, leading to a spondylolisthesis with intact or unilateral pars fractures.

Fig. 38-5 demonstrates different patterns of stress fracture seen on the reverse-gantry CT views. These fractures may be unilateral or bilateral, and there are usually marked differences between the left and right sides. The fracture may range from a thin lucent line that is usually, but not always, adjacent to the tip of the inferior articular facet of the most cranial vertebra to almost complete lysis of the pars interarticularis. This asymmetry between the left and right sides is due to the effect of abnormal rotatory and compressive forces. Right-arm bowlers rotate to the right, and the maximum compression forces are also on this side. The lysis occurs on the right side with these bowlers, and on the opposite side there is often abnormal thickening or sclerosis of the pars, as well as a small lucent fracture. The direct opposite is seen in left-arm bowlers. However, with unilateral fractures the defect is on the opposite side of the bowling arm, and it is thought to result from abnormal repetitive rotation. Thus two mechanisms may cause isthmic fractures.

Fig. 38-5, *D,* shows a more chronic stress fracture in a young fast bowler without symptoms. There is no abnormal stress reaction adjacent to the fracture in this view, and the tip of the inferior articular facet is not directly adjacent to the fracture, as it is in Fig. 38-5, A to C. An anteroposterior (AP) radiograph of this bowler's pelvis is seen in Fig. 38-4, *A.* Note the relationship between L5 and the iliac crests; this pars fracture is probably a relatively stable one without excessive abnormal movement.

Fig. 38-6 shows abnormal stress concentration in the

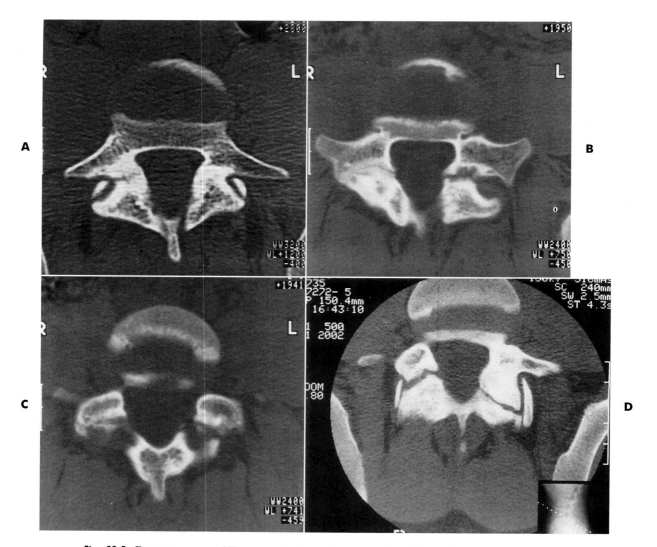

Fig. 38-5. Reverse-gantry CT scans. **A,** Scan demonstrating bilateral pars stress directly adjacent to the inferior tip of the inferior articular facet of the cranial vertebra. An early stress fracture is apparent on the right, which will probably heal with appropriate treatment. **B,** Scan demonstrating asymmetric pars interarticularis changes in a left-arm fast bowler. On the right, considerable sclerosis with a linear defect is seen in contradistinction to the opposite side, where considerable lysis has occurred. The left side was subject to repetitive compression and rotation forces. This type may heal with conservative treatment. **C,** Scan demonstrating changes that are more symmetric but unlikely to heal without surgical measures. **D,** Scan demonstrating a different pattern of fracture at a stable lumbosacral junction (iliac crests clearly seen) where the fractures are not adjacent to tips of the inferior cruciate articular process nor is there any adjacent lysis of the pars. These fractures are potentially more stable than those in **A** to **C,** but they are unlikely to heal, and treatment is symptomatic.

pars interarticularis in a young international fast bowler. Analysis of his action demonstrated a poor technique, and he is probably at risk of developing a stress fracture similar to those seen in Fig. 38-5, *A* and *B.*

Using the above facts, one can usually determine whether one is dealing with a stable or an unstable mobile segment, which is important in making treatment decisions.

DIAGNOSIS AND TREATMENT

Management of low back pain consists initially of making as accurate a clinical diagnosis as possible of the cause of the pain. Some players may have recurrent hamstring strains without back pain. Careful clinical assessment may demonstrate a lesion in the lumbar spine that is causing reduced lumbar movement, and appropriate treatment may resolve this recurring problem.

Once the diagnosis is established, local measures are usually successful. These include rest, immobilization,

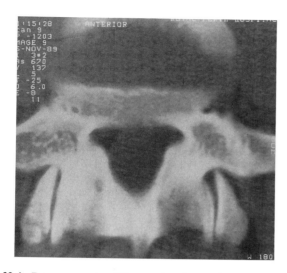

Fig. 38-6. Reverse-gantry CT scan showing early stress reaction in the pars interarticularis. Note the narrowing of the spinal canal directly adjacent to this stress reaction.

joint mobilization, manipulative treatment, local physiotherapy, or local cortisone injection, depending on the cause of the pain. It is suspected that the soft tissue pain a bowler often experiences may in some cases be due to an underlying discogenic or facet pain source, but treatment of the trigger point can still resolve the pain. Treatment of more resistant problems is discussed later.

Early recognition of the stress fracture is mandatory; the clinical signs that must be observed have already been discussed, and any fast bowler who complains of pain should be fully investigated even if the symptoms are minor. A ^{99m}Tc scan is done, and then a reverse-gantry scan should be done of any hot spots. Standard CT scans (perpendicular to the disc space) may miss a fracture, since they do not always scan through the pars interarticularis. In some cases no fracture is present, but pars stress with sclerosis is found on the CT scan (see Fig. 38-6). If a stress fracture is discovered by ^{99m}Tc or reverse-gantry CT scanning, the bowler should cease bowling. If the fracture is a recent one, treatment is aimed at initially getting the fracture to heal with immobilization and avoidance of fast bowling. An exercise program can be begun, and once union of the fracture has occurred, an analysis of the patient's bowling action can be undertaken. If the fracture is long-standing, then treatment initially is symptomatic, followed by a strengthening program and assessment of the patient's bowling action.

Generally, true stress fractures are unstable only in extension and rotation, and provided that these movements are avoided, the fracture may heal spontaneously. A recent study[13] of L5 pars fractures showed that immobilization could increase movement at L5-S1; therefore immobilizing an L5 stress fracture in this situation should not be considered unless incorporation

of the thigh is included in the orthosis, or flexion and extension radiographs are taken in and out of the brace to assess the effectiveness of the brace.

If the fracture or spondylolisthesis is long-standing, then treatment is symptomatic, with a period of rest or even a local cortisone injection. Once the pain has resolved, the player's action is assessed and rehabilitation is undertaken with a graduated return of the player to the sport; he can resume bowling when the CT scan shows evidence of healing of the most recent fracture.

The other major problems that can occur are facet dysfunction syndromes, either in the thoracodorsal or low lumbar areas, or an intevertebral disc protrusion. Conservative management is recommended initially with local measures, cortisone injection (including facet injections and epidural steroids), and attention to a player's physical fitness. Cryoanalgesia can be performed if a specific area of local tenderness is found and fails to respond to the previous techniques. Occasionally, surgical management is necessary, and this is described later in the chapter. Another common problem complained of by fast bowlers is pain either over the twelfth rib or over one of the lateral aspects of the transverse process, usually on the side opposite the bowling arm. This is thought to be a musculotendinous strain, and local treatment, initially by physiotherapy and followed in resistant cases by local injections of cortisone, usually proves effective in its management.

It is advisable for players returning after an injury to wear a trunk support. These are well tolerated by players. In lesions involving L5, it is sometimes necessary to include a thigh support to control lumbosacral movement. These thigh supports can be stitched to the trunk support. Either thigh can be used, depending on the injury and which forces need to be modified.

Although conservative treatment may relieve the symptoms, it is vital that a player's action be analyzed and that an appropriate strengthening program be instituted to prevent further problems.

SURGICAL MANAGEMENT

Surgical management is considered if a player fails to respond to an adequate trial of conservative treatment and has a well-defined pathologic lesion. If a fusion is being considered, a routine MRI scan is essential to assess the status of the intervertebral discs above and below the main pathologic level. Surgical techniques used for discectomy, repair of the pars fracture, and spinal fusion are described in this section. It should be remembered that the repair of the pars fracture is the only spinal operation that can restore not only normal anatomy but also normal biomechanics.

Discectomy

Chymopapain and percutaneous discectomy have been popular in the past, but these techniques have not been found to be useful with fast bowlers. However, in the presence of a disc protrusion without sequestration or spinal stenosis, it is not unreasonable to try one of these techniques. Percutaneous discectomy often has less associated postoperative pain and is probably preferable to chymopapain, although there is no objection to the latter.

Open discectomy and microdiscectomy are similar techniques, and the most important aspect in both is to remove the entire nucleus pulposus. Otherwise, the player is at risk of recurrent protrusion on returning to the sport, given the forces he places on his spine. There is no evidence to suggest that total or partial removal of the nucleus pulposus has a higher incidence of low back pain or instability, and removal of the entire degenerate nucleus is believed to be mandatory. The nucleus is nonfunctional once it has degenerated but can cause problems with recurrent protrusion. Also, it is worthwhile to consider removing any adjacent degenerate nucleus. If a player has an L5-S1 protrusion causing sciatica and there is evidence of degenerative disease at the L4-5 level, removing the entire nucleus at both levels in a single procedure is favored as a preventive measure against future disc replacements given the forces to which these bowlers subject their spines. The postoperative management is very important, with isometric exercises started immediately once the acute pain has resolved. Swimming is allowed 3 weeks postoperatively, and running can begin 3 to 6 weeks postoperatively, with a formal isotonic strengthening program. Bowling can begin 8 to 10 weeks after the operation.

Repair of the Pars Fracture

Two techniques are available. One is the modified Buck technique,[3,22] with a compression screw passed across the fracture to compress it, and the second is the Scott wiring technique[18] wherein a wire is passed around the transverse process and lamina as a tension band, once again in combination with bone grafting.

Modified Buck technique. The standard midline approach is used, and the soft tissues are dissected off the spine to expose the L4-5 and the L5-S1 facet joints for the L5 pars, and the L3-4 and L4-5 facets for the L4 pars. The inferior part of the facet capsule directly cranial to the fracture is removed, and 3 to 4 mm of the inferior tip of the inferior facet joint is removed with an osteotome. This serves two purposes: it removes a possible impingement of the inferior facet on the pars fracture and also allows a much better operative exposure of the fracture, as well as a wider graft area. All possible soft tissue is removed from the dorsal, lateral, and interior aspects of the fracture. Then a small piece of bone is removed from the inferior edge of the lamina of the involved level. A 3.2-mm drill is then passed between the cortical surfaces of the lamina across the fracture and into the base of the pedicle. Cancellous bone graft taken from the right iliac crest is then packed on the interior of the fracture and over its dorsal and lateral surfaces, extending up onto the transverse process and lateral aspect of the superior facet. Bone graft is also run caudally over the lamina. A 40- or 45-mm-long AO malleolar screw is then passed across the fracture to stabilize it on each side. Usually it is not possible to see the screw on the sclerotic side, and a radiograph can be taken if any doubt exists about the placement of the screw (Fig. 38-7).

Patients are mobilized 2 to 3 days postoperatively while wearing a Jewett brace or a corset. Preoperative flexion/extension views, taken with and without the Jewett brace, demonstrate the effectiveness of this thoracodorsal orthosis in immobilizing the particular segment. If there is in fact increased movement, particularly at L5, when the flexion/extension radiographs

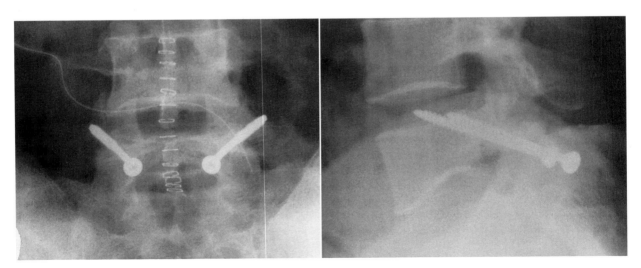

Fig. 38-7. Postoperative AP and lateral radiographs showing the position of the AO malleolar screws after bone grafting of a pars fracture.

are taken with the Jewett brace, then a corset is used. Isometric exercises are begun in the first week, and swimming is allowed 3 to 4 weeks postoperatively. Reverse-gantry CT scans are taken at 3 months (Fig. 38-8), and if union has occurred at this stage, the exercise or rehabilitation program is increased. Usually it takes up to 6 months for these fractures to unite, and once there is radiologic evidence of union, full activities, including bowling, can be resumed. Roca et al.[22] reported union in 14 of his patients 6 months postoperatively, with 13 returning to full sporting activity.

The pars fractures that are not suitable for fixation are as follows:

1. An associated congenital anomaly causing marked pars narrowing so that it is not technically possible to pass the screw (in these cases the Scott wiring technique, or even a spinal fusion, needs to be considered)
2. Spondylolisthesis with more than 3 mm of forward displacement
3. Very wide defects on the reverse-gantry CT scans

Spinal Fusion

Spinal fusion is reserved for those players who have segmental instability syndromes. Preferably, fusion should be confined to one level, and certainly no more than two levels should be fused if the player is contemplating a return to the sport. Fusion can be anterior, posterior, or a combination, depending on the underlying problem. With posterior fusions, internal fixation with spinal plates or a Hartshill rectangle is important.[5,9] The Hartshill rectangle is preferred, since it is a relatively simple form of internal fixation and provides excellent stability with high-fusion rates. For spondylolisthesis, a formal intertransverse fusion technique is recommended in combination with spinal plates, since sublaminal wires are nonfunctional in these situations.

Where the lamina is intact, a modified fusion technique is used. The facet joints are excised, and all soft tissue is denuded from the interfacet area to display the pars interarticularis and also expose the transverse process and lateral aspect of the superior facet at the most cranial portion of the fusion mass. A Hartshill rectangle is then secured over the level or levels to be fused with sublaminal wiring (1.1-mm gauge wire), and corticocancellous bone graft is packed between the facet joints and up to the transverse process and lateral aspect of the superior facet, which have been denuded. This limited fusion, combined with the stability of the Hartshill rectangle, allows less muscle stripping and less muscle retraction, which reduces the amount of postoperative muscle scarring, a factor very important with athletes. Fig. 38-9 shows a postoperative radiograph of the Hartshill rectangle; the anatomic specimen demonstrates not only the rectangle but also the area of the fusion mass.

Patients are mobilized 2 days postoperatively without a corset, and an isometric exercise program is begun. Swimming and hydrotherapy can begin 3 weeks postoperatively, and bike riding is introduced 4 to 6 weeks postoperatively. A formal muscle-strengthening program can begin at approximately 6 to 8 weeks, and running can begin at 12 weeks, provided that x-ray and CT scan findings are satisfactory. Once there is radiologic evidence of union, usually best seen on the CT scan

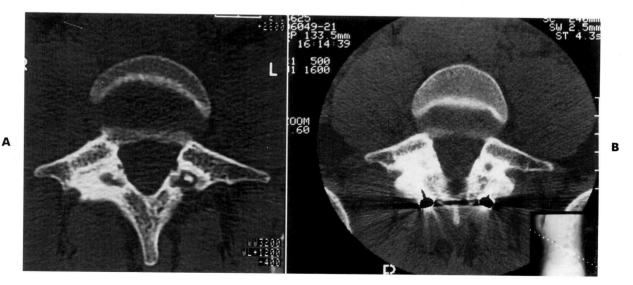

Fig. 38-8. A, Reverse-gantry CT scan of an L5 pars fracture before surgery (same patient as shown in Fig. 38-9). **B** Reverse-gantry views of the L5 pars 6 months after surgery showing union of the fractures. The fast bowler returned to full sporting activity with no recurrence of his fractures 2 years postoperatively and has continued to play cricket.

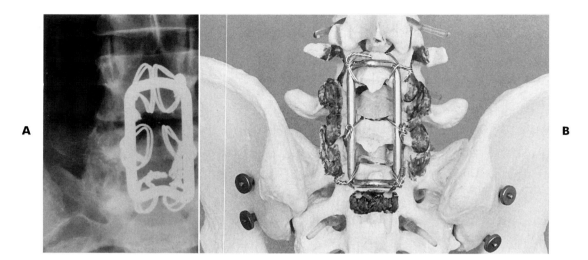

Fig. 38-9. A, AP radiograph of a Hartshill rectangle used to stabilize L4-5 and L5-S1 in an international fast bowler. **B,** Fusion area for L4-S1 fusion. The lateral aspect of the superior facet of the most cranial vertebra to be fused and the medial aspect of the adjacent transverse process are decorticates (see **A**), and the fusion gutter is continued down to the superior sacral facet, or most caudal level to be fused.

or tomography, then bowling can begin, provided that the player's level of physical fitness allows it.

PREVENTION OF INJURY

The radiologic study of 22 high-performance young fast bowlers in Western Australia referred to earlier revealed a 50% incidence of stress fractures or spondylolisthesis. Four of this group stopped bowling because of pain and had surgical repairs of the defects. Ten of the 11 bowlers with isthmic defects had pain; 10 of the 11 were also assessed as bowling with a "mixed" action, which studies have concluded is more likely to cause injury than either the "front-on" or "side-on" bowling techniques. A lot of young potential fast bowlers have to give up the sport because of these stress fractures, and there is usually a fault in their bowling action. It is believed that proper coaching methods must be instituted early in a player's career in an attempt to reduce this very high incidence of stress fractures.

Principles for the Preparation of Fast Bowlers

Educating coaches to detect potential problems in the action of young players, encouraging players to do strengthening exercises to prevent fatigue while bowling, and perhaps even having a limit on the number of "overs" schoolboys can bowl in each match will help prevent stress fractures to the pars interarticularis. Proper training methods, attention to footwear, and limbering-up exercises before bowling are also important preventive measures.[7] Detailed programs for preparing fast bowlers can be found in a textbook by Elliott, Foster, and Blanksby.[7]

Bowling actions (Figs. 38-10 to 38-12). Fast bowlers have traditionally been classified as bowling with either a side-on or front-on delivery action. Research has, however, indicated that neither of these actions is closely associated with an increase in injuries to the back. A prospective study by Foster et al.[10] on 82 high-performance young male fast bowlers (mean age = 16.8 years) clearly showed that specific technique and overuse factors were linked to stress fractures to lumbar vertebrae. This study revealed that 30% of players sustained a stress fracture, primarily to L4 and L5, and 27% sustained a soft tissue injury to the back that caused them to miss at least one match, although a more recent study has shown the incidence of stress fractures to be 50% in fast bowlers under 19 years of age.[14] Cinematographic data indicated that a mixed action produced a greater potential for injury; that is, bowlers who had the lower body (foot and hip) alignment of a front-on bowler and the upper body (shoulder and head) alignment of a side-on bowler were more likely to suffer a back injury than bowlers who used either a side-on or front-on delivery action. The group most prone to back injury were those bowlers who used a mixed technique and rotated the trunk to realign the shoulders by more than 40 degrees to a more side-on orientation between back foot impact and front foot impact. Compare Fig. 38-11, *A* and *B*, with Fig. 38-10, *A* and *B*, and Fig. 38-12, *A* and *B*. Note how this extra rotation and the position of the head force the spine into a hyperextended position at front foot impact (Fig. 38-11, *C*).

A greater release height when expressed as a percentage of standing height was also significantly related

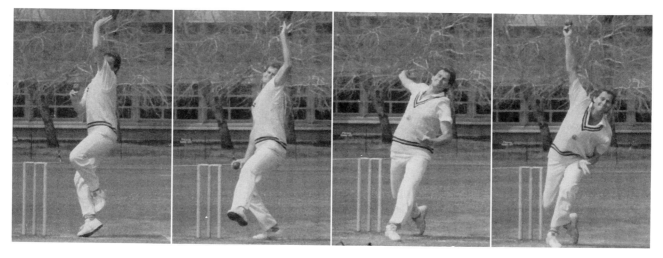

Fig. 38-10. Side-on action.

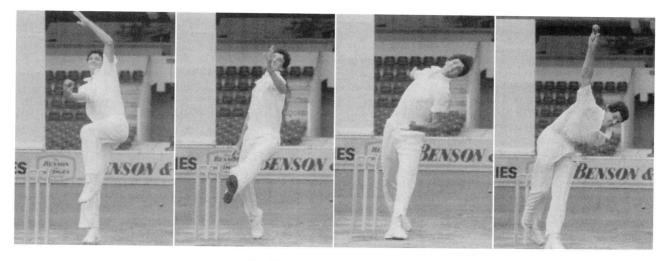

Fig. 38-11. Mixed bowling action.

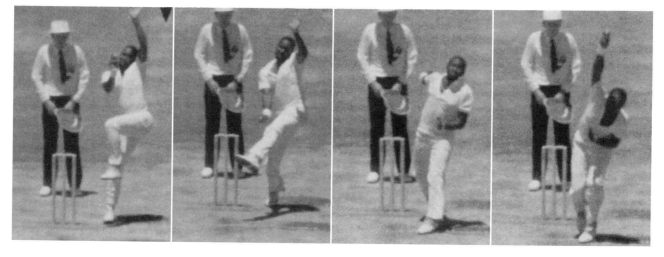

Fig. 38-12. Front-on bowling action.

to back injuries. The authors suggested that this may be related to a lower limb that is further extended at front foot impact through to delivery, which may not dissipate force as effectively as with the bowler who marginally flexes the front knee joint between front foot impact and delivery. The key features associated with each of these three bowling actions is outlined here; a comprehensive review of these techniques can be found in the book by Elliott, Foster, and Blanksby.[7]

Side-on bowling technique (see Fig. 38-10)

Back foot impact. The back foot should be approximately parallel to the rear crease, and lines drawn through the shoulders and through the hips should point down the pitch (i.e., the body should be at right angles to the stumps at the bowler's end of the wicket). The bowler should look behind the front arm (that should be held high in the air) with his eyes focused on the base of the striker's off-stump.

Back foot impact to front foot impact. The hips and shoulders should begin to rotate toward the batsman. The elbow of the nonbowling limb is accelerated into the side of the body, and the front lower limb should be thrust outward and downward to land on the bowling crease. The front foot should land pointing straight down the pitch or slightly oriented to the on-side of the wicket and in general alignment with the back foot. A delivery stride of 75% to 85% of the bowler's height is a good rule of thumb.

Front foot impact to release. The hips and shoulders continue to rotate so that at release the bowler is almost perpendicular to the line of delivery, and the upper limb rotates vigorously forward as the nonbowling elbow is pulled into the side. The trunk leans slightly forward, and the upper limb should be relatively upright at release.

Mixed bowling technique (see Fig. 38-11).

It is this technique that produces abnormal forces on the spine, allowing abnormal rotation. The bowler has a front-on foot placement and hip alignment but attempts to attain a side-on upper body position, causing considerable stress to be applied to the low lumbar spine. Compare the action in Fig. 38-11, *C* and *D*, with the actions of Terry Alderman and Malcolm Marshall, shown in Figs. 38-10, *C* and *D*, and 38-12, *C* and *D*, respectively. Fig. 38-11 shows that the bowler has rotated his shoulders by an angle of approximately 40 degrees to attain a more side-on position between back foot impact and front foot impact. He also initially views the batsman from outside his nonbowling arm and therefore has to hyperextend his spine at the point just before release to be able to see where he is bowling, causing a forced hyperextension and thus additional stress on the lumbar spine.

Front-on bowling technique (see Fig. 38-12)

Back foot impact. The back foot should face down the pitch or to the on-side of the wicket. Lines drawn through the hips and shoulders should be aligned diagonally across the pitch, with the bowler focusing on the off-stump from inside the raised nonbowling arm.

Back foot impact to front foot impact. The hips and shoulders rotate through a smaller arc than was recorded in the side-on technique. Malcolm Marshall demonstrates the ideal front-on action in Fig. 38-12, *A* to *C*, whereas Terry Alderman demonstrates the classic side-on action in Fig. 38-10, *A* to *C*. Recent radiographs of Terry Alderman's back, after a long and distinguished career with the Australian team, failed to demonstrate degenerative disease in the lumbar spine, and there was complete absence of any abnormal stress reaction or degenerative disease except for some minor changes at the T12 area.

Good technique, of either a front-on or a side-on nature but not a mixture of both, together with a logical approach to the number of overs bowled at practice and in a match, as well as a physical training program developed for the individual needs of the fast bowler, will not only produce superior match statistics but will also protect the bowler from injury.

Physical Fitness and Fast Bowling

Physical fitness and a proper technique are essential ingredients for success with a minimal risk of injury. These two aspects of fast bowling must also be linked to a sensible approach to the length and number of bowling spells if the risk of injury is to be reduced. Foster et al.[10] reported that 59% of bowlers out of a sample of 82 fast bowlers who bowled in excess of the mean number of matches for the group suffered a stress fracture or soft tissue injury to the back compared with an injury frequency of 38% for the total group.

Proper assessment of muscle strength so that the individual athlete can be given a specific strengthening program in the off-season is also vital to a player's preparation. It is essential for the experienced fast bowler to attain high levels of aerobic and anaerobic fitness, muscular endurance, and strength, in addition to retaining adequate levels of flexibility. The well-prepared fast bowler will then be able to operate at a high level of intensity over repeated spells without becoming unduly fatigued. According to Dennis Lillee,[16] "Natural ability will carry you just so far. . . . It is literally survival of the fittest in the sphere of fast bowling."

As our life-style becomes more sedentary, the specific fitness requirements for fast bowling become even more important. For the young fast bowler in particular, graduated fitness training is of vital importance. His technique must also be monitored, not only at practice but also during a game. Coaches also must ensure that an individual is not over-bowled and fatigued, thus placing abnormal stress on his spine and increasing the potential for injury.

CASE HISTORIES

CASE 1

A 26-year-old right-arm fast bowler had a 16-month history of low back and right thigh pain. The back pain began after intense training for cricket. Some months later he developed episodes of lower right abdominal pain for periods of up to a few hours. His left leg was not involved except for a 3-week period of numbness involving the anteromedial aspect below the knee. His symptoms improved at the end of the cricket season but returned some months later when he returned to training.

It is noteworthy that the patient's acute pain was often worse immediately after delivery of the ball as the (right) delivery arm and the trunk reached maximum rotation about his fixed front (left) foot. To avoid this, he took to placing his left foot in a more externally rotated position, thereby effecting less restraint to rotation following delivery. This was beneficial.

Examination

There was no abnormality on clinical examination; the patient had a full range of motion of his lumbar spine and no abnormal neurologic findings.

Diagnostic Studies

Conventional straight radiographs showed no abnormality, apart from sclerosis of the right L4 pedicle on the anteroposterior (AP) view (Fig. 38-13). An isotope bone scan, however,

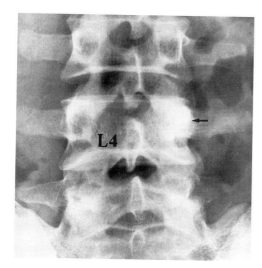

Fig. 38-13. AP radiograph of the lumbar spine showing sclerosis of the right L4 pedicle *(arrow).* (From Weatherley CR, Mehdian H, Vanden Berghe L: *J Bone Joint Surg* 73B:990, 1991.)

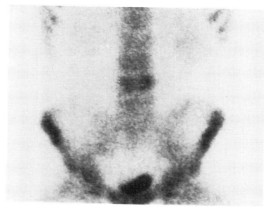

Fig. 38-14. Bone scan showing increased uptake on both sides at the L4 level. (From Weatherley CR, Mehdian H, Vanden Berghe L: *J Bone Joint Surg* 73B:990, 1991.)

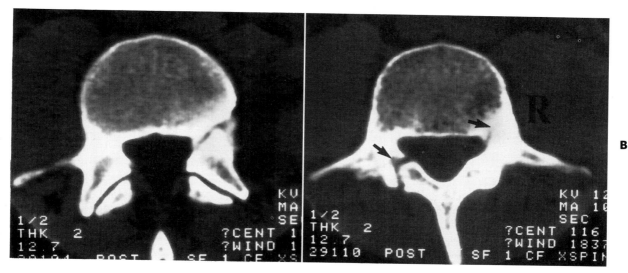

Fig. 38-15. A, CT scan at L4 showing fracture and sclerosis of the base of the right pedicle. **B,** CT scan at L4 (a different section from that in **A**) showing a unilateral spondylolysis on the left side in addition to the changes noted on the right. (From Weatherley CR, Mehdian H, Vanden Berghe L: *J Bone Joint Surg* 73B:990, 1991.)

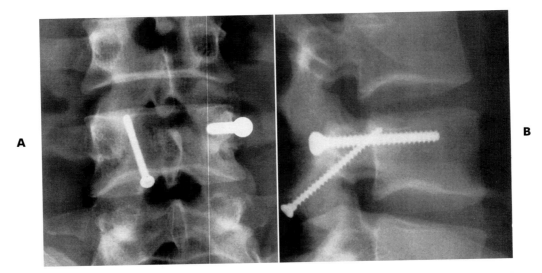

Fig. 38-16. A, AP radiograph at 1 year showing placement of the screws. **B,** Lateral radiograph at 1 year. (From Weatherley CR, Mehdian H, Vanden Berghe L: *J Bone Joint Surg* 73B:990, 1991.)

showed increased uptake on both sides at the L4 level (Fig. 33-14). A CT scan revealed a fracture of the base of the right pedicle with sclerosis and a unilateral pars defect on the left at the same level (Fig. 38-15).

Treatment

The patient was treated surgically. The fracture of the right pedicle was considered a hypertrophic nonunion and fixed simply with a pedicle screw to effect compression and stabilization. The point of entry was lateral to avoid possible impingement against the screw head during lumbar extension. The contralateral pars defect was also treated in a direct manner using the screw fixation technique described by Buck[3] for spondylolysis. Postoperatively he wore a molded polyethylene lumbar support for 6 weeks.

He was symptom free from the time of the operation and returned to fast bowling 6 months postoperatively. Straight radiographs revealed no displacement or breakage of the screws at 1 year (Fig. 38-16), and a CT scan showed union of both defects.

Case 2

A 22-year-old right-arm fast bowler gave a history of low back pain on the right side that had begun 6 years previously while the patient was bowling. The pain resolved completely some weeks later when the cricket season finished. The following year it returned, and he was unable to play. The year after that, he had some back pain during training but nonetheless completed a full season. In the fourth year, however, the pain returned and never resolved, and the patient was forced to abandon a promising career.

When the patient was bowling, the pain would extend upward and to the right buttock, and also down the outer side of the right thigh. He also noted that his back pain could be avoided to some extent while bowling by changing to medium-pace bowling and thereby diminishing the force and extent of the involved movements.

There was no abnormality on clinical examination. The AP radiograph showed, as in Case 1, an obvious sclerosis of the right L4 pedicle, but in this case the sclerosis was associated with a deviation of the spinous process (Fig. 38-17). Somewhat surprisingly, there was no obvious abnormality on either side at the L4 level on a ^{99m}Tc high-density proton (HDP) bone scan. A CT scan revealed an obvious enlargement of the right L4 pedicle with a dense sclerosis extending into the postero-lateral corner of the vertebral body on this side (Fig. 38-18). It also showed a spondylolytic defect at this level on the other side.

The patient was treated surgically in the same manner as the patient in Case 1, with the same success.

Evaluation of Cases

Both of these men, of similar age, developed low right-sided back pain in the course of being right-arm fast bowlers, and each was demonstrated to have a sclerotic right L4 pedicle. The fact that in each case the pain was on the side of the sclerotic pedicle and was relieved immediately by its fixation suggests strongly that the sclerotic pedicle was the pain source. It also suggests that in both cases the sclerosis was associated with a fracture; otherwise it is difficult to understand why in Case 2 internal fixation should also be associated with relief of symptoms. It is postulated that in each case the sclerosis or nonunion developed secondarily to an asymptomatic defect in the contralateral neural arch at that level.

Furthermore, the history in each case suggests that other factors may be important in the development of a pseudoarthrosis of the pedicle, including repetitive moments, body rotation, and speed (force) of delivery. Thus stopping bowling, turning the left foot out to reduce the constraint to body rotation, or slowing the

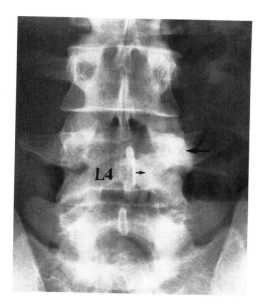

Fig. 38-17. AP radiograph showing sclerosis of the right L4 pedicle associated with a deviated spinous process.

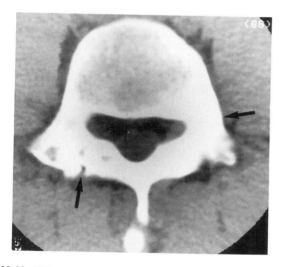

Fig. 38-18. CT scan at L4 showing sclerosis of the right L4 pedicle and posterolateral area of the vertebral body associated with a unilateral spondylolysis on the left side.

speed (force) led to a symptomatic improvement. Some idea of the specificity of movements responsible, however, may be obtained from the fact that both were able, despite the fracture, to pursue other sports and activity with little or no pain. The obliquity of the bilateral lesions may be further evidence that rotation is an important etiologic factor.

In each of these bowlers the L4 level was involved. This is in keeping with a review of 15 other published cases of a fractured or sclerotic pedicle associated with a contralateral spondylolysis in which 13 occurred at one

Table 38-1. Level and Side of Pedicle Sclerosis or Fracture in 15 Published Cases

	Left	Right
L1		
L2		1
L3		1
L4		5
L5	2	6

of the lower two levels[1,11,12,24] (Table 38-1). This may reflect the fact that in any one individual it is either L4 or L5 (depending on the deep-seatedness of L5 and its lateral attachments) that represents the last link in the segmented chain permitting axial rotation against the unsegmented sacrum. Furthermore, since axial rotation may be increased in flexion,[15] the forces generated in fast bowling will be even further increased at the end of follow-through, when the lumbar spine may be both rotated and flexed. Translatory movements[20] may also be important, especially in the presence of an existing discontinuity in the neural arch.

In both these bowlers the pedicle fracture was on the right side. Once again, this correlates with the literature, with 13 of 15 cases reviewed being on this side (see Table 38-1). Although this may reflect right-handedness, Stewart,[25] in his classic paper on neural arch defects in the skeletons of Alaskan natives, found 12 examples of pedicle fractures associated with contralateral defects. The majority were on the left side and in female skeletons. He, too, considered that this might reflect handedness but did not stipulate which side. The possibility may exist that Eskimo women played cricket and had left-arm fast bowlers; however, the terrain would not seem to lend itself to this activity, so an alternative explanation may need to be sought.

It may be that a stress fracture of a pedicle is a more common cause of back pain than is currently realized. Roche and Rowe[23] noted that in a series of 183 neural arch separations more than one sixth were unilateral. If, as seems likely, the unilateral lysis is the precursor of the contralateral and symptomatic pedicle fracture, then there is clearly a population at risk, especially in certain athletic pursuits, such as fast bowling. Failure to diagnose the condition even when it has become symptomatic may reflect not only a lack of awareness of the condition but also the paucity of changes that may be present on straight radiographs—the most common supplementary diagnostic study for back pain.

In these two cases the obvious finding on the AP radiograph was the sclerotic pedicle. This has led in the past to a provisional diagnosis of an osteoid osteoma or osteoblastoma. Exactly how long is needed for the sclerosis to be manifested radiologically is not known, but in these two cases it was well established on AP radiographs taken 13 months and then 5 years after the initial symptoms. It is probable, however, that early in the history there is less sclerosis, with the result that the diagnosis may be missed.

In studies on isolated vertebrae, Roche and Rowe[23] noted that a unilateral spondylolysis may be associated with a deviation of the spinous process away from the lysis. The combined findings on an AP radiograph of a sclerotic pedicle and a deviated spinous process should therefore raise suspicion that there may be a contralateral lysis and alert one to the diagnosis (see Fig. 38-17). In both of these cases the unilateral lysis was not seen on the AP or lateral views and was at best only suggested on an oblique view.

CT would seem to be the investigative tool of choice for this condition, with the hypertrophic and sclerotic pedicle and the contralateral lysis showing up either on one section or on serial sections. Whether or not a fracture line is visible within the sclerosis, however, may depend on such factors as the plane of the section, the thickness of the section, and, of course, the size of the fracture gap. Thus in Case 1, although the fracture line is gross on one section (see Fig. 38-15, *A*), it is much less in evidence among the sclerosis in another (see Fig. 38-15, *B*). It is not difficult to appreciate, therefore, that dense sclerosis without a clear break does not exclude a fracture, even on CT examination. Porter and Park[21] reported similar difficulties in identifying a unilateral spondylolysis.

The findings of the bone scan in these two cricketers are interesting. In Case 1 there was increased uptake associated with both lesions, whereas in Case 2 no increased uptake was observed. Factors accounting for this difference may include the size and duration of the lesions, as well as the sensitivity of the scanning technique. Thus although the findings taken alone may be unreliable, the bone scan may still be a useful supplementary investigation.

The treatment of this condition if conservative measures fail is surgical. In the article that first defines the clinical condition,[24] 11 cases were described; of these, 7 patients were treated surgically. Two of the initial patients had excision biopsy of the sclerotic pedicle in combination with spinal fusion. When the benign nature of the lesion was identified, however, the recommended operation changed to a three-level fusion. In 1986 Garber and Wright[11] restricted the surgery to the pathologic level. They described a case in which the spondylolytic defect was grafted and the sclerotic pedicle was drilled and grafted. One-level fixation was then carried out using the Scott wiring technique for spondylolysis.[18]

In 1991 Gunzburg and Fraser[12] and Weatherley, Mehdian, and Vanden Berghe[26] reported two cases treated along similar lines. In managing the pedicular pseudarthrosis, however, Gunzburg and Fraser osteotomized the transverse process to expose and excise and graft the lateral half of the pseudarthrosis before inserting a screw across the defect. They reported the patient to be almost symptom free at 6 months postoperatively. Although this is a logical way to approach and graft, the latter would not seem to be necessary. The lesion is in effect a hypertrophic nonunion, and in keeping with the surgical management of similar lesions elsewhere in the body, fixation alone should be adequate. This view certainly seems to have been borne out in the two cases described here.

ACKNOWLEDGMENT

Thanks go to Mrs. Joan Williams of the Department of Human Movement and Recreation Studies, The University of Western Australia, for the typing of a major portion of this manuscript.

REFERENCES

1. Aland C et al: Fracture of the pedicle of the fourth lumbar vertebra associated with contralateral spondylolysis, *J Bone Joint Surg* 68A:1454, 1986.
2. Bradman D, Foreword. In Frith D: *A pictorial history of test matches since 1879,* Cambridge, UK, Lutterworth Press, 1981.
3. Buck JE: Direct repair of the defect in spondylisthesis: preliminary report, *J Bone Joint Surg* 52B:432, 1970.
4. Cyron BM, Hutton WC: The fatigue strength of the lumbar neural arch in spondylolysis, *J Bone Joint Surg* 60B:234, 1979.
5. Dove J: Internal fixation of the lumbar spine: the Hartshill rectangle, *Clin Orthop* 203:135, 1986.
6. Elliott BC, Foster DH: A biomechanical analysis of the front-on and side-on bowling techniques, *J Hum Move Stud* 10:83, 1984.
7. Elliott BC, Foster DH, Blanksby B, editors: *Send the stumps flying—the science of fast bowling,* Nedlands, 1989, University of Western Australia Press.
8. Elliott BC, Foster DH, Gray S: Biomechanical and physical factors influencing fast bowling, *Aust J Sci Med Sport* 18(1):16, 1986.
9. Fidler M: Posterior instrumentation of the spine, *Spine* 11:367, 1986.
10. Foster DH et al: Back injuries to fast bowlers in cricket: a prospective study, *Br J Sports Med* 23:150, 1989.
11. Garber JE, Wright MA: Unilateral spondylolysis and contralateral pedicle fracture, *Spine* 11:63, 1986.
12. Gunzburg R, Fraser RD: Stress fracture of the lumbar pedicle, *Spine* 16:185, 1991.
13. Hardcastle P, Miller R: The effect of spinal braces in reducing sagittal plane movement in the low lumbar spine, Unpublished manuscript, 1990.
14. Hardcastle P et al: The incidence of degenerative disc disease and stress fractures in Western Australian fast bowlers, Unpublished manuscript, 1986.
15. Hindle RD et al: Twisting of the human back in forward flexion, *Proc Inst Mech Engrs* 203:83, 1989.
16. Lillee DK: *The art of fast bowling,* Sydney, 1977, Collins.
17. Micheli LJ: Overuse injuries in children's sports: the growth factor, *Orthop Clin North Am* 14:337, 1983.
18. Nicol RO, Scott JH: Lytic spondylolysis: repair by wiring, *Spine* 11:1027, 1986.
19. Payne WR, Hoy G, Carlson JS: What research tells the cricket coach, *Sports Coach* 10(4):17, 1987.
20. Pearcy MJ, Tibrewal SB: Axial rotation and lateral bending in the normal lumbar spine measured by three-dimensional radiography, *Spine* 9:582, 1984.

21. Porter RW, Park W: Unilateral spondylolysis, *J Bone Joint Surg* 64B:344, 1982.

22. Roca J et al: Direct repair of spondylolysis, *Clin Orthop Rehabil Res J* 246:88, Sept 1989.

23. Roche MB, Rowe GG: The incidence of separate neural arch and coincident bone variations, *J Bone Joint Surg* 34A:491, 1952.

24. Sherman FC, Wilkinson RH, Hall JE: Reactive sclerosis of a pedicle and spondylolysis in the lumbar spine, *J Bone Joint Surg* 59A:49, 1977.

25. Stewart TD: The age incidence of neural-arch defects in Alaskan natives, considered from the standpoint of etiology, *J Bone Joint Surg* 35A:937, 1953.

26. Weatherley CR, Mehdian H, Vanden Berghe L: Low back pain with fracture of the pedicle and contralateral spondylolysis, *J Bone Joint Surg* 73B:990, 1991.

◆

Chapter Thirty-Nine

Basketball

Harry N. Herkowitz
Benjamin J. Paolucci
Michael A. Abdenour

Because it requires running, jumping, twisting, and direct contact between individual players, playing basketball places considerable stress on the spinal column. These maneuvers affect the thoracic and lumbar spine more often than the cervical region. Injuries to the cervical area occur more often from impact injuries (e.g., the player falling to the floor). Unlike the paralysis-producing injuries that occur from cervical spine trauma in football players, the vast majority of cervical injuries in basketball players are soft tissue trauma.

The challenge to the clinician is not only to relieve the pain, but also to enable the player to return to the sport, with its competitive demands. Most back injuries are usually self-limited and minor, and lead to minimal alteration in function and activity. However, the basketball player with a more severe back problem or recurrent disorder will require a thorough evaluation and may require the assistance of additional health care personnel for treatment and rehabilitation.

For the weekend athlete, the usual causes of injury are (1) lack of conditioning, followed by an intense, competitive "pick-up game," or (2) a predisposing spinal abnormality, such as a degenerative lumbar disc or spondylolisthesis.

In organized competition, conditioning tends to be less of a factor as the athlete progresses from the high school to the professional level. However, although these athletes tend to be aerobically conditioned, back strengthening is often ignored. Thus injuries to the spine are usually soft tissue strains or sprains rather than disc abnormalities.

College and professional basketball is a physically demanding game played by large athletes. Although basketball is traditionally thought of as a noncontact sport, in reality considerable contact occurs, especially under the basket (Fig. 39-1). Often the players are airborne with their spines rotated and/or extended, which places considerable stress on the back (Fig. 39-2). In this compromised position players may also encounter direct blows to the back or neck region (Fig. 39-3).

The presence of spinal canal stenosis increases the likelihood of spinal injury (Fig. 39-4). Although stenosis does occur in the cervical region, the thoracic and lumbar regions accept the brunt of trauma to the spinal column. Most often the presentation appears to be that

of a strain or sprain. Occasionally a protruded or herniated disc occurs in an already-narrowed stenotic spinal canal (Fig. 39-5). Therefore, with a lack of reserve space within the spinal canal, minor degrees of protrusion may cause radicular symptoms and signs. Spinal stenosis appears to occur more frequently in the taller athletes than in the general population.

During the initial evaluation a complete history should be taken and a physical examination performed. The clinician must be aware of any underlying conditions that may contribute to the player's complaints. Depending on the history and physical findings, additional diagnostic studies may be indicated at that time. These may include radiographic examination, laboratory studies, bone scanning, computed tomography (CT), magnetic resonance imaging (MRI), myelography, and electromyography.

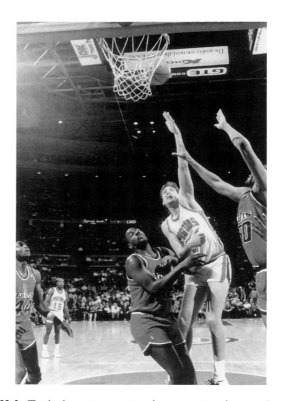

Fig. 39-1. Typical contact among players attempting to rebound under the basket. (Courtesy Einstein Photo.)

STRAINS AND SPRAINS

The most common spinal injuries in basketball players are soft tissue trauma to the lumbar, thoracic, and cervical regions. The ligament and joint capsules are vulnerable to injury in these areas, as are the musculotendinous units. The spectrum of injury in the musculotendinous units ranges from stretching to a partial tear, with complete rupture being rare. These injuries usually result from mechanical overloading aided by severe external forces, including hyperextension, hyperflexion with rotation, and ipsilateral side bending.

When only muscle tissue has been injured, the time-related response to soft tissue damage is usually characteristic. Generally, there is local pain and tenderness with localized inhibition of voluntary muscle contraction. Severe injuries may appear quite benign initially, with limitation of spine motion reaching a maximum only after several hours of swelling. Sometimes these athletes do not notice discomfort until the

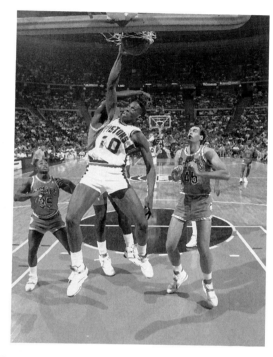

Fig. 39-2. Considerable stress is placed on the lumbar spine as the player hyperextends following a "dunk." (Courtesy Einstein Photo.)

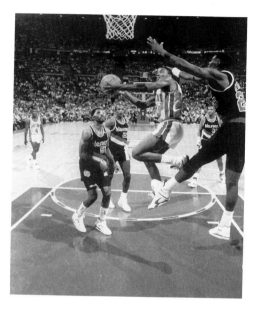

Fig. 39-3. As the player becomes airborne for the lay-up, he is susceptible to contact from the opposing team, risking injury to the spine. (Courtesy Einstein Photo.)

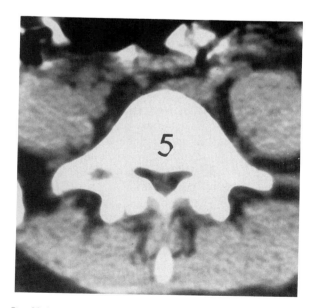

Fig. 39-4. Trefoil canal with severe spinal stenosis at L5.

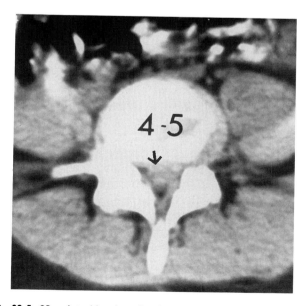

Fig. 39-5. Herniated lumbar disc *(arrow)* within a stenotic spinal canal at L4-5.

morning after the injury. The swelling of the soft tissues, pain level, and degree of limitation of motion at 24 to 72 hours indicate the degree of soft tissue damage. Negative x-ray findings in the absence of neurologic deficits and radicular symptoms, along with a pain-free range of motion, allow one to reasonably predict a swift return to competition.

Initial treatment consists of rest, immobilization, and cryotherapy within the first 48 hours, antiinflammatory agents, ultrasound, and massage. Physical therapy may begin when tolerated because muscle flexibility is necessary before the player can return to competition. Returning to competition too early will usually result in recurrent injury. The mechanism of injury must be remembered, and stretching the back should be approached carefully during the acute injury phase. The athlete's general condition and training program should also be addressed, with alterations made during the healing phase. Stationary cycling and stair climber–type exercising to maintain cardiovascular and muscle tone are important at that time. Dynamic back strengthening, which should be started once the acute injury is healed, is helpful in preventing repeat injury.

Chronic sprains and strains present a different picture. The concern that some other condition may be causing the athlete's complaints must be considered. The importance of repeated, careful physical examinations cannot be overlooked. Imaging studies, such as CT scanning and MRI, may be required to aid in the diagnosis.

FRACTURES

Spinal fractures in basketball players are usually lumbar in origin and are nondisplaced, occurring at the transverse or spinous processes. Rarely, compression fractures of the vertebra body occur. Plain radiographs are usually sufficient to make the diagnosis. A bone scan may be helpful in suspected pars interarticularis fractures or vertebral end-plate fractures. The treatment is symptomatic, with athletic inactivity necessary until healing is complete. Aerobic conditioning activity is started as soon as the pain becomes tolerable.

SPONDYLOGENIC BACK PAIN

Spondylogenic back pain is usually associated with hyperlordotic posturing of the lumbar spine, tight hip flexors, and tight hamstrings. Abdominal strengthening, lumbodorsal and hamstring stretching, and antilordotic posturing of the lumbar spine are usually the only treatment required. High-grade spondylolisthesis is generally not seen at the professional level of competition.

DISCOGENIC BACK PAIN

The presentation of discogenic back pain is quite variable in basketball players. Back pain may be the predominant component, but more frequently, evidence of

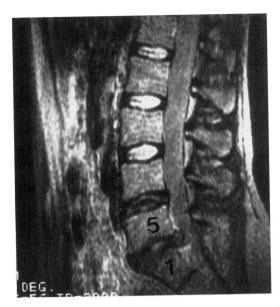

Fig. 39-6. Sagittal MRI scan demonstrating a herniated disc at L5-S1.

nerve root irritation is present. A positive straight leg raising test, loss of reflexes, or frank muscle weakness may not be present initially. Limitations of forward flexion or backward extension usually occur. MRI is recommended when a disc herniation is suspected (Fig. 39-6).

Treatment is primarily conservative. Over 50% of basketball players with discogenic low back pain are able to return to full sports activity without significant pain after nonoperative therapy. However, if the athlete is unable to resume preinjury activity after a reasonable course of nonoperative treatment, surgical alternatives can be considered.

OTHER CAUSES OF BACK PAIN

As indicated earlier, other causes of back pain may need to be considered, including tumor, blood dyscrasias, metabolic disorders, or inflammatory arthritides. In this age group, benign spinal tumors such as eosinophilic granuloma or osteoid osteoma should be considered (Fig. 39-7), as well as more serious systemic illnesses, such as lymphoma or leukemia, which may also present with back pain as the initial complaint. The inflammatory syndromes include rheumatoid arthritis, ankylosing spondylitis, ankylosing spondylitis associated with inflammatory bowel disease, and Reiter's syndrome. Although these causes of back pain are rare, they should be considered in the differential diagnosis.

Athletes with some of these causes of back pain may be allowed to participate when the underlying condition is well controlled and when it is shown that the condition will not impair the athlete in the future if he or she is allowed to continue to play.

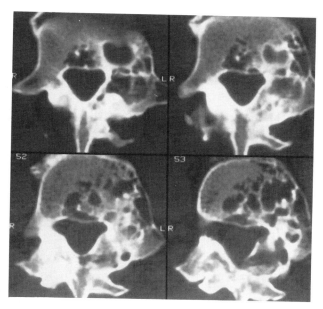

Fig. 39-7. CT scan of a 27-year-old college athlete with progressive low back pain. Confirmation of an osteoblastoma of L3 was made at surgery.

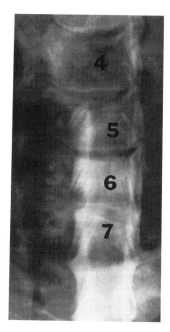

Fig. 39-8. AP myelogram of a 32-year-old male weight lifter demonstrating an extradural defect due to a herniated disc at C6-7 on the right.

OPERATIVE TREATMENT

The overwhelming majority of players respond to nonoperative intervention. When these measures fail, surgery may be contemplated. The indications for surgery in this select population group are the same as those in the nonathlete population (i.e., a clinical picture consistent with the imaging studies without a satisfactory response to nonoperative treatment). For the vast majority of patients, the decision to undergo surgery is an elective one. The only indication for aggressive surgical intervention is a progressive neurologic deficit.

The incidence of cervical spine disc herniations or spondylotic spurs causing significant radiculopathy are much less frequent in basketball players than in football players (Fig. 39-8). For those players who have persistent radicular pain with or without deficit, the study of choice is MRI. Surgical intervention may be undertaken if the MRI scan confirms an extrinsic lesion (e.g., a herniated disc). In the case of a unilateral single-level disc herniation, the surgical procedures that can be considered are a posterior foraminotomy or an anterior discectomy with fusion (Fig. 39-9). The question as to which procedure would ensure that the athlete may return to the court "as good as new" is not answerable with scientific data. Both procedures provide significant relief of radicular pain. However, a study comparing anterior fusion with posterior foraminotomy for cervical soft disc herniation demonstrated better long-term results with anterior fusion.[3]

Our preference is an anterior discectomy with iliac autogenous horseshoe graft fusion (Smith-Robinson

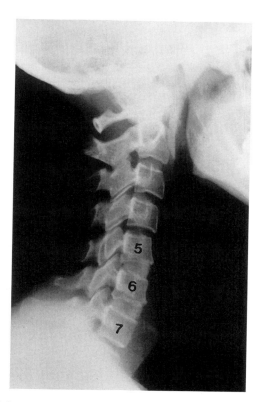

Fig. 39-9. Postoperative radiograph of a two-level anterior discectomy and fusion (Smith-Robinson) at C5-6 and C6-7.

type). This procedure provides relief of symptoms along with long-term stability. The player is allowed to return to competition when (1) solid fusion is present, (2) there is painless range of motion, (3) a neck–strengthening and conditioning program has been completed (in 6 weeks to 3 months), and (4) there is radiographic proof of a solid arthrodesis.

Lumbar Spine Surgery

Radiographic confirmation of a surgical lesion in the lumbar spine requires an MRI scan or myelogram with or without a CT scan (Fig. 39-10). A CT scan is also indicated for cases in which spinal stenosis is suspected in order to directly visualize the lateral recesses. In cases of developmental spinal stenosis, the CT scan provides a more accurate view of the canal dimensions than the MRI scan.

The principles of surgical intervention are to deal with the pathologic condition and at the same time cause the least amount of trauma to the normal, surrounding areas. In addition, surgery should be confined to the specific cause of the player's pain, even though a more global problem may exist. An example of this is seen in the 31-year-old professional basketball player with intractable low back and right leg pain shown in Fig. 39-5. This player's myelogram and CT scan demonstrated developmental spinal stenosis of the entire lumbar spine. However, the clinical findings pointed to the herniated disc present between the fourth and fifth lumbar vertebrae. Therefore surgery was performed *only* at the L4-5 level to remove the herniated disc.

The procedure for a herniated lumbar disc is as follows:

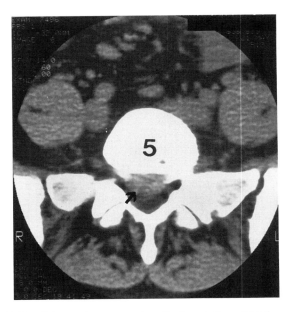

Fig. 39-10. CT scan demonstrating disc herniation at L5 *(arrow)*.

1. The skin incision is 1 to $1\frac{1}{2}$ inches in length.
2. A laminotomy is performed to the level of the window of yellow ligament.
3. The lateral one third of the ligament is removed, leaving the majority of the ligament intact and covering the dural sac.
4. The nerve root is identified, along with its lateral border.
5. The compressive problem (e.g., a herniated disc) is removed while the remaining "normal" portion of the disc is left alone.

The postoperative management following hospital discharge in 2 to 3 days is as follows:

First 2 weeks—Walk for exercise 30 minutes twice a day.

Third week—Add stationary cycling and/or swimming.

Fourth week—May begin weight exercise for upper and lower extremities.

Fifth week—Begin back flexibility and abdominal strengthening.

Sixth to eighth week—Begin dynamic back and abdominal strengthening using weight resistance training machines.

Second to third month—Begin running and basketball conditioning drills.

Is there a role for chemonucleolysis or percutaneous discectomy in the management of lumbar disc herniations? Following a renewed interest in chemonucleolysis in the early 1980s, this procedure has waned in popularity because of its unpredictable clinical results and the occurrence (although infrequent) of severe neurologic injury.

Percutaneous discectomy may be considered when a disc protrusion is superimposed on a patient with concomitant spinal stenosis at that level by reducing the pressure produced by the disc on the narrow canal. Percutaneous discectomy may also be considered when a significant central disc protrusion is causing back and sciatic pain.

In both situations MRI and/or myelography and/or CT may be used to differentiate a protrusion from an extruded or sequestered disc herniation. A protrusion is usually present if (1) disc herniation is confined to the level of the disc space and (2) a CT scan demonstrates the abnormality on fewer than three consecutive CT scan cuts.

FACTORS SPECIFIC TO THE ATHLETE

The treatment rendered athletes for injuries to the neck and back must follow the principles and practices used for all persons with similar problems. However, there are differences between the athlete and the general population that may influence treatment outcome and prognosis:

Physical fitness—Athletes work out regularly in aerobic and weight-training exercise. This places their bodies at peak physical fitness and shortens healing time in many cases.

Mental attitude — Physical fitness leads to a mental toughness and puts the athlete in the "right frame of mind" to recover from injuries quickly.

Motivation — The livelihood of the professional athlete (in this case basketball player) depends on the ability to play the sport, which is motivation in itself to return to the court whenever it is medically safe.

Pressures may exist for the player, trainer, and physicians to get a basketball player back on the court as quickly as possible by taking treatment shortcuts or allowing unproven therapeutic modalities in the hope that the player will improve faster. In the treatment of injuries to the spine, there are no "quick fixes." Most injuries heal within a short time period, however, allowing the player to return to competition quickly. It is the responsibility of the medical team to provide the appropriate treatment and to advise the player as to when it is safe to return to competition so that persistent or further injury is prevented.

It is encouraging to note that the vast majority of injuries to the neck and back can be treated expediently so that the athlete can return to competition. In most cases of surgical intervention, return to the prior level of competition is a reasonable expectation.

SUGGESTED READINGS

Herkowitz HN: Current status of percutaneous discectomy and chemonucleolysis, *Orthop Clin North Am* 22:327, 1991.

Herkowitz HN, Kurz LT, Overholt DP: Surgical management of cervical soft disc herniation, *Spine* 15:1026, 1990.

MacNab I, McCulloch J: *Backache,* ed 2, Baltimore, 1990, Williams & Wilkins.

Wroble RR, Albright JP: Neck and low back injuries in wrestling, *Clin Sports Med* 5:295, 1986.

Chapter Forty

◆

Baseball

Robert G. Watkins

CATCHING AND INFIELDING

At the Kerlan-Jobe Orthopaedic Clinic the initial thrust of our evaluation of spinal problems in baseball players in 1984 involved examining and interviewing every catcher in the National League (Fig. 40-1), none of whom reported having low back pain. Findings on physical examinations and histories were normal, and the complete lack of symptoms was unexpected in baseball players or even in the general population. We could only conclude either that catchers were screened closely early in their career to eliminate those with back problems or that squatting is a good position for backs. Certainly, the low incidence of lumbosacral pain and degenerative disease and the population groups for whom squatting is a common practice would lead one to believe that the squatting position puts no undue stress on the lumbar spine.

Infielders (Fig. 40-2) are the players who most commonly seek help for back pain, which is not unexpected because of the bending involved in this position. As in any activity that requires bending, participants with proper bending techniques usually have fewer problems than those whose technique is faulty. In a rigorous practice day, infielders often have to take 100 ground balls, which requires repeated bending. Under game conditions, infielders stand, bend over in ready position, and are relatively inactive for periods of time. Then they are suddenly forced to perform extreme torsion and twisting motions of the lumbar spine, as well as unusual off-balance bending, lifting, and torso-twisting maneuvers. Luckily, proper fielding mechanics are protective of the low back. Although good coaching and good technique reduce the risk of low back spasm, it is often unavoidable. A number of infielders in major league baseball have dealt with lumbar spine problems over an entire career.

HITTING

Hitters, who make up another interesting group of players, include any player who has to swing a bat (Fig. 40-3). Hitters who take a lot of batting practice, swing with great velocity, and swing with a heavy bat are subject to lumbar spine injury. However, an infrequent hitter,

such as a pitcher, who does not have good hitting mechanics is also vulnerable to injury. Lumbar spine problems in hitters begin with their eyes; that is, the ability to see the ball is a critical factor in swing mechanics. Abnormal swing mechanics involve a loss of control between the hips and shoulders, essentially a loss of body synchrony. Irregular and uncoordinated motion of the upper extremity and upper torso puts undue rotational strain on the lumbar spine. Injury of the lumbar spine in someone required to engage in this type of torsional activity further compounds the problem by producing stiffness, weakness, and asymmetry that add to the pain and prevent satisfactory healing. The biomechanics of hitting can be considered an ocular-muscular reflex, a reference to the fact that the triggering of the bat mechanics (the triggering of the muscles) is a split-second response to what the hitter is able to see. A hitter who is not picking up the ball well tends to open the hips too early. With the bat and upper torso lagging behind, there is a sudden torsional stress to catch the shoulders and the bat up with the rest of the body. Poor visualization of the ball produces delays in hand and arm responses.

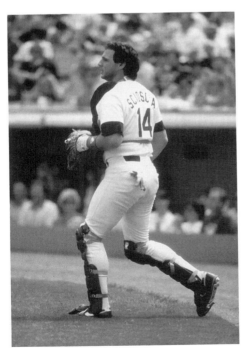

Fig. 40-1. National League catcher in action.

Portions of this chapter are modified from Watkins RG: Baseball. In White AH, Schofferman JA editors: *Spine care,* vol 1, *Diagnosis and conservative treatment,* St Louis, 1995, Mosby; and Watkins RG et al: Dynamic EMG analysis of torque transfer in professional baseball pitchers, *Spine* 14:404, 1989.

Hitting Mechanics

To diagnose and treat lumbar spine problems in hitters, the physician should understand hitting mechanics. Proper swing mechanics require power in the legs and trunk, a rigid, solid cylinder of torque transfer, and fine muscle control of the arms and wrists.

Test design. For a scientific look at hitting mechanics, electromyographic (EMG) studies of trunk musculature in hitters were done in our laboratory and included 18 professional baseball players at the Los Angeles Dodgers' instructional training camp in Phoenix, Arizona. Among the batters 13 were right-hand dominant and 5 were left-hand dominant. Ages ranged from 19 to 44, averaging 22 years.

The Basmajian technique[4] was employed to insert fine-wire electrodes into the muscles of the supraspinatus, triceps (lateral head), posterior deltoid, and middle serratus anterior (sixth rib) of each subject's lead (forward) arm, as well as the lower gluteus maximus of his trail (back) leg. Surface electrodes monitored muscles of the right and left erector spinae, abdominal obliques, vastus medialis obliques (VMO), semimembranosus, and biceps femoris (long head) of the trail leg. A lightweight belt pack allowed transmission of the EMG signals via frequency modulation (FM) telemetry to a recording console. Resting and maximum manual muscle test (MMT) recordings were made for each muscle.

Each subject was allowed to warm up until comfortable and then hit six pitched fast balls (approximately 75 miles per hour). Simultaneous high-speed motion picture photography using 16-mm film at 400 frames per second captured each swing. An electronic pulse marked the film and EMG record, which facilitated film synchronization with the recorded EMG data.

The film was examined and divided into four discrete phases (Fig. 40-4), as follows:

Phase I—The windup began as the lead heel left the ground and ended as the lead toe reestablished ground contact.

Phase II—The preswing began as the lead forefoot struck the ground and ended as the swing began.

Phase III—The swing was subdivided into early, middle, and late, as determined by the bat position.
  A. Early swing began as the bat moved forward until it was perpendicular to the ground.
  B. Middle swing continued until the bat was parallel with the ground.
  C. Late swing continued until ball contact.

Phase IV—The follow-through began with ball contact and ended as the lead shoulder reached maximum abduction and external rotation.

The EMG data were then converted from analog to digital data by sampling 2500 times per second and were integrated by averaging groups of 200 samples per second. By means of a resting signal as baseline and a peak 1-second MMT as the 100% level, these records were then processed by computer to yield a relative activation figure. Activity patterns were assessed every 5 msec and expressed as a percentage of the activity recorded during the MMT. The mean percentage of MMT and standard deviations were obtained for each muscle throughout the swing. An analysis of variance

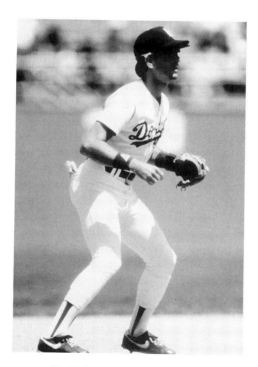

Fig. 40-2. Infielder in position.

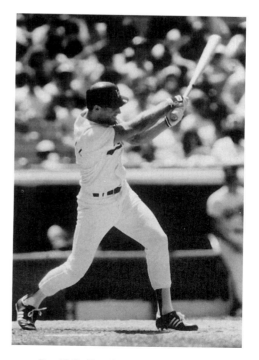

Fig. 40-3. Baseball hitter in action.

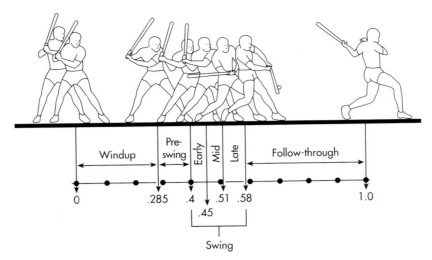

Fig. 40-4. Four discrete phases of the baseball swing: windup, preswing, swing, and follow-through (see text).

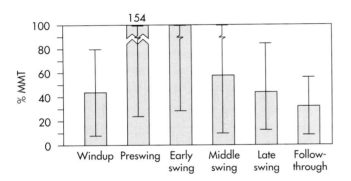

Fig. 40-5. Biceps femoris activity (trail leg).

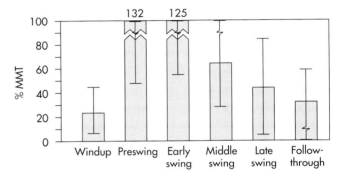

Fig. 40-6. Lower gluteus maximus activity (trail leg).

(ANOVA) (p < 0.5) was performed to determine statistically significant differences between phases for each muscle and between specific muscle groups. When the ANOVA revealed such differences, a posthoc sequential Tukey multiple comparison test was completed.

Test results

Lower extremities. Hamstring activity (biceps femoris and semimembranosus muscles) was below 50% MMT in the windup (Fig. 40-5). During the preswing, however, activity increased significantly to 154% and 157% MMT, respectively. Activity decreased significantly in the early swing to 100% and 90% MMT, respectively, and continued declining throughout the remainder of the swing to its lowest level (<4% MMT) in the follow-through.

Lower gluteus maximus activity was lowest during the windup (25% MMT) and increased significantly during the preswing to 132% MMT. Activity remained high in the early swing (125% MMT), decreased thereafter in the middle swing (65% MMT), and decreased again in the late swing (45% MMT). Activity decreased in the follow-through to a low of 26% MMT (Fig. 40-6).

VMO activity increased significantly from the windup (26% MMT) to the preswing (63% MMT) and again from the preswing to the middle swing, during which it peaked at 107% MMT. It diminished thereafter through the late swing (97% MMT) and follow-through (78% MMT).

Trunk. During the windup, activity in both erector spinae was low (24% MMT) but increased significantly to more than 90% MMT throughout the preswing, early swing, and middle swing. Activity then decreased in the late swing (98% MMT lead, 85% MMT trail) to significantly lower levels during the follow-through (58% MMT, 68% MMT). There was no significant difference in activity between the lead and trail erector spinae during any phase.

As in the erector spinae, both abdominal oblique muscles demonstrated relatively low levels of activity during the windup (<30% MMT). Activity jumped significantly to greater than 100% MMT in the preswing and remained elevated throughout the remainder of the phase (Fig. 40-7). No significant differences in activity were found between lead and trail oblique muscles.

Comparison of the abdominal oblique and erector

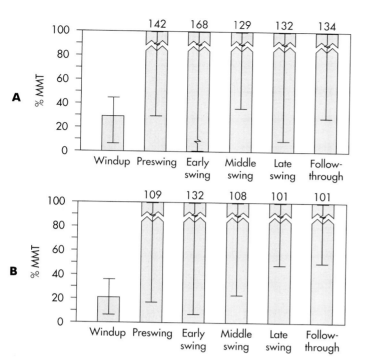

Fig. 40-7. **A,** Right abdominal oblique muscle activity (trailing side). **B,** Left abdominal oblique muscle activity (lead side).

spinae muscles revealed a statistically significant difference in activity level only during the follow-through phase, during which the abdominal oblique activity remained high (101% MMT, 134% MMT) relative to the decreasing erector spinae level (58% MMT, 68% MMT).

Upper extremities. Posterior deltoid activity increased significantly from a low in the windup phase (17% MMT) to a high in the preswing (101% MMT). Signal intensity subsequently decreased throughout the remainder of the swing, and this decrease was significant between the late swing (76% MMT) and follow-through (25% MMT).

The triceps demonstrated low activity in the windup (25% MMT), which increased significantly in the early (92% MMT) and middle swing (73% MMT). Activity then declined significantly between the middle swing and follow-through (23% MMT).

Supraspinatus muscle activity remained relatively low (<32% MMT) throughout the swing. The lowest activity occurred during the windup (13% MMT), which revealed significantly less activity than during the preswing, midswing, or late swing (32% MMT each).

Middle serratus muscle activity remained low throughout the swing (<40% MMT), particularly during the windup (18% MMT), which showed significantly less activity than either the middle or late swing (39% MMT each).

Test evaluation

Windup. Activity levels during the windup were relatively low except in the trail leg hamstrings. During this period of single-leg stance, hamstring activity maintained hip extension as weight shifted to the trail leg in preparation for the swing.

Preswing. The high level of activity in the hamstrings and lower gluteus maximus muscles during the preswing indicated their role in hip stabilization and initiation of power. Both lead and trail erector spinae and abdominal oblique muscles were also quite active at this time for trunk stabilization and power transmission. As the body was lowered during the preswing and early swing, posterior deltoid and triceps activity increased markedly to maintain lead shoulder elevation.

Swing. During the preswing and early swing, there was increased activity in the VMO, which prevented collapse of the increasingly flexed trail leg and promoted push-off to facilitate force transfer. When weight was transferred to the lead leg, hamstring and gluteus maximus activity in the trail leg declined. Trunk activity in both erector spinae and oblique muscles remained high throughout the swing, with erector spinae activity declining just before ball contact. This demonstrated the importance of the trunk in power transmission as the body uncoils.

Swing progression yielded decreasing, albeit relatively high, activity in the posterior deltoid and tricep muscles, suggesting their likely positional role. Although they may contribute to power generation, their consistently decreasing levels throughout the swing suggest they are not the main "drivers." The trunk muscles (erector spinae and obliques) play an important role not just in power transmission but also in coordinating upper to lower extremity muscle function.

Follow-through. Activity levels in the lower and upper extremities were low during follow-through except for the VMO, which maintained an extension force on the flexed trail knee. Back and abdominal oblique muscle activity levels remained high, maintaining trunk rotation and stabilization.

Overall assessment. In summary, a distinct pattern of muscle activity was observed during the batting swing. Lower extremity groups appear important in early pelvic stabilization and power generation. The hamstrings maintain hip stabilization in addition to contributing to the "thrust" provided to initiate rotation (uncoiling mechanism). VMO activity increased throughout swing as the lower extremity pushed against the ground and through the bent knee to contribute the forward thrust of the pelvis and trunk.

The erector spinae and abdominal oblique muscles were extremely active in trunk stabilization and rotation for smooth power transfer. The lack of discernible activity differences between lead and trail spinae or oblique muscle muscles suggest their premier importance in torso stabilization and rotation, rather than power generation per se. However, it is also possible that our use of surface electrodes for the oblique muscles recorded information from both the internal and external oblique muscles inasmuch as these are relatively thin adjacent muscles. This may preclude the ability to discern a "coupling force" between the internal and external fibers and thus the lead and trail sides as well. Differences between the lead and trail erector spinae muscles may have been similarly masked because of their close proximity.

The posterior deltoid and tricep muscles appeared to be more important in positioning than in power generation. The middle serratus anterior and supraspinatus muscles did not significantly contribute to the swing.

The uncoiling of the wound-up pelvis, trunk, and upper extremities on a stable base provides the power of the baseball batting swing. Of the muscles tested, there appears to be a sequence of activity, from the lower extremities (most active group in preswing) through the trunk (highest in early swing) to the upper extremity muscle groups. This sequence appears nearly identical to that observed in the golf swing, in which initiation of the swing begins in the hip.[10] As in batting analysis, EMG studies of the golf swing show the importance of the trunk in stabilization and power transfer.[15] In the golf swing, the serratus anterior and supraspinatus muscles were more active than during the batting swing, and the posterior deltoid was less active.[9,16] This is most likely due to the higher position of the golf club, which requires scapular protraction and humeral abduction. The baseball bat is held in a position of more horizontal abduction and thus initiates relatively more activity in the posterior deltoid. The pectoralis major and latissimus dorsi muscles in the golf swing may contribute to the power by internally rotating and abducting the humerus. This position places the arm in a stable position to transmit the power to the ball. However, this study did not monitor activity in these muscles. Future studies of additional upper extremity muscle groups will be of great interest in furthering our present understanding.

The following conclusions were drawn:

1. Hamstring and lower gluteus maximus activity contributes significantly to the stable base and the "power-of-the-thrust" form that the torso "uncoils" during the swing.
2. Skilled baseball batting relies on a coordinated transfer of muscle activity from the lower extremities to the trunk and finally to the upper extremity.
3. The high level of activity in the erector spinae and abdominal oblique muscles throughout the swing suggests the importance of emphasizing abdominal and back exercises in a comprehensive exercise and conditioning program for baseball batters.
4. Unlike previous study conclusions, the triceps and other muscles of the upper extremity studies appear most important in positioning the swing. Contribution of other upper extremity muscles to power generation remains an area for future study.
5. This study provides a baseline on which further

investigation of the baseball batting swing can be performed. Prevention and rehabilitation of batting injuries can be more specifically focused, given an understanding of the biomechanics of the batting swing.

Evaluation from the athlete's perspective. For a more practical understanding of hitting, we turned to a hitting coach and a skilled batter.[8,17]

The swing starts with the stance, which relies on balance. Every player will be a little different: open or closed, feet further apart, feet closer together. The ideal is probably placement of the feet at shoulder width, but the key is balance. The batter can fashion a hole for the back foot to use in pushing off, changing the stance slightly from closed to opposite-field open for an inside pitch. No matter where the player is and what he is doing before initiating the hitting motion, control is based on balance in the stance and proceeds to the forward stride. As a pitcher begins the windup and approach to the plate, the hitter coils up. This coiling maneuver brings the bat to the position necessary to initiate the swing. Again, regardless of the amount of motion activity, most bats come to a relatively standard position in relation to the strike zone just before the forward stride is initiated.

The hitter assumes the correct body position: the coiled hips and head are approximately parallel to the ground, and the knees are slightly bent. There is some flexion of the lumbar spine, the shoulders are level, and the head is turned as the hitter looks directly at the pitch, chin against shoulder. Hand position varies slightly according to each player. A reasonable amount is 4 to 8 inches from the body, letters high to shoulder high. In the coiled position the hitter holds the bat at approximately 45 degrees, with the elbow parallel to the ground and out from the body. Hands held too far from the body may reduce power, whereas if they are too close to the body or too low, the bat speed will be reduced. In most missed pitches, especially the fast ball, the hitter swings below the ball. Holding the hands too low not only reduces the bat speed but, except in exceptional cases, may reduce the contact zone. In this coiled position, the hitter begins moving with the forward arm motion of the pitcher, picking up the ball from the pitcher's hand and beginning to time his stride forward and swing.

The number one key to hitting, obviously, is vision. The hitter who does not see the ball can only guess and will not be able to make contact. Not only is visual acuity a critical factor, but eye control and eye function are of equal importance. The hitter must have clear binocular focus to be able to visualize the ball and to predict its location. The speed of the ball makes it virtually impossible to completely follow the ball to the bat. The ideal is to follow the ball as far as possible and then make a prediction as to its line of projection. Without visualization, concentration, and focus, the hitter will fail to project the arrival point of the ball, and inadequate ball contact is the consequence. In addition, balance and control are determined by eye focus, as in any coordinated muscle activity. If the eyes and head are locked and focused on a point, the body has a much greater chance of reproducing a coordinated, balanced motion than if the eyes are closed or poorly focused.

Thus the key in the stance and coil position is balance, eye focus, and body readiness to start the stride. What happens before this coiling mechanism is not of great importance, but body and head position in the coiled portion of the swing should at least place the bat in a position that will facilitate the stride.

Ben Hines,[8] the Dodgers' batting coach, indicates that there are five basic aspects of the swing starting with the stride, as follows:

1. Back foot rotation, in which the heel is rotated out and the body pivots on the ball of the back foot
2. Forward stride with the left foot
3. Rapid hip and trunk rotation that takes the navel from a position parallel with the pitch to being perpendicular to the pitch
4. Triangulation of the arms and extension of the arms
5. Lateral flexion of the wrist

Stride. Efficiency of motion is essential to the hitter.[17] The hitter must avoid needless motion. Motion must be balanced and coordinated in the forward stride. The backward motion in the coiling position precedes the forward motion. The front leg internally rotates, and the coil position will externally rotate in the stride. The stride should be directly toward the pitcher. The weight shift in a hitter is very important. With the forward stride the weight stays back on the back foot as the forward foot strides forward lightly on the ball of the foot. The front leg now rotates externally, and the knee goes into extension. The ability to lock the knee of the front leg, providing firm rigid resistance to body motion, is important in keeping the axis of rotation of the body centered. If the knee flexes, the body weight shifts forward, and the proper axis of rotation is lost. As the foot lands evenly, it may be slightly open. The knee, of course, is initially slightly flexed as the foot lands and then locks in extension as the hips come through. This rotation around a center axis is important.

The midsection is the core of the swing action from which the hitter generates power.[17] Maintaining a center axis of motion and balance plays a critical role in maintaining head position. Too much head motion equals loss of both coordination and visualization of the ball. Locking the head to the center of axis of rotation is a key to the stride and swing positions. The bat in the coiled position is approximately at a 45-degree angle. As it comes through, there is a relative leveling of the bat, usually with less than 10 degrees of angulation. The pitch starts high because the pitcher

is on the mound and throwing downward, whereas the bat comes through level. There will be a difference of a certain number of degrees of angulation between the ball and the bat. The bat comes down as the ball comes down.

Rotation. The forward stride of the legs and the rotation of the hips are reasonably standard in speed and approach. Large muscles of this type cannot be controlled quickly enough to allow the hitter to adjust to the speed at which a pitch is thrown. Therefore the stride, at a fairly standard distance, with standard open or closed length, allows compensation. One of the important parts of batting-training technique is a rapid, sudden hip twist in which the navel goes from 90 degrees to the pitch to directly parallel to the pitch. A rapid, swift twist of the hips is what, in many ways, determines the bat speed and allows the hitter to be in a prime position to adjust to the speed and type of pitch. Therefore stride length and hip rotation, with the navel toward the pitcher, are the same in virtually every pitch and must be a standardized, balanced, well-coordinated motion.

After this sudden hip rotation occurs, adjustments to various speed pitches and pitch locations become crucial. As in golf (see Chapter 47), there is a ratio of derotation of the body as it leaves the coil position to the point of contact. In hitting there is an adjustable ratio of derotation. With the power generated through hip and belly rotation, the fine control comes with the speed of (1) the upper body uncoiling, (2) elbow extension, and (3) wrist lateral flexion. Location of the pitch, of course, will vary tremendously, and the fine adjustment takes place in these latter three aspects. Therefore the upper body trails behind the derotation of the hips. Trailing behind does not imply a helter-skelter, uncoordinated motion. Because the ratio of derotation of upper body to lower body must vary with the pitch, it requires even more muscular trunk control to allow the proper rotation to take place, depending on the pitch. Therefore the hitter must visualize the ball and, in less than a second, determine the ratio of derotation of the upper body, as well as the position of the head, elbows, and hands for the point of contact with the ball. This requires excellent muscle control, balance, and coordination. Proper hitting depends on retraining muscles to fire and respond to changes in balance and coordination and retraining trunk muscles to maintain a tight, rigid, but mobile control between the upper and lower body. Lumbar pain that prevents proper rotation or that causes muscles to stop, to work improperly, or to work in an uncoordinated fashion can have a devastating effect on the player's ability to deliver the bat to the ball.

After hip rotation, with the upper body trailing behind slightly under maximum muscle control at a specific ratio of derotation determined by the pitch, the upper body rotates through to the point of ball contact. The head is level, going down with the pitch while the eyes focus on the ball. The chin of the right-handed batter, which is against the left shoulder in the coiling position, will end up against the right shoulder after ball contact. (The opposite, of course, is true for the left-handed hitter.) Again, head motion equals poor efficiency. At this point, with the bat coming through the strike zone, the shift is to the shoulders and upper arms, with triangulation of the arms: the chest as the base and the two arms parallel as they extend out. Locking the lead shoulder is of critical importance. Stabilization of the lead shoulder allows extension of the lead elbow and proper generation of bat speed. The bottom hand pulls and anchors the bat: the top hand pushes and guides the bat. As the arms and elbows extend, the bat is still trailing behind, with the wrists still in the cocked position.

Obviously, proper technique—including the weight shift from the back foot to the forward foot and the position of the elbows, hands, wrists and the bat—allows the hitter to delay the final commitment of bat position as long as possible. It provides longer visualization of the ball and a better prediction of the point of contact—all taking place at the same time the body is generating tremendous torsional force. Therefore the reproducible bat swing must generate the power and force necessary for the swing while delaying final commitment of bat position, allowing the wrists and hands to provide fine bat control and bat position at the point of contact. It is certainly possible to make contact with the ball with neither trunk rotation nor power but without sufficient results on the field. The follow-through after ball contact is not of major consequence. Weight will be shifted to the front foot, and the left knee will be locked. Adequate control of quadriceps function of the front leg is imperative. The arms will be extended; the top hand will

roll over at an appropriate time and should not be rushed too early. Follow-through is a natural part of the swing and not of major consequence.

In summary, stance, balance, control, head in proper position, stride, standardized lower body stride and position, and uncoiling of the upper body require maximum trunk control and balance to produce the correct ratio of derotation that will allow the bat to arrive at the appropriate place. The locked lead shoulder provides a rigid upper arm for proper elbow extension. Tight wrist control is obtained with proper lateral flexion of the wrist. The head rotates from the lead shoulder in the coiled position to the trailing shoulder in the follow-through.

PITCHING

Some of the most difficult cases of lumbar spine problems are seen in baseball pitchers (Fig. 40-8). It is extremely common in spring training to see throwers, especially baseball pitchers, having pain in the opposite-side sacroiliac (SI) joint. This is due to unaccustomed torsional strain, probably in the lower facet joints, after the winter break. There is a high incidence of back stiffness in throwers as they start to regain peak mechanical functioning and begin throwing again. A common occurrence is referred discogenic or facet joint pain in the typical pattern (i.e., through the facet joint, across the posterior superior iliac spine, SI joint, posterior ilium, and into the area of the greater trochanter). A concomitant problem is the development of secondary contractures, weakness, bursitis, tendinitis, and inflammations in the referred pain area. Often a pitcher will have greater trochanteric bursitis or SI joint pain that produces its own secondary effects.

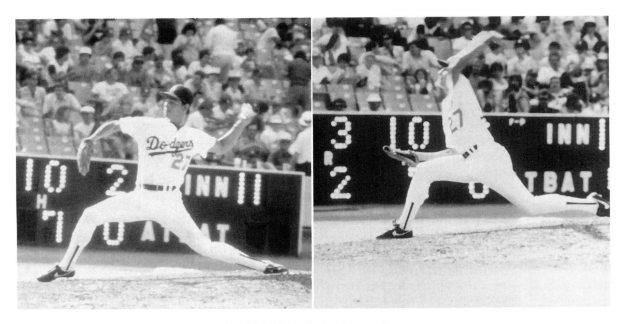

Fig. 40-8. Typical pitching motion.

A key aspect of a pitcher's rehabilitation is not only the resolution of the back problem; the secondary inflammatory effects of referred pain can produce the same biomechanical abnormalities in the pitching motion, thus leading to further injury. Indeed, the pain itself may prevent proper pitching and performance and thus cause additional injury. True sciatica and muscle weakness in a leg result in a critically important dysfunction in a pitcher: severe abnormalities of pitching motion that place the arm, shoulder, and elbow in jeopardy. Sciatica, especially with associated pain of increasing intradiscal and interabdominal pressure, can result in severe dysfunction during the throwing motion. Trunk stability is critical to a pitcher's throw, and any pain that produces weakness and stiffness can lead to a potentially catastrophic injury.

Dynamic EMG Analysis of Torque Transfer

EMG evaluation of trunk muscle activity during participation in sports is a well-recognized technique that provides insight into performance and injury. In an effort to better study the role of trunk musculature and lumbar injury in the professional baseball pitcher—who engages in one of the most demandingly precise high-speed torsional activities in sports—we turned to EMG evaluation of trunk musculature in the Centinela Hospital gait laboratory.

With help from Harry Farfan, M.D., and from professional pitchers, coaches, and trainers, we initially postulated that trunk fatigue produces increased lordosis of the lumbar spine and therefore places the shoulder and arm behind in the throwing motion. This leads to a high release point, and the ball rises in the strike zone and becomes easier to hit. Also, arm strain can result from using the arm muscles to try to catch the arm up to the trunk.

In an attempt to evaluate this phenomenon of the "slow arm" secondary to timing changes, we had to understand the normal patterns. First, 20 nonprofessional athletes underwent EMG analysis of trunk musculature while pitching. This evaluation indicated a basic pattern of firing sequences needed for the pitching motion. The contrasting patterns indicated a sequence necessary for skilled performance. Fifteen professional baseball pitchers from the Dodgers' staff volunteered to be tested. The objective of this study was to document the firing sequence and intensity of contraction of the trunk musculature during the baseball pitch in the professional pitcher. Our goal was to provide a foundation for the analysis of pitching biomechanics, trunk conditioning, and rehabilitation that could be used to improve the efficiency of the athlete and decrease the incidence of injuries.

The 15 volunteers underwent EMG activity amplitude evaluation via surface electrode telemetry of their trunk musculature, including the abdominal obliques, rectus abdominis, lumbar paraspinous, and gluteus maximus bilaterally. These activity levels were collected during the pitching sequences, with the players using proper biomechanics at approximately 60% to 70% of maximum velocity, as measured by radar gun. After an evaluation by a physical therapist, with the aid of computerized telemetry, ensured proper electrode placement, all the players warmed up before the study pitches.

Then each player was asked to do four runs consisting of 40 pitches; adequate telemetry recording of each muscle group was obtained with the use of high-speed film (450 frames per second) and a speed gun. Two separate series of runs were conducted, as delineated by the individual muscle groups tested.

The signals from the leads were transmitted by means of an FM-FM telemetry system capable of transmitting data from four muscles simultaneously. Correct electrode placement was confirmed via MMT specific to the tested muscle, as documented on an oscilloscope. Each subject wore a battery-operated FM transmitter belt pack designed to prevent restriction in bodily movement. Muscle activity patterns were synchronized with high-speed film (450 frames per second) to obtain muscle activity values at each phase of the pitching motion. The film was then synchronized for computer analysis in terms of the following phase of pitching:

1. Trunk movement to hands apart
2. Hands apart to foot touch (leading leg)
3. Foot touch to maximum external rotation (dominant shoulder)
4. Maximum external rotation to ball release
5. Ball release to end of follow-through

Results. The key factor in evaluating even a homogeneous group of subjects is determining the consistency of trends and reproducible changes. Even with exclusively professional pitchers, we found wide variance of delivery styles, physical characteristics, and techniques, which produced a wide range of absolute values but consistent and predictable trends in muscle activity.

The nondominant rectus abdominis, lumbar paraspinous, and abdominal oblique muscles all showed consistent and significant increases in activity over their dominant-side partners at predictable phases. The glutei demonstrated bilateral increases consistent with the phases of pitching.

The nondominant rectus exhibited individual increases into the active phase of fivefold to twentyfold, with sustained increases throughout the active phase as high as tenfold. The mean increase over the active phase through ball release for the nondominant rectus abdominis was 40% higher than that of the dominant side. In the actual cocking phase (foot touch to maximum external rotation), individual activity levels increased from 5 to 100, and from 12 to 114 (2000% and 950% increases, respectively) from the prior phase on the nondominant side. At this same point the dominant side was 35.5 and 11.5 (compared with 100 and 114, respectively).

Four players demonstrated slight dominant-side predominance in cocking, two were reversed or balanced in delivery, and all pitchers were in nondominant-side control at the time of ball release and follow-through (Fig. 40-9).

The nondominant lumbar paraspinous demonstrated individual increases of 100% to 400% during the active phases, with an occasional subject showing dominant-side increases as well. During the maximum cocking phase, through and including ball release, this nondominant muscle demonstrated a mean of 50% increase in activity over the dominant side. The dominant lumbar paraspinous was much more active than the rectus abdominis counterparts at an earlier phase. However, in

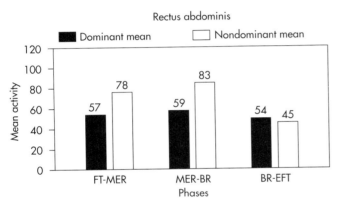

Fig. 40-9. Rectus abdominis activity during pitching phases from foot touch *(FT)* through end of follow-through (EFT). *D,* Dominant side; *ND,* nondominant side; *MER,* maximum extended rotation; *BR,* ball release. (From Watkins R et al: Dynamic EMG analysis of torque transfer in professional baseball pitchers, *Spine* 14:404, 1989.)

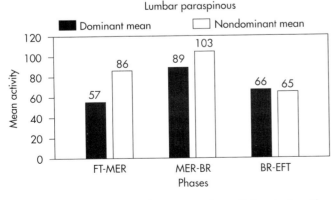

Fig. 40-10. Lumbar paraspinous muscle activity during the pitching phases from foot touch *(FT)* through end of follow-through *(EFT). D,* Dominant side; *ND,* nondominant side. (From Watkins R et al: Dynamic EMG analysis of torque transfer in professional baseball pitchers, *Spine* 14:404, 1989.)

every subject, during each of the active phases through ball release, the nondominant side demonstrated increased activity. In the cocking phase the mean increase was 51%, whereas in the delivery phase the mean was only 16%, with generalized increases overall on both sides and individual increases on the nondominant side from 6% to 250% (Fig. 40-10).

The abdominal oblique muscles demonstrated consistent increases in the nondominant side as opposed to the dominant side during the active phases. Increases of 300% to 500% activity were seen in 9 of 16 pitches in the active phases, with increases in all pitchers on the nondominant side over the dominant side. Mean increases of 85% in the nondominant abdominal oblique muscles of all subjects and all runs occurred in the final three phases, a greater increase than in any other muscle or pair of muscles. A mean increase of 98% in the cocking phase alone is the largest mean increase of any pair of muscles—nondominant versus dominant—in any phase (Fig. 40-11).

The glutei are firing bilaterally in an expected pattern, as seen by stance phases of the pitching motion. The dominant side bears all the weight initially as rotation begins, and as the stride begins during the cocking and acceleration phases, the nondominant side becomes equally active and must balance as the dominant side pushes through hip extension in the "controlled falling" of delivery. The nondominant side remains flexed at the hip, the gluteus stabilizing the pelvis as the trunk derotates, and delivery and ball release follow (Fig. 40-12).

Evaluation. The concept of trunk strengthening and control is not a new one. Over the years, however, most of the data have been collected in regard to the failed back, discogenic disease, and spondylolisthesis[9] as opposed to athletic performance. Most EMG data have focused on posture, loading, and muscle effects on ligamentous and bony structures. Until recently, no reliable, accepted measurement of trunk strength and coordination has been available. We hoped the results of our study would lead to multiple applications. Our first objective was to document the firing sequence and activity levels of the trunk musculature in pitching at the professional level. These baseline data provide trends and patterns that can be used to evaluate faulty biomechanics and thus to develop a successful rehabilitation tool. With continued refinement and growth of the data base, we hope to be able to effectively evaluate prospective athletes and potential professionals.

A phase of coiling or rotational loading immediately before the cocking phase is one of the most important load components in the pitching motion. This phase loads the body so that the arm can both load and release with maximum power and efficiency. During this phase the dominant gluteus maximus muscle is the key factor, first working in neutral and slight extension for balance to allow maximum coiling as a stabilizer of the pelvis and

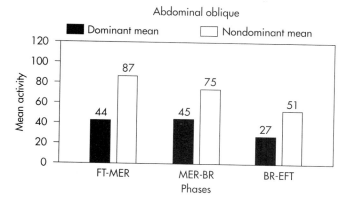

Fig. 40-11. Abdominal oblique muscle activity during pitching phases from foot touch *(FT)* through end of follow-through *(EFT)*. *D*, Dominant side; *ND*, nondominant side. (From Watkins R et al: Dynamic EMG analysis of torque transfer in professional baseball pitchers, *Spine* 14:404, 1989.)

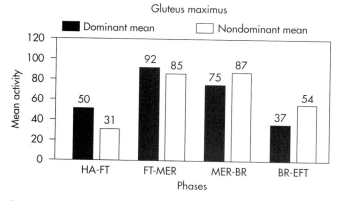

Fig. 40-12. Gluteus maximus activity during pitching phases from foot touch *(FT)* through end of follow-through *(EFT)*. *D*, Dominant side; *ND*, nondominant side; *MER*, maximum extended rotation; *BR*, ball release. (From Watkins R et al: Dynamic EMG analysis of torque transfer in professional baseball pitchers, *Spine* 14:404, 1989.)

trunk and, immediately following, as a powerful extensor to provide maximum power transmitted through the leg. During these cocking and acceleration phases, which take less than 0.3 seconds,[5] the player goes through the phenomenon of "controlled falling."[14] This controlled falling sequence is a combination of deceleration and derotation of the trunk during maximum cocking and subsequent acceleration of the pitching arm to ball release and follow-through. These oppositional forces cause an imbalance and result in the pitcher's "falling" toward the dominant side. This action must be resisted to maintain body position for both power and accuracy and to prevent injury in the trunk and arm.

It is during this transition that the nondominant-side trunk muscles become most important. The predominance of contralateral muscles to control rotation is a

well-documented concept.[1,11] These paraspinal muscles act as stabilizers while the oblique muscles act to initiate further flexion or rotation.[11] In other posture and loading studies of EMG back muscle activity using asymmetric loading on an increased angle at a fixed point, higher activity was found on the contralateral side in the lumbar region.[1]

In this situation of controlled falling, both rotational forces and gravity must be resisted. Asmussen[2] and Asmussen and Klaussen[3] documented the counteraction of gravity to be maintained (primarily by one set of back muscles). The abdominal muscles affect posture only 20% to 25% of the time.[3] Previous data support our findings in applying this concept of trunk support and the rotational component involved. Donisich and Basmajian's work[7] also documented this paradoxic activity of increased lumbar contralateral EMG function in axial rotation. All of the previous work based on a form of external load have been lifting studies, studies of resisted movements, or studies of static postures.[1] To evaluate trunk muscle function during active motion, the subject is measured in various postures and in transition, resisting his own acceleration and deceleration and generating power through the trunk as in lifting. Previous studies have shown that during rotation or transition, the contralateral rotations and trunk stabilizers have been most active.[1-3,7,11]

In analyzing the pitching data, we find the same patterns of muscle activity, and therefore power, that is seen in simple postural loading activities. Thus it should be possible to apply the concept of trunk strengthening to improved function and decreased injury. Chaffin and Moulis[6] proposed that strengthening the deep back muscles relieves pressure on the intervertebral discs and should therefore decrease injury during loading. Parnianpour et al.[13] documented the effect of fatigue on both the motion output and patterns of trunk movements, showing that fatigued muscles are slower and subsequently take longer to respond to change in loads. This demonstrated the phenomenon of compensation by secondary muscle groups causing loading in some injury-prone patients. Nordin et al.[12] have shown that after discectomy male patients have a loss of 55% to 71% of isometric strength in flexion and extension, respectively. These data applied to athletic injury show that it is crucial for a pitcher to have maximum strength to maintain his level of performance and avoid injury. Thus maintaining a strong trunk helps avoid stressing the shoulder and elbow by protecting them from the overuse and abnormal motion seen with poor trunk mechanics.

In terms of our initial objective, we demonstrated a reproducible and consistent pattern despite delivery and physical variations. Figs. 40-13 to 40-18 illustrate our evaluation of faulty biomechanics in three players. Player O.H. is an experienced player at the top of his craft and ability. Although his actual activity levels often

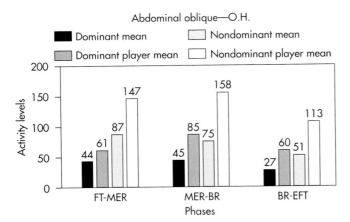

Fig. 40-13. Abdominal oblique muscle activity in O.H., an experienced and consistent major league pitcher. Comparison of activity levels; mean versus individual player. (From Watkins R et al: Dynamic EMG analysis of torque transfer in professional baseball pitchers, *Spine* 14:404, 1989.)

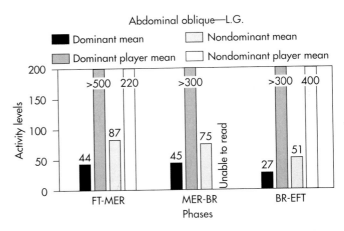

Fig. 40-14. Abdominal oblique muscle activity in L.G., a minor league pitcher who had played an infield position. Comparison of activity levels; mean versus individual player. (From Watkins R et al: Dynamic EMG analysis of torque transfer in professional baseball pitchers, *Spine* 14:404, 1989.)

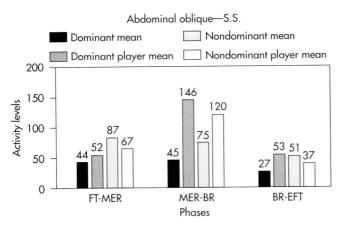

Fig. 40-15. Abdominal oblique muscle activity in S.S., an outfielder. Comparison of activity levels; mean versus individual player. (From Watkins R et al: Dynamic EMG analysis of torque transfer in professional baseball pitchers, *Spine* 14:404, 1989.)

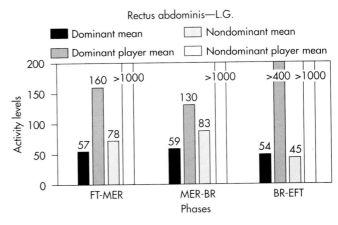

Fig. 40-16. Rectus abdominis muscle activity in L.G. Comparison of activity levels; mean versus individual player. (From Watkins R et al: Dynamic EMG analysis of torque transfer in professional baseball pitchers, *Spine* 14:404, 1989.)

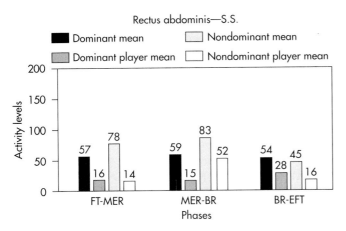

Fig. 40-17. Rectus abdominis muscle activity in S.S. Comparison of activity levels; mean versus individual player. (From Watkins R et al: Dynamic EMG analysis of torque transfer in professional baseball pitchers, *Spine* 14:404, 1989.)

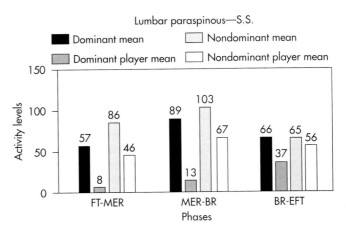

Fig. 40-18. Lumbar paraspinous muscle activity in S.S. Comparison of activity levels; mean versus individual player. (From Watkins R et al: Dynamic EMG analysis of torque transfer in professional baseball pitchers, *Spine* 14:404, 1989.)

are higher than the mean, they are highest in the nondominant oblique muscles in all phases and in the nondominant paraspinous and rectus abdominis muscle in the torque phase of unloading before ball release. In comparison, with L.G., a rising young player who was recently made a pitcher and who is developing his pitching biomechanics, one notes extremely irregular activity levels that are off the scale and in no reproducible pattern consistent with the subject mean (Fig. 40-16).

The third player, S.S., a professional outfielder who volunteered for the study, participated as a pitcher, using the mound and attempting his best pitching biomechanics. His data, represented in Figs. 40-15, 40-17, and 40-18, indicate the vast differences in his values compared with either those of O.H. or the mean patterns. These values are of particular significance in that this player is also a professional baseball player, yet shows none of the fine-tuned biomechanics associated specifically with pitching.

One might question the importance of demonstrating (1) a mean firing sequence of trunk musculature and (2) the differences in firing sequence among a top-level pitcher, a strong outfielder, and a rookie pitcher. In our short study all three athletes are strong and have good musculature. The point is that trunk muscle coordination is as important as trunk muscle strength in the ability to perform as a top-level baseball pitcher. When coordination and strength are combined, the player is more effective and experiences less fatigue. Therefore a logical conclusion is that a trunk-strengthening program that incorporates balancing and coordination is more effective and provides a shorter route to good training. On this basis we have considered the possibility of using gait laboratory analysis in decision making as a predictive indicator for success in terms of biomechanics and muscle activity. Obviously, there is a need for a larger sampling of pitchers, with particular emphasis on those who have had continued success over time and the fewest injuries. It is our hope that gait analysis will be added to the current methods of pitcher evaluation. The most important practical application is to aid the athlete through use of the complete data package, muscle activity levels, firing patterns, with their trends and timing, and the aforementioned high-speed photographic techniques. By means of careful laboratory analysis, coupled with evaluation by coaches and trainers, we can aid in the detection of biomechanical changes and, through rehabilitation or changes in technique, improve the athlete's efficiency.

The use of gait analysis for the injured athlete in need of rehabilitation is an important concept. The significant association of the injured shoulder or elbow with the weak or injured lumbar spine needs further documentation. Unfortunately, under laboratory conditions, we could not replicate a pitcher's fatigue and study the

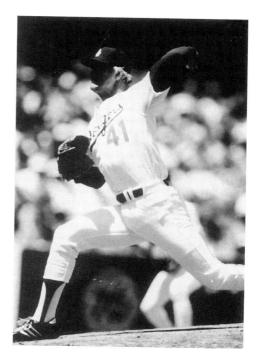

Fig. 40-19. Throwing motion.

resultant interaction of the arm and spine. It is an accepted concept in baseball that fatigue causes an early release point in the throwing motion, which in turn causes the ball to rise at the batter, making it easier to hit. This fatigue originates in a weak trunk and increased lumbar lordosis that places the arm behind the body, causing the arm to work harder and predisposing it to injury (Fig. 40-19). By using laboratory evaluation, we hope to aid in rehabilitation programs by emphasizing the role of trunk strength in shoulder rehabilitation.

Implications. The documentation of trunk activity in the dynamic stage of baseball pitching clearly demonstrates a reproducible pattern of muscle function based on strength combined with coordination. This pattern directly affects the biomechanics of the throwing arm by controlling the stability and loading characteristics responsible for maximum power and control. The implication of such a pattern is that the play of athletes can be objectively analyzed to maintain peak technique or to improve biomechanics.

The rehabilitation of an injured athlete, whether for shoulder, elbow, or back problems, can be better assessed with gait analysis. The use of objective physical data for goals and program documentation can improve a rehabilitation program. In addition, it may be possible to predict a successful outcome on the basis of expanded data correlated with productivity evaluation.

DIAGNOSIS OF INJURIES

Most baseball injuries are similar to those encountered in a general practice devoted to spinal problems.

Torsional injuries to the cervical and lumbar spine produce injuries to the joints in that area: advanced degenerative changes and changes related to the patient's age, as well as minimal findings on the basic x-ray film, magnetic resonance imaging (MRI), or computed tomography (CT). The essential injury is to the joint, defined as a neuromotion segment. The disc, the two facet joints, the nerves, blood vessels, ligaments, tendons, and muscles are part of that joint complex. The exact pathomechanics usually involve an injury to the intervertebral disc that results in abnormal motion in the disc, with inflammation and pain. There may be muscle and fascial tears, compression fractures, and disc herniations.

The torsional stress that athletes experience can cause mechanical neck problems because of unilateral muscular activity. Contractures and weakness can develop from constant rotation in the same direction. Certainly, injuries can result from head-first slides, sudden twists, or sudden bursts of muscular activity. Our initial approach to treatment is specificity in the diagnosis: is disc herniation, foraminal stenosis, or radiculopathy present? The answer often leads to the recommendation of nonoperative care or the need for surgical intervention in cases of radiculopathy.

Cervical myelopathy is rare but can occur in baseball players as it does in all groups of athletes. For lumbar spine problems, the situation is much the same. Athletes who experience torsional stress sustain rotatory annular disc lesions that produce mechanical pain. Often these injuries can be managed nonoperatively (e.g., severe discogenic injuries to the end-plate and even disc herniations with degenerative disease and spondylolisthesis).

A disc herniation that presents with radiculopathy, although it may be treated nonoperatively, often requires surgery. The operation of choice for an extruded disc fragment is a microscopic lumbar discectomy.[17] Certain congenital abnormalities of formation produce mechanical problems in the spine. Facet joint trophism, stress fractures, fused segments—all can produce undue strain on adjacent joints in the lumbar spine and lead to premature degeneration, pain, and stiffness in high-performance athletes. It is only through sheer hard work and determination that these problems can be conquered to allow the player a full, productive career. Spondylolysis and spondylolisthesis are common occurrences in baseball players.

TREATMENT OF LUMBAR SPINE PROBLEMS

Standard treatment of lumbar spine problems includes decreased inflammation, strengthening, stretching, and conditioning, with one important addition. Hitters typify the athlete to whom a cardinal rehabilitation rule applies: take the instrument out of the

player's hands. Like tennis players or any athlete who uses a racquet, hitters, when they have the bat in hand, are going to swing the bat basically the same way they have always swung the bat. If they have developed poor trunk mechanics over a period of time in response to an injury that is still painful, or as a compensation for contractures and weaknesses, they will not be able to change those mechanics as part of their rehabilitation as long as they are holding the bat. It is too inbred a learned response. Something that occurs in a split second and involves muscle performance of the entire body is very difficult to change.

1. Take the bat out of their hands. Take them away from home plate, out of baseball, onto the gym floor or the therapist's table, and begin a muscle-retraining process that teaches muscles to fire and contract in response to trunk and upper extremity stimuli.
2. Start the trunk stabilization program. Progress to level III stabilization training (see Chapter 27).
3. Teach muscles to maintain a tight muscle contraction throughout a full rotation.
4. Teach trunk musculature to relock the shoulders to the hips in a controlled, tight fashion.
5. Reestablish flexibility through contractures and provide full range of motion for the spine throughout the normal degrees of motion required to perform the activity.
6. Institute resistive proprioceptive neuromuscular facilitation (PNF) techniques in which the hitter is rotating against resistance from the therapist or at the full range of motion. Use isometric muscle control in a push-pull pattern for reestablishing muscle function, and restore symmetry of muscle balance by strengthening the muscles on the opposite side.
7. Do rotational resistive exercises in the opposite direction.
8. Reevaluate the batting stance just as you reevaluate the approach for a golfer.
9. Ensure balance and control—that the hitter is able to establish a tight, neutral spine position, holding the spine in an appropriate posture to produce a coordinated, balanced, strong swing.
10. Progress to an aerobic conditioning program toward maximum aerobic shape.

First the trainer supervises floor work that consists of exercises for stability, balance, coordination, and the proprioceptive neuromuscular facilitation (PNF) techniques while the therapist establishes strong, tight, trunk control, good flexibility, balance, and restored aerobic conditioning. Then the therapist and the trainer work initially to institute the basics of bat mechanics while emphasizing the muscle-strengthening and conditioning program. At this point the hitting coach can play a major role by collaborating with the trainer to teach the hitter to translate the acquired strength, flexibility, and coordination into sport-specific activity—in this case, translating total body coordination into the batting swing. However, the hitter is returning to the groove that made him successful. At this point the hitting coach's experience can prove invaluable in suggesting slight changes in hand position on the bat, opening the stance, emphasizing a more effective type of eye control, and improving technique for hitting various types of pitches.

It is, of course, difficult to change the basic swing of a baseball player who has attained success as a major league hitter. Rehabilitation can include shortening the swing, changing the hand position, emphasizing head control, recommending going to right field with an outside pitch, changing the bat size, and teaching other techniques. However, the basic rehabilitation principle remains: establishing a strong, functional trunk that can transfer power from the legs to the end of a bat within a rehabilitation program that reestablishes balance and coordination, as well as pain-free function, with the proper coordination needed to decrease undue strain on the lumbar spine. A friction-free, coordinated swing is often compared with a well-oiled, friction-free machine and is less likely to break down.

Rehabilitation of the infielder is much like rehabilitation in any lifting job. Proper infield techniques are designed to protect the spine. The simple concept of squatting to gather a ground ball is good for backs. Bending over at the waist with the knees straight is poor lifting technique and very bad fielding technique. The infielder requires strengthening of the quadricep muscles and the legs. The ability to work in a bent-forward position is more proportional to quadriceps strength than back strength. Of course, abdominal and extensor strengthening is important. Without strong legs and the ability to work in a squatted position, the back will be unduly stressed. Even the use of an abdominal binder in an infielder is not inappropriate if it does not restrict range of motion; it might provide an added bit of support in this sometimes necessary off-balance, forward-bending position. Usually, however, muscle control and strengthening techniques are adequate. Good fielding technique, use of the legs in squatting, and maintaining strength in the legs and quadriceps are paramount.

CASE ILLUSTRATIONS

Figs. 40-20 to 40-30 illustrate cases involving spinal injuries in baseball players.

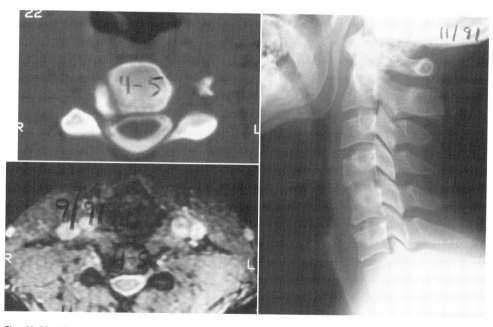

Fig. 40-20. Transverse section of the contrast CT scan in a 31-year-old professional baseball player with weak right shoulder abduction and a clinical C5 root lesion. He underwent a successful anterior cervical fusion. Although he had some problems with nerve root irritation after returning to play, the fusion was solid and the C5 nerve root showed full return of strength.

Fig. 40-21. This 32-year-old outfielder had a history of mechanical back pain for several years. Radicular pain developed in his upper leg, and subsequent tests showed bilateral spondylotic defects and degenerative disc disease at L3-4. The patient underwent an intensive trunk stabilization rehabilitation program for 2 years and returned to full, productive major league play.

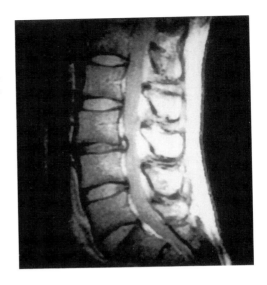

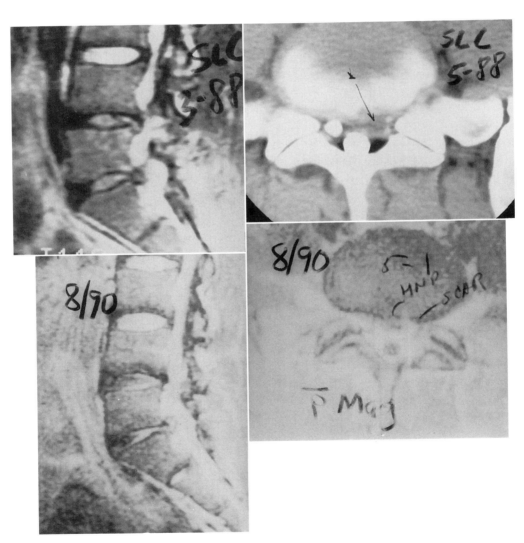

Fig. 40-22 This 30-year-old major league outfielder had undergone lumbar discectomy for radicular leg pain. Two years later he had a recurrent disc herniation that was removed and found to be an extruded fragment. The patient returned to full normal, function in sports.

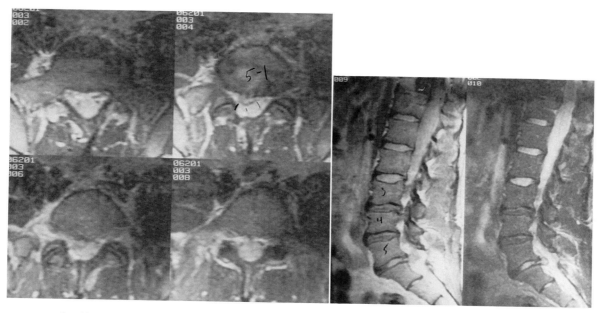

Fig. 40-23. This 26-year-old major league outfielder had S1 radiculopathy, with a large extruded disc fragment on L1 and L2, in addition to three-level degenerative disc disease. Although 4 years later the patient underwent a percutaneous discectomy at L3-4 for a central bulge and upper lumbar root disturbance, he continued to play at the major league level throughout the entire period.

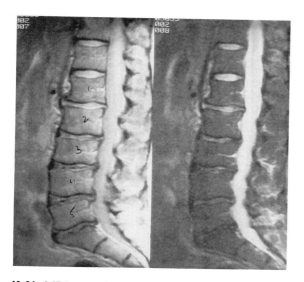

Fig. 40-24. MRI scan of a 34-year-old starting American League third baseman. This patient suffered multiple episodes of mechanical back dysfunction without significant radicular symptoms.

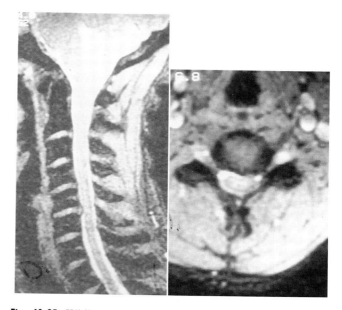

Fig. 40-25. While turning to make a catch, this 29-year-old professional baseball player experienced a sudden onset of excruciating neck pain and radiating pain in the left arm that radiated into the thumb and index finger in a C6 distribution, producing numbness of the thumb and weakness in wrist dorsiflexion. The severity of the pain required him to stand in the outfield with his arm on top of his head. His rehabilitation program consisted of aggressive antiinflammatory medications, 10 days of rest, and chest-out posture-correcting exercises. His symptoms slowly decreased, and he returned to play on a limited basis for approximately a week, continuing the strengthening program, and returned to full activity within 3 weeks after initiation of treatment (6 weeks after onset of symptoms). At 1 year he had had no further recurrence.

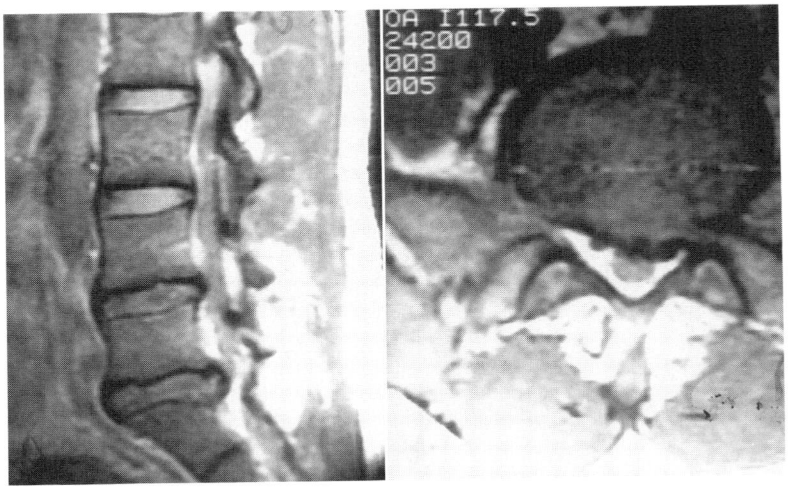

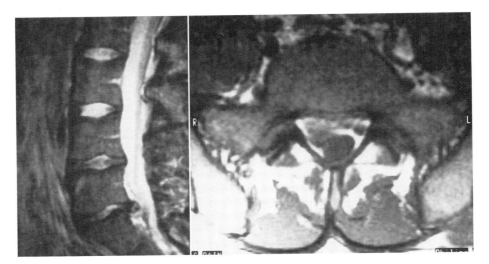

Fig. 40-26. This 22-year-old minor league professional outfielder experienced radicular pain in the left leg for 6 months, with positive findings on straight leg raising and an S1 distribution of symptoms (20% back pain, 80% leg pain). He underwent microscopic lumbar discectomy. Postoperative residual radicular pain responded to intensive rehabilitation, and he returned to minor league play.

Fig. 40-27. This 21-year-old infielder, who was completing his first year at full major league play, had L5-S1 radiculopathy. The treatment recommendation was a one-level microscopic lumbar discectomy and postoperative rehabilitation. It can be seen that the patient suffered from two-disc degenerative disease and significant degenerative changes in the L5-S1 disc space. It was predicted that the patient would need significant postoperative rehabilitation if he were to make an effective return to his sport.

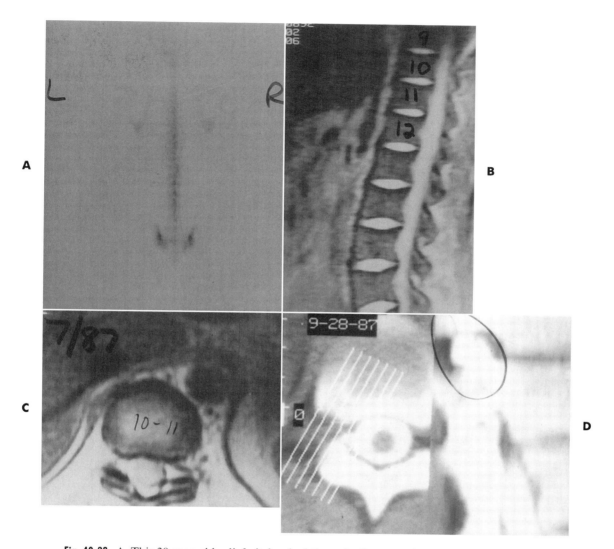

Fig. 40-28. A, This 30-year-old relief pitcher had thoracic rib cage pain that typically occurs in the nonthrowing arm of throwers and torsionally stressed athletes. Symptoms may indicate a rib stress fracture, a costovertebral articulation problem, torn soft tissue of the muscle or fascia, or injury to the cartilaginous tip of the rib. Because the throwing athlete experiences tremendous pull of the off-side abdominal oblique muscles, local modalities, physical therapy and rehabilitation, and antiinflammatory medications provided no relief. Results of a bone scan obtained to reveal a possible stress fracture were negative. **B,** MRI showed no evidence of thoracic disc herniation or a lumbar spine problem. The transverse sections suggested findings in the intervertebral foramen at T10-11 on the left, but this wisp was inconclusive for a pathologic lesion. The patient was advised to undergo a myelogram and contrast CT scan. **C,** The scan demonstrated a calcification, probably an avulsion fracture off the tip of the superior facet in the T10-11 intervertebral foramen. **D,** A nerve root block in that area provided relief of pain. The patient underwent a microscopic foraminotomy and returned to play without the radicular pain.

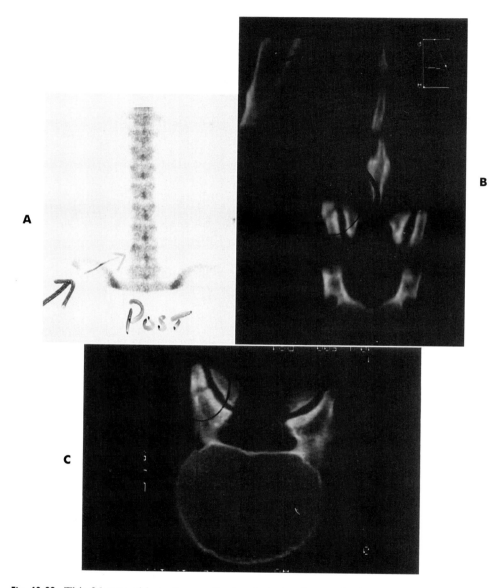

Fig. 40-29. This 26-year-old starting professional pitcher in a major league developed pain in his flank and back on the side opposite his pitching arm. A bone scan was obtained that identified a hot spot in the area of the facet joint on the left side at L4-5. A follow-up CT scan of that area showed a fracture in the superior facet. After 2 weeks of strengthening exercises, he attempted to return to play but developed more pain as soon as he started to throw. He required 6 months of rest and rehabilitation and returned the next season. **A,** Initial bone scan. **B,** Initial CT scan. **C,** CT scan at 4 months.

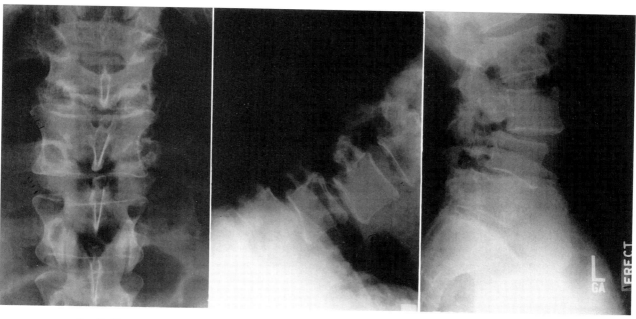

Fig. 40-30. This infielder played for 10 years in the major leagues with no appreciable low back pain. After retirement, his participation in martial arts resulted in symptoms. Investigation revealed structural abnormalities that did not limit his performance.

REFERENCES

1. Andersson GBJ et al: Quantitative electromyographic studies of back muscle activity related to posture and loading, *Orthop Clin North Am* 8:85, 1977.
2. Asmussen E: The weight-carrying function of the human spine, *Acta Orthop Scand* 29:276, 1960.
3. Asmussen E, Klausen K: Form and function of the erect human spine, *Clin Orthop* 25:55, 1962.
4. Basmajian JV: *Muscles alive: their functions revealed by electromyography,* Baltimore, 1967, Williams & Wilkins.
5. Braatz JH: The mechanics of pitching, *J Orthop Sports Ther* 9(2):56, 1987.
6. Chaffin DB, Moulis EJ: An empirical investigation of low back strains and vertebral geometry, *J Biomech* 2:88, 1969.
7. Donisich EW, Basmajian JV: Electromyography of deep back muscles in man, *Am J Anat* 133:25, 1972.
8. Hines B (Los Angeles Dodgers batting coach): Personal communication, 1992.
9. Jobe FW, Moynes DR, Antonelli DJ: Rotator cuff function during the golf swing, *Am J Sports Med* 14:388, 1986.
10. Jobe FW, Schwab DR: *30 exercises for better golf,* Inglewood, Calif, 1986, Champion Press.
11. Morris JM et al: An electromyographic study of the intrinsic muscles of the back in man, *J Anat* 96:509, 1962.
12. Nordin M et al: A comparative analysis of postoperative discectomy trunk strength and endurance. Paper presented at the meeting of the Federation of Spine Associations, Atlanta, Ga, Feb 15, 1988.
13. Parnianpour M et al: The effect of fatigue on the motor output and pattern of isodynamic trunk movement. Paper presented at the annual meeting of the International Society for the Study of the Lumbar Spine, West Palm Beach, Fla, April 1988.
14. Perry J: Personal communication, 1983.
15. Pink M: *The biomechanics of golf.* Paper presented at the 1990 PGA teaching and coaching summit, Nashville, Tenn, Nov 1990.
16. Pink M, Jobe FW, Perry J: EMG analysis of the shoulder during the golf swing, *Am J Sports Med* 18:137, 1990.
17. Winfield D (New York Yankees baseball player): Personal communication, 1991.

◆

Chapter Forty-One

Gymnastics

Peter R. Kurzweil
Douglas W. Jackson

There has been a significant increase in the popularity of gymnastics in the United States over the past two decades, and as a result, more injuries are being seen by physicians. Children begin participation in private clubs at an age before school gymnastics programs are available, and nearly all preelite and elite gymnasts are preteenagers and adolescents. However, interscholastic participation has decreased dramatically during the last 10 years as a result of soaring equipment costs and insurance premiums. High schools can no longer offer enough training for the serious gymnast. Private gymnastics clubs, on the other hand, have flourished and are the source of most high-level gymnasts. Private club programs have supplied most of the members of our U.S. Olympic gymnastics teams.

To excel in gymnastics at a national or international level takes tremendous commitment on the part of the athletes. The typical junior elite female gymnast (ages 10 to 14 years) works out twice a day, training up to 5 hours daily, and may be in the gym 5 or 6 days a week.[3,10] Many gymnasts seek particular coaches and clubs for special training not available near their homes. In one study, 16 of 50 female gymnasts lived away from home.[3] As the time spent in the gym increases, the gymnasts have certain demands that determine where they may attend school, leaving little time for other activities. The commitment to excellence and requirements to excel place great physical, and at times emotional, burdens on these children.

EPIDEMIOLOGY

Gymnastics is associated with a high injury rate. This association in part stems from the extensive media coverage given to catastrophic head and neck injuries. In the past many of these mishaps occurred on the trampoline, an event that was significantly restricted in 1976. Any sport in which high-speed maneuvers are performed, often at substantial height, has the potential for a high injury rate. In addition, the long hours of intense training, often 20 to 30 hours a week, increase the athlete's exposure to potential injury and overuse syndromes.[10,26,36]

INJURY RATES

In comparison with other interscholastic sports, gymnastics consistently has one of the highest rates of injury.[6,7] One of the factors that influences this rate is the particular gymnastics event. In women's gymnastics, floor exercises are responsible for the most injuries, followed in order by the balance beam, uneven bars, and vaulting.[8,19,26,29,31] Vaulting consistently has the fewest injuries, which may be due to the fact that less time is spent practicing and competing in this event. Although floor exercises carry the highest injury rate, this event should not be considered the most hazardous. The statistics reflect the fact that gymnasts spend most of their time practicing floor exercises and therefore have a greater exposure to potential injury during this event. Most of the injuries resulting from floor exercises are relatively minor. In contrast, although use of the trampoline before its elimination resulted in less than one fifth of the injuries, these injuries were often the most severe.[8]

Another factor affecting the rate of injury is the gymnast's level of skill. Elite gymnasts have a significantly higher injury rate than less highly skilled athletes.[18,26,28,31] Top-level gymnasts spend more time practicing than novices and subsequently have greater exposure time during which an injury may occur. They also routinely perform more difficult maneuvers that carry higher risk.

Most injuries occur in the first hour of practice and during the first few months of the season.[3] Ninety-five percent of injuries happen in training, which is not surprising, since gymnasts spend much more time working out than competing. However, competition may actually carry a higher risk than training. Although competition occupies only 0.4% of the athlete's time, it is responsible for 5% of the injuries.[8]

INCIDENCE OF BACK INJURIES

The incidence of low back pain in gymnasts varies widely, but most authors agree it is fairly common. In an early study by Jackson, Wiltse, and Cirincione,[16] low back pain significant enough to interfere with training was found in 25 of 100 young female gymnasts. Oseid[25] reported low back pain in 75% of 41 young female gymnasts.

Goldstein et al.[10] prospectively investigated spinal injuries in top-level female gymnasts. Magnetic resonance imaging (MRI) scans were performed in 33 athletes to document disc or bony abnormalities. Of these, 9% (1/11) preelite, 43% (6/14) elite, and 63% (5/8) Olympic-caliber gymnasts had lumbar spine changes on

MRI. The average number of hours spent in training per week and the age of the gymnast were found to be associated with abnormal MRI findings. More than half of the athletes who trained more than 15 hours a week had positive MRI findings, whereas 87% of those who trained less than 15 hours a week had negative MRI findings. This study suggests that intense training over a period of time predisposes the female gymnast's spine to chronic changes.

Caine et al.[3] prospectively followed 50 young female gymnasts over one season. Of the 33 girls who sought medical attention during the year before the study, a third had problems with the lower back, which was the most frequently injured site. At the start of the surveillance period, more than half of the gymnasts reported aches and pains during workouts, with the wrist and lower back being the most frequently affected areas. The most common diagnosis was "nonspecific pain" in the lower back, which was attributed to an overuse syndrome.

FLEXIBILITY AND SPINAL MOBILITY

The five most commonly performed women's gymnastics skills include front and back walkovers, front and back handsprings, and the handspring vault. The back handspring and back walkover require the greatest amount of hyperextension (Fig. 41-1). During front and back walkovers and the back handspring, maximum lumbar hyperextension occurs very close to the time that impact is sustained by the hands or feet.[11,16]

Given this routinely performed complex bending,

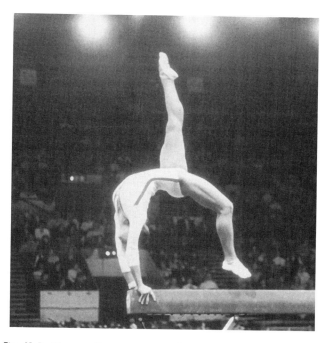

Fig. 41-1. Gymnastic maneuvers often require significant lumbar hyperextension.

Kirby et al.[17] set out to determine whether female gymnasts were more flexible than nongymnasts. They found that gymnasts were more flexible in some, but not all, areas. The gymnasts studied had greater shoulder flexion and abduction, lumbar flexion, hip extension, and toe-touching ability. There was no significant difference in lumbar, knee, or elbow extension. The lack of any difference in lumbar extension was surprising, since gymnasts have a higher incidence of lumbar symptoms and use the extended lumbar position frequently, which has been linked to spondylolysis in several reports.[16,38]

Jackson, Wiltse, and Cirincione[16] compared the flexibility of female gymnasts with that of male high school football players. The ability to place and hold both palms on the floor with the knees fully extended was recorded in these two groups; 137 (93%) of 147 gymnasts and 39 (36%) of 108 football players were able to perform this maneuver without a warm-up or stretching. This comparison considered factors other than innate flexibility, including arm and leg length and training effects.

DIAGNOSTIC TESTS

Most episodes of low back pain are self-limited and resolve spontaneously in 3 to 6 weeks. Pain lasting longer than that in a young gymnast merits consideration for a thorough work-up. Establishing a diagnosis and initiating proper treatment early will often prevent a more long-term disabling condition from developing. The physician should be selective in deciding which tests will be most beneficial in managing the gymnast's low back symptoms.

Routine lumbosacral radiographs seldom contribute to the management of low back pain in the general population. However, radiographic changes in young athletes are more common and have been shown to correlate with back pain.[13,33] Male gymnasts and wrestlers have the highest incidence of abnormalities.[33] Schmorl's nodes are found more frequently in athletes than in nonathletes,[7] leading some to speculate that these nodes may represent traumatic intraosseous disk herniation.[20] Abnormalities of the vertebral ring apophysis occurred exclusively in athletes in one study.[32]

Jackson[14] found radiographic changes in almost all athletes with back pain persisting more than 3 months. Radiographic changes in the lumbar spine in 22 of 52 (42%) male and female gymnasts had positive findings that included reduced disc height, Schmorl's nodes, spondylolysis, and alterations in the configuration of the vertebral body. There was a significant correlation between the severity of back pain and the number of radiographic abnormalities. These findings were suggestive of a causative relationship between vigorous athletic activity, radiographic abnormalities, and back pain.

The technetium bone scan is usually very helpful in evaluating suspected acute or healing osseous injuries in

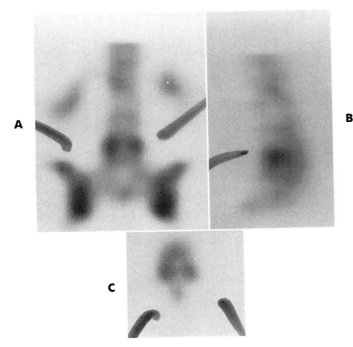

Fig. 41-2. Single photon emission computed tomography (SPECT) demonstrating bilateral pars interarticularis injury at L5-S1. **A,** Coronal plane image. **B,** Sagittal plane image. **C,** Axial plane image.

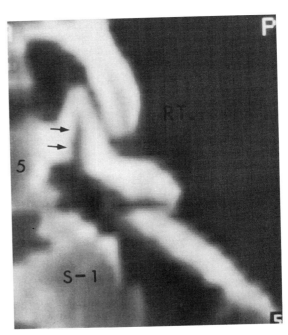

Fig. 41-3. Three-dimensional CT reconstruction showing fracture of the pars at L5 *(arrows).*

the gymnast. It is particularly useful with problems in the posterior elements (facet joints, pars, and pedicles). In cases where clinical suspicion of spondylolysis is high but plain radiographs appear normal, radionuclide bone scanning using single photon emission computed tomography (SPECT) is helpful[4] (Fig. 41-2).

A computed tomography (CT) scan is useful for delineating fractures of the lumbar spine. It is our test of choice to demonstrate bony problems of the posterior elements. Because of the radiation required for this test, however, we use it very selectively in young gymnasts. It may also be coupled with a three-dimensional reconstruction (Fig. 41-3).

MRI has been a real asset in evaluating young gymnasts, especially if serial evaluation is needed. It is highly sensitive and specific for disc lesions, which previously required myelography and/or CT scanning to be demonstrated.[10] Subtle, early degenerative changes of the discs and damage to the annulus and neural elements are more clearly delineated by MRI than by other techniques. Osseous abnormalities, including posterior element fractures, may be visualized with MRI, but CT scans are still preferable (Fig. 41-4).

In the study of top-level female gymnasts by Goldstein et al.,[10] low back pain was found in 73% of those with MRI results positive for spondylolysis or a disc problem. Only 14% of the athletes with negative MRI results had back symptoms, and most of these were mild and

intermittent. Although it is expensive, MRI involves no ionizing radiation and is an excellent method for screening and following athletes with low back problems.

DIFFERENTIAL DIAGNOSIS OF BACK PAIN

Our experience with young gymnasts suggests that over half the cases will resolve before a definitive diagnosis is attained. The sequence of the work-up is guided by the gymnast's age, level of competition, and suspected problem.

We prefer to categorize gymnastic injuries around the spine into three areas: (1) soft tissue, (2) disc, and (3) bone. Soft tissue injuries encompass sprains and strains of the paraspinous muscles and ligaments. Discogenic problems include injury to the discs, as well as anterior and posterior extrusions. Bony problems generally involve the posterior elements—pars interarticularis (reaction or fracture), facet joint (chondromalacia), and spinous/transverse processes (avulsion)—but they may involve the vertebral end-plates, compression fractures, and the related apophysis.

STRAINS AND SPRAINS

The most common back injuries in gymnasts involve the soft tissue structures of the spine. The musculotendinous units, ligaments, and joint capsules are all vulnerable to injury in the back, just as they are in the rest of the body.

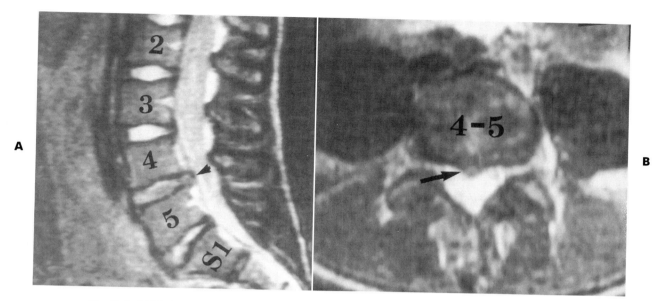

Fig. 41-4. MRI demonstrating a herniated nucleus pulposus at L4-5. **A,** T2-weighted sagittal image. **B,** T2-weighted axial image.

Physical examination is usually unremarkable except for secondary changes of tenderness and muscle spasm. Limitations in range of motion and trigger points may be present. A lumbar list and reduced lumbar lordosis may be observed in more severe cases. Patients should also be evaluated for possible leg length discrepancies.[9] An extensive work-up is usually not required.

The key to initial treatment is rest. We prefer a program of "relative rest," which avoids aggravating activities. The gymnasts are encouraged to seek alternate forms of fitness that avoid loading the back, such as stationary biking, using stair-climbing machines, or swimming. This maintains conditioning and is usually more acceptable to the gymnasts, who are unlikely to tolerate a trial of complete rest. Nonsteroidal antiinflammatory agents and muscle relaxants may be prescribed when appropriate. Injection of trigger points with an anesthetic and corticosteroid can be considered if the acute symptoms persist and are highly localized.[30]

The healing phase for soft tissue injuries may take as long as 6 to 8 weeks for full return of function. During this time the gymnast should be started on a program of reconditioning of the lower back and abdominal muscles, stretching exercises, and spinal mobilization techniques. It is helpful to have this treatment coordinated by a qualified physical therapist or athletic trainer, who can work more closely with individual athletes and their coaches. Increases in endurance, strength, and flexibility are gradual and cannot be rushed. Return to unrestricted competition is done in stages as the gymnast's condition improves and symptoms subside. It is important to emphasize to all involved in the gymnast's care that a full return to competition and training should not occur until all symptoms have subsided and the athlete has had time to recondition. With this philosophy, reinjury and the development of a chronic problem can be minimized.

LUMBAR DISC DISEASE

Changes in the lumbar discs occur as part of the natural aging process.[14,17,22,27] Because the peak age for disc herniation is in the third and fourth decades,[15] this condition is rarely seen in young gymnasts. However, gymnasts who train for more than 15 hours a week may be at risk for developing changes at an earlier age than the general population.[10]

Tertti et al.[34] investigated the incidence of disc degeneration and its relationship to low back pain in young gymnasts. MRI studies were performed on 35 gymnasts, 11 of whom reported low back pain with exercise. The images showed evidence of degenerated discs in only three of these gymnasts. Subsequent radiographs demonstrated that these latter cases were associated with Scheuermann's disease or abnormalities of the lumbosacral junction. The authors concluded that despite the excessive range of motion and repetitive loading of the lumbosacral spine, back pain in gymnasts is not suggestive of damage to the intervertebral discs.

The most limiting lumbar disc changes in a gymnast or other young athlete are usually associated with posterior and posterolateral herniation that affects the adjacent neural elements. The referred pain is often unilateral and may radiate down the buttocks and posterior thigh. Lesions mimicking discogenic problems in this young population are unusual. Physical findings vary and may include paraspinous muscle spasm, limited thoracolumbar motion, loss of lumbar lordosis, and a trunk list. The sitting straight leg knee extension test and contralateral supine straight leg raising test are quite reliable signs of a herniated disk.[35]

If focal neurologic abnormalities are found or symptoms become overly restrictive, further diagnostic tests may be needed to define the extent of the problem. MRI is the procedure of choice to screen for abnormalities of the discs or other causes of nerve root irritation in the young gymnast. With this information the physician can provide realistic expectations to the athlete regarding appropriate restrictions, return to sports, and some insight into the long-term prognosis.

Restriction of activity and use of analgesics have been the mainstays of treatment of symptomatic discs. Conservative care usually resolves the lumbar disc symptoms within a month or two. Traction and manipulation are not routinely used in the treatment of sciatica.[2] If corsets or braces are used for external support during the early recovery phase, they should be abandoned as early as possible to prevent atrophy of the abdominal and paraspinous musculature. Epidural cortisone injections have been helpful in hastening the recovery of about 40% of our young athletes with more chronic radicular symptoms.[15,16] A gymnast with persistent radicular pain that does not respond to conservative

treatment becomes a candidate for further diagnostic studies.

The majority of discogenic problems do not require surgical intervention, although it is reasonable to consider surgery when no improvement is seen for several weeks.[2] Prolonged irritation of the neural elements may not allow return to the same performance level. Chronic changes may persist even after successful lumbar decompression of the extruded disk material. Whether the athlete can and should return to his or her sport after surgery is also a consideration. Surgical techniques that do not require extensive exposure and denervation of paraspinous musculature are highly desired if the gymnast is planning to return to competition.

Herniation of the disc through the anterior growth plate may be another source of low back pain in the skeletally immature gymnast[32] (Fig. 41-5). This entity has been linked to hyperflexion injuries and is most commonly seen at the thoracolumbar junction. Subsequent narrowing at the disk space and irregularities of the anterior vertebral body may be seen on radiographs (Fig. 41-6). This entity may be accompanied by altered disc mechanics among adolescent and preadolescent gymnasts. It differs from Scheuermann's apophysitis, which is characterized by a decrease in the anterior vertebral height (wedging) and undulation of the vertebral end-plate. Herniation through the growth plate often skips vertebral levels and usually involves less than three vertebrae. This entity may also be an incidental finding in an athlete without pain.[30]

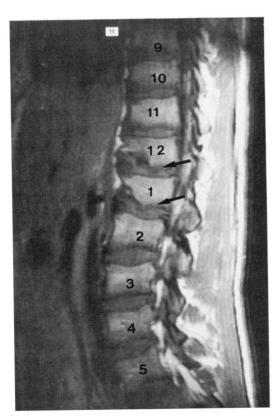

Fig. 41-5. T2-weighted MRI scan showing anterior herniation of the disc through the growth plates of vertebral bodies T12 and L1 *(arrows).*

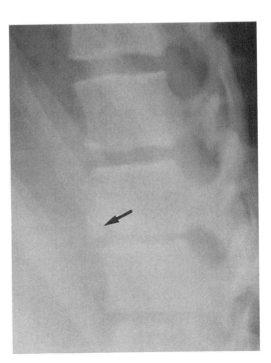

Fig. 41-6. Radiograph showing irregularity of the anterior vertebral body of T12 with slight narrowing of the T12-L1 disc space.

Sward et al.[32] emphasized the importance of delayed radiographic follow-up of gymnasts with back pain following trauma. They reported two female gymnasts (ages 13 and 16) with lower thoracic back pain following a jump. Both landed in a position of hyperflexion with possible axial rotation. Radiographs obtained soon after the injury showed no abnormalities. Since the pain persisted, technetium bone scans were obtained. A scan at 4 months showed negative findings in one case. Focal uptake in the neural arch of T12 was seen in the other gymnast at 6 months. Neither study demonstrated uptake in the anterior corner of the T12 vertebral body, where abnormalities were seen on radiographic examination in the vertebral ring apophysis at 1 year. The lack of correlation between the bone scan and plain radiographs was not adequately explained. Traumatic injury of the anterior vertebral ring apophyses may result from hyperflexion injuries with subsequent reduction of disc height, disc degeneration, and prolapse of disc material. Radiographic changes may not be present for several months, and the sensitivity of technetium bone scans for detecting this injury may be low. Repeating plain radiographs during follow-up visits may be important in certain circumstances.

LUMBAR FACET SYNDROME

Abnormalities of the facet joints are another potential source of back pain, as well as gluteal and thigh pain, in the gymnast.[1,12,23,30] The synovial lining of the facet joint capsule is innervated by the posterior primary ramus, and irritation or inflammation of this lining may give rise to back pain and sciatica-type symptoms. There has been some difficulty in classifying patients with this syndrome because there is no characteristic pain pattern and frequently no obvious radiographic abnormality. Four clinical criteria are correlated with this entity: (1) back pain associated with groin or thigh pain, (2) well-localized paraspinal tenderness, (3) reproduction of symptoms with extension-rotation, and (4) radiographic evidence of significant facet changes.[23]

On physical examination pain is generally aggravated by lumbar extension (which compresses the joint) and relieved by flexion (which separates the joint surfaces). Well-localized paravertebral tenderness and limitation in spinal movement are characteristic findings. In most cases the neurologic examination is normal.

Plain radiographic evaluation in the young gymnast with lumbar facet syndrome usually reveals no abnormalities. Subtle facet changes such as narrowing, irregularity, or sclerosis are best documented by CT scans. A bone scan may help confirm a facet problem by demonstrating increased uptake exclusively in the facet joints. Diligent palpation and placement of radiographic markers over the point of maximal tenderness may also help localize the problem.

Injection of the facet joints may be diagnostic and therapeutic.[23,24] The pressure from the injection may initially provoke the symptoms, with subsequent relief following infiltration of a local anesthetic. If a corticosteroid is included, the inflammation of the joints may be relieved on a long-term basis. Interestingly, Mooney and Robertson[23] reported three cases where depressed deep tendon reflexes returned to normal following injection of the facet joints with lidocaine (Xylocaine). However, the success rate with facet joint injections is only 50% to 60%.[5,23,24]

The cause of facet joint problems varies. There may be cartilage problems similar to those of chondromalacia of the patella or frank arthritis. Synovitis of the lining of the facet joints may occur. Hypermobility between vertebral bodies may cause abnormal tracking and be another source of pain. These nonspecific lumbar facet joint problems are often difficult to treat, as is the case with similar problems in other joints in the body. This syndrome frequently does not respond to conservative measures. Injection of the facet joints is usually considered when symptoms persist despite 2 months of treatment with rest, antiinflammatory medication, and physical therapy.[12] Most gymnasts are able to return to competition once symptoms subside.

SPONDYLOLYSIS AND SPONDYLOLISTHESIS

Spondylolysis in gymnasts is often an acquired defect in the pars interarticularis. Repetitive hyperextension maneuvers put the gymnast's spine at risk for developing this entity, although genetic predisposition may also play a role. The lumbar spines of 100 young female gymnasts were screened radiographically[16]; 11% had a pars interarticularis defect compared with 2.4% in the nonathletic female population, and spondylolisthesis was found in 6%. Most gymnasts early in their career

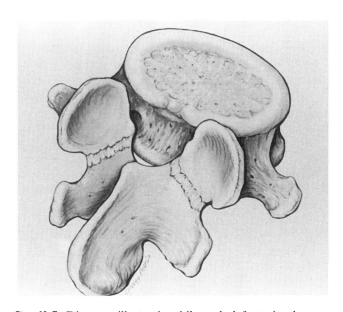

Fig. 41-7. Diagram illustrating bilateral defects in the pars interarticularis in spondylolysis.

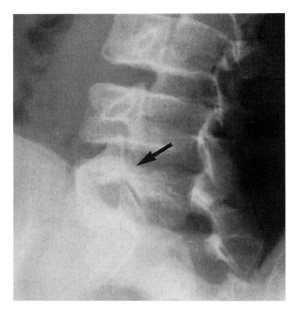

Fig. 41-8. Radiograph showing sclerosis and elongation of the pars interarticularis in pars stress reaction. This may be a precursor to spondylolysis.

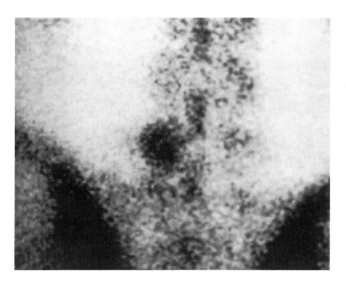

Fig. 41-9. Technetium pyrophosphate bone scan. Marked, unilateral uptake of the radiotracer indicates a recent injury to the pars interarticularis.

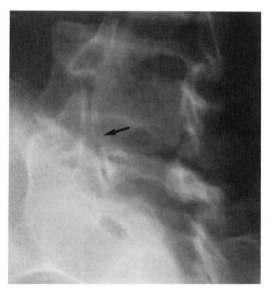

Fig. 41-10. Radiograph demonstrating a bony defect of the pars interarticularis in spondylolysis.

were unaware of these findings. The treating physician must remember that the presence of a radiographic change does not necessarily explain the cause of the patient's lumbar pain.

Persistent lumbar pain in a gymnast that is aching in nature, unilateral, and exaggerated by hyperextension should alert the clinician to a possible posterior element problem. The one-legged hyperextension test is helpful in diagnosing unilateral problems. Early lesions are usually unilateral but may progress to bilateral pars involvement (Fig. 41-7). Most gymnasts with a symptomatic pars defect without vertebral slippage are able to place their fingertips to the floor and do not have signs of nerve root irritation.

Early in this process radiographic findings will be negative, although subtle changes such as sclerosis and attenuation of the pars interarticularis may occur (Fig. 41-8). This stress reaction in the pars results in increased bone turnover and is best documented by technetium pyrophosphate bone scanning (Fig. 41-9). If a pars defect does appear on initial radiographs (Fig. 41-10), it is important to determine whether this represents an acute or chronic process, since the former have a greater healing potential. Acute defects appear fuzzy and are well delineated, whereas chronic changes usually demonstrate bone resorption and smooth, sclerotic borders. A bone scan may be helpful in distinguishing whether another level is involved, whether the involvement is unilateral or bilateral, and whether the lesion is old or acute. If the scan is negative, it can be assumed that the defect has less chance for bony healing. Symptoms may subside

even without bony healing. Return to gymnastics is dependent on the resolution of pain.

The bone scan is not necessary in all cases, since the diagnosis can usually be suspected from physical examination and radiographic studies. However, it is helpful in counseling the young athlete who is facing a considerable period of disability. Once the findings of the scan are positive, usually a minimum of 3 months and an average of 6 months are needed for the athlete to be able to return to pain-free competition. Some youngsters have been unable to return for considerably longer periods of

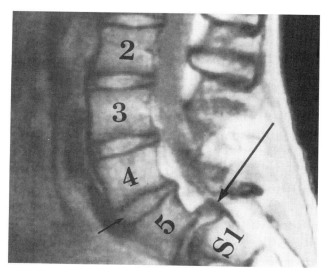

Fig. 41-11. MRI scan showing spondylolisthesis at L5-S1 *(big arrow)*. There is a herniated nucleus pulposus at L4-5 *(small arrow)*.

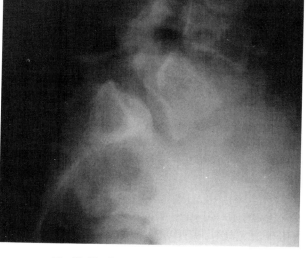

Fig. 41-12. Grade II spondylolisthesis.

time. The resolution of pain predates the resolution of activity demonstrated on the bone scan. The athlete can usually return to competition before the bone scan activity resumes normal levels.

The physician caring for the young gymnast with a symptomatic pars defect is primarily concerned with eliminating the lumbar pain and preventing vertebral slippage. Spondylolisthesis usually develops in childhood unrelated to athletic participation.[37] It is present before gymnasts enter their period of increased training. Because the age of rapid slippage is between 9 and 13 years, athletes should be followed closely during this time.[14] Slippage rarely increases after skeletal maturity. In our experience with the young gymnast, progression of grade I slippage of more than 1 degree is rare. Grade I slips at the L5-S1 level are usually incidental findings and are not uncommonly found in asymptomatic young gymnasts (Fig. 41-11). The physician should not assume that this radiographic abnormality is the cause of pain but should look for other causes. A bone scan may be helpful in evaluating the associated pars interarticularis defects, the levels above, the facet joints, or other bony lesions of the lumbar spine.

Most gymnasts with symptomatic spondylolisthesis complain of pain with activity. The pain may be unilateral or bilateral and is frequently associated with paraspinous muscle spasm. Gluteal and thigh pain may be present, although neurologic deficits and nerve root tension are rarely found. If the gymnast develops symptoms from a degenerative disc, it is usually at the level above the slip. The physician may find tight hamstrings and a vertical sacrum in the higher-degree slips. The altered lumbar function of a high-degree slip

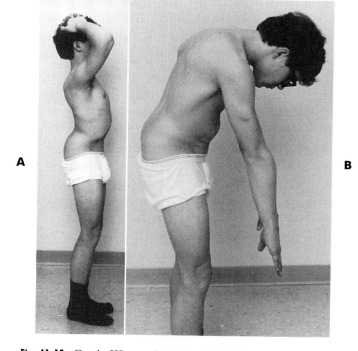

Fig. 41-13. Grade III spondylolisthesis. **A,** Exaggerated lumbar lordosis (swayback) is seen on standing erect. **B,** The vertical sacrum becomes pronounced with forward flexion, which is also limited by tight hamstrings.

eliminates the gymnast from competition. The pain from the altered posterior elements may be exacerbated by hyperextension maneuvers.

Treatment of low back pain in a symptomatic gymnast with low-grade spondylolisthesis should start with conservative measures. Restriction of aggravating activities and an appropriate course of medication are often enough to enable the athlete to return to gymnastics. Otherwise, a temporary trial of antilordotic bracing may be considered.[21,30]

With more significant olisthesis (grade II or greater) structural changes, such as disc degeneration, facet arthritis, and altered posterior element loading, may result in persistent, chronic symptoms (Figs. 41-12 and 41-13). Surgery may be considered but is not always successful in returning the athlete to the same level of competition. A 1- or 2-year layoff postoperatively makes it difficult for athletes to catch up to their peers in their competitive careers. Participation in gymnastics should not be the sole indication for fusion in a young athlete. Many will have satisfactory resolution of their symptoms by selectively giving up gymnastics.

It has been the policy of one of us (DWJ) to discourage gymnasts from competition if they have grade II or greater spondylolisthesis. Secondary structural changes, such as a vertical sacrum, loss of hip extension, and hamstring tightness, usually eliminate these gymnasts from elite competition. However, although the risk of subsequent degenerative damage may be high, not all athletes are deterred from participation. Some do continue to perform with multiple-level involvement and back pain.

REFERENCES

1. Badgely CE: The articular facets in relation to low back pain and sciatic radiation, *J Bone Joint Surg* 23A:481, 1941.
2. Bell GR, Rothman RH: The conservative treatment of sciatica, *Spine* 9:54, 1984.
3. Caine D et al: An epidemiologic investigation of injuries affecting young competitive female gymnasts, *Am J Sports Med* 17:811, 1989.
4. Collier BD, Johnson RP: Painful spondylolysis or spondylolisthesis studied by radiography and single photon emission computerized tomography, *Radiology* 154:207, 1985.
5. Dory M: Arthrography of the lumbar facet joints, *Radiology* 140:23, 1981.
6. Eisenberg I, Allen WC: Injuries in a women's varsity athletic program, *Physician Sportsmed* 6(3):112, 1978.
7. Garrick JG, Requa RK: Girls' sports injuries in high school athletics, *JAMA* 239:2245, 1978.
8. Garrick JG, Requa RK: Epidemiology of women's gymnastics injuries, *Am J Sports Med* 8:261, 1980.
9. Giles LGF, Taylor JR: Low back pain associated with leg length inequality, *Spine* 6:510, 1981.
10. Goldstein JD et al: Spine injuries in gymnasts and swimmers: an epidemiologic investigation, *Am J Sports Med* 19:463, 1991.
11. Hall SJ: Mechanical contribution to lumbar stress injuries in female gymnasts, *Med Sci Sports Exerc* 18:599, 1986.
12. Helbig T, Lee CK: The lumbar facet syndrome, *Spine* 13:61, 1988.
13. Hellstron M et al: Radiological abnormalities in the spine of athletes, *Acta Radiol* (in press).
14. Jackson DW: Low back pain in young athletes: evaluation of stress reaction and discogenic problems, *Am J Sports Med* 7:364, 1979.
15. Jackson DW, Rettig A, Wiltse LL: Epidural cortisone injections in the young athletic adult, *Am J Sports Med* 8:239, 1980.
16. Jackson DW, Wiltse LL, Cirincione RJ: Spondylolysis in the female gymnast, *Clin Orthop* 117:68, 1976.
17. Kirby RL et al: Flexibility and musculoskeletal symptomatology in female gymnasts and age-matched controls, *Am J Sports Med* 9:160, 1981.
18. Lowry CB, Leveau BF: A retrospective study of gymnastics injuries to competitors and noncompetitors in private clubs, *Am J Sports Med* 10:237, 1982.
19. McAuley E et al: Injuries in women's gymnastics: the state of the art, *Am J Sports Med* 15:558, 1987.
20. McCall IW et al: Acute traumatic intraosseous disc herniation, *Spine* 10:134, 1987.
21. Micheli LJ, Miller E: Use of modified Boston brace for back injuries in athletes, *Am J Sports Med* 8:351, 1980.
22. Miller JAA, Schmatz C, Schultz AB: Lumbar disc degeneration: correlation with age, sex, and spine level in 600 autopsy specimens, *Spine* 13:173, 1988.
23. Mooney V, Robertson J: The facet syndrome, *Clin Orthop Rel Res* 115:149, 1976.
24. Moran R, O'Connell D, Walsh MG: The diagnostic value of facet joint injections, *Spine* 13:1407, 1988.
25. Oseid S: Unpublished data, Oslo-1, Norway, Pediatric Research Institute, University Hospital.
26. Pettrone FA, Ricciardelli E: Gymnastic injuries: the Virginia experience 1982-1983, *Am J Sports Med* 15:59, 1987.
27. Pritzker KPH: Aging and degeneration in the lumbar intervertebral disc, *Orthop Clin North Am* 8:65, 1977.
28. Silver JR, Silver DD, Godfrey JJ: Injuries of the spine sustained during gymnastic activities, *Fr Med J* 293:861, 1986.
29. Snook GA: Injuries in women's gymnastics: a 5-year study, *Am J Sports Med* 7:242, 1986.
30. Spencer CW, Jackson DW: Back injuries in the athlete, *Clin Sports Med* 2:191, 1983.
31. Steele VA, White JA: Injury prediction in female gymnasts, *Br J Sports Med* 10:31, 1986.
32. Sward L et al: Acute injury of the vertebral ring apophysis and intervertebral disc in adolescent gymnasts, *Spine* 15:144, 1990.
33. Sward L et al: Back pain and radiologic changes in the thoracolumbar spine of athletes, *Spine* 15:124, 1990.
34. Tertti M et al: Disc degeneration in young gymnasts: a magnetic resonance imaging study, *Am J Sports Med* 18:206, 1990.
35. Troup JDG: Straight leg raising and the qualifying tests for increased root tension: their predictive value after back and sciatic pain, *Spine* 6:526, 1981.
36. Walsh WM, Huurman WW, Shelton GL: Overuse injuries of the knee and spine in girls' gymnastics, *Orthop Clin North Am* 16:2, 1985.
37. Wiltse LL, Jackson DW: Treatment of spondylolisthesis and spondylolysis in children, *Clin Orthop* 117:92, 1976.
38. Wiltse LL, Widell EH, Jackson DW: Fatigue fracture: the basic lesion in isthmic spondylolisthesis, *J Bone Joint Surg* 57A:17, 1975.

Chapter Forty-Two

◆

Dance

Hamilton Hall
Jo-Anne Piccinin

Of all the forms of dance, classical ballet is the most physically demanding. To study the impact of dance on the spine, there is no better subject than the professional ballet dancer. Ballet is dance and more. Classical ballet is the rhythmic progression of precise and rigidly defined body positions linked by specific steps, turns, and jumps.

The movements of the dancer are highly stylized and exceedingly complex. Beginning with the five basic leg positions, incorporating the recognized postures for the head, trunk, and arms—allowing for positioning to the right or left and adding the accepted derivatives—there is a total of 47 possible positions in the ballet repertoire. These can be combined in 13,284 different ways, and when each is performed with one of three different foot placements, there are 39,852 possibilities.[29]

Fairbank and Hall[8] note that "in most human endeavors, a certain degree of incompetence is tolerable, perhaps even enhancing, since errors, within limits, sometimes have a way of inducing a kind of approval for one who is trying very hard and isn't quite perfect. But in the ballet, anything much less than perfection comes perilously close to absurdity." To make what is unnatural and exceedingly difficult appear both natural and effortless requires extraordinary physical effort. Four hundred years of tradition and an obsession to excel over past performances challenge both the limits of the dancer's endurance and the spine's ability to withstand the strain.

WHY DANCERS ARE DIFFERENT

By temperament and training, the elite ballet dancer is an atypical professional athlete. Dancers train for over a third of their brief careers, perfecting skills and physical abilities to equal and, in many instances, exceed those required of a professional football, baseball, or hockey player. The dancer is further unique in that these often herculean efforts must be carried out in front of a live audience that has no tolerance for even minor mistakes and that expects a performance to reflect grace, apparent ease, and charisma. A dancer's career, like that of many professional athletes, is brief. It is also solitary, obsessively introspective, and, except for the extremely rare principal artist, lacking in the adulation and financial rewards that are so much a part of modern professional sport.

For little more than personal satisfaction and the approval of their peers, dancers will sacrifice much of

their life to their art. They do this in the knowledge that when their career is over, there may be little left. How many dancers can sell their name and face as part of a national advertisement campaign or go on to provide color commentary for televised performances?

Overall hangs the threat of sudden serious injury and a premature end to the already fleeting dream. The specter of back injury can be banished only through better medical understanding of the unique demands on the dancer's spine, a more scientific, active, and coordinated approach to treatment, and greater emphasis on proper training and prevention.

TRAINING

Training for a career in ballet often starts before the age of 10 years. There is general agreement that it takes 10 years to train a dancer to advanced levels of classical ballet technique.[20] The careers of most professional dancers last about two decades, with very few going on for 30 years. Many dancers are forced to stop performing because of injuries or accidents. Subjecting the developing, growing spine to repeated stress and impact may create more long-lasting, less treatable pathologic conditions.[10]

Beginning and basic ballet training for children 8 to 11 years old focuses on correct placement of the head, arms, body, and legs. Emphasis is placed on the five school positions of the lower limbs and on turnout of the legs from the hips down. Little can be done to increase turnout after the early years, and proper early training can decrease the later need to create an apparent increase in external rotation through exaggerated lordosis of the lumbar spine (Figs. 42-1 and 42-2).

Intermediate ballet training usually starts at age 14 years. Female dancers may begin pointe work, whereas young male dancers begin studying the rudiments of partnering, with little lifting permitted.

A schedule of five classes or more a week is normal for advanced students. The Canadian National Ballet School holds three classes a day. Most artists will make their professional debut by the time they are 18 years of age. After joining the company, a typical dancer continues with several hours of daily classes for his or her entire career. A dancer may move abruptly from an off-season routine of 2 hours' daily training to a rehearsal schedule of 10 or more hours a day.[5] The maintenance of strength, stamina, and flexibility is countered by the stress of

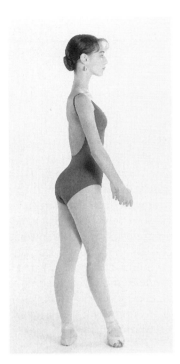

Fig. 42-1. In the fourth position, the feet are turned outward so that the heels and toes are in line, forming a square.

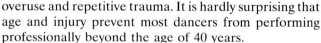

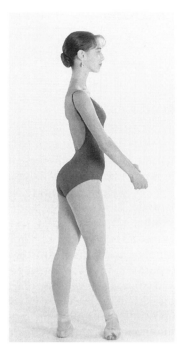

Fig. 42-2. By increasing the lumbar lordosis, the external rotation of the forward leg can be significantly increased.

overuse and repetitive trauma. It is hardly surprising that age and injury prevent most dancers from performing professionally beyond the age of 40 years.

Thirty minutes of work at the barre, usually consisting of warm-up and stretching exercises, is followed by center work, often the same pattern of exercise performed without the support of a rail. All ballet movements and variations begin and end with the five basic leg positions: "Through them, all other movement is strained; to them it all returns."[16] Movements of the arms and trunk are carefully controlled and modified in terms of the particular school of ballet. Jumps, lifts, and turns place additional and variable loads on the dancer's spine. Studies indicate that classical ballet exceeds even professional football in terms of the mental and physical demands of athletic performance.[15,28] Sammarco[33] describes the dancer "as highly conditioned as the gymnast, as controlled as a high wire artist, as powerful as a weightlifter, and as agile as a running back." In dance, however, the emphasis on artistic effect takes precedence over the physical requirements, and dancing through pain is expected. Ballet dancers see themselves as artists, not athletes, and that can lead to injury.[11]

PATTERNS OF BACK INJURY

Most mechanical back pain in the general population is aggravated by postural strain, weak abdominal muscles, and poor trunk support. In the well-conditioned athlete, low back pain tends to relate more to the

particular sport.[31] Back injuries occur in all stages of a dancer's career. Although difficulties with the hip and knee are typical of the young dancer, and leg and foot complaints are heard most frequently from older performers, back problems affect all ages and levels of skill. They are common in both male and female dancers, although male dancers show a slightly higher incidence.

Dancers are committed to hazard. With every performance there is the risk of artistic failure, momentary loss of control, or the danger of an accident. Although injury can result from a single twist, lift, or fall, most dancers report problems related to repeated minor trauma. Even when the degree of physical damage is limited, the impact of a back injury can curtail performances for months or even an entire season.

Young dancers present a specific problem. There is a decrease in flexibility during the adolescent growth spurt, and in the spine this may create an increased tendency to lordosis. When these factors are combined with poor training, inadequate trunk muscle endurance, and an overly demanding schedule, back pain becomes almost inevitable.

Paradoxically, the hypermobility sought so aggressively by the dancers may be part of the problem.[9] Poor posture with excessive lordosis, particularly in the novice, is commonly associated with low back pain. This curvature of the low back is not fixed; rather, it occurs dynamically with attempts to increase external rotation of the hip or with a poorly controlled lift. These dancers can hold a pelvic tilt when instructed to do so, but excessive spinal mobility, poor muscle control, and a lack of proper posture training permit the lordosis to return during lifts, turns, and jumps.

The effect of hypermobility on a dancer's future remains unclear. In a study of ballet dancers in South Africa, Klemp and Chalton[17] found significantly more hypermobile persons among dancers who had continued dancing than among those who had stopped. However, only 2 of 12 dancers who had progressed in their careers were hypermobile. Back pain in professional dancers cannot be attributed merely to loose joints.

The precise localization of any pathologic condition producing back pain is controversial, and the literature on soft tissue back injury and the specific causes of back pain presents a varied and confusing picture.[12,18,19,21,24] Specifically relating the problem to ballet is further hampered by the fact that most orthopaedic interest in this group has centered on injuries to the lower limbs and feet. Back pain is often relegated to the discussion of "other injuries" or may not be mentioned at all. Yet back pain remains a significant problem in the dance population.[23] The strain of maintaining extremes of posture with apparent ease while repeatedly leaping and, more significantly, landing and twisting takes its toll. In ballet the spine plays primarily a supporting role, particularly for the male dancer involved in frequent partnering. For this group, low back pain is a common complaint.

According to Ende and Wickstrom,[7] most injuries occur when the dancer is older, overtired, ill, out of practice, or coping with poor working conditions. Typically, dancers are at greatest risk when they attempt difficult maneuvers while still perfecting the technique. Wright,[41] in a 4-year review of dance injuries at the National Ballet of Canada, found back problems constituted 27% of all injuries. He noted that most back injuries occurred during rehearsals. Dancers typically attributed the pain to an inadequate warm-up or overuse. Bowling,[3] in a survey for the National Organization of Dance and Mime in the United Kingdom, found the back and neck to be the single most common site of injury, accounting for 15% of the total. Again, dancers blamed overwork, fatigue, and insufficient warm-up. Poor floors, drafty environments, demanding choreography, and the repetition of difficult movements were also mentioned. As in Wright's series, half the dancers who suffered back injuries reported continuing difficulties after returning to regular performances.

There appears to be little to be gained by reviewing the accepted or disputed sources of back pain. By focusing not on specific spinal problems but on the typical patterns of pain, a clearer picture begins to emerge.[8] Documenting the nature of onset, duration of attack, and location of the dominant pain is of greater practical value than establishing a radiologic or even anatomic diagnosis.[26,27] Identifying the common mecha-

nisms of injury, such as faulty lifting techniques, provides immediate direction to the management of the problem. Understanding the aggravating factors inherent in the performance of classical ballet is essential to understanding the complaints of the individual dancer. Discovering the postures, positions, or activities that provide relief is the first step in formulating effective treatment.

Discogenic Back Pain

Discogenic back pain is typically back dominant and aggravated by flexion or lifting. Attacks persist for weeks or months before gradually subsiding. Although the specific problem within the disc is still subject to controversy, there is agreement that large portions of the disc and the adjacent ligaments are pain sensitive.[37] It is generally accepted that repetitive stress on the disc is associated with an increased incidence of pain, although there is no correlation between individual episodes of back pain and the radiologic evidence of disc degeneration.

Thomasen,[36] discussing 20 years of experience as an orthopaedic surgeon for ballet dancers, reports that the average age for onset of symptomatic lumbar disc degeneration is 30 years. He notes an equal incidence in male and female dancers. Micheli[22] believes that discogenic low back pain is a problem predominantly in male dancers and is associated with lifting. Dunn[4] considers

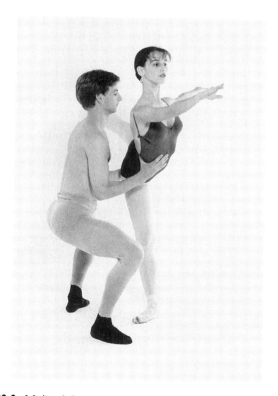

Fig. 42-3. Maintaining an erect posture by using the abdominal and thigh muscles not only improves the appearance of the performance, but also reduces strain on the low back.

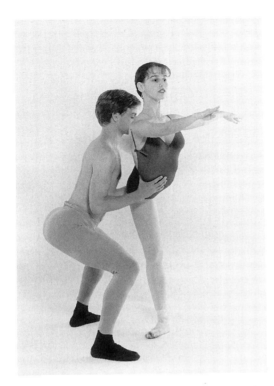

Fig. 42-4. Excessive forward bending while the back is arched compensates for weakness in the trunk and lower limbs. Frequent lifting from this position has been identified as a cause of back pain in male dancers.

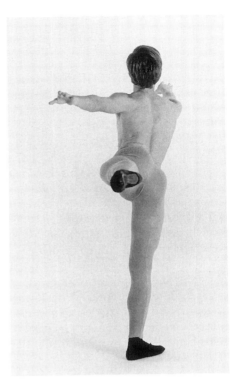

Fig. 42-5. The arabesque requires external rotation of the elevated leg while the torso is held forward from the waist.

discogenic problems more common in male dancers because of their need to lift repetitively from a forward bent position. Although back injury can result from a single event, most back problems in dancers develop more gradually through repetitive minor trauma. Continual overuse places recurring stress on the disc and may be a factor in accelerating the degenerative process (Figs. 42-3 and 42-4).

Facet Syndrome

There is a group of dancers in whom back-dominant pain is produced primarily by repetitive extension. The pattern of pain in this group, sudden short-lived attacks separated by periods of normal function, is significantly different from the pattern in those considered to have discogenic problems. Currently there is again debate about the role of the posterior element complex as an alternate site of back pain, but there is no doubt that more than one discrete pattern of pain exists within the population of professional ballet dancers.[14]

Again, focusing on the pattern, rather than on the presumed anatomic site of the pain, provides a clearer picture of dance-related back injuries. Bachrach[1] notes that repeated hyperextension produces typical "pinching" pain in the low back. He also notes that this is most common in those dancers who have already developed a

hyperlordosis to compensate for restricted external rotation of the hip. Both Dunn and Thomasen describe similar episodic low back pain associated with frequent hyperextension.[6,36]

Ironically, a balanced lumbar lordosis not only is beneficial in reducing excessive load on the apophyseal joints, but also is essential for a correct performance appearance. Particularly in movements such as the arabesque or attitude, or in lifting a partner, proper technique demands a "neutral" lumbar curve. An apparent increase in turnout of the leg can be effected by increasing the lumbar lordosis (Figs. 42-5 and 42-6). Cheating in this fashion not only increases the risk of injury to the posterior elements and the incidence of low back pain, but also prevents the development of good basic techniques, which, in turn, will restrict future progress.

Bony Lesions

With the demands of classical ballet on the spine, it is not surprising that the incidence of spondylolysis and spondylolisthesis is greater in dancers than in the general population.[35] The reported frequency among dancers approaches that seen in elite gymnasts.[34] The sudden onset of back pain while the spine is held in forced extension, particularly if the dancer is standing on one

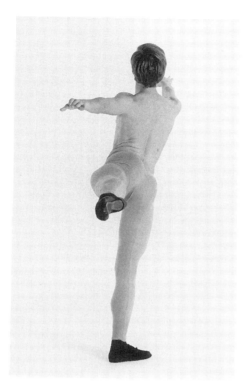

Fig. 42-6. Hyperextension can be used to compensate for limited external rotation at the hip. This "trick" may interfere with further improvement in the dancer's techniques.

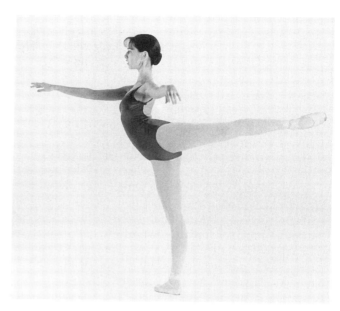

Fig. 42-7. The performance of an arabesque requires the extension of the lumbar spine, which places stress on the posterior elements. The sudden onset of pain while the dancer holds this position is typical of an acute traumatic spondylolysis.

foot, such as in the arabesque position, is highly suggestive of an acute traumatic spondylolysis (Fig. 42-7). The dancer with a unilateral defect finds that standing on the ipsilateral leg produces the most pain. A reduced range of forward movement, localized back pain increased with extension, and normal findings on neurologic examination support the diagnosis.[30] In contrast to the patterns of pain considered to arise in the disc or facet, for which no pathologic condition can be objectively demonstrated, acute spondylolysis can be verified on x-ray film or with a bone scan.

Micheli[22] notes that although other types of dance place less physical demand on the spine, all dancers share an increased incidence of spondylolysis. He attributes this in part to the role of classical ballet in most dancers' training. Thomasen anecdotally reports on 17 dancers with spondylolysis and spondylolisthesis. In his small series the lesion is twice as common in women and occurs most often at L4.

The presence of an acute unilateral and even bilateral spondylolysis does not necessarily indicate instability. It is not unusual to identify an old, symptom-free lysis in the x-ray film of a mature dancer. The acute episode, associated with positive findings on bone scan, will make dancing difficult and is an indication for treatment but does not mark the inevitable end of a dancer's career.

Fractures of the pars interarticularis are a relatively common cause of low back pain in dancers, but stress fractures can occur in other areas. Ireland and Micheli[13] reported a stress fracture of both pedicles of the second lumbar vertebra in an 18-year-old female dancer. Weiker[40] reported that dancers in the American Ballet Theater have more stress fractures than those dancers who performed with the New York City Ballet. He attributes this to the fact that dancers with the American Ballet have a more aggressive style and spend more time on the road, dancing on hard, unsprung floors.

An increased incidence of scoliosis has been identified in female dancers. Warren[38] believes there is a relationship between delayed menarche and secondary amenorrhea. She also notes a high familial incidence. Decreased upper-to-lower body ratios and a long arm span—features that are coveted as representing the ideal body form in classical ballet—may be inherited traits associated with scoliosis. Warren et al.[39] point out that these physical characteristics are not as marked in the mothers and nondancing sisters of ballet artists.

Nerve Root Involvement

Unlike the back-dominant pain pattern that typifies presumed disc or posterior element involvement, the leg-dominant pain accompanying direct nerve root compression is frequently associated with a documented pathologic condition. Still, many dancers suffering primarily leg pain receive no definitive diagnosis, and their management is equally nonspecific. Thomasen gives a personal account of 53 dancers with acute sciatica. The levels of involvement and response to treatment were similar to those expected in the general population. Micheli[21] does not make a significant differentiation between discogenic problems with or without sciatica. He reports that both are more common in male dancers. Standard treatment is recommended.

This conventional management of acute sciatica illustrates the typical inconsistency in the medical approach to dance injuries. If a pathologic condition of the spine can be objectively identified, the diagnosis and treatment follow conventional lines, with no special relevance to the demands of the art form. Only when the trauma is less well defined are the unique mechanisms of dance injury and the special character of the dancer taken into account. Neither conventional nor dance-oriented management is optimal. With so many divergent opinions, there will be no consensus on any etiology that cannot be demonstrated irrefutably. Without a proven diagnosis, the practitioner's personal preference and the dancer's immediate subjective response may be the only relevant factors.

Muscular Strain and Sacroiliac Pain

A tradition of performance has bred a tradition of injury. Ligament sprains and strains, muscle pulls, chronic tendinitis, and abnormal painful sacroiliac movement are the classic unproven diagnoses. Miller et al.[23] note that minor spinal injuries are frequent and that degeneration of the sacroiliac joint and low back pain are commonly identified problems. No definitive etiology is indicated. Wright found that all the back injuries recorded in his study of the National Ballet of Canada, except for one case of spondylolysis, were diagnosed as trauma to the soft tissues. Half of those dancers treated for back pain continued to complain of recurrent problems after returning to a full schedule.

Typical of the uncritical reporting of nonspecific back pain in dancers is this account of Thomasen, who describes sacroiliac pain in a 20-year-old female dancer. Radiographic findings were normal, and an injection of local anesthetic produced no relief: "Later she had a myelogram in Norway and after the injection of contrast fluid she had an epileptic fit. When she woke up, the pain had disappeared and she was able to dance again."[36]

Micheli[22] notes that undifferentiated pain in the low back is the most frequent back disorder encountered in the young dancer and that the source of this pain is usually a diagnosis of exclusion. He also notes an association between nonspecific low back pain and hyperlordotic posturing that may reflect both an anatomic malalignment and muscle-tendon imbalance.

Bachrach attributes most dance injuries to overuse and believes they are frequently associated with pro-

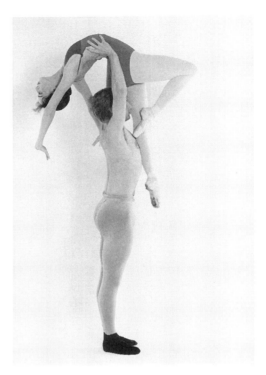

Fig. 42-8. A combination of strength and flexibility make a difficult maneuver appear graceful and effortless. The demands on the lumbar spines of both dancers are obvious.

found weakness of the iliopsoas. The condition that he calls "the psoas insufficiency syndrome" is accompanied by an increased lumbar lordosis and fixed flexion of the hips. Depending on whether the lower limb is fixed or free, the psoas functions as either an internal or an external rotator of the femur. A tight iliopsoas restricts external rotation of the hip during weight bearing, a deficiency for which the dancer compensates through increased lumbar lordosis (Fig. 42-8). The action of the psoas is countered on the posterior pelvis by the pull of the gluteus maximus and the hamstrings, and anteriorly by the abdominal muscles. Maintaining muscle balance becomes an important aspect in minimizing low back strain.

As a resident physiotherapist for the Royal Ballet Company of London, Dunn believed that muscle strain or tear was by far the most common injury causing low back pain in dancers. In her work she also mentions overstretching of the spinal ligaments but describes no specific anatomic pathology.

Both the extreme specificity of psoas insufficiency and the vague generality of a muscle tear or ligament strain are typical of back pain diagnoses in the dancer. In the absence of any opportunity for objective measurement or histologic examination, the experience and bias of the observer take precedence in formulating a diagnosis.

TREATMENT

The same lack of objectivity that typifies diagnosis of dance-related back injuries is reflected in the standard approach to treatment. In the absence of a clear pathologic condition, symptom relief becomes the only objective. Although this is not an inappropriate goal, it is an approach open to easy abuse.

The demands of ballet on the dancer's back are not generally appreciated within the medical community. Not every physician understands the total commitment required to excel in this profession nor the impact that this obsession has on the dancer's life-style. Advice on modifying the job or increasing physical fitness, suitable for the general population or in an industrial setting, is often inappropriate when applied to the professional dancer.

The void created by general medical disinterest in dance-related back injury and the lack of definitive information is filled with a variety of conflicting opinions. With little or no objective confirmation, trainers, exercise therapists, kinesiologists, physical therapists, chiropractors, and osteopathic physicians present the dancer with a seemingly endless array of contradictory information. In the United States it is estimated that 20,000 dance students audition each year for schools affiliated with professional companies. With growing interest in dance and ballet, and with no uniformity to the treatment approach, the field of back care for dancers is fertile ground for self-proclaimed gurus and experts.

Typical of these contradictions are the discussions on the relationship between scoliosis and ballet. Does dance training cause the deformity? Is there a relation to the dancer's intense level of physical activity before puberty? Dancers with scoliosis have been shown to have a significant increase in delayed menarche compared with those without a curvature of the spine. A link, although not verified statistically, has been noted between scoliosis and secondary amenorrhea in dancers. Other related factors include increased height, deviant eating behavior, and, perhaps most significantly, a 28% incidence of scoliosis in the families of the affected dancers. This compares with a familial incidence of 4% for those who had no abnormal curvature.

Because of their ability to control posture and body movement and their extreme motivation, many dancers with mild to moderate degrees of scoliosis continue to perform while completely masking the spinal deformity. Although there is no evidence to relate specific ballet movements to the development or elimination of scoliosis, it has nevertheless been suggested that ballet could be used as part of the management for patients with a slight curvature.[2] When scoliosis must be treated, conventional therapies range from intermittent bracing to instrumented fusions. Unfortunately, the latter will, in all probability, end the dancer's career.

The world of the classical ballet artist is a circum-

scribed one.[32] Through training, extreme motivation, and absolute commitment to their art, professional dancers learn that they are unique and different from other people. Peer pressure is a major influence. Medical intervention is viewed at best as a necessary intrusion. Dancers within a company are very quick to share information regarding successful therapies. Individual practitioners may find themselves suddenly in vogue and equally rapidly out of favor on the basis of their success in the management of a single performer. This dissemination of information also leads to the widespread use of self-administered medication, principally nonsteroidal antiinflammatory agents. Dancers will avoid formal medical contact for fear, often justified, that the physician's recommendations will include instructions to stop dancing. Any choice between accepting a medically imposed limitation and continuing to perform is no choice at all.

Objectives

Given the dancer's intense devotion to perfection, the required level of physical activity, and the typically heavy schedule, a primary objective of treatment is immediate pain control with no loss of performance time. This short-term demand focuses attention on short-term goals, occasionally to the detriment of long-term health concerns. The liberal use of antiinflammatory drugs, both oral and injectable, and regular reliance on analgesic medication are commonplace. Satisfying the immediate professional needs of these artists while protecting them from lasting injury is the challenge of dance medicine. When the medical profession cannot fill the demand, the dancer turns quickly to other sources, often discarding various opinions until finding one that satisfies an established preconception. With their somatic preoccupation, dancers require physical explanations for their pain and loss of ability. Providing a clear, concise, and mechanistic answer is an important objective. Dancers accept pain as an inevitable accompaniment of their art. Understanding makes it bearable.

Methods

Good dance medicine is beneficial compromise. Convincing the dancer to accept proper treatment implies agreement between the artist and the physician on what is "proper." The dancer's desire to continue dancing without interruption must be balanced against valid medical concerns.

Because most back pain is a self-limiting problem, with most cases showing spontaneous recovery within a matter of weeks, the treatment of back pain abounds with placebo cures. With the emphasis on rapid pain relief, modalities offering only transient comfort may be imbued with unjustified healing properties. Dancers lack medical sophistication and readily accept quasiscientific explanations. There is scant need for treatment selectivity inasmuch as there appears to be little or no correlation between the presumed diagnosis, the physical problem, and the effect of therapy. The indiscriminate and repetitive use of ice, ultrasound, and interferential current is the norm. A variety of electrical devices and various forms of cold laser have their advocates. In the absence of any clear guidelines and recognizing the unique nature of the demands on the dancer's back, one clinic recommends the application of ultrasound well above the manufacturer's recommended levels. There is, of course, no way to know whether this procedure produces a therapeutic response well above the manufacturer's expectations. On the basis of peer pressure and anecdotal reporting, most dancers demand a pragmatic approach. They have no interest in the lack of evidence that any of this equipment has benefit beyond the placebo effect. Refusing to employ passive modalities serves no purpose except to send the dancer to another practitioner. Combining passive modalities with appropriate stretching and therapeutic exercise can be effective. Something as simple as heat, cold, and firm bandaging may reduce the dancer's symptoms to a point where performance is possible.

Medication is frequently taken in excess. The reasoning is that if a little is good, more is clearly better. With the short-term objective in sight, physicians often recommend brief courses of an antiinflammatory agent or intermittent use of an analgesic to maintain high performance levels. The dancers themselves readily accept medication as a means of sustaining their abilities. Like the physical modalities, drugs are often taken well above recommended levels. Miller and colleagues describe a dancer who was taking 21 self-prescribed medications and had been using phenylbutazone continuously for 5 years.

For dancers whose problem is more back than leg pain and whose symptoms are aggravated by forward bending or lifting—classically a discogenic pattern—treatment should include both passive and active extension exercise. Bed rest has little appeal, and there is little compliance with the prescription. Exercise to increase the strength and endurance of the trunk muscles is more readily accepted. A lack of success with manipulation has been attributed to the dancer's normally increased spinal mobility. Although there is no biomechanical rationale, Dunn reports anecdotally cases of symptom relief with repeated manual traction on one or both of the dancer's legs.

Although dancers train for many hours a day, they do not spend all their time in the studio. It may be possible to alter a forward-flexed posture to minimize symptoms during classes and rehearsals, but changes in the actual performance are considerably more difficult to achieve. Symptom relief may be possible only after the performance is over. Education in good back care, the use of a small roll or cushion when sitting, and an awareness of the relationship between low back posture and pain can help to reduce the duration of a painful episode and promote recovery in spite of an uninterrupted schedule.

Whether or not the posterior elements are the source, repetitive hyperextension can produce back pain. As with the common discogenic pattern—namely pain produced by repetitive flexion—altering posture and strengthening support muscles should be integral components of treatment for extension pain. In this group good basic dance training is essential. The use of increased lumbar lordosis to gain apparent external rotation at the hip is a self-defeating strategy.

The identification of a traumatic spondylolysis is often possible on clinical grounds with the typically sudden onset of back pain aggravated with extension, particularly when the dancer is standing on one leg. This acute injury, verified with positive findings on bone scan, should be treated with what Weiker described as "aggressive protection," including the use of a total contact orthosis and a modified exercise program emphasizing abdominal strengthening and antilordotic posturing. The intensity of treatment depends on the age of the dancer and the duration of symptoms. The younger performer with a recent onset of pain should receive the most active therapy.

The treatment of acute sciatica in the professional dancer follows conventional lines. Direct nerve root compression, with or without clinical evidence of conduction loss, generally produces symptoms felt most acutely in the leg. Because most patients with nerve root involvement will recover fully without surgery, an extensive conservative program is warranted. This includes relative rest with limited performances, modified classwork, and, for the male dancers, no lifting. Brief periods of bed rest, short-term bracing, and medication all have a role. As the acute episode subsides, the nonoperative treatment expands to a closely supervised physical rehabilitation program with emphasis on strengthening the torso muscles and maintaining a neutral lordosis.

Muscular sprains and strains are the most common sources of the dancer's painful back. In the absence of any structural damage and with no evidence of neurologic involvement, the management of muscular backache reflects the prevailing diversity of opinion. Heat, cold, and the entire gamut of modalities are called into play. Traction and manipulation vie with training and exercise as the treatments of choice. In dealing with such a transient capricious problem, the acceptance of any treatment depends largely on the enthusiasm of the practitioner and the prevailing opinion among the dancers. In the absence of any objective criteria, there can be no single solution. Regardless of the "definitive" therapy, however, treatment must also include extended warm-up and cool down periods, ample stretching routines, the liberal use of counterirritants and massage, and convincing psychologic support.

The contact forces of the facet joints on the two sides of the body change, as seen in cadaver studies. As the spine rotates to the right (thoracic spine counterclockwise and lumbar spine clockwise), the left facet joints are in tight contact; and as the spine rotates to the left (thoracic spine clockwise and lumbar spine counterclockwise), the right facet joints are in tight contact. Farfan[3] has shown that the resistance of the facets to torsional loads equals the entire torsional load of the annulus. The annulus must be designed to survive the rhythmic load presented to it. Gracovetsky[6] has shown that the orientation of the annulus collagen fibers is ideally designed to resist torsional loads. A pressurized nucleus is not essential to maintenance of the compression strength of the spinal motion segment. Traditional thought on the role of the annulus has been that of a retaining wall of a high-pressured nucleus. However, in vitro studies have shown that the role of the annulus is more important in resisting torsional stresses.[1,2] Farfan[3] found that by removing a 2-cm portion of the posterior annulus, there was a concomitant 25% decrease in its torque strength.

Lateral bending of the spine also varies with the running cycle. It bends to the left between the left foot heel strike and right foot toe-off, and to the right between the right foot heel strike and left foot toe-off. The strong, springlike facet joints help to derotate the spine even in light of the relatively high coefficient of disc viscosity. Potential energy is converted to kinetic energy (resulting in motion) between the heel strike and toe-off. Concomitantly, there is loss of energy between the toe-off and heel-strike. Cappozo[1,2] and then Thurston and Harris[9] observed the motion of the lumbar spine in the lateral and sagittal plane and divided the motion by 5 to obtain the average displacement of each lumbar segment. (Their assumption that there is equal motion at all the spinal segments was partially incorrect.) These results correlated with the average mechanical work needed to overcome inertia during locomotion. There were minimal changes in axial inertia during the running cycle; there were slightly more changes in sagittal inertia. The most significant changes were in lateral inertia. For example, at the L4 level the body had to produce 8 W of power to overcome the sagittal inertia from heel strike to toe-off. However, there was a release of 2 W of power during the remainder of the cycle as a result of the spring motion of the facet joints.

The recovery of the facet joints is coupled to the viscosity of the intervertebral disc. Farfan correlated the intervertebral disc viscosity to facet motion in vitro. With the high disc viscosity, as in runners with young healthy discs, there was more energy-absorbing capacity of the annulus to loads in axial, lateral, and sagittal planes. This helps the facet joints in their springlike action. With low disc viscosity, as in runners with degenerated or injured discs, the energy-absorbing capacity is decreased (although it never reaches zero), and this interferes with the facet joints' spring action. Although it cannot be determined where the power lost during portions of the gait goes, most of it must be used in the elastic deformation of the lumbodorsal fascia and used to help rotate the pelvis during the coupled motion. It is clinically relevant that with injury to the spinal motion segment, such as with an injured facet joint or disc, the carefully balanced segmental motion of the spine is disrupted and performance must be deaminized.

The back muscles play a critical role during gait. Although in vivo data on the exact tension in the ligamentous structures versus the tension of muscles are not available, electromyographic (EMG) data suggest that several important changes occur during running. At right heel strike, the right multifidus, rotators, iliocostalis lumborum, longissimus thoracis, iliocostalis thoracis, rectus abdominis, external oblique, gluteus maximus, and left psoas muscles are firing. These same groups of muscles on the opposite side of the body are firing as the foot on that side hits the ground. It is important to note that the psoas has two distinct peaks in the EMG at heel strike that correspond with the two actions of this muscle: to restore the rotational spinal position and to correct spinal lordosis. The multifidus and longissimus act as lateral flexors of the spine. For example, the left multifidus and longissimus have peak activity at left heel strike. This acts to bend the spine to the left. After toe-off, lateral bending changes direction and the opposite multifidus and longissimus fire strongly. During midswing, however, there is activity in the multifidus and longissimus on both sides—the spine is relatively neutral. The importance of these observations is obvious, since an injury or weakness of the back muscles can impair running. Rehabilitation of a runner is dependent on restoration of proper trunk muscle strength.

By allowing greater flexion of the lumbar spine, the relative extension of the hips is increased during midsupport—when the supporting leg is directly under the body. The lumbar spine effectively participates in the coordinated extension of the hip, knee, ankle, and foot; and this provides the extension thrust during the takeoff part of the stance phase of running. Therefore the lumbar spine starts in a relatively flexed position during the time of midsupport. During landing the lumbar spine is in a relatively extended position. In addition to sagittal motion, there is axial rotation of the spine during running. The spine undergoes axial rotation in a manner wherein the lower spinal segments rotate backward with extension of the trailing leg (takeoff); concomitantly, the upper spinal segments rotate forward. A pattern has been described in which axial rotation is combined with lateral bending so that the spinous processes point in the same direction as the lateral bending. If the spinal motion were axial rotation alone without any lateral bending, then greater efficiency would be provided by the spine in a relatively straight, rodlike contour.

However, because the motion of the spine is lateral bending coupled with axial rotation, there must be a curvature or lordosis to the lumbar spine. Lowett first described this in 1903. During rehabilitation from injury, it is important to regain this lordosis either surgically or by exercises such as pelvic tilt exercises.

BODY POSTURE

The body's posture during different periods of running changes to accommodate for track conditions, endurance, and speed. In a pure track speed race, only speed and endurance are necessary. Therefore the center of gravity of the runner is not affected by frequent turning, tackling, or changing cadence. The trunk posture is upright, and the feet are relatively close together under the body and in line with the progression of motion. The trunk muscles play an important role in maintaining an erect posture. In a contact sport such as football, on the other hand, the center of gravity is constantly changing with contact and with the changing direction of movement. In these latter circumstances the trunk is relatively low, with the lumbar spine in more flexion. The feet are more widely spaced to allow greater stability in meeting the needs of lateral motion and in changing the direction of motion. It is important to note that the direction of movement can change only when one foot is in contact with the ground. Therefore when the particular requirements of a sport require continuously changing direction or cadence, relatively greater time must be spent in the stance phase of running.

The position of the pelvis has been described as controlling not only the motion of the hip relative to the ground, but also the motion of the lumbar spine. Forward rotation of the pelvis (clockwise on lateral view) results in extension of the lumbar spine to a swayback, lordotic position. There is a concomitant increase in internal rotation of the thighs, a lowering of the longitudinal arch of the foot, a decrease in the ability to flex the hip, and a shift in the center of gravity, allowing the metatarsal heads to bear more weight. This is important in the touchdown part of the stance phase of running. However, the more erect posture with the flexed, flat-backed position of the lumbar spine is accompanied by a backward rotation of the pelvis and extension of the foot and ankle. This is important in the lift-off part of the stance phase of running, since it allows maximum backward thrust by the trailing leg.

FOOTWEAR

The importance of the biomechanics of the spine during running has been stressed. In particular, the rotation of the pelvis is the key to proper counterrotation of the spine during running. For all practical purposes, the lower limb rotation is directly translated to the pelvis during heel strike. The locking and unlocking mechanism of the hind foot is related to the degree of supination and pronation: during supination the hind foot is locked and rigid, and during pronation it is flexible and soft. The locking and unlocking process is principally responsible for the impact absorption during running. Proper footwear should allow good heel cushion during impact yet also allow good heel control. Shoes should have flexibility at the natural midfoot break. Any deficiency in footwear that causes the lower limb to malrotate the pelvis can alter the tightly coordinated spinal motion, resulting in low back pain or decreased performance. Leg length inequalities that significantly alter the level of the hemipelvis can alter the spinal mechanics. Many authors have suggested that minor leg length inequalities need correction. They base this suggestion on the fact that long-distance marathon runners with low back pain often have a slight leg length inequality. However, if we consider that leg length inequality of up to 2 cm is physiologic, this correction may not help the runner with back pain, and other sources should be explored.

BACK INJURIES

As previously mentioned, running differs from walking in that during running, an airborne phase alternates with a support phase. Because of the airborne phase, considerable impact must be absorbed at foot strike. Each foot essentially collides with the ground 50 to 70 times/min or 800 to 2000 times/mile. Depending on the running speed, each of these collisions results in a force equal to two to four times the body weight that must be absorbed. Failure to absorb this force properly through external (shoes) and internal (sequential biomechanics of the lower limb, pelvis, and back) means is likely to result in an overuse injury. Variations in the anatomic structure, anthropometric proportions, muscle strength, state of training, and posture account for many individuals being more susceptible to shock absorption injuries than others.

During running, the initial impact is absorbed by the foot, ankle, and knee joint, as well as by the supporting musculotendinous units. Segmental articulation of the lower extremity to a mobile lumbar spinal-pelvic unit functions to continue absorption and dissipation of the forces. An erect trunk favors mobility of the lumbar spinal-pelvic unit to maintain postural equilibrium. Sequential timing allows the body to control a smooth, undulating sagittal path for the center of gravity. Any interference with sequential timing, particularly of foot supination and pronation, transfers abnormal stress up the chain and may result in a back injury.

A well-cushioned shoe and a heel-toe gait offer the best absorption. Conversely, forefoot running on concrete and running up and down curbs exaggerates the shock to the feet, legs, and back. Uphill and downhill running may both have detrimental effects on the back. During uphill running, flexion of the lumbar spine tilts the pelvis anteriorly, thereby limiting hip flexion and putting greater stress on the low back muscles. Downhill running results in hyperextension of the lumbar spine and a posterior pelvic tilt that may cause low back pain. Downhill running also increases the impact at heel strike.

During walking, the inability to dissipate forces at one location has been shown to result in overload at the next joint as the forces ascend toward the skull. These forces can be expected to be magnified with running. An initial injury to a distal area, such as an ankle or foot in runners, may interfere mechanically with the dissipation of locomotor forces, thereby contributing to the development of more proximal injuries. In runners, back injury is commonly seen in combination with at least one other injury. In one study it was found that 87% of triathletes with a back injury also had a knee, thigh, ankle, or foot injury. Since triathletes frequently continue to train despite being injured, a case can be made for the progression of injury up the kinetic chain. If an alteration is made in body alignment because of injury, the ability to dissipate forces is also altered. Most reports of overuse injuries in runners find no clear association with training distances or pace, suggesting that training practices by themselves are unlikely to cause a back injury in a previously healthy runner. Conversely, it seems likely that once an injury has occurred, continued running will exacerbate the primary condition and contribute to additional injuries. Thus both intrinsic (body alignment and shock absorption) and extrinsic (training-related) factors play a role in the pathogenesis of overuse injuries to the back in runners.

A prevailing concept is that most low back pain and sciatica are the result of degenerative disc disease. Back pain in runners is no different and can most often be attributed to some previously existing condition, to age-related degenerative changes in the lumbar spine, or to poor conditioning of the musculotendinous structures, all of which limit the ability to cope with the repeated mechanical stress of running. It is not unusual for back pain to become manifest in the middle-aged runner,

particularly after increasing mileage or hill training. Running, with its inherent need for shock absorption, cannot protect against the degenerative process and may very well accelerate the process. This finding is consistent with the observation that running exacerbates the problem of low back pain in most athletes.

PREVENTION OF INJURY

As with prevention of any overuse injury, common sense is the most important factor. An individual with a preexisting back problem would be well advised to choose an activity other than running for the maintenance of fitness and perhaps as a competitive outlet. For example, swimming has been reported to maintain fitness of triathletes without worsening an existing back injury. Likewise, a more distal injury, such as an ankle tendinitis, may alter running biomechanics and interfere mechanically with the appropriate dissipation of forces. Running should be avoided until the distal injury has completely healed.

REFERENCES

1. Cappozzo A: The forces and couples in the human trunk during level walking, *J Biomech* 16:265, 1983.
2. Cappozzo A: Compressive loads in the lumbar vertebral column during normal level walking, *J Orthop Res* 1:292, 1984.
3. Farfan H: The torsional injury of the lumbar spine, *Spine* 9:714, 1984.
4. Farfan H, Kirkaldy-Willis W: The present status of spinal fusion in the treatment of lumbar intervertebral joint disorder, *Clin Orthop* 158:198, 1981.
5. Floyd W, Silver P: The function of erector spinae muscles in certain movements and postures in man, *J Physiol* 120:184, 1955.
6. Gracovetsky S: An hypothesis for the role of the spine in human locomotion: a challenge to current thinking, *J Biomed Eng* 7:205, 1985.
7. Inman T, Ralston J, Todd F: *Human walking,* Baltimore, 1981, Williams & Wilkins.
8. Silver P: Direct observation of changes in tension in the supraspinous and interspinous ligaments during flexion and extension of the vertebral column in man, *J Anat* 88:550, 1954.
9. Thurston A, Harris J: Normal kinematics of the lumbar spine and pelvis, *Spine* 8:199, 1983.
10. Thurston A, Whittle M: Spinal and pelvic movement during walking—a new method of study, *N Engl J Med* 10:219, 1981.

Chapter Forty-Four

Track and Field

Jeffrey A. Saal

Although track and field participants frequently have low back pain, only sporadic reports about their injuries have appeared in the medical literature. At present there are no data on the incidence of lumbar spine injuries in athletes participating in track and field events. However, low back pain appears to contribute to loss of competition time for these athletes.

Track and field–related lumbar spine injury subtypes are determined by the biomechanics required by the athletic event coupled with the pathologic state. Repetitive motions that combine flexion and rotation can lead to annular tears of the intervertebral disc. These tears may evolve into gradual disc prolapse or may lead to internal degeneration of the disc. Annular injuries of the intervertebral disc cause altered functional biomechanics of the spinal segment, resulting in nociceptive input that will synapse in the dorsal root ganglion (DRG). This synapsing may then lead to efferent discharges from the DRG, causing erector spinal contraction. Moreover, DRG stimulation is capable of producing spinal zone pain that radiates into regions of the back, buttocks, hips, thighs, calves, ankles, and feet, resulting in soft tissue contractures of the gluteal musculature, hip rotators, hamstrings, hip flexor, and calf musculature. Torsional disc injuries can cause a lumbar list and create pelvic torsion. When these phenomena are coupled with musculotendinous contractures, an obvious alteration in spinal biomechanics will ensue. Asymmetric stride lengths and unbalanced axial rotation of spinal segments result in synchronous motion patterns that may lead to a decrement in competitive efficiency and to the persistence of lumbar pain syndromes.

The intervertebral disc is more likely to be injured during training for track and field events than in competition. The major culprit is probably the technique used in weight training. In my experience, improperly performed free bar squats and seated, low-pulley cable rows are the most problematic for athletes. Problems result from inadequate attention to technique, and overzealous training regimens may also be responsible.

Repetitive hyperextension or repetitive torsion, coupled with hyperextension, causes the posterior spinal elements to be injured. Improper pole planting during a pole vaulting attempt can cause facet injuries or neural arch stress fractures (e.g., spondylolysis). Javelin competitors are also at risk for posterior-element injuries because of repetitive hyperextension and rotation.

Lower extremity stretching exercises are a potential cause for intervertebral disc injury. Improper technique during the hamstring stretch can lead to excessive flexional loading of the intervertebral disc. Repetitive flexional loading, of which the classic hurdle stretch is a particularly good example, can lead to fatigue breakdown of the annular collagen. Therefore alternative stretching exercises that are spine-safe must be taught.

Injury prevention starts with an adequate understanding by the coaching staff of dynamic lumbar muscle stabilization. Stabilization is a technique that helps avoid most of the low back injuries encountered in track and field athletes. Clinics on injury prevention enable coaches to learn this valuable technique (Fig. 44-1).

CASE STUDIES

Each case study presented in this section provides an example of a lumbar injury subtype in typical track and field athletes. The case studies consist of a description of the history and physical examination, the identification of a mechanism of injury, a description of the differential diagnostic work-up, and a presentation of the rehabilitation plan.

CASE 1

History

A 21-year-old discus thrower had a 4-month history of left-sided lumbar pain in the waist that radiated to his buttocks during prolonged sitting (i.e., longer than 30 minutes). The athlete also experienced posterior thigh pain. Standing and walking relieved the pain in his buttocks, and he reported no night pain. After a warm-up period the intensity of the pain was reduced and the discus thrower was able to practice and compete. However, 2 or 3 hours after competition, he developed low back stiffness and buttock pain. Eventually his pain worsened, and he was unable to practice effectively. He was vying for a spot on the Olympic team, and the competitive season was only 8 weeks away. He reported three previous episodes of low back and buttock pain in the preceding 18 months, each of which persisted for 2 weeks. Each of the previous episodes was accompanied by a lumbar list to the right that the athlete described as the hip or pelvis "going out," causing him to lean to one side and develop a feeling that the left leg was shorter than the right. Although the previous episodes responded to manipulative treatment, this last occurrence did not respond, and he thought that the thigh pain developed subsequent to the manipulative treatment.

The first episode began 3 weeks after the athlete felt a pop in his back while he was performing a squat with moderately heavy weights. He thought that his spotter did not assist him

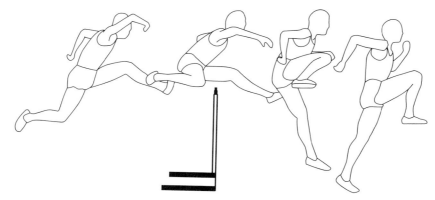

Fig. 44-1. Hurdler. Adequate hamstring and iliopsoas flexibility allows the athlete to hurdle while eliminating excessive lumbar flexion.

quickly enough, because he got too far forward on the left side and had difficulty correcting his position.

Findings of the remainder of the review of systems, past medical history, and surgical history were negative.

Physical Examination

Inspection during the physical examination revealed a slight pelvic list to the left with a loss of lumbar lordosis. Repetitive testing of forward flexion in the standing position reproduced the patient's back and buttock pain on the left side. There was no reversal of the lumbar curve during forward flexion. Lumbar extension caused back pain; however, list correction resulted in centralizing the pain when the athlete performed repetitive extension in the standing and prone positions. Straight leg raising to 90 degrees was painless on the right side, but straight leg raising to 60 degrees on the left side reproduced the patient's back pain. Concomitant ankle dorsiflexion caused tugging and burning sensations in the patient's posterior thigh and slight tingling in the dorsum of the left foot.

Sensory, reflex, and motor test results were normal. However, the gluteus medius and maximus muscles in the left extremity were weaker than those muscles in the right extremity. Poor flexibility was found in the left hip flexors, adductors, and hamstrings. The hip's range of motion was full and painless, and assisted internal and external rotation of the hip was painless. Findings on the femoral stretch test were negative.

Differential Diagnosis

The history and physical examination showed the probability of a contained, left-sided, paracentral herniation of the L4-5 intervertebral disc. The athlete's previous episodes of back pain were essentially prodromal episodes of annular collagen breakdown in the posterior lateral annular wall. However, with repetitive combined flexion and rotational loads on the spine, the annulus began to progressively fail. Therefore the athlete continued to injure himself.

As the posterolateral annular wall began to fail and the herniation occurred, manipulative treatment could not provide any substantial relief from pain. The patient's sitting intolerance and relief when standing and walking were consistent with a disc lesion. His asymmetric strength and flexibility were clues

to the altered biomechanics that needed to be addressed in his rehabilitation program.

Diagnostic Studies

Findings of the studies obtained and reviewed were as follows:

Lumbosacral spine radiographic findings—No left lumbar list, spondylolysis, or spondylolisthesis was noted. The L5 vertebra was sacralized, and facet tropism was noted, with no arthropathy at the L4-5 level. No disc space narrowing was noted.

Magnetic resonance imaging (MRI) findings—Moderate desiccation of the disc was noted at L4-5, with a left posterolateral, contained, herniated nucleus pulposus. No nerve root or thecal sac effacement was noted. A hyperintense zone was noted in the periphery of the herniation on the T2 sequence. There was no central lateral or intervertebral canal stenosis at any level. Moderate disc herniation was noted at L3-4 and L2-3, with posterior annular degeneration.

Electromyographic (EMG) findings—There was electrophysiologic evidence of a left L5 radiculopathy and no significant axonal loss.

Rehabilitation Plan

Extension exercises increased the patient's lower back pain and did not reduce his buttock and leg pain. Because nonsteroidal antiinflammatory agents had not provided any relief, an epidural cortisone injection was administered. The procedure was performed by means of fluoroscopic guidance, and the medication was instilled on the left paracentral epidural space after needle placement was confirmed by nonionic contrast dye. The next day the athlete began a dynamic lumbar muscle stabilization program with extension bias. Special attention was paid to strengthening the gluteus medius and maximus that had been noted to be weaker on the left side but that were neurophysiologically normal on EMG testing. Contractures of the patient's left hip flexors, hamstrings, and adductors were also targeted for attention. The athlete's weight-training program was reviewed, and faulty weight-lifting techniques were corrected. The athlete's discus-throwing technique was also evaluated.

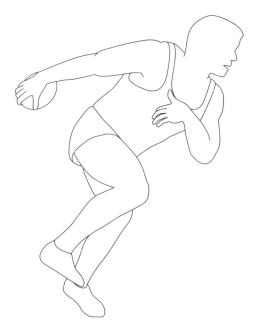

Fig. 44-2. Discus thrower. Early in the throwing motion the trunk's balance point must be maintained. This allows acceleration and propulsion to occur explosively without damaging the spine.

The patient displayed an uncoupling of his pelvis and shoulder rotations very early into the acceleration phase of a throw. His center of gravity demonstrated obvious vertical and lateral displacement during the preparation phase. He was taught how to stabilize his spine while throwing by maintaining a steady center of gravity and not allowing his pelvis to lead his shoulder into the acceleration of the throw too early (Fig. 44-2).

Rehabilitation Summary

The condition of the athlete was diagnosed, the injury was localized, and the inflammation was immediately treated. Specific strength and flexibility deficiencies were pinpointed and highlighted in the rehabilitation program. Weight-training faults and the biomechanical faults in the athlete's sports technique were evaluated and corrected. The core of the rehabilitation program is dynamic lumbar muscle stabilization extended to include revised sports-specific techniques.

This case study raises a number of questions:

1. Of what concern are the L3-4 and L2-3 discs that were desiccated?
2. What caused the high-intensity zone in the L4-5 disc?
3. What role did the sacralization of L5 play in this injury?
4. What role did the facet tropism at L4-5 play in this injury?
5. Why did the athlete respond to the cortisone injected in the epidural space but not to the nonsteroidal antiinflammatory agents?
6. Why was fluoroscopic guidance helpful for the efficacy of the epidural injection?
7. What information did the EMG findings contribute to the diagnostic process?
8. Why was the athlete not just allowed to do extension exercises?

CASE 2

A 16-year-old pole vaulter reported low back pain of 8 weeks' duration, which began after he attended a pole-vaulting camp to improve his technique. He felt the pain only in his back and had no accompanying pain in the buttocks or legs. Prolonged standing, rapid walking, and running worsened the patient's pain. Although sitting was not painful, rising from a seated position was. The pain occurred when he rolled over from side to side at night, occasionally waking him up. He had no previous episodes of back pain.

Physical Examination

Inspection revealed no scoliosis, pelvic obliquity, or skin lesions, but there was increased lumbar lordosis. All motions of the lumbar spine were painless other than extension, which caused low back pain. When the examiner initiated passive assisted extension combined with rotation and axial loading, the patient's low back pain was reproduced. No leg or buttock pain was produced from any maneuver. Straight leg raising was limited by hamstring flexibility at 45 degrees. The femoral stretch test was limited by quadriceps flexibility, and it reproduced the patient's low back pain. Hip range of motion was full and painless, but poor bilateral flexibility was noted in the iliopsoas and hip external rotator. On palpation there was diffuse paraspinal spasm in the lumbar region. Tenderness was noted at L5-S1 over the facet regions. Test results for sacroiliac joint mobility were normal. Neurologic examination findings were normal.

Radiographs of the spine, taken by a sports medicine physician the patient had consulted 3 weeks previously and that had been interpreted as normal, also were reviewed. Careful review of the x-ray films raised the suspicion of a bilateral lucency in the region of the pars interarticularis.

Differential Diagnosis

The history and physical examination results were consistent with a posterior element pain syndrome. Pole vaulting with improper technique that resulted in a late pole plant would force the lumbar spine into hyperextension. Repetitive hyperextension of the lumbar spine can injure facet joints or can cause a neural arch stress fracture. Hyperextension can also exacerbate preexistent spondylolysis or spondylolisthesis. Therefore differentiation between acute and chronic lesions is necessary.

Diagnostic Studies

Oblique x-ray films were obtained, which demonstrated bilateral pars interarticularis fractures. No spondylolisthesis was noted. End-plate defects were noted at L3, L4, and L5 with concomitant disc-space narrowing. No scoliosis was noted.

A technetium-radionuclide bone scan was undertaken,

which demonstrated no focal areas of increased activity. No other studies were obtained or reviewed.

Rehabilitation Program

The athlete and his parents were informed that he had a bilateral spondylolysis at L5-S1 without an accompanying spondylolisthesis. The lesion was described as existing before the current pain syndrome. The current pain syndrome was thought to be due to an exacerbation of the preexistent spondylolysis, resulting in a local inflammatory response at the lytic defect coupled with probable dorsal root ganglion stimulation. The athlete and his family were advised that he could safely participate in pole vaulting but that specific treatment was necessary.

The rehabilitation program initially focused on the flexibility of the patient's lower extremities. Poor hamstring, quadriceps, and iliopsoas flexibility leads to an anteverted pelvis with an accentuation of lumbar lordosis. This postural position increases posterior-element loading, especially at the L5 junction. Ultrasound and passive assisted stretching facilitated the patient's transition to spine-safe stretching of the lower extremities. The athlete was instructed to stretch at least twice a day, as well as before and after pole-vaulting practice.

Strength training initially stressed the lower abdominal oblique musculature, which, along with the lower lateral latissimus dorsi, was found to be deficient. Dynamic lumbar muscle stabilization training taught the athlete to find and hold a spinal posture that reduced his lumbar lordosis, as well as reducing hyperextension and uncoupled pelvis and shoulder rotation.

The patient's general leg and upper body strength were increased with a 12-week program of progressive resistance training.

When the athlete's flexibility, balance, coordination, and strength were adequate, he was coached in proper pole-vaulting technique. His coach was also trained to enhance his awareness of the risk of injury from faulty mechanics and from progressing through the exercise program too quickly.

Rehabilitation Summary

An accurate diagnosis was arrived at rapidly, and the athlete and his family were counseled regarding the findings. Specific areas of soft tissue flexibility and inadequate strength were addressed.

The athlete was trained in dynamic lumbar muscle stabilization and was taught how to incorporate stabilization into his athletic training and pole vaulting. Braces, corsets, and medications were not used. A corticosteroid injection into the lytic defect could have been used if necessary, but in this case, as in most cases in my experience, it was not necessary. Bracing would have led only to disuse atrophy of the known sequelae of immobilization and was therefore not used. Alternatively,

active dynamic bracing of the support musculature, coupled with appropriate spinal biomechanics, was used to promote pain relief and provide a long-term program of spinal safety for this developing athlete.

RECOMMENDATIONS FOR TRACK AND FIELD ATHLETES

These cases illustrate two straightforward and relatively uncomplicated low back syndromes typically found in participants of track and field events. The biomechanical stresses on the lumbar spine are clearly more problematic in field events than in track events, although training errors and weight from injuries play a significant role in the development of injury in athletes participating in these sports. Runners have no specific risk factors for the development of a lumbar pain syndrome. However, leg-length discrepancies, patterns of asymmetric lower extremity flexibility, facet tropism, disc degeneration, intraosseous disc herniation, and segmentation anomalies may predispose high-level runners to mechanical pain syndromes.

The key to successful treatment of low back injuries in athletes participating in track and field events include the following:
1. Early intervention
2. Accurate diagnosis
3. Goal setting
4. Time-line management
5. Aggressive, dynamic, lumbar muscle stabilization

SUGGESTED READINGS
Injury Mechanisms

Saal JA: Rehabilitation of sports-related lumbar spine injuries, *Phys Med Rehabil State Art Rev* 1:649, 1987.

Saal JA: Lumbar injuries in gymnastics, *Phys Med Rehabil State Art Rev* 4:426, 1990.

Saal JS et al: High levels of inflammatory phospholipase A₂ activity in lumbar disc herniations, *Spine* 15:674, 1990.

Dynamic Lumbar Muscle Stabilization

Saal JA: The rehabilitation of football players with lumbar injury, II, *Physician Sportsmed* 16(1):117, 1988.

Saal JA: Dynamic muscular stabilization in the nonoperative treatment of lumbar pain syndromes, *Orthop Rev* 14:691, 1990.

Saal JA, Saal JS: Nonoperative treatment of herniated lumbar intervertebral disc with radiculopathy: an outcome study, *Spine* 14:431, 1989.

General Athletic Rehabilitation

Saal JA: Rehabilitation of the injured athlete. In DeLisa JA, editor: *Principles and practice of rehabilitation medicine*, Philadelphia, 1988, JB Lippincott.

Chapter Forty-Five

◆

Weight Lifting

Joseph D. Fortin

Sports that feature weight lifting as a primary element have enjoyed a meteoric rise in popularity over the past 20 years. There are at present approximately 10,000 active powerlifting competitors and more than 20,000 bodybuilding participants in the United States. The advent of the cross-training concept (i.e., weight training to boost performance) has secured a role for weight lifting in most athletic endeavors. Each year roughly 1.5 million youths participate in the sport of football. In preparation for playing this sport, most of these youths are involved in some type of weight-training program.

As weight training becomes an integral part of athletic conditioning, it is essential that the physician who treats these athletes understand the nature of the training program for two important reasons: (1) to determine if the injury is related to the weight-training program and (2) to determine if the program can be altered to prevent injury.

Many studies substantiate the need to investigate the relationship of strength-training techniques to sports injury occurrence. Brady, Cahill, and Bodnar,[8] in a study of 80 high school athletes, reported a causal relationship between the development of lumbosacral pain and weight training in 29 students. Seven of the 29 students required hospitalization: two for lumbar discectomy and two for lumbar fusion because of spondylolisthesis. In 37 of the 80 athletes it was difficult to determine the exact cause of injury. Among collegiate football players 30% have missed playing time because of a lumbar spine complaint,[31] whereas a 12% incidence of spinal injuries necessitating time lost from play was disclosed in a 7-year National Football League (NFL) survey.[85] Yet the incidence of pars defects has been reportedly higher in weight lifters[18,66] than in football players[31] or the general population. There may be a higher incidence of degenerative lumbar spine changes in weight lifters than in track and field athletes who use weight lifting for performance enhancement.[1]

Moreover, no other sport imposes such tremendous loads on the spine as weight lifting.[27] Notwithstanding the impact of repetitive loading, a normal lumbar motion segment may fail at compressive loads not higher than 10 to 12 kN; yet some weight-lifting feats exceed these magnitudes (e.g., 18.4 to 36.2 kN).[56] Thus it is likely that some complaints of spinal pain attributed to a given sport may result from the strength-training conditions rather than the athletic endeavor.

Several studies indicate that the nature of weight-lifting injuries depends on the type of weight-training routine used. In Olympic weight-lifting activities, the wrist, shoulder, and knee regions account for more injuries than the low back as a result of the athlete's forcefully "rotating out" from the weight and rapid acceleration into the low squatting position.[67] In contrast the low back is likely the most common site of injury in the weight-training[8] and powerlifting populations. Brown and Kimball[10] reported 50% of all injuries in adolescent powerlifters were to the low back.

Although the kinematics and kinetics of skilled versus unskilled weight-lifting performance have been investigated in many studies, few attempts have been made to relate these differences to patterns of injury. The lack of rigid scientific validation of strength-conditioning methodology does not obviate the need to apply sound biomechanical principles to prevent weight-lifting injuries. Thus this chapter explores the role of spinal injury in skilled versus unskilled weight-lifting execution, and a kinesiologic perspective is developed and adapted to address common rehabilitation issues.

WEIGHT-LIFTING CATEGORIES
Olympic Weight Lifting

In Olympic weight lifting the athlete attempts to lift his or her maximum amount of weight in two overhead lifts: the snatch, and the clean and jerk. The snatch involves pulling the weight from the floor, catching it overhead in a squatting position, and then driving it upward to a standing position. The clean and jerk is a two-movement maneuver. In the clean, the athlete pulls the weight from the floor, catches it at shoulder height in a squatting position, and then assumes an erect position. The jerk consists of accelerating the weight from the shoulders to an overhead position.

Powerlifting

In powerlifting the athlete's aim is to lift the maximum weight possible in the squat, the bench press, and the deadlift. The squat consists of holding the weighted bar behind the neck on the shoulders while coming to a squatting position in which the thighs are parallel to the floor, and then returning to a standing position. The bench press involves lowering a weight to the chest in a supine position and then lifting the weight to arm's length. The deadlift is explained in detail later.

Bodybuilding

The goal of bodybuilding is muscular hypertrophy, definition, symmetry, and artistic presentation. Although many bodybuilders use powerlifts as an integral part of their training, strength is achieved but is not the primary objective.

Weight Training

Some athletes use a weight-training program to supplement and enhance their performance in another sport—most often through repetitive action against submaximum resistance. Weight trainers who seek explosive power and muscle hypertrophy may use powerlifting and weight-lifting maneuvers in addition to their other training with free weights and machines.

"CORE" AND ASSISTANCE EXERCISES

Primary, or core, movements are those that require the greatest recruitment of muscle mass in their execution. They complement many sports activities well, and the exercises include the deadlift, squat, snatch, and clean lifts.[32,33,42,47,94] Core exercises allow the highest power output[46] and overall strength gains. Intermediate-level movements (bench press, behind-neck press, bent-over-row, and leg press) are likewise kinesthetically congruent with athletic motion but incorporate fewer muscle groups and joints.

Ancillary or assistance exercises, such as leg extension, hamstring curls, calf raises, arm or biceps curls, and flies, further isolate (one or two) muscle groups and joints. Ancillary exercises allow athletes to concentrate on sport-specific muscle groups (e.g., the calves of a dancer or forearms of a tennis player).

BIOMECHANICAL OBJECTIVE OF WEIGHT LIFTING: A PHYSICAL MEDICINE PERSPECTIVE

An essential mechanical objective in weight lifting is the transference of loads from the shoulders to the ground. The inextricable link of soft tissues from the hips to the shoulders allows this transfer of weight vis-à-vis its continuity.[50] Muscle fibers of the hip extensors are contiguous with the lumbodorsal fascia, which in turn blends into the tendinous portion of the latissimus dorsi muscle and eventually inserts on the humerus.[50,51] The tension on this "cable" of interwoven connections is regulated by active muscle control and passive tensile ligamentous forces (resulting from postural dynamics as the pelvic tilt).[52]

Maximizing the amount of weight lifted while minimizing the loads on the spine necessitates awareness of a basic postural strategy.[55] Postural equipoise for the core exercises entails (1) staying as upright as possible throughout the lift, (2) maintaining the head carriage over the shoulders, (3) balancing the shoulders over the base of support, (4) using the posterior rotation of the ilium (i.e., pelvic tilt) as the primary force to approxi-

mate the weighted bar to the long axis of the body, except in the double-knee bend (discussed later), and (5) maintaining a balanced load as close to the center of gravity line as feasible throughout the lift, thus diminishing lever arm distances.

Successful rehabilitative and preventive measures provide education on the fundamental concepts of strength conditioning (such as periodization), various lift techniques, and the principles of elastic energy storage and stretch-reflex facilitation. The muscles of the trunk and extremities are balanced to length and strength, and dynamic postural control is maintained throughout all lifting motions by the application of stabilization exercises.[89]

THE DEADLIFT
Biomechanical Analysis

Fig. 45-1 depicts a weight lifter who leans forward to lift a weighted bar from the floor in front of him. Tensile forces, applied by the weight to the upper extremity together with forces from contributing body segments, generate anterior shear forces across the planes of the lumbar discs.[96] These anterior forces are opposed by posterior restraining ones supplied by concentric contractions of the hips and spine extensors. Attempts to assume an upright posture are aided also by extension at the knee and ankle. Most of the muscle power for maintaining the trunk in an upright posture is afforded by the hips and thighs. Regardless of the degree of hip flexion, some extension power is supplied by the gluteal

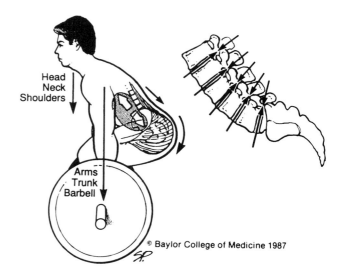

Fig. 45-1. Operative forces affecting spinal loads in the deadlift. **A,** The superincumbent weight generates large anterior shear forces across the lumbosacral motion segment. These forces are opposed by the concentric contractions of the hip and spinal extensors *(curvilinear arrow)*. The intraabdominal pressure mechanism diminishes the effects of the superincumbent loads *(open arrows)*. **B,** The forces are concentrated at the neural arch. (Courtesy Baylor College of Medicine, Dallas, Tex.)

muscles, inasmuch as the relatively long anteverted femoral neck places their attachments well posterior to the lumbosacral axis of rotation. To appreciate the importance of gluteal muscles, consider the fact that they are capable of generating a moment of 15,000 inches/pound—enough for a 150-pound man to manage a weight three times his body weight above his pelvis.[25-28] In contrast, the spinal extensor attachments are closer to the axis of rotation and are often incapable of generating a posterior shear force adequate to oppose the anterior shear elicited by the body and barbell weight. The interaction of these forces is concentrated at the neural arch.[29,96]

Sequential Analysis

A study of the deadlift provides a cogent reference point to gain insight into the biomechanics of all weight-lifting maneuvers. The deadlift involves lifting a barbell from the floor to an erect position in one continuous motion (Fig. 45-2). To initiate the lift, the lifter assumes a position in which the center of gravity is over the base of support. The back is flat or slightly flexed, and this position is held throughout the lift (thereby reducing motion and shear across the planes of the discs while still maintaining optimal tension on the posterior lumbar ligamentous system). The attitude of the trunk to the vertical is not greater than 45 degrees, which allows the hips and knees optimal leverage. The ultimate amount of trunk flexion will, of course, vary as a function of the relative length and flexibility of contributing body segments.

The largest moment is attained as the weight clears the knees, because the weight is farthest from the lumbosacral axis of rotation. At this critical moment the weight lifter is simultaneously extending the hips and

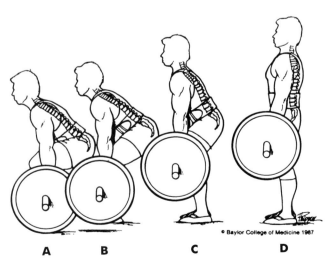

Fig. 45-2. Deadlift motion. **A,** Starting position. **B,** Lift-off. **C,** Knee passing. **D,** Lift completion. (Courtesy Baylor College of Medicine, Dallas, Tex.)

© Baylor College of Medicine 1987

knees in approximating the weighted bar to the long axis of the body. Otherwise, the lifter would be relying on the inefficient spinal extensors at the cost of increased stress on the intervertebral joints. In completing the movement, the athlete continues extending the hips and knees while retracting the scapula to assume an upright position.

Execution

The athlete in Fig. 45-3 has a superb deadlift style both in magnitude and in form. A dynamic functional analysis discloses an excellent approximation throughout the lift of the centers of mass of the head, torso, and pelvis with the base of support and weighted bar.[56] The lifter assumes a relatively upright posture at lift-off (Fig. 45-3, *A*) and stabilizes his spine in a consistent alignment, which reduces the overall spinal excursion and torque. The hip extensors are effectively used in posteriorly accelerating the torso as the long axis of the body moves closer to the barbell (Fig. 45-3, *B*). Finally, the lifter does not hyperextend on completion of the lift (Fig. 45-3, *C* and *D*).

On lift initiation the skilled athlete has obviated the need to rely on the weaker erector spinae muscles (versus the gluteal muscles) while maintaining sufficient tension on the posterior lumbar ligamentous system throughout until the moment is small enough for the back muscles to balance it.[25,27,28,55,68]

In contrast to the first lifter, the athlete in Fig. 45-4 initiates the lift in a round-back style and with a significantly less erect trunk (Fig. 45-4, *A*). Because he is less upright, his hips are more flexed and not as advantageously placed for optimal torque.[26] This necessitates that his lumbar spine undergo a greater excursion to complete the lift while sustaining substantial flexion in this bending moment. The application of inordinate forces may cause nuclear contents of the disc to be forced through the end-plates or posterolateral corners of the annulus (which act much like stress risers).[30] If the lifter pulls the weight unevenly or loses control, turning to one side or the other, torsional stress across the intervertebral joints is intensified. If the posterior arch is forced beyond 2 to 3 degrees of deformation, concomitant damage to the facet and annulus may occur[29,30,71] (Fig. 45-5, *A*). Fig. 45-4, *B,* illustrates the athlete leaning backward early in the lift sequence because he is extending his knees without simultaneous hip extension. Intradiscal pressure increases if the athlete lifts with the knees extended rather than flexed.[78] The athlete completes the lift by hyperextending through the lumbosacral axis (Fig. 45-4, *C* and *D*).

Predominant erector spinae activity during great moments also is detrimental because the lumbodorsal fascia—to transmit the force of the hip extensors—must stay taut and the lumbar spine must remain flexed.[25] Extension causes the tip of the inferior articular process

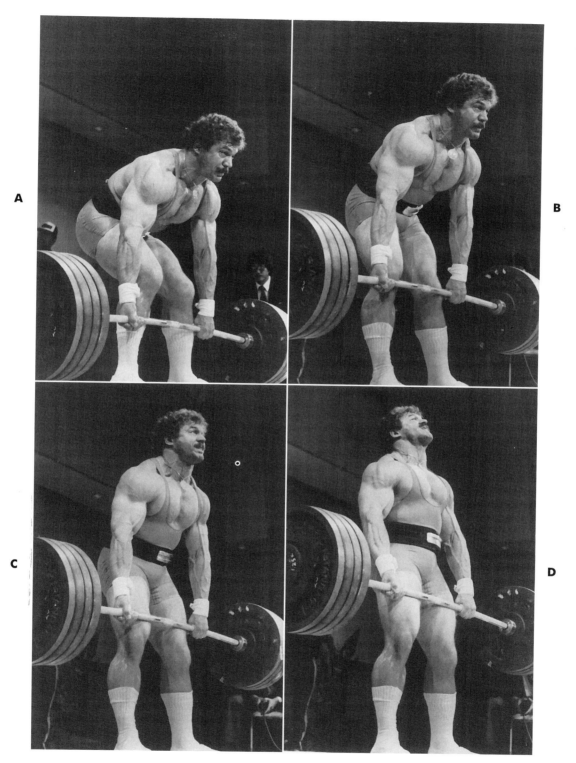

Fig. 45-3. Superb deadlift technique in a World Class powerlifter. **A,** Lift-off. **B,** Knee passing. **C,** Approaching lockout (the final position). **D,** Lift completion. (Courtesy Mike Lambert, editor, *Powerlifting, USA.*)

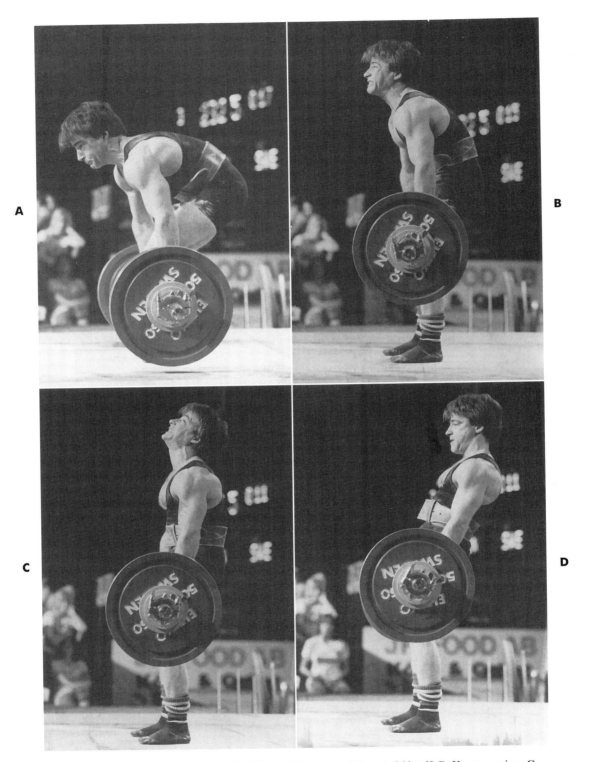

Fig. 45-4. Poor deadlift technique in a World Class powerlifter. **A,** Lift-off. **B,** Knee passing. **C,** Approaching lockout. **D,** Lift completion. (Courtesy Mike Lambert, editor, *Powerlifting, USA.*)

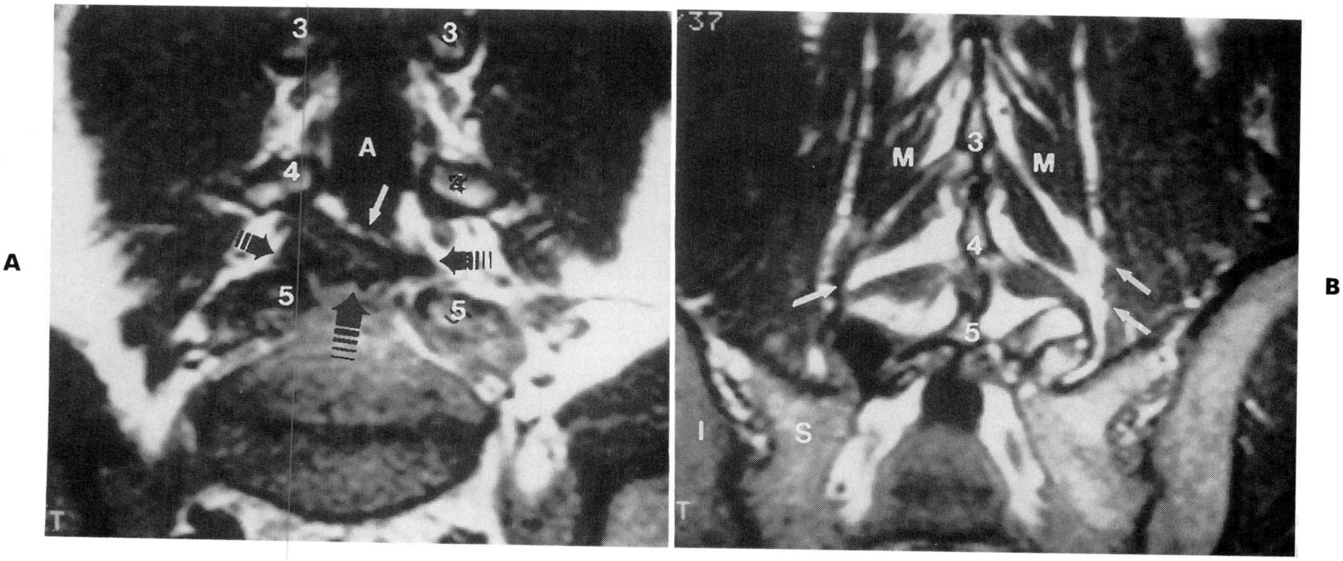

Fig. 45-5. Magnetic resonance imaging (MRI) scan of coronal lumbar T1. **A,** MRI scan at the level of the pedicles of a 30-year-old bodybuilder with a cauda equina syndrome. A massive sequestered disc fragment occupies most of the central canal and right L4 nerve root entry at midzone *(arrows)*. Posterior joint hypertrophic arthropathy was also present (on axial section, not shown). These pathologic changes are the result of large, repetitive axial and torsional loads. *3,* Pedicle of L3; *4,* pedicle of L4; *5,* pedicle of L5. **B,** MRI scan at the level of the spinous processes of the athlete in **A.** Note the marked atrophy of the multifidus muscle *(M)* as demonstrated by the fatty replacement *(arrows)*. *3,* Spinous process of L3; *4,* spinous process of L4; *5,* spinous process of L5; *S,* sacrum; *I,* ilium.

to impact the subjacent lamina. If the load continues to be applied to the extended joint, the upper vertebra undergoes axial rotation, which may lead to capsular strain or rupture, erosion of the periosteal lamina, or annular disruption.[103] The increased incidence of neural arch defects in athletes involved in sports requiring repeated forceful hyperextension has been well established.* Kotani and associates[66] found a 30.7% incidence of spondylolysis in a group of 25 weight lifters.

Cinematographic Analysis

It is generally accepted that athletic injury prevention and rehabilitative measures do not always correlate with the actual kinetics and kinematics of performance. To this end I examined data from a previous motion analysis study of the deadlift and compared it with the aforementioned postural strategy used for injury prevention and rehabilitation.[9,35] Brown and Abani's study of 10 skilled and 11 unskilled adolescent powerlifters[9] used cinematographic analysis to develop a multisegmental model of the deadlift motion in the sagittal plane.

Fig. 45-6 represents a reconstruction of the deadlift motion of one of the skilled subjects. The horizontal moment arm of the ankle, knee, and hip is plotted on a time line. The area under the diagonal lines represents lift-off. The time at which the weight "clears" the knees

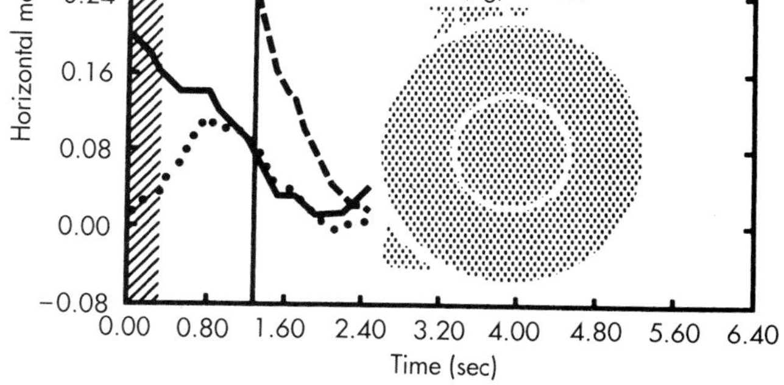

Fig. 45-6. Skilled lifter. Sagittal-plane reconstruction of the deadlift. Horizontal moment arm of the hip, knee, and ankle over time. (Modified from Brown EW, Abani K: *Med Sci Sports Exerc* 72:554, 1985.)

---

* References 21, 31, 38, 65, 72, 88, 96.

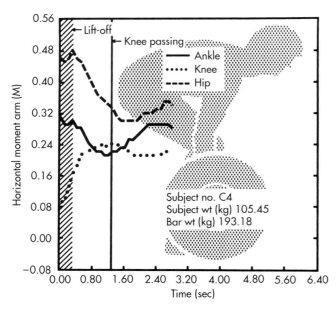

Fig. 45-7. Unskilled lifter. Sagittal-plane reconstruction of the deadlift. Horizontal moment arm of hip, knee, and ankle over time. (Modified from Brown EW, Abani K: *Med Sci Sports Exerc* 72:554, 1985.)

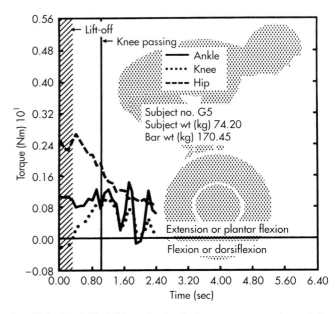

Fig. 45-8. Unskilled lifter. Sagittal-plane reconstruction of the deadlift. Torque over time. (Modified from Brown EW, Abani K: *Med Sci Sports Exerc* 72:554, 1985.)

(knee passing) is indicated by a vertical line. A comparison of Figs. 45-6 and 45-7 demonstrates that the skilled lifter starts with the trunk in a more upright position than the unskilled lifter, as evidenced by a smaller horizontal moment arm at lift-off. At knee passing, the horizontal moment arm of the hip rapidly approaches zero in the skilled lifter who takes effective advantage of the hip extensors.

In contrast to unskilled subjects, all of the skilled subjects in Brown and Abani's study achieved a positive angular trunk acceleration commensurate with the moment the barbell cleared the knees. The hip extensors, vis-à-vis the posterior pelvic tilt, accelerate the trunk in extension, thus allowing the lifter to assume an upright posture.[52] This early burst of hip extensor recruitment (while the erector spinae are relatively silent) allows the weighted bar to gain velocity at knee passing.[47] An athlete who chooses a stooped posture at lift-off may be unable to coordinate this acceleration with knee passing. Accordingly, kinematic studies to date demonstrate that skilled lifters attain a higher vertical bar velocity at sticking points.[9,73]

Fig. 45-8 represents torque forces occurring at the hip, knee, and ankle in an unskilled lifter performing a deadlift. Attempts to jerk the weight upward by repeated hip, truncal, head, and neck flexion—followed by rigorous extension in a whiplash motion—are represented by the erratic lines. Tremendous forces are necessary to rapidly accelerate and decelerate the barbell. Skilled deadlifters and squatters apply consistent vertical forces

to the bar, thereby minimizing acceleration and inertial forces.[9,73,74]

THE SQUAT

McLaughlin, Dillman, and Lardner,[73] using cinematographic analysis, noted significant technique differences between skilled and unskilled powerlifters. The unskilled lifters approached the low position at a faster bar velocity and therefore "bounced" or recoiled more. The inertial effects of "bouncing" causes increased shear forces across the lumbar discs—a potential axial overload situation[27]; it also affords less control over the weight and a greater propensity for injury. A slow, controlled descent allows elastic energy to be stored, which can be used in assisting the concentric contractions of the hip and knee extensors on the ascent.[74,83] In this study the unskilled lifters, in contrast to the skilled athletes, leaned farther forward in the ascent. Leaning forward increases the flexion moment (hence spinal compressive loads).[12] Leaning forward also disables the lifter's proprioceptive control; thus the athlete may lose control of the weight to one side or another. Forward flexion with rotation (without any superincumbent load other than body weight) may increase disc pressure by 400%.[78] Athletes should be trained to descend slowly and drive the hips forward through extension while simultaneously extending their knees (without leaning forward in the early ascent) (Fig. 45-9).

Many lifters perform squats with their heels on a 2 × 4 block, placing their lumbar spine in hyperlordosis.

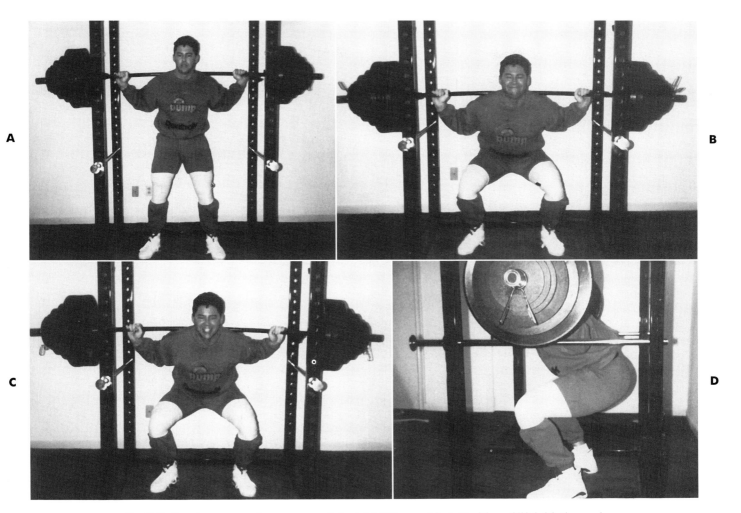

Fig. 45-9. Squat maneuver in a power rack (weight 470 pounds). **A,** Position of lift initiation and completion. **B,** Approaching the low squatting position (just before the final "dip"). **C,** Early ascent phase. **D,** Lateral view of the early ascent phase. Note that the torso inclination is not excessive (approximately 40 degrees to the vertical).

This technique, some body builders claim, enhances quadriceps recruitment (as the load is shifted during forward lean), but this extensor activity is merely offset by opposing flexor torque.[84] The shim is also used by some lifters (who may actually lean more without it) to compensate for inflexible extensor groups at the hip, knee, or ankle. Proper form and muscle balancing prevent hyperlordosis and inordinate forward lean/ flexion load. Newly developed devices that place the weight closer to the lumbosacral axis of rotation may significantly diminish spinal compressive loads during squatting.[69]

The effect of the squat exercise on knee stability continues to be a concern for physicians, coaches, and athletes. Previous admonitions of detrimental and destabilizing ligamentous disruption have been refuted.[13-15] Chandler and Stone[13] (members of the National Strength and Conditioning Association Research Com-

mittee) carefully illuminated the facts versus myths associated with the squat exercise and delineated prudent guidelines for performance of the maneuver.

OLYMPIC WEIGHT LIFTING

Competitive Olympic weight lifting is a stunning spectacle for sports enthusiasts and biomechanists alike. A well-executed Olympic lift displays optimal biomechanics; once the second pull has occurred, lifting the barbell overhead involves not balancing larger moments, but rather achieving tremendous neuromuscular coordination in subjugating moments near zero. The double-knee bend is the style of weight lifting associated with lower stress on the lumbar spine.[22,23] The double-knee bend engages the hip extensors (initially) and the knee extensors (subsequently) through both knee joints' strongest range of motion (Fig. 45-10). This style involves reflexing the knees and rotating the

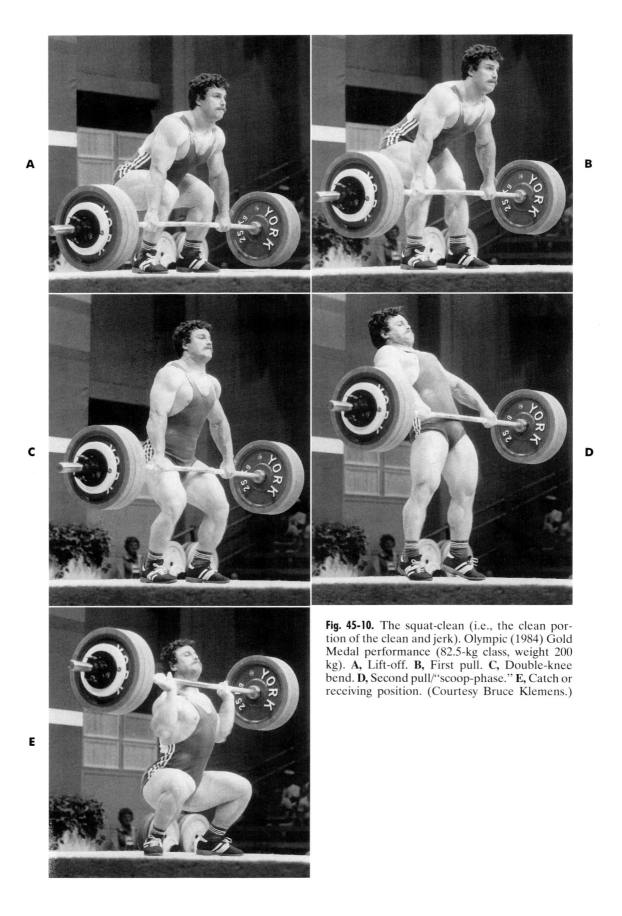

Fig. 45-10. The squat-clean (i.e., the clean portion of the clean and jerk). Olympic (1984) Gold Medal performance (82.5-kg class, weight 200 kg). **A,** Lift-off. **B,** First pull. **C,** Double-knee bend. **D,** Second pull/"scoop-phase." **E,** Catch or receiving position. (Courtesy Bruce Klemens.)

torso closer to the vertical, after the barbell has cleared the knees (first pull). The rapid but controlled eccentric flexion of the knees reportedly enables the storage of viscoelastic kinetic energy and stretch reflex facilitation for the second pull.[45] The final explosive knee extension (second pull) leads to the top-pull (full-extension) position when the lifter begins to move under the bar to catch it overhead. Comparable to other lifts (already discussed), mechanical stress on the lumbar spine during the clean and jerk increases with load, speed of movement, and forward torso lean.[59] Olympic lifts require blazing speed (5 and 6 m/sec^2 for clean and snatch, respectively) and the swift application (0.6 to 0.9 seconds) of great forces—all while many joints are loaded through a wide range of motion.[40,41,48,49] Training must therefore enable the musculoskeletal system to endure rapid loading over the sport's specific spectrum of joint angles.

Variable-resistance equipment can be used to fortify the eccentric strength of the hamstring and gluteal muscles, which are vital in determining torso inclination in the first pull.[45] Plyometric exercises provide a controlled medium for Olympic-style lifters to develop fast-twitch strength and enhance the viscoelastic properties of connective tissue.[16] Tilt boards, balance beams, and dissociative (dancelike) exercises are excellent tools to build coordination and enhance dynamic postural control. The stabilization concept trains the lifter to effectively use antagonists (e.g., gluteus/psoas muscle, hamstring/quadriceps muscles) to reduce loads on the spine—throughout all phases of a lift.[89]

Integrating strength and coordination drills into a therapeutic exercise prescription for Olympic lifters is essential but does not obviate the need for careful scrutiny of the lift technique itself.

INJURIES, SYNDROMES, REHABILITATION, AND STRENGTH CONDITIONING

Many injuries to the low back from weight lifting or weight training are chronic, with an insidious onset. The athlete, who is often engaged in other sporting activities, may be unable to precisely identify the time of onset. The adolescent athlete with well-localized, unilateral, aching low back pain exacerbated by repetitive hyperextension lifting maneuvers may have underlying neural arch defects. Early detection, as well as proper joint protection and immobilization, in this young athlete with spondylolysis may prevent slippage (i.e., spondylolisthesis), and allow dramatic pain relief, as well as return to activity within several months.

It is essential to distinguish this athlete from the far more commonly seen athlete who has chronic low back pain, an uncertain diagnosis, normal findings on conventional imaging and diagnostic studies, no signs of nerve root irritation, and little pain when not training. The latter athlete may have the beginnings of posterior ele-

ment changes and altered discovertebral joint or sacroiliac joint mechanics. These pathologic changes may consist of facet or sacroiliac joint synovitis, focal cartilage necrosis or fibrillation, and small circumferential tears of the annulus (unimpressive on routine studies).[3,20,87,99] This differential can be assayed by the employment of provocative injection techniques.[19,37,93,101] Unless predisposing structural imbalance and technique factors are considered as part of the overall rehabilitation equation, the athlete may incur further damage or continue to have chronic pain. Although most of the more common spinal afflictions resulting from weight lifting are amenable to a conservative approach, problems that require surgical intervention (such as cauda equina syndrome) (see Fig. 45-5, A) or those that may contraindicate some type of therapy (such as spinal instability) must be identified. The aim of treatment is to decrease pain to a tolerable level and increase spinal range of motion, stability, and strength to a functional level.

Neck and Shoulder Problems

Some weight trainers perform an inordinate number of exercises (such as cable crossovers, bench presses, bicep curls, forward and lateral flies) to the exclusion of other complementary movements (such as the incline press, deadlifts, reverse flies, pullovers, reverse cable crossovers, and overhead presses). The resultant imbalance includes tight pectoralis minor and external rotary shoulder muscles, as well as weak rhomboids, lower trapezius, serratus anterior, and external rotary shoulder muscles. Inspection reveals a protracted scapula; poorly developed posterior deltoid, serratus anterior, and rhomboid muscles; and relatively overdeveloped pectoral and anterior deltoid muscles.

The resultant inequity can lead to cervicothoracic facet dysfunction (tired neck syndrome), shoulder impingement, and hyperlordosis. At the end range of shoulder flexion in overhead lifts, compensatory hyperextension occurs through the lumbosacral spine as a result of the tight pectoralis minor muscles. A graphic expression of a force couple imbalance about the shoulder girdle is a case report of a fractured first rib caused by the overhead position of the jerk.[67]

Adjunctive therapeutic exercises include wall slides, eccentric strengthening of the external rotary shoulder muscles, and rows. Eccentric strengthening of the shoulder's external rotary muscles and rhomboids is not addressed in most strength-training programs despite their role in indirectly determining the horizontal moment arm of the loads transferred from the shoulder to the torso. These muscles, by kinetically "checking" the anterior displacement of the glenohumeral axis—in the first pull (Olympic lifts) and lift-off/knee passing (deadlift)—influence the cervicothoracic loads. Well-balanced shoulder girdle musculature will enhance a lifter's longevity and symmetry.

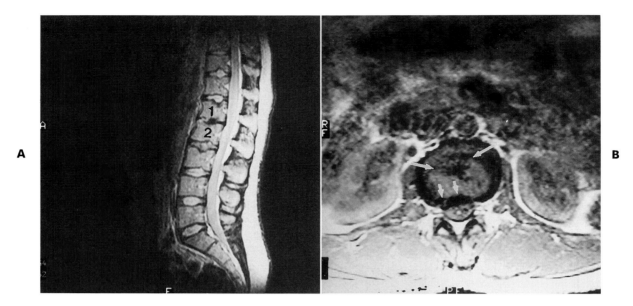

Fig. 45-11. MRI scan of a 31-year-old powerlifter with a thoracolumbar syndrome. **A,** T2 midline sagittal section. Marked L1-2 disc-space collapse and desiccation, combined with end-plate reactive changes and a small, contained disc prolapse, is apparent. (*1,* L1 vertebral body; *2,* L2 vertebral body.) **B,** T1 axial section (L1-2). A right paracentral/posterolateral disc prolapse with spondylotic ridging is evident *(shorter arrows).* The large end-plate/Schmorl's lesion *(longer arrows)* attest to the enormous compressive loads this motion segment has sustained.

Thoracolumbar Syndrome

The thoracolumbar region is a vulnerable point of stress concentration[102] (stiffness properties of the spine abruptly change); yet it receives little or no attention in conventional strength conditioning. Compressive and large flexion moments are enormous in the early phases of the deadlift and Olympic lifts, as well as in the early ascent phase of the squat—when the superincumbent center of mass and barbell is well anterior to the axis of rotation.

Fig. 45-11 shows an MRI scan of the lumbar spine of a powerlifter with a thoracolumbar syndrome. The cause of her flexion injury became readily apparent after a dynamic analysis of her lifting motions. Poor coaching (combined with inflexible hip flexors, quadriceps, and heel cords) did not lend itself to timely and explosive initiation of the pelvic tilt (i.e., forward and upward hip thrust) in the deadlift and early ascent phase of the squat. Thus the lumbodorsal fascia and posterior "cable" were not taut enough to counterbalance the anterior thoracolumbar load.

Atrophy of Erector Spinae Muscles

Spinal extensors such as the multifidus play an important role in assisting extension and in opposing small flexion and possibly torsional loads at the completion of lifts.[55] Yet these extensors are sometimes atrophic in weight lifters because of muscle imbalance (see Fig. 45-5, *B*). Strengthening exercises for the spinal extensors may be needed.

Sacroiliac Joint Dysfunction

Superincumbent and ground reaction forces must be transferred to and from the spine (as a load-bearing mechanism) and lower extremities (as the base of support) by means of the sacroiliac joints (as the final pathway between the spine and lower extremities).

The keystone/interdigitating configuration of the sacrum and the pelvis, together with balanced transiliac ligamentous and muscular tension, allows a complex, dynamic transfer of tremendous loads—without sacrificing the athlete's ability to attain or maintain an erect posture while locomoting or lifting.[51-55,99]

Muscle-balancing work for patients with sacroiliac joint dysfunction should concentrate on the powerful two-joint muscles around the sacroiliac joint (i.e., gluteus maximus, biceps femoris, piriformis, and psoas) as they exert shear and torsional loads proportional to the strength of their contraction.[58,75,76,98]

The clinical presentation, diagnosis, and rehabilitation of patients with SI joint dysfunction are detailed elsewhere.[6,36,37]

Balancing Lower Extremity and Pelvic Girdle Musculature

In addition to back development, the lower extremity and pelvic girdle musculature should be incorporated into the rehabilitation prescription for prevention of spinal injuries to weight lifters. Tight hip flexors and quadriceps, as well as weak hamstrings, limit the power and range of hip extension and, secondarily, posterior trunk acceleration.[80]

Abdominal Development

The erector spinae muscles are mechanically unable to balance loads exceeding roughly 20 kg.[51] Current mathematic and clinical constructs suggest that the abdominal muscles provide a substantial "missing moment" required for heavy lifting. Further rigid scientific validation is necessary to establish a resolute model that depicts the precise interactions between intraabdominal pressure, the posterior ligamentous system, and spinal compressive loads throughout various phases of a given lift.* Nonetheless, abdominal muscles appear to be essential in counterbalancing large axial and torsional spinal loads. Their conditioning should be a basic element in any weight lifter's prevention or rehabilitative program.

An electrophysiologic examination of the sit-up exercise underscores the value of stringent form in abdominal strengthening.[80,86] The initial 40 to 50 degrees of trunk flexion (the trunk curl) is associated with the greatest abdominal activity—specifically the upper rectus and to a lesser degree the oblique muscles. Oblique and lower rectus muscles are recruited with a weight held in the upper thorax region. Rotation of the trunk during the trunk curl will augment the oblique musculature activity. Parenthetically, the significance of the oblique abdominal muscles (particularly the transverse abdominis) in weight lifting cannot be understated inasmuch as they represent a much longer lever arm to oppose lumbar torsion loads than do the short rotary muscles of the spine.[54,55]

The second phase of the sit-up relegates the abdominal muscles to an exclusively isometric role. In the early stages of rehabilitation of the spine, isometric abdominal activity performed while in a position of optimal spinal function avoids excessive compressive loads, but such activity needs to be increased before the athlete returns to play.

Abdominal-strengthening exercises should be performed with the hips flexed and an anterior pelvic tilt avoided, thereby achieving optimal abdominal isolation and preventing lumbosacral hyperextension (psoas paradox). A rapid succession of repetitions, with the head and trunk curled, physiologically obscures abdominal muscle isolation via central pathway irradiation or a mass flexion synergy effect.[63] To minimize compression and torsional forces, patients with lumbar spine pain (especially of discogenic cause) must maintain neutral spinal alignment while performing abdominal exer-

cises.[78] Some patients with deconditioned abdominal muscles will need assistance initially to maintain proper spinal alignment.

Treatment Protocol

The application of fundamental biomechanical concepts to the rehabilitation of weight lifting–related spinal injuries is not an objective of this chapter. The four-phase treatment protocol presented here for a power-lifter with a lumbar posterior joint dysfunction[35] provides a framework that is congruent with the general principles already described:

I. Phase I (week 1)
  A. Goal—To decrease inflammation and pain
  B. Nonsteroidal antiinflammatory medication
  C. Local application of ice for 15 to 20 minutes to the lumbosacral region three times daily
  D. Deep cross-fiber massage after icing
  E. Postural education that emphasizes co-contraction of gluteal and abdominal muscles in maintaining optimal spine mechanics
II. Phase II (week 2)
  A. Goal—To increase range of motion
  B. Segmental mobilization or muscle-energy techniques to improve lumbar motion segmental mechanics
  C. Stretching of hip flexors, quadriceps, iliotibial bands, and lumbar posterior ligaments
III. Phase III (week 3)
  A. Goal—Strengthening and conditioning
  B. Abdominal strengthening (isometric to advanced rotary)
  C. Strengthening rotary and extensor muscles of the spine
  D. Stabilization exercises, including progressive plyometrics and the body cycle
  E. Calisthenics (e.g., push-ups and squat-thrusts)
  F. Plyometrics[16]
IV. Phase IV (week 4)
  A. Goal—Progressive return to lifting, focusing on biomechanical efficiency in the deadlift motion
  B. Placing the center of gravity over the base of support
  C. Avoiding a "stooped" round-back position in the initiation of the lift (keeping the torso as upright as possible throughout the lift)
  D. Using the power of the hip extensors in the early phases of the lift combined with simultaneous knee extension
  E. Avoiding hyperextension in lift completion
  F. Emphasizing a controlled fluidity of motion versus sudden starting and stopping

This protocol was individualized for a specific patient.[35] The timing and focus of therapy will, of course, vary according to the athlete and his or her condition.

---

* References 4, 53-55, 57, 69, 77, 97.

Resistance: How Much?

Training with heavy loads may facilitate neuromuscular patterns that are inapparent with lighter loads.[17] Therefore excessive training at low resistance to the exclusion of high resistance may be detrimental to performance (requiring large loads) and can cause injury. The number of repetitions and the amount of resistance should be tailored to achieve specificity of training. Thus a continuum of athletes who would benefit, respectively, from low-resistance/high-repetition up to high-resistance/low-repetition Olympic-style training (or subdivisions thereof, such as high pulls and push jerks) might include the following: runners (halfbacks, receivers, and sprinters), jumpers (volleyball, high jump, basketball, and hurdlers), throwers (shot put, javelin, and hammer), pushers (linemen, fullbacks, sumo wrestlers), and weight lifters. Preliminary data from studies of volunteers (with and without symptoms) demonstrate that as maximal deadlift loads are exceeded, posterior angular trunk velocity is curtailed.[51] This finding is consistent with the stress-strain properties of collagen and may provide a reasonable index of a safe load for some lifts. The magnitude of the weight and fatigue should be considered to prevent injury when optimal form is compromised in any lifting situation.

The objective is to decrease injury potential while simultaneously maximizing peak power and varying training stimuli. Because current data are insufficient to determine the exact resistance for any athletic goal, Garhammer[48] has suggested emphasizing lifts in the 70% to 90% range of a one-repetition (maximum) movement. The physiologic concept of periodization or cyclic training is also paramount in determining the frequency, duration, variation, and specificity of any weight-lifting program.[2,33,47,82,93]

Machines Versus Free Weights

The controversy surrounding the superiority of isokinetic or variable-resistance weight training over free weights (dynamic training) is frivolous. Manufacturer claims that (1) isokinetic equipment (such as Cybex) allows muscles to shorten at a constant velocity at all speed settings and (2) variable-resistance equipment (e.g., Nautilus) can match the resistance to the user's maximal force-production capability curve have been refuted.* The challenge in strength conditioning is to tailor the benefits of the various methodologies to the needs of each athlete. Dynamic weight training is unparalleled in enhancing neuromuscular coordination and explosive power.† Warnings of a high injury potential associated with rapid overloading exercises[79] are ill founded, because the viscoelastic properties of bone and connective tissues allow them to absorb greater energy

when subject to rapid (versus slow) loading. Moreover, properly executed free-weight exercises can accommodate any muscle tension and the concomitant lifting force by accelerating at variable rates in unconstrained patterns.[42]

Isokinetic equipment may allow torque and power measurements at appendicular joints, but the reliability of data on the spine is uncertain.[51] These machines have a useful application in charting strength gains, measuring effort consistency, and providing feedback for explosive contractions at high-speed movements.

Variable-resistance equipment advantages include the following: (1) joint and muscle group isolation, (2) reduction of injury potential through a controlled/constrained system, and (3) ease of resistance adjustment.

Equipment

Weight-lifting belts afford an increase in intraabdominal pressure,[62] which most likely varies with the belt size. When positioned immediately above the greater trochanters, some belts may act by harnessing sacroiliac motion.[11,100] They may also aid the athlete by providing proprioceptive awareness of the attitude of the trunk to the horizontal in maintaining the optimal position of the spine for a given lift.

Power racks can be used to prevent injury in some lifting situations (such as squatting) at submaximal loads but should not take the place of experienced spotters at maximal or burnout (submaximal repetitions to failure) efforts (see Fig. 45-9).

Force plate analysis has documented that the position of the foot indirectly determines the relationship of the barbell to the lifter and to torso inclination.[23,39,43,44] Thus weight-lifting shoes are important in preventing spinal injury; they should have a strong counter and medial and longitudinal arch support, as well as a heel that affords mediolateral stability.

A basic understanding of the sport-specific spinal mechanics is essential in outlining injury prevention and rehabilitative management. The widespread practice of weight-lifting demands further investigation of the nature of weight-lifting injuries relative to biomechanical strategies and technique differences. The synchronization of recently advanced technologies, such as three-dimensional film analysis, force plate dynamics, electromyography, and cineradiography, holds great promise for the future.[5,51,61,91]

---

* References 34, 60, 64, 70, 79, 81, 90.
† References 7, 24, 42, 82, 92, 94, 95.

REFERENCES

1. Aggrawal ND et al: A study of changes in the spine in weightlifters and other athletes, *Br J Sports Med* 13:58, 1979.
2. Atha J: Strengthening muscle, *Exerc Sport Sci Rev* 9:1, 1981.
3. Ayres CE: Further case studies of lumbo-sacral pathology with

consideration of involvement of intervertebral disc and facets, *N Engl J Med* 213:716, 1935.

4. Bartelink VL: The role of abdominal pressure in relieving the pressure on the intervertebral disc, *J Bone Joint Surg* 39B:718, 1957.
5. Baumann W et al: *Int J Sports Biomech* 4(1):68, 1988.
6. Bernard PN, Cassidy JD: Sacroiliac joint syndrome: pathophysiology, diagnosis and management. In Frymoyer J, editor: *The adult spine: principles and practice,* New York, 1991, Raven Press.
7. Bhanot JL, Sidhu LS: Comparative study of reaction time in Indian sportsmen specializing in hockey, volleyball, weightlifting, and gymnastics, *J Sports Med Phys Fitness* 20:113, 1980.
8. Brady TA, Cahill BR, Bodnar LM: Weight training–related injuries in the high school athlete, *Am J Sports Med* 10(1):1, 1982.
9. Brown EW, Abani K: Kinematics and kinetics of the dead-lift in adolescent powerlifters, *Med Sci Sports Exerc* 72:554, 1985.
10. Brown EW, Kimball RG: Medical history associated with adolescent powerlifting, *Pediatrics* 72:636, 1983.
11. Buyruk HM: Effective pelvic belt application on sacroiliac joint mobility. In Vleeming A, Snijders CJ, Stoeckart R, editors: *Progress in vertebral column research: first international symposium on the sacroiliac joints—its role in posture and locomotion,* Rotterdam, 1991, European Conference Organizers.
12. Cappozzo A et al: Lumbar spine loading during half pike squat exercises, *Med Sci Sports Exerc* 17:613, 1985.
13. Chandler TJ, Stone MH: The squat exercise in athletic conditioning: a position statement and review of the literature, *Natl Strength Cond Assoc J* 13(5):51, 1991.
14. Chandler TJ, Wilson GD, Stone MH: The effect of the squat exercise on knee stability, *Med Sci Sports Exerc* 21:299, 1989.
15. Chandler TJ, Wilson GD, Stone MH: The squat exercise: attitudes and practices of high school football coaches, *Natl Strength Cond Assoc J* 11(1):30, 1989.
16. Chu DA: *Jumping into plyometrics,* Champaign, Ill, 1992, Leisure Press.
17. Connan A, Moreaux A, VanHoecke J: Biomechanical analysis of the two-hand snatch. In *Biomechanics,* vol 7B, Baltimore, 1981, University Park Press.
18. Dangles CJ, Spencer DL: Spondylolysis in competitive weight lifters. Paper presented at the annual meeting of the American Orthopaedic Society for Sports Medicine, Orlando, Fla, July 1, 1987.
19. Dwyer A, Aprill C, Bogduk N: Cervical zygapophysial joint pain patterns. I. Study in normal volunteers, *Spine* 15:453, 1990.
20. Eisenstein SM, Parry CR: The lumbar facet arthrosis syndrome, *J Bone Joint Surg* 69B:3, 1987.
21. Ende LS, Wickstrom J: Ballet injuries, *Physician Sportsmed* 10(7):105, 1982.
22. Enoka RM: *Biomechanical analysis of the pull in Olympic weightlifting,* master's thesis, Seattle, 1976, University of Washington.
23. Enoka RM: The pull in Olympic weightlifting, *Med Sci Sports* 11:131, 1979.
24. Everson J: Variable resistance vs. isotonic weight training in monozygotic male twins, *Natl Strength Cond Assoc J* 5(5):31, 1983.
25. Farfan HF: Muscular mechanism of the lumbar spine in the position of power and efficiency, *Orthop Clin North Am* 6:135, 1975.
26. Farfan HF: The biomechanical advantage of lordosis in hip extension for upright activity, *Spine* 3:336, 1978.
27. Farfan HF: Biomechanics of the lumbar spine. In Kirkaldi-Willis WH, editor: *Managing low back pain,* New York, 1983, Churchill Livingstone.
28. Farfan HF, Gracovetsky S, Lamy C: Mechanism of the lumbar spine, *Spine* 6:249, 1981.
29. Farfan HF, Osteria V, Lamy C: The mechanical etiology of spondylolysis and spondylolisthesis, *Clin Orthop North Am* 117:40, 1976.
30. Farfan HF et al: The effects of torsion on the lumbar intervertebral joint: the role of torsion in the production of disc degeneration, *J Bone Joint Surg* 52A:468, 1970.
31. Ferguson RJ, McMaster JH, Stanitski CL: Low back pain in college football linemen, *J Sports Med* 2(3):63, 1974.
32. Fleck SJ, Falkel JE: The value of resistance training for the reduction of sports injuries, *Sports Med* 3:61, 1986.
33. Fleck SJ, Kraemer WJ: *Designing resistance training programs,* Champaign, Ill, 1987, Human Kinetics Books.
34. Fleming LK: Accommodation capabilities of Nautilus weight machines to human strength curves, *Natl Strength Cond Assoc J* 7(6):68, 1985.
35. Fortin JD: Low back pain in weight lifters, *Arch Phys Med Rehabil* 68:642, 1987.
36. Fortin JD: The sacroiliac joint: a new perspective, *J Back Musculo Rehab* 3(3): 31, 1993.
37. Fortin JD et al: Sacroiliac pain referral maps. I. Asymptomatic volunteers. II. Clinical evaluation, *Spine* 19:1475, 1994.
38. Gainor BJ, Hagen RJ, Allen WC: Biomechanics of the spine in the pole vaulter as related to spondylolysis, *Am J Sports Med* 11(2):53, 1983.
39. Garhammer J: Force plate analysis of the snatch-lift, *Int Olympic Lifter* 3:22, 1976.
40. Garhammer J: Power production by Olympic weightlifters, *Sci Sports Exerc* 12:54, 1980.
41. Garhammer J: Biomechanical characteristics of the 1978 world weight-lifting champions. In *Biomechanics,* vol 7, Baltimore, 1981, University Park Press.
42. Garhammer J: Free weight equipment for the development of athletic strength and power, *Natl Strength Cond Assoc J* 3:24, 1981.
43. Garhammer J: Balance on the feet during weightlifting. In *American weightlifting yearbook,* Chicago, 1984, American Weight-lifting Coaches Association.
44. Garhammer J: Center of pressure movements during weightlifting. *Proceedings of the second international symposium of biomechanics and sports,* Delmar, Calif, 1984, Academic Publishers.
45. Garhammer J: Power clean: kinesiologic evaluation, *Scand J,* 16:6, 1984.
46. Garhammer J: Biomechanical profiles of Olympic weightlifters, *Intl J Sports Biomech* 1:122, 1985.
47. Garhammer J: *Sports illustrated strength training,* New York, 1986, Harper & Row.
48. Garhammer J: Weight lifting and training. In Vaughn CL, editor: *Biomechanics of sports,* Boca Raton, Fla, 1988, CRC Press.
49. Garhammer J, Whiting WC: A comparison of three data smoothing techniques in the determination of weightlifting kinematics, Unpublished manuscript.
50. Gracovetsky S: A hypothesis for the role of the spine in human locomotion: a challenge to current thinking, *J Biomed Eng* 7:205, 1985.
51. Gracovetsky S: *The spinal engine,* New York, 1988, Springer-Verlag.
52. Gracovetsky S: The importance of pelvic tilt in reducing compressive stress in the spine during flexion-extension exercises, *Spine* 14:412, 1989.
53. Gracovetsky S, Farfan HF: The optimum spine, *Spine* 11:543, 1986.
54. Gracovetsky S, Farfan HF, Helleur C: The abdominal mechanism, *Spine* 10:317, 1985.
55. Gracovetsky S, Farfan HF, Lamy C: A mathematical model of the lumbar spine using an optimal system to control muscles and ligaments, *Orthop Clin North Am* 8:135, 1977.
56. Granhed H, Jonson R, Hansson T: Loads on the lumbar spine during extreme weightlifting, *Spine* 12:146, 1987.

57. Grillner SJ, Nilsson J, Thorstensson A: Intra-abdominal pressure changes during natural movements in man, *Acta Physiol Scand* 103:275, 1978.

58. Gunterberg B, Romanus B, Stener B: Pelvic strength after major amputation of the sacrum: an experimental approach, *Acta Orthop Scand* 47:635, 1976.

59. Hall SJ: Effective attempted lifting speed on forces and torque exerted on the lumbar spine, *Med Sci Sports Exerc* 17:440, 1985.

60. Harman E: Resistive torque analysis for five Nautilus exercise machines, *Med Sci Sports Exerc* 15:113, 1983 (abstract).

61. Harman EA: A 3-D biomechanical analysis of the bench press exercise, *Med Sci Sports Exerc* 16:159, 1984.

62. Harman EA et al: Effects of a belt on intra-abdominal pressure during weightlifting, *Med Sci Sports Exerc* 21:186, 1989.

63. Harris FA: Facilitation techniques and technological adjuncts in the therapeutic exercise. In Basmajian JV, editor: *Therapeutic exercise,* ed 9, Baltimore, 1984, Williams & Wilkins.

64. Hinson MN, Smith WC, Funk S: Isokinetics: a clarification, *Res Q* 50:30, 1979.

65. Jackson D, Leon W, Circincione R: Spondylolysis in the female gymnast, *Clin Orthop* 117:68, 1976.

66. Kotani PT et al: Studies of spondylolysis found among weight-lifters, *Br J Sports Med* 6:4, 1971.

67. Kuland DN et al: Olympic weightlifting injuries, *Physician Sports-med* 5:89, Nov 1978.

68. Kumar S: Physiologic responses to weightlifting in different planes, *Ergonomics* 10:987, 1980.

69. Lander JE, Bates BT, Dezita P: Biomechanics of the squat exercise using a modified center of mass bar, *Med Sports Sci Exerc* 18:469, 1986.

70. Lander JE et al: Comparison between free-weight and isokinetic bench pressing, *Med Sci Sports Exerc* 17:344, 1985.

71. Liu YK et al: Torsional fatigue of the lumbar intervertebral joints, *Spine* 10:894, 1985.

72. McCarrol JR, Miller JM, Ritter M: Lumbar spondylolysis and spondylolisthesis in college football players, *Am J Sports Med* 14:404, 1986.

73. McLaughlin TM, Dillman CJ, Lardner TJ: A kinematic model of performance in a parallel squat by champion powerlifters, *Med Sci Sports Exerc* 9:128, 1977.

74. McLaughlin TM, Lardner TJ, Dillman CJ: Kinetics of the parallel squat, *Res Q* 49:175, 1978.

75. Miller C: Rotary action of legs and hips common to many sports, *Natl Strength Cond Assoc J* 1:20, 1979.

76. Miller JAA, Schultz AM, Anderson GBJ: Load displacement behavior of the sacroiliac joints, *J Orthop Res* 5:92, 1987.

77. Morris JM, Locas DB, Bresler B: Role of the trunk in stability of the spine, *J Bone Joint Surg* 43A:327, 1961.

78. Nachemson A: The influence of spinal movements on the lumbar intradiscal pressure and on tensile stresses in the annulus fibrosis, *Acta Orthop Scand* 33:385, 1963.

79. Nautilus: a concept of variable resistance (Nautilus Sports/Medical Industries), *Natl Strength Cond Assoc J* 3:48, 1981.

80. Noe D: Myoelectric activity and sequencing of selected trunk muscles during isokinetic lifting, *Spine* 17:225, 1992.

81. Noffroid MR et al: A study of isokinetic exercise, *Phys Ther* 59:735, 1969.

82. O'Shea JP: *Scientific principles and methods of strength fitness,* Reading, Mass, 1969, Addison-Wesley.

83. O'Shea JP: The parallel squat, *Scand J,* 17(2):20, 1985.

84. Plaenhoef FC: *Patterns of human motion—a cinematographic analysis,* Englewood Cliffs, NJ, 1971, Prentice Hall.

85. Powell JW: Summary of injury patterns for seven seasons 1980-1986. In *NFL injury surveillance program,* San Diego, 1987, San Diego University (Department of Physical Education).

86. Rasch PJ, Burke RK: *Kinesiology and applied anatomy,* ed 6, Philadelphia, 1978, Lee & Febiger.

87. Reilly J et al: Pathological anatomy of the lumbar spine. In Helfet AJ, editor: *Disorders of the lumbar spine,* Philadelphia, 1978, JB Lippincott.

88. Rossi F: Spondylolysis, spondylolisthesis and sports, *J Sports Med Phys Fitness* 18:317, 1978.

89. Saal JA: Rehabilitation of sports-related lumbar spine injuries, *Phys Med Rehabil State Art Rev* 1(4):58, 1987.

90. Sawhill JA: *Biomechanical characteristics of rotational velocity and movement complexity in isokinetic performance,* doctoral dissertation, Eugene, 1981, University of Oregon.

91. Simms D, Fortin JD: 3-D biomechanical analysis of a lifting movement, Unpublished manuscript.

92. Starr B: *The strongest shall survive: strength training for football,* Annapolis, Md, 1976, Fitness Products.

93. Steindler A: Differential diagnosis of pain low in the back: allocation of pain by procaine hydrochloride method, *JAMA* 110:106, 1983.

94. Stone MH: Consideration in gaining a strength, power training effect, *Natl Strength Cond Assoc J* 4:22, 1982.

95. Stone MH, O'Brien HS: *Weight training: a scientific approach,* Minneapolis, 1987, Burgess.

96. Troup JG: Mechanical factors in spondylolisthesis and spondy-lolysis, *Clin Orthop* 117:59, 1976.

97. Troup JG: Dynamic factors in the analysis of stoop and crouch lifting methods: a methodological approach in the development of safe materials handling standards, *Orthop Clin North Am* 8:201, 1977.

98. Vleeming A, Stoeckart TR, Snijders SJ: The sacrotuberous ligament: a conceptual approach to its dynamic role in stabilizing the sacroiliac joint, *Clin Biomech* 4:201, 1989.

99. Vleeming A et al: Relationship between form and function in the sacroiliac joint. I. The clinical anatomic aspects. II. The biome-chanical aspects, *Spine* 15:130, 1990.

100. Vleeming A et al: Towards an integrated therapy for peripartum pelvic instability: a study based on biomechanical effects of pelvic belts. In Vleeming A, Snijders CJ, Stoeckart R, editors: *Progress in vertebral column research: first international symposium on the sacroiliac joints: its role in posture and locomotion,* Rotterdam, 1991, European Conference Organizers.

101. Walsh PR et al: Lumbar discography in normal subjects: a controlled, prospective study, *J Bone Joint Surg* 72A:1081, 1990.

102. White AA, Panjabi MM: *Clinical biomechanics of the spine,* Philadelphia, 1978, JB Lippincott.

103. Yang KH, King AI: Mechanism of facet load transmission as a hypothesis for low back pain, *Spine* 9:557, 1984.

Chapter Forty-Six

◆

Tennis

Jeffrey A. Saal

Clinical work on tennis injuries to date has focused primarily on the upper extremities, with little attention paid to the spine. However, the lumbar spine forms the base of support that allows a fluid transmission of force to the extremities. Practitioners in sports medicine are well aware that a poor base of support will not allow significant power to be generated by the upper extremities. Consider the biomechanical requirements of throwing a baseball or serving a tennis ball.[6] Rotator cuff musculature is principally active during deceleration. Major propulsion forces are generated from the torso and legs, and positional control of the body's center of gravity located anterior to the L2 and L3 vertebrae, just below the umbilicus, is a determining factor in impulse generation.[2,3] If the center of gravity is allowed to rise and fall, power generation is dissipated.

The unique aspects of the tennis stroke can place the lumbar spine in jeopardy. Much of the force generated during tennis strokes is torsional in nature. The rotational action of all tennis strokes has the potential to place stress on the spinal structure. Torsion is often accompanied by spinal flexion. The combined forces of flexion and rotation can cause fatigue-related disruption of the collagen fibers in the posterior annulus. Excessive loads may be placed on the articular cartilage surfaces of the lumbar and thoracolumbar facet joints. These repetitive forces on the disc may lead to annular tears, disc protrusions, or disc herniations. Long-standing repetitive overload delivered by microtrauma may lead to adaptive changes in the intervertebral disc biochemistry. This may manifest as multilevel lateral disc protrusions as a result of changes in the annulus collagen and nuclear proteoglycan ratios.

Figures for the incidence of disc, facet joint, and neural arch damage from playing tennis are not currently available. In my experience, posterior element pain syndromes (i.e., facet synovitis, facet capsular injury, and spondylolysis with or without spondylolisthesis) compose the injury subset most frequently seen in young tennis players. I have observed a 3-to-1 ratio of disc to postelement syndromes in national and world class tennis players. Soft tissue injuries to the thoracic lumbar region are also seen in this group of athletes. When present, these injuries usually involve the iliopsoas, the gluteal musculature, and/or the thoracolumbar fascia.[11] The upper lumbar facet joints and thoracolumbar junctional facet joints appear to be more prone to injury.

This weakness may be due to their sagittal geometry, which is more vulnerable to excessive torsional force. In my experience, these are the most common facet joint and soft tissue (i.e., ligamentous capsule) injuries suffered by tennis players.

FACTORS IN LUMBAR SPINE INJURY
Tennis Serve

Frequently I see young tennis professionals with lumbar spine and/or rotator cuff injuries that are the result of common biomechanical defects. The serve causes most lumbar injuries in tennis players, although at present there are no data to substantiate this clinical observation. In the serve, the ball toss, the position of the lower extremities, and power generation determine the load placed on the lumbar spine. If the ball toss occurs behind the serving shoulder of the player, the player must rotate and hyperextend the spine to make racquet contact. This essentially uncouples the shoulder and pelvis. Ball impact is accompanied by a rapid reversal of the rotation of the lumbar spine, literally throwing the spine from hyperextension and counterclockwise rotation to clockwise rotation and hyperflexion. This corkscrewing motion transfers the force of its torque to the spinal segments (Figs. 46-1 and 46-2).

In preparation for a serve, a player's knees must flex and a dipping motion must occur that includes pelvic rotation coupled with shoulder rotation. However, with an improperly placed ball toss, uncoupled pelvic motion occurs. The dipping motion and pelvic shoulder turn prepare the server to move into the ball at impact. The legs supply the driving force as the pelvis and shoulders turn to face the target at full impact. The racquet-bearing arm is essentially used as a whip that is accelerated by the reversal of torso rotation (i.e., the corkscrew effect). The body's center of gravity, having been lowered by the dipping motion, then moves forward along the same vector as the ball. This creates impulse generation. Insufficient leg drive, uncoupling the lower body from the upper body, will lead to spinal rotation. In addition, significant racquet power will be lost, resulting in excessive arm acceleration. Although the forces of deceleration on the rotator cuff have always been a focal issue, in my opinion this extreme arm acceleration is a major factor in the generation of rotator cuff injury. After all, the forces of deceleration actually counterbalance the forces of acceleration.

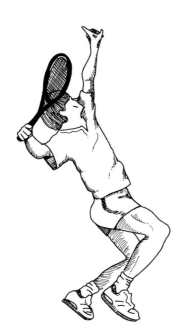

Fig. 46-1. The deep knee bend allows a dipping motion to facilitate trunk rotation and avoids thoracolumbar hyperextension. Note the shoulder and pelvic position coupled in the same angle of rotation.

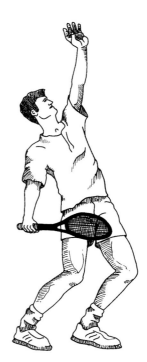

Fig. 46-2. The shoulders and pelvis begin to rotate as a coupled unit. Excessive spinal rotation is avoided while total trunk rotation is accomplished.

Backhand

The backhand serve, with use of a two-handed technique, can place significant force on the lumbar spine and hip. The closed stance and long follow-through required by this technique cause a high degree of spinal rotation and do not allow spinal release at follow-through. Instructing the player to slightly open the front foot toward the hitting target can reduce the rotational stress on the spine and hip. Leg drive and a deep stance will additionally assist in power generation and will decrease spinal load.

Forehand

Currently a common style is to hit topspin, the racquet going from low to high, with a wide-open stance. A wide-open stance keeps the shoulder parallel, rather than perpendicular, to the net. This style requires the generation of force to come principally from the upper body, thereby robbing the player of any significant leg drive and torso impulse generation. The topspin hitting style requires that the pelvis and shoulder be uncoupled, which results in a load transmission to the lumbar spine. Clinically the resulting load transmission often manifests as a lateral and far-lateral disc herniation at L3-4 and L4-5 ipsilateral to the side of hand dominance. Adaptive changes in these players often demonstrate changes in disc morphology that may remain asymptomatic for

prolonged periods of time. A partial open stance appears to be the most rational way to optimize tennis performance and still not jeopardize the lumbar spine.

Equipment

One of the goals in the design of tennis racquets has been to decrease forces to the upper extremity while maximizing power and maintaining ball control. An updated racquet design may have contributed to the reduction in lumbar injuries by facilitating power generation for the recreational player. Given new racquet designs, players do not need to try to overpower the ball, which invariably leads to poor form and, ultimately, to excessive spinal loads.

Court Surface

There are theoretic considerations concerning the effect of the court surface on the lumbar load. Clay is a more shock-absorbing and forgiving surface and requires a sliding step. Composite courts are less forgiving and transfer higher loads to the lower extremities and spine. Grass courts share some of the shock-absorbing capabilities of clay courts, but they can be rock hard and therefore even worse than composite courts. Tennis professionals often tell me they can feel the difference in their low backs when they switch from one court surface to another. For the recreational player, playing on different court surfaces is not a significant issue.

Player's Age

Degenerative changes of the spine often predispose middle-aged recreational players to low back injury. The degenerative spinal segment becomes hypomobile, and with an increased load bearing on the facet articular cartilage, accompanying stenosis may also present. A degenerative segment in the hypermobile phase (i.e., early degenerative spondylolisthesis at L4-5 or the early retrospondylolisthesis at L3-4 or L4-5) will cause excessive strain on annular fibers, facet capsules, and restraining ligaments. Subpar physical conditioning will lead to poor soft tissue flexibility and inadequate muscular strength. When this is accompanied by a lack of ability to stabilize the spine, excessive forces will be placed on the spinal structures. These phenomena are further complicated when faulty tennis technique places the trunk in improper positions and angles. Exacerbating preexistent asymptomatic spinal stenosis, which results in intermittent radicular pain and back pain, is a common complaint in older players.

ASPECTS OF REHABILITATION

The basic principles of athletic rehabilitation have been discussed elsewhere.[8] Therefore only principles specifically related to treatment of the lumbar spine in tennis players are presented in this section.[12]

Flexibility

Contracture and shortening of the iliopsoas and the hip rotator must be reversed. Tight hip flexors lead to increased lumbar lordosis, especially while the player is running. Asymmetric hip-flexor contractures may lead to lumbar rotation and extension with running and reaching. Tight hip rotators will cause the lumbar spine to absorb all of the deceleration forces and may predispose the players to injury. In addition, attention to the gastrocsoleus, quadriceps, and hamstring musculature (Fig. 46-3) is necessary.

The thoracolumbar fascia and shoulder complex are additional focal areas in a stretching program. Adequate extensibility of the fascia and shoulder complex will facilitate coupled shoulder motion. If the soft tissues in the anterior shoulder remain tight, they will force players to hyperextend the thoracic spine to make ball contact during a tennis serve. This chronic hyperextension and rotation may lead to facet joint pain, exacerbation of spinal stenosis, or shearing of the outer annular disc fibers.

Joint Mobility

The functional range of motion of a spinal segment should be maximized, as should that of the hips, knees, ankles, and shoulders. Manual therapy is an important adjunct in the accomplishment of this task. However, the mobility of a spinal segment by itself without stability and strength is worthless and may even be deleterious.

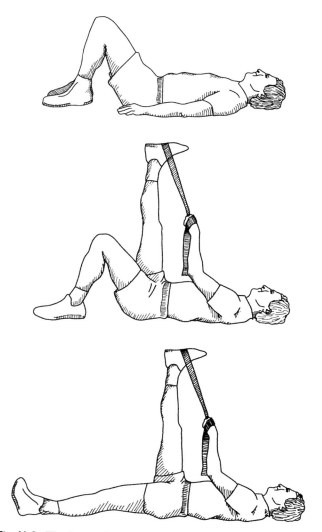

Fig. 46-3. The hamstring stretch will increase the flexibility that is necessary to stabilize the spine properly.

Therefore manual techniques that maximize mobility must be accompanied by exercise and neuromuscular education. Severely degenerative segments will become more symptomatic when their range is pushed, and hypermobile segments (i.e., spondylolisthesis) should not be mobilized at all.

Strength

The internal oblique abdominal muscles, the latissimus dorsi, and the serratus anterior, coupled with the thoracolumbar fascia, are necessary to stabilize the spine against repetitive rotational forces. Therefore strategies that strengthen these muscle groups in a spine-safe fashion are necessary[9,12,15] (Fig. 46-4). In addition, players must be taught how to use these muscle groups in a consolidated fashion to dynamically stabilize the spine.[7,10]

Lower extremity musculature, including the quadriceps, gluteus maximus, and medius, must be strength-

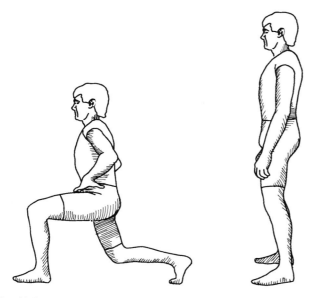

Fig. 46-4. Forward lunges are one of the many exercises that strengthen the abdominal, leg, and buttock muscles and help the individual practice balance and stabilization.

ened to ensure an adequate base of support. To eliminate lumbar lordosis, an anterior pelvic tilt coupled with a lowered stance (i.e., lowering the center of gravity) is necessary. This position is similar in principle to the basic horse stance used in martial arts training. The gluteal muscles are often overlooked in rehabilitation programs. These muscles may require special rehabilitation techniques to resume normal firing patterns of neurophysiologic motor units.[4] Poor gluteus medius strength will lead to excessive lateral hip deviation and sway in the single-legged stance phase of running, walking, and so on. Weakness in the gluteus maximus will lead to an overdependence on the lumbar spine extensors to promote trunk extension.

Neuromuscular Education

After flexibility and strength are attained, players must be taught dynamic lumbar muscular stabilization (DLMS).[9,13,14] This process of muscular reeducation coordinates muscle groups in the control of the pelvis and lumbar spine, thereby making available sufficient power generation and transfer of torso torque. DLMS eliminates repetitive microtrauma to the lumbar motion segments, thereby encouraging healing of spinal injuries. It also may alter the progression of degenerative processes of the spine.

In DLMS the musculature braces the spine, a state identified as muscle fusion. This muscular bracing protects the motion segments against repetitive microtrauma and excessively high single-occurrence loads.[5] The abdominal mechanism, which couples the midline ligament and the dorsolumbar fascia—combined with a

slight reduction in lumbar lordosis—can eliminate shear stress to the lumbar intervertebral segment. The abdominal musculature may flex the lumbar spine through its action on the superficial portion of the dorsolumbar fascia. It may also extend the lumbar spine through its action on the deep portions of the fascia that form the alar interspinal ligaments. This coupled action enables the abdominal muscles to corset the lumbar region in concert with the latissimus dorsi, which also acts on the dorsolumbar fascia. The lowering of the center of gravity through slight knee flexion, facilitated by adequately strong quadriceps muscles, is an important element in the bracing of the spine.[5,7,12]

Control of lordosis during flexion and extension is extremely important because of the changes in axial rotation that are possible at intervertebral segments at different degrees of lordosis. The control of lordosis and muscular stabilization are two mechanisms that demonstrate how flexibility and balanced muscular function permit the management of stresses applied to lumbar intervertebral segments.

Adequate flexibility and spinal range of motion (ROM) must be attained in order to apply muscle fusion. In an interesting study regarding diurnal variations and stresses on the lumbar spine, Adams, Dolan, and Hutton[1] described a daily pattern of changes in lumbar disc and ligament extensibility. These changes, based on the creep of soft tissue structures, lead to increased spinal ROM. Adams and colleagues noted that bending and lifting activities performed early in the morning, when ligamentous and annular fibers are less extensible, are more likely to cause fatigue damage to the disc than similar activities performed later in the day. Thus flexibility of the structures eliminates this repetitive fatigue stress to the intervertebral joint. Muscles that attach to the pelvis as "guy wires" can effectively change the pelvic position and symmetry.

Pelvic positioning is the key to postural control of the lumbar spine. Therefore adequate flexibility of the hamstring, quadriceps, iliopsoas, gastrocsoleus, hip rotator, and iliotibial band muscles is important, as are flexible neural elements.

Stabilization Training Routines

Stabilization training routines can be divided into basic and advanced programs (see box on p. 503).[9] The regimen commences with exercises performed in the supine or prone position, then advances to exercises performed in the kneeling position, then standing, and finally to movements of position transition (i.e., standing to sitting, sitting to standing, and supine to sitting). The athlete must have meticulous technique while performing these exercises; therefore supervision by an experienced physical therapist or exercise trainer is important. The basic-level exercises are first taught with one-on-one instruction and then in a group. Each exercise is

Exercise Training for Lumbar Disc Disorder

Soft Tissue Flexibility

Hamstrings musculotendinous unit
Quadriceps musculotendinous unit
Iliopsoas musculotendinous unit
Gastrocsoleus musculotendinous unit
External and internal hip rotators

Joint Mobility

Lumbar spine segmental mobility
Hip ROM
Thoracic segmental mobility

Stabilization Program

Finding neutral position (standing, sitting, jumping, prone)
Prone gluteal squeezes with:
    Arm raises
    Alternate arm raises
    Leg raises
    Alternate leg raises
    Arm and leg raises
    Alternate arm and leg raises
Supine pelvic bracing
Bridging progression
Basic position:
    One leg raised with ankle weights
    Stepping
    Balancing on gym ball

Quadruped (alternating arm and leg movements with ankle and wrist weights)
Kneeling stabilization (double knee, single knee, lunges with and without weight)
Wall-slide quadriceps strengthening
Position transition with postural control

Abdominal Program

Curl-ups
"Dead bugs" (supported, nonsupported)
Diagonal curl-ups
Diagonal curl-ups on incline board
Straight leg lowering

Gym Program

Latissimus pull-downs
Angled leg press
Lunges
Hyperextension bench
General upper body weight exercises
Pulley exercises to stress postural control

Aerobic Program

Progressive walking
Swimming
Stationary bicycling
Cross-country ski machine
Running (initially supervised on a treadmill)

---

designed to develop isolated and co-contraction muscle patterns to stabilize the lumbar spine in its neutral position. A neutral spine position is not necessarily a total absence of lordosis but rather the most comfortable position for the patient on the basis of biomechanical principles discussed later.

Each patient should be monitored during the exercise program to define the optimal spine position. Care should be taken to ensure proper form and exercise repetition speed. The neurophysiologic principle of central pathway irradiation secondary to increased amplitude of effort must be kept in mind.[4] Engram motor programming is the goal of the exercise program; therefore careful repetition of the exercises with precise movements is required. Once engram motor programming has occurred, the exercise routine is patterned in the motor cortex—available without conscious effort.

When proper exercise form and technique have been achieved, the program can be advanced. Balancing on a large gym ball will make the floor exercise more challenging. The addition of wrist and ankle weights or theraband also intensifies the effort required, thus requiring a greater degree of dynamic stabilization. These principles also can be applied to the weight-

training portion of the program.[15] The patient is taught how to mount and dismount weight-training equipment while maintaining stabilization principles. Patients should be educated as to the safe methods of changing the weight stack–resistance pin on the machines and lifting and racking free weights, as well as how to use free weights, pulleys, and single-station weight machines. This resistance equipment requires contraction of the lower abdominal musculature to maintain optimal anteverted pelvic positioning, with the lower back flattened against a back support while a stabilized neutral spine is maintained. Therefore all gym routines become functional stabilization exercises.[11]

Sport-specific stabilization routines are used in the advanced portion of the program. The use of pulleys and elastic tubing for resistance training in a variety of positions is taught. The gym ball can be used to challenge balance while the athlete attempts single-arm and double-arm exercises[10] (Fig. 46-5).

The baseline side-shuffle drill trains the player to shuffle step on the baseline from side to side while maintaining neutral position. The volley setup drill trains the player to sit up in proper volleying position while maintaining a stabilized spine. The ball toss drill is

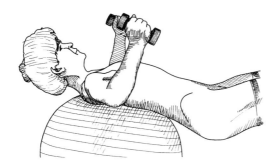

Fig. 46-5. Chest flies performed while on a Swiss gym ball.

coupled with serving practice to train proper ball-toss position to facilitate a coupled shoulder and pelvic motion pattern.

I supervise the on-court stabilization training in which the principles of injury prevention (discussed in the stroke-technique section) are reinforced. Players are encouraged to seek out a teaching professional to work on specific tennis technique flaws.

Exercise training is the core of the athletic rehabilitation process. However, pain and inflammation must be adequately controlled to allow the athlete to participate in the sport-specific exercise training.[16] Acupuncture is a useful adjunctive treatment for this purpose. Its drugless, nontoxic nature provides an ideal aid in sports medicine. In addition, it is considered to be most effective on younger and constitutionally stronger persons. Not only can acupuncture treatments reduce pain and inflammation, but they can also reduce muscle hypertonicity, thus facilitating stretching of the specific muscles that may be central to the rehabilitation process.[5]

REFERENCES

1. Adams MA, Dolan P, Hutton WC: Diurnal variations in the stresses on the lumbar spine, *Spine* 12:130, 1987.
2. Ariel G: Biomechanical analysis of shotputting, *Track Field Q Rev* 79:27, 1980.
3. Ariel G: Biomechanical analysis of the hammer throw, *Track Field Q Rev* 80:41, 1980.
4. Harris FA: Facilitation techniques and technological adjuncts in therapeutic exercise. In Basmajian JV, editor: *Therapeutic exercise,* Baltimore, 1984, Williams & Wilkins.
5. Saal JA: Rehabilitation of sports-related lumbar spine injuries, *Phys Med Rehabil State Art Rev* 1:613, 1987.
6. Saal JA: Rehabilitation of throwing and tennis related shoulder injuries, *Phys Med Rehabil State Art Rev* 1:597, 1987.
7. Saal JA: Rehabilitation of football players with lumbar spine injuries, *Physician Sportsmed* 16(9):61, 1988.
8. Saal JA: Rehabilitation of the injured athlete. In DeLisa JA, editor: *Principles and practice of rehabilitation medicine,* Philadelphia, 1988, JB Lippincott.
9. Saal JA: Dynamic muscular stabilization in the nonoperative treatment of lumbar pain syndromes, *Orthopedics* 19:691, 1990.
10. Saal JA: Intervertebral disc herniation: advances in nonoperative treatment, *Phys Med Rehabil State Art Rev* 4:175, 1990.
11. Saal JA: Lumbar injuries in gymnastics, *Spine State Art Rev* 4:426, 1990.
12. Saal JA, Saal JS: Nonoperative treatment of herniated lumbar intervertebral disc with radiculopathy, *Spine* 14:431, 1989.
13. Saal JA, Saal JS: Initial stage management of lumbar spine problems, *Phys Med Rehabil State Art Rev* 2:187, 1991.
14. Saal JA, Saal JS: Later stage management of lumbar spine problems, *Phys Med Rehabil State Art Rev* 2:205, 1991.
15. Saal JS, Saal JA: Strength training and flexibility. In White AH, Anderson R, editors: *Conservative care of low back pain,* Baltimore, 1991, Williams & Wilkins.
16. Saal JS et al: High levels of inflammatory phospholipase A_2 activity in lumbar disc herniations, *Spine* 15:674, 1990.

Chapter Forty-Seven

Golf

Brett Fischer
Robert G. Watkins

Golf is an athletic sport! It takes athletic ability to consistently hit a No. 3 iron 200 yards and land near the hole. With this swing the golfer may generate a club-head speed of around 100 mph in less than one fifth of a second.[10] With this amount of power and speed, as well as the repetitive nature of golf, it is obvious that injuries to the spine will occur. In fact, the majority of injuries to players with the Professional Golf Association (PGA) Tour have involved the spine.[1]

Effective rehabilitation of athletes with these injuries requires that the medical practitioner not only be educated in the use of trunk stabilization exercises but also have working knowledge of the physical mechanics of the golf swing. Insight into how the body functions in a proper golf swing can enhance the golfer's swing, as well as restore spinal function and prevent further injury.

This chapter focuses on the following aspects of the golf swing: the basic mechanics, the important trunk and hip muscles involved, and specific exercises for stability and mobility of the spine.

BASIC MECHANICS OF THE GOLF SWING

The essence of a mechanically sound golf swing is strength, balance, proper posture, and flexibility. For many years it was believed that strength in the arms and shoulders generated the power and speed in the golf swing; actually, however, the trunk generates the power, and the hip and trunk muscles transmit this power and speed.[7] This is not to say that the shoulders (rotator cuff muscles) and arm muscles do not play integral roles. The rotator cuff muscles are responsible for providing a coordinated and harmonious movement to protect the glenohumeral complex.[8]

The purpose of trunk stabilization exercises is to retrain the musculature to control, coordinate, and optimize function—especially that of the spine—in sport-specific movements.[9] Again, these exercises not only assist in the rehabilitation of the player's spinal injuries but also enhance a golfer's ability to perform an "athletic golf swing." An athletic golf swing is a swing that uses the large trunk muscles to provide the needed power and speed while supporting the lumbar spine in a relatively constant neutral position throughout the swing. This is believed to be the safest way to swing.

For many years golfers were taught a swing in which the hips slid (rather than rotated) from side to side, with the lumbar spine finishing in extreme hyperextension or

a reverse C (Fig. 47-1). However, the reverse C swing is not only harmful but also inefficient because the off-balance golfer loses the power generated by the trunk and hip muscles.

In contrast, the athletic swing is a golf swing in which the larger muscles of the trunk dictate the golf swing. David Leadbetter,[4] world-renowned golf teacher, describes the athletic swing as "the efficient coiling and uncoiling of one's torso in a rotary or circular motion which maximizes centrifugal force. Centrifugal force is the force created away from the center of one's swing, transmitting from your body (trunk and hips) out through your arms and hands. This creates clubhead speed and maintains the club on a steady orbit or arc." This is an important concept in the rehabilitation of the golfer's spine, because if the neutral position of the lumbar spine is lost (excessive lumbar flexion or extension) during the golf swing, power and speed also will be lost and, more important, the steady arc of the club head will be disrupted as it travels on an incorrect plane.

The athletic golf swing not only maximizes the power generated but also causes less stress on the lower back. Furthermore, the athletic swing can be imitated by an amateur or a patient with a spinal injury, because it does not require excessive flexibility in the trunk and hip

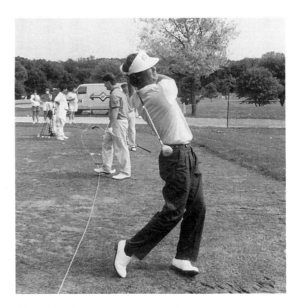

Fig. 47-1. A commonly seen swing among amateurs.

region. The finish in an athletic golf swing is much more upright (although the lumbar spine is still neutral) (Fig. 47-2) than the reverse C swing.

The five basic phases of the athletic golf swing are as follows:

1. *Setup/address*—Posture of the golfer, ready position (Fig. 47-3, *A*)
2. *Take-away/move-away*—From ball address to the top of the back swing (Fig. 47-3, *B*)
3. *Transition*—From the end of the backswing until the arms return to horizontal (Fig. 47-3, *C*)
4. *Acceleration*—From the arms horizontal to ball contact (Fig. 47-3, *D*)
5. *Follow-through*—From ball contact to the end of the golf swing (Fig. 47-3, *E*)

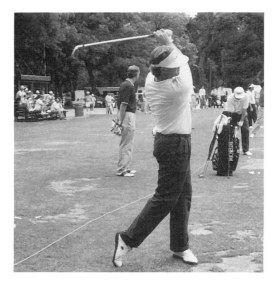

Fig. 47-2. The athletic golf swing finish is a balanced swing with minimal stress on the lower back.

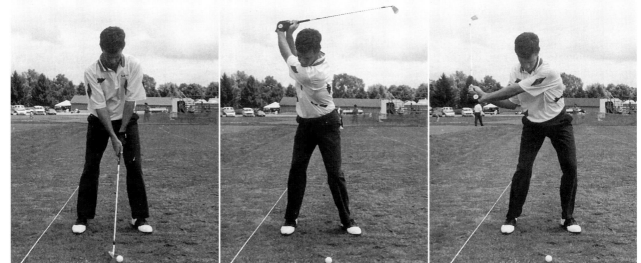

Fig. 47-3. Five phases of the athletic golf swing. **A,** Setup/address. **B,** Take-away/move-away. **C,** Transition. **D,** Acceleration. **E,** Follow-through.

EXERCISES FOR THE ATHLETIC GOLF SWING

All exercises are explained for right-handed golfers and should be performed bilaterally.

Phase 1: Setup/Address

In phase 1, balance and posture are the most important factors in preparing and allowing the body to make a powerful and safe swing. Theoretically, if a perpendicular line were dropped from the shoulder, it would intersect the patella. The golfer should be in a ready and balanced position. Many golfers rock forward and then backward to find the middle, or balanced, position on the balls of their feet.

Fig. 47-4 shows a golfer with too much weight on his heels, and Fig. 47-5 shows a golfer with weight too far forward on his toes. Both setups are incorrect because they throw the golfer off balance and will cause a problem in the swing. More important, they place the golfer at a higher risk for injury.

Phase 1 exercises

Postural exercises (Figs. 47-6 and 47-7)

Balance exercises (Figs. 47-8 and 47-9) — An efficient method of improving the patient's ability to control movement and posture. While balancing on a rocking board, the patient relearns smooth, coordinated movement, apparently by improving proprioceptive function. A poor movement pattern can also develop with deconditioning, and in this case it is the neglect of healthy movement that could cause harm.[3]

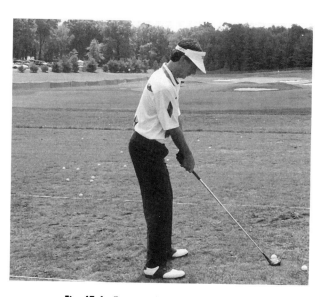

Fig. 47-4. Stance that is too upright.

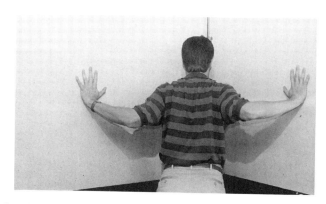

Fig. 47-6. Pectoralis stretch, which prevents shoulder protraction, thus allowing the golfer to increase the depth of the take-away.

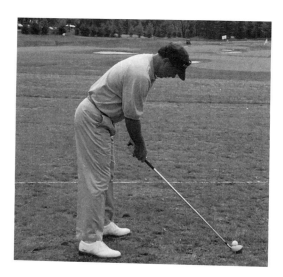

Fig. 47-5. Stance that is bent over too far.

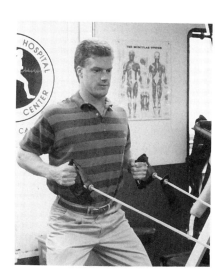

Fig. 47-7. Rowing.

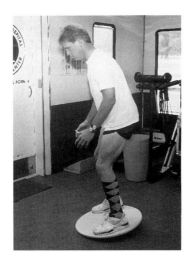

Fig. 47-8. General balance exercise.

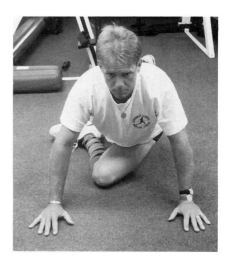

Fig. 47-10. Piriformis stretch.

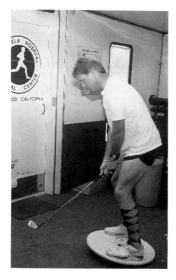

Fig. 47-9. Balance exercise with club in setup position.

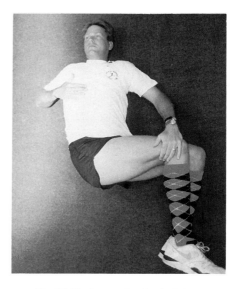

Fig. 47-11. Lower back stretch.

Quadriceps-strengthening exercises — Allow the golfer to assume a semisquat position with the lumbar spine in neutral.

Phase 2: Take-Away/Move-Away

Phase 2 covers the period from ball address to the top of the backswing (see Fig. 47-3, *B*). Here, proper coiling in the backswing is mandatory for maximum power.[11] Many golfers believe they are coiling when they turn their hips, shoulders, and chest the same amount during the back swing. They are certainly turning, but they are not coiling, and therefore they lose a lot of power. Ideally, a golfer needs a 2:1 ratio (shoulder turn to hip turn). This coiling is needed to put the trunk muscles (lumbar rotators, abdominal obliques) in an optimal

stretch position to achieve maximal firing of those muscles. For example, if two ends of a rubber band are moved in the same direction and one end is let loose, there will be little, if any, recoil from the rubber band. On the other hand, if one end is taken farther away from the other end, there will be a considerable recoil once the one end of the rubber band is released. This example holds true for the trunk muscles.

Phase 2 exercises

Internal hip and hamstring stretch — Hamstring stretch with internal rotation of the hip to enhance the amount of flexibility in the backswing (especially the right leg).

Piriformis stretch (Fig. 47-10)

Lower back stretch (Fig. 47-11)

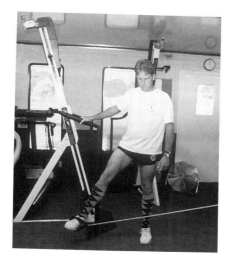

Fig. 47-12. Abductor exercise.

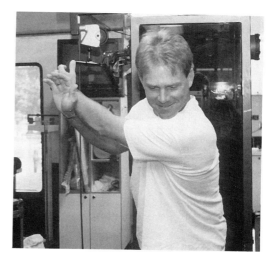

Fig. 47-14. Standing trunk twist.

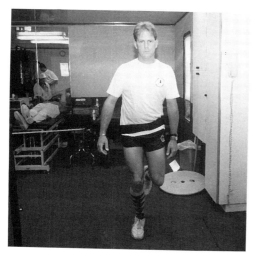

Fig. 47-13. Right abductor exercise. This exercise is a co-contraction of the right hip with emphasis on the right abductor. It is performed by keeping the trunk "neutral" while executing a semisquat with resistance pulling from the right.

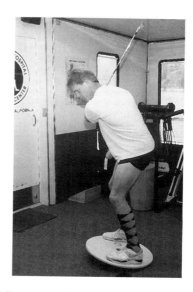

Fig. 47-15. Balance exercise with club in take-away position.

Right abductor exercises (Figs. 47-12 and 47-13)—Important exercise to support and balance the weight as the body shifts to the right side.

Standing trunk twist (Fig. 47-14)—Stretch involving both the trunk and the shoulders.

Balance exercise (Fig. 47-15)—Trains the patient to stay balanced, with the spine neutral, at the top of the backswing (balancing anterior to posterior).

Phase 3: Transition

Phase 3 covers the period from the end of the backswing until the arms are horizontal. A smooth transition from backswing to downswing depends on the movement in the lower portion of the body, specifically the legs.[4] The hips begin the swing as the left leg pulls and the right leg pushes the pelvis forward. In the right leg the gluteus, biceps, femoris, and semimembranosus muscles push the pelvis forward for power.[7] Tightness in the hip flexor muscles can hinder the amount of this hip extension. Therefore it is imperative that the hip flexors be loosened (e.g., by stretching, massage, myofascial release) on a regular basis. In the left leg, the adductor magnus is most active as it pulls the pelvis forward. This pushing and pulling results in pelvis rotation.[7]

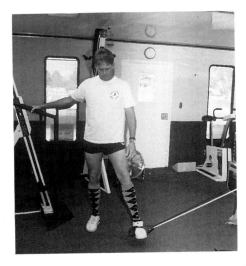

Fig. 47-16. Leg adduction exercise (in this example the left leg).

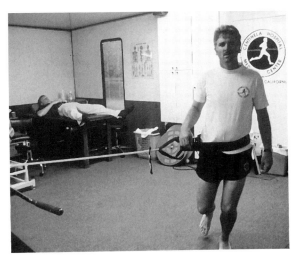

Fig. 47-17. Left adductor exercise. This exercise is a co-contraction of the left hip with emphasis on the left adductor and quadriceps. It is performed by doing a semisquat, as in Fig. 47-13.

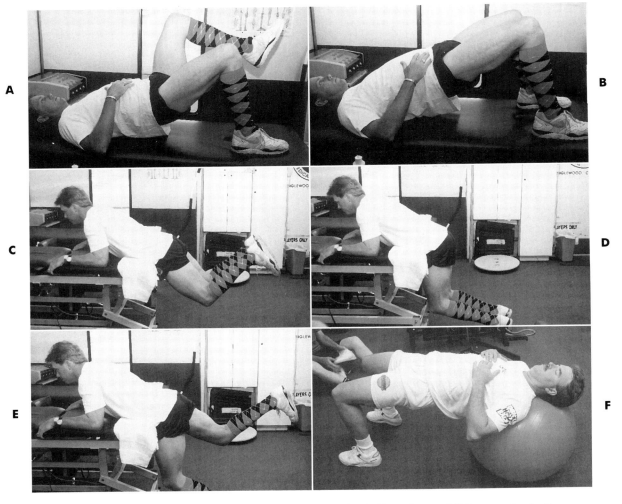

Fig. 47-18. A to **E,** Hip extension exercises. The exercise in **E** can be used if the exercise in **C** and **D** is too difficult. **F,** Static hip extension exercise. This exercise works on the endurance capabilities of the hip extensors. Patients keep their spine "neutral" while trying to stay in that position as long as they can.

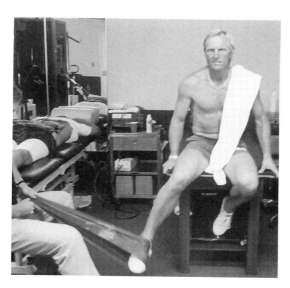

Fig. 47-19. Hip external rotation.

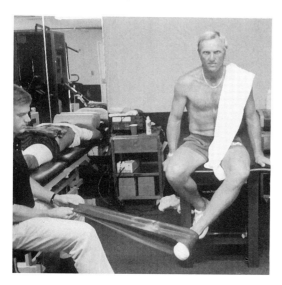

Fig. 47-20. Hip internal rotation.

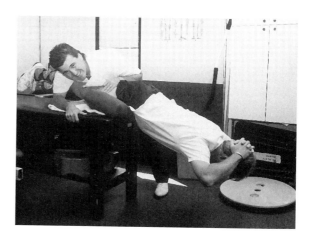

Fig. 47-21. Reverse sit-up.

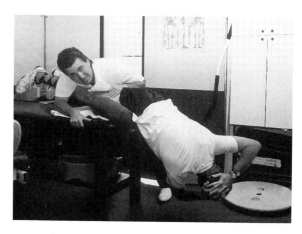

Fig. 47-22. Reverse sit-up with rotation.

Phase 3 exercises
Left leg adduction (Figs. 47-16 and 47-17) — Pulls the pelvis forward.
Left leg abduction
Right leg adduction
Hip extensor exercises (Fig. 47-18)
Hip external exercises (Fig. 47-19)
Hip internal exercises (Fig. 47-20)
Hip flexor stretching
NOTE: Research at the Centinela Fitness Institute, Inglewood, California, revealed that, of the golfers on the PGA Tour who were tested, the internal rotators of the left hip of the average right-handed PGA player were stronger than those of the right, and the external rotators

of the right hip were stronger than those of the left. A possible explanation of these findings is that a highly repetitive, reproducible pattern develops strong right hip external rotators and left hip internal rotators during the transitional and acceleration phases.

Phase 4: Acceleration

Phase 4 covers the period from when the arms are horizontal to the moment of ball impact. There is continued power transmission from the trunk and hip region, with controlled weight shifting from the right to the left side. At impact, the angle of the lumbar spine should be at neutral.
Phase 4 exercises
Reverse sit-up (Fig. 47-21) — All movement is centered at the hip joints.
Reverse sit-up with rotation (Fig. 47-22)
Seated rotations (Fig. 47-23)
Standing rotation (Fig. 47-24)

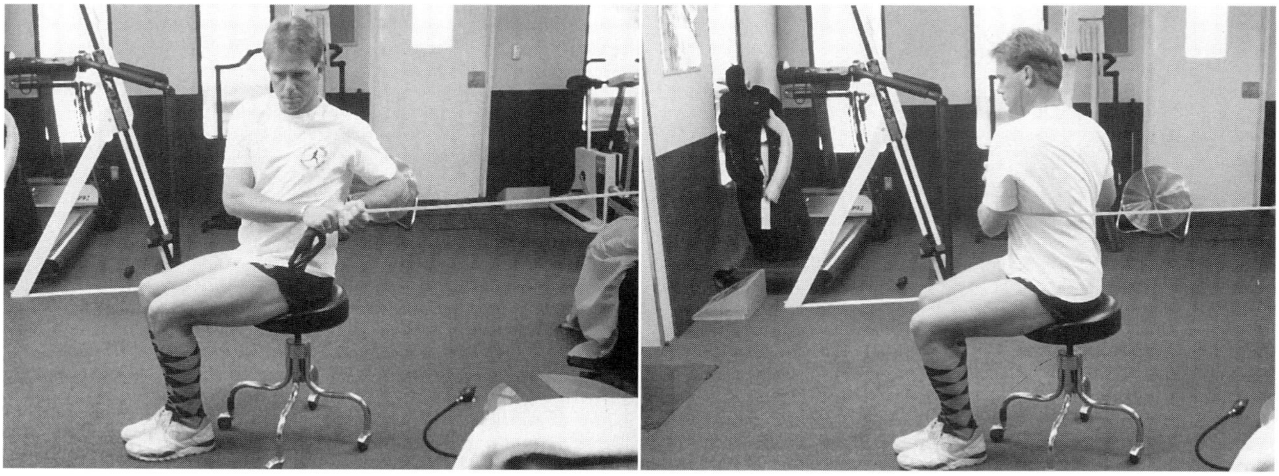

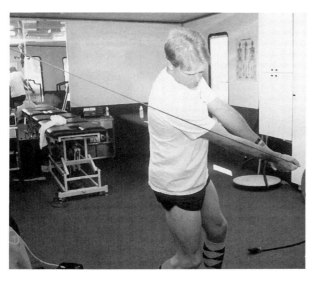

Fig. 47-24. Standing rotation.

Fig. 47-23. Seated rotation.

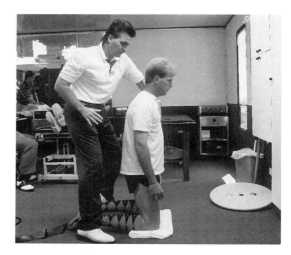

Fig. 47-25. Balance and trunk-strengthening exercise. Here the patient is instructed to stay neutral as the therapist pushes the patient in all directions.

Abdominal exercises
Balance/trunk-strengthening exercise (Fig. 47-25)

Phase 5: Follow-Through

Phase 5 covers the period from ball contact to the end of the golf swing. Just after impact, the golfer should feel the left side "firm up" because the hip muscles are used to stabilize the hip and pelvis as the weight and torque are transferred to the left side.[7] Weakness in the left hip region increases the risk of injury to the left sacroiliac joint and lumbar spine because there is no control or support as the body rotates through the swing. Leadbetter[4] adds that if the player uses the lower body to support the hip and pelvis, the upper body will be able to rotate through the ball.

Many times golfers complain of "not being able to stay down on the ball" or of having a "hard time getting through the ball." This is sometimes due to problems in the hips. Some patients with hip problems (e.g., restrictive capsule, muscular tightness) may find it easier to swing by turning the left foot outward (externally rotating) to allow for more freedom and less stress on the hips during the follow-through phase.

Phase 5 exercises
Left hip exercises (see Figs. 47-16 and 47-17)
Multidirectional balance exercises (Fig. 47-26)

AEROBIC CONDITIONING

Because golf is not an aerobic sport, aerobic conditioning should be included in any effective lower back

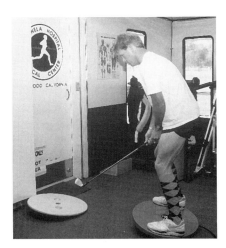

Fig. 47-26. Multidirectional balance exercise.

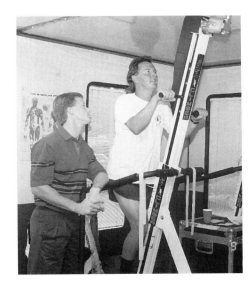

Fig. 47-27. Stair climber exercise.

rehabilitation program. Nutter[6] showed that higher aerobic fitness shows a strong negative correlation with the incidence of both lower back pain and disc herniation. Exercise results in increased aerobic metabolism in the outer annulus and the central portion of the nucleus pulposus, bringing about reduction of lactate concentration.[2]

Also, aerobic conditioning plays a significant role in muscle coordination during periods of fatigue. Fatigue can produce abnormal muscle function and overcompensation and thus resultant injury. Fatigue obviously can affect performance through a lack of proper balance and coordination as a result of inappropriately, selective, weak muscles.

Unfortunately, some patients cannot tolerate certain types of aerobic conditioning that have high levels of loading to the spine, such as jogging. However, several types of aerobic conditioning exercises are highly effective without loading the spine (e.g., water exercises[12] and the stair climber [Fig. 47-27]).

EVALUATION, TREATMENT, AND REHABILITATION

As structure governs function, similarly, abnormal structure governs dysfunction.[2,5] Thus a thorough evaluation must be undertaken before strengthening and stretching exercises are begun. The examination is completed by use of x-ray films, magnetic resonance imaging, computed tomography scanning, muscle testing, range of motion, segmental testing of vertebrae for hypomobility and hypermobility, postural evaluation, palpation, and various other methods and/or tests.

Once the dysfunction is identified, appropriate treatment techniques must be used to correct the structural abnormality. This will allow for enhanced function and therefore improve the rehabilitation process in which trunk strength, muscle coordination, and balance are stressed. Trunk strength involves the muscles of the

thighs, hips, and trunk. The trunk muscles include the rectus abdominis, oblique abdominis, paraspinal musculature, latissimus dorsi, and, further up the spine, the scapular stabilizers. The muscles that insert into the lumbodorsal fascia play a key role in providing adequate balance and strength for the lumbar spine and the trunk during the golf swing. Trunk strength provides a synchrony of motion between the upper and lower extremities in that there is a controlled unwinding of the upper body relative to the trunk. The power of the golf swing is transferred from the strong leg and hip musculature through the trunk and out to the end of the club head.

Trunk fatigue produces a loss of this synchrony between the upper and lower extremities. This reduction in muscle strength prevents a proper transfer of force and leads to compensations by the body. Thus the improvement of muscle strength, coordination, the firing sequence of muscles, and body balance underlies the entire rehabilitation process and facilitates the golfer's achieving a consistent, reproducible, effective swing.

An injury to the spine can cause pain, which produces weakness and a loss of muscle control. This loss of muscle control, which can lead to further injury because the joint is now unsupported, is similar to quadriceps weakness and its cause-and-effect relationship to a knee injury. As soon as referred pain begins, muscles in the area of referred pain become weak. Any attempt to reproduce a proper golf swing under these circumstances can be difficult and can lead to continued pain, poor swing mechanics, and subsequently poor performance. Obviously, just as in a knee injury, the solution to this problem is to first correct the structural or damaged area and then strengthen that area by use of golf-specific exercises.

ACKNOWLEDGMENTS

Special thanks to Centinela Hospital Medical Center, Paul Azinger, Chuck Cook, Nolan Henke, Paul Hopenthal, David Leadbetter, Larry Mize, Greg Norman, Mark O'Meara, Marilyn Pink, Dan Pohl, and Payne Stewart for their help with this chapter.

REFERENCES

1. Duda M: Golfers use exercise to get back in the swing, *Physician Sportsmed* 17(8):109, 1989.
2. Holm S, Nachemson A: Variations in the nutrition of the canine intervertebral disc induced by motion, *Spine* 8:866, 1983.
3. Hubka M: Conservative management of idiopathic hypermobility and early lumbar instability using proprioceptive rehabilitation: a report of two cases, *Chiropract Techn* 1(3):88, 1989.
4. Leadbetter D: *The golf swing*, Lexington, Mass, 1990, Stephen Greene Press.
5. Martinke D: The philosophy of osteopathic medicine. In DiGiovanna, Schiowitz, editors: *An osteopathic approach to diagnosis and treatment*, Philadelphia, 1991, JB Lippincott.
6. Nutter P: Aerobic exercise in the treatment and prevention of low back pain, *Occup Med State Art Rev* 3:1, 1988.
7. Pink M: Biomechanics of Golf. Lecture presented at PGA meeting, Nashville, Tenn, Nov 1990.
8. Pink M, Jobe F, Perry J: Electromyographic analysis of the shoulder during the golf swing, *Am J Sports Med* 8(2):137, 1990.
9. Saal J: Advances in nonoperative treatment, *Phys Med Rehabil State Art Rev* 4(4):339, 1990.
10. Stover C, Wiren G, Topaz S: The modern golf swing and stress syndromes, *Physician Sportsmed* 4(9):43, 1976.
11. Tomasi TJ: Are you coiling or just turning? *Golf Illust*, p 43, Aug 1991.
12. Watkins R, Buhler B, Loverock P: *The water workout recovery program*, Chicago, 1988, Contemporary Books.

Chapter Forty-Eight

◆

Soccer

Pieter F. van Akkerveeken

Because soccer players may have body contact with their opponents, soccer is considered a contact sport. This aspect of soccer is responsible for the majority of injuries. During contact, players may suddenly change direction in their movements and collide; a collision between two players running at maximum speed may result in a fractured tibia or a rupture of knee ligaments. In skilled and well-trained soccer players the rate of injuries is strongly related to the level of play[11]; although an amateur player will avoid high-risk contact, professional players are willing to take those risks because of the large amounts of money involved.

EPIDEMIOLOGY

No studies on the relationship between spinal disorders and soccer have been published. However, publications on soccer and injuries in general are abundant. Unfortunately, the majority of publications are difficult to compare because they lack uniform terminology.

Under the auspices of the Counsel of the European Community, in 1986 a task force defined a sports injury as one that must be acquired during a match or training and must reduce the activity of the athlete, require treatment or medical advice, and/or result in social and economic consequences.[23] Ekstrand and Gillguist[5] gave a more tangible definition: the injury must cause a player to miss at least the next game or practice session. To classify the injuries according to their severity, they defined three categories: "minor," resulting in absenteeism from training and/or games of less than 1 week; "moderate," causing absenteeism from 1 week to 1 month; and "major," causing absenteeism of more than 1 month.

The rate of injuries is usually expressed per 1000 hours of games or training. Injuries are differentiated according to injuries occurring in men, women, or youth; in indoor or outdoor soccer; and in professional or amateur soccer. Furthermore, the type and location of injury (see box at right), the source of the injury, and whether the injury is due to a specific, well-defined trauma or to "overuse" are considered. The latter may be questionable because symptoms due to "overuse" may well be caused by mechanisms other than soccer. This is of particular significance in entities not well defined, such as low back pain.

Ekstrand and Gillguist[5] studied an amateur division with 12 teams and 180 players for 1 year. They reported 256 injuries in 124 players. Of these 256 injuries, 12 (5%)

were located in the "back." Nine of these were "minor"; three were "moderate." No major injuries of the neck or back were observed. Of all injuries, 88% were located in the lower extremity; the majority of "major" injuries were located in the knee, and the majority of "moderate" injuries were located in the knee, ankle, and thigh. They concluded that 184 of the 256 injuries were due to factors that could have been prevented, such as joint laxity, inadequate rehabilitation after a previous injury, muscle tightness, lack of training, unsatisfactory equipment, and foul play. Muscle tightness was related to muscle ruptures and tendinitis and not to ligamentous injuries of the knee and ankle. Whether these factors are also of significance to neck and back injuries has not been reported.

Jörgensen[13] compared the rate and location of injury in 480 soccer players and 288 handball players. He broadened the definition of a sports injury by including injuries to players who were able to continue playing after special bandaging or medical attention. Of 521 injuries in 355 soccer players, he reported 10 incidences of back pain, representing only 2% of the total number of injuries. None of these required medical attention. Of all soccer injuries, 82% were located in the lower extremities.

Nielsen and Yde[20] reported 37 injuries in 34 professional soccer players in one season. Seven of these (19%) were classified as "other" (not being located in the lower extremity). In the 59 amateur soccer players these authors studied, this figure was 11%, and for adolescents it was 19%. Because upper extremity injuries are included in the category "other," the incidence of neck and back problems was probably less than 10%.

In an overview of the literature in 1987, Keller, Noyes,

Soccer Injuries	
Type of Injury	**Location of Injury**
Strain	Foot
Contusion	Ankle
Sprain	Knee
Fracture	Thigh
Dislocation	Groin
Bursitis/tendinitis	Leg, other
Other	Back, other

and Buncher[14] reported a lack of solid epidemiologic data. These authors questioned the rate of severe injuries, the greater frequency of head and facial injuries among youths as compared with adult players, and the reported correlations; according to them, the lack of statistical evaluation in a number of studies had resulted in vagueness and possibly bias. They considered it remarkable that two thirds of traumatic injuries occurred during a match, whereas 84% of overuse injuries were the result of training, and they concluded that muscle strength, flexibility and endurance, cardiovascular endurance, and, to a lesser degree, balance, coordination, and skill were significant in the prevention of injuries. Neck or back disorders were not mentioned.

Engström et al.[6] observed back symptoms in some 2% of the 64 professional soccer players they studied over a 1-year period, and these injuries were considered "overuse" caused by training. Again, a great majority of injuries were located at the lower extremity (95%) and occurred predominantly during a match (47%).

Weineck[28] reported injuries of the "torso" in 7% of players studied, of the lower extremity in 56% of players studied, of the upper extremity in 23% of players studied, and of the head in 14% of players studied.

Part of the study by Ekstrand and Gillguist[5] dealt with female soccer players: in 1 year 150 players sustained 248 injuries. Of these, 12 were located in the back and 7 were in the "other" category (including the neck). Of the 12 back injuries, 5 were considered of traumatic origin; the other 7 were due to overuse. In 2 of the 7, symptoms were persisting.

In an in-depth study on etiology and prevention of sports injuries, Backx[2] observed the following incidence of injuries in 7468 schoolchildren; neck 2.8%, trunk 1.4%, and low back 6.1%. He did not specify the incidence in the 1340 children participating in soccer. However, he described an excellent intervention strategy based on behavior modification and also proved its efficacy in the largest subgroup—children playing soccer.

During 1 year 4018 children and adolescents between the ages of 8 and 18 were studied by McCarrol, Meany, and Sieber,[19] who reported 176 injuries. Of these, only one was located in the neck and three were in the lower back. Details were not given. One very serious injury was described: a child acquired a rupture of the abdominal aorta as a result of blunt trauma.

During an international youth soccer tournament in Norway in 1984, 1116 male teams and 332 female teams were studied.[16] During the 6 days of the tournament 411 injuries and "hyperventilatory conditions" were documented. Of these, the trunk was involved in 16 incidences in boys and in 15 in girls, averaging 7.5% of the total number of injuries. All of these injuries were minor. Details of location and nature were not given.

Schmidt-Ollson et al.[23] reported 312 injuries in 1 year in 496 youth players aged 12 to 18. Of these, 14% were

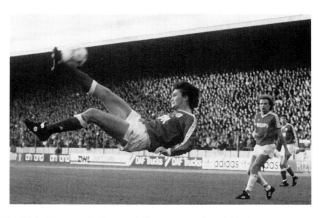

Fig. 48-1. Forward player giving an overhead kick. During such a maneuver the player has to land on his shoulder blades to avoid serious injury to the cervical spine.

related to the back. This is rather high in comparison with the other studies. Unfortunately, data related to the gravity of the injuries are not given.

Thus it could be concluded that neck and back disorders constitute a problem particular to soccer players. On the contrary, the incidence is even lower than in the general population.[10] One may speculate that this is due to the good physical condition of soccer players. Nevertheless, severe trauma may occur.

CASE 1

During an overhead kick (Fig. 48-1) a forward player of Nantes, France, fell on his occiput during a European cup match in 1978. Because of hyperflexion he acquired a bilateral fracture dislocation at C5-6, resulting in total quadriplegia.[11]

TRAUMATIC INJURIES
Neck Injuries

Trauma to the cervical spine during soccer may occur in scrimmages (encounters with the opposition to gain or retain possession of the ball) and as a result of an incorrect heading maneuver, caused by the body being pushed out of balance by an opponent.

Major injuries such as fractures and fracture dislocations are extremely rare. Usually these injuries result from a fall on the occiput forcing the cervical spine into hyperflexion. A sprained neck occurs more frequently, although it is still relatively rare. A sprain is defined as an injury to the neck resulting in pain and stiffness; at orthopaedic, neurologic, and radiologic examination, including extension/flexion views, no pathologic condition is found. Symptoms usually disappear in a couple of days and seldom last longer than 1 week. If symptoms persist for more than 2 weeks, the diagnosis should be questioned and ancillary diagnostic procedures should be carried out.

Back Injuries

Major trauma to the lumbar spine is also extremely rare. During the last 10 years no spinal fracture occurring during soccer has been reported. Less serious injuries to the lumbar spine may be classified as compression or torsion injuries, depending on the type of impact suffered.[7] An overload in compression may result in a massive annular rupture in the median line, usually of the L5-S1 segment and often leading to an immediate cauda equina syndrome. In the growing spine it may result in small impression fractures of the end-plate. Although these lesions are indeed observed in older children and adolescents, no case caused by a soccer injury has been reported. As a result of torsion, a sprain of the back, or in more severe cases a small annular rupture, may occur, sometimes in combination with ruptures of the facet joint capsule. In a considerable torsion overload, fractures of the neural arch have been described.

Asymmetric impacts to the trunk occur with great frequency during soccer games. When the player is out of balance because of body contact with an adversary, the motion is not well controlled and a torsional injury to the back may occur. Because the impact is usually minor, the result is only a sprained back. The soccer player is asymptomatic in a couple of days, whereas a more severe sprain may last a couple of weeks.

A sprained back is defined as acute pain after injury in combination with some stiffness and tenderness in the paraspinal muscles. At orthopaedic, neurologic, and radiologic examination, including standing extension and flexion views, no pathologic condition of the spine is observed. It is widely assumed that trauma to the muscles is responsible for the symptoms of a sprained back, although no evidence is available to support this assumption.

An indirect injury to a muscle is usually located at the myotendinous junction and is caused by excessive tension, stretching, or a combination of the two.[8] Although back muscle injuries have not been studied systematically, detailed knowledge of muscle injuries has accumulated through study of injuries of the extremities.[8,21] The incidence is higher in persons with fatigue, weak muscles, unconditioned muscles, inadequate warm-up, or an overstretched muscle. In muscle injuries of the extremities, it has been clearly demonstrated that the muscle is the site of the lesion that causes pain. Computed tomography has documented areas of edema within the muscle, whereas circumscript areas indicating a hematoma were not observed.[8,9] Other studies of extremity injuries indicate that the injury occurs predominantly at the junction of the tendon and the muscle belly, and at the osseotendinous junction.[1,8]

It has been suggested that eccentric contractions of slightly fatigued muscles, particularly multisegmental muscles, are the cause of small ruptures. Intersegmental muscles deep in the back meet these criteria and may therefore be subject to injury.[8]

Symptoms due to muscle injury of the back usually disappear within a couple of days or may last for 1 to 2 weeks. During that period muscle strength returns to normal and swelling, as observed in the case of muscle injuries to the extremities, is resolved. These lesions can be defined by magnetic resonance imaging (MRI). Until now, however, no study on acute muscle injuries of the back has been reported.

Case 2

A 36-year-old amateur soccer player who had formerly played in the top amateur league and was still in good physical condition ran into an opponent who blocked his way. This collision resulted in a flexion-rotation injury to the trunk.

Shortly after the incident the player had severe backache and was blocked in a flexed position. He could not continue playing. After examination by a club physician and later by his general practitioner, he was treated with bed rest and was referred to a physical therapist after 2 weeks. He was treated with diathermy and massage. The stiffness gradually decreased, but pain persisted. After 4 weeks he was referred to an orthopaedic surgeon.

Although the player had pain in his leg, the pain pattern was clearly not radicular, and signs of nerve root irritation were absent. Radiologic examination, including standing extension/flexion views, did not reveal any pathologic condition. At quantitative examination of his trunk muscle function (Fig. 48-2), he demonstrated a significant decrease in strength, speed, and coordination and an even bigger decrease in endurance.

A plan to condition his trunk muscles and, in particular, to enhance endurance was carried out. Gradually his symptoms disappeared, and after 4 months the player was completely symptom free and with normal trunk muscle function.

Lesson to be learned: Because of bed rest followed by lengthy passive therapy, the function of the player's trunk muscles decreased, resulting in impending chronicity. This protracted course could have been avoided by initiation of an exercise program as soon as symptoms decreased.

OVERUSE INJURY

An overuse injury is one with a gradual onset of symptoms in which the sufferer cannot recall a specific traumatic event. Overuse injuries occur more frequently at the end of each competitive season and during the off-season.[12,22] The relationship with a repetitive activity is self-evident in the case of a clearcut problem, such as a prepatellar bursitis. In low back pain, however, a specific condition to account for the symptoms is difficult to demonstrate. Therefore the term *overuse* may be used incorrectly in many instances.

On the other hand, the term *overuse* may be applied correctly even in cases where a pathologic condition is present. For example, a soccer player with an isthmic defect of a lumbar arch can be completely symptom free but become symptomatic after a soccer match. The

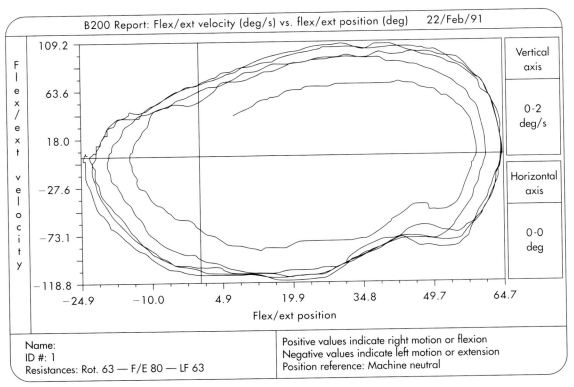

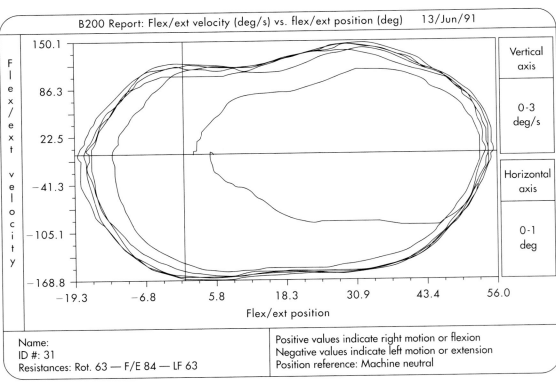

Fig. 48-2. A number of different back function criteria can be measured and plotted against each other with the use of automated dynamometers. Here velocity is plotted against position during flexion/extension. The bottom graph was obtained nearly 4 months after the top graph. Note the improvement in angular velocities from about maximum 110 to about 160 degrees/sec. Also, the different cycles have become more consistent. Finally, a dip observed in the top graph at around 45 degrees of flexion coming up from the bended position to neutral has disappeared completely. This dip is hypothesized to be a result of a coordination disorder due to a small muscular lesion. In this patient a correlation was observed between the gradual disappearance of the dip and improvement of speed and torque on the one hand and the decrease of symptoms on the other.

explanation for this phenomenon is speculative: because of the lesion the player's spine has a diminished load-sharing capacity; therefore muscles have to bear more of the load during activity, and they become exerted and painful. Also, it is conceivable that the lesion itself gets "overloaded" and fires nociceptive impulses. In these cases the term *overuse* may be used to indicate a contributing factor that in combination with a preexisting lesion causes symptoms.

Case 3

At the age of 15 an active soccer player had a period of low back pain without trauma. He was seen by a general surgeon who could not find any pathologic condition. Radiographic findings were reported as normal, although retrospectively a lytic defect seemed to be present. Years later he acquired low back pain, again without trauma. The following year he again had a spell of low back pain radiating to the buttocks and the posterolateral aspect of the thighs, in particular on the left side. Symptoms occurred again 2 years later, but only after a match or heavy training. At examination his trunk and lumbar spine motion proved to be normal. During motion no pain was elicited. Signs of nerve root compression were absent. Radiologically a bilateral lytic defect of L5 was observed, followed in later years by degenerative changes of the L5-S1 disc, resulting in decreased height and a slight olisthesis (Fig. 48-3).

It was recommended that the player strengthen his trunk muscles and boost muscle endurance to provide a compensatory mechanism. In doing so, he has been able to perform well in the top professional soccer league in the Netherlands.

The majority of soccer players with a lytic defect become asymptomatic when they increase the strength and endurance of their trunk muscles. The condition of the musculature must be checked quantitatively to ensure progress. The direct aim of an exercise program is the dynamic performance of the trunk muscles and not the reduction of pain.[17] Similarly, measurement of trunk function also has to be dynamic (see Fig. 48-2).

When symptoms persist, it has to be proved that the lytic defect is indeed causing the symptoms; to that purpose, the lytic defect is injected with a small amount of lidocaine (Xylocaine) to obtain a selective block. When the symptoms are subsequently relieved, the lytic defect is considered symptomatic. Direct repair according to Buck[4] is indicated in those cases where the disc is proved to be normal by MRI or discography.

Dysfunction of the trunk or a pathologic condition of the spine may cause symptoms at a distance; referred pain is a well-known phenomenon.[15,24] The majority of patients with shoulder blade pain that is referred pain of cervical degeneration also have neck pain. Similarly, patients with referred pain radiating down the buttock and thigh also have low back pain. However, some persons may have only referred pain. When the location of pain is restricted to a small area (e.g., the anterolateral aspect of the knee), diagnosis may be difficult. This pain pattern has been observed occasionally in persons with an isthmic defect.

Case 4

A 23-year-old soccer player had pain at the lateral aspect of the right knee. Because of persisting symptoms a diagnostic arthroscopy was performed but revealed no pathologic condi-

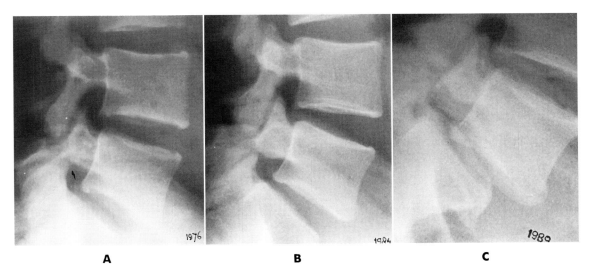

| A | B | C |

Fig. 48-3. A, An interruption in the cortex (*arrow*) may represent a lytic defect in this lateral radiograph of a 15-year-old soccer player with low back pain. **B,** The lesion seems unchanged in this view taken 8 years later. **C,** Definite degenerative changes can be seen in this view taken 13 years after the original radiograph. The disc height has decreased, and a small osteophytic reaction is visible anteriorly. The lytic defect is more obvious, and degeneration has resulted in a grade I olisthesis.

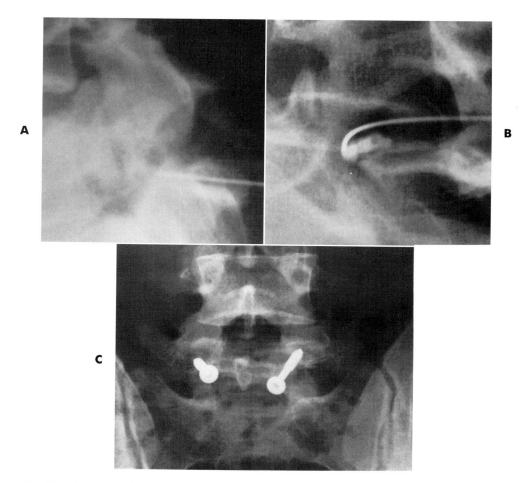

Fig. 48-4. A, Lateral view of low lumbar segments showing a needle positioned in the lytic defect of L5. **B,** Oblique view of the same area after injection of 0.2 ml of contrast medium. During injection the patient's knee pain was provoked and was subsequently completely relieved after injection of 0.3 ml of lidocaine for about 3 hours. **C,** Posteroanterior radiograph of the low lumbar spine after direct repair of the lysis. Screws were directed from a distal point through the lamina and the defect into the pedicle, and cancellous chips were placed in the defect after removal of the fibrous tissue.

tion. Although he had no back pain, his lumbar spine was examined radiologically. The radiographs demonstrated a bilateral lytic defect in the arch of L5.

After invasive radiodiagnostic procedures (Fig. 48-4), this defect proved to be symptomatic, and because the lumbosacral disc was normal on MRI, a direct repair of the lytic defect according to Buck[4] was performed. Three months postoperatively the player regained full soccer activities, and at follow-up 2 years later he still had no back or knee pain.

Because knee injuries are the predominant injury in soccer players, knee pain is in many cases explained as overuse when no lesion can be observed at diagnostic arthroscopy. In these cases it is recommended that the lumbar spine be examined radiologically even when the patient has no back pain.

Adductor overuse is a common cause of medial thigh pain. One of the causes could be the back; it has been demonstrated by Morrenhof[20] in a biomechanical study that overuse of thigh muscles, in particular the adductors, may be related to insufficient stabilization of the pelvis and may be caused by insufficient trunk muscle function. However, this relationship has not been proved clinically.

SPORTS MEDICINE EXAMINATION

A network of sports medicine consultancies has been set up in the Netherlands. These attempt to prevent sport injuries by providing information, education, and medical examinations before the sport is played. These examinations are meant to be sport specific, and sports medicine exclusions are defined for a number of sports. For soccer, no exclusions on the basis of spinal disorders have been defined. However, recommendations may be made in individual cases in relation to timing and/or the level of play. This may imply a temporary exclusion for competitive games in order to build up strength during training and to prevent reinjury.

After a period of low back symptoms, and in particular after a radicular syndrome regardless of whether the treatment has been surgical, it is imperative that a professional soccer player be sure that the load-bearing capacity of his trunk and back is normal. In other words, the timing of regaining full professional activities is dependent on the condition of the trunk muscles after healing of the spinal lesion. During the conditioning program, the progress of the trunk muscles needs to be checked at regular intervals with automated strength-testing instruments (see Fig. 48-2). Not so much the maximum isometric strength but the dynamic endurance is of significance.

In the case of persisting symptoms in the presence of well-conditioned trunk muscles, a spinal specialist should be consulted to answer the question of whether a symptomatic pathologic condition is present. Also, the question of whether continuing to play soccer will be harmful needs to be answered.

REFERENCES

1. Bach BR Jr, Warren RF, Wickiewicz TL: Triceps rupture: a case report and literature review, *Am J Sports Med* 15:285, 1987.
2. Backx FJG: *Sports injuries in youth,* thesis, University of Utrecht, Utrecht, The Netherlands, 1991.
3. Brynhildsen J et al: Previous injuries and persisting symptoms in female soccer players, *Int J Sports Med* 11:489, 1990.
4. Buck JE: Direct repair of the defect in spondylolysis, *J Bone Joint Surg* 52B:432, 1970.
5. Ekstrand J, Gillguist J: The avoidability of soccer injuries, *Int J Sports Med* 4:124, 1983.
6. Engström B et al: Does a major knee injury definitely sideline an elite soccer player? *Am J Sports Med* 18:101, 1990.
7. Farfan HF: *Mechanical disorders of the low back,* Philadelphia, 1973, Lea & Febiger.
8. Frymoyer JW, Gordon SL, editors: *New perspectives on low back pain,* Park Ridge, Ill, 1989, American Academy of Orthopaedic Surgeons.
9. Garrett WE Jr, et al: The effect of muscle architecture on the biomechanical failure properties of skeletal muscle under passive extension, *Am J Sports Med* 16:7, 1988.
10. Haanen HCM: *Een epidemiologisch onderzoek naar lage rugpijn,* thesis, Erasmus Universiteit Rotterdam, Rotterdam, The Netherlands, 1984.
11. Inklaar H: Personal communication, 1991.
12. Johansson C: Injuries in elite orienteers, *Am J Sports Med* 14:410, 1986.
13. Jörgenson U: Epidemiology of injuries in typical Scandinavian team sports, *Br J Sports Med* 18:59, 1984.
14. Keller CS, Noyes FR, Buncher CR: The medical aspects of soccer injury epidemiology, *Am J Sports Med* 15:230, 1987.
15. Kellgren JH: Observations on referred pain arising from deep somatic structures with charts of segmental pain areas, *Clin Sci Mol Med* 4:35, 1939.
16. Maehlum S, Dahl E, Daljord OA: Frequency of injuries in a youth soccer tournament, *Physician Sportsmed* 154:73, 1986.
17. Mayer TG, Gatchel RJ: *Functional restoration for spinal disorders,* Philadelphia, 1988, Lea & Febiger.
18. Mayer TG et al: A prospective two-year study of functional restoration in industrial low back injury, *JAMA* 258:1763, 1987.
19. McCarrol JR, Meany C, Sieber JM: Profile of youth soccer injuries, *Physician Sportsmed* 12:113, 1984.
20. Nielsen AB, Yde J: Epidemiology and traumatology of injuries in soccer, *Am J Sports Med* 17:803, 1989.
21. O'Donoghue DH: Injuries to the muscle-tendon unit. In O'Donoghue DH, editor: *Treatment of injuries to athletes,* Philadelphia, 1984, WB Saunders.
22. Orava S, Puramed J: Exertion injuries in adolescent athletes, *Br J Sports Med* 12:4, 1978.
23. Schmidt-Olsen S et al: Injuries among youth soccer players, *Am J Sports Med* 19:273, 1991.
24. van Akkerveeken PF: *Lateral stenosis of the lumbar spine,* thesis, University of Utrecht, Utrecht, The Netherlands, 1989.
25. Weineck J: Sportanatomie, *Perimed Verlag,* 9:122, 1979.

Chapter Forty-Nine

Volleyball

Lytton Williams

Volleyball has gained international popularity second only to soccer since its introduction in the United States 100 years ago at Holyoke, Massachusetts, by William Morgan. It was exported abroad by American servicemen and has continued to gain popularity ever since.

The game was originally a recreational activity at family outings. Now, however, volleyball is played not only on beaches around the world, but has also become a fast-paced power game played in high schools, colleges, the Olympics, and professionally. Participants include men and women of all ages and at all levels. Because of the jumping, diving, and torque involved in the game, injuries relative to the level of play and age tend to affect the spine and axial skeleton.

The indoor game is played on a court 5 feet long and 2½ feet on each side, with a net dividing the court, which at its highest point is 8 feet across the court. It is played by 12 players, 6 on each side, with 3 in the front row and 3 in the back row. The ball is served from one end of the court to the other side, and the volley begins.

The outdoor version is played on a slightly smaller court, with only two players on each side. Although the technique of the game is the same, fewer injuries with moves such as diving occur because of the soft sand. Generally, moves such as rolling are not part of the game in the sand.

TYPES OF INJURIES

The sport of volleyball, whether at the recreational, amateur, or professional level, produces many rotational, flexion, and hyperextension forces on the spine, knees, and shoulders. The ball has to be played over an 8-foot net, which compels the players to do a great deal of jumping, thus placing a lot of axial loading on the spine, knees, and hips. The ball is also hit and received at speeds of 60 to 100 miles per hour. Consequently, sudden changes in position place torque, acceleration, and deceleration forces on the player's spine. In addition, certain offensive and defensive plays can cause injury to the spine.

Offensive Play Injuries

Serving. The floater serves a top-spin serve, and the jump service, in which the server jumps to hit the ball, produces flexion, hyperextension, and rotational forces on the cervical, thoracic, and lumbar spine (Fig. 49-1). This sudden movement can cause ligament and or disc injury.

Passing the ball and setting. This offensive play includes passing the ball to a setter who sets the ball for the hitter (Figs. 49-2 and 49-3). This sequence involves running, squatting, and jumping, which if performed in an off-balance position can cause uneven loading and torque on the spine. Any resultant injury mostly affects the cervical and lumbar spine, causing pulled ligaments and occasionally jammed facet joints or a herniated disc that can result in neck, back, arm, and or leg pain, with symptoms of sciatica or radicular pain.

Hitting. Ineffective setting of the ball can make it harder for the hitter to efficiently execute the hit. If the ball is set behind the hitter or too far in front, the hitter has to twist or stretch too far. This can cause pulled ligaments and muscles, especially if the player is inexperienced or out of shape and has not done enough stretching before the game. Stretching exercises before and after the game should be done to lessen injuries (see Fig. 49-5).

Defensive Play Injuries

Defensive play in volleyball places the player at increased risk for injury. In attempting to stop the

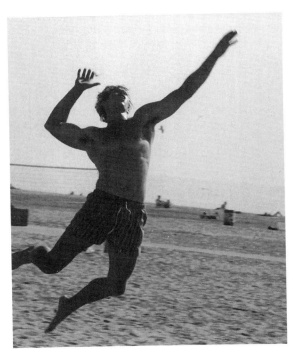

Fig. 49-1. Jump service.

opponent from scoring, the player—often while stretching—winds up in awkward, off-balance positions. This can cause neck, low back, disc, and facet joint injury.

Digging. Digging is a defensive play in which the player has to stop the ball from touching the floor and get the ball to the setter for a perfect hit (Fig. 49-4).

The digger has to be positioned to make sudden changes—from erect to sudden squatting, sprawling, diving, or rolling on the court to defend the ball and make a good pass. In diving, rolling, and sprawling, the player can sustain fractures of the spinous process or the cervical, lumbar, and thoracic spine, as well as fractures of the facet and transverse process. Ligamentous muscle pull and frank disc herniation can also occur.

DIAGNOSIS AND TREATMENT

The amount of axial load from jumping and rotational forces placed on the spine, whether the game is played at the amateur, recreational, or professional level, can cause minor or serious injuries to the cervical, thoracic, or lumbar spine. Most sprains and strains that occur in the professional athlete are pulled muscles and ligaments and jammed facets. These can be treated conservatively with rest, antiinflammatory drugs, muscle relaxants, and occasionally injections at trigger points with lidocaine (Xylocaine) and a corticosteroid agent. Then the patient is placed on an exercise and reconditioning program.

If there is no improvement of back, neck, arm, or leg pain and the positive tension signs of root irritation persist, a work-up with a complete physical examination and diagnostic tests may be necessary to identify the area of abnormality. X-ray films of the affected area should be done, followed by a computed tomography (CT) scan and/or bone scan if a bony injury, such as

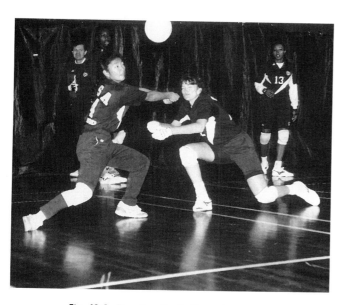
Fig. 49-2. Passing the ball to the setter.

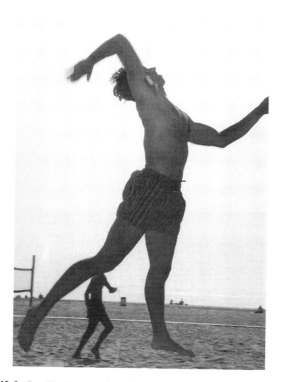
Fig. 49-3. Ineffective setting that causes the hitter to miss the ball can lead to back injury.

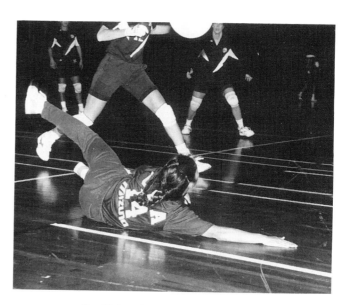
Fig. 49-4. Digging, a defensive play.

a fracture or tumor, is suspected. If soft tissue or nerve involvement is suspected, magnetic resonance imaging (MRI) is indicated.

Minor injuries, such as sprains, strains, and pulls, in the recreational athlete can be treated by rest, antiinflammatory agents, or a short-term change in sports activities to one that is less traumatic to the spine.

Professional volleyball players rarely have very serious spinal injuries because of their regularly performed conditioning and weight program. Minor injuries of sprains and strains are treated with temporary rest and supervised reconditioning and education of the muscles by the coach and the trainer. If no improvement in

symptoms occurs, then the trainer and patient should consult a physician and undergo a complete examination and, if necessary, diagnostic studies and appropriate treatment.

Spinal Deformities

Persons with spinal deformities may be involved in the sport but not at the professional level, unless the deformity is mild and the extreme forces of hyperextension, rotation, and axial loading will not affect the athlete.

Scoliosis. Scoliosis is a rotational deformity of the spine, and volleyball at a professional level will cause

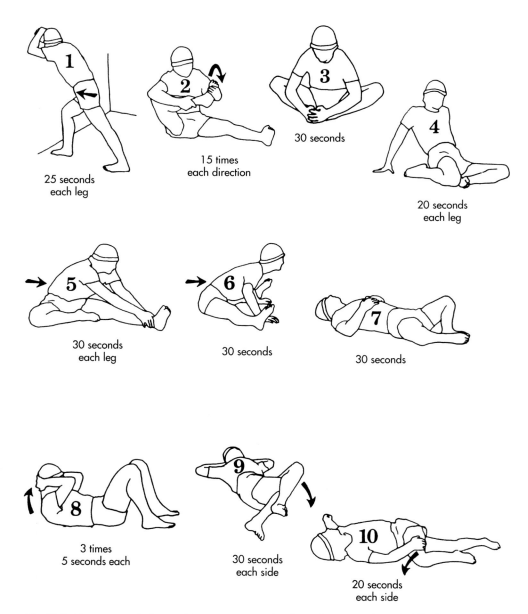

Fig. 49-5. Recommended stretching program to be done for approximately 15 minutes before and after volleyball. (Excerpted from *Stretching.* © 1980 by Bob and Jean Anderson. $13.00. Shelter Publications, Inc., P.O. Box 279, Bolinas, CA 94924. Distributed in bookstores by Random House. Reprinted by permission.)

frequent injury to the facet joints because of the extreme range of motion on the cervical, thoracic, and lumbar spine. The sport may be played at the recreational or amateur level but not at the intensity of the professional level.

Kyphosis. Kyphosis is a flexion deformity of the thoracic spine. In the adolescent there is inflammation of the end-plates, with retarded growth or uneven growth of the end-plate that results in wedging of the disc spaces over three or more levels. This causes the deformity that is seen with increased roundness of the dorsal spine and

occasional pain. This deformity does not lend itself to hyperextension, rotational, and extreme forces. Defensive moves, such as digging, diving, rolling, and blocking, will eventually cause repeated injuries in these athletes even if the sport is played at the amateur or recreational level.

Fractures and Spondylolisthesis

Pars fractures in the spine and spondylolisthesis, which can occur in the adolescent and younger athletes with persistent back pain, require attention. The

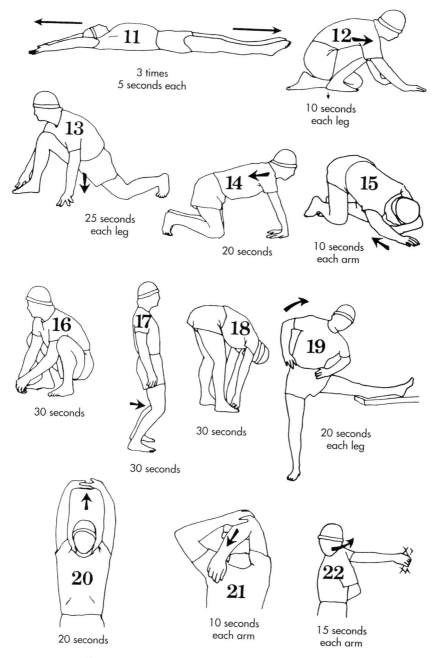

Fig. 49-5, cont'd. For legend see opposite page.

work-up should include x-ray films, a bone scan, and CT scan. Treatment should include rest, antiinflammatory agents, and bracing. If there is no improvement in symptoms, surgical fusion may be considered as a last resort.

Conditioning and Other Nonspinal Injuries

Athletes, whether recreational or professional, must be involved in some form of conditioning and stretching exercises both before and after play (Fig. 49-5). Other joint injuries that may mimic neck, dorsal, and lumbar spine injury are those of the shoulders, elbows, hips, knees, and ankles. Injury to the shoulder ranks highest in frequency of occurrence in the sport. Next is the knee, which is prone to "jumper's knee," or patellar or quadriceps tendinitis. Treatment of these injuries is conservative (rest, stretching, physical therapy, and antiinflammatory medication). Surgery is rarely performed except for a severe pathologic condition that is documented on diagnostic MRI studies.

ACKNOWLEDGMENTS

Special thanks to coaches Terry Liskevych and Greg Giovanazzi, of the U.S. Olympic women's volleyball team, Wilt Chamberlain, and Butch May for their time and assistance.

Chapter Fifty

Equestrian Sports

W. Carlton Reckling
John K. Webb

People have been riding horses for the last 50 centuries. The Scythians domesticated the horse circa 3000 BC[110] and rode horses on territorial conquests across the steppes of what is now Europe and Asia. Through the ages, the horse has been an indentured servant, a military machine, a transportation vehicle, a ceremonial showpiece, and a sporting partner. The horse has been selectively developed to perform certain tasks and to look a certain way. From those early ponies ridden by "the warriors of the steppes," the modern horse has evolved into a 19-hand jumping, racing, and show machine. The horse, by selective breeding, has become a highly specialized and also highly stressed creature.[52]

TYPES OF EQUESTRIAN ACTIVITIES

Equestrian sports encompass a broad range of organized and unorganized activities. The rider and horse interact in such diverse arenas as the rodeo ground and the dressage arena, and in capacities as varied as therapeutic riding for the handicapped to the cross-country adventures of the hunt. A variety of activities are available to the riding enthusiast.

Hacking is simple riding for pleasure and recreation. This type of riding most often takes place near the home and often occurs on public roads. Thoughtless drivers and the horse's fear of the mechanical are a dangerous combination. In addition, this type of riding is usually unsupervised and is always unregulated, and riders rarely wear protective helmets. For all of these reasons, hacking is the equestrian activity with the highest risk for serious injury.[47,59,84,129]

In *trekking,* which takes place in rough country and over long distances, a rider is paired with an unfamiliar mount. Avoidance of the animal's hindquarters is paramount in avoiding injury when a person is walking.[55] A potential for medical complications results from an unfit population exposed to arduous conditions.

Racing may take place over long ranges, cross-country, or over formal courses. Long-distance (endurance) events can cover up to 50 miles. Average speeds are 8 mph. Riders follow designated routes and race against the clock. The British Horse Society* organizes and monitors all competitors from the local qualifying races to the national championships. Protective helmets meet-

ing British Standards Institute (BSI) standards are required of all competitors.[51] There is a low incidence of serious injury in endurance events. This probably reflects the age and experience of both the riders and the mounts. The requirement of head protection, the "safe" nature of the course routes, and the overall low speeds of the riders also contribute to the low injury rate.

Course racing differs from other forms of riding in that large sums of money are wagered on the outcomes of individual races. High stakes demand fair play and high standards. In both the United Kingdom and the United States, government regulation and a legal framework are in place to deal with nearly all aspects of racing, including medical aspects. Safety is accepted as being in the interests of all parties involved.

In Great Britain racing occurs in three forms: flat racing, over-the-fence racing (National Hunt), and point-to-point racing. The first two disciplines take place at permanent sites dedicated to the given events. Routine maintenance of the course, slopes, fence, rails, paddocks, and areas for mounting and dismounting is performed under the auspices of the Race Courses Association,[128] as well as the Jockey Club.[78] These types of racing are performed by professional jockeys.

Point-to-point racing is performed by amateur riders. Local clubs organize events at temporary local venues. Courses challenge the riders and their mounts, combining vigorous cross-country riding with demanding jumps. There are no specific qualifications for the rider, and many are inexperienced.

The Jockey Club operates an annual licensing system of all professionally involved trainers, jockeys, and stable hands. This is kept under continuous review. A jockey's license requires an initial medical examination by the individual's general practitioner, which is reinforced by an annual medical examination by Jockey Club physicians for jump jockeys who are over 35 years of age and flat-race jockeys who are over age 40. A protective (BS 4473) helmet is required, and a Kevlar Body Protector meeting British Equestrian Trade Association (BETA) standards is recommended. Each individual jockey, whether professional or amateur, operating under Jockey Club rules has to carry and keep a personal medical record or log in which all accidents are recorded in red. The place, time, and details of the accident, together with the medical observations and recommendations, which may include suspension of racing for an

---

* British Equestrian Centre, Kenilworth, Warwickshire CV8 2LR, UK.

appropriate period, are entered. At the start of each meeting, the logs of all jockeys intending to race are reviewed by the course physician. Only then is clearance given to ride in the races that day. After an accident a jockey cannot ride again without formal medical review, appropriate clearance, and the red entry in his record. Suspension for a minimum of 21 days is customary following a skull fracture with an associated period of unconsciousness. All injuries are referred to the various compensation funds, where the individual's records are again reviewed for possible cumulative injury.[5,25,63,78]

Accident report forms are filled out by the course physician after each encounter. These forms are collected and analyzed by the Jockey Club. In addition, video records from every professional race are collected and preserved in a central archive for further analysis.

Show jumping is the art of surmounting any obstacle on horseback in public. There were more than 30,000 competitive entries in Great Britain in 1994.[55] The low accident/injury rate in competitive show jumping reflects the precision, control, and relatively slow speeds required of the competitors. It is the aspiring jumpers who push both their own and their mounts' limits of experience and ability who are most at risk for injury. The British Show Jumping Association[26] requires the wearing of appropriate helmets and provides guidelines for course safety.

Dressage involves set patterns of maneuvers on the spot, in a circle, and at the walk, trot, and canter. Relatively low speeds and the wearing of protective headgear combine to provide a low competition injury rate. Dressage groups' rules in the United Kingdom require a "hard hat," and BS standard protection is compulsory in the show jumping phase.[49,111] Low back ache is experienced by a majority of competitors. Poorly described and reported only anecdotally,[55] this low back pain is thought to reflect the loss of lumbar lordosis resulting from the riding styles of this discipline, compounded by the continuous demand for extreme pelvic obliquity.

Horse trials and eventing combine the skills of dressage, road and track, steeple chase, and cross-country racing. These courses are designed with a variety of challenging obstacles. The most direct route is the most difficult. Alternative routes are less demanding but more time consuming. The rider must continually make split-second decisions about how to best surmount each approaching obstacle. Guidelines for course construction are available from the British Horse Society.[73] The wearing of a standard helmet is mandatory. The high level of individual competence, the wearing of helmets, and the relatively low speeds involved have limited the traumatic outcome of many spectacular incidents during competitions. However, fatalities and serious injury continue to occur.[55]

Hunting is an event of local clubs. These clubs belong to no parent organization, and there are no rules for minimum equestrian competence, required protective equipment, or accident reporting. Studies evaluating emergency room visits and hospital admissions have shown a high incidence of injury. Imperfect mount-rider bonds, the distraction of numbers, rough country, variable conditions, individual euphoria, crowd hysteria, and the wide variety of rider fitness, age, competence, experience, and practice all contribute to the high injury rate.[60,64,67] Often the hunt is combined with alcohol consumption, which is a particularly deadly combination.[4,55]

Polo has a low injury rate. Head, knee, knuckle, and shin protection are the rule, and face masks are commonly worn. However, use of the face mask is controversial; antagonists claim that the face guard may catch in a mallet, causing the rider to be flicked off a horse and sustain severe neck injuries. The game is governed by the Huringham Polo Association.[74]

In the *tetrathalon,* an equestrian cross-country course under Pony Club rules[106] is added to air pistol marksmanship, cross-country running, and swimming.

Riding for the mentally and physically disabled continues to expand in popularity. All forms of disability are involved. Enthusiasm is matched by improving techniques and benefits.[112]

Nonriding equestrian sports include in-hand showing of breed and show classes. Although the hazards of long reins and lack of control from the rear of the animal can be a dangerous combination,[108] head and spinal injuries have rarely been described in horse driving trials.[83] *Driving trials* are a horse-powered vehicular activity judged on presentation and dressage, and set on cross-country, marathon, and cone-defined obstacle courses. The emphasis is on precision and skill rather than speed. This is reflected in the low injury rate. Injuries are more common in *trotting,* which is a long-established major activity similar to flat racing, but which has the added risk of collision between the light, two-wheeled rigs.[77]

The various *rodeo events* require many different skills from the cowboy-horse team. Calf roping requires rapid acceleration/deceleration and rapid dismount from the horse.[99] In steer wrestling, the cowboy leaps from the galloping horse onto the neck of a speeding steer. In bronc riding, the rider attempts to maintain his position on a bucking horse: one hand firmly grips a rope positioned around the animals' withers; the other hand must remain in the air. The energy of the horse and its bucking are transmitted to the rider. A vigorous and repetitive flexion/extension (whiplash motion) of the entire spine takes place. Serious injuries are not uncommon in these and other nonequestrian rodeo events.[62,100] Organized rodeo competition takes place at the junior level under the auspices of the Little Britches and the High School Rodeo associations. Intercollegiate rodeo is governed by intercollegiate mandates, and the Professional Rodeo Cowboys Association* governs the men's professional circuit. Accident report forms are variably required and collected. All organizations have safety committees, which review accident report data, monitor the health of their members, and make recommendations regarding policy and practices.

BASIC FEATURES AND EQUIPMENT

Throughout the various riding disciplines, certain common features are found. Primary control of the animal is through the reins, bridle, and bit. Secondary communication is given through the saddle and stirrup.[15,17,31] The stirrup-boot combination has evolved to a precision piece of equipment. The stirrup must properly fit the boot; the stirrup should be only 2 cm wider than the boot.[29] The heel of the boot must prevent the foot and ankle from prolapsing through the stirrup,[114] to prevent the foot from becoming locked in the stirrup in the event of a fall. The British stirrup also has a break-away feature. Often the young child is not heavy enough to spring the release mechanism, resulting in additional danger. The proper stirrup-boot combination allows for rapid dismount, a safety technique that itself requires teaching.

All of the equipment or tack required for riding is subject to repeated application of high stresses. For this reason, equipment may rapidly fatigue, and most equipment should be thought of as temporary. It is essential to perform premounting and dismounting checks of all tack.[9,64]

BIOMECHANICS

To understand the nature of spinal injuries in equestrian sports, it is necessary to understand the energy of the horse and rider and the envelope of hazard surrounding the horse-rider pair. A horse weighs up to 500 kg (1100 lb) and travels at a speed of up to 65 km/hr (40 mph). The rider's head may be poised up to 4 m (12 feet) from the ground.[98] The force of a kick through a steel-shod shoe exceeds 10 kN.[31] When 15 cm^2 of shoe contacts the body, it can generate 10 mPa of force. This is certainly enough to fracture the skull, ribs, vertebral processes, and other bones.

The rider is mounted in unstable equilibrium above the horse's centers of mass and gravity. The horse and rider behave in classic newtonian terms as an asymmetric couple. When the horse decelerates abruptly, the energy of the entire system (horse and rider) is transferred to the rider; this causes a near-instantaneous acceleration of the rider to a velocity above that of the initial horse-rider system. The velocity is imparted in an extended arc or trajectory as a function of position of the horse-rider system at the moment of deceleration of the horse.

The "jockey style" head-forward stance predisposes to a forward-directed trajectory and a forward roll on landing (Fig. 50-1). This has previously been described as Becker's principle.[12] The classic riding style, with the feet thrust out and the head held high, often leads to a backward somersault.

If any portion of the rider fails to disengage from the horse or the tack, the trajectory arc may be tightened considerably. Additional radial acceleration is added to the rider in the direction of the ground. Any combination of force vectors may be applied to the spine during a fall and on contact with the ground, obstacles, or other riders or horses. The forces imparted to the rider may exceed 300 G,[29] which is far above the amount of energy necessary to cause fracture and/or dislocation in any region of the spine.

MECHANISMS OF INJURY

A fall is the usual mechanism of spinal injury. In addition to high-energy impact with the ground, riders may be thrown onto and into objects starting from a height of up to 4 m (12 feet) and from initial velocities of 65 km/hr (40 mph).[98]

A rider may be dragged if the arm or leg becomes entangled in the reins or other tack, or if the feet fail to disengage from the stirrups.[59,114] Repeated impact injuries to the soft tissues, as well as traction injuries to the brachial and lumbar plexus, are common with this mechanism of injury.[29]

A rider may be crushed or compressed between the horse with its massive weight and the ground. Such compression injuries to the chest, abdomen, and pelvis may be life-threatening and at times fatal.[90]

A thrown rider may be trampled by his or her own horse or by other horses (Fig. 50-2). Injuries to the head, ribs, and vertebral transverse or spinal processes are

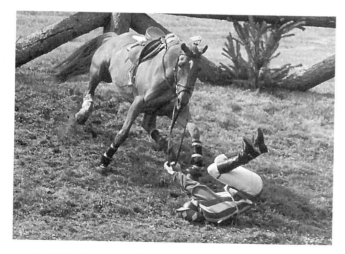

Fig. 50-1. Forward roll on landing. (© Kit Houghton.)

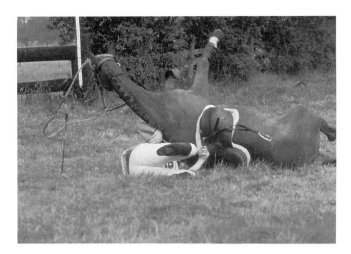

Fig. 50-2. Rider crushed by horse. (© Kit Houghton.)

common. Serious spinal injuries can occur from this mechanism of injury.

Kicking most often occurs during handling and grooming.[42,109,123] The combined spaces of the stable and the trailer diminish the safety zone in which to work with and around the animal. Minimum forces of 10 kN are imparted at a height typically 1 m from the ground. This places the ribs, pelvis, and head at risk for significant injury.[79]

Other equestrian injury mechanisms have been described. Butting, biting, and other related mechanisms are well detailed elsewhere.[18,48,55]

STATISTICS

Equestrian sports are ever-increasing in popularity. In the United States up to 30 million will ride in a given year.[4,16,29] In the United Kingdom, the riding community exceeds 3 million.[35] Accident and mortality data are incomplete. There is no national collection or archival registry in either the United States or the United Kingdom. Several organizations in both countries record injury data and compile statistics; however, this information is incomplete, since it pertains only to riders falling under the umbrella of these organizations.

In the United Kingdom the Office of Population Census and Surveys (OPCS)[103,104] collects data from coroners and death certificates (an imperfect practice at best) and compiles fatality statistics for various high-risk sports. In 1992 the office listed 12 equestrian-related fatalities in 2.87 million participants. The calculated fatality rate for equestrian sports is 0.48 per 100,000 participants per year, which compares favorably with the calculated fatality rates of motor sports (9.2 per 100,000 per year), air sports (15.5 per 100,000 per year), and climbing (28.8 per 100,000 per year). Equestrian sports have been compared, in terms of risk, with high-risk sports such as motorcycle riding.[43] These data show that the calculated risk is much lower for equestrian sports.

The incidence of injury has been calculated by other authors in a variety of manners.* Mortality studies have been presented by Pounder[107] and by others.[75] Pounder estimated death rates as 1 per 1 million population per year in southwestern Australia. In these studies young female riders constituted the majority of those injured.

Hospital admission studies show similar statistics.† The riders involved in these studies are predominantly female (68% to 85%). Head injury occurs in 55% to 100%, with spinal injury occurring in 10% to 20%.

Emergency department studies[43,59,71,76,101] again show a preponderance of female riders being injured (52% to 87%) and a younger population (10 to 25 years of age) sustaining the majority of the injuries.‡

Inexperience is often cited as a cause of accidents.[47,61,84] However, a review of U.S. Pony Club data by Bixby-Hammett and Brooks[18] shows that the rider at greatest risk is the child with only D-level (very minimal) knowledge and skill, but who has more than 5 years of riding experience. (This young amateur rider may be pushing his or her ability with increasingly challenging riding activities and may have recently begun riding a horse that is more spirited.) Others have recorded that in fox hunting, those with the most experience have had the most injuries.[67] Studies have shown that 25% of injured riders have been injured before.

Injury rates have been estimated by various methods as <1 per 1000 lessons,[43] 0.7 per 1000 rides,[59] and 2 per 1000 riding hours.[94] Each of these studies employs a different denominator in the calculation of the injury rate, which makes meaningful comparison impossible.

Equestrian organizations that have compiled accident and injury data include the U.S. Pony Club,§ the U.S. Combined Training Association, the American Horse Shows Association, the American Horse Council, Horse Industry Directory,‖ the National Park Service,¶ and the Horsemanship Safety Association.#[16,17,101] Female riders are disproportionately represented in the data records, constituting up to 92% of those injured. The preponderance of young girls in all of these studies is just slightly greater than the proportional gender representation in the respective organizations and age groups. The U.S. Pony Club is one of the few organizations that make note of gender in their data records. Membership in this organization is 88% female.

Additional studies have been made of spinal cord and head injury patients.[65,82,93] These studies show that the

---

* References 14, 30, 36, 40, 43, 50, 76, 88, 89, 91, 96, 97, 102, 103.
† References 10, 17, 29, 33, 93, 101.
‡ References 7, 10, 12, 14, 17, 20, 21, 43, 59, 75, 84, 93, 94. 101, 116.
§ 893 S. Matlack Street, Suite 110, West Chester, PA 19382.
‖ 1700 K Street NW, Suite 300, Washington, DC 20006.
¶ P.O. Box 37127, Washington, DC 20013-7127, attention D.F. Herring, Chief, Division of Engineering and Safety Services.
# 5304 Reeve, Mazomanie, WI 50560, attention Betty Talbot.

patients with spinal cord and head injuries as a result of equestrian accidents are 80% female. This is in complete contradistinction to the usual statistics in spinal cord and head injury units, where patients are typically 80% male.

All of the above studies and data represent amateur riders. The Jockey Club[78] in Great Britain monitors all professional race jockeys and amateur jockeys involved in point-to-point racing. These injury statistics give a somewhat different demographic picture. Jockey Club unpublished data (on 700 consecutive fractures in National Hunt and flat-course jockeys) show that most of these injuries involve riders who are male and over the age of 30 years. Injury incident rates range from 1 per 720 rides for flat-course racing to 1 per 88 rides for National Hunt (over-the-fence) racing to 1 per 42 rides (2.4%) for amateur cross-country point-to-point racing. Injury patterns are also different for this population.

The amateur rider is typically female and under age 25. Typical injury patterns are upper extremity injury (24% to 33%), lower extremity injury (18% to 24%), head and neck injury (13% to 22%), and trunk injury (10% to 20%). Fractures represent 15% to 30% of injuries in the reported series. One may compare the data on the 700 consecutive fractures in flat-course and National Hunt professional jockeys with the large series of fractures (513) in amateur riders from Whitlock.[126] In professional riders, fractures of the clavicle, shoulder, and ribs make up 382/700 fractures (54.6%); this compares with only 90/513 fractures (17.5%) in amateurs. Clavicle fractures make up 296/700 fractures (42.3%) in professional riders, but only 41/513 fractures (8%) in amateur riders. Spinal fracture was reported in 9/700 fractures (1.3%) in professionals but in 39/513 fractures (7.6%) in amateur riders. These data would certainly support the premise put forth by Firth, Fu, and Stone[55] that professional riders "know how to fall." They are able to quickly disengage from their mounts and roll clear. The greater proportion of shoulder girdle injuries in professional riders indicate that the energy of the fall is absorbed by the upper extremities, whereas the lower incidence of spinal fractures in these riders is indicative of their controlled impact with the ground. The higher proportion of spinal fractures in amateur riders is indicative of falls with landings on the buttocks.[29] An uncontrolled emergency dismount with a subsequent uncontrolled impact with the ground results in considerable force applied in a variety of vectors to the spine.

SPINAL INJURIES

The most common spinal injury in equestrian riders is a fracture of the transverse process or spinous process of the vertebra. This fracture may occur during a fall, although it is much more likely to occur during a kicking or trampling episode.[70,72] Fracture or fracture-dislocation of the spine can occur at any spinal level. In some series thoracolumbar and lumbar fractures are more common[126]; in other series cervical fractures predominate.[19,29,119,120]

Cervical spine injuries are usually the result of a flexion force, which is secondary to Becker's principle,[12,124] and the traditional head-forward jockey-style stance. Less common are cervical injuries involving extension, lateral flexion, and rotatory forces. Axial loading is a distinctly uncommon mechanism of cervical spine injury in equestrians. Spinal cord injury is common in cases of cervical spine fracture or fracture-dislocation.[45,54] The severity of these injuries is again a representation of the large amount of energy transferred to the rider from the combined horse-rider system.

Cervical spine injuries at every level have been reported in equestrians. These injuries range from occipitocervical dissociation and odontoid fractures[85] (Fig. 50-3) to cervicothoracic dislocation. The majority occur in the lower portion of the cervical spine (Fig. 50-4).

Cervical spine injuries may also be entirely soft tissue in nature, and these injuries may easily be missed on initial examination.[125] Complete and careful evaluation is necessary to diagnose soft-tissue injuries; in particular, the "hidden tetrad" should be considered on cervical radiographs (Fig. 50-5). Latent instability of the cervical spine is a contraindication to continued participation in equestrian events.

Any combination of forces can cause fracture in the thoracic spine, although the common mechanism is flexion. As in the cervical spine, there is little tolerance to compression in the thoracic cord; thus spinal cord injuries are common. Translocation of the thoracic spine without cord injury has been reported,[118] but this type of injury is extremely rare.

Fractures of the cervical and thoracic spine are often unstable and result in compression of the neural canal. Instability of the spine is an indication for surgical stabilization. Evidence of cord injury from proven compression is another indication for surgery (Fig. 50-6). In fact, these are the two major indications for surgery.

Thoracolumbar and lumbar injuries are usually compression fractures.[29] The mechanism of injury is usually an axial load with a flexion element secondary to a fall of the rider on the buttocks; these injuries are usually stable. If more energy is involved in the injury, a burst fracture results. These injuries are often accompanied by neurologic injury to the conus medullaris or cauda equina. If a rotatory or shear force vector is present in the injury, a severe unstable fracture-dislocation may occur. Isolated facet dislocation has been described in the lumbar spine secondary to a fall from a horse.[22]

Sacral fractures can be a result of either a direct axial impact[86] or a crush/compression injury.[127] Symphyseal disruption has also been described in equestrian-related injuries.[56]

A few words must be said about the other major

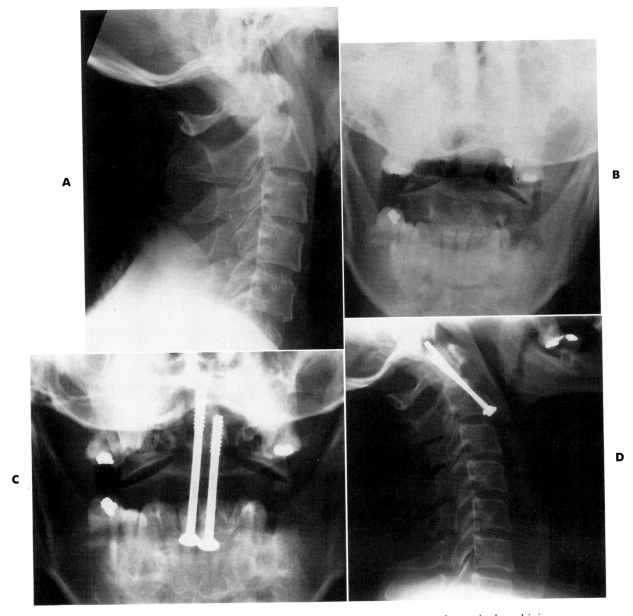

Fig. 50-3. Type II odontoid fracture sustained by a jockey, with a complete spinal cord injury. It was stabilized with odontoid screws. **A,** Lateral cervical spine radiograph showing an odontoid fracture. **B,** Open-mouth anteroposterior (AP) radiograph showing a fracture at the base of the odontoid peg. **C,** Postoperative AP radiograph showing screws in place. **D,** Postoperative lateral radiograph showing screws in place.

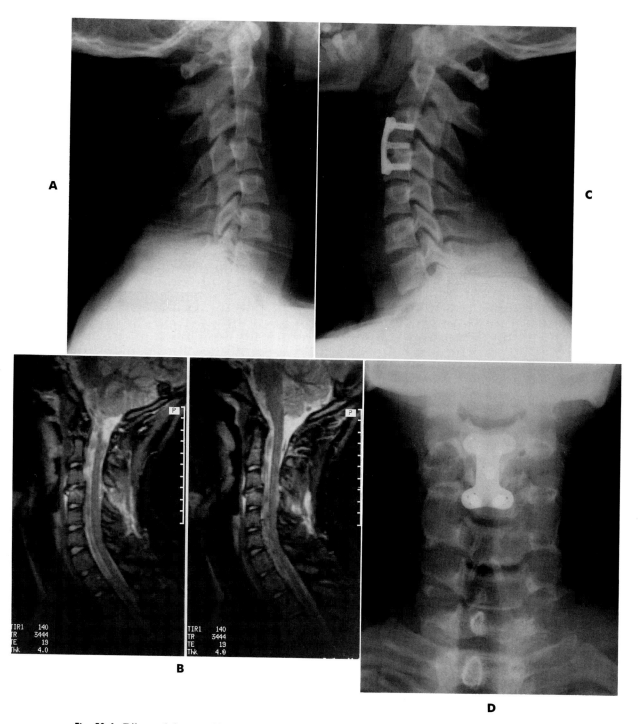

Fig. 50-4. Bilateral facet subluxation of the cervical spine with severe posterior ligamentous damage. **A,** Lateral cervical spine radiograph showing subluxation of C4 on C5 with fracture of the body of C5. **B,** MRI sagittal images showing significant soft tissue injury posteriorly at C4-5 interspinous spaces. The scan also shows stripping of the posterior longitudinal ligament from the body of C5. **C,** Postoperative lateral cervical spine radiograph showing the plate, screws, and graft in place. **D,** Postoperative AP radiograph showing the plate and screws in place.

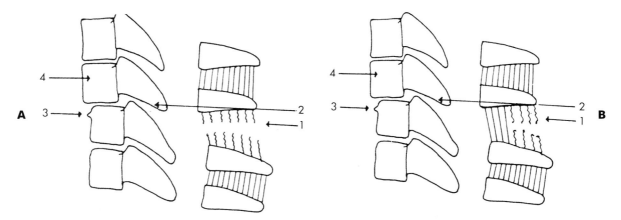

Fig. 50-5. Radiologic "hidden tetrad," denoting ligamentous instability of the spine. **A,** Complete tear of the posterior cervical complex. *1,* Widening of the interspinous space; *2,* intervertebral subluxation with opening of the apophysial joints; *3,* vertebral compression fracture; *4,* loss of cervical lordosis. **B,** Incomplete tear of the posterior cervical complex. *1,* Widening of the interspinous space; *2,* intervertebral subluxation with opening of the apophysial joints; *3,* vertebral compression fracture; *4,* loss of cervical lordosis.

injuries encountered in equestrian sports. Injuries of the head and crush injuries to the chest, abdomen, and pelvis are relatively common and often accompany spinal injuries. A race course physician must be aware of these potentially devastating injuries, as well as experienced and knowledgeable in their on-course management. The surgeon treating the patient with an equestrian-related spinal injury will often find that the patient has one or more of these injuries accompanying the spinal injury.

Head injury occurs in up to 70% of the injured riders in some series. It has been reported that up to 40% of head injuries in equestrians occur with an associated spinal injury.[65] It behooves the race-course physician to treat the unconscious patient as having a spinal injury until it has been proved otherwise.

Compression and crush injuries are a result of the rider being caught between the horse (weighing 500 kg [1100 pounds], with a center of mass over 5 feet off the ground) and the ground during a fall. Major injuries to the chest, abdomen, and pelvis are common. Hemopneumothorax is frequent. One must be aware that a widened mediastinum may be a result of a thoracic vertebral fracture and the resultant hematoma. This should not preclude eventual investigation of the great vessels with an arch aortogram to rule out injury to the great vessels.

Crush injuries also involve the abdomen and pelvis. A ruptured spleen and liver with associated hemorrhagic shock is common in children.[55] Rupture of other viscera is not uncommon. Pelvic fractures are often accompanied by massive retroperitoneal blood loss and hemor-

rhagic shock. Possible injury to the urethra and bladder should be kept in mind.

SCIWORA (spinal cord injury without radiographic abnormality) is an acronym for a constellation of injuries to the pediatric spinal cord. There are several anatomic differences in the pediatric spine that make it more flexible and prone to traction-type injuries.[53] The facet joints are more horizontal in the child. The soft tissues of the spine, and particularly the neck, are more elastic in children than in adults. Spinal cord injury without radiographic evidence of fracture or dislocation has been described in many series.* No one mechanism of injury has been implicated in these injuries; flexion, hyperflexion, hyperextension, and rotation have all been cited as causes.[37]

The etiology of SCIWORA is not known. Longitudinal traction injury to the spinal column and cord, cord rupture, traumatic infarction, end-plate separation, transient disc herniation, and vascular compromise have been hypothesized as being causative.[39] SCIWORA constitutes 20% to 35% of spinal cord injuries in children.[46,105,115] In cases of SCIWORA, the cord injury is more often complete (44% of cases are complete injuries[39] versus only 30% in cases of spinal cord injury with known osseous injuries).[46,105] This injury has been described in children up to 16 years of age,[105] which is the average age at which the child's spine reaches adult configuration and properties. SCIWORA is much more common in children younger than 8 years of age.

* References 3, 32, 34, 38, 80, 81, 87, 105.

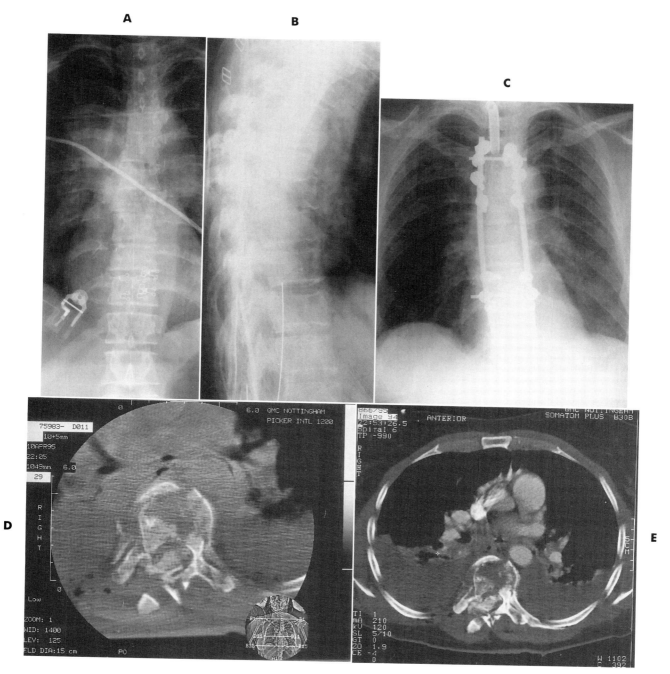

Fig. 50-6. Thoracic fracture with severe cord compression. **A,** AP thoracic spine radiograph showing burst fracture at T8. **B,** Lateral radiograph of the thoracic spine showing fracture at T8. **C,** Postoperative chest radiograph showing instrumentation in place and the presence of a temporary tracheostomy tube. **D,** CT scan of the T8 vertebra showing a burst fracture of the lamina and complete canal occlusion. **E,** CT scan of the chest showing a fractured vertebra, mediastinal hematoma, and bilateral hemothoraces.

The most common location of the lesion is controversial; the C2 level,[115] the C5 to C8 level,[105] and the thoracic spine[3,32,38,80,81] have all been mentioned as the most common level of injury.

Although most patients display neurologic signs and symptoms immediately after the injury, up to 54% of patients have a delayed onset of neurologic signs and symptoms.[105] This delayed onset has been reported as ranging from 30 minutes to 4 days. Most patients with delayed onset will recall mild, transient tingling or numbness at the time of initial injury.

Diagnosis depends on a significant element of suspicion. Careful questioning of the patient is necessary to elucidate the mechanism of injury and any subtle neurologic symptoms or signs. Immediate immobilization is necessary. Magnetic resonance imaging may confirm injury to the spinal cord. Controlled dynamic x-ray studies may document instability. Treatment of instability requires immobilization in an orthosis or surgical stabilization. The role of steroids in preventing progressive deficit has not been studied.

The prognosis of a child with SCIWORA is grim. The initial presentation is usually one of a complete injury, and improvement is the exception. It is important that the course physician's maneuvers avoid further damage to the injured spinal column and be directed toward early immobilization, correct diagnosis, and appropriate treatment.

Traction injuries to the brachial and lumbar plexus are rare. These injuries occur when the rider fails to disengage from the reins or saddle when falling, resulting in a stretch injury to the brachial or lumbar plexus. Avulsion of cervical roots has been reported.[29] Injuries to the lumbar plexus can be minimized by a proper boot-stirrup match, proper safety release mechanisms, and break-away stirrups.

MANAGEMENT

The course physician must be aware of the possibility of any injury combination. There are no set injury patterns. One should presume that each casualty will result in head, spinal, and visceral injuries compounded by pneumothoraces and internal hemorrhage into the head and abdomen. Initially one must assume that unstable spinal injury is present, and move the head, neck, and body as one piece.

Initial medical management follows the ABCs of advanced trauma life support (ATLS) and European Resuscitation Council guidelines[1,11,41]:

Airway — Use the jaw lift/head tilt (in that order). Do not use the neck lift/jaw lift. The first 10 to 15 degrees of head tilt is at the base of the skull — not the neck.

Breathing — Clear the airway as the victim lies (in the position found). Position the victim supine (unless

the person is trapped) so that the diaphragm is not splinted. Support ventilation (provide mouth-to-mouth, mouth-to-mask, bag-and-mask, or mechanical resuscitation/ventilation).

Circulation — Apply external cardiac compression and/or provide fluid replacement as indicated. Control hemorrhage with direct pressure.

Detection of neurologic injuries is the next concern. The conscious level is defined and recorded on the Glasgow Coma Scale,[121] and limb and motor power (legs as well as arms) are noted on the Medical Research Council motor scale (0-5).[95] Pupil size and reaction, pulse, and blood pressure complete the basic recordings required for brain, spinal cord, and systemic injury management. Such injury has to be presumed to be present until it has been proved otherwise. The Medical Equestrian Association,* the European Resuscitation Council, and ATLS courses are recommended to provide the basic knowledge and expertise required in initial trauma assessment and management.[1,11,41]

The initial position of the victim should be maintained unless danger, airway, breathing, circulation, and/or unconsciousness dictate otherwise. In equestrian events the fallen rider may be trapped under fencing or intertwined with the unstable remnants of a fence. The physician must weigh the advantages of a controlled move with as much horizontal component as possible against the need for an earlier move than one would wish because of the risk of the fence remnants collapsing and causing an uncontrolled massive movement in several directions at once. This is a matter of judgment. The former is preferred to the latter. The calculation is to assess whether or not the fence will collapse and then remove the rider as best as one is able in a manner compatible with the fallen rider's safety and one's own safety.[8]

After initial stabilization, the rider with serious spinal injuries should be evacuated to a major medical center capable of dealing expeditiously with spinal injuries. The rider should be transferred to this center within "the golden hour" — the time that may mean the difference between neurologic recovery and no recovery. High-dose steroids have proved to be effective in saving levels in both complete and incomplete spinal cord injuries.[23] Other agents active on spinal cord receptors and antioxidants that decrease the concentration of free radicals at the site of cord injury are currently being investigated.[57] For high-dose steroid therapy to be effective, it must be instituted within 8 hours of injury. Patients are initially given a 30-mg/kg bolus of methyl-

---

* In care of The Medical Commission on Accidental Prevention, Royal College of Surgeons, Lincoln's Inn Fields, London, WC2A 3PN, UK. American Medical Equestrian Association: 103 Surrey Road, Waynesville, NC 28786.

prednisolone, followed by a continuous infusion of 5.4 mg/kg/hr for 23 hours.

Surgical decompression of the spinal canal at the cervical, thoracic, and lumbar levels has been shown to have a beneficial effect on the eventual long-term neurologic outcome.[2,13,24,92] There has been a trend toward better results with early decompression[2]—hence the need for rapid transfer to a major center.

It is the policy of the Centre for Spinal Studies and Surgery in Nottingham to decompress and stabilize spinal fractures as early as possible because the patient will often deteriorate medically after admission, secondary to associated pulmonary, abdominal, and head injuries. Often the patient is the most fit immediately on arrival.

MEDICAL CONTRAINDICATIONS TO RIDING

The following medical conditions should be considered contraindications to riding: (1) congenital absence of the odontoid process of the axis, (2) temporary paralysis of any cause, (3) head injury with permanent impairment, and (4) latent instability of the cervical spine.

Relative contraindications are conditions that require the patient to be evaluated on a case-by-case basis before participating in equestrian events. These include the following:

1. Previous cervical fracture or dislocation. Stability must be documented before the patient is allowed to ride. The patient who has previously undergone spinal fusion and/or has one or more immobile segments of the cervical spine may be at increased risk for neurologic injury.
2. Congenital narrowing of the cervical spinal canal. Torg[122] has shown that flexion injuries to the cervical spine are likely to cause transient cord neurapraxia in the presence of degenerative changes, congenital anomalies, instability, and congenital stenosis of the spinal canal. This large review of cervical spine injuries did not reveal a relationship between those patients suffering permanent spinal cord injury and the presence of underlying congenital stenosis of the cervical spinal canal.
3. Brachial injury.
4. Lumbar injury.
5. Untreated herniated intervertebral disc.
6. Recurrent injury to the cervical or lumbar ligaments or muscles.

PREVENTION OF INJURY

Prevention of injury begins with proper equipment. The most important piece of gear is a properly fitted riding helmet designed according to the accepted American[7] or British[28,29] standards. This helmet must be securely fastened at all times and should be replaced after any significant impact.[44] The components and specifications of a well-constructed helmet are extensively detailed.[55]

Properly matched boot-stirrup combination are paramount. Appropriate breeches, gloves, and jacket are a necessity. The Kevlar Body Protector[78] can theoretically protect the ribs and soft tissues but has no effect on the incidence or severity of spinal injuries.

Responsible course construction and adequate casualty preparation[66,98] are significant factors in reducing the rate of injury and the severity of any injuries that occur. Collection and analysis of data regarding equestrian injuries will help in preventing further occurrences.[68,69] A standardized incident form for detailing the incident, total hours ridden, and local conditions is essential to define problems and effect change.[58,113]

The most important step in accident prevention is sound training of horse and rider.[54,127] Proper supervision of inexperienced riders by certified instructors should be the standard. Riding instructors should be qualified, certified, and subject to periodic recertification.

REFERENCES

1. Advanced Life Support Working Party of the European Resuscitation Council: Guidelines for advanced life support: a statement, *Resuscitation* 24:111, 1992.
2. Aebi M et al: Indication, surgical technique and results of 100 surgically-treated fractures and fracture dislocations of the cervical spine, *Clin Orthop* 203:244, 1986.
3. Ahmann PA, Smith SA, Schwartz JF: Spinal cord infarction due to minor trauma in children, *Neurology* 25:301, 1975.
4. Alcohol use and horseback riding associated fatalities—North Carolina, 1979-1989, *MMWR* 41(19):335, 1992.
5. Allen WMC: Racing accidents in Great Britain—a review of their frequency, nature and the preventive measures for their control. In *Medicine in equestrian sports*. Abstracts. First European third national conference, Saumur, France, Sept 18-20, 1981.
6. American Society for Testing and Materials: Standard specification for headgear used in horse sports and horseback riding (F1163-88). In *Annual book of ASTM standards*, Philadelphia, 1988, American Society for Testing and Materials.
7. Avery JG: *Fact sheet: horse riding accidents in children*, London, 1986, Child Accident Prevention Trust.
8. Baker JH: The first aid management of spinal cord injury, *Ambulance* 3(1):2, 1988.
9. Barclay WR: Equestrian sports, *JAMA* 240(17):1892, 1978 (editorial).
10. Barone GW, Rodgers BM: Paediatric equestrian injuries: a 14-year review, *J Trauma* 29:245, 1989.
11. Basic Life Support Working Party of the European Resuscitation Council: Guidelines for basic life support: a statement, *Resuscitation* 24:103, 1992.
12. Becker T: Das stumpfe Schadel trauma als sportunfall, *Mschr Unfallheilkd* 62:179, 1959.
13. Benzel EC, Sanford JL: Recovery of nerve root function after complete quadriplegia from cervical spine fractures, *Neurosurgery* 19(5):809, 1986.
14. Bernhang AM, Winslett G: Equestrian injuries, *Physician Sportsmed* 11:90, 1983.

15. Bivar ADH: Cavalry equipment and tactics on Euphrates, *Dumbarton Oaks Papers* 22:273, 1972.

16. Bixby-Hammett DM: Accidents in equestrian sports, *Am Fam Physician* 36:209, 1987.

17. Bixby-Hammett DM: Pediatric equestrian injuries, *Pediatrics* 89:1173, 1992.

18. Bixby-Hammett DM, Brooks WH: Common injuries in horseback riding: a review, *Sports Med* 9:36, 1990.

19. Bixby-Hammett DM, Brooks WH: Neurologic injuries in Equestrian sports. In Jordan BD, Tsairis P, Warren RF, editors: *Sports neurology,* Rockville, Md, 1989, Aspen.

20. Bjornstig U: *Skador vid ridsport,* Stockholm, 1982, Konsument-verket.

21. Bjornstig U, Eriksson A, Ornehult L: Injuries caused by animals, *Injury* 22(4):295, 1991.

22. Boger DC et al: Unilateral facet dislocation at the lumbosacral junction: case report and literature review, *J Bone Joint Surg* 65A:1174, 1983.

23. Bracken MB et al: A randomized, controlled trial of methylpred-nisolone or naloxone in the treatment of acute spinal cord injury, *N Engl J Med* 322(20):1405, 1990.

24. Bradford DS, McBride GG: Surgical management of thoracolum-bar fractures with incomplete neurologic deficits, *Clin Orthop* 218:201, 1887.

25. British Horseracing Board and The Jockey Club: *The orders and instructions of the British Horseracing Board and the rules of racing and instructions of The Jockey Club,* London, 1993, The Board and The Club.

26. British Show Jumping Association: *The rules and yearbook 1993,* Kenilworth, UK, 1993, British Equestrian Centre.

27. British Standards Institution: BS6473: 1984 with Amendment 1 (AMD 4731 29 March 1985), Amendment 2 (AMD 5423 31 Dec 1986), London, 1984-1986, The Institution.

28. British Standards Institution: *Protective skull caps for jockeys,* BS4472: 1988, London, 1988, The Institution.

29. Brooks WH, Bixby-Hammett DM: Prevention of neurologic injuries in equestrian sports, *Physician Sportsmed* 16:84, 1988.

30. Brote L, Skau A: Horse riding accidents in western Oster-gotland—a prospective study 1978-1980, *Lakartidningen* 78(24):2356, 1981.

31. Brown PN, Silver IA: Calculations. Cited in Firth JL: Equestrian injuries. In Scheider RC, Kennedy JC, Plant ML, editors: *Sports injuries: mechanisms, prevention and treatment,* Baltimore, 1985, Williams & Wilkins.

32. Burke DC: Traumatic spinal paralysis in children, *Paraplegia* 11:268, 1974.

33. Busch HM et al: Blunt bovine and equine trauma, *J Trauma* 26:559, 1986.

34. Campbell J, Bonnett C: Spinal cord injury in children, *Clin Orthop* 112:114, 1975.

35. Cannon P. Cited in Regan PJ et al: Hand injuries from leading horses, *Injury* 22:124, 1991.

36. From the CDC: injuries associated with horseback riding—United States, 1987-88, *JAMA* 264:18, 1990.

37. Chambers HG, Akbarnia BA: Thoracic, lumbar, and sacral spine fractures and dislocations. In Weinstein SL, editor: *The pediatric spine: principles and practice,* New York, 1994, Raven Press.

38. Cheshire DJD: The pediatric syndrome of traumatic myelopathy without demonstrable vertebral injury, *Paraplegia* 15:74, 1978.

39. Choi JU et al: Traumatic infarction of the spinal cord in children, *J Neurosurg* 65:608, 1986.

40. Clarke KS: Calculated risk of sports fatalities, *JAMA* 197:894, 1966.

41. Committee on Trauma: *Advanced trauma life support,* Chicago, 1992, American College of Surgeons.

42. Cone TE Jr: Book of accidents (1830). Excerpt XI. Riding a wild horse, *Pediatrics* 47:947, 1971.

43. Danielsson LG, Westlin NE: Riding accidents, *Acta Orthop Scand* 44:597, 1973.

44. De Loes M, Goldie I: Incident rate of injuries during sport activity and physical exercise in a rural Swedish municipality: incident rates in 17 sports, *Int J Sports Med* 9:461, 1988.

45. Depassio J et al: Spinal injuries with neurological signs while practicing a sport, *Semaine Hopitaux Paris* 59(45):3131, 1983.

46. Dickman CA et al: Pediatric spinal cord injury without radio-graphic abnormalities: report of 26 cases and review of the literature, *J Spinal Disord* 4:296, 1991.

47. Dittmer H: The injury pattern in horseback riding, *Lagenbecks Arch Chir Suppl Kongressbd,* p 466, 1991.

48. Dittmer H, Wubbena J: An analysis of 367 riding accidents, *Unfallheilkd* 80:21, 1977.

49. Dressage Group: *Dressage rules and official dressage judges panel,* Stoneleigh, UK, 1993, British Horse Society.

50. Edixhoven P, Sinha SC, Dandy DJ: Horse injuries, *Injury* 12:279, 1981.

51. Endurance Riding Group: Rules and omnibus schedule 1993, Stoneleigh, UK, 1993, British Horse Society.

52. Equus caballus, *N Engl J Med* 293:665, 1975.

53. Fesmire FM, Luten RC: The pediatric cervical spine: develop-mental anatomy and clinical aspects, *J Emerg Med* 7:133, 1989.

54. Firth JL: Equestrian injuries. In Schneider RD, Kennedy JC, Plant MI, editors: *Sports injuries: mechanism, prevention and treatment,* Baltimore, 1985, Williams & Wilkins.

55. Firth JL, Fu FH, Stone DA, editors: *Sports injuries: mechanism, prevention and treatment,* Baltimore, 1994, Williams & Wilkins.

56. Flynn M: Disruption of symphysis pubis while horse riding: a report of two cases, *Injury* 4:357, 1973.

57. Geisler FH, Dorsey F, Coleman WP: Recovery of motor function after spinal cord injury—a randomized, placebo-controlled trial with GM-1 ganglioside, *N Engl J Med* 326(26):1829, 1991.

58. Gerberich SG: Sports injuries: implications for prevention, *Public Health Rep* 100:570, 1985.

59. Gierup J, Larsson M, Lennqvist S: Incidence and nature of horse riding injuries—a one-year prospective study, *Acta Chir Scand* 142:57, 1976.

60. Gleave JR: The impact of sports on a neurosurgical unit. Paper presented at the British Institute of Sports Medicine, Cambridge, UK, April 1975.

61. Gratz RR: Accidental injury in childhood: a literature review on pediatric trauma, *J Trauma* 19:551, 1979.

62. Griffin R, Peterson KD, Halseth JR: Injuries in professional rodeo, *Physician Sportsmed* 12:130, 1984.

63. Gronwall D, Wrightson P: Cumulative effects of concussion, *Lancet* ii:995, 1975.

64. Grossman JA et al: Equestrian injuries: results of a prospective study, *JAMA* 240:1881, 1978.

65. Hamilton MG, Tranmer BI: Nervous system injuries in horseback riding accidents, *J Trauma* 34:227, 1993.

66. Hannah HW: The veterinarian's duty to foresee animal-inflicted injury, *J Am Vet Assoc* 169:570, 1976.

67. Harrison CS: Fox hunting injuries in North America, *Physician Sportsmed* 12:130, 1984.

68. Heipertz W, Steinbruck K: Analysis of riding accidents and proposition for their prevention. In *Medicine in equestrian sports.* Abstracts. First European third national conference, Saumur, France, Sept 18-20, 1981.

69. Henggeler J: The riding accident—meaning and prevention. *Medicine and equestrian sports.* Abstracts. First European third national conference, Saumur, France, Sept 18-20, 1981.

70. Hipp F et al: Fracture of the vertebrae due to riding accidents, *Fortshr Med* 95:1567, 1977.

71. Hobbs GD, Yealy DM, Rivas J: Equestrian injuries: a five-year review, *J Emerg Med* 12:143, 1994.
72. Holdsworth F: Fractures, dislocations and fracture-dislocations of the spine, *J Bone Joint Surg* 52A:1534, 1970.
73. Horse Trials Group: *Rules* 1993, Stoneleigh, UK, 1993, British Horse Society.
74. Hurlingham Polo Association: *Yearbook 1993,* Kirtlington, UK, The Association, 1993.
75. Ingemarson H, Grevsten S, Thoren L: Lethal horse-riding injuries, *J Trauma* 29:25, 1989.
76. Injuries associated with horseback riding—United States, 1987-88, *MMWR* 39:329, 1990.
77. Ives W, Brotman S: A review of horse-drawn buggy accidents, *Pa Med* 93:22, 1990.
78. Jockey Club: *Regulations for point-to-point steeple chases,* London, 1994, The Club.
79. Kadish H, Schunk J, Woodward GA: Blunt pediatric laryngotracheal trauma: case reports and review of the literature, *Am J Emerg Med* 12:207, 1994.
80. Kewalramani LS, Kraus JF, Sterling HM: Acute spinal cord lesions in a pediatric population: epidemiological and clinical features, *Paraplegia* 18:206, 1980.
81. Kewalramani LS, Tori JA: Spinal cord trauma in children: neurologic patterns, radiologic features, and pathomechanics of injury, *Spine* 5:11, 1980.
82. Kiwerski AU, Ahmad SH: Paraplegia in women, *Paraplegia* 21(3):161, 1983.
83. Kiwerski J: Spinal injuries caused by falling from horse carriages, *Pol Tyg Lek* 39:1063, 1984.
84. Klasen HJ: Accidents with saddle horses, *Ned Tijdschr Geneeskd* 125:136, 1981.
85. Kraususki M, Kiwerski E: Results of the treatment of fracture of the odontoid process of the axis, *Ortop Travmatol Protez* 3:52, 1990.
86. LaFollette BF, Levine MI, McNiesh LM: Bilateral fracture dislocation of the sacrum: a case report, *J Bone Joint Surg* 68A:1099, 1986.
87. LeBlanc HJ, Nadell J: Spinal cord injuries in children, *Surg Neurol* 2:411, 1974.
88. Lei HR, Lucht U: Horseback-riding accidents. I. Frequency of accidents in a horseback-riding population, *Ugeskr Laeger* 139:1687, 1977.
89. Lennqvist S: Is horseback riding a dangerous sport? *Lakartidningen* 74:4608, 1977.
90. Lloyd RG: Riding and other equestrian injuries: considerable severity, *Br J Sports Med* 21:22, 1987.
91. Lucht U, Lie HR: Horseback-riding accidents. II. A prospective hospital study, *Ugeskr Laeger* 139:1689, 1977.
92. McAfee PC, Bohlman HH, Yuan HA: Anterior decompression of traumatic thoracolumbar fractures with incomplete neurological deficit using a retroperitoneal approach, *J Bone Joint Surg* 67A:89, 1985.
93. McGhee CN, Gullan RW, Miller JD: Horse riding and head injury: admissions to a regional head injury unit, *Br J Neurosurg* 1:131, 1987.
94. McLatchie GR: Equestrian injuries—a one year prospective study, *Br J Sports Med* 13:29, 1979.
95. Medical Research Council: *Aids to the examination of the peripheral nervous system,* London, 1976, HMSO.
96. Metropolitan Life Insurance Co: Competitive sports and their hazards, *Stat Bull Metropol Life Insur Co* 46:1, 1965.
97. Metropolitan Life Insurance Co: Fatalities in sports 1970-78, *Stat Bull Metropol Life Insur Co* 60:2, 1979.
98. Miles JR: The racecourse medical officer, *J R Coll Gen Pract* 19(93):228, 1970.
99. Morgan RF et al: Rodeo roping thumb injuries, *J Hand Surg* 9:178, 1984.
100. Myers MC et al: Injuries in intercollegiate rodeo athletes, *Am J Sports Med* 18:87, 1990.
101. Nelson DE, Bixby-Hammett D: Equestrian injuries in childhood and young adults, *Am J Dis Child* 146:611, 1992 (review).
102. Office of Population Censuses and Surveys: *General household survey 1986,* London, 1989, HMSO.
103. Office of Population Censuses and Surveys: *Fatal accidents occurring during sporting and leisure activities 1982-92,* DH4 84/3, 85/5, 87/2, 88/3, 88/6 and 89/4, London, 1992, HMSO.
104. Office of Population Censuses and Surveys: *VS3 mortality statistics for England and Wales,* Titchfield, UK, 1992, OPCS.
105. Pang D, Wilberger JE Jr: Spinal cord injury without radiographic abnormalities in children, *J Neurosurg* 57:114, 1982.
106. Pony Club: *Yearbook 1993,* Stoneleigh, UK, 1993, British Horse Society.
107. Pounder DJ: "The Grave Yawns for the Horseman": equestrian deaths in South Australia 1973-1983, *Med J Aust* 141:632, 1984.
108. Regan PJ et al: Hand injuries from leading horses, *Injury* 22:124, 1991.
109. Reich L: Head and neck injuries in equestrian accidents, *HNO* 27:416, 1979.
110. Rice TAT: *The Scythians,* London, 1957, Thames and Hudson.
111. Riding Clubs Office: Official rules: riding test, equitation, jumping, show jumping, dressage and horse trials competitions, Kenilworth, UK, 1993, British Horse Society.
112. Riding for the Disabled Association: *Annual report and accounts 1993,* Kenilworth, UK, 1993, The Association.
113. Robey JM, Blyth CS, Mueller FO: Athletic injuries: application of epidemiologic methods, *JAMA* 217:184, 1971.
114. Robson SEE: Some factors in the prevention of equestrian injuries, *Br J Sports Med* 13:33, 1979.
115. Ruge JR et al: Pediatric spinal injury: the very young, *J Neurosurg* 68:25, 1988.
116. Schmidt B, Hollwarth ME: Sports accidents in children and adolescents, *Z Kenderchir* 44:357, 1989.
117. Silver JR, Lloyd-Parry JM: Hazards of horse-riding as a popular sport, *Br J Sports Med* 25:105, 1991.
118. Simpson AH et al: *Thoracic spine translocation without cord injury,* J Bone Joint Surg, 72B:80, 1990.
119. Steinbruck K: Spine injuries due to horse-riding, part 1, *Unfallheilkd* 83:366, 1980.
120. Steinbruck K: Spine injuries due to horse-riding, part 2, *Unfallheilkd* 83:373, 1980.
121. Teasdale G, Jennett B: Assessment of coma and impaired consciousness: a practical scale, *Lancet* ii:81, 1974.
122. Torg JS, editor: *Athletic injuries to the head, neck and face,* Philadelphia, 1981, Lea & Febiger.
123. A treatise on the blood, inflammation and gunshot wounds, *Clin Orthop* 28:3, 1963 (first published in 1794 by G Nichol, London).
124. Vigouroux RP, Guillermian P, Verando R: Neurotraumatology of sportive origin, *Neurochirurgie* 24:247, 1978.
125. Webb JK et al: Hidden flexion injury of the cervical spine, *J Bone Joint Surg* 58B:322, 1976.
126. Whitlock MR: Horse riding is dangerous for your health. In *Proceedings of the second international conference on emergency medicine,* Brisbane, Australia, 1988, Australian College for Emergency Medicine.
127. Whitlock MR, Whitlock J, Johnston B: Equestrian injuries: a comparison of profesional and amateur injuries in Berkshire, *Br J Sports Med* 21:25, 1987.
128. Yates JJ: A survey of British racecourses in respect of falls. In *Medicine in equestrian sports.* Abstracts. First European third national conference, Saumur, France, Sept 18-20, 1991.
129. Zachariae L: Dog bites and other lesions caused by animals, *Ugeskr Laeger* 135:2817, 1972.

Chapter Fifty-One

Skiing

Courtney W. Brown
Michael E. Janssen
Linda C. Tiefel

Epidemiologic analysis of a large number of ski injuries has been used over the past 40 years in an attempt to identify trends and problem areas, as well as to evaluate progress in the reduction of injuries.[6] The incidence of skiing injuries has decreased during the past few decades,[8] with the injury rate now approximating two to three injuries per 1000 skier days. However, the injury risk rate has been estimated to be about 25 times higher in Alpine competitions than in Alpine training.[5] The higher the competitive level, the greater the risk of injury to the elite athlete. An estimated 85% of skiers who have participated in Alpine World Cup races have experienced a serious injury during their careers.

The types of injuries suffered by competitive Alpine skiers appear to be similar to those experienced by noncompetitive Alpine skiers, but a higher percentage of the injuries are located in the lumbar spine. The lower leg remains the most common area injured in skiers of all types.

Although skiing is often considered a risky sport, it is not generally considered a possibly fatal endeavor. In fact, the risk of death as a result of a skiing injury is very low. In a 10-year review (1973 to 1983) the U.S. Consumer Product Safety Commission found that only 117 death certificates revealed a relationship to skiing.

No deaths were found in a review of 458 patients hospitalized at St. Anthony Hospital in Denver, Colorado (1980-1991), for skiing injuries. Of these patients, 58 were diagnosed with a spinal injury. Cervical trauma was most common (n = 24), whereas lumbar (n = 21) and thoracic (n = 13) spinal injuries were less common. Injury patterns ranged from isolated transverse process fractures to unstable burst fractures and/or fracture dislocations. Neurologic injury with quadriplegia occurred as a result of 3 of 24 cervical spine injuries.

POTENTIAL FOR INJURY

As a referral center for skiing injuries, we have had the opportunity to manage a variety of spinal injuries, from the recreational weekend skier to the Olympic competitor. Most of these injuries have been atraumatic and have resulted from an overuse syndrome. Skiing technique and style appear to correlate with the type of spinal problem in most patients.

Loads on the spine are produced primarily by body weight, muscle activity, and externally applied loads.

Because the lumbar region is the main load-bearing area of the spine in the downhill ski racing position and the area in which the pain most commonly occurs, loads in this region are of great interest. Flexion of the trunk increases the load by increasing the forward-bending moment. The forward inclination of the spine results in an eccentric annular bulge on the concave side of the flexed spine. In this flexed position the lumbar disc is depressed anteriorly while protruding posteriorly as both compressive and tensile stresses increase (Fig. 51-1). In our experience, the most common levels of involvement in premature disc degeneration in this competitive skiing population are L4-5 and L5-S1.

Competitive downhill racers assume a tuck position similar to the shape of an egg to reduce wind resistance (Fig. 51-2). This flexed spinal position results in an increase in both interosseous lumbar pressure[4] and interdiscal pressure.[7] Single- or multiple-level degenerative disc disease can occur from years of performing in this position. Numerous downhill skiers have these problems, although slalom skiers axially load and rotate their spines and thus risk the same injury. Usually this occurs at a single level rather than at multiple levels.

Herniated Discs

Figs. 51-3 to 51-6 illustrate disc herniation injuries in skiers.

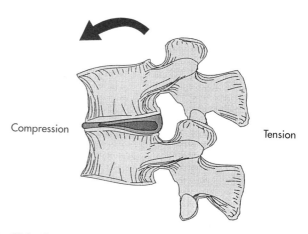

Fig. 51-1. Compressive and tensile stresses in the flexed spine.

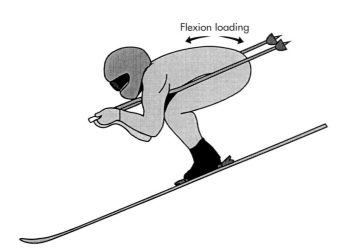

Fig. 51-2. Tucked position with flexed spine.

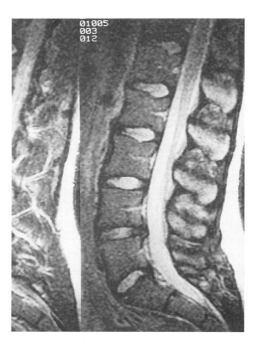

Fig. 51-3. This 21-year-old member of the U.S. downhill team for 6 years sustained an injury while training for technical events. Diagnosis by magnetic resonance imaging (MRI) revealed an L4-5 disc herniation. She responded to vigorous trunk stabilization, nonoperative treatment, and she continued on the team, skiing in the 1992 Winter Olympics, without having had surgery.

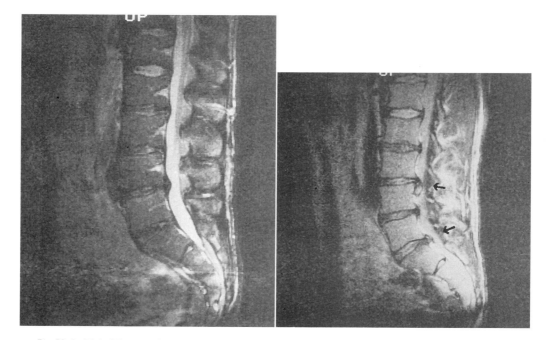

Fig. 51-4. This 25-year-old member of the U.S. downhill team for 4 years experienced repetitive back pain and was treated independently with massage and antiinflammatory agents. Rehabilitation of an injured knee failed because of severe radiculitis and radiculopathy. MRI and a myelogram revealed L3-4 and L5-S1 disc herniations. He underwent surgery at both levels. He was able to return to the World Cup circuit but competed with only moderate success. Herniation at the L4-5 disc led to a secondary surgery. Afterward, he was unable to return to the World Cup circuit.

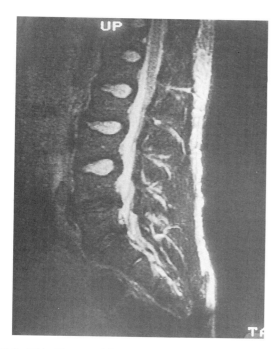

Fig. 51-5. This 31-year-old member of the U.S. Alpine men's slalom team for 13 years experienced repetitive episodes of low back pain with mild radiculitis. Evaluation revealed L4-5 and L5-S1 degenerative disc disease. He was treated nonoperatively with a trunk stabilization exercise program. He remained competitive without having surgery.

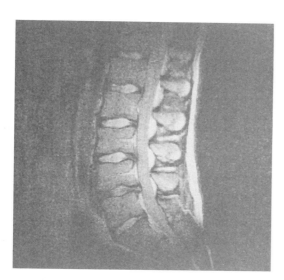

Fig. 51-6. This 21-year-old member of the U.S. Alpine men's slalom team suffered from severe back pain, restricted motion, and radiculitis. L4-5 disc herniation was revealed by MRI study. After failure of a nonoperative treatment program, he underwent a percutaneous discectomy at L4-5. He won the Canadian National Championship 3 months later and competed in the 1988 Olympics.

Spondylolysis and Spondylolisthesis

Competitive slalom and giant slalom racers appear to have an abnormally high incidence of spondylolysis and spondylolistheses. In 1988 three out of five members of the U.S. Alpine men's slalom team had this problem. We extrapolated two potential causes. First, the racers are more likely to be in an erect position when executing turns (Fig. 51-7). Second, when they are in this erect position, they are taught to perform a jet turn to produce more acceleration through the gate. This produces extension loading of the spine, driving the inferior edge of the superior facet into the pars interarticularis of the lower vertebrae. Repeat executions of this position tend to result in a stress fracture, which may eventually produce an acquired spondylolysis defect.

The skiers complain of low back pain, usually in extension. Occasionally they may exhibit radiculitis. Plain x-ray films sometimes show bony defects. Bone scan findings have been positive, unilaterally and bilaterally, and at different levels. Older racers with a history of repetitive pain have shown significant bony defects on both plain x-ray films and computed tomography (CT) scans. Some have shown a forward slip.

Figs. 51-8 and 51-9 illustrate spondylolisthesis in skiers.

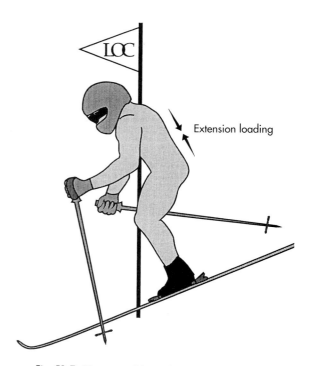

Fig. 51-7. Erect position with neutral spine.

Fractures

Traumatic injuries to the spine customarily are collision injuries involving immovable objects, such as trees, lift towers, rocks, fences, and buildings. Occasionally, severe falls can have similar results. The common de-nominator is excessive speed. Slick ski clothing and icy snow conditions can also contribute to these injury potentials, resulting in unstable fractures with paraplegia. Figs. 51-10 to 51-12 illustrate fractures in skiers.

◆   ◆   ◆

In other styles of skiing, such as freestyle, mogul skiing, or simply recreational skiing, any of the aforementioned injuries can occur, with mogul skiers tending to have a higher instance of spondylolysis or spondylolisthesis secondary to extension loading.

In conclusion, the incidence of spinal problems appears to be high in both professional and recreational skiers. In 1988 the entire U.S. slalom team had either spondylolysis or disc problems. At the same time several members of the U.S. downhill team demonstrated disc problems.

NONOPERATIVE TREATMENT
Principles

When a nonoperative spinal injury has occurred and a diagnosis has been established, early physical therapy intervention is appropriate. There are three components to treatment.

1. Design a set of exercises that modifies pain, increases mobility, and maintains or improves trunk strength.
2. Maintain cardiovascular conditioning by any method with which the athlete is comfortable.
3. Educate the athlete regarding the appropriate postural alignment and biomechanics to optimize healing and prevent further injury. This third component is often overlooked.

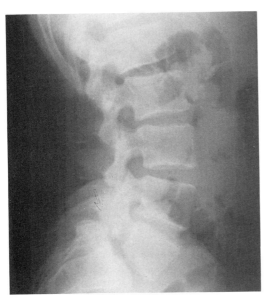

Fig. 51-8. This 26-year-old member of the U.S. Alpine men's slalom team for 11 years was found to have a well-established grade I spondylolisthesis at L5, with degenerative disc disease at L5-S1. He was treated with antiinflammatory agents and a thermal, molded brace in slight flexion for many years without surgical intervention and continued to perform well on the professional circuit.

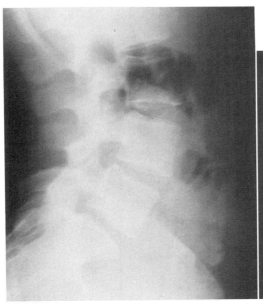
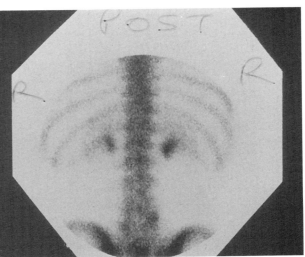

Fig. 51-9. This 18-year-old member of the U.S. development team was evaluated for acute low back pain. The work-up revealed positive findings on a bone scan but no lytic defect on a CT scan. He was treated with antiinflammatory agents and a thermal, molded brace in slight flexion. He was able to compete within 1 week of his injury.

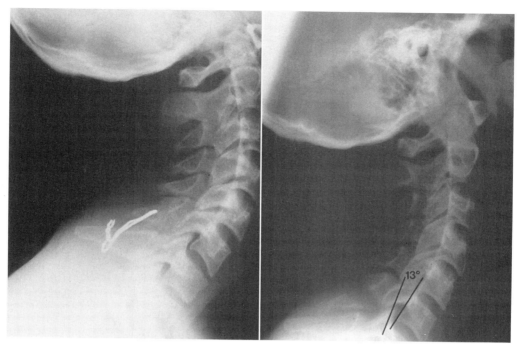

Fig. 51-10. This member of the U.S. downhill team sustained a C6-7 fracture subluxation, which was found to be unstable. This was successfully treated with open reduction, internal fixation, and fusion. He returned to downhill racing.

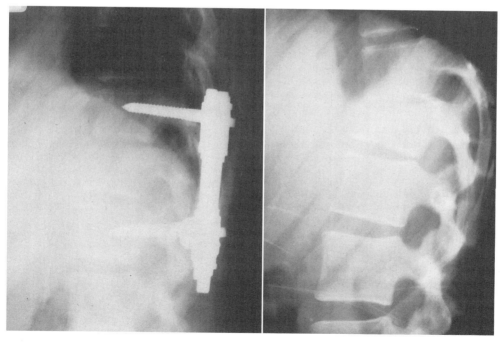

Fig. 51-11. This 23-year-old member of the Canadian National Ski Team sustained an unstable T12-L1 burst fracture during downhill training. She was successfully treated with AO fixateur interna. Because of additional injuries, she did not return to competitive ski racing.

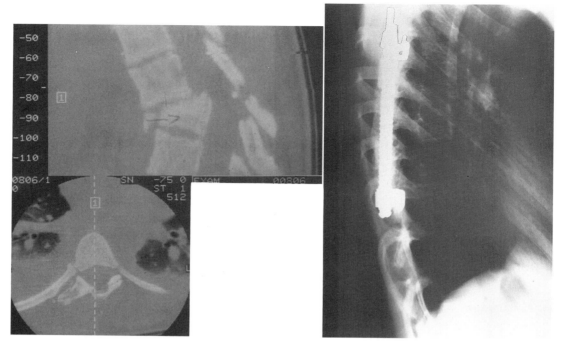

Fig. 51-12. This 23-year-old recreational skier was injured in a tree collision after sliding on ice. She suffered significant neurologic loss. She was treated with open reduction, internal fixation, and spinal fusion. There was complete resolution of all neurologic deficits. She has returned to normal activities, although, as of this writing, not skiing.

The use of modalities such as heat, ice, ultrasound, traction, electrical stimulation, and massage have a relatively limited and short-term benefit but may enhance the conditioning program.

Herniated Discs

An active conditioning program for a herniated disc usually begins with passive extension exercises and gradually moves to an active exercise program as tolerated by the athlete. As pain is reduced, there is gradual inclusion of full back–and abdominal-strengthening exercises (Fig. 51-13). This should also include emphasis on "closed-chain" activities, such as standing balance routines to enhance strength with proprioceptive responses. These closed-chain exercises keep the distal part in contact with a surface (in this case, feet on the floor), using postural mechanisms and producing accelerating, decelerating, and stabilizing core muscle contractions throughout the entire musculoskeletal system.

Therapy should use tools such as a balance board (Fig. 51-14), balance beam, and gymnastic ball (Fig. 51-15); trunk-resisted forward/backward and lateral (theratube) exercise; and plyometrics (progressive, explosive jumping routines that involve concentric, eccentric, and stabilization contractions of the trunk musculature) (Fig. 51-16). Trunk stabilization exercises in a swimming pool, which use extremity movement to produce resistance, are also helpful. The athlete may return to skiing when symptoms have subsided and

agility drills, sport-specific exercises, and running are well tolerated and pain free, criteria that indicate that range of motion with strength and without pain has been achieved.

Spondylolisthesis

Spondylolisthesis, although it causes acute pain, may be managed quite well with bracing and limited exercise. A thermal, molded brace in slight flexion may be used, thus allowing the skier to return to the sport as pain decreases. As healing occurs, a full physical therapy

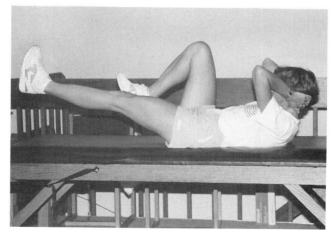

Fig. 51-13. Traditional abdominal-strengthening exercise.

evaluation is useful to determine if muscle imbalances are present and if there is a need for back and abdominal exercises to improve trunk stability. If so, the exercises discussed in the preceding section on disc problems are used (see Fig. 51-15). Note that these exercises may need to be modified to prevent further extension loading for a spondylolisthesis type of injury.

Fractures

When a spinal fracture occurs and is determined to be stable, the athlete is usually supported by a brace or a cast. It is important during this healing period that a physical therapist evaluate the athlete and design a cardiovascular program, as well as a full exercise program for maintaining extremity strength. Trunk strength can be addressed with isometric, stabilization exercise within the brace or cast. Balance activities may also be used. When the cast or brace is removed, the athlete is given a full back and abdominal strengthening and conditioning program similar to the herniated disc program. Once again, the exercises may need to be modified to match the tolerance of the athlete.

SURGICAL TREATMENT AND REHABILITATION
Herniated Discs

Surgical removal should be performed with as little soft tissue and bone trauma as possible; therefore a microdiscectomy with loops or a microscopic approach is indicated. The patient undergoing disc surgery benefits

from the same progressively rigorous spinal rehabilitation program as those treated nonsurgically. This treatment program accelerates recovery and results in decreased scarring. On the first postoperative day, the patient should be ambulatory and walking with a high-step gait pattern to begin mobilization of the lumbar spine. Posture and biomechanical training for activities of daily living (ADLs) are also initiated.

During the brief hospital stay, this program progresses to include gentle flexion/extension mobility exercises and an exercise program for spinal stabilization. The cardiovascular conditioning program is initiated but is contingent on pain tolerance.

Outpatient physical therapy should continue for approximately 6 weeks, progressing to a program that includes full back and abdominal strengthening and spinal stabilization. This should include mat exercises, the balance board/beam for proprioceptive response, theratubing for forward/backward and lateral resistance, and swimming pool exercises. Other strengthening equipment may be used as available. The athlete may return to skiing only after full spinal mobility and strength have been attained, as well as the ability to perform sport-specific drill and plyometric activities without pain (see Fig. 51-16).

Spondylolysis and Spondylolisthesis

Surgical intervention for spondylolysis and spondylolisthesis is rarely indicated. However, if symptoms do not resolve with a nonoperative approach, surgery should be considered. This can include reducing and bone grafting the defect with ASIF spondylolysis screws or single-level spinal fusion. Athletes who develop disc

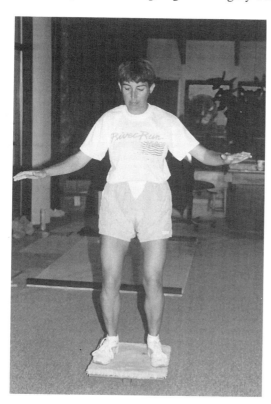

Fig. 51-14. Proprioception training on a balance board.

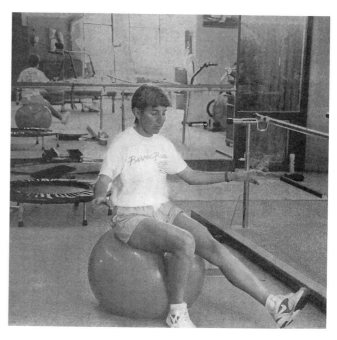

Fig. 51-15. Initiating trunk stabilization on a gym ball.

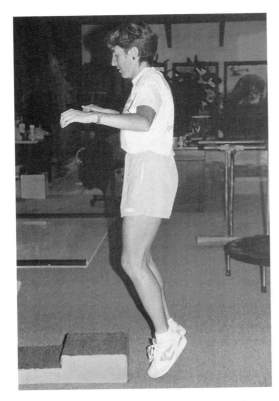

Fig. 51-16. Plyometric exercise. Jumping from the floor surface to different heights.

degeneration with a subsequent further slip as a result of repetitive trauma may also require a fusion. This may be achieved with pedicle screws to maintain lumbar lordosis and to ensure an increased fusion rate.

After lumbosacral fusions, a chairback thermal, molded, restrictive brace is used. The athlete is maintained in a brace for 3 or more months. As pain resolves, early posture and biomechanics training, as well as cardiovascular conditioning, is initiated. Extremity exercises begin with an emphasis on correct trunk posture. Trunk isometrics are performed until good, mature fusion is attained. As soon as there is evidence of a developing fusion, activity is increased and time in the brace is decreased. Stress is increased on the spine with an active loading program. When the fusion is mature, trunk musculature is addressed with a progression of various exercises that emphasize mobility. Beginning with mat exercises, the program gradually progresses to include all closed-chain exercises in the standing position, as described in the section on nonoperative treatment for a herniated disc. The athlete may return to the sport when the fusion mass is mature and strength

and range of motion are near normal. The patient must demonstrate the ability to perform and tolerate agility drills, plyometrics, and running without significant pain.

Fractures

Spinal fractures that are proved unstable are treated by reduction fusion in the thoracic, thoracolumbar, or lumbar region with posterior instrumentation such as Edwards rods, hooks, and sleeves or the new AO fixateur interna.[2] In our experience the indication for anterior surgery in acute injury is limited. Cervical spine injuries may be treated with either an anterior approach using the new ASIF titanium plates, a posterior approach using lateral mass plates, or a halo vest if alignment is satisfactory.[1,3]

Postoperative rehabilitation of spinal fracture is similar to that described for spondylolisthesis. Depending on the level fractured and the type of brace used, physical therapy progresses within the limited maturity of the healing fracture. Isometric trunk exercise can be introduced early, while the patient is still braced, by initiating a standing closed-chain program using balance activities to enhance trunk stability. As always, it is crucial to emphasize posture, biomechanics of ADLs, and cardiovascular conditioning. When the fusion is solid, the athlete can progress through the full spinal rehabilitation program.

After a spinal fusion, the skier must recognize the increased theoretic risk of injury at the terminal levels of fusion, although we have not observed this complication. Skiing ability may be limited. In our experience, several competitive skiers have been able to return to and excel in their specialty after simple disc excision. However, patients who have undergone fusion and have returned to competition have not routinely been able to achieve their preinjury competitive level.

REFERENCES

1. Abital JJ, Garfin SR: Surgical management of cervical disc disease: anterior cervical fusion, *Semin Spine Surg* 1:223, 1989.
2. Dick W: *Internal fixation of thoracic and lumbar spine fractures,* Toronto, 1989, Hans Huber.
3. Edwards C: Thoracolumbar trauma: posterior reduction and fixation with a modular spinal system, *Semin Spine Surg* 2:8, 1990.
4. Esses S: Interosseous vertebral body pressures, *Spine* 17(6), 1992.
5. Margreiter R, Raas E, Lugger LJ: The risk of injury in experienced Alpine skiers, *Orthop Clin North Am* 7:51, 1976.
6. Moritz JA: Ski injuries: a statistical and analytical study, *JAMA* 121:97, 1943.
7. Nachemson A: Towards a better understanding of back pain: a review of the mechanics of the lumbar disc, *Rheumatol Rehabil* 14:129, 1975.
8. Tapper EM: Ski injuries from 1939-1976: the Sun Valley experience, *Am J Sports Med* 6:114, 1978.

Chapter Fifty-Two

◆

Ice Hockey

Steven C. Dennis
Robert G. Watkins

Ice hockey is one of the most exciting sports for both participants and spectators. It is an extremely fast-paced and aggressive sport, as well as one of the most potentially dangerous to play. Whether the level of play be the 5-year-old "minimight" in a nonchecking league, the elite international amateur, or the professional player, the risk of catastrophic injury is extremely high.

INCIDENCE OF SPINAL INJURIES

Fortunately, injuries to the spine are not among the most common injuries suffered in ice hockey. They are, however, frequently the most devastating and disabling, all too often ending in quadriplegia or significant neurologic deficits. The literature is sparse in discussions of general spinal injuries in hockey, primarily because they tend to be considered part of the game. Such injuries are generally expected in a sport that seemingly rewards hard hitting and aggressive play as much it does the perfect shot or perfect pass. The most detailed data have involved injuries of the cervical spine, primarily fracture dislocations, that have resulted in neurologic deficits, including quadriplegia. These injuries are discussed in detail later in the chapter, particularly with regard to the mechanism of injury.

In recent years, possibly the most notable—although not the most devastating—spinal injuries have been those associated with elite professional players. Although these injuries have been publicized in the newspapers rather than reported in the medical literature, the attention has emphasized the significance of lumbar spine problems that afflict many sports professionals. The injuries sustained by these players have resulted not only in missed practices but also in missed important games, including play-off games. Some of these professional athletes have undergone lumbar spine surgery and have returned to the game. Other National Hockey League (NHL) players have been sidelined for treatment of disc disease.

In discussing these injuries with physicians and trainers who see these professional athletes on a day-to-day basis, we find that back injuries are common, although usually not disabling. In a 3-year Swedish study of an elite amateur team, lumbar spine injuries accounted for almost 16% of injuries, but only one fifth resulted in any limitation of playing ability.[3] Other European data include the occurrence in elite play of lumbar vertebral injury in the former Czechoslovakia,

but no specific information has been made readily available regarding frequency, loss of playing time, or any long-term disability.[1] In a Danish study, "back problems" accounted for 7% of lost playing time because of disability, averaging 16 days per injury, with three players absent for more than 3 weeks.[4] To keep disability time in perspective, however, in this same study, knee and elbow injuries resulted in periods of disability that averaged more than 1 month per injury.[4]

A 7-year longitudinal study of injuries among high school hockey players in Minnesota noted a 5% incidence of back injuries, predominantly of the lumbar spine, with almost a 30% risk of residual symptoms after recovery and a thirtyfold risk of future symptoms that would prohibit play.[2]

A 20-year review of Canadian hockey provided the most extensive study of spinal injuries in the sport. On the basis of data from 1966 through 1987, a total of 117 major injuries were reported.[11] All minor injuries, which comprise most spinal injuries, were specifically excluded, such as sprains, strains, whiplash, and flexion/extension injuries. Because of the difference in the objectives of various studies, it is difficult to use their data as a baseline or reference point. The greatest difficulty, however, lies in the fact that none of the studies to date has dealt with injuries that could be documented radiographically or neurologically or that suggested the possibility of permanent disability. None has given any attention to the minor injuries that prohibit play for a practice or two or possibly a game or two.

According to Lorentzon's data[4] on both elite-level and experienced amateur players, approximately one fifth of the reported injuries kept players from participating, although only 8% had major noncervical injuries. Tator et al.[11] documented approximately 20% of injuries to the thoracic or the lumbar spine that involved instability and/or neurologic damage. Therefore the risk of serious spinal injury below the C7 level limited to serious fractures and/or fracture dislocations of the spine is no greater statistically than 0.2% to 0.5% of total injuries. The physics of such a trauma suggest that it must be inflicted by means of tremendous speed and/or mass carried through a precise vector on or toward an unyielding end point. In terms of hockey this describes faster, larger players using aggressive checking against the boards and other players.

Data from the aforementioned studies are not exact,

but several attempts at both retrospective and prospective analyses are currently being considered or have already been undertaken to better define these risks and the actual probability, frequency, or occurrence of such injuries, as well as any relationship to playing ability.

CHECKING AND SPINAL INJURY

In an Olympics hockey contest between the United States and Sweden, which was televised internationally, an infamous check came from behind, drew blood, and resulted in a concussion, as well as a missed game and practice for a notable U.S. defenseman. In that game the player was penalized for boarding. However, in the observation of this event by one of us (S.C.D.), the only thing that distinguished this particular check was the unfortunate position of the defenseman in relationship to the bar supporting the Plexiglas that he struck with his face. In essence, there was nothing illegal about the check itself—just the unfortunate results for the U.S. player, providing even more support to the argument that checking from behind, even when "legal," is a very dangerous practice. Injuries as a result of contact are predominantly those that are inflicted from behind, usually with the player directly facing the boards.

Another aspect of checking involves acute hyperextension through a focal point of impact as the opponent checks from directly behind the player attempting to clear the puck with the hip, shoulder, or stick. The opponent then accelerates that player into an abnormal biomechanical position and then subjects him to a very sudden secondary impact against the boards, usually in a semifixed position as a result of the orientation of the skates on the ice and the attempted resistance by the struck player.

An additional mechanism of injury is that which often occurs when a player is ridden to the boards in a flexed-rotated or extended-rotated position as a check is thrown several steps away from the boards themselves but the player is held until impact to keep him out of the play and the puck cleared. Because of the increase in momentum through the two players moving together against the boards, this type of check can be as dangerous as a blind boarding type of check. The initial impact is almost always from behind or predominantly from behind, with the check itself originating from the stick and/or upper body. Such direct trauma followed by sudden impact can result in a pars interarticularis or transverse process fracture, or even in an acute disc injury as a result of the flexed-rotated or the extended-rotated position preceded by high-velocity direct force.

The last major check, commonly extolled on television and in the sports journals, which all too frequently results in injury, is the classic *hip check*. As an offense player rushes into the attack zone, the defense player, while skating backward, uses the angle of approach to his advantage and slides into the opponent about waist- or thigh-high with his own hip and leg as he himself accelerates to keep up his own speed. This motion allows the defensive player to continue his momentum, stay on his skates, search the ice for his teammates, and possibly control the puck. The offensive player, however, who is moving at a very high rate of speed, is launched into the air as he attempts to evade the check, almost always twisting at this point to stay on his skates and continue his momentum toward the net. The offensive player is almost always in a forward-flexed position to maximize his stride and speed. As a result, he eventually lands on his low back or buttocks or, as he attempts to remain skating, hyperextends as he rotates and lands chest first, or even hip or face first, on the ice in an acutely hyperextended position. This is a spectacular play to watch from either perspective, whether the defenseman is successful in his hip check or the offensive player is successful in evading the check. However, the potential for injury to either player is extremely high—although rare—because of the high-speed impact and rotational positions that result from such multiple-vectored motion coming to such an abrupt end point.

LUMBAR SPINE INJURIES AND BEGINNING PLAYERS

One of the major issues in injuries to the lumbar spine is the preparation of ice hockey players who are to be involved in such an aggressive sport. Several considerations must be dealt with in terms of the player's age, size, and level of play.

Grouping of Youngsters

For younger players, learning to skate and the rules of the game is not the most significant consideration; the major problem is that not all children of the same age or even the same size necessarily have the same level of physical development. Although nonchecking leagues are currently sanctioned for children younger than 13 years of age, the fact that their skating skills are not always controlled produces frequent collisions between players, as well as between players and the boards. A solution recently employed in youth football is to classify the players not only by age but by age and weight as a precaution against excessively high load impacts on contact. This approach, however, presents several problems for the younger, less mature, and less muscularly developed child who is overweight and therefore also physiologically underdeveloped in regard to growth plates and ligamentous development but is expected to compete with the older child on the basis of weight alone. Conversely, a slim but more mature and more developed child of lesser weight might participate with younger children, which could cause a similar problem. This older child would be able to generate significantly more force and could possibly collide with a younger child at a higher-impact speed, which could result in a more serious injury.

These arguments apply to all young people of either

sex until they are skeletally and physiologically mature. A significant number of reports in the literature have noted the risk of injury to the growing child as a result of training and competing in ice hockey, with its higher speeds, rigid boundaries, the constant impact of ice on skates, and the repetitive trauma not only to the lower extremities and hips but also to the upper extremities and spine.

Strength and Trunk Stabilization Training

On reaching maturity, young people are capable of acquiring the kind of physical conditioning needed to help protect them from lumbar spine injuries. The principles of trunk control and strengthening cannot be overemphasized in preventing injury and decreasing the potential severity and disability of injury to the lumbar spine. The key muscle groups of the rectus, obliques, lumbar paraspinals, gluteals, and quadriceps have paramount importance for lumbar spine function. The "rigid cylinder" concept is one in which the muscles of the trunk are fully strengthened. Thus the rigidity of the vertebral column serves to protect the neural elements and increase the stability of the annular portion of the disc by shifting certain rotational and flexing-rotational force vectors to stronger muscles without sacrificing flexibility. Also, increased gluteal and quadriceps strength and improved resistance to fatigue protect the spine and contribute to a stronger trunk through improved biomechanical posture. The extremities also are protected from fatigue and overuse injuries by the improved efficiency of better trunk position and strength. This concept is well documented in several articles concerning baseball pitchers and better protection against overuse of the upper extremities as a result of improved trunk efficiency and strengthening.[13]

Posch et al.,[5] in a study of a Swedish amateur team, documented decreased peak leg muscle strengthening over the course of the season despite two games and two practices per week. Although the rate of major injuries did not increase, the authors indicated that this was not an elite professional team. Even though the players' oxygen uptake, an indication of aerobic function, remained stable, it was significantly lower than that of an elite team. Sim et al.[6] noted that injuries increased early in the season, most notably as a result of players being hit by the stick about the head and face. Overall, injuries decreased over the course of the season, although the cause was indeterminate and possibly a result of experience, practice, or more efficient use of aggressive play as opposed to indiscriminate hitting.

Unfortunately, no study to date has reported the relationship of a specific type of injury to a specific period in the season or to its frequency or severity in terms of conditioning and strength. Because most lumbar injuries are simply noted as minor, current hockey statistics do not allow accurate predictions concerning how the disability may be minimized, if not

avoided. The inference from team physicians is that conditioning is the single most important factor, yet is objectively difficult to document.

CERVICAL SPINE INJURIES
Incidence

The most severe spinal injuries involve the cervical spine. Although the studies by Tator et al.[8-11] are the most extensive of those published, unfortunately, they do not quantify true injury rates. The most significant statistic is that major spinal injuries have increased significantly in frequency through the 1980s.[11] At that point rule changes were made in an effort to prevent this increase from continuing. One of the most alarming aspects of these statistics is that approximately 75% of major cervical injuries involve a neurologic deficit.[11] Gerberich[2] noted that of all injuries in Minnesota high school hockey, which interestingly enough constitutes 20% of all high school hockey in the United States, 22% involved the head and neck, with 4% confined to the neck alone. Of the total injuries 18% were considered major, including three cervical fractures.

The most extensive study on neck injuries in hockey was undertaken by Tator et al.[11] and published in the *Canadian Journal of Surgery* in February 1991. This long-term 20-year review by the Committee on Prevention of Spinal Cord Injuries Due to Hockey is an exhaustive search through the records of the Canadian Amateur Hockey Association. An alarming finding is that 85% of the injuries reported occurred in the last 7 years of the study. Final statistics cover the last season under study only until March 1990, yet show the greatest percentage of injury up to that point of any year studied.

Age as a Factor

A significant finding is that it is not the advanced amateur or professional who is sustaining cervical spine injuries but rather the adolescent, the developing, growing child playing in amateur leagues. Of the age-documented cases 64% involved players between the ages of 12 and 20 years, whereas only 19% involved players between 21 and 30 years of age.[11] Of the neurologically injured players, 80% of the injuries affected the cervical spine, with 50% of the total injuries affecting the vertebrae between C4 and C6. These statistics are consistent with reports in the literature on the cervical spine, which indicate that C5-6 and C4-5 are the most commonly compromised levels in all contact sports. In contrast, Torg's landmark work[12] on quadriplegia in football players revealed that injury at the C3-4 level most commonly resulted in actual quadriparesis, or quadriplegia.

The environment in which cervical or neurologic injury most often occurs is during an organized game, with more than 75% of the injuries occurring in supervised, refereed, organized league play. This arouses suspicion about the quality of supervision, not only during the game but also during training. One questions the methods that are being taught, as well as the teaching and enforcement of the rules both before and during league play. A common theme in the studies of Tator,[11] Sim,[7] Torg,[12] Jorgensen,[3] and others is that although serious injuries occur in all sports, hockey and football place the player at greater risk because contact is a basic element and the tendency is to emulate the professional player without regard for the rules or the participant's level of play (i.e., the harder one hits and the more frequently one hits, the better the player one is). Although it is common to reward the expert player for roughness in hockey, successful play is not based on brute force. The accomplishments of the truly great players are based on their talents in skating, passing, shooting, and avoiding the check.

Causes

In more than 54% of cervical injuries, the initiating event was a check, with 30% occurring from behind.[11] In 65% of the documented major injuries, the resultant impact was with the boards. Impact with another player was responsible for another 10% of injuries overall. The mechanism of injury is analogous to neck injuries in football, (i.e., actual loading in a slightly flexed position of the cervical spine). Subsequently, the motion segment of bone-disc-bone is crushed with retropulsion of the elements posteriorly, with or without rupture of the interspinous and capsular ligaments. Most often an incomplete cord lesion or root lesion evolves, depending on the rotation of the head at the time of impact. In the study by Tator et al.,[9,10] however, five deaths occurred as a result of severe spinal cord injury at an upper cord segment level. In the boarding type of check or in one that "rides" the player to the boards, the cervical spine is at risk as the head is forced against the glass or boards into an acutely hyperextended position. In the elite player the neck is more commonly extended; the player at this level tends to remain aware of the game around him and tries to clear the puck despite the impact as he attempts to keep playing. In this position, more soft tissue injuries tend to occur rather than bone injuries.

However, as players look to the ice for the puck or attempt to avoid the check by skating out of the play, the neck usually remains flexed; the risk now is for acute flexion with axial loading injuries. This position potentiates a secondary risk for a "clay shoveler's" avulsion fracture of the cervical spine, a compression or burst fracture, or a fracture dislocation. Obviously these are the most serious types of injury to occur and the ones most likely to result in neurologic sequelae.

Popularity of the Sport

The epidemiology of the injuries in hockey raises considerable concern about the marked increase in the popularity of this sport in the United States. Even in an

area such as southern California, hockey participation is growing dramatically at the youth and adult amateur levels, primarily for the beginner or early intermediate skater. On the basis of Tator's statistics in hockey versus Torg's statistics in football, in terms of per capita figures hockey in Canada carries approximately three times the risk of quadriplegia as does football in the United States. However, a hopeful distinction between U.S. amateur hockey leagues versus those in Canada, particularly for the years during which the statistics were collected, is that in the United States, leagues for players younger than 13 years of age—and in some areas leagues for those younger than 16 years—have remained nonchecking, as have almost all adult beginner and intermediate leagues. Canadian hockey has traditionally been "checking hockey" even in youth leagues, but this approach has been studied and modified and is being considered for permanent change at some time in the future.

Psychologic Factors

An interesting commentary that emerged from the study of injuries among Minnesota high school players was that the purpose of playing hockey was to decrease tension and release aggressive tendencies.[2] The individual risk of concussion to the players who gave this reason for participation was actually four times greater statistically, as shown retrospectively at the season's end. At the professional level, however, the risk of neck and back symptoms was 12 and 30 times greater, respectively, for those players who had had previous injury.[2] The predominant result appears to be that rather than relieving tension, the use of force stops other players from establishing the tempo and tone of the game. This level of play certainly takes on different meanings when one considers the financial rewards for winning. A leading sports magazine recently highlighted a greatly talented player, beginning with his development as a youth player, then an elite amateur, and then a young professional. Although the athlete's skill as a skater was noted, he was particularly lauded for his adeptness with a hockey stick. The focus of this skill was not on the player's scoring ability but on tripping, holding, and other acts bordering on the illegal for which he was known (i.e., using his hockey stick against other players without being penalized). Numerous publications have featured the hard-hitting play. More recently, however, there has been concern over injury and lack of enforcement of the rules, as well as considerable criticism of inconsistent handling of discipline by NHL administrators and the referees themselves. It is interesting to note that in a game that moves at such a high rate of speed over such a large surface, there is only one official on the ice who actually can call penalties. This provides a great contrast to professional basketball, which has fewer players, a smaller surface, and slower speeds but has three officials, each of whom can call any penalty at any time.

PREVENTION OF INJURY

It is inappropriate to find fault with hockey at the professional level exclusively or to place blame exclusively on administrative and officiating personnel or the players. Of course, standards and examples must be set and enforced, and these professionals have the best opportunity to improve the image of hockey, but the elite-level players whose actual living depends on a performance cannot be held totally responsible for certain concerns about physical safety.

Most serious spinal injuries are occurring in young players, and this problem must be addressed at several levels. Because today's players are taller and heavier and able to skate faster, these physical attributes must be considered in assigning teams and in competition among youth leagues. No longer can age be the only criterion; ability, experience, and size must be included in the decision-making process. There is an obvious desire to emulate the professional player, and in turn the aggressiveness and often dirty play also are copied. In addition, helmets, face shields, and complete protective gear make these young players feel invulnerable, which helps contribute to the aggressiveness of their play. Tator et

al.[11] and Torg[12] have shown decreases in head injury as a result of better helmets, but there is no statistical documentation of a decrease in neck injuries. It is of note that no studies to date have dealt with minor injuries or have established a meaningful overall injury rate.

A great responsibility falls on the leagues and the officials who establish and enforce new and existing rules. The key is to prevent the increasing number of injuries, particularly those resulting from cross-checking (i.e., checking from behind, boarding, and illegal use of the stick, all of which obviously can and do lead to unexpected collisions with either the boards or other players). Better conditioning and training, particularly for the older child and adolescent—but not to the point of risking the growing bone from overuse and developmental problems—must also be encouraged. Further, there is a need for improved statistics and data collection for injuries with a better reporting system to increase awareness of the risks and how to avoid them.

CASE ILLUSTRATIONS

Figs. 52-1 to 52-5 illustrate cases involving spinal injuries in hockey players.

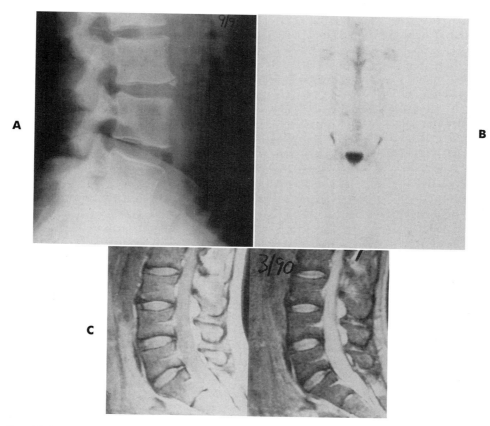

Fig. 52-1. This patient suffered a hyperextension injury of the lumbar spine when he was cross-checked from behind, high and low, hyperextending the spine. The apparent avulsion fracture or unfused apophysis (**A**) does not really show evidence of this injury on the bone scan (**B**) or MRI scan (**C**). Nevertheless, a considerable period of time elapsed before the player was allowed to return to play.

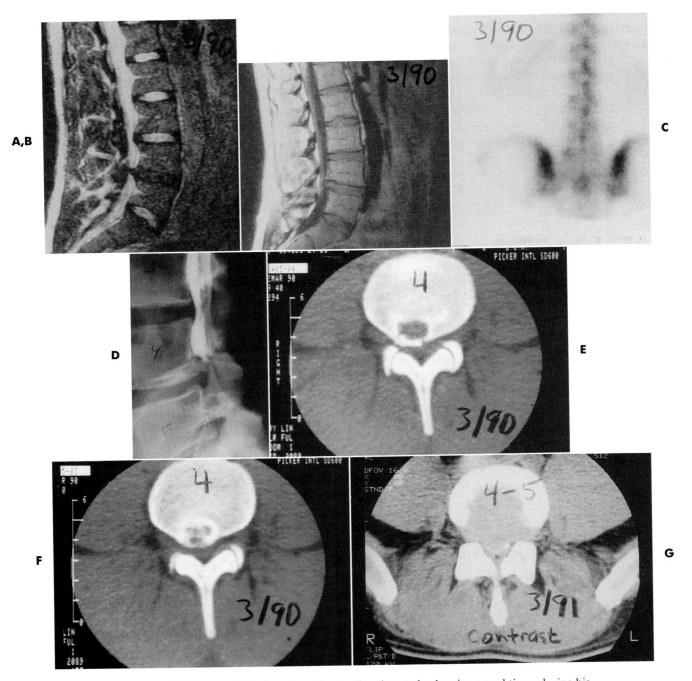

Fig. 52-2. This 28-year-old hockey player had suffered acute back pain several times during his career. Suddenly both legs became weak, and he had severe pain in the buttocks that radiated to both legs. Findings on straight leg raising were positive for severe back and leg pain, with no evidence of bowel and bladder dysfunction. **A** and **B,** MRI scans show a significant posterior obstruction; the posteroinferior end-plate of L4 is seen to be involved, probably as Smorl's node. **C,** The bone scan shows no excessive uptake at the midline on the anterior view but does show this increase on the facet joint or lateral pars area. There was no documented pars defect, but increased warmth indicated a strain in that area. **D,** The myelogram shows not only a block but also what appears to be bone posteriorly in the spinal canal off the caudal surface of L4. **E** to **G,** Three CT scans show the significant posterior protrusion of material. The noncontrast study shows a significant Smorl's node and posterior bony edge. Subsequent deterioration **(G)** a year after the initial evaluation **(E** and **F)** indicated the need for surgery.

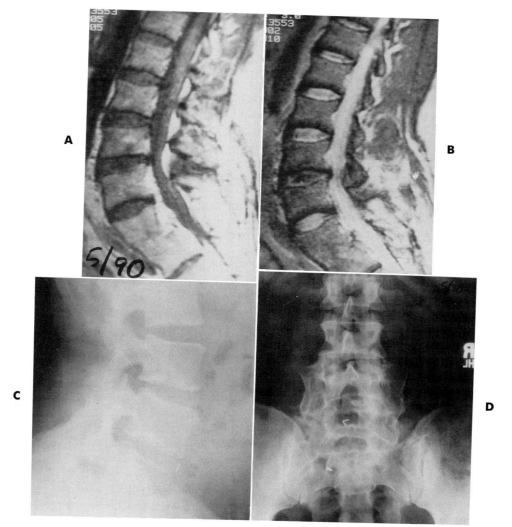

Fig. 52-3. A retired hockey player sought evaluation for back pain. **A** and **B,** The results of his old fusion are clearly visible. **C** and **D,** These views show evidence of disc degeneration and stenosis at the level above the old fusion. The athlete was able to return to play for 3 years after his spinal fusion and had only intermittent problems thereafter.

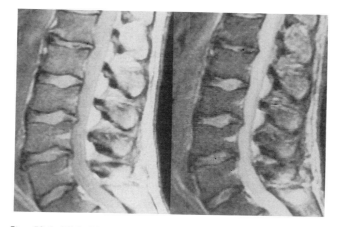

Fig. 52-4. This 32-year-old hockey player was forced to retire because of mechanical back pain that occurred only during play. There was no evidence of radiculopathy; his complaint was purely back pain.

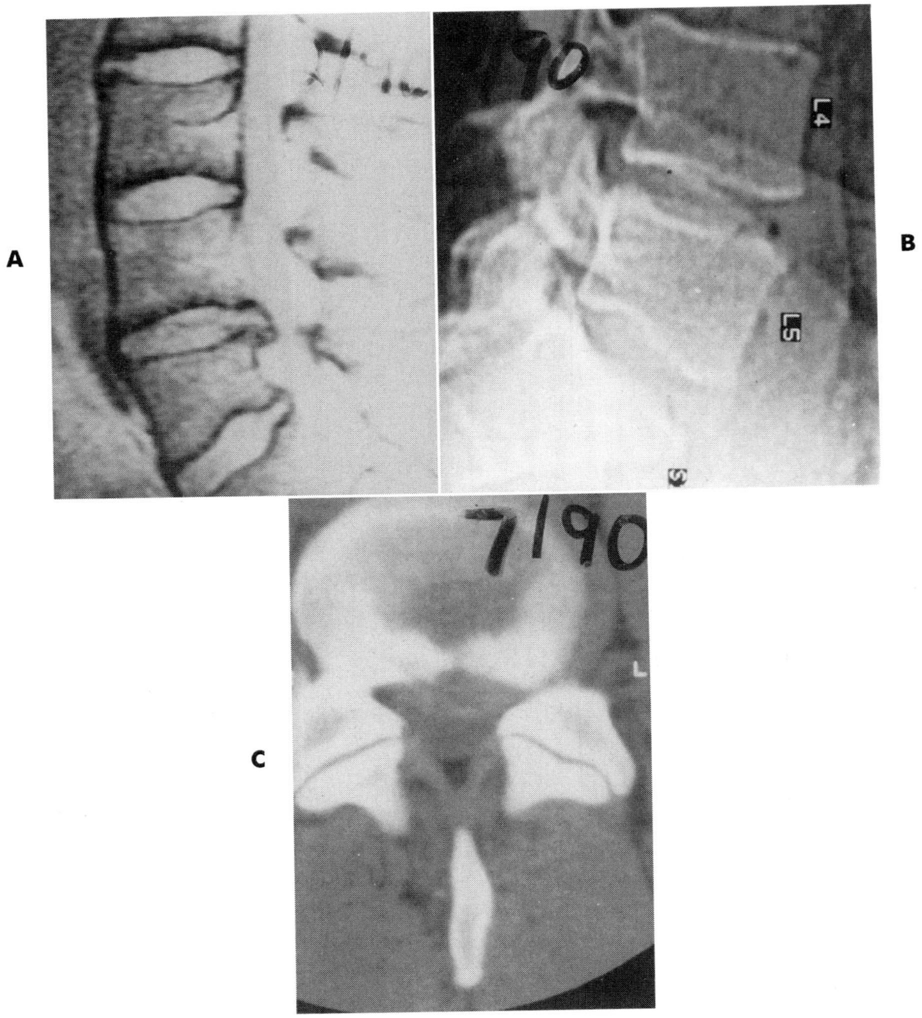

Fig. 52-5. This 24-year-old hockey player was diagnosed with a disc herniation (**A**). He was treated with an aggressive nonoperative rehabilitation program. He ultimately underwent surgery the following year (**B** and **C**) because of recurring symptoms and had a microscopic lumbar discectomy. It is of note that he had a spondolytic defect at L5-S1, along with a clear-cut disc herniation at L4-5. The preferred treatment is a one-level discectomy at that level.

REFERENCES

1. Feriencik K: Trends in ice hockey injuries: 1965 to 1977, *Physician Sportsmed* 7(2):81, 1979.
2. Gerberich SG et al: An epidemiological study of high school hockey injuries, *Childs Nerv Sys* 3:59, 1987.
3. Jorgensen U, Schmidt-Olsen S: The epidemiology of ice hockey injuries, *Br J Sports Med* 20(1):7, 1986.
4. Lorentzon R et al: Injuries in international ice hockey, *Am J Sports Med* 16:389, 1988.
5. Posch E et al: Prospectus study of concentric and eccentric leg muscle torques, flexibility, physical conditioning, and variation of injury rates during one season of amateur ice hockey, *Int J Sports Med* 10:113, 1989.
6. Sim FH, Simonet WT: Ice hockey injuries, *Physician Sportsmed* 16(3):92, 1988.
7. Sim FH et al: Ice hockey injuries, *Am J Sports Med* 15:86, 1987.
8. Tator CH: Neck injuries in ice hockey: a recent, unsolved problem with many contributing factors, *Clin Sports Med* 6(1):101, 1987.
9. Tator CH, Edmonds VE: National survey of spinal injuries in hockey players, *Can Med Assoc J* 130:875, 1984.
10. Tator CH et al: Spinal injuries due to hockey, *Can J Neurol Sci* 11(1):34, 1984.
11. Tator CH et al: Spinal injuries in ice hockey players, 1966-1987, *Can J Surg* 34(1):63, 1991.
12. Torg JS: Epidemiology, pathomechanics, and prevention of athletic injuries to the cervical spine, *Med Sci Sports Exerc* 17:295, 1985.
13. Watkins RG et al: Dynamic EMG analysis of torque transfer in professional baseball pitchers, *Spine* 14:404, 1989.

Chapter Fifty-Three

◆

Figure Skating

Lyle J. Micheli
Claire F. McCarthy

Recognition of figure skating as a major sport came with the inclusion of figure skating events for men, women, and pairs in the Olympic Winter Games. Ice dancing was officially recognized in the World Championships in 1952 and in the Olympics in 1976. Most recently, precision team skating was officially recognized by the International Skating Union (ISU) at the 1994 Council Meeting held in Boston. Precision team skating as an event in the World Championships is anticipated for the near future.

Figure skating is a high-performance sport in which athletic and artistic movements are intrinsically entwined to produce exciting and esthetically pleasing performances. Skaters are expected to perform difficult movements in unison with accompanying music in individually interpreted expressions of style. Separate scores are awarded for both the athletic and the artistic components of an event. The more difficult the content in terms of selection of elements and the more accurate the execution, the higher the score in "technical merit." Artistic components, such as carriage and line, creativity, originality, and music interpretation, are reflected in the scores on "presentation and style." Competitive skating is fast, strenuous, and, at times, dramatic and very exciting. High degrees of strength, endurance, flexibility, agility, coordination, and balance are required, as are personal discipline and diligence.

There are five categories of figure skating: compulsory, or school figures; free skating; pair skating; ice dancing; and, most recently, precision team skating.

THE COMPETITIVE SKATER IN RELATION TO GROWTH AND MATURATION

The age range of serious competitors is from late school age to late adolescence or early adulthood. Some of our best competitors are still adolescents, and some of the "comers" are preadolescents or young adolescents. The majority of competitive skaters, particularly at the lower levels, are actively involved in the dynamic process of growth and maturation. During this process a number of physical and emotional changes occur that need to be understood by individual skaters, professional instructors, parents, and health-related personnel.

A period of skeletal growth occurs that results in changes in bone structure and content, alterations of the tensile strength at the insertions of tendons into bone, and alterations at the epiphyseal-metaphyseal junction (growth plate). In addition, a loss of flexibility is frequently experienced as the muscles and tendons accommodate to the increasing length of the long bones. Concurrently, the ratio of leg length to trunk length increases. Unfortunately, during this period, training timetables frequently include plans to escalate the levels of difficulty to be achieved by the skater, particularly in jumping skills. The early period of adolescence, or acceleration phase of growth, represents a time of high risk for injury. It is significant that the spine continues to grow throughout adolescence. Skaters need to become sensitive to their aches and pains and help to recognize problems early.

FIGURE SKATING AND THE SPINE

The nature of figure skating dictates the importance of the spine to performance, both athletically and artistically. Skating challenges the structural design of the spine. Falls of any kind, and particularly those with landings on the ischium, test the ability of the spine to absorb compression forces. The reverberations of hard landings are also felt in the lumbar spine. The various adjustments made by the spine in support of the extremities to achieve an esthetic line require flexibility. The many lifts in pair skating and ice dancing challenge the stability of the spine. Knowing the position of the center-of-gravity line through the spine and the location of the center of mass within the pelvis are key to learning the skills of figure skating.

An erect posture and good body alignment are essential ingredients to success. Spins can be faster, jumps can be higher with more revolutions, spirals can be controlled for longer periods of time, and intricate footwork and steps are easier. A deviation in postural control during the performance of compulsory figures is reflected in the tracing. A less-than-perfect circle, a flattened edge, or a wiggly line is easily seen. A continued degradation of performance on simple figures can be an early sign of a beginning musculoskeletal problem.

Skating Technique and the Spine

The posture of increased lordosis and anterior pelvic tilt is a common finding in skaters both on and off the ice and is frequently thought to be the correct one by the young competitor. This posture is sometimes compounded by the temporary decrease in flexibility that occurs during the adolescent growth spurt mentioned

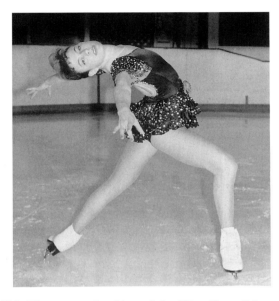

Fig. 53-1. The posture/position of the "Ena Bauer" is one of marked hyperextension of the lumbar spine and anterior tilt of the pelvis to accommodate bilateral hip external rotation. (Courtesy Anna-May Walker.)

earlier. In skaters this decrease in flexibility is particularly notable in anterior hip structures, the hamstring muscles, and the gastrocsoleus muscle group, with secondary tightening of the lumbodorsal fascia.

Most movements in skating place a heavy demand on the skater's postural and motor systems (Fig. 53-1). If a skater is not able to achieve a corrected posture and preferably maintain it, then many of the standard elements of free skating will place undue stress throughout the lumbar and thoracolumbar regions of the spine. For example, a spiral done with the nonskating leg extended high behind and the arms stretched parallel to the ice requires at least 90 degrees of straight leg raising of the weight-bearing leg (Fig. 53-2). Inability to obtain this position easily places an extension moment on the spine because of the need to right the head. Another example is the beautiful lay-back spin (Fig. 53-3); full extension of the hip and a forward movement of the pelvis are required for the head and thorax to be extended. The lay-back spin also requires full extensibility of the abdominal musculature.

Jumps inherently have only an indirect impact on the spine, in terms of falls, aborted attempts, and hard landings. A skater usually has a preferred landing leg and a preferred spinning leg. Few skaters jump to both directions; therefore the stresses involved in landing occur unilaterally. Landings occur only on one foot; double-footed landings are not allowed. The muscular

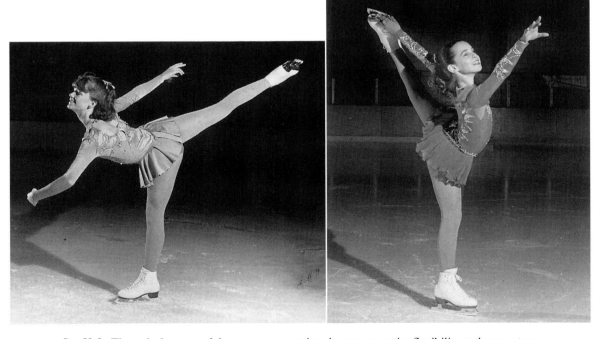

Fig. 53-2. The spiral, a graceful maneuver, requires lower extremity flexibility to lessen stress across the lumbar spine. Maintenance of position and line places a demand on extensor musculature. (Courtesy Anna-May Walker.)

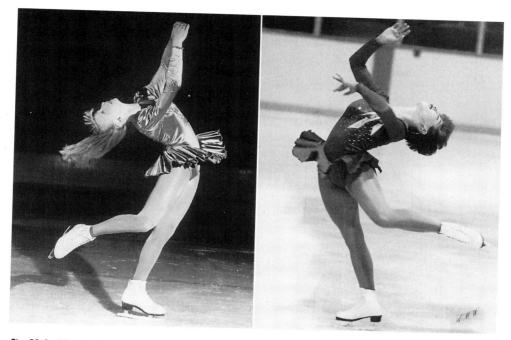

Fig. 53-3. The lay-back is a spin variation that increases the level of difficulty. Positional control and balance are challenged by the posterior position of the thorax and increased extension of the lumbar spine. (Courtesy Anna-May Walker.)

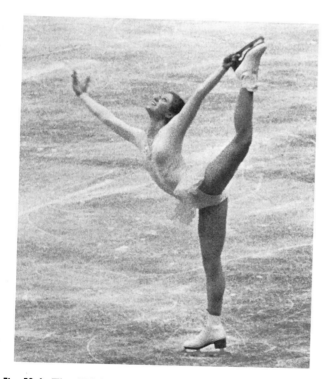

Fig. 53-4. The "Biellmann spin," performed here by its originator, Denise Biellmann, is characterized by upright posture and an overhead hand-to-skate blade connection. The fulcrum of the closed loop at the lumbar spine demands a moderate to high degree of lumbar hyperextension. (Courtesy Anna-May Walker.)

pattern used to check rotations and land upright and in control is a consistent one.

The Axel-Paulson jump requires a powerful forward swing of the potential landing leg (iliopsoas concentric contraction) to gain height and distance. The weight of the boot and blade adds to the rate of acceleration of the swing leg. The heavier the boot, the greater the acceleration and the more energy and control needed to decelerate. As the skater lands, the hip musculature controls deceleration and body alignment (laterally, posteriorly, and anteriorly), as well as pelvic rotation.

Skaters are encouraged to be creative. One way of being creative is by designing a movement that becomes the skater's "signature," such as the "Biellmann spin," described as a grab-hold spin (Fig. 53-4). Standing on her spinning leg (left), the skater extends her back, grabs her free leg (right), and pulls it high over her head. This position is held throughout the spin, which must be at least six revolutions. Depending on the skater's structural flexibility, the fulcrum for the closed-loop bend falls within the lumbar spine, and there is marked extensibility of the abdominal muscles and the hamstring muscles of the support leg. Because this spin is known to be extremely difficult, young skaters practice it, but few achieve the ability to do it, and even fewer do it in competition (Fig. 53-5).

Some freestyle moves in pair skating and ice dancing increase the risk of injury because of added speed and the design of the movements (Fig. 53-6). In senior pair

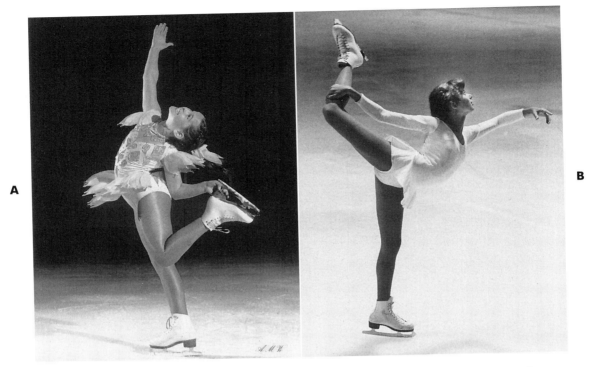

Fig. 53-5. Modified positions of the lay-back (**A**) and Biellmann (**B**) spins. (Courtesy Anna-May Walker.)

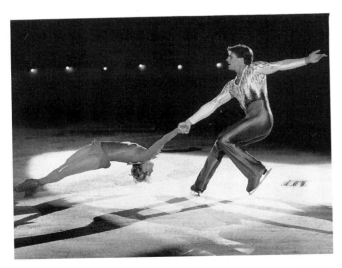

Fig. 53-6. The "death spiral," a required element in pair skating competitions, places a heavy demand on spinal musculature of the male and female skaters for postural and positional control. (Courtesy Anna-May Walker.)

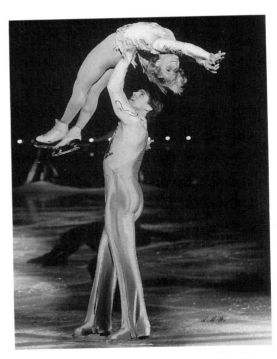

Fig. 53-7. Overhead lift. The male skater lifts his partner, maintains her in an overhead stretch, and lowers her gently to the ice while moving and at times turning. Lift assist and postural and positional control by the female skater are essential to achieve the maneuver, minimize expected stress on the lumbar spine, and protect her partner during failed maneuvers. (Courtesy Anna-May Walker.)

skating, the male skater lifts his partner overhead in a variety of patterns and then must also lower her to the ice (Fig. 53-7). Lifts are generally made from the front. Although a lift done perfectly results in substantial stress to the lumbar spine of the male skater, the same lift with no assist from the female skater, or an awkward, aborted one, multiplies the amount of stress and certainly challenges the protective function of the spinal column. There are restrictions to overhead lifts in the lower skating classifications, but a late-maturing male skater at a level of competition that allows overhead lifts will still be at risk.

Female pair skaters are at risk from falls, which can occur from a variety of heights; the fall can occur from as high as the outstretched overhead position of the skater's partner. In the throw axel, the female skater is thrown up and away from her partner. The higher and longer the throw, the more spectacular the movement. To achieve consistency in this movement requires a lot of practice and a lot of falls.

In ice dancing there is a tendency to develop an accentuated lordotic posture. The performance of the compulsory dances and original set-pattern dance causes no significant additional stress to the spine unless the swing of the free leg into extension is done without control. In free dance, the speed made possible by two skaters in close position adds another dimension. Lifts are also allowed to the level between the waist and shoulder of the male skater. Posturing is allowed. It is the swift entrance in and out of some postures that presents

risk (e.g., repeated quick extension of the trunk and extension or lateral flexion with a rotation [Fig. 53-8] particularly to the lumbar spine).

Posture, body alignment, and control of the body's center of mass begin with the spine. When creating new movements or altering old ones, one should begin with the position and control of the spine and pelvis. A careful analysis will help identify potentially harmful stresses.

BACK INJURIES

Back injuries are relatively uncommon when judged against the total of all injuries in figure skating. The majority of injuries encountered by figure skaters involve the knee or foot and ankle. A survey of the overall complaints of patients seen in our sports medicine clinic who were figure skaters or ice dancers between 1981 and 1990 revealed that of 175 skating injuries, 14 were back injuries (Table 53-1). Several of these were acute traumatic injuries and were diagnosed most often as back strain. Seven injuries occurred to the hip and pelvis, and included in this group were traumatic injuries to the base of the buttocks and sacrum; such injuries can be acutely painful, and on one occasion the skater was eliminated from training competitions for over a month. These injuries were diagnosed as buttock contusions and sacrococcygeal strains.

While back injuries accounted for only 8% of the skating and ice dance injuries, they had a relatively higher level of severity, often seriously limiting performance and at times resulting in the ending of a promising career.

As with most sports injuries, these injuries have been conveniently divided into acute traumatic injuries and overuse injuries. Certainly, the most common overuse injury to the lumbar spine encountered in young athletes is that of spondylolysis of posterior elements in overuse syndromes. This appeared to be the case in the skaters

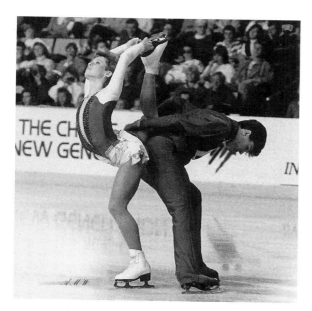

Fig. 53-8. Biellmann position used in a pair maneuver. The partner is a source of external force, which increases the hyperextension moment. With such posturing, a high level of program technical difficulty is achieved. (Courtesy Anna-May Walker.)

Table 53-1. Skating and Ice Dance Injuries, 1981 to 1990 (Sports Medicine Division, Children's Hospital, Boston)

	Number	%
Head/neck	4	2.3
Shoulder	6	3.4
Upper extremity (other)	4	2.3
Back	14	8.0
Discogenic	5	2.9
Posterior element/spondylolysis	7	4.0
Sprain	2	1.1
Hip/pelvis	7	4.0
Upper leg	5	2.8
Knee	77	44.0
Lower leg	15	8.6
Ankle/foot	43	24.6
TOTAL	175	100.0

seen in our clinic. Seven of these skaters had incapacitating spondylolysis and were ultimately treated with bracing and exercises to relieve these symptoms. Six of the seven were able to return to full skating and competition with no further symptoms.

A relatively high incidence of complaints of back pain, particularly in the girls, was found among a group of elite young skaters in 1985. Of the 33 girls in the study, 11 had scoliosis and 5 also complained of lower back pain. Only 1 of the 19 boys in the study complained of back pain.

Of greater significance, physical examination revealed that 5 skaters were noted to have very tight lumbodorsal fascia, 11 more were unable to reverse their lumbar lordosis on forward bending, and only 3 of the skaters examined demonstrated a normal range of motion of the lumbar spine in both flexion and extension.

These findings are consistent with observations of skating training and technique. A number of skating techniques demand sustained posturing into a lordotic alignment of the lumbar spine. In addition, there is little systematic attempt to ensure full range of motion and strength of the lumbar spine, pelvic, and hamstring areas in off-ice training techniques. As a result, many young skaters are at risk from techniques to combat this tendency. In our experience, many young skaters develop extension contractions of the lower back and tight hamstrings.

Studies of injuries in figure skating and ice dancing are relatively uncommon. Most studies have been site-specific, including specific studies of foot and ankle injuries, injuries of the patellofemoral mechanism and their association with relative muscle tightness, and overviews of injuries as a whole.

The figure skater who complains of back pain in association with training techniques and who describes an injury that appears to be of the overuse pattern type should be carefully assessed for the possibility of posterior element overuse. As with any complaint of back pain, careful and systematic history taking is important to determine the pattern of onset of pain, particularly in maneuvers that may exacerbate the pain, and any referral of pain.

ASSESSMENT AND TREATMENT

A thorough assessment is required in the case of a figure skater who complains of back pain in association with training techniques and who describes an injury that appears to be of the overuse pattern type. As with any complaint of back pain, a careful and systematic history will help determine the pattern of onset of pain. Of particular interest is the history before the onset of pain and the period between the onset of pain and the present appointment. Was there a single incident specifically remembered by the skater? If so, the skater should be asked to describe the incident in detail. Was there a change in training schedule? In the type of movements

practiced? In intensity? In duration? Which movements hurt the most? Which hurt the least? Skaters can be asked to list major movements in the order of the degree of pain felt, or list the movements in their competitive programs and assign a pain score. When combined with a recent history, a careful comparison of pain-free movements with painful movements can help determine the cause and type of injury and focus the physical examination. Depending on the skater's category, a separate history on jumps, lifts, or throws can be valuable. Efforts expended on performing lifts, throws, and posturing are sensitive to the location of the body's center of mass, which is affected by changes in the body/trunk ratio and weight increases.

A physical examination includes an assessment of posture, range of motion, strength, leg length, psychosocial aspects, and functional aspects, both on and off the ice. A postural analysis in the sagittal plane will identify poor alignment; the line should fall from the tip of the ear, through the tip of the shoulder, through the greater trochanter, behind the axis of the knee, and through the midfoot. The pelvis should be in neutral position; an anterior tilt of the pelvis or a lordotic posture can be easily seen. Determining the range of motion of the trunk, the lower extremities, and the shoulders and elbows of the upper extremities is necessary to establish treatment programs and to monitor progress. At a minimum, a skater should be able to assume the long sitting position with the pelvis level, a hip angle of 90 degrees, and the ankles at neutral. Forward flexion of the spine should show an even curve of the spine forward, and all spinous processes should be easily palpated, particularly in the lumbar spine. From the right-angle sitting posture to the forward-flexed position, an excursion of approximately 2½ to 3 inches can be measured. Trunk rotation, with the pelvis held in position, is 180 degrees. Trunk rotations and lateral bends should also be symmetric. Straight leg raising of 90 degrees should be easily achieved, as well as negative Thomas, Ober, and Ely test results. The Achilles tendon should be at an angle of at least 90 degrees, if not 100 degrees. At the shoulder, full abduction combined with extension is necessary for pair skaters, ice dancers, and precision team skaters.

Strength tests of the trunk, hip, and shoulder musculature are not possible with significant back pain or complaint. Asymmetry of abdominal contraction and observation of muscle atrophy should be noted. Weakness of musculature in the lower extremities and descriptions of sensory changes should be noted.

Discrepancy in real leg length does not represent a problem to the skater on ice. An apparent leg length discrepancy, as a sign of asymmetry, however, could predispose a skater to injury.

Imaging techniques can be helpful in establishing the diagnosis. New techniques of SPECT bone scanning to rule out the possibility of overuse posterior element stress fracture or spondylolysis, as well as magnetic resonance imaging (MRI) to determine discogenic components of pain, are helpful.

Once the diagnosis has been established, every attempt is made to begin a treatment program that will allow the injured tissues to heal and yet, at the same time, allow the skater to continue conditioning and training.

If a skater is diagnosed as having spondylolysis stress fracture of the lumbar spine, we usually institute a program of antilordotic bracing and specific exercises to reverse these components. We do however, allow the skater to continue skating while under treatment for this condition. Skaters are allowed to do figures and simple techniques that do not involve jumping or hyperextension of the spine in the brace. Once skaters become totally asymptomatic, they are allowed short periods of training out of the brace. But, again, any technique that has a potential for hyperextending the spine or increasing the load on the posterior elements is not allowed for 6 months. The skater is generally treated with a program of bracing 18 to 20 hours a day, the out-of-brace period being confined to technique training and relatively light training, while the aforementioned injuries or acute traumatic injuries to the back are avoided.

In our experience, injuries have been relatively less serious. We have had several cases of back strain that appeared to be associated with torsion and twisting rotational maneuvers to the spine. These patients have been treated with an operative period of rest and therapeutic modalities and techniques, and have been able to return to full training in 2 to 3 weeks.

Traumatic impact of the buttocks and sacrococcygeal joint due to falls on the ice has also been encountered.

This can be extremely painful to the skater and can sometimes result in loss of ice time. These patients are treated as having acute traumatic injuries, with initial periods of icing, relative rest, and, of course, a careful assessment to rule out the possibility of a specific injury. The skater is allowed to resume progressive activities as tolerated and in the range of comfort. Once again, it has been our experience that most skaters are able to return to the ice in 2 or 3 days, but in several instances, strains of the sacrococcygeal joint and contusions of the buttocks resulted in the skater's being off the ice for a period of 6 weeks.

The psychosocial aspects of figure skating and competition are many and need to be considered during the evaluation of an injury and the planned management of a skater with a spinal injury. Jumping is the major athletic component, and the spine is an essential element in the style, line, and successful landing.

PREVENTION OF INJURY

Correction of the overuse injuries to the posterior elements of the lumbar spine would appear to be readily addressed with programs of off-ice training, specifically those that include antilordotic and flexibility exercises to build abdominal strengthening. Attention to abdominal strengthening should be part of every office program for skaters, in addition to programs of flexibility of the hip flexors, hip adductors, iliotibial band, and hamstrings.

For the younger skater, special protective equipment is available with pads in the gluteal regions, which will minimize or decrease the possibility of traumatic sacrococcygeal or gluteal injuries in this age group in particular. These have been used effectively in the past with a number of skaters.

Chapter Fifty-Four

Wrestling

Thomas C. Tolli

Spinal injuries are common among wrestlers.[13] Fortunately many of these injuries are sprains or strains and rarely are fatal or cause permanent paralysis.* Few studies evaluating spinal injuries in wrestlers are available. However, the increasing popularity of the sport makes it essential for coaches, trainers, and team physicians to have a thorough understanding of these problems.

The three types of competitive wrestling are international freestyle, intercollegiate freestyle, and international Greco-Roman. International freestyle is the style used in Olympic and World Cup competition. The contest consists of three rounds each that are 3 minutes in length with 1-minute rest periods between rounds. The rounds begin with both wrestlers on their feet. Holds on any body part are permitted, with points scored for takedowns, back points, and pins. No points are awarded for escapes or for dominating an opponent (riding time).

Intercollegiate freestyle was developed from the Lancashire style of wrestling in England and is practiced in American high school and collegiate competition. The competition consists of three rounds, with the first lasting 3 minutes and the second and third rounds each 2 minutes in length. There are no rest periods between rounds. The last two rounds begin with one wrestler in a position of advantage. This style is similar to international freestyle, but points are allowed for escapes and riding time. Thus mat wrestling is more commonly encountered in intercollegiate freestyle wrestling. International Greco-Roman wrestling, which began more than 100 years ago in France, has no relationship to classic Greek or Roman wrestling.[11] The lower extremities cannot be used to trip or hold the opponent, and no holds below the waist are allowed. Thus the upper body is more involved, and throws are more often utilized.

EPIDEMIOLOGY

A review of collegiate wrestling injuries revealed that the shoulders, knees, and spine are commonly injured (Table 54-1). Studies evaluating high school and Olympic wrestlers yielded slightly different results. Regua and Garrick[9] studied 231 high school wrestlers over a 2-year period and found that spinal injuries were the most frequently reported. Of all injuries reported in this study, 34% were to the spine. Upper and lower extremity

injuries accounted for 29% and 33%, respectively. Estwanik et al.[5] studied the most highly skilled wrestlers at the 1976 Olympic trials and evaluated two different tournaments employing the international freestyle and Greco-Roman style of wrestling. The international freestyle competition involved 313 wrestlers and resulted in 83 injuries. Spinal problems accounted for 14.5% of all injuries, with the neck (10.8%) being more commonly injured than the lower back (3.6%).

The Greco-Roman competition involved 146 participants and only 17 injuries. Spinal injuries occurred frequently and were reported in 17.6% of all injuries. Surprisingly, neck injuries (5.8%) were less common than lower back injuries (11.7%).

Although it is obvious that spinal injuries are common among wrestlers, these studies indicate that more experienced and more skilled wrestlers suffered fewer injuries to the spine. This is evident when high school wrestlers are compared with collegiate or Olympic athletes.[4,9]

Although the frequency of spinal injuries remains fairly consistent, the degree of severity is highly variable. Sprains and strains to the neck and lower back are most common; however, catastrophic injuries and fatalities have been reported.[1,8,15] Less commonly, temporary nerve root injury from traction or compression of the neck may also occur.[5,14] Spinal concussion resulting in transient quadriparesis, as well as cervical fracture dislocation, has also been reported.[12,15] Fortunately, the more severely debilitating injuries occur infrequently.

CERVICAL SPINE INJURIES

Studies published in the 1980s indicate that cervical sprains and strains account for 46% to 87.5% of all neck injuries.[5,9,10,12,14] Neurogenic pain syndrome (pinched nerves, "stingers") caused by traction or compression of the neck have been reported in 21% to 44% of all neck injuries.[5,8,10,14]

Wroble and Albright[14] found that injuries resulting from neurogenic pain syndromes resulted in an average of 17.9 days lost from wrestling. In contrast, wrestlers with sprains or strains missed an average of only 6.3 days. Overall, the average time lost from all neck injuries was 10.7 days. In addition, 25% of wrestlers lost no time from competition, and 38% were absent for 7 or more days. Wroble and Albright,[14] as well as other investigators,[2,3] also discovered that a wrestler with a previous neck injury had a 50% chance of recurrence, whereas a

* References 4, 5, 7, 9, 10, 12, 14.

Table 54-1. Percentage of Injuries by Body Location in Collegiate Wrestling

Reference	No. of Players	No. of Injuries	Knee (%)	Neck (%)	Shoulder (%)	Back (%)	Head and Face (%)	Hand and Arm (%)	Other (%)
Wroble and Albright[14]	464	866	24	12	12	5	11	5	31
Kersey and Rowan[7]	353	110	20		12.7		36.4*	8.2	22.7
Roy[10]	115	276	15.2	10.1	12.7	4.7	18	13.4	25.9
Snook[12]	129	901	20	5.5	17.7	3.3	8.8	13.3	31.4

*Indicates head, face, and neck injuries.

previously uninjured athlete risked only a 20% chance of injury.

LOWER BACK INJURIES

Sprains and strains are common injuries and in some studies were responsible for 50% to 100% of all back problems.[5,12,14] In contrast, stress fractures and herniated nucleus pulposus are rarely encountered.[5,12,14] Wroble and Albright[14] found that wrestlers lost an average of 5.3 days of competition as a result of lower back injury. Sprains and strains resulted in an average loss of only 3.8 days. These researchers concluded that recurrent sprains and strains were a concern but were less common than recurrent neck injuries. Overall, a wrestler had an 8% chance of sustaining a back injury and a 30% chance of having at least one recurrence.[14]

MECHANISM OF INJURY

Takedowns have been associated with a high injury rate.[4,9] The review by Regua and Garrick[9] showed that 50% of all injuries occurred during takedowns. Forcing the neck into hyperextension to block or attempt a takedown may lead to neck injuries.

Forced lateral deviation may lead to neurologic injury with compression on the ipsilateral side and traction on the contralateral side (Fig. 54-1). Hyperflexion can result in compression fractures, disc lesions, and fracture dislocations, as well as C1-2 ligamentous injuries. There are multiple mechanisms of injury for the low back. Low back extension along with forceful torsion may also contribute to injury. Forceful extension against resistance, as occurs when a wrestler attempts to lift an opponent off the mat, also places the lower back at risk for injury (Fig. 54-2). Although these events may lead to an acute injury, repetitive trauma may cause a significant degree of disability.

The rate of injury may be related to fatigue. Kersey and Rowan[7] of Oregon State University showed that the injury rate increased with each period. Of 110 injuries 52% occurred in the final period. Injuries reported in the first and second periods accounted for 19% and 28%, respectively. On the other hand, Estwanik, Bergfeld, and Canty,[4] did not find fatigue to be a factor in the injury rate among Olympic wrestlers.

The most severe injuries reported were a result of illegal body slams or throws to the mat (Fig. 54-3). Roy[10] reported two severe injuries that resulted from illegal slams. Neither athlete suffered permanent neurologic loss; however, both required several weeks to fully recover. Wu, Wo, and Lewis[15] described three high school wrestlers who suffered injuries caused by illegal holds and throws. In a nonregulation match one wrestler was injured by an unacceptable hold, the full Nelson. The other two athletes were engaged in regulation matches and were illegally thrown. The first wrestler suffered a fracture dislocation at the C5-6 level, whereas the second had a fracture dislocation at the C3-4 level.

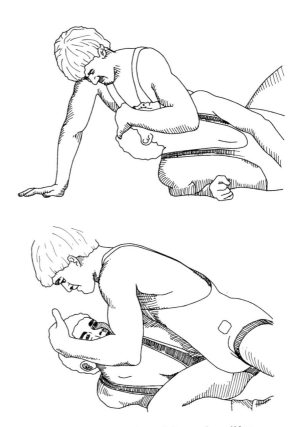

Fig. 54-1. Wrestler *(on top)* applying a face lift to opponent. Excessive force by first wrestler's left arm may result in hyperextension and hyperlateral flexion of opponent's neck. Nerve traction or compression injuries may result.

Thus the most catastrophic injuries reported were a result of illegal holds or throws.[14,15]

TREATMENT

Treatment in the acute setting requires strict adherence to the "ABCs" of emergency medical care—airway, breathing, and circulation. Responsible personnel (coaches, trainers, physicians) should be familiar with appropriate methods used to move patients with suspected spinal injuries.[3] Such techniques should be practiced in a controlled setting until the maneuver is perfected. A complete history and physical examination are essential in establishing an accurate diagnosis. When neurologic deficits are present, special attention should be directed toward identifying the specific nerve root lesion. Thus a comprehensive understanding of neuroanatomy is indispensable.

Radiographic evaluation should include plain roentgenograms in both the anteroposterior and lateral projections. Lateral views in flexion and extension are useful for identifying spinal instability. Bone scans are recommended when pain persists and plain roentgenograms show normal findings. A positive bone scan finding indicates a possible stress fracture, pars defect, or acute spondylosis and should be followed by computerized tomography scans for further evaluation of the bony structures. Soft tissue injury may exist despite negative bone scan results. Therefore a magnetic resonance imaging study should precede a normal bone scan to eliminate the possibility of a soft tissue (disc or ligamentous) injury. It is important to remember that the spinal radiographs of many uninjured wrestlers show abnormal findings. Thus radiographic abnormalities are considered pertinent only when they correlate with appropriate clinical signs and symptoms.

Treatment at the mat side requires caution. Any wrestler complaining of neck pain or showing any neurologic deficit should be removed from competition. At the mat side, one should be able to make arrangements for appropriate management and transport of a patient with a spinal injury. The responsible person delivering medical care should be able to evaluate the range of motion, as well as neurologic involvement. A wrestler with any neurologic involvement should not return to competition unless all deficits have resolved, and then only if the patient has full range of motion without neck pain. For example, a wrestler who has an episode of a stinger can return to competition if all symptoms and deficits have resolved and if the neck range of motion is full. However, wrestlers who continue to have dysesthesias or show a deficit should not return to competition. Even after resolution of these problems, the wrestler should not compete as long as range of

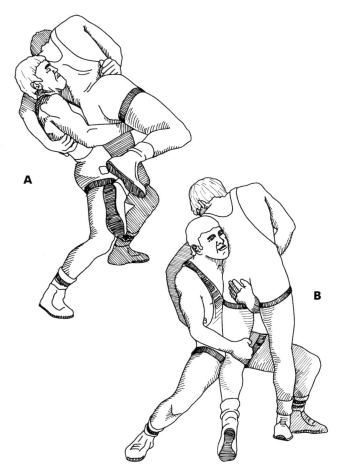

Fig. 54-2. A, Improper lifting may result in low back injury. Proper lifting involves squeezing with the arms and lifting with the hips. Pulling up with the arms puts severe stress on an extended lumbar spine and may result in a looser hold and potential back injury. **B,** Wrestler *(at left)* demonstrates proper techniques by keeping his arms low and tight on the waist and using his hips to produce lifting power.

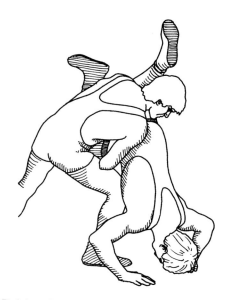

Fig. 54-3. Driving the opponent's head and shoulder into the mat may result in devastating injuries. Wrestler *(at left)* throws opponent to the mat. Had opponent not absorbed the force of the throw with his arms, a serious injury might have resulted.

motion is limited. Wrestlers should be discouraged from competition if they have recurrent episodes involving stingers or other neurologic injuries. Reinjury or further neurologic damage may result from a premature return to competition. Determining when an athlete may return to a sport after an episode of transient quadriparesis continues to be an area of controversy. A wrestler who suffers one episode of quadriparesis because of spinal cord concussion may return to competition if all symptoms resolve. However, a wrestler who has two or more episodes of transient quadriparesis is prohibited from further participation in contact sports.

A spinal injury without neurologic deficit also requires very close attention at the scene. Athletes with limited range of motion or pain that persists should be considered to have sustained a fracture until proved otherwise.

PREVENTION OF INJURY

Injury prevention should begin with proper physical conditioning inasmuch as fatigue may have a role in wrestling injuries. A specific trunk stabilization program with an emphasis on balance and coordination should be included in the training routine. Back and neck exercises that emphasize positions of extreme flexion or extension

should be avoided, and efforts should be concentrated more on isomeric muscle strengthening rather than on heavy isotonic exercises. In general, strengthening of the shoulders and the trapezius and latissimus dorsi muscles enhances neck and back stability. Deadlifts with extreme weight, which place excessive stress on the lower back, should be avoided. Instead, strengthening should be directed toward the buttocks and thighs. Barbell squats with use of proper techniques or the safety bar[6] place more emphasis on the buttocks and thighs and less stress on the lower back. Partial deadlifts with use of power racks are effective and may result in fewer injuries to the lower back.

Rules that prohibit illegal throws and holds should be strictly enforced. Severe penalties, including immediate disqualification and team penalization, may improve rule compliance. Proper coaching is essential to avoid injuries and prolong a wrestler's career. Power techniques should emphasize the buttocks, thighs, and legs. Forceful hyperextension of the neck and back increases the risk of injury (Fig. 54-4) and should not be used as a routine wrestling maneuver. Such techniques should be rarely used and only in desperation to avoid a pin. Instead, emphasis should be placed on proper technique, which will minimize injuries, prolong the athlete's career, and produce a more highly skilled wrestler.

REFERENCES

1. Acikgoz B et al: Wrestling causing paraplegia, *Paraplegia* 28:265, 1990.
2. Albright JP et al: Head and neck injuries in college football: an eight year analysis, *Am J Sports Med* 13:147, 1985.
3. Andrish JT, Bergfeld JA, Romo L: A method of management of cervical injuries in football: a preliminary report, *Am J Sports Med* 5:89, 1977.
4. Estwanik JJ, Bergfeld J, Canty T: Report of injuries sustained during the United States Olympic wrestling trials, *Am J Sports Med* 6(6):145, 1978.
5. Estwanik JJ et al: Injuries in interscholastic wrestling, *Physician Sportsmed* 8(3):111, 1980.
6. Hatfield FC: Squats—a king of all exercises. In *Power—a scientific approach,* Chicago, 1989, Contemporary Books.
7. Kersey RD, Rowan L: Injury account during the 1980 NCAA wrestling championships, *Am J Sports Med* 11:147, 1983.
8. Mueller FO, Cantu RC: Catastrophic injuries and fatalities in high school and college sports, fall 1982–spring 1988, *Med Sci Sports Exerc* 22:737, 1990.
9. Regua R, Garrick JG: Injuries in interscholastic wrestling, *Physician Sportsmed* 9(4):44, 1981.
10. Roy SP: Intercollegiate wrestling injuries, *Physician Sportsmed* 7(11):83, 1979.
11. Sayenga D: Wrestling. In *Encyclopedia Britannica,* vol 19, Chicago, 1979, Macropedia.
12. Snook GA: Injuries in intercollegiate wrestling, *Am J Sports Med* 10(3):142, 1982.
13. Watkins RG: Neck injuries in football players, *Clin Sports Med* 5:215, 1986.
14. Wroble RR, Albright JP: Neck and low back injuries in wrestling, *Clin Sports Med* 5(2):295, 1986.
15. Wu WQ, Lewis RC: Injuries of the cervical spine in high school wrestling, *Surg Neurol* 23:143, 1985.

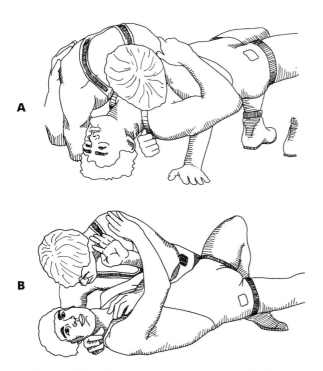

Fig. 54-4. A, Wrestler *(on bottom)* uses a head bridge to avoid getting pinned. Such a technique places extreme stress on the cervical spine. **B,** Wrestler *(on bottom)* eludes a pin by using an alternate maneuver, which places less stress on the neck. Wrestler brings his elbow in under opponent to clear opponent off of him. As wrestler turns off his back, he uses the hip-heist twisting of his hips to obtain a prone position, thereby avoiding a pin.

Chapter Fifty-Five

Boxing

Curtis W. Spencer III

The specialty of sports medicine has developed not only for the treatment of athletic injuries but for their prevention as well. Nowhere is this responsibility for prevention as pronounced as it is the world of boxing, the last of the gladiator, or "blood," sports. To win is to draw blood by battering the competition into submission. More than 330 deaths have occurred in the sport since 1945.[21] Brain damage, both acute and chronic, retinal detachment, facial lacerations, and skeletal injuries are an accepted part of the sport. Because of the serious nature of the injuries, the actual continuation of boxing as a sport at all is at stake. One camp demands a total ban on the sport[13,18]; the other believes that with modifications the sport can be made safe.[3] In between is the public itself, which fills the stadiums to watch the modern gladiators fight to the death.

SAFETY

The United States has dominated the world of professional boxing for the last century. In the last 50 years very few world champions in the various weight classifications have not been citizens of the United States. American boxers are aggressive: head blows receive the only points, and the knockout is the measure of achievement. In Europe, where some countries have actually banned the sport altogether, the trend has been to modify the rating system. Judges are now looking at the finesse of the boxer, giving points equally for body blows and trying to deemphasize the overall importance of the knockout. The Olympic games have adopted this model as well. However, it may prove difficult to gain popular support for this model in the United States. Boxing, with its roots in ancient history, including its Olympic heritage, has great worldwide appeal as it is played in this country. It is hoped that use of the sports medicine model to identify training techniques, conditioning patterns, and potential types of injuries can help shape a safer sport.[8]

Although no one can deny that boxing is a dangerous sport, there are actually few acute injuries outside of the widely publicized killings that occur in the ring. For example, acute injuries of the spine are almost unknown.[13] The reasons for this remain unclear. During training, boxers do little in the way of neck conditioning or strengthening of the axial muscles. Yet, there is little doubt that the forces delivered during a knockout blow should be able to produce deforming injury to the spine. Two possible conclusions can be drawn. One is that the

boxer's head-protecting instincts lessen the impact of those blows, thus reducing the actual force of impact. The second is that the cerebrum is more sensitive to knockout blows, so that the boxer is knocked out before his spine can be injured.

The number-one risk, outside of death, appears to be the insidious chronic neurologic problems that occur as a result of cumulative head blows. This trauma can progress even after the termination of the boxer's career.[20] Physicians have tried to control the incidence of neurologic deficit in several ways, including limiting the number of fights, modifying the equipment used, and screening fighters more closely for signs of neurologic damage.

Exposure to Blows

There is no ideal number of bouts a fighter can box before neurologic compromise occurs. Casson et al.[2] believe that after 25 fights boxers begin to show brain changes on electroencephalograms (EEGs) and computed tomography (CT) scans. They state that by the time 50 fights have occurred, the outward clinical signs of neurologic deterioration are beginning to show. Therefore, limiting the boxer's exposure in terms of number of bouts and time spent in the ring is suggested as a method of controlling the long-term sequelae of boxing. Although this approach is still controversial, it has been gaining the support of many state boxing commissions. Proposals to limit head strikes, as in the chest boxing currently practiced in The Netherlands, have been supported by many. The new Olympic rules of rewarding body strikes and head blows equally will most probably change the nature of the sport.

Equipment

Equipment changes may affect the nature of injuries. The use of head gear, as in amateur boxing, protects against cuts and eye injuries but probably does not diminish injuries to the brain.[8] Developing better head gear might prevent concussive forces to the brain. Lighter, softer gloves that decrease knockout power may be beneficial. However, some believe that the larger gloves provide a bigger shield and greater protection overall, thereby diminishing the chances of receiving any head blows.[7] It is obvious that as long as a knockout is the goal of the professional, then equipment that prevents knockouts is counterproductive. If improved head gear were introduced into professional boxing, as it has been in the amateur sports, perhaps injuries could be prevented.

Medical Supervision and Regulation

Uniform screening regulations and closer medical supervision are vital. In New York, which, along with California, Nevada, and New Jersey, dominates the sport, the Boxing Commission has strict regulations governing the issuance of professional fighting permits. Annual CT scans, EEGs, electrocardiograms, and dilated eye examinations are mandatory.[8] The New York Boxing Commission has granted medical examiners the complete authority to suspend a boxer if too many knockouts or consecutive losses have occurred, or if the boxer demonstrates poor boxing proficiency. The New York Boxing Commission has also empowered the ringside physician to terminate the fight at any time, giving him absolute and ultimate authority over the referee. Regulations such as these should be made universal.

The demands for a national boxing authority to monitor boxers is growing. This would be beneficial, especially in preventing boxers from jumping from one state to the next to avoid medical disqualification. The reciprocity among the states of California, New Jersey, and New York has been instrumental in achieving a national data bank for the professional pugilist.

HISTORICAL PERSPECTIVE

The first historical reference to boxing was in the Olympic games in 688 BC. The contestants fought barehanded in those matches, and the contest continued until one boxer was defeated. Eventually the Greeks developed leather thongs to protect the hands, and two centuries later a prefabricated leather device consistent with the modern glove became standard equipment. During the Roman Empire era, fighters wore leather gloves reinforced with lead and metal spikes, and boxing became a brutal sport until the dawn of the Christian era. During the rise of Christianity, the Romans banned boxing. It went into a decline until it was reintroduced into the seventeenth-century British Empire. Boxing's popularity rose during the early nineteenth century, leading to the start of the modern age of boxing begun in 1882, when John L. Sullivan defeated Paddy Ryan for the heavyweight championship. Boxing eventually became legal in the United States in 1896, when the New York legislature took action to regulate boxing. At present, boxing is legal throughout most of the world. Only the Scandinavian countries, Poland, Czechoslovakia, and Nicaragua have banned it.

EPIDEMIOLOGY

The exact number of fighters in the world is unknown, although the Amateur Athletic Union estimates that 65,000 participants are enrolled in their programs. *Ring* magazine claims 13,000 professional boxers in North America, with approximately 25,000 boxers worldwide.

The incidence of trauma obtained from multiple studies indicates that the panic associated with boxing's acute injuries may perhaps be unfounded. McCunney's reported estimates[17] reveal boxing to be somewhat safer than college football and motorcycle racing (Table 55-1). Estwanik, Boitano, and Ari[7] studied acute amateur boxing injuries in the 1981 and 1982 USA National Championships. All contestants were examined before and after each fight so that injuries sustained in each bout were isolated from other injuries. During these tournaments there were 547 bouts (1094 participants). There were 85 injuries of varying degrees of severity, with an overall rate of injury of 4.75% (Table 55-2). During these bouts only one injury occurred that was specifically related to the spine, and that injury was an acute lumbar strain.

Jordan and Campbell,[9] in a study of acute injuries among professional boxers in New York State, identified more than 376 injuries in 3110 rounds of boxing (Tables 55-3 and 55-4). Of these, 262 were head injuries, showing a frequency of 0.8 head injuries per 10 rounds fought. Permanent neurologic dysfunction was rarely noted in any of these boxers.

In the instructional boxing program at West Point Military Academy, approximately 7000 cadets sustained 315 injuries, of which 68 resulted in neurologic dysfunc-

Table 55-1. Fatality Rates of High-Risk Sports

Sport	No. of Deaths per Year	No. of Participants	Rate per 1000
Horse racing (jockeys and sulky drivers)	23	1,800	12.8
Sports parachuting	370	30,000	12.3
Hang gliding	169	30,000	5.6
Mountaineering	308	60,000	5.1
Scuba diving	1,100	1,000,000	1.1
Motorcycle racing	77	115,000	0.7
College football	11	40,000	0.3
Boxing	10	78,000	0.13

From McCunney RJ: *Physician Sportsmed* 12:57, 1984.

Table 55-2. Specific Injuries to Boxers at the 1981 and 1982 USA/ABF National Championships*

Injury	No.
Hand, Soft Tissue	**19**
Sprained thumb metacarpophalageal collateral ligament	7
Subungual hematoma	1
Contusion and/or sprained hand	10
Sprained wrist	1
Facial Lacerations	**14**
Sutured	14
Fractures	**7**
Nose	3
Ribs	1
Fifth metacarpal	2
Lunate	1
Miscellaneous	**4**
Knee effusion	1
Ankle sprain	1
Acromioclavicular sprain	1
Acute lumbar strain	1
Ear	**3**
Perforated tympanic membrane	2
Subperichondrial hematoma	1
Eye	**3**
Corneal abrasion	2
Subconjunctival hematoma	1
Mouth	**2**
Fractured teeth	2

From McCunney RJ: *Physician Sportsmed* 12:57, 1984.
*ABF, Amateur Boxing Federation.

tion.[12] Blondstein and Clarke[1] assessed boxing injuries in 3000 amateur boxers over a 7-month period and found that only 29 boxers sustained severe concussions or were knocked out more than once. Neurologic and EEG evaluations were normal in all.

McCown[16] studied acute injuries among professional boxers in New York State during the 1950s and observed 325 knockdowns and 789 technical knockouts among 11,173 participants. Only 10 of these boxers required hospitalization.

This summary of acute trauma is incomplete without mention of cervical spine injuries. The various cervical spine injuries that have been reported are noteworthy both in their low frequency and in their profound severity. Neck injuries are so rare that we must ask ourselves why. The force necessary to injure the spine is most likely greater than the knockout punch. The force transmitted by a punch is directly proportional to glove mass and velocity of the swing, and inversely proportional to the total mass, or size of the boxer opposing the punch.[19] The force, once generated, first concusses the brain with its direct blow and then concusses with a contrecoup in the rebound (Fig. 55-1). The brain absorbs the energy of the blow before enough energy is transmitted to the bony structures of the spine. Therefore the spine is usually spared a significant injury.

It is noted that a blow forceful enough in the axial or compressive manner to produce the classic Jefferson fracture (burst to the ring of the atlas) is rare. However, this fracture has been reported by Strano and Marais.[22]

Flexion injuries occur when a boxer falls on the back of his head or sustains a punch to the neck or upper chest. If forceful enough, a blow can rupture the transverse ligaments with a resultant atlantoaxial dislocation. This injury can present with tingling in the feet and occipital headaches. This type of injury probably occurs more frequently than has been diagnosed, but it is still quite rare. It is known that when the distance

Table 55-3. Acute Boxing Injuries per Year for 2 Years

	Aug 1982 to July 1983	Aug 1983 to July 1984	Mean
Total licensed boxers (906)	484	422	453
Total rounds fought (3110)	1,636	1,474	1,555
Total craniocerebral injuries (262)	138	124	131
Total other injuries (114)	53	61	57
Total injuries (376)	191	185	188
Head injuries per 10 boxers	2.9	2.9	2.9
Other injuries per 10 boxers	1.1	1.1	1.25
Total injuries per 10 boxers	4.0	4.3	4.15
Craniocerebral injuries per 10 rounds fought	0.8	0.8	0.8
Other injuries per 10 rounds fought	0.3	0.4	0.35
Total injuries per 10 rounds fought	1.1	1.2	1.15

From Jordan BD, Campbell E: *Physician Sportsmed* 16:88, 1988.

Table 55-4. Noncraniocerebral Boxing Injuries Over a 2-Year Period

Injury	No.
Facial lacerations	66
Hand	8
Eye	8
Abdomen	7
Orbital hematoma/contusion	5
Nose	5
Jaw	4
Exhaustion	3
Ribs	3
Ear	1
Shoulder	1
Testicle	1
Abrasion	1
Muscle strain	1
TOTAL	114

From Jordan BD, Campbell E: *Physician Sportsmed* 16:88, 1988.

between the odontoid and the anterior arch on a lateral x-ray film exceeds 4 mm, the supporting structures have probably failed. If the distance exceeds 7 mm, all ligamentous stability is suspect.[6] Because there is a moderate degree of normal anatomic variation in the atlantoodontoid distance, routine baseline cervical flexion/extension lateral films might be beneficial in screening professional boxers to detect occult instabilities and to provide baseline reference after injury.

Flexion and compression forces that are significant enough to produce the classic teardrop fracture have been reported only once. Although Kewalramani and Krause[11] could not prove the mechanism of the injury, the boxer in their report, injured at the C6 level, became quadriplegic. Flexion-rotation injuries that result in a broken or locked facet must be exceedingly rare because no injuries of this nature have been reported in the English literature.

Hyperextension injuries, which overwhelm the weaker anterior cervical muscles, may cause momentary tingling and numbness in the lower extremities, possibly

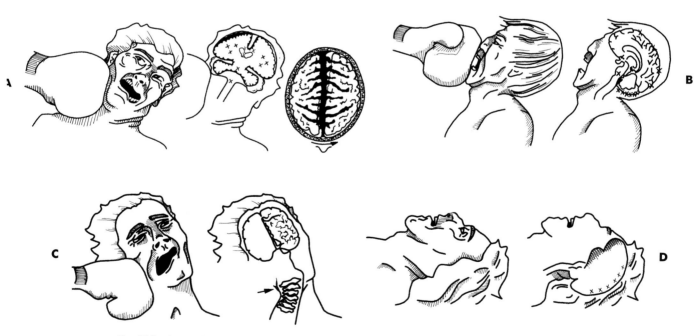

Fig. 55-1. Acute brain damage induced by the following. **A,** Rotational (angular) acceleration causes rotational movement of the brain resulting in a subdural hematoma by tears of stretched veins and diffuse axonal injury by damage to long fiber tracts in the white matter, corpus callosum, and brainstem. **B,** Linear acceleration of the head causes gliding contusions in parasagittal regions of the cerebral cortex, ischemic lesions in the cerebellum, and axonal damage in the brainstem. **C,** Injury to the carotid artery and compression of the carotid sinus cause generalized ischemia of the brain. **D,** Impact deceleration of the head by falls against the ropes or mat causes contrecoup lesions of the orbital surface of the frontal lobes and tips of the temporal lobes, as well as gliding contusions. (Redrawn from Lampeat PW, Hardman JM: *JAMA* 251:2676, 1984.)

a result of vertebral artery spasm or ischemia. Hyperextension of the neck can also result in laminar fractures, as reported by Jordan et al.[10] in a fighter who struck the posterior portion of his neck on the back of a ring rope.

It is the chronic injuries in boxing that are high in frequency and profoundly debilitating. The most common is the chronic brain injury or, as Martland[14] described it, "that punch drunk state." Roberts[20] evaluated 250 boxers randomly chosen from the professional ranks of the British Board of Control, and of these, 224 were examined. Of these, 37 boxers, or 17%, demonstrated evidence of central nervous system problems that could be attributed to their boxing career. The most predominant findings were those of cerebellar and extrapyramidal symptoms that could be directly linked to head blows. Mawdsley and Ferguson[15] evaluated 10 ex-boxers, all of whom had progressive neurologic deterioration, and Critchley[5] reported on 69 boxers who had various stages of chronic neurologic disease, including pronounced tremors and parkinsonian types of disorders. Corsellis, Brujon, and Freeman-Browne[4] determined that chronic brain injury had a pathologic basis, with a loss of tissue in the substantia nigra, as well as septal and hypothalamic abnormalities, that would account for the parkinsonian and ataxic disequilibrium.

PHYSICAL EVALUATION OF BOXERS

The physical evaluation of the boxer consists of a routine medical evaluation plus a detailed neurologic examination. The physician must be able to evaluate the fighter in the prefight, intrafight, and postfight periods.

The neurologic examination must test the routine functions of cranial nerves, strength, reflexes, and coordination. However, the mental status is an important component of the fighter's overall well-being. This component must be tested quickly because it is instrumental in the intrafight evaluation, and it must be approached at the fighter's educational level and in his native language.

Any fighter with an abnormal finding on the prefight examination needs an in-depth diagnostic work-up. During the fight the physician must be alert for signs of deteriorating coordination, observing also as the fighter returns to his corner. Any signs of incoordination, altered mental status, or spinal injury should alert the physician to terminate the bout.

TREATMENT

With all acute spinal injuries, immediate immobilization of the involved area is necessary for safe transfer to a medical facility. Resuscitation equipment should be available at ringside at all fights. This is especially important because subdural hematoma is the most common acute structural neurologic lesion in boxing. Subdural hematoma requires immediate intravenous administration of mannitol and hyperventilation of the injured boxer. Transfer to a medical facility should follow immediately. All boxers with acute nonstructural injury to the central nervous system (i.e., amnesia or concussion) should be medically suspended and observed. They should be brought back to boxing slowly. Any spinal injury of magnitude will end a boxer's career, and rehabilitation to his sport is moot.

REFERENCES

1. Blondstein JL, Clarke E: Further observations on the medical aspects of amateur boxing, *Br Med J* 1:362, 1957.
2. Casson IR et al: Neurological and CT evaluation of knockout boxers, *J Neurol Neurosurg Psychiatry* 45:170, 1982.
3. Committee on Medical Aspects of Sports: Statement on boxing, *JAMA* 181:158, 1962.
4. Corsellis JAN, Brujon CJ, Freeman-Browne D: The aftermath of boxing, *Psychol Med* 3:270, 1973.
5. Critchley M: Medical aspects of boxing, particularly from a neurological standpoint, *Br Med J* 1:357, 1957.
6. Dvorak J, Panjabe MM: Functional anatomy of the atlas ligament, *Spine* 12:183, 1987.
7. Estwanik JJ, Boitano M, Ari N: Amateur boxing injuries at the 1981 and 1982 USA/ABF National Championships, *Physician Sportsmed* 12:123, 1984.
8. Jordan BD: Medical and safety reform in boxing, *J Natl Med Assoc* 80:407, 1988.
9. Jordan BD, Campbell E: Acute boxing injuries among professional boxers in New York State: a two year survey, *Physician Sportsmed* 16:87, 1988.
10. Jordan BD et al: Brain contusion and cervical fracture in a professional boxer, *Physician Sportsmed* 16:85, 1988.
11. Kewalramani LS, Krauss JF: Cervical spine injuries resulting from collision sports, *Int Med Soc Paraplegia* 19:303, 1981.
12. Legwold G: Few head injuries found in Academy boxing study, *Physician Sportsmed* 10:43, 1982.
13. Lundberg GD: Boxing should be banned in civilized countries—round 3, *JAMA* 266:2483, 1986.
14. Martland HS: Punch drunk, *JAMA* 91:1103, 1928.
15. Mawdsley C, Ferguson FR: Neurological disease in boxers, *Lancet* 2:795, 1963.
16. McCown IA: Boxing injuries, *Am J Surg* 98:509, 1959.
17. McCunney RJ: Brain injuries in boxers, *Physician Sportsmed* 12:53, 1984.
18. Morrison RG: Medical and public health aspects of boxing, *JAMA* 255:2475, 1986.
19. Parkinson D: The biomechanics of concussion, *Clin Neurosurg* 29:131, 1982.
20. Roberts AH: *Brain damage in boxers,* London, 1969, Pitman Medical Scientific Publishing.
21. Rogers T: Canadian boxer dies after fight injury, *New York Times,* July 8, 1980.
22. Strano SD, Marais AD: Cervical spine fracture in a boxer—a rare but important sporting injury: a case report, *S Afr Med J* 63:328, 1983.
23. Unterharnscheidt F: About boxing: review of historical and medical aspects, *Tex Ref Biol Med* 28:421, 1970.

Chapter Fifty-Six

Rugby

David Jaffray

Rugby football, both Union and League forms, is a game played mainly in Britain, Ireland, France, and many countries of the old British Commonwealth, although its popularity is spreading quickly to other countries, especially after the advent of the World Cup trophy. Rugby Union traditionally has been an amateur sport, and it still is, although the degree of commitment now demanded of the players makes it as physically challenging as most professional contact sports. The speed of the game has increased as a result of recent changes in the rules of the game, and the size of the players is ever increasing. The players of even two decades ago begin to resemble midgets in comparison.

Rugby is a contact sport, and it is this contact, both static in scrums and dynamic in tackles and mauls, that predisposes players to injuries of the cervical spine in particular. The focus of this chapter is injury to the cervical spine, particularly quadriplegia. Broken legs may heal. Ligaments can be repaired. Quadriplegia is permanent and often regarded as a living death. It not only destroys the victim's life, it can drastically affect the lives of a player's immediate family. Whereas the person who becomes quadriplegic as a result of a vehicular accident usually finds economic salvation through the courts, the rugby player at the moment has no similar financial recourse. Some players may have the foresight to take out personal insurance, but this is not always the case. Perhaps in the future, laws will compel rugby clubs to adequately insure their players. At present in the United Kingdom quadriplegia as a result of a vehicular accident would attract an award between 1 and 2 million pounds. Amateur though rugby football may be, there is nothing amateur about the effects of quadriplegia.

INCIDENCE OF QUADRIPLEGIA

Cervical spine injury is not peculiar to rugby football, but in the United Kingdom, rugby is the main cause of cervical spine injuries, with equestrian sports a distant second.[7,12,13,23,25]

The true incidence of these injuries is not known because accurate recordkeeping has never been introduced or enforced. For example, the four cases of quadriplegia in Oswestry (Shropshire, England) during the 1991 season were not even known to the Rugby Football Union. Available statistics may not be reliable. Studies of small, well-defined groups of rugby players in Wales[28] suggested that there was no increase in the number of quadriplegics. However, other reports differ

and suggest an increase.[11] Canadian experience[22] supports my belief in the need for a reliable central register.

At the moment we rely on many anecdotal incidents rather than the true occurrence, and some of these anecdotes are horrific. For example, on one Saturday in 1979 in New Zealand there were four neck injuries on one day, which caused three cases of quadriplegia, two complete and one incomplete, and one death. For a country the size of New Zealand, such an incidence is incredible. During a 7-year period in the 1970s in New Zealand, 64 rugby players became quadriplegics. Silver,[20] in a survey of cervical cord injuries through rugby football in England and Wales between 1952 and 1982, documented 48 cases in the 30-year period. Of these, 21 injuries caused complete quadriplegia and 27 caused incomplete quadriplegia; thus in England and Wales during this period there was an average of one case of complete quadriplegia a year. In recent years in Oswestry there have been an average of two per year; in 1991 there were eight hospitalizations, four of which were for quadriplegia. In New Zealand in the 1970s for 3 years, more cases of quadriplegia in spinal injury units were caused by rugby football than by vehicular accidents. The incidence of neck injuries in New Zealand is again on the increase as the game has changed. Many authors in the past have stressed the need for central registers of quadriplegia. The establishment of such registers is achievable, but reluctance on the part of the governing bodies has been a deterrent. Although it may be possible to discover the true incidence of quadriplegia, it will never be possible to know the many near-misses that must exist.

TYPES AND CAUSES OF INJURY

It is always a flexion injury that causes quadriplegia. Such injuries can result from the scrum collapsing (Figs. 56-1 and 56-2); heads crashing together as the scrum forms[16] (Fig. 56-3); head-on tackles; the player charging with the neck flexed[15] (Fig. 56-4); or the player striking the ground in mauls or rucks (Fig. 56-5). Traditionally these injuries were confined to the front-row forwards and scrums, in which the players are locked together like dueling reindeer. When they collapse with the weight of their colleagues behind them, their necks are hyperflexed. This configuration used to be the main cause of injury until the laws were changed to modify scrums and, in particular, to prevent collapse of the front row. However, even before these law changes, many cases of quadriplegia were the result of injuries in rucks and mauls.

Now the injuries appear to occur more in the tackles than in the scrums. As the game speeds up and the weight of the players increases, the number of collisions at high speed, with players going in head first, will increase. These injuries, in my experience, are always soft tissue injuries. There are seldom any fractures. Those that do occur are inevitably at the C5-6 level and vary on x-ray film from a bifacet injury or a unifacet dislocation to the hidden injury described by Webb et al.[27] using data from Oswestry. The degree of disruption required to produce a bilateral dislocation is remarkable. All the soft tissue structures are ruptured (Fig. 56-6), including the anterior and posterior longitudinal

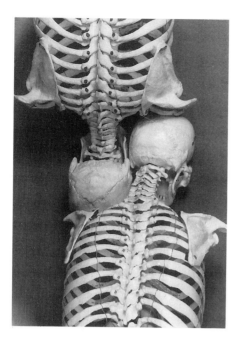

Fig. 56-1. Looking down on the position adopted by opposing forwards in a scrum.

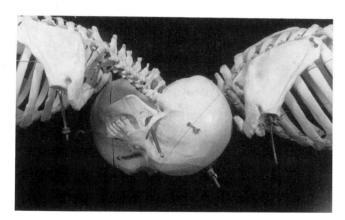

Fig. 56-2. Observation from the side makes it obvious that the neck is easily forced into flexion.

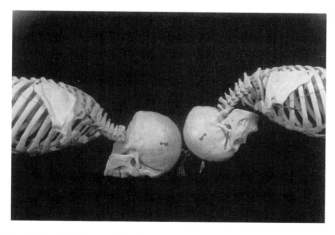

Fig. 56-3. Crashing of the heads together as the scrum forms or even during broken play.

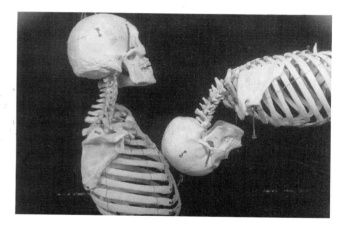

Fig. 56-4. Collision with the neck in a flexed position.

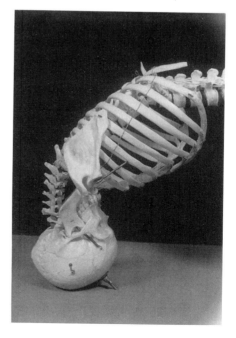

Fig. 56-5. The position adopted when a scrum collapses or a player is thrown to the ground (a "spear" tackle).

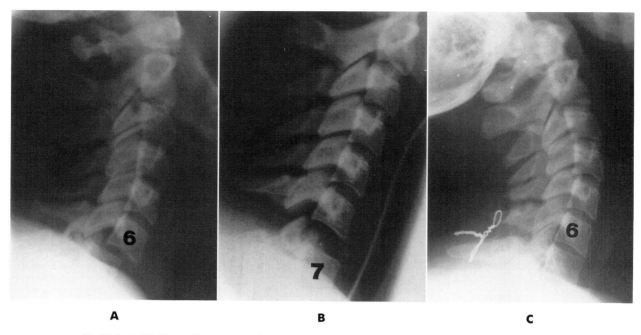

A   **B**   **C**

Fig. 56-6. A, Unifacet dislocation with no neurologic abnormality (not a rugby player). **B,** X-ray film taken with the patient under minimal traction and general anesthesia while other injuries were being treated. These neck injuries, whether unifacet or bifacet dislocations, result from complete soft tissue disruptions as shown here. **C,** The dislocation has been safely reduced and fused.

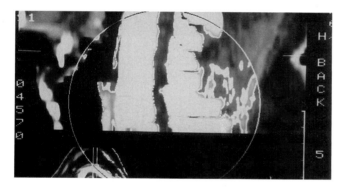

Fig. 56-7. CT scan of a rugby player with a spinal stenosis from previous injuries. He became quadriplegic from another injury (bifacet dislocation) at this level.

ligaments and the capsules of the facet joints, as well as the intraspinous ligaments.[14] Beatson[3] described the tissues required to produce such injuries in 1963. The spinal cord is invariably severed in bifacet and unifacet dislocations, although the player who is lucky enough to have a congenitally wide spinal canal may be spared. This is not common. Like American football players and soccer players, the rugby player can be a victim of repeated injuries that lead to spinal stenosis. Should the player with spinal stenosis suffer a facet dislocation, he is certain to be paralyzed (Fig. 56-7).

Acute disc prolapses[26] can result in the same mechanism of injury but would appear to be uncommon. Probably many such injuries resolve, but a few are treated by anterior discectomy and fusion. Unfortunately, many players return to the game after such surgery and have been encouraged to do so by clinicians. This may be suicidal because the neck is now even more prone to injury, just as in a congenital condition such as Klippel-Feil syndrome.[19] Bailes et al.[2] offer guidelines on who can return safely to sport. I prefer to play safe. Rugby players, especially front-row forwards, can suffer temporary paralysis through subluxation of the cervical spine. When asked to advise players that suffer such injuries, I have no hesitation in advising retirement from the game. One such player (see Fig. 56-7) did not heed this advice and became quadriplegic after another injury.

Chronic damage to the cervical spine probably occurs in rugby Union forwards just as in American football players and soccer players. Fortunately, this may prove to be more of a radiologic problem than a clinical problem. A review of the x-ray films of retired rugby forwards would probably prove quite rewarding. Repeated heading of the ball in soccer players has been noted to produce changes in the cervical spine.[10] As already mentioned, spinal stenosis can be a real hazard in active players, but probably in retired players it may well prove to be innocent.

TREATMENT

Those injuries that produce damage to the cervical cord are instant and irreversible.[1] A few injuries, such as those experienced by players with congenitally wide spinal canals, may not produce a neurologic condition, and it is vital that these patients receive appropriate first aid—that is, immobilization of the cervical spine with a collar and confinement of the player to a horizontal position. It would appear that such basic information would be commonsense knowledge, but in a recent international match between England and Scotland, one forward who had suffered temporary quadriplegia was assisted by attendants to walk off the field rather than being carried on a stretcher. The lack of familiarity with basic first aid for potential neck injuries in rugby is reinforced by a South African report.[8] At the moment it would appear that surgery has little to offer these patients apart from stabilization of these ligamentous injuries by fusion. Reversal of neurology is a long way off.

PREVENTION OF INJURY

Can these injuries be prevented? Not totally. These injuries are caused by the very factors that make the game attractive to watch: speed, contact, and size. There will always be cervical spine injuries in rugby Union football. They will inevitably increase as the game develops from an amateur sport to a highly competitive sport. They are more common in adolescence in those players whose bodies are immature but heavy (and perhaps they are less likely to think in an adult fashion). The abolition of scrums and the decrease of speed in the game in adolescence might be worth thinking about. Awareness of the dangers could perhaps be made more obvious to the players whose lives are particularly at risk, namely the front-row forwards. Widespread awareness of the effects of quadriplegia and the cost to society may encourage the players to take out the appropriate personal insurance. Changes in the laws of the game have reduced quadriplegia in American football by two thirds.[7] Heavy tackling by two opponents was responsible for two serious neck injuries in South Africa.[17] The recent World Cup competition illustrated the new trend of tackling opponents ferociously. Such behavior invites serious injury. High tackles, described in another South African report,[18] are equally dangerous.

Significant prevention of serious injuries could be effected by the modification of controllable behavior, about which there have been numerous warnings.[4-6,9,21,24,27]

REFERENCES

1. Bailes JE, Maroon JC: Management of cervical spine injuries in athletes, *Clin Sports Med* 8(1):43, 1989.
2. Bailes JE et al: Management of athletic injuries of the cervical spine and spinal cord, *Neurosurg* 29:491, 1991.
3. Beatson TR: Fractures and dislocations of the cervical spine, *J Bone Joint Surg* 45B:21, 1963.
4. Burry HC, Calcinai R: The need to make rugby safer, *Br Med J* 296:149, 1988.
5. Carvell JE et al: Rugby football injuries to the cervical spine, *Br Med J* 286:49, 1983.
6. Cervical spine injuries and rugby union, *Lancet* 1:1108, 1984.
7. Epidemiology, pathomechanics and prevention of athletic injuries to the cervical spine, *J Med Sci Sports Exerc* 17:295, 1985.
8. Glaun R et al: Are high schools adequately prepared to cope with serious rugby injuries? *S Afr Med J* 66:768, 1984.
9. Horan FT: Injuries to the cervical spine in schoolboys playing rugby football, *J Bone Joint Surg* 66B:470, 1984.
10. Kurosawa H, Yamanoi T, Yamakoshi K: Radiographic finds of degeneration in cervical spines of middle aged soccer players, *J Skeletal Radiol* 20:437, 1991.
11. McCoy GF et al: Injuries of the cervical spine in schoolboy rugby football, *J Bone Joint Surg* 66B:500, 1984.
12. Oh S: Cervical injury from skiing, *Int J Sports Med* 5:268, 1984.
13. Paley D, Gillespie R: Chronic repetitive unrecognized flexion injury of the cervical spine, *Am J Sports Med* 14:92, 1986.
14. Pullicino VC et al: Is uni-facetal dislocation of the cervical spine a stable injury? *Clin Radiol* (in press).
15. Scher AT: Vertex impact and cervical dislocation in rugby players, *S Afr Med J* 59:227, 1981.
16. Scher AT: "Crashing" the rugby scrum—an avoidable cause of cervical spinal injury, *S Afr Med J* 61:919, 1982 (case report).
17. Scher AT: The "double tackle"—another cause of serious cervical spinal injury in rugby players, *S Afr Med J* 64:595, 1983 (case report).
18. Scher AT: Rugby injuries of the upper cervical spine, *S Afr Med J* 64:456, 1983 (case report).
19. Scher AT: Cervical vertebral dislocation in a rugby player with congenital vertebral lesion, *Br J Sports Med* 24:167, 1990.
20. Silver JR: Injuries of the spine sustained in rugby, *Br Med J* 288:37, 1984.
21. Silver JR: *Injury* 19:298, 1988 (letter).
22. Sovio OM, Van Peteghem PK, Schweigel JF: Cervical spine injuries in rugby players, *Can Med Assoc J* 130:735, 1984.
23. Tator CH, Edmonds VE: National survey of spinal injuries in hockey players, *Can Med Assoc J* 130:875, 1984.
24. Taylor TK, Coolican MR: Rugby must be safer—preventative programmes and rule changes, *Med J Aust* 149(4):22, 1988.
25. Torg JS, Das M: Trampoline and minitrampoline injuries to the cervical spine, *Clin Sports Med* 4(1):45, 1985.
26. Tysvaer AT: Cervical disc herniation in a football player, *Br J Sports Med* 19:1, 1985.
27. Webb JK et al: Hidden flexion injury of the spine, *J Bone Joint Surg* 58B:322, 1976.
28. Williams P, McKibbin B: Unstable cervical spine injuries in rugby—a 20 year review, *Injury* 18:329, 1987.

Chapter Fifty-Seven

Rowing

Joel S. Saal
Timothy M. Hosea

Rowing has maintained a dedicated following in the United States since its initial introduction into intercollegiate athletics. As a sport for both teams and individuals, rowing is a physically demanding athletic challenge. The physiologic requirements of the rowing athlete include the highest levels of aerobic fitness and peak anaerobic power. Demands placed on the musculoskeletal system are also high. The intensity of rowing exercise and the rigors of rowing form generate repetitive stress to joint and connective tissues. Although little data are available that precisely define the rate of injuries that involve the spine, there is general concern among physicians and trainers caring for rowers about the inordinately high rate of low back injuries among competitive rowers. The biomechanics of rowing generate high levels of stress across the lumbar spine. The training demands of competitive rowing are also a source of injury to the lumbar spine and must be carefully evaluated in the injured rower.

Rehabilitation of the rowing athlete with a spinal injury involves careful consideration of training room and boat techniques. Repetitive loading is the primary cause of lumbar spine injuries, and because more time is spent in the training room than in competition, the importance of proper training room techniques should be emphasized. Modification of the methods to incorporate a spine-protective mechanism through coordinated muscular stabilization of the spine, combined with efficient delivery of force to the oar-water interface, can be accomplished with a systematic and specific rehabilitation approach.

HISTORICAL PERSPECTIVE

The first boat race probably occurred shortly after the second canoe or boat was built. Paddles were used for propulsion until sometime after 1000 BC when human beings discovered that an oar working against a fulcrum was more mechanically effective. Along with the oar came the discovery that greater efficiency in levering an oar through the water occurs when the rower is facing the stern. The seated position with a sliding seat was found to allow even greater force to be exerted against the oar.

The first intercollegiate boat race was held in 1829 between Oxford and Cambridge universities. The crews rowed more than 2¼ miles from Hamilton Lock to Henley Bridge as a trial of strength and skill. In the United States, boat racing began at the intercollegiate level in 1843 with the formation of the first boat club at Yale University. In 1852 Harvard and Yale universities began racing each other's six-man shells. It was not until the yearly race in 1876 that the eight-man shell with coxswain became the standard. Until this time, a fixed-seat stroke, in which the pull primarily used the backs and arms, had traditionally been used. Then a sliding seat and swivel oarlock were developed, which made it possible to harness the greater power of the legs for the stroke.

BASIC ROWING TECHNIQUES

Rowing involves maneuvering either one oar—sweep (Fig. 57-1)—or two—sculling (Fig. 57-2)—through the water for propulsion. Persons sculling or rowing are seated facing the stern of the shell on a seat that moves fore and aft on a set of tracks. Along with the swivel oarlocks, this seat increases the mechanical advantage and propulsion of the shell. The following sequence is the same for all rowing events from individual sculling to the eight-man shell.

The rowing stroke is divided into two events—catch and finish—and two phases—drive and recovery. The *catch* occurs with the placement of the oar into the water, initiating the *drive*. In the drive phase the shell is accelerated through the water. The drive is completed with the *finish,* when the oar is removed from the water. The *recovery* phase (or return) of the position of the next catch for the next stroke then occurs.

At the catch, the knees are flexed, the shoulders and elbows are extended, and the back is forward-flexed (Fig. 57-3). Movement at this time consists of lifting the hands and firming the lower back for the drive phase.

The drive phase is divided into three stages—the leg drive, the back swing into the bow, and the hands brought into the body. The linkage between the upper and lower back acts as a braced cantilever (Fig. 57-4). The drive phase involves aggressive knee and hip extension, as well as trunk and shoulder extension with scapular adduction and elbow flexion. It concludes by dropping the hands and dorsiflexing the wrists to flip (i.e., feather the oar and remove it from the water [Fig. 57-5]).

The recovery phase begins by moving the hands away from the body and flexing the knees and then sliding the seat and making a back swing into the stern to stretch the body for the next catch (Fig. 57-6). Elbow extension and

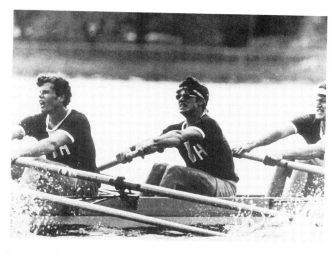

Fig. 57-1. Sweep oarsmen in middrive. Sweep rowing indicates one oar per person on either the port or starboard side of the shell. The sweep races are in two-, four-, or eight-man shells.

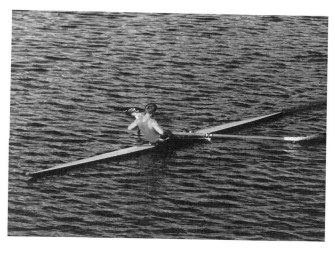

Fig. 57-2. Sculler at the finish. Sculling involves one oar for each hand, with oars used simultaneously.

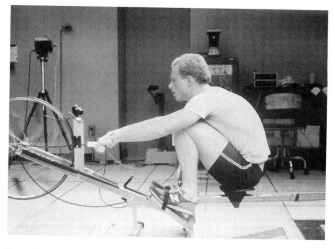

Fig. 57-3. Olympic sculler at the catch on a Concept II ergometer. The knees and back are flexed, with the elbows and shoulders extended.

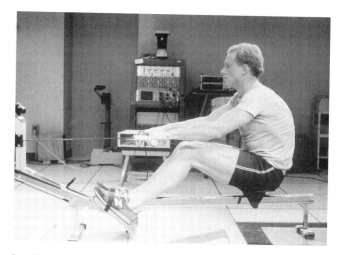

Fig. 57-4. During the drive phase, the knees are extended, with the back acting as a braced cantilever, transferring the leg drive through the shoulders and arms to the oar handle.

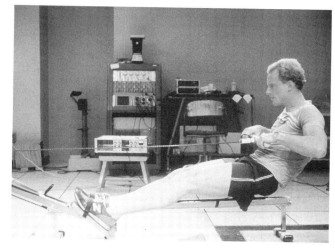

Fig. 57-5. At the finish, the elbows bend, bringing the oar handle into the body, while the knees essentially are fully extended. The seat stops at this point with the back extended.

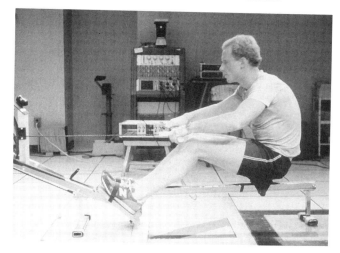

Fig. 57-6. The recovery phase is led by the hand moving away from the body, with the elbows extending and the back and knees flexing to resume the position at the catch.

scapular adduction promote the swing of the hands away from the body. Trunk, hip, and knee flexion all promote proper positioning for the catch.

EPIDEMIOLOGY

Only limited data are available specifying the rate of spinal injuries in competitive rowers. It is, however, the common experience of sports and spine physicians to see rowers with low back pain and a lesser number with thoracic pain. The lumbar spine is clearly at risk, from a biomechanical standpoint, in the rowing athlete. The requisite loaded lumbar flexion in the catch position theoretically delivers very high loads to the lower lumbar discs.

Howell[12] reported on the musculoskeletal profile of lightweight women rowers with musculoskeletal injuries. Measurement of the trunk and pelvic strength and flexibility demonstrated relative hyperflexion of the lumbar spine in the athletes with low back pain. A causal relationship was suggested, but not proved, in this study. This may reflect a higher incidence of hyperflexion as a physiologic requirement for an efficient rowing stroke. Idealized anthropometric profiles for elite women rowers were suggested by Hebbelinck et al.[9] on the basis of their analysis of anthropometric data from university student control subjects compared with Olympic rowers.

The physiologic profiles and the optimum state of cardiovascular and anaerobic fitness have also been studied in detail.[8] Roy et al.[14] attempted to isolate the cause of low back pain in varsity rowers by studying the electromyographic evidence of paraspinal surface characteristics. Spectral analysis of trunk muscle activity revealed a significant relationship between muscle asymmetry and fatigue, especially in those features that related to recovery. A clear difference was noted in the signal analysis of the port versus starboard rowers, allowing a blinded observer to correctly identify into which group the rower belonged. However, the relationship of these factors to the incidence of low back injuries has not been evaluated, and a clear direction toward the prevention of low back injuries in elite and collegiate oarsmen has not been achieved. The high perceived rate of low back injuries in elite rowers has raised concern in the physicians who care for the U.S. national team.[18] As in other groups of rowers, clear incidence data are lacking. A 2-year review we completed of a local National Collegiate Athletic Association (NCAA) division I female rowing class revealed 7 low back injuries, which included 6 disc herniations in a pool of 18 athletes.[11] Although this is a narrow sample in numbers and time period, the implication matches the experience of sports medicine and spine physicians who frequently treat rowing athletes.

PATTERNS/TYPES OF INJURIES

Because of the large increase in the number of intercollegiate rowing programs and the growing use of

rowing machines for physical fitness, the injury patterns of rowing need to be identified.

Hosea et al.[11] reviewed the incidence of various injuries to rowing athletes at two universities: Harvard and Rutgers. The medical records of every athletic injury are kept by the sports medicine staff of these two universities. This survey revealed 180 injuries to oarsmen and oarswomen over a 3-year period. At Harvard, 47% of male rowing participants and 62% of female rowing participants were injured. The knee was the most common injury site (29%), followed by the back (22%) (Fig. 57-7). The vast majority of injuries seen in this population of rowers were related to stress or overuse (Table 57-1). Rowing involves a continuous, repetitive motion during which stresses are continually increased or decreased, depending on the stroke phase. Off-water training also involves similar activities, such as weight lifting, running, stair running, cross country skiing, rowing in water tanks, and using a rowing ergometer. Such activities predispose participants to stress fractures, such as those noted in our rowing population, and to injuries involving the spine, ribs, femur, tibia, and fibula.

The association between rowing and stress fractures of the ribs has been described.[10] In our survey, eight rowers (five women and three men) had stress fractures that were confirmed by bone scan. Biomechanical analysis of rib stress fractures predicted that the highest bending stresses occurred at the posterolateral segments of the rib.[7] It is believed that the serratus anterior muscle is the major contributor to this bending stress across the rib and that the forces applied by this muscle, as well as the major and minor rhomboids, exert significant stress across the posterior aspect of the ribs.[7,10]

During the drive phase of the stroke, maximum forces are transmitted across the ribs as the muscles contract to transmit the power of the legs and torso through the arms to the oar. By using wire and surface electrodes, we

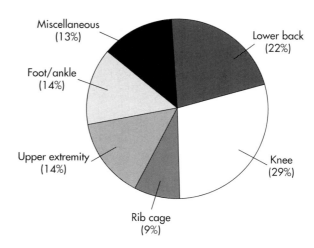

Fig. 57-7. Rowing injuries, 1983 to 1986, at Harvard and Rutgers universities.

have found that the serratus anterior muscle fires maximally at the catch. This activity continues through the drive phase of the stroke, with the muscle "turning off" at the finish through the recovery.

The rhomboids, the latissimus dorsi, and the erector spinal muscles at T4 and T7 activate just after the catch

Table 57-1. Crew Injury Survey of 180 Harvard University and Rutgers University Rowers

Site of Injury	No. of Injuries
Knee	**52**
Chondromalacia	22
Iliotibial band (ITB) syndrome	15
Patellar tendinitis	7
Meniscal tear	3
Pes bursitis	2
Hamstring tendinitis	2
Midclavicular line sprain	1
Back	**39**
Mechanical	29
Herniated nucleus pulposus	5
Spondylolysis	5
Rib Cage	**16**
Stress fracture	8
Costochondritis	4
Strain	3
Contusion	1
Upper Extremity	**25**
Extensor tensosynovitis	8
Shoulder impingement	4
Flexor sheath tenosynovitis	4
Biceps tendinitis (elbow)	3
Thumb sprain	2
Carpal tunnel syndrome	1
Acromioclavicular separation	1
Anterior shoulder dislocation	1
Olecranon bursitis	1
Foot/Ankle	**25**
Ankle sprains	12
Plantar fasciitis	3
Heel pain	3
Metatarsalgia	2
Peroneal tendinitis	2
Achilles tendinitis	1
Tarsal coalition	1
Clubfoot	1
Miscellaneous	**21**
Femur stress fracture	1
Greater trochanter bursitis	1
Shin splints	3
Hamstring strain	4
Fibular stress fracture	1
Plantaris rupture	1
Achilles tendinitis	1
Cervical strain	6
Quadriceps strain	3

Data from Hosea TM et al: Myoelectric and kinematic analysis of the lumbar spine while rowing, *Am J Sports Med* (in press).

and also continue to the finish[13] (Fig. 57-8). The oarsman or oarswoman thus experiences a forceful maximum muscle firing pattern starting at the catch and ending with the finish of the stroke. This on-and-off muscle pattern involving the ribs leads to a fatigue mode of loading.

Rib stress fractures generally occur during periods of intense training. They most often occur in intercollegiate populations after the holiday season and during early spring, just before the racing season when rowers are attempting to earn their seats in the boat by seat racing. The pain is generally sharp and stabbing and of sudden onset, usually occurring with rowing. The pain is discretely localized along the spinal aspect of the scapula to the midaxillary line. It is exacerbated during the drive phase. Because of the proximity of pain close to the spine, a lesion in the thoracic spine must be ruled out in these cases.

Diagnosis by bone scans, with increased uptake in the posterolateral aspect of a rib versus the thoracic spine as seen with an osteoid osteoma of the posterior elements, is diagnostic for rib stress fracture. Occasionally the stress fracture may appear acutely on x-ray examination.

Rib stress fractures generally heal within 6 to 8 weeks. In the meantime, athletes can utilize other modes of aerobic exercise, such as a bicycle ergometer. Running and jumping activities tend to accentuate the discomfort experienced by persons suffering from these fractures.

Low Back Pain

In our survey of intercollegiate oarsmen and oarswomen, low back pain was a common complaint. Howell's study of 17 elite lightweight oarswomen[12] revealed an 82.2% incidence of low back pain compared with a sex-matched incidence in the general population of 20% to 30%. According to Stallard,[17] "backache is suffered by almost all those in serious rowing training nowadays."

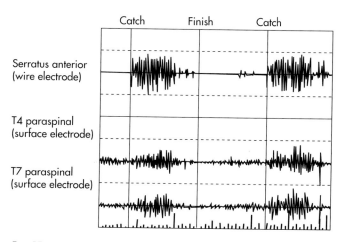

Fig. 57-8. Myoelectric activity of the serratus anterior and the thoracic paraspinal musculature during the rowing stroke.

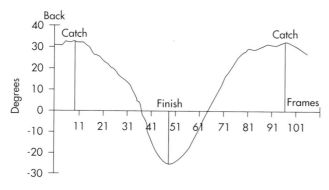

Fig. 57-9. Typical example of trunk motion during the rowing stroke, with approximately 30 degrees of flexion at the catch, a smooth transition to extension at the finish, and then return to the flexed position at the catch.

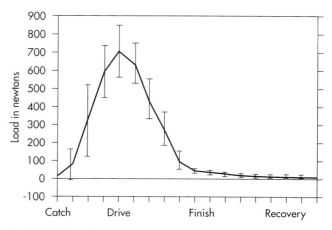

Fig. 57-10. The force at the oar measured with a strain gauge shows a rapid acceleration to a peak during the middrive phase, followed by a tapering to the finish.

Because of the high number of lower back injuries in this sport, a study was undertaken to identify the loads placed on the lumbar spine during rowing.[11] Seven elite rowers participated in this study—three men and four women who, among them, had competed in a total of 18 international and Olympic events. The men averaged 9 years of competitive rowing, the women 7½ years. All reported a history of low back pain that required complete cessation of all training activities for at least 1 week. Kinematic data were obtained with use of five infrared cameras arranged to allow stereoscopic visualization of all data points while the subjects rowed at a rate of 33 strokes per minute. The average power per stroke for each subject was calculated along with the resistance against the oar handle. Myoelectric data were obtained from eight major muscle groups by use of MCI surface electrodes. With mathematic equations derived from Cappozzo[4,5] and Schultz,[16] biomechanical analysis was performed to identify the loads at the L3-4 lumbar motion segment.

The men in this study generated an average of 8.7 W per stroke compared with 4.62 W per stroke for the women. For the men, the peak load at the oar was 850 N versus 616 N for the women. The data, normalized for body weight, indicated that the men pulled 16% harder than the women. The trunk moved from approximately 30 degrees of flexion at the catch to 28 degrees of extension at the finish. The men had a flexion angle of the trunk at the catch more forward than that of the females—34 degrees versus 27.5 degrees. Both populations finished with essentially the same amount of extension. A representative sample of the trunk flexion and extension through the rowing stroke is shown in Fig. 57-9.

PHYSIOLOGY AND MECHANISM OF INJURY
Loads on the Spine

At the catch, there is rapid generation of significant force at the oar. This force accelerates to a peak near the

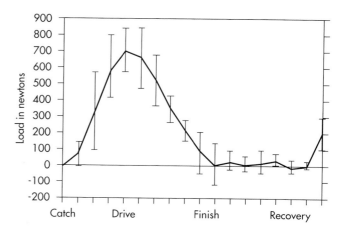

Fig. 57-11. The shear load on the lower back mirrors the load applied to the oar. With the acceleration of the knees and the back, the shear load peaks at middrive and tapers to the finish. There is minimal shear load on the lumbar spine during the recovery phase.

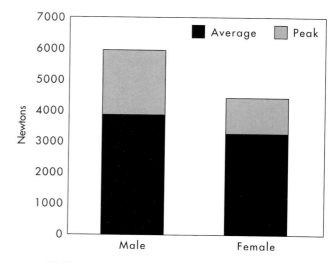

Fig. 57-12. Mean compression load at L4 while rowing.

middle of the drive phase and tapers to the finish. This pattern was seen in both men and women (Fig. 57-10). The anterior shear force at the L3-4 motion segment mirrors the resistance applied to the oar. With the significant load applied at the oar and the acceleration of the knees and back, the shear load peaks at middrive and then tapers to the finish (Fig. 57-11). Again, this same pattern was exhibited by male and female rowers. Peaks of anterior sheath at the L3-4 motion segment for the men were $848 + 133$ N and for the women, $717 + 69$ N. These are essentially the same when normalized for body weight.[11]

Compressive loads averaged 3919 N for the men and 3330 N for the women. The peak compression load occurs in the latter part of the drive phase as the upper torso extends over the lower back. At this point there was an average peak compressive load of $6066 + 186$ N for the men and $5031 + 694$ N for the females (Fig. 57-12). When normalized for body weight, the compressive loads for both sexes were nearly the same, with a peak of 7 times body weight for men and 6.85 times body weight for the women. On average, both groups were subjected to an average compressive load of 4.5 times body weight throughout the rowing stroke. The forces in the lateral bending plane while the rowers were sculling never reached a magnitude greater than 40 to 50 N in either direction. This probably is not the case in sweep rowing, however, in which there is lateral bending and twisting of the spine as the shoulders attempt to stay parallel to the oar.

Myoelectric Analysis

At the catch, the rectus femoris and thoracic paraspinal musculature fire nearly simultaneously as they initiate the drive phase. As the knees and hips begin to extend, the gluteus maximus and hamstrings fire, controlling the drive and stabilizing the pelvis. This muscular effort of the legs is transferred through the back to the oar. The back acts as a braced cantilever and provides an additional source of power by extending. This is demonstrated by the marked increase in L3 myoelectric activity shortly after the catch (Fig. 57-13).

The force generated by the legs and back is then transmitted to the oar through the shoulders, which are stabilized by the latissimus dorsi and serratus anterior muscles. With peak acceleration of the oar at midline, these muscles function maximally and in unison. During the latter part of the drive, the rectus femoris continues firing to keep the knees extended while the arms pull the oar into the body.

At the finish the aforementioned major muscle groups are essentially "off." The rectus abdominis fires to flex the trunk, and the arms push the oars back to the catch.[13] During the recovery there is little or no activity of the paraspinal musculature. The compressive load is balanced by the anterior musculature and posterior passive restraints. The medial hamstrings fire submaximally to

flex the knee, propelling the seat up the slide so that the rowing sequence can be repeated.

Our biomechanical analysis of the rowing stroke revealed the existence of significant loads in the lower lumbar spine. Similar to loads that produced pathologic changes in cadaver studies,[1-3] these loads can produce not only herniated nucleus pulposus but defects of the pars interarticularis (i.e., spondylolysis and spondylolisthesis).[6] All the etiologic factors that may produce low back pain must be kept in mind during the evaluation of an oarsman or an oarswoman with low back pain.

REHABILITATION OF INJURED ATHLETES

The unique mechanics of competitive rowing can place inordinately high stresses on the lumbar spine. The required training for the event and the competition itself present different physical risks to the lumbar spine and

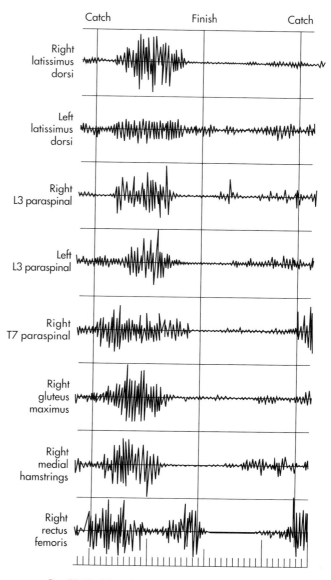

Fig. 57-13. Myoelectric activity while rowing.

therefore must be considered individually. The effort required by an individual rowing athlete is to equalize full-force, high-velocity passage of the oar through the water in synchronization with the other members of the rowing team. Although the rehabilitation methods have an underlying basic protocol designed for specific injury subsets, the injured athlete's physical strengths and limitations must first be assessed.

The initial step in rehabilitation is the establishment of an accurate diagnosis. Lumbar disc injury subsets are very frequently encountered in rowers, but the contribution of posterior element pathology and pain generation should not be overlooked. As a result of the forced attainment of a forward-flexed posture in sitting, the frequency of disc herniation and annulus tears in rowers appears to be quite high. These injuries may occur suddenly, during a competition or during training in the weight room. Frequently the athlete complains of pain over several days, which increases while he or she is sitting. The threshold for pain in rowing athletes may be elevated as a result of the extraordinary levels of aerobic challenge they endure. The higher levels of circulating endorphins may contribute to this phenomenon. The initial complaints of back pain and hamstring pain in the rower must be evaluated with a high degree of suspicion for a disc lesion, instead of the common assumption of back sprain or strain.

Early initiation of rehabilitation can prevent a more serious degree of injury, as well as limit the degree of deconditioning and injury time loss. A disc herniation is an easy diagnosis to establish in the presence of leg pain and the classic clinical features of sciatica. Appropriate clinical suspicion and adequate imaging studies can clearly establish the structural diagnosis. However, a primary complaint of low back pain, significant midline tenderness, and sitting intolerance suggests that a central small disc protrusion on imaging studies is indeed the pain generator. Persistent complaints of low back pain and sitting intolerance, with normal findings on

imaging studies, suggest an annulus tear that is not self-limited as the source of pain. This diagnosis of exclusion is frequently ascribed to a persistent lumbar sprain. This injury can be debilitating because of the characteristic limitation of tolerance to axial loading, especially in sitting. Whereas the conclusive diagnosis requires the use of discography, rehabilitation can be carried out on the basis of clinical diagnosis. Discography can be withheld while the option of surgery is contemplated.

Disc Injury Subsets

The unifying feature of the rehabilitation of disc injury subsets in rowers with low back pain is resolution of flexion loading. The combination of flexion and torsion loading is common in rowing technique. The essence of the rehabilitation program is to allow for an effective rowing stroke with limitation of the degree of flexion and torsion, combined with a muscle-protective mechanism to reduce shear forces during the executed rowing stroke. The method we have used to a high degree of success in athletes and nonathletes alike is the dynamic lumbar muscle stabilization program[15] (Figs. 57-14 to 57-19). The lumbar spine is considered to be supported by combined action of the abdominal oblique musculature and the latissimus dorsi muscles via their insertion to the thoracolumbar fascia. Co-contraction of these muscle groups, with the primary role for trunk extension placed on the gluteus group, shifts the point of rotation in the sagittal plane to the hips instead of repetitive flexion extension at the spine. In many sports it is possible to achieve this action purely through paying strict attention to details of the given physiognomy of the individual athlete. However, in rowing, there is an inherent and irrevocable degree of flexion/extension in the lumbar spine necessary to achieve efficiency and power in the stroke. Careful attention to strength and flexibility deficits in the injured rower, as well as substitution of latissimus power for a portion for the

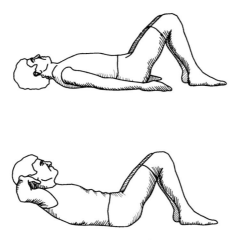

Fig. 57-14. Partial sit-ups.

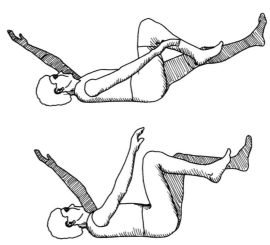

Fig. 57-15. Abdominal bracing with arms and unsupported legs.

spine-generated moment, can achieve a good clinical and functional outcome in many cases of lumbar disc herniation with radiculopathy, annulus tear, and disc protrusion without radiculopathy.

An important element to this dynamic posture control is the limitation of torsional forces commonly encountered by the rower. Starboard and port rowers face opposite but repetitive unidirectional torsional loading. The development of lateral or paracentral disc herniation opposite the side of pull of the stroke is not uncommonly seen in clinical practice. Adaptation to these forces with improved trunk strength, and especially with strength and coordination of the contralateral abdominal oblique and serratus anterior muscles, is important. Most of these patients do not need surgical treatment for these problems. The physical requirements of rowing are so great that even with a surgical

treatment plan, substantial rehabilitation is necessary. Pain control can be achieved quite effectively with the judicious and precise use of epidural corticosteroid injection. These types of measures can facilitate the exercise regimen and allow for much more effective rehabilitation. Even a small surgical procedure in this type of athlete can have extensive ramifications because of the demands of the sport. Surgery in these athletes may mean the end of their competitive career. Therefore aggressive rehabilitation, with careful attention to the individual athlete's strengths and weaknesses, is recommended before surgery is considered for the rowing athlete (Fig. 57-20).

Posterior Element Subsets

The degree of spinal extension that occurs at the completion of the rowing stroke can result in increased force placed on the posterior elements. There are no precise data on the prevalence or incidence of spondylolysis or spondylolisthesis in rowing athletes. In practice it appears that pars interarticularis fractures and abnormalities are not as frequently encountered in rowers as they are in gymnasts or football players. By nature of the rowing stroke, greater loads are placed in flexion (i.e., the position at the catch phase) than in extension. However, during the gym training and endurance activities used in preparation for rowing, the posterior elements can be placed at risk for injury. Weight-training methods can result in sudden excessive loads, causing

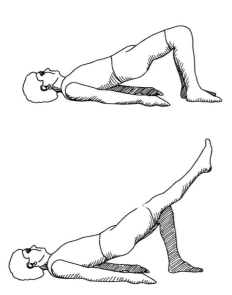

Fig. 57-16. Bridging with leg extension.

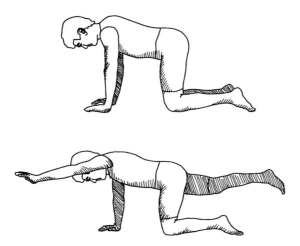

Fig. 57-17. Quadruped arm and leg raises.

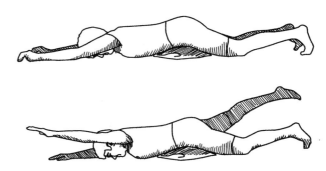

Fig. 57-18. Prone arm and leg lifts.

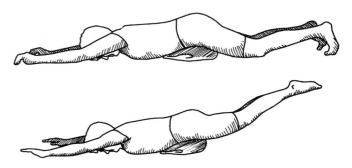

Fig. 57-19. Prone double–arm and leg lifts.

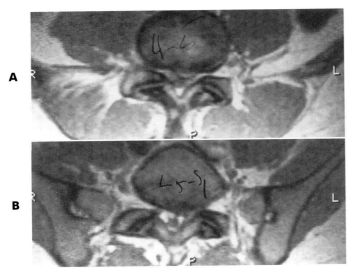

Fig. 57-20. A, MRI scan of the lumbar spine of an 18-year-old rower injured in division I finals, who reported increased leg and back pain in the sitting position. Treatment with dynamic lumbar stabilization training and a sport-specific program allowed for return to rowing competitively at 6 months from the time of injury. **B,** Broad-based herniated nucleus pulposus at left paracentral L5. An L4-5 focal protrusion is also demonstrated.

facet-mediated pain referral. The athlete with this injury complains of low back pain that may be unilateral or bilateral (i.e., increased while sitting and relieved somewhat while standing). In this instance rehabilitation exercises directed at a reduced lumbar lordosis while standing and training can be helpful. In situations that require further intervention, facet injection with corticosteroid and anesthetic can result in a successful

outcome and return the athlete to activity (Figs. 57-21 to 57-30).

Return to Training and Competition

After initial presentation following the injury, the athlete is evaluated by the athletic trainer, who may initiate acute pain control intervention. After evaluation by the consulting physician, a clinical diagnosis is established and a treatment and rehabilitation plan is designed and implemented. When reduction in pain level and increased functional capacity for training exercises are accomplished, return to competition and training guidelines must be instituted. In dealing with injured athletes, especially high-level athletes, it is important to specifically state the levels of progressive return to activity. When the athlete is feeling better, he or she will invariably ask about returning to the boat. Assessment of the competition schedule and delineation of realistic goals should be undertaken early in the course of treatment. The initial limitation of pain is usually not enough for return to activity. Completion of a program of back education, as well as an adequate skill and strength level in dynamic stabilization exercises, is necessary.

The initial return to activity consists of gym training and progressive running. Distance running tends to be less stressful on the spine than sprinting. Both types of training—aerobic and short and intermediate anaerobic—are necessary for rowers. Running at 75% pace is instituted, initially for ½ mile, then 1 to 2 miles. This is followed by an increase in pace to 100% over the same distance. Once this is achieved, sprints are begun at 50%, progressively increasing to maximum speed with some supervision of style. Return to training in the boat begins only after careful review of the adapted stroke on a

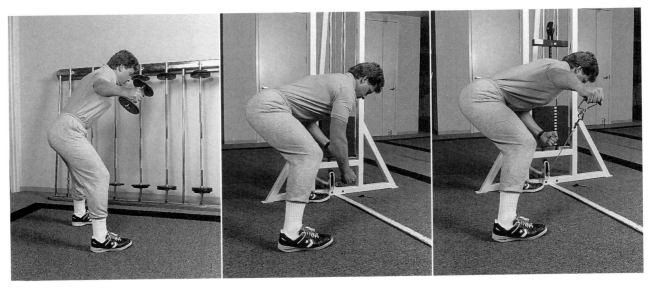

Fig. 57-21. Posterior deltoid raises.

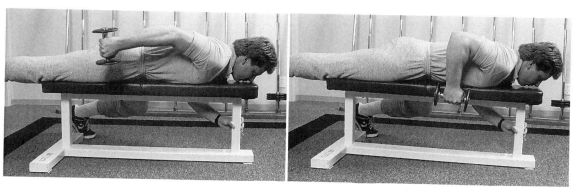

Fig. 57-22. Dumbbell extensions.

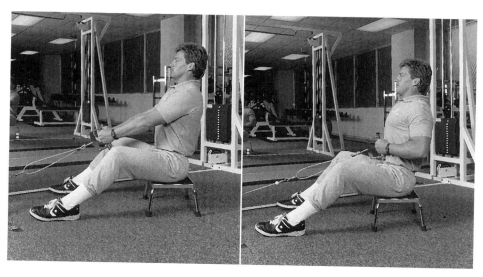

Fig. 57-23. Seated rowing.

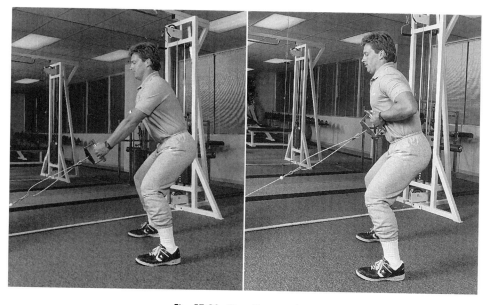

Fig. 57-24. Standing rowing.

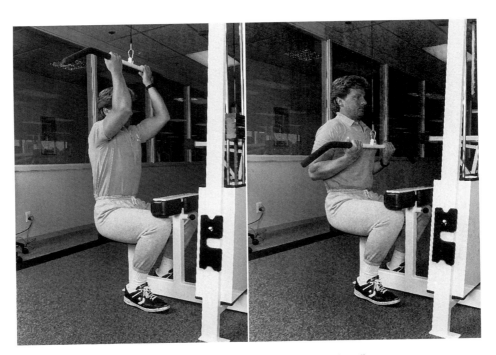

Fig. 57-25. Latissimus pull-downs (underhand).

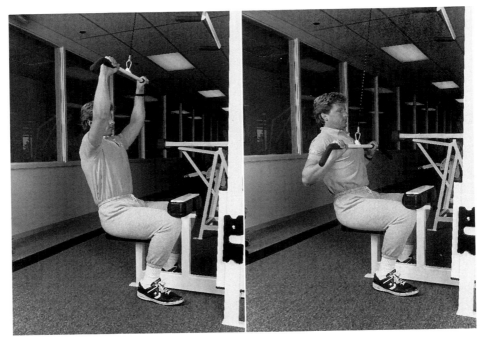

Fig. 57-26. Latissimus pull-downs (overhand).

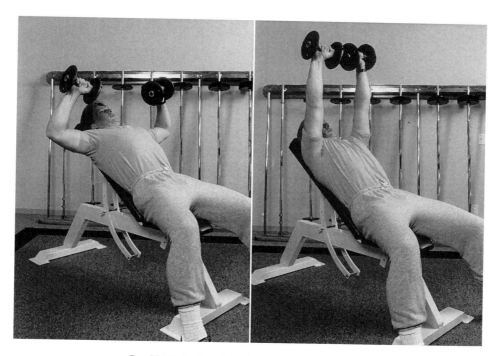

Fig. 57-27. Incline bench press with dumbbells.

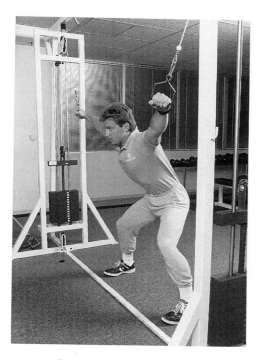

Fig. 57-28. Cable crossovers.

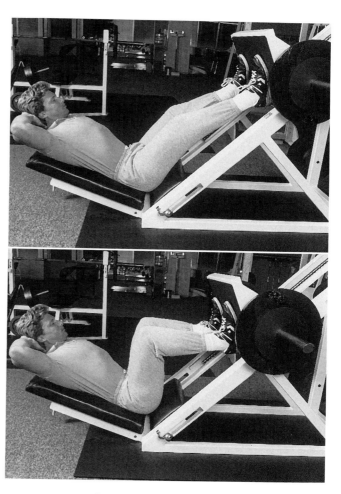

Fig. 57-29. Angled leg press.

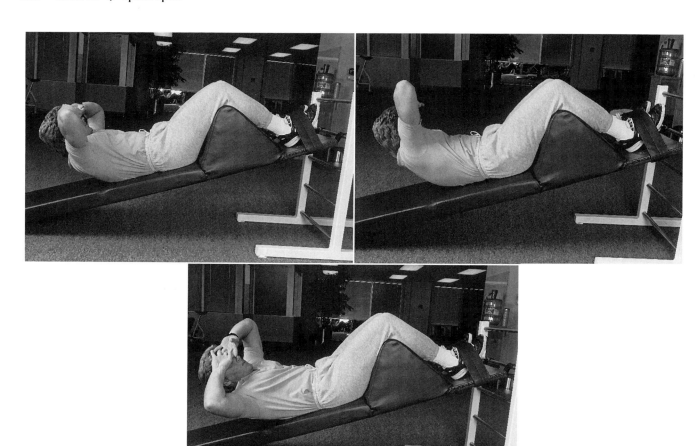

Fig. 57-30. Incline board curl-ups.

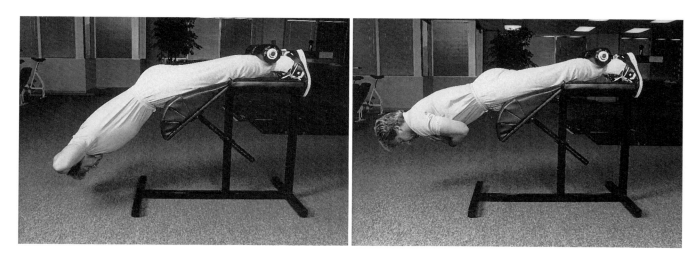

Fig. 57-31. Hyperextension bench.

rowing ergometer and on land simulation. Training in boat activities at lower levels of endurance is undertaken before the rower's eventual return to sprint training, which is the most physically demanding component.

REFERENCES

1. Adams MA, Hutton WC: Prolapsed intervertebral disc: a hyperflexion injury, *Spine* 7:184, 1982.
2. Adams MA, Hutton WC: The effect of fatigue on the lumbar intervertebral disc, *J Bone Joint Surg* 65B:199, 1983.
3. Adams MA, Hutton WC: Gradual disc prolapse, *Spine* 10:524, 1985.
4. Capozzo A: The forces and couples in the human trunk during level walking, *J Biomech* 16:265, 1983.
5. Capozzo A: Compressive loads in the lumbar vertebral column during normal level walking, *J Orthop Res* 1:292, 1984.
6. Cyron BU, Hutton WC: The fatigue strength of the lumbar neural arch in spondylolysis, *J Bone Joint Surg* 60B:234, 1978.
7. Derbes VJ, Harran T: Rib fracture from muscular effort with particular reference to cough, *Surgery* 35:294, 1954.
8. Hagerman F: Applied physiology of rowing, *Sports Med* 1:303, 1984.
9. Hebbelinck M et al: Anthropometric characteristics of female Olympic rowers, *Can J Appl Sports Sci* 5:255, 1980.
10. Holden DL, Jackson DW: Stress fractures of the ribs in female rowers, *Am J Sports Med* 13:342, 1985.
11. Hosea TM et al: Myoelectric and kinematic analysis of the lumbar spine while rowing, *Am J Sports Med* (in press).
12. Howell DW: Musculoskeletal profile and incidence of musculoskeletal injuries in lightweight women rowers, *Am J Sports Med* 12:278, 1984.
13. Mickelson TC, Hagerman FC: Functional anatomy of the rowing stroke, *Oarsman* 11:6, 1979.
14. Roy SH et al: Musculoskeletal profile and incidence of musculoskeletal injuries in lightweight women rowers, *Med Sci Sports Exerc* 22:463, 1990.
15. Saal JA, Saal JS: Nonoperative treatment of herniated lumbar intervertebral disc with radiculopathy: an outcome study, *Spine* 14:431, 1989.
16. Schultz AB, Anderson GBJ: Analysis of loads on the lumbar spine, *Spine* 6:76, 1981.
17. Stallard MC: Backache in oarsmen, *Br J Sports Med* 14:105, 1980.
18. Strayer L: Personal communication, 1991.

Chapter Fifty-Eight

Cycling

Edmund R. Burke

The popularity of cycling as a competitive and recreational activity continues to grow in the United States. In 1990 the National Sporting Goods Association reported that more than 56 million persons rode their bicycles six or more times within the year.[4] Also in that year there were 4.1 million participants in mountain biking, a gain of 28% over 1989 and a meteoric 174% rise since 1987. The increase in cross-training and triathlon events has led to many more bicyclists. Increased participation has also resulted in a growing number of avid and recreational cyclists with musculoskeletal problems. Thus medical personnel are challenged to make helpful recommendations to their patients in terms of an understanding of the biomechanics of cycling and proper positioning on the bike.

The medical literature has provided us with much information about accidental trauma in cycling[3,28,29] but only limited information on nontraumatic injuries. Kuland and Brubaker[20] studied the prevalence of bicycle tourist riding across the United States. They found that knee pain, back pain, and saddle soreness were among the most cited injuries reported by the cyclists.

Weiss[30] reported on 132 participants in an 8-day bicycle tour. The most common nontraumatic injury was buttock pain (32.8%), knee pain (20.7%), and neck/shoulder pain (66.4%), with significant symptoms occurring in 20.4% of the participants. Nearly all riders (95%) with neck and shoulder symptoms reported pain in the region of the trapezius muscle; 5% complained of numbness in the area. Some of these cyclists suggested possible causes of back and shoulder pain, including road vibration transmitted through the handlebars and arms to the shoulder girdle, hyperextension of the neck in the normal riding position, and the wearing of a bicycle helmet, which obstructed part of the upper field of vision, necessitating excessive neck hypertension.

Hill and Mellion[17] have suggested that neck and back problems are caused by the increased load placed on the arms and shoulders to support the rider, especially the weight of the upper chest and head. This is accentuated with the use of drop handlebars. This type of constant load is very fatiguing; overextension of the upper body (reaching because of improper position) is the primary position problem causing these overuse syndromes.

In competitive athletes the incidence of back injuries and pain can be quite high. In a survey investigating the training and injury patterns of competitive triathletes it was found that 17% experienced lower back pain.[31] In a

study of competitive cyclists Bohlman[3] reported a 10% incidence of "pain and discomfort" in the lower back.

Many of the nagging pains associated with lower back pain in cycling are caused simply by tension in the low back muscles. The basic racing position on the bicycle, coupled with the way cyclists use their backs under effort, produces tension in the hip and low back region. It usually starts with an ache in the lumbar region and in the deep muscles of the buttock. This ache is in the muscles (gluteus maximus) used for driving the pedals; these muscles are especially stressed when big gears are used in climbing or time trialing.

Other published articles have attributed bicycling-related problems to development of Scheuermann's disease, especially in young (under 20 years of age) cyclists who cycle extensively. Some authors also mention the incidence of dorsal arthritis in 13% of bicycle racers, usually older than 40 years of age.[11,19] Chrestian[9] reinforces the idea that position on the bike and gearing used are probable causes of lumbar pain. In addition to mechanical concerns, long hours in the saddle can result in low back pain and fatigue. The best prevention for these problems is gradual acclimation and conditioning to the sport and proper adjustment of the bicycle.[23] In addition, stretching, both before and during long rides, helps relieve discomfort. (See Sheets and Hochschuler[26] for additional information on the prevention of back discomfort and pain in cycling.)

POSITION ON THE BIKE

Low back, shoulder, and neck pain often results from an improper position on the bike. Discomfort and pain also can be caused by excessive or too-rapid changes in saddle height position. The rider should check to see that the saddle-to-pedal position is correct (Fig. 58-1). If the saddle is too high, it will cause excessive sacroiliac joint movement, which could provoke low back and buttock pain. Lowering the position of the saddle may alleviate the pain.

A correct position on the bike allows use of the gluteus maximus and biceps femoris muscles for full leg extension. According to LeMond,[22] "the optimal saddle height for the most effective power output and efficient oxygen consumption is 0.883 of the inseam." This is determined by measuring from the floor to the crotch of the cyclist who is standing in bare feet (pubic symphysis height) (Fig. 58-2). This inseam measurement is multiplied by 0.883. The result is an optimal saddle height, measured from the center of the bottom bracket to the top of the seat (the part where the cyclist sits, not the part that rises in the back). For example, if a person's inseam length is 32 inches (81.3 cm), the ideal saddle height would be 28.3 inches (71.8 cm).

This method assumes that the cyclist rides in cycling

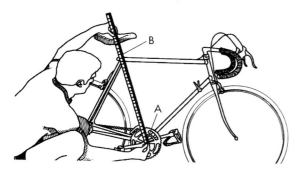

Fig. 58-1. Measuring the frame size. A tape measure is used to determine the distance from the center of the bottom bracket *(A)* to the top of the saddle *(B)*.

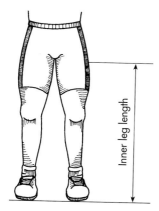

Fig. 58-2. Measuring the leg length. The inseam length is measured while the cyclist is standing barefoot.

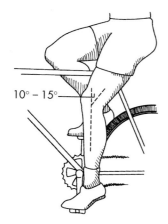

Fig. 58-3. Determining correct knee flexion. When the seat height is set properly, the knee angle is 10 to 15 degrees when the cyclist is seated on the bike and pedaling with the ball of the foot.

shoes that are about ½ inch (1.2 cm) thick; thicker shoes will require adding a few millimeters to the height. With the use of clipless pedals, 2 to 3 mm are subtracted from the saddle height. The cyclist is encouraged to experiment within a few millimeters of "ideal" height to find the most comfortable position. A simple rule of thumb is that the saddle height should allow approximately 15 to 25 degrees of knee flexion when the ball of the foot is on the pedal and the pedal is in the 6 o'clock position (bottom dead center)[12] (Fig. 58-3). For persons recovering from knee injuries, the American Academy of Orthopaedic Surgeons recommends starting with a 15-degree bend in the knee joint.

If the saddle must be raised or lowered substantially, the changes should be made gradually—no more than 3 mm per week. Furthermore, the top of the saddle should be horizontal or tilted up slightly. The nose of the saddle should not point down because the cyclist will tend to slide off the front of the saddle. This places more weight and stress on the hands, arms, and shoulders.

Several investigators have estimated optimal seat height on the basis of caloric expenditure and power output.[16,24,27] These researchers generally agree that oxygen consumption is minimized at approximately 100% of trochanteric height, or 106% to 109% of symphysis pubis height (measured from the ground with the cyclist in bare feet). Seat height in these studies was established by measuring from the center of the pedal axle aligned with the seat tube to the top of the saddle where the cyclist sits. This is different from the formula established by LeMond.[22]

Muscle activity patterns, joint force and moment patterns, and pedal force effectiveness have also been reported for various seat heights.[5,6,10,12-14,18] Rugg[25] analyzed muscle activity, joint moment patterns, muscle length changes, and moment arms of trained cyclists at the ankle across seat heights. A complex relationship emerged in which seat height changes influenced muscle

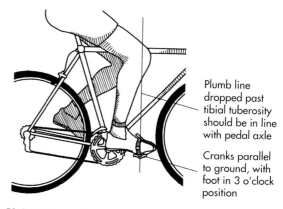

Fig. 58-4. Determining correct seat position relative to the pedals. A plumb line is dropped from the middle of the forward knee (patella) and should drop through the center of the pedal axle.

activity patterns, joint moment profiles, force velocity, and length-tension operating conditions for the triceps surae muscle group. (See Gregor, Broker, and Ryan[15] for an excellent review of the biomechanics of cycling.)

The saddle's fore and aft position should be checked. The pedals should be in the 3 o'clock and 9 o'clock positions, with the ball of the foot firmly on the pedal. A plumb line dropped from the front of the knee at the middle of the kneecap should drop through the center of the pedal axle (Fig. 58-4). If it does not, the seat-post clamp should be loosened and the saddle slid forward or backward as necessary.[17]

If the cyclist is suffering from sore, aching muscles in the neck after a long ride, the riding position should be checked first. If the distance from the saddle to the handlebars is too short, the cyclist will really have to stretch his or her neck to see the road ahead. Generally, the correct combination of top tube–stem length enables a cyclist in the normal riding position to look down and have the handlebars obscure the stem. A longer stem will be required to push the handlebars out where they belong. Too long a stem can also cause problems. The cyclist may be too far stretched out on the bike, which causes the person to hold the head back, thus placing undue stress on the neck and shoulder muscles. The top of the stem should also be level with the top of the saddle, or no more than 1 inch below the top of the saddle.

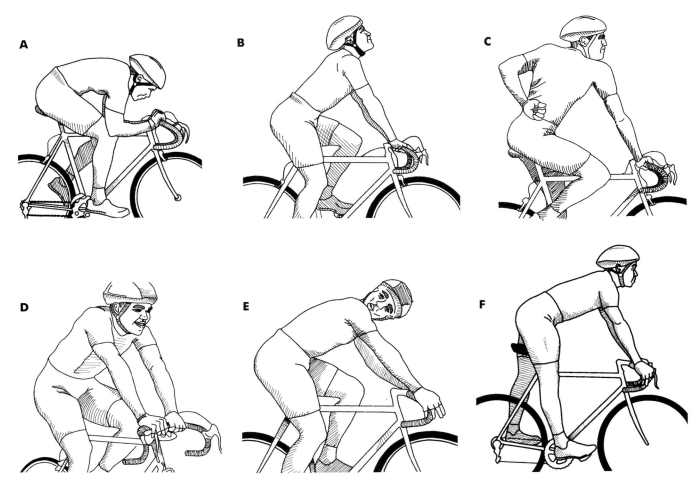

Fig. 58-5. On-the-bicycle stretches. **A** and **B,** Middle and upper back: While on the saddle with the hands on the bar, round the back while lowering the head slightly. Hold for 5 seconds and then straighten the back, lifting up from the breastbone and looking slightly upward to extend the spine. Hold for 5 seconds or more. **C,** Lower and middle back: While keeping one hand on the bar next to the stem, reach around and place the back of the hand and forearm across the lower back. Twist the upper body toward the arm that is behind the back. Hold for 5 seconds. Repeat several times. **D,** Shoulder and neck: Lift both shoulders toward the ears until tension is felt. Hold for 5 seconds and then slowly lower to the original position. **E,** Neck: Turn the chin toward the shoulder for a few seconds. Repeat to the other side. **F,** Gluteus maximus and hamstrings: With the forward pedal in the 9 to 10 o'clock position, stand up, raise the hips, straighten the legs, and drop the heels. Hold for 5 seconds. Then rotate the crank 180 degrees and repeat.

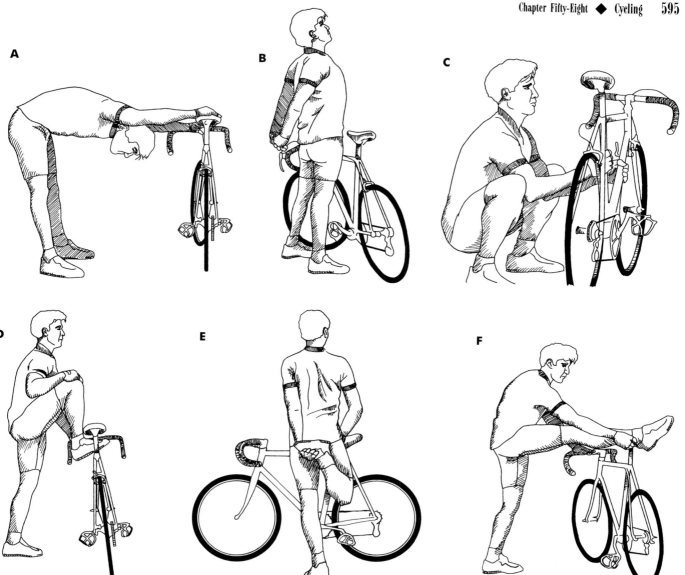

Fig. 58-6. Stretches before and after cycling. **A,** Arms, back, shoulders, back of the neck, and hamstrings: Stand 3 to 4 feet from the bicycle with the feet shoulder width apart. Place one hand on the saddle and one on the stem. Keeping the knees slightly bent and the hips directly over the feet, slowly lower the upper body and move the chin toward the chest until tension is felt. Hold for 20 to 30 seconds. Repeat several times. **B,** Shoulders, spine, and upper back: Let the bike lean against the hips, or rest it against a wall or tree. Interlace the fingers behind the back, palms up. Slowly lower the hands to straighten the arms and then carefully rotate the arms backward until a stretch is felt through the front of the shoulders. Hold for 15 to 20 seconds. Repeat several times. **C,** Knees and lower back: Stand about 2 feet from the bike with the feet about shoulder width apart and the toes pointed slightly outward. Grasp the middle of the seat tube and down tube. Slowly squat, keeping the heels planted and the middle of the knees above the feet. Hold for 20 to 30 seconds. Be careful when knee problems are present. **D,** Hip and groin: Hold the bar top with one hand. Bend and lift one leg, bringing the knee toward the chest, and place the foot on the saddle, top tube, or rear tire. Keep the other leg fairly straight and the other foot pointed forward. Hold for 15 to 20 seconds. Repeat with the other leg. **E,** Quadriceps: Stand on the left side of the bike and place the right hand on the saddle for balance. Reach behind with the left hand and grasp the top of the right foot. Slowly pull the foot toward the middle of the buttocks until the stretch is felt in the quadriceps and knee. Hold for 15 to 30 seconds. Grasp the handlebar stem with the left hand and reverse the procedure for the left leg. **F,** Hamstrings: Place one ankle atop the seat or the rear tire while keeping one hand on the back edge of the saddle and the other on the stem. The other leg should almost be straight (but not locked), with the foot pointed directly ahead. Slowly bend over until a stretch is felt in the hamstrings of the elevated leg. Keep the quadriceps of this leg relaxed. Hold for 15 to 30 seconds. Repeat with the other leg.

The posture should be varied while the cyclist is riding. A periodic change of position helps muscles relax. The cyclist should allow the neck to be held at various angles by moving the grip on the handlebar from the tops, to the brake lever hoods, to the drops. In addition, rolling the head from side-to-side reduces fatigue.

STRETCHING

Pedaling requires a limited, repeated motion, and the muscles are never fully contracted or extended. This can cause tightness and pain in the hamstrings, quadriceps, and lower back. Thus, stretching during longer rides will lessen fatigue and improve performance.[1,8] The exercises shown in Figs. 58-5 and 58-6 will help reduce tightness and pain in the neck, shoulders, limbs, and back.

While on the bike, the cyclist is advised to stretch only when riding alone (not in a group) at a manageable speed—certainly not in heavy traffic or on rough roads. A high level of concentration is required for the cyclist to do these stretches correctly while maintaining safe riding habits.

Stretches performed before the ride will help the body warm up, increase muscle blood flow, and prepare the body for the tasks ahead.[2] Stretching at rest stops during a long ride will relieve muscular tension and help postpone fatigue. Doing stretches after cycling will assist the body in cooling down and may prevent soreness.

One of the keys to a healthy back is a strong back. Because cycling does not work the abdominal muscles, specific exercises are required to strengthen them. Weak stomach muscles allow the lower back to curve inward, straining the muscles, ligaments, and discs of the back. The clinician should recommend bent-knee sit-ups and other abdominal exercises to patients with lower back pain.[7,21]

As is true of most sport injuries, prevention of spine and back injuries in the cyclist is not always easier than the treatment, but it is certainly more conducive to more productive and enjoyable hours on the bicycle.

REFERENCES

1. Anderson B, Burke ER: Loosen up, *Bicycling,* p 129, April 1990.
2. Anderson B, Burke ER: Scientific, medical, and practical aspects of stretching, *Clin Sports Med* 10:63, 1991.
3. Bohlman JT: Injuries in competitive cycling, *Physician Sportsmed* 9(5):117, 1981.
4. Breakaway news, *Bicycle Dealer Showcase,* p. 10, May 1991.
5. Broker JP et al: Effects of seat height on force effectiveness in cycling, *Med Sci Sports Exerc* 20:583, 1988.
6. Browning RC et al: Effects of seat height changes on joint force and movement patterns in experienced cyclists, *J Biomech* 21:871, 1988.
7. Burke ER: Back: the overlooked cycling muscles, *Bicycling,* p 84, Jan/Feb , 1990.
8. Burke ER, Anderson B: Fast and loose, *Bicycling,* p 80, July 1991.
9. Chrestian R: Lombalgies et pubalgies chez le cycliste, *Cinesiologie* 27(118):88, 1988.
10. Desipres M: An electromyographic study of competitive road cycling conditions simulated on a treadmill. In Nelson RC, Morehouse C, editors: *Biomechanics,* vol 4, Baltimore, 1974, University Park Press.
11. Elegem P: Cyclisme et pathologie chronique, *Acta Orthop Belg* 49(1-2):88, 1983.
12. Ericson MO: On the biomechanics of cycling: a study of joint and muscle load during exercise on the bicycle ergometer, *Scand J Rehabil Med* 16:1, 1986.
13. Ericson MO et al: The forces on ankle joint structures during ergometer cycling, *Foot Ankle* 6:135, 1985.
14. Ericson MO et al: Muscular activity during ergometer cycling, *Scand J Rehabil Med* 17:53, 1985.
15. Gregor RJ, Broker JP, Ryan MM: The biomechanics of cycling. In Holloszy JO, editor: *Exercise and sport science reviews,* vol 19, Baltimore, 1991, Williams & Wilkins.
16. Hamley EJ, Thomas V: Physiological and postural factors in the calibration of the bicycle ergometer, *J Physiol* 191:55, 1967.
17. Hill WJ, Mellion BM: Bicycling injuries: prevention, diagnosis, and treatment. In Morris MB, editor: *Sports injuries and athletic problems,* Philadelphia, 1988, Hanley & Belfus.
18. Jorge M, Hull ML: Analysis of EMG measurement during bicycle pedaling, *J Biomech* 19:683, 1986.
19. Judet H: Pathologie micro-traumatique et inflammatoire. In Judet H, Porte G, editors: *Médicine du cyclisme,* Paris, 1983, Masson.
20. Kuland DN, Brubaker CE: Injuries in bike centennial tour, *Physician Sportsmed* 6(6):74, 1978.
21. Legwold G: Look back, *Bicycle Guide,* p 10, Oct 1989.
22. LeMond G: *Greg LeMond's complete book of bicycling,* New York, 1988, Perigee.
23. Mayer PJ: Helping your patients avoid bicycling injuries, *J Musculoskel Med* 2(5):31, 1985.
24. Nordeen KS, Cavanagh PR: Simulation of the lower limb kinematics during cycling. In Komi PA, editor: *Biomechanics,* Baltimore, 1975, University Park Press.
25. Rugg SR: *Muscle mechanics of the triceps surae and tibialis anterior muscles during ankle dorsi- and plantarflexion,* doctoral dissertation, Los Angeles, 1989, University of California.
26. Sheets CG, Hochschuler SH: Considerations in cycling for persons with low back pain. In Hochschuler SH, editor: *Back in shape: a back owner's manual,* Boston, 1991, Houghton Mifflin.
27. Shennum PL, DeVires HA: The effect of saddle height on oxygen consumption during bicycle ergometer work, *Med Sci Sports Exerc* 8:119, 1976.
28. Tucci JJ, Barone JE: A study of urban bicycling accidents, *Am J Sports Med* 16:181, 1988.
29. Watts CK, Jones D, Crouch D: Survey of bicycling accidents in Boulder, Colorado, *Physician Sportsmed* 14(3):99, 1986.
30. Weiss BD: Nontraumatic injuries in amateur long distance bicyclists, *Am J Sports Med* 13:187, 1985.
31. Williams MM et al: Injuries amongst competitive triathletes, *NZ J Sports Med* 16(1):2, 1988.

Chapter Fifty-Nine

Motor Sports

Terry R. Trammell

One of the fastest-growing sports in the United States today is motor racing. The premiere form of this sport is the Indy Car PPG World Series, which includes the Indianapolis 500, probably the best known motor race in the world. Although the sport would appear to be exceedingly dangerous and the risk of injury inordinately high, that has not proved to be the case. In Indy car events from 1985 through 1989, 367 crashes occurred that involved 413 drivers, 38 of whom sustained 48 injuries. Of these 48 injuries, 29.2% were closed head injuries, 31.1% were injuries to the lower extremities, 27.1% were injuries to the upper extremities, and 12.5% were injuries to other systems. Three involved the cervical spine for an incidence of 6%.[2,4]

In the decade from 1981 to 1991, approximately 50 drivers were injured driving Indy cars. Nine of these drivers sustained injuries to the axial skeleton for an incidence of approximately 20%.

The data collected regarding Indy car racing have shown that on the average one injury occurs per 9.7 crashes.[5] Although the likelihood of a crash per mile driven is 30 times greater in an Indy car at speeds in excess of 145 mph, the likelihood of injury is only 1.2 times that seen in passenger car crashes.[4] When one considers the forces at play in a motor racing crash, it is fortunate that injury to the axial skeleton is relatively rare in motor racing.

Car design is credited with protecting the driver from serious injury in most circumstances. An Indy car is designed to dissipate energy by shedding parts in an accident, which takes away energy from the crash, preventing its transmission to the driver (Fig. 59-1). Injuries to the torso are unusual and have accounted for fewer than 10% of injuries sustained by drivers of Indy cars during the last 10 years.

CAR DESIGN FACTORS

Car design is largely responsible for protecting the driver, who is cocooned in a monocoque (tub) that in most cases protects his torso from injury. The driver is restrained in this tub by a five-way lap belt (Fig. 59-2) that prevents his ejection from the car in an impact.

The head and neck are protected by a roll bar that prevents the head from contacting the ground in a rollover situation. The use of a horseshoe collar, as well as custom-built pads added to the inside of the cockpit, offers additional protection (Fig. 59-3). The driver wears a specially designed full-face helmet that can sustain a

10-G impact and, in most cases, can prevent injury to the upper cervical spine. A disadvantage is that it may function as an increased weight, increasing the load on the lever arm (i.e., the lower cervical spine).

EXTRICATION PROCEDURES

Of tantamount importance in protecting the cervical spine is the technique by which the driver is extricated from a crashed race car. In Indy car racing the helmet is full faced; thus it must be removed to establish an airway. In an unconscious driver the helmet itself frequently adds enough weight to occlude the driver's airway. This creates a different situation from motor sports in which an open-faced helmet is worn. In the latter case it is probably safer to leave the helmet in place and stabilize the cervical spine beneath the helmet, extricate the driver from the car, and then remove the helmet after the driver has been secured to a backboard and his neck braced. With an open-faced helmet an adequate airway can be established without the helmet being removed.

In Indy car racing the removal of the full-faced helmet requires two persons. The head and neck must be stabilized by one member of the team, who also has to remove the chin restraint straps while the second member of the team maintains gentle traction on the helmet to keep the neck in a neutral position. The person

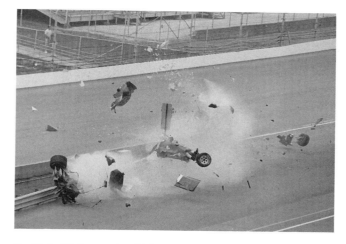

Fig. 59-1. High-speed collision results in explosive dissipation of kinetic energy. As parts are shed from the car, energy is expended, diverting its potentially injurious effect on the driver. This driver sustained multiple foot injuries but no injury to the torso. (© 1991 John Frame.)

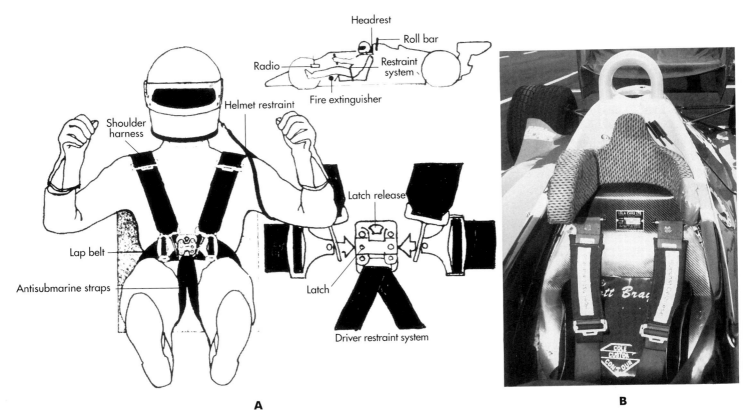

Fig. 59-2. A, Five-way safety harness. B, Padded five-way belt in the monocoque.

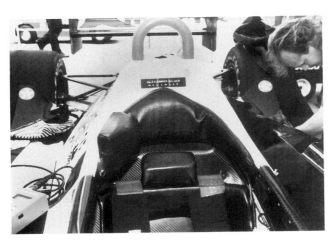

Fig. 59-3. Custom padding to protect the driver's head and neck. Note the roll bar extending well above the top of the cockpit to protect the driver's neck in the event of a rollover.

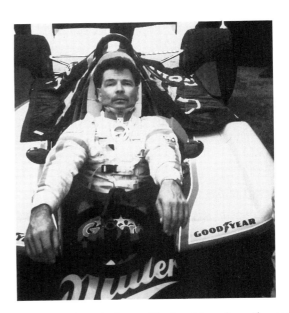

Fig. 59-4. Extrication device to lift the driver from the car. It consists of a cervicothoracic brace that attaches to a specially designed lumbar corset (part of a rigid metal scoop) to immobilize the head and the thoracic and lumbar spine. The head is supported by the cervicothoracic brace.

in front of the driver who has removed the helmet strap then stabilizes the cervical spine while the second person gently removes the helmet, pulling it directly off in line with the neck. Further stabilization is achieved by application of a specially designed cervicothoracic brace to maintain the neck in a neutral position and provide very slight traction.

The driver is removed from the car by application of a specially designed shovel type of torso backboard that is fastened to the driver with a corset brace that goes around the chest and waist to facilitate extrication from the car. The driver is then placed onto a standard spinal board, and his head, neck, and the remaining portion of his trunk are immobilized (Fig. 59-4).

The specially designed extrication equipment is necessary because of the narrow width of an Indy car, which is frequently less than 16 inches and therefore precludes the use of the type of board for driver immobilization that is the preferred means of extricating victims of a passenger car crash. The proper application of the spinal board and neck brace is extremely important in preventing further injury should a cervical spine fracture be present. The board and brace are always used to extricate an unconscious driver. In some circumstances a cervical collar is used for a driver who is fully conscious and has no neck pain but has sustained other injuries. The collar is worn until adequate x-ray evaluation of the neck can be completed.

INJURIES

My involvement with Indy car racing has provided an unusual opportunity to view, firsthand, accidents that result in injury. Also, extensive nationwide media coverage of professional motor sports has provided an opportunity to acquire and review videotapes of these events. The ability to study in detail accidents that resulted in injury and to ascertain the mechanisms and forces involved is unusual in the study of trauma. Normally the treating physician sees only the aftermath of the collision and rarely, if ever, views the responsible forces evolving at the time of impact or is present on site immediately after the crash.

Cervical Spine Injuries

The most frequent injury to the cervical spine in Indy car racing is a sprain/strain of the left-sided neck musculature. To counteract the G forces, which are anywhere from 3 to 6 G at a high-speed oval, drivers for years have worn a helmet strap that fastens to the left side of the helmet and is passed beneath the axilla on the left side. Because the ovals are run counterclockwise, the driver is always turning left. The centrifugal force tends to throw the driver's head to the right in the corners, and the axillary strap helps maintain the neck in an upright position (Fig. 59-5, A). This, however, frequently produces compression of the axillary area, as well as paresthesias

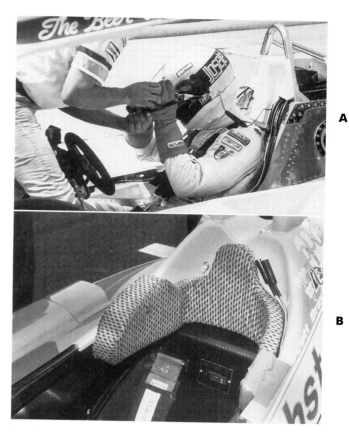

Fig. 59-5. A, Left-sided axillary strap that passes beneath the driver's left axilla and fastens to the left side of the helmet to counteract G forces, which cause the driver's head to tilt to the right. **B,** Right-sided helmet pads have replaced axillary straps, preventing a right-headed tilt and strain of the muscles on the left side of the neck.

in the driver's left arm. Most drivers have abandoned the axillary strap in favor of a specific right-sided pad that is applied to the car to help maintain the head in an upright position and counteract the G forces of turning left at high speeds (Fig. 59-5, B).

Fractures. Fractures of the cervical spine occur infrequently. Direct frontal impact rarely produces neck injury because the driver is accelerated forward against his belts and there is little excursion of the neck. On the other hand, a rear-ended impact usually produces a flexion/extension type of injury as the driver is accelerated backward against the cowling and head support and ricochets off the headrest forward. This sequence produces a flexion moment that is amplified because the torso is still moving backward at the time of impact as the head is accelerated forward in a contrecoup motion. The weight of the helmet is an additional factor, and the driver is vulnerable to flexion/compression injury.

Although this mechanism can produce significant injury, it rarely does. Commonly, the sudden flexion movement produces avulsion of the spinous processes and/or simple compression fracture of the cervical vertebral bodies. However, this mechanism can cause fracturing of the vertebral body and disruption of the posterior ligaments.

The most common mechanism of significant cervical spine injury occurs in a high-speed violent rollover in which the driver's head is accelerated centrifugally out of the car, resulting in a distraction force on the neck that then can be coupled with either a forward or a lateral flexion moment to produce resultant injury to the cervical spine. More rarely, the result is a rebound phenomenon that produces axial loading of the cervical spine and causes an axial loading injury. Extension is prevented by the headrest and cockpit cowling. In most cases actual contact with the ground as a result of a rollover is prevented by the roll bar. However, in rare circumstances, if the driver is exceptionally tall, his head

may approach the level of the roll bar so that in a violent rollover his restraining straps can stretch, which, coupled with distraction on his neck, can actually produce contact of the vertex of the skull through the helmet with the ground. This can result in some degree of direct loading on the skull that is then transmitted to the cervical spine.

The following are specific examples of injury to the cervical spine.

C1 and C2 injuries. Injury to the upper cervical spine (fractures of C1 and C2) are usually related to rollover, as already noted. Fig. 59-6 involves a patient who was driving a Formula Ford, an open-wheeled roadster that is lighter in weight and smaller than an Indy car, and rolled over at high speed. Because of the driver's height, the angle of the roll bar, and the fact that the contact was made in a soft dirt area, the roll bar sank into the ground

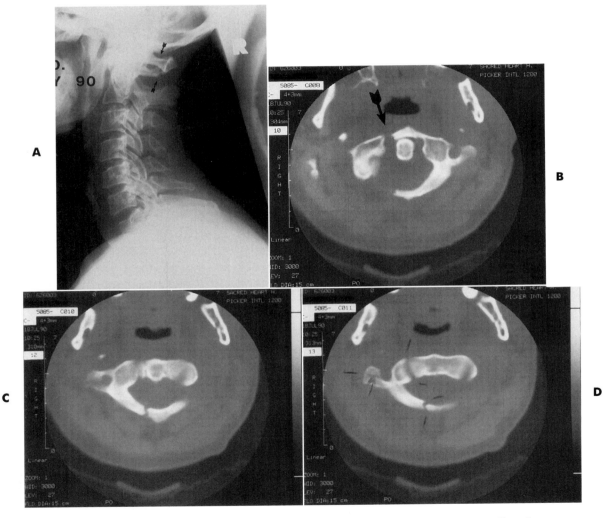

Fig. 59-6. Fracture ring of C1—Jefferson fracture as a result of direct axial loading that occurred when the driver's head made contact with the ground as the roll bar sunk into the ground when the car went off course in a rollover. **A,** Lateral x-ray film showing C1 fracture. **B,** CT scan showing fracture of the right anterior aspect of C1. **C** and **D,** CT scans further delineating injury to C1.

and the driver's helmet contacted the ground. The direct application of force to his neck caused a fracture of the ring of C1. This is the classic Jefferson fracture that results from direct axial compression applied to the skull with the cervical spine aligned neutrally or in slight extension.[1]

Fig. 59-7 demonstrates an injury sustained in a high-speed collision with subsequent rollover at the Indianapolis Motor Speedway. The result was a fracture of the body of C2, a type III fracture of the base of the odontoid, with extension into the body of C2 without displacement. The mechanism of this injury is one of axial compression associated with some degree of horizontal shear applied in the sagittal plane.[6] This injury most likely occurred when the forehead portion of the driver's helmet made contact with the side of his car during the rollover. The forces generated may also have been great enough to produce some degree of the rebound phenomenon discussed earlier.

Another example of an injury to C2 is the classic traumatic spondylolisthesis (hangman's fracture). Fig. 59-8, *A*, illustrates a violent, multiple-impact accident that involved a high-speed rollover. The left side of the anteroinferior portion of the driver's helmet contacted the left wall of the cowling during the rollover, producing a hyperextension right lateral flexion moment, while the centrifugal force of the rollover produced traction on the neck, which resulted in this fracture (Fig. 59-8, *B*).

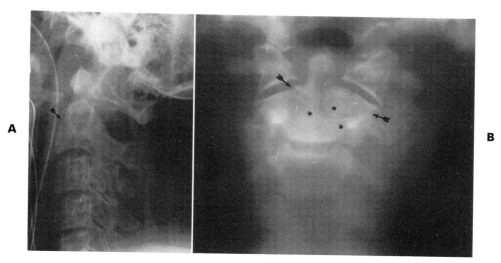

Fig. 59-7. C2 fracture resulting from a high-speed collision and subsequent rollover. **A,** Lateral cervical spine film indicating fracture of the anterior cortex of C2 *(arrow)*. **B,** Anteroposterior (AP) tomogram demonstrating the degree of extension into the body of C2.

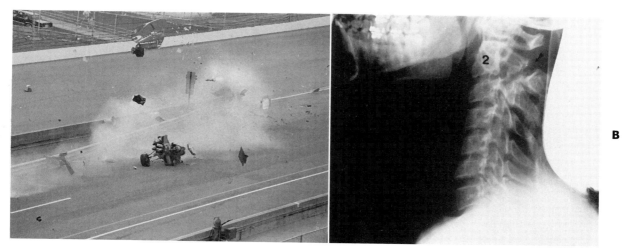

Fig. 59-8. C2 fracture—traumatic spondylolisthesis. **A,** Violent multiple-impact accident with rollover. The driver struck the left side of his helmet on the cowling of the car at the moment of rollover, producing C2 injury. **B,** Lateral x-ray film showing C2 injury. (**A** © 1991 John Frame.)

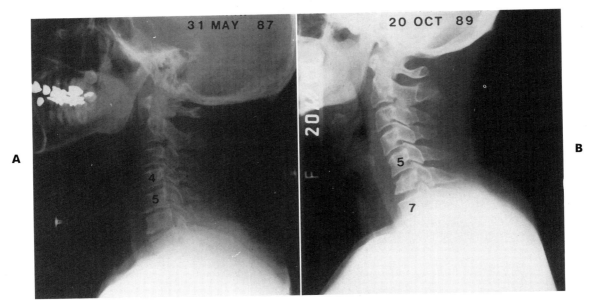

Fig. 59-9. **A,** Avulsion fractures of the spinous process of C4 and C5 resulting from a rear-end impact with the concrete barrier. **B,** Compression fracture at C6 as a result of a similar rear-end collision.

At the moment of impact with the ground, the roll bar functioned to prevent driver contact with the ground. Examination of the driver's helmet showed no markings on the top of the helmet, only along the left mandibular portion anteriorly.

C3 to C7 injuries. Injuries to the lower cervical spine are usually related to flexion/extension moments. They range from the simple avulsion of the cervical spinous processes to simple compression fractures of the lower cervical spine. Fig. 59-9, *A*, shows the avulsion fracture of the C4 and C5 spinous processes that this driver sustained when he slammed, tail first, into a concrete barrier. His injury was typical of a clay shoveler's fracture.[6] The driver, anticipating the impact from the image in his rear-view mirror, set his shoulders and rigidly gripped the wheel as the accelerating car left the asphalt surface and passed over the intervening grass.

A similar rear-end collision resulted in a compression fracture of C6 as demonstrated in Fig. 59-9, *B*. This injury was clearly associated with a contrecoup force that was applied to the occiput when the driver smashed into a concrete barrier, end around, at high speed. His head struck the headrest, propelling his head forward while his torso continued backward. This resulted in a mild concussion that rendered the driver unconscious and caused the injury to C6. The mechanism was clearly delineated, both from the videotaped footage of the crash and the fact that the only area of damage was to the driver's helmet directly at its point of contact with the headrest.

At higher speeds, more violent forces are applied when the direct posterior impact occurs, resulting in fractures of the midcervical spine, with fracturing of the vertebral body and disruption of the posterior ligaments because of a more severe flexion force. This is an example of how increased force can produce more significant injury. The injury shown in Fig. 59-10 occurred at two levels, both due to the forward acceleration of the head in the flexion moment, which produced disruption of the interspinous ligaments between C4 and C5, as well as compression fracturing in the anterior aspect of the body of C4. Also, the deceleration forces resulted in axial loading of the lower cervical spine with a bursting type of fracture of the body of C7. This injury, initially treated with an orthosis, demonstrated the progressive development of kyphosis at the C4-5 level, eventually necessitating posterior instrumentation and fusion.

A similar injury is shown in Fig. 59-11. This driver sustained a compression fracture of C5 during a violent rollover in a stock-type hill-climb car. Rollover forces and the centrifugal force generated were so great that the driver's belts stretched and his head impacted the roll cage from the inside. Because the injury resulted from axially applied forces, with the neck in slight flexion and the posterior ligamentous stability intact, this driver was successfully treated in an orthosis.

Fracture dislocations of the lower cervical spine associated with quadriplegia occur rarely in open-wheeled racing. Such an injury is demonstrated in Fig. 59-12. In this case a top-fuel drag race car, involved in a collision with a retaining barrier, rolled over at the moment of impact. In spite of the fact that the roll bar functioned and prevented the driver from actually

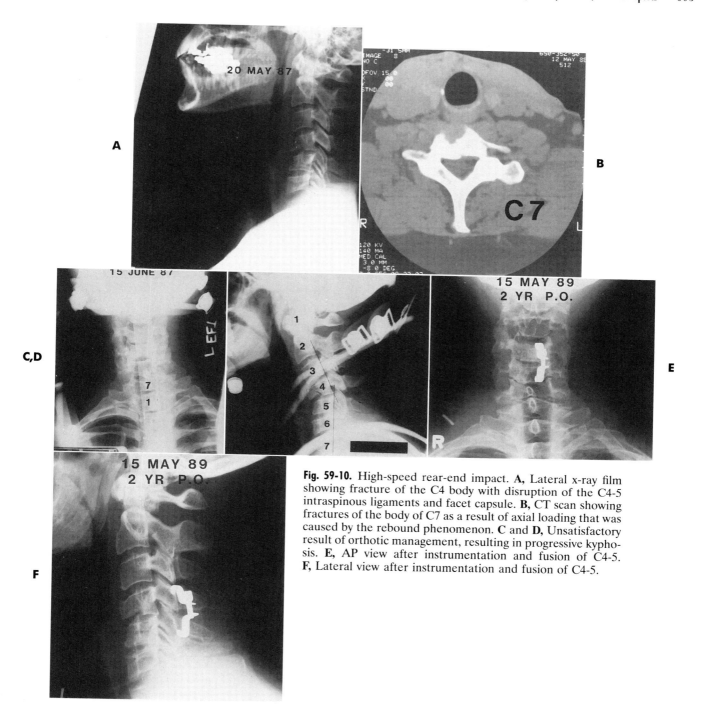

Fig. 59-10. High-speed rear-end impact. **A,** Lateral x-ray film showing fracture of the C4 body with disruption of the C4-5 intraspinous ligaments and facet capsule. **B,** CT scan showing fractures of the body of C7 as a result of axial loading that was caused by the rebound phenomenon. **C** and **D,** Unsatisfactory result of orthotic management, resulting in progressive kyphosis. **E,** AP view after instrumentation and fusion of C4-5. **F,** Lateral view after instrumentation and fusion of C4-5.

contacting the ground with his head, a flexion injury occurred. The injury was caused by a combination of the forces applied to the head when the car impacted the barrier, suddenly decelerating the head and rolling over, and thus accelerating the head in the distraction mode while in a forward-flexed position. The weight of the head, plus the weight of the helmet, acted as a weight at the end of the cervical spinal lever arm, producing the injuries demonstrated. Fig. 59-12 further demonstrates

the complex nature of fractures that can occur because of the violent forces applied to the cervical spine in a racing accident. The mechanism of injury may have several components: the result of multiple forces applied to the neck at varying rates and the duration of application from different directions with the neck in varying positions during the application of those forces.

Accidents associated with frontal impacts and subsequent rollover can apply a flexion moment to the cervical

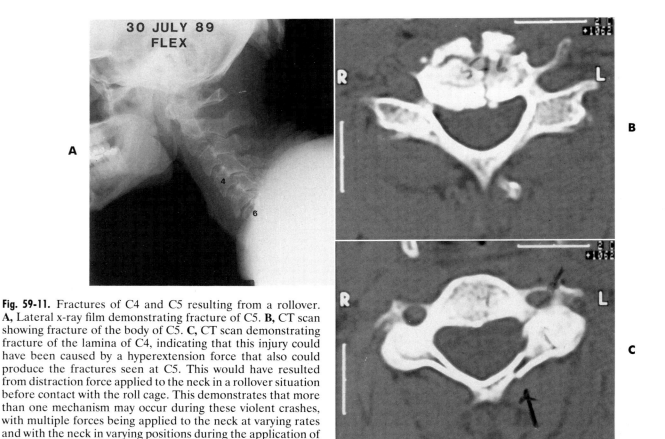

Fig. 59-11. Fractures of C4 and C5 resulting from a rollover. **A,** Lateral x-ray film demonstrating fracture of C5. **B,** CT scan showing fracture of the body of C5. **C,** CT scan demonstrating fracture of the lamina of C4, indicating that this injury could have been caused by a hyperextension force that also could produce the fractures seen at C5. This would have resulted from distraction force applied to the neck in a rollover situation before contact with the roll cage. This demonstrates that more than one mechanism may occur during these violent crashes, with multiple forces being applied to the neck at varying rates and with the neck in varying positions during the application of those forces.

spine followed by a flexion/extension moment as the head is accelerated away from the torso and then rebounds back toward the torso. This causes an axial loading phenomenon to a spine that may already have fractured in flexion or undergone fracture or ligamentous injury in distraction and extension before the application of the axial load.

Fortunately, the most common mechanism of injury to the cervical spine in a high-speed impact with a barrier is with the car moving backward. This results in collision of the driver's head with the cowling of the car. The head is then suddenly accelerated forward in a flexion moment, producing injury to the spinous processes in most cases or minor compression fracturing of the midcervical spine as demonstrated in Fig. 59-9. Severe injuries of the cervical spine, with or without cord injury, are almost exclusively the result of violent rollover. They are more commonly the product of distraction on the upper cervical spine or axial loading in a flexed moment on the lower cervical spine.

Thoracolumbar Spine Injuries

Injuries to the thoracolumbar spine, which are relatively rare because the driver is securely cocooned in his car, almost always result from direct frontal impact. The mechanism of injury to the thoracolumbar spine is the result of the car striking a barrier with a direct frontal impact. The rear end of the car rises off the racing surface and slams back to the ground, producing an axial load that is transmitted to the driver's buttocks, pelvis, and thoracolumbar spine. This mechanism of injury can also result when the bottom of the car buckles under direct frontal impact as a result of the tub's bending. The buckled bottom of the tub lifts up against the driver's buttock and pelvis, again applying a direct axial load to the torso. The driver is unable to move away from this load because he is harnessed into the car with heavy, broad shoulder straps and pads that prevent his torso from rising out of the car in an impact situation. Furthermore, the seating arrangement places the driver in a semireclining position, with the thoracolumbar spine fixed in a flexed position, so that, depending on the driver's size, the axial load to the spine is transmitted slightly anterior to the vertebral body. This produces more of a flexion moment on the thoracolumbar spine than would occur if a normal, direct axial load were applied to the spine as, for example, in a fall from a height.

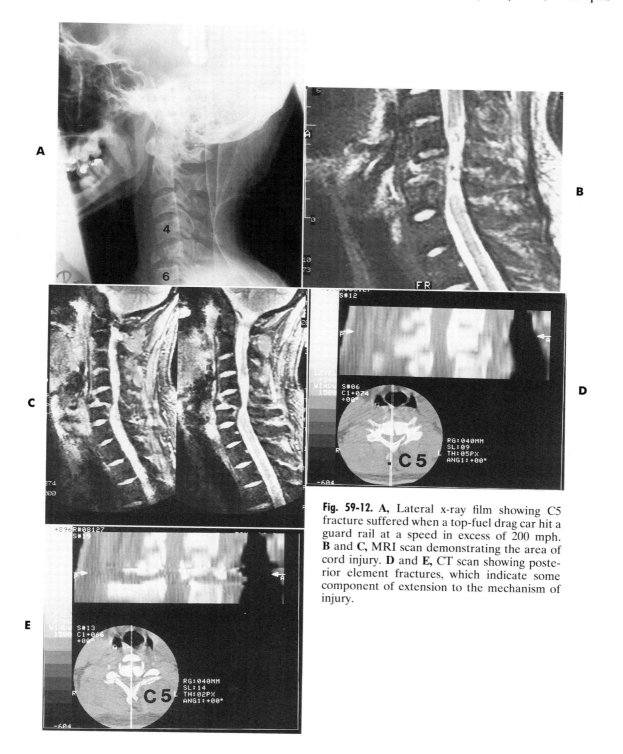

Fig. 59-12. A, Lateral x-ray film showing C5 fracture suffered when a top-fuel drag car hit a guard rail at a speed in excess of 200 mph. **B** and **C,** MRI scan demonstrating the area of cord injury. **D** and **E,** CT scan showing posterior element fractures, which indicate some component of extension to the mechanism of injury.

Figs. 59-13 and 59-14 provide examples of simple compression fractures associated with direct frontal impact at high speed. In both cases the driver hit an immovable barrier with the car's rear end lifting off the track surface and slamming back down against the track surface, which applied the load directly to the buttock and pelvis and was then transmitted to his axial skeleton.

Fig. 59-13 demonstrates a compression fracture 1 year after an injury that was treated with a rigid orthosis. Because of the driver's size and the fact that he was belted into the car in a semireclining posture, the injury occurred in a flexed position, producing a compression fracture, as opposed to the expected burst fracture seen with axial loading.

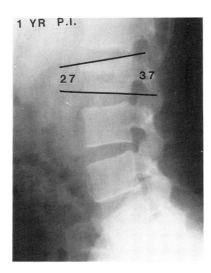

Fig. 59-13. Compression fracture of L2 resulting from a frontal impact — load applied exactly along the thoracolumbar spine. The driver was seated in a semireclining posture that forced the thoracic/lumbar junction in slight flexion, accounting for this flexion type of fracture.

In Fig. 59-14 the driver had a history of a previous back injury and had minimal symptoms at the time of this accident. Although a CT scan suggested some degree of hematoma around the vertebra, it was not very helpful in establishing the acute nature of the injury; however, a bone scan clearly showed acute injury not only to L1, but to T12 as well. This has great prognostic significance.

The final situation in which fracturing of the thoracolumbar spine occurs in racing accidents is a frontal impact of such force that the entire car shortens and buckles as the driver is straightened up in his seat. This straightening results from acceleration of the engine and monocoque against the back, which reduces the flexion of the thoracolumbar spine. Then the applied load to the pelvis due to shortening of the underbelly of the car results in a more typical burst fracture.

In summary, injury to the thoracolumbar spine in an Indy car is usually the result of a direct frontal impact that produces an axial load type of injury. Because the driver is securely restrained into the tub, which prevents rotational and lateral bending and provides no opportunity for extension, these fractures usually occur as a result of direct axial loading in slight flexion.

Injury to the cervical spine in motor sports usually results from the head being accelerated inside the cockpit as a result of violently applied forces, the weight of the head, and the helmet acting as a weight on the end of the cervical lever arm. The forces applied can be violent enough to produce distraction forces that combine with bending forces to produce fracture. Severe

fractures, fracture dislocations, and cord injury are almost always the product of a rollover situation. The more common injury sustained is in forward flexion and is usually the result of a direct backward impact in which the driver's head strikes the cowling and is propelled forward in a contrecoup movement, producing a flexion injury to the cervical spine. This mechanism is seen in other forms of auto racing, and in those forms injury to the cervical spine is also usually due to a rollover situation. In certain circumstances, however, impact from a lateral or "T-bone" type of crash in a stock car can produce lateral motion of the neck associated with sudden deceleration or flexion. This is combined with distraction resulting from the sudden deceleration of the car while the driver's head is continuing along with the weight of his helmet. Although this mechanism is unusual, it is known to have produced a hangman's fracture without rollover and has resulted in a fatality in at least one stock car accident.

Injuries to the axial skeleton seem to be confined to accidents in an open-cockpit car, such as a roadster, in which the driver's torso is restrained tightly inside a tub or monocoque and is prevented from moving. Thus the head, which is relatively free, is accelerated away from the torso during impact or rollover. In the last 25 years the National Association for Stock Car Auto Racing (NASCAR) has reported only three fractures of the cervical spine, two of which occurred in the recent past.[3] There has been one severe ligamentous injury. Data are not available as to what percentage of the total number of injuries these three fractures represent or what percentage of the NASCAR crashes resulted in injury. Certainly, the perception is that the accident rate is at least as high as in Indy cars and that the injury rate is slightly higher. But because of the larger, enclosed cab of a stock car, injury to the axial skeleton would appear to be rare in a NASCAR accident.

The roll cages of open-cockpit cars are well designed and, in every case, have prevented the driver's head from actually striking the pavement. In some situations the inferior aspect of the driver's helmet can contact the cowling of the car, particularly in a violent rollover, and this has resulted in fracture of the upper cervical spine. The usual case, however, is that injury to the cervical spine is the result of the violent forces applied to the neck because of the weight of the head and helmet, resulting in injury to the cervical spine, which acts as the lever arm fastening the head to the torso.

REHABILITATION

Fractures of the cervical and thoracic spine are treated no differently in professional race drivers than in any patient group, and a discussion of treatment specifics is not germane here. It is recommended, however, that any driver who has undergone fusion of the cervical spine, particularly an anterior fusion, be advised not to

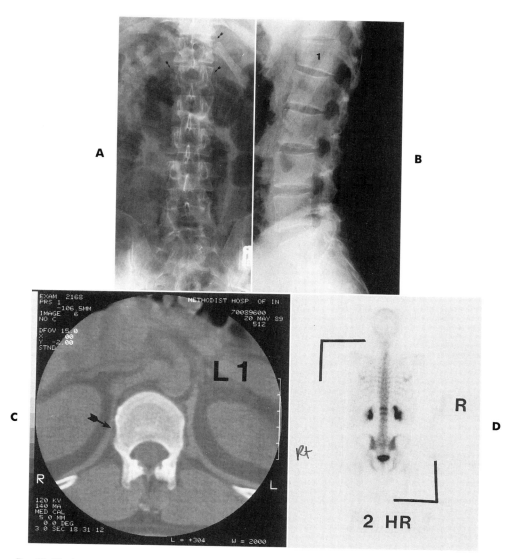

Fig. 59-14. A and **B,** AP and lateral x-ray films showing L1 fracture resulting from a frontal impact. The patient had a history of prior injury and minimal symptoms. **C,** CT scan, which was not very helpful in discerning if the injury was acute. **D,** Bone scan clearly demonstrating the acute nature of the T12 and L1 fractures; this is of great prognostic significance.

return to driving for a minimum of 6 months. After the removal of any postoperative orthosis, the driver should undergo 6 to 12 weeks of neck-strengthening exercises, beginning with isometric exercises, particularly of the sternocleidomastoid muscles, the anterior paravertebral muscles, and the posterior muscle complex. Then some resistive exercises can be added.

It is also recommended that no driver who has sustained a cervical fracture resulting in instability of the cervical spine and/or who has required surgery should return to competition any sooner than 9 months, and preferably 12 months, after injury. If a driver has undergone an anterior cervical fusion and is relatively tall, so that his head protrudes somewhat from the cockpit, it is suggested that the driver be discouraged

from returning to competition at all. The risk is that a second injury could result in more severe fracture or that a lesser degree of application of forces could result in fracture dislocation at the level above the fusion because of the change in the mechanics of the cervical spine. Shorter drivers who sit lower in the car are at less risk for this kind of injury because their head is more protected and cocooned in the car.

For drivers who have sustained a minor fracture (i.e., minimal compression fracture or avulsion of the spinous processes), it is strongly recommended that when they return to driving, which is usually possible within 8 to 12 weeks after injury, they wear a horse collar beneath their helmet to decelerate the head more gradually during an impact situation.

It is usually possible for drivers who have sustained compression fractures of the thoracolumbar spine that have been treated by orthosis to return to driving without any restriction or special caution 3 months after injury. It is recommended, however, that they have their car seat modified to provide for reduced flexion moment at the thoracolumbar spine.

Drivers who have undergone instrumentation and fusion of the thoracolumbar spine are kept out of competition for a full year but are usually allowed to return to some testing in a low-risk situation out of the brace at about 9 months. Once the lesion is healed, at 1 year to 18 months after injury, they are allowed to return to full and unrestricted driving activities and are believed to be at no higher risk than before injury.

Fortunately, injury to the axial skeleton in professional racing, which is predominantly seen in open-cockpit cars, is reasonably rare and to date has resulted in only one permanent cord injury.

REFERENCES

1. McAfee PC: Cervical spine trauma. In Frymoyer JW et al: *The adult spine: principles and practices,* New York, 1991, Raven Press.
2. Olsen C: Personal communication, NHRA.
3. Punch J: Personal communication, National Association of Stock Car Auto Racing.
4. Trammell, TR, Olvey SE: Crash and injury statistics from Indy-car racing 1985-1989. In *Proceedings, Association for the Advancement of Automotive Medicine, 34th annual conference,* Des Plaines, Ill, 1991, The Association.
5. Trammell TR, Olvey SE, Reed DB: Championship car racing accidents and injuries, *Physician Sportsmed* 14(5):114, 1986.
6. White AA III, Panjobe MM: *Clinical biomechanics of the spine.* ed 2, Philadelphia, 1990, JB Lippincott.

Chapter Sixty

◆

Sumo Wrestling

Masamitsu Tsuchiya

Sumo wrestling, a 2000-year-old fighting sport, has evolved into a very popular sport in Japan with about 850 active professional sumo wrestlers. There are six official tournaments a year; these are held every 2 months, and each tournament lasts 15 days.

Although there is a wide range in weight among the wrestlers, there is no classification by weight. Wearing only a loincloth, or *Mawashi,* the wrestlers fight each other within a circular, sand-covered ring 4.55 m in diameter. The bout ends when one wrestler forces his opponent outside of the ring or when any part of the body of a wrestler except the soles of his feet touches the floor of the ring. The one pushed out of the ring or thrown down in contact with the surface of the ring is the loser.

The wrestlers are extremely heavy, and since sumo is a hand-to-hand fighting sport, many injuries occur. In particular, low back pain is a very common problem among sumo wrestlers.

INCIDENCE OF LOW BACK PAIN

Between December 1982 and December 1993, 2008 injuries in 688 patients were treated in our orthopaedic department. The locations and numbers of injuries were as follows: trunk lesions, 558 (27.8%); upper extremity lesions, 406 (20.2%); lower extremity lesions, 1026 (51.1%); and others, 18 (0.9%). The trunk lesions were as follows: head contusions or neck sprains, 128 (6.4%); chest or back contusions, 52 (2.6%); low back pain, 350 (17.4%); and others, 28 (1.4%). The upper extremity lesions were as follows: shoulder lesions, 114 (5.7%); hand or wrist lesions, 95 (4.7%); elbow lesions, 87 (4.3%); acromioclavicular joint lesions, 63 (3.2%); upper or forearm contusions, 21 (1.0%); and others, 26 (1.3%). The lower extremity lesions consisted of knee lesions, 510 (25.4%); ankle joint lesions, 156 (7.8%); foot lesions, 136 (6.8%); phlegmons, 105 (5.2%); muscle strains, 85 (4.2%); and others, 34 (1.7%). The knee lesions were as follows: ligament and/or meniscus lesions, 279 (13.9%); knee sprains, 104 (5.2%); knee contusions, 43 (2.1%); patellar dislocations, 36 (1.8%); and others, 48 (2.4%). Based on these numbers, low back pain is the greatest problem in sumo wrestlers after knee injury. Low back pain included 76 (3.8%) cases of acute low back pain and 274 (13.6%) cases of chronic low back pain. Included with the chronic low back pain cases were 74 (3.7%) cases of lumbar disc herniation.

The average age of sumo wrestlers with low back pain was 20.2 years; the average length of experience was 3.9 years; the average height was 180.6 cm (6 feet), and the average weight was 119.9 kg (264 pounds). A comparison of all active sumo wrestlers at the beginning of 1994 found that the younger and less experienced sumo wrestlers were more susceptible to low back pain (Table 60-1). There has been no correlation among age, length of experience, height, and weight in terms of acute versus chronic low back pain (Table 60-2).

RADIOGRAPHIC FINDINGS

Abnormal radiographic findings were found in 234 (76%) of 308 radiographs. The most common finding was spondylolysis in 135 cases (43.8%). Other findings were as follows: ballooning of the disc space, 121 (39.3%); spina bifida occulta, 46 (14.9%); narrow disc space, 40 (13%); Schmorl's node, 40 (13%); and irregular vertebral body, 31 (10.1%). The vertebral body ratio is calculated by dividing the mean value of the vertebral height by the length of the upper rim of the vertebral body in lateral view (Fig. 60-1). The ratio of sumo wrestlers is 0.71, whereas that of ordinary people is 0.76. There is a statistical significance to the fact that the vertebral body of sumo wrestlers is flatter than that of ordinary people (Table 60-3).

Spondylolysis has no correlation with age, length of experience, height, or weight (Table 60-4). However, the high incidence of spondylolysis in sumo wrestlers is probably related to the high load on the lumbar spine during other sports activities before they became sumo wrestlers. There is no clear explanation why the vertebral body is flatter than that of ordinary people. There

Table 60-1. Comparison of Sumo Wrestlers: Low Back Pain Sufferers Versus Controls

	Wrestlers With Low Back Pain	Controls†
Age (years)	20.2* ± 3.2	21.2 ± 4.0
Length of experience (years)	3.9* ± 3.3	4.8 ± 4.0
Height (cm)	180.6 ± 5.7	181.1 ± 5.4
Weight (kg)	119.9 ± 23.6	121.7 ± 26.6

*p < 0.001.
†All active sumo wrestlers at the beginning of 1994.

Table 60-2. Comparison Between Sumo Wrestlers With Acute Low Back Pain and Those With Chronic Low Back Pain

	Acute Low Back pain	Chronic Low Back Pain	Significant Difference
Age (years)	20.1 ± 3.5	20.3 ± 3.6	None
Length of experience (years)	3.6 ± 3.4	4.0 ± 3.5	None
Height (cm)	180.2 ± 6.4	180.3 ± 5.8	None
Weight (kg)	122.4 ± 30.3	122.0 ± 23.5	None

Table 60-3. Vertebral Body Ratio in Sumo Wrestlers and in Ordinary People

	Wrestlers	Ordinary People
Vertebral body ratio	0.71* ± 0.07	0.76 ± 0.08

*p < 0.001.

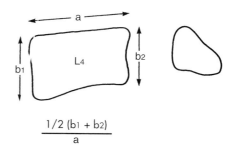

$$\frac{1/2\ (b_1 + b_2)}{a}$$

Fig. 60-1. Vertebral body ratio.

Table 60-4. Comparison Between Sumo Wrestlers With Spondylolysis and Those Without Spondylolysis

	Spondylolysis (−)	Spondylolysis (+)	Significant Difference
Age (years)	20.6 ± 3.9	19.8 ± 3.0	None
Length of experience (years)	4.2 ± 3.9	3.6 ± 3.0	None
Height (cm)	181.1 ± 6.0	180.3 ± 5.7	None
Weight (kg)	124.1 ± 24.5	119.6 ± 25.0	None

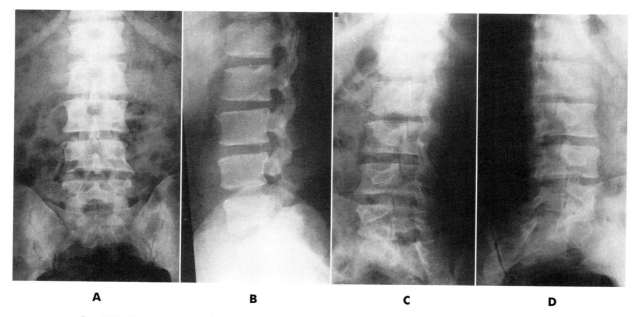

A   B   C   D

Fig. 60-2. Spondylolysis of the fourth and fifth lumbar vertebrae. **A,** Frontal view. **B,** Lateral view showing Schmorl's nodes in the first, second, and third vertebral bodies. **C,** Left anterior oblique view. **D,** Right anterior oblique view.

is some correlation with the high incidence of ballooning of the disc space. However, the correlation of this ballooning with low back pain and the vertebral body ratio is unclear.

TREATMENT

All sumo wrestlers are advised to tie their belts tightly and to contract the abdominal muscle forcefully at the beginning of a bout in order to increase the abdominal pressure that decreases the stress on the lumbar spine. In addition, abdominal and back muscle–strengthening exercises are practiced.

Pain killers and muscle relaxants are taken by wrestlers suffering from low back pain. If there is a clear tender point, a local block of the paravertebral muscle or a facet block is performed. Most cases of low back pain improve to a tolerable limit within a few weeks. However, there is a tendency for residual pain in cases of spondylolysis. In the case of lumbar disc herniation, an epidural block using caudal puncture and a root block are performed after magnetic resonance imaging (MRI). Surgery has been performed in three cases of lumbar disc herniation.

CASE 1

On March 1, 1987, a 25-year-old, 175-cm, 115-kg, Makuuchi (high-ranked) sumo wrestler felt acute low back pain with bilateral numbness and muscle weakness of the leg after sumo training. After visiting several facilities, he was admitted to our orthopaedic department on March 26. He couldn't walk because of muscle weakness, and he complained of severe low back pain. Physical examination revealed severe stiffness of the back, positive bilateral Valleix tenderness, positive straight leg raising (right, 45 degrees; left, 60 degrees), positive femoral

nerve stretch test, findings, disappearance of deep tendon reflexes of the leg, and $\frac{9}{10}$ hypoesthesia below the L2 level and $\frac{8}{10}$ below the S1 level. A manual muscle test revealed severe muscle weakness below the L2 level, especially below the S1 level. He could not flex his ankles at all. Spondylolysis of the fourth and fifth lumbar vertebrae was found on plain radiographs (Fig. 60-2). Nothing was revealed by magnetic resonance imaging (MRI). Myelography revealed a total block between the second and third vertebral bodies (Fig. 60-3). Discography at the disc between the second and third vertebrae resulted in reappearance of dull pain on injection of contrast medium, and epidural leakage of contrast medium was found (Fig. 60-4).

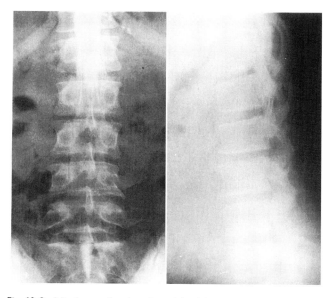

Fig. 60-3. Myelography showing a block between the second and third vertebral bodies of the lumbar spine.

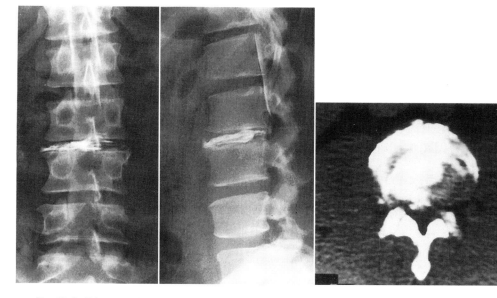

Fig. 60-4. Discography between the second and third vertebral bodies of the lumbar spine showing leakage of contrast medium into the epidural space.

On April 1, a bilateral partial laminectomy of the second lumbar vertebra was performed. From the epidural space, a mass of prolapsed disc tissue the size of the tip of a little finger was removed. After the operation, severe low back pain dramatically decreased, and the patient was able to move his ankle slightly. After 2 weeks of bed rest, gait exercise was begun. Until then, muscle power of the ankle had recovered only to a poor level. At 1 month after the operation, muscle power of the thigh had improved to a good level and that of the ankle had reached a fair level. The patient's recovery of muscle power was excellent; however, he could not stand on his toes. Therefore he could not return to the ring and retired in January 1988.

CASE 2

A 15-year-old, 181-cm, 109-kg Jonidan (low-ranked) sumo wrestler entered the sumo stable in May 1987. After 1 month of training, his low back pain rapidly increased. On September 3, 1987, he was admitted to our department because of severe low back pain and right leg numbness. Physical examination revealed low back stiffness, motion pain at trunk flexion, negative straight leg raising test results, and a decreased deep tendon reflex. There was no motor or sensory disturbance.

Plain radiographs showed no particular findings (Fig. 60-5). Myelography revealed protrusion of the disc between the fourth and fifth lumbar vertebrae, as well as flattening and widening of the right fifth root (Fig. 60-6). Discography between the fourth and fifth lumbar vertebrae caused a reappearance of leg pain and revealed leakage of contrast medium into the spinal canal (Fig. 60-7).

On September 17, 1987, a right partial laminectomy of the fourth lumber spine was performed. During the operation protruding disc tissue was removed. After the operation severe

low back pain decreased. However, 2 months later, right leg pain recurred after sumo training. Several root blocks provided relief from the pain. The wrestler returned to the ring for the May official tournament in 1988. Because his leg pain continued, he retired from sumo wrestling in September 1988.

CASE 3

In December 1988 low back pain began in a 15-year-old, 182-cm, 90-kg Jonokuchi (lowest ranked) sumo wrestler. He

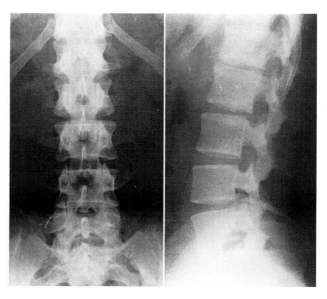

Fig. 60-5. Plain radiographs showing no particular findings to account for low back pain.

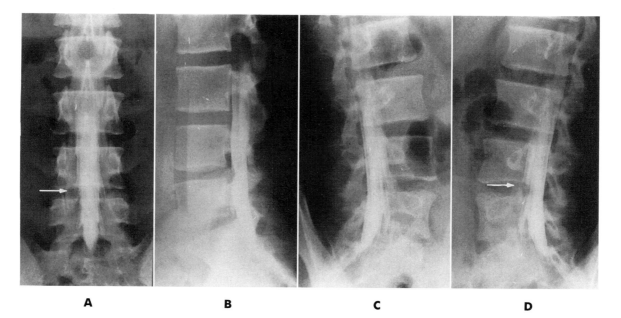

Fig. 60-6. Myelography showing flattening and widening of the fifth lumbar nerve root (*arrow*) (**A**), indenting between the fourth and fifth lumbar disc levels (**B**), a normal left lumbar nerve root (**C**), and a defect of the right fifth lumbar nerve root (*arrow*) (**D**).

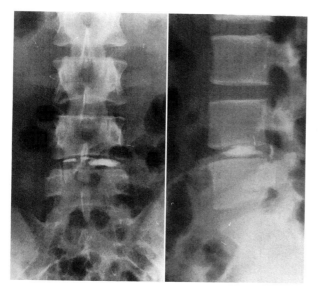

Fig. 60-7. Discography of the fourth and fifth vertebral bodies of the lumbar spine showing leakage of contrast medium into the spinal canal.

entered the sumo stable in March 1989. Because his low back pain continued, he was admitted to our hospital on April 10, 1989. Physical examination revealed pain in his back on forward flexion and right side bending, pain at the fourth spinous process of the lumbar spine, and positive straight leg raising test results (right, 30 degrees). MRI revealed protrusion of the disc between the fourth and fifth lumbar processes. After lumbar disc herniation was diagnosed, several epidural blocks were performed. However, the low back pain could not be controlled. Myelography showed a defect of the contrast medium at the fifth right lumber nerve root. Discography showed protrusion of the contrast medium into the spinal canal; however, there was no reappearance of the leg pain. The fifth right lumbar nerve block caused a reappearance of the leg pain and improvement in the straight leg raising test from 30 degrees to 60 degrees. On June 14, 1989, a bilateral partial laminectomy was performed. Prolapsed and degenerative disc tissue was removed. After the operation straight leg raising improved to 70 degrees; however, numbness of the leg and mild low back pain continued. Unfortunately, the wrestler could not return to the ring and retired in November 1990.

Although the results of the cases presented here were unsatisfactory, these were severe cases, with the difficulties compounded by the heavy weight and hard training of sumo wrestling. In addition, a possible lack of ability to adapt to the sumo world might have played a part, especially in the younger sumo wrestlers.

There are several problems in regard to treating sumo wrestlers. Extremely heavy wrestlers cannot be checked by MRI because they are unable to enter the instrument. We prepared long needles for lumbar puncture; however, in some cases it was very troublesome to perform this procedure. In addition, we gave up on some cases because of the inability to perform discography.

Patient History and Examination Forms

FORMS TO BE COMPLETED BY THE PATIENT

Patient History

Please take time to fill out the appropriate spaces

Name _____ Date _____

Age _____ Medication allergies _____ Current Rx'd medicine _____

Present job _____

Type of work done _____

When did your back or neck pain originally start? _____

When did your arm or leg pain originally start? _____

When did your current episode begin? _____

Did your pain start gradually? _____ Suddenly? _____ Injury _____

What type of injury? _____

What time of day is your pain worse? Morning _____ Later in the day _____

Middle of the night _____

Do you have numbness or tingling in an arm or leg? Please describe.

_____

Are there any recent changes in bowel or bladder habits? Please describe.

_____

Do you feel stiffness in the morning? _____

My pain is: check the appropriate column:	Better	Worse	No different
With cough or sneeze	_____	_____	_____
With straining	_____	_____	_____
Sitting in straight chair	_____	_____	_____
Sitting in soft, easy chair	_____	_____	_____
Bending forward to brush teeth	_____	_____	_____
Walking up stairs	_____	_____	_____
Walking down stairs	_____	_____	_____
Lying flat on stomach	_____	_____	_____
On side with knees bent	_____	_____	_____
When bending	_____	_____	_____
When lifting	_____	_____	_____
When working overhead	_____	_____	_____
Lying on back	_____	_____	_____
Standing	_____	_____	_____

	Yes	No
My back sometimes gets stuck when I bend forward.	_____	_____
After walking, bending forward relieves my pain.	_____	_____
My back feels like giving way when I bend forward.	_____	_____
Do you have headaches?	_____	_____

Continued.

Patient History — cont'd

	Yes	No
Have you had a change in hearing, vision?	_____	_____
Have you had dizzy spells?	_____	_____
My pain stops me when I walk a certain distance.	_____	_____
Have you been in a hospital for back, leg, or neck pain?	_____	_____

Number of times hospitalized _____ Please give dates. _____

How long can you sit? _____

How long can you walk? _____

If you have to stop walking, how long does the pain last?_____

Have you had myelograms? _____

Number of times _____

Have you had neck or back surgery? _____

Number of times _____ Please give dates and types. _____

Have you been in the hospital with other medical problems?_____

Number of times _____ Please describe. _____

What treatments have made your pain better? _____

What treatments have made your pain worse? _____

Who referred you to this office? _____

Do you have an attorney helping you? _____

Do other members of your family have significant back trouble? _____

Who? _____

Did you have to change jobs? _____ To what? _____

Are you under any pressure at home? _____ At work? _____

Mild _____ Moderate _____ Severe _____

What can you not do because of your pain that you want to do? _____

_____

What was the date of your last physical exam and the name of the M.D.?

Who did it? _____

Pelvic done? _____ Rectal done? _____

Patient Pain/Sensation Chart

Date _____

Please give this paper to the doctor at the time of examination

Mark the areas on your body where you feel the described sensations. Use the appropriate symbol. Mark areas of radiation. Include all affected areas. Just to complete the picture, please draw in your face.

NUMBNESS — PINS AND NEEDLES ○○○○ BURNING XXXX STABBING ////
                              ○○○○   XXXX   ////
                              ○○○○   XXXX   ////

Have you had prior back or neck surgery? ( )Yes ( )No

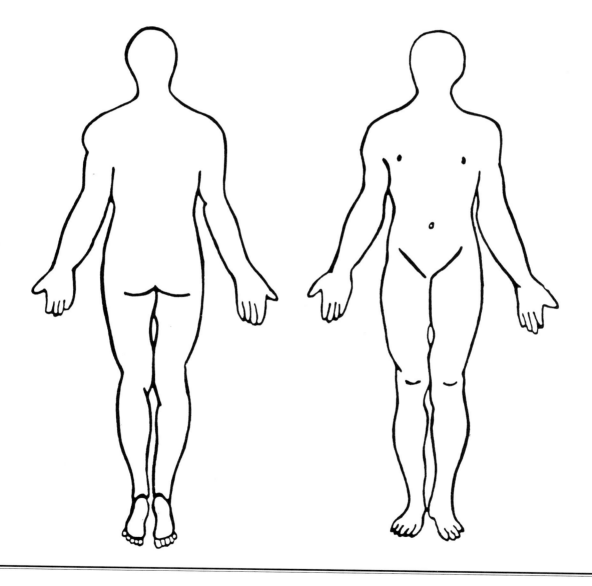

Oswestry Function Test

Please choose one answer only

Pain Intensity

1. I can tolerate my pain without having to use pain killers.
2. My pain is bad, but I manage without taking pain killers.
3. Pain killers give me complete relief from my pain.
4. Pain killers give me moderate relief from my pain.
5. Pain killers give me very little relief from my pain.
6. Pain killers have no effect on my pain, and I do not use them.

Personal Care

1. I can look after myself normally without causing extra pain.
2. I can look after myself normally, but it causes extra pain.
3. It is painful to look after myself, and I am slow and careful.
4. I need some help, but I manage most of my personal care.
5. I need help every day in most aspects of self-care.
6. I do not get dressed, wash with difficulty, and stay in bed.

Lifting

1. I can lift heavy objects without causing extra pain.
2. I can lift heavy objects, but it gives me extra pain.
3. Pain prevents me from lifting heavy objects off the floor, but I can manage light to medium objects if they are conveniently positioned.
4. I can lift only very light objects.
5. I cannot lift anything at all.

Walking

1. Pain does not prevent me from walking any distance.
2. Pain prevents me from walking more than 1 mile.
3. Pain prevents me from walking more than 1/2 mile.
4. Pain prevents me from walking more than 1/4 mile.
5. I can only walk using a cane or crutches.
6. I am in bed most of the time and have to crawl to the toilet.

Sitting

1. I can sit in any chair as long as I like.
2. I can sit only in my favorite chair as long as I like.
3. Pain prevents me from sitting more than 1 hour.
4. Pain prevents me from sitting more than 1/2 hour.
5. Pain prevents me from sitting more than 10 minutes.
6. Pain prevents me from sitting at all.

Standing

1. I can stand as long as I want without extra pain.
2. I can stand as long as I want, but it gives me extra pain.
3. Pain prevents me from standing more than 1 hour.
4. Pain prevents me from standing more than 1/2 hour.
5. Pain prevents me from standing more than 10 minutes.
6. Pain prevents me from standing at all.

Sleeping

1. Pain does not prevent me from sleeping well.
2. I can sleep well only by taking medication for sleep.
3. Even when I take medication, I have less than 6 hours' sleep.
4. Even when I take medication, I have less than 4 hours' sleep.
5. Even when I take medication, I have less than 2 hours' sleep.
6. Pain prevents me from sleeping at all.

Sex Life

1. My sex life is normal and gives me no extra pain.
2. My sex life is normal but causes some extra pain.
3. My sex life is nearly normal but is very painful.
4. My sex life is severely restricted by pain.
5. My sex life is nearly absent because of pain.
6. Pain prevents any sex life at all.

Social Life

1. My social life is normal and gives me no extra pain.
2. My social life is normal but increases the degree of pain.
3. Pain has no significant effect on my social life apart from limiting my more energetic interests, like dancing, etc.
4. Pain has restricted my social life, and I do not go out as often.
5. Pain has restricted my social life to my home.
6. I have no social life because of pain.

Traveling

1. I can travel anywhere without extra pain.
2. I can travel anywhere, but it gives me extra pain.
3. Pain is bad, but I manage journeys over 2 hours.
4. Pain restricts me to journeys of less than 1 hour.
5. Pain restricts me to short necessary journeys of less than 1/2 hour.
6. Pain prevents me from traveling except to the doctor or hospital.

FORMS TO BE COMPLETED BY THE PHYSICIAN

History and Present Status of the Back/Neck Problem

Patient's name _____ Date _____

CHIEF COMPLAINT (Major items only) _____

_____

ONSET: Time—sudden or gradual—Date and time of day _____

*Cause—injury, sickness, etc. _____

_____

†Immediate symptoms _____

_____

_____

_____

COURSE: Detailed chronologic study of symptoms and medical care and reaction to each procedure

_____

_____

_____

_____

_____

_____

_____

_____

PAST RELEVANT HISTORY: Previous and recent attacks, etc. _____

_____

	1	2	3	4
Pain	1	2	3	4
Function	1	2	3	4
Occupation	1	2	3	4

PROGRESS: Better, worse, stationary _____

Relation to Activity

Lying down—position of greatest comfort: _____

Does rest or activity relieve? _____

Awakened often and why? _____

Sitting—one side, or shifts _____ How most comfortable? _____

Getting up from sitting—need assist?_____ Hard or soft _____ Driving _____

Standing—one side or shifts _____ Time, and what happens? _____

Walking—distance _____ What happens? _____

Stairs, inclines, irregular ground _____

Bending—degree _____ Pain and assist returning to erect position ___

Lifting: Wt. _____ lbs. _____ Fatigue _____

Working _____ Type _____ Date discontinued _____ Returned _____

Effect of manipulation _____ Support: type and effect _____

Effect of exercise _____

*Describe carefully just how forces of the accident affected the patient, how he or she was thrown, fell, landed: twists to back or limbs. Just mechanical factors. (Don't include extraneous material, such as who was to blame.)

†How patient felt immediately: unconscious—how long; ache, severe pain, gradual increase, inability to walk or use certain joints, numbness, and/or paralysis.

Continued.

History and Present Status of the Back/Neck Problem — cont'd

Neurologic Effects

Ratio of neck/arm pain: _____ / _____

Radiation of pain: Where? _____ When? _____

Effects of coughing, sneezing, and straining during bowel movements: On back, where? _____

On referred pain, how far? _____

Areas of skin tingling, numbness, coldness_____ Muscle weakness? _____

Chronic Inflammatory Factors

Stiffness after rest: Getting out of bed _____ After sitting _____

Effect of change of weather _____ Cold, damp weather _____ Hot _____

Effect of heat to part _____ Type of heat _____

(Women) Relation to menstrual periods _____

Remarks: _____

Physical Examination

Review of Systems
HEENT
Chest
Cardiovascular
Abdomen
Rectal
Fundi
Prostate

Pulses	Right	Left
Femoral		
Popliteal		
Pedal		
Bruits		

Back and Lower Extremity Examination

Range of motion	Right	Left
Flexion		
Extension		
Left lateral flexion		
Right lateral flexion		

Muscle strength	Right	Left
Hip abduction		
Hip adduction		
Hip flexion		
Hip extension		
Knee flexion		
Knee extension		
Ankle dorsiflexion		
Ankle plantar flexion		
Ankle inversion		
Ankle eversion		

Physical Examination — cont'd

	Right	Left
Muscle strength — cont'd		
Toes dorsiflexion		
Toes plantar flexion		
Big toe dorsiflexion		
Reflex grades	Right	Left
Patella		
Achilles		
Posterior tibia		
Pain radiation	Right	Left
Thighs		
Calves		
Feet		
Foot top		
Foot bottom		
Heel		
Big toe		
Little toe		
Sensory function	Right	Left
Light touch		
Pinprick		
Vibratory		
Tests	Right	Left
Leg lengths		
Thighs		
Calves		
Muscle spasm		
Convexity scoliosis		
Kyphosis		
Lordosis		
Tests	Right	Left
Babinski		
Clonus		
Laségue		
Flip		
Bowstring		
Cram		
Foot dorsiflexion		
Neck flexion		
Faber		
Hip range of motion		
Femoral stretch		

Point tenderness

Thoracic spine
L1
L2
L3
L4
L5
S1
S2 to S5
Coccyx
Anterior spine

Continued.

Physical Examination — cont'd

Point tenderness — cont'd	Right	Left
Sacroiliac joint		
Sciatic notch		
Greater trochanter		
Ischial tuberosity		
Paraspinous		

Straight leg raising	Right	Left
Supine — leg pain		
Sitting — leg pain		
Contralateral — leg pain		
Sitting — low back pain		
Contralateral — low back pain		

Neck and Upper Extremity Examination

Muscle strength	Right	Left
Trapezius		
Cuff		
Deltoid		
Rhomboid		
Serrant		
Pectoralis		
Biceps		
Triceps		
Forearm supination		
Forearm pronation		
Wrist extension		
Wrist flexion		
Thumb		
Grip		
Intrinsics		

Sensory function

Light touch
Pinprick
Vibratory

PERRLA

Gag
Tongue
Smile
Hearing
Sight
Thyroid
Neck mass
Bruits:
    Carotids
    Subclavicular
    Axillary
Torticollis

Range of motion	Right	Left
Flexion		
Extension		
Left flexion		
Right flexion		
Left rotation		
Right rotation		

Index